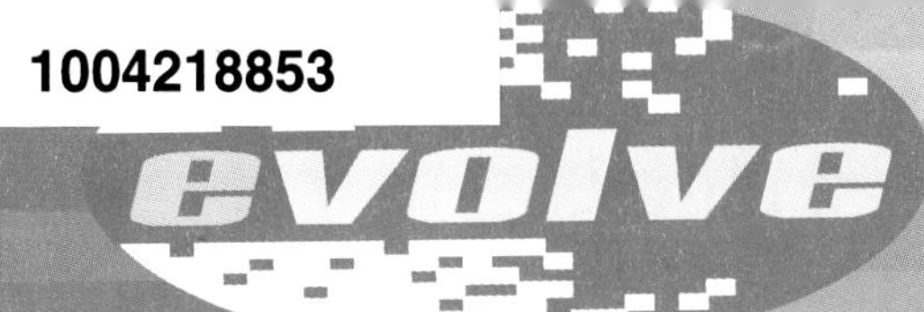

The Latest Evolution in Learning.

Evolve provides online access to free resources designed specifically for you. The resources will provide you with information that enhances the material covered in the book and much more.

LOGIN: http://evolve.elsevier.com/Ulrich/

Evolve Online Courseware for Ulrich and Canale: *Nursing Care Planning Guides: For Adults in Acute, Extended, and Home Care Settings,* sixth edition, offers the following features:

- **Online Care Planner**
  Create, edit, and print a customized care plan by choosing from 40 care plans from the sixth edition of NURSING CARE PLANNING GUIDES. You may also select from the description of the disease condition/surgery and the nursing diagnoses or collaborative problems with desired outcomes and nursing interventions.

  Care plans included on the Online Care Planner are denoted with a evolve next to the care plan on the inside cover list and next to the care plan in the text.

Think o... evolve.

NURSING CARE PLANNING GUIDES

For Adults in Acute, Extended, and Home Care Settings

NURSING CARE PLANNING GUIDES

For Adults in Acute, Extended, and Home Care Settings

Sixth Edition

SUSAN PUDERBAUGH ULRICH, BSN, MSN
Nurse Educator and Legal Nurse Consultant
Lane Community College
Eugene, Oregon

SUZANNE WEYLAND CANALE, BSN, MSN
Nurse Educator and Legal Nurse Consultant
Lane Community College
Eugene, Oregon

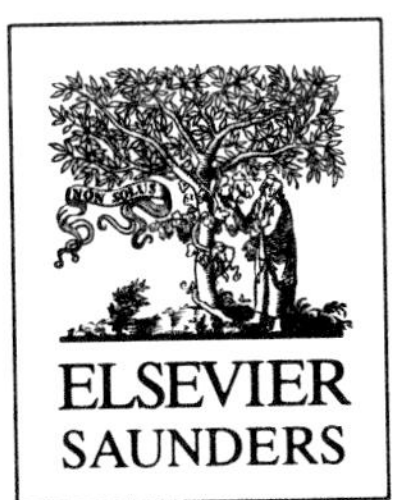
ELSEVIER
SAUNDERS

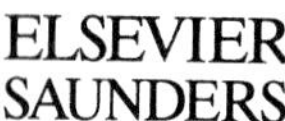

11830 Westline Industrial Drive
St. Louis, Missouri 63146

Nursing Care Planning Guides for Adults in Acute, Extended, and Home Care Settings ISBN 0-7216-3923-2

Previous editions copyrighted 2001, 1998, 1994, 1990, 1986

International Standard Book Number 0-7216-3923-2

Acquisitions Editor: Sandra Clark Brown
Senior Developmental Editor: Cindi Anderson
Publishing Services Manager: John Rogers
Senior Project Manager: Beth Hayes
Senior Designer: Amy Buxton

Printed in the United States of America

Last digit is the print number: 9 8 7 6 5 4 3 2 1

Reviewers

Rosemary Macy, RN, MS
Assistant Professor
Department of Nursing
Boise State University
Boise, Idaho

Charlotte A. Wisnewski, PhD, RN, BC
Assistant Professor
School of Nursing
University of Texas Medical Branch
Galveston, Texas

Preface

Nursing Care Planning Guides for Adults in Acute, Extended, and Home Care Settings is a comprehensive reference to guide the planning of nursing care for adults with commonly recurring medical-surgical conditions. The scope of the book has been broadened to include information that is applicable to clients receiving nursing care in acute care, community, extended care, and home care settings. The book has been updated to include the most recent North American Nursing Diagnosis Association (NANDA)-approved nursing diagnoses and Nursing Outcomes Classification (NOC) and Nursing Interventions Classification (NIC) labels.

This book contains care plans for 70 medical-surgical conditions. Each of the care plans includes a description of the medical condition or surgery and identifies the nursing diagnoses/collaborative diagnoses that would be relevant. For each diagnosis there is a specific etiology statement, desired outcome and a complete list of nursing actions. There is a continued focus in this edition on comprehensive etiology statements, comprehensive coverage of potential complications (collaborative diagnoses), and thorough client teaching. The content represents standards of nursing care and is intended to be a guide for students and practitioners to use in planning individualized client care.

Unit I provides guidelines on how to modify and individualize the care plans. It uses a case study approach to demonstrate the collection of data; selection of pertinent nursing diagnoses; and individualization of etiology statements, desired outcomes, and nursing actions.

Unit II addresses 24 commonly used nursing diagnoses. The key component of this unit is the inclusion of the rationale for each nursing action, which provides the nursing student and practitioner with a clear understanding of how each action helps to achieve the outcome for the specific nursing diagnosis. In addition to actions and rationales, the following information is included for each nursing diagnosis in this unit: NANDA-based definition, related factors or risk factors, defining characteristics, desired outcomes, documentation criteria, and suggested NIC interventions. This unit also facilitates the planning of care for the client with a medical-surgical condition that is not addressed in this text.

Unit III focuses on care of the elderly client. It includes the nursing diagnoses that reflect the biopsychosocial changes that commonly occur with aging and are intensified with the stressors of illness. The information is applicable to care of the elderly in all health care settings. It can be used independently and in combination with care plans appropriate to the client's concurrent medical condition(s) and/or surgical situation.

Units IV through VII include care plans that provide information regarding conditions or treatment modalities. The standardized care plans in Unit IV on Preoperative and Postoperative Care should be used with each surgical care plan in the text. The care plans on Immobility and Terminal Care (Units V and VI) are applicable to a wide range of conditions and should be utilized whenever appropriate. The care plans in Unit VII cover treatment modalities for neoplastic disorders and are referred to when appropriate in subsequent care plans involving neoplastic disease. Each of the standardized care plans in these units can be used to plan care for a client with a condition not covered in this text. When care plans in Units IV through VII are to be used with a care plan in Units VIII through XIX, the authors indicate this at the beginning of the plan by the phrase **Use in conjunction with** or **Refer to.**

Units VIII to XIX are divided according to body systems. Care plans within each unit deal with conditions that are frequently seen in health care settings.

The content in each care plan is organized in a traditional nursing care plan format that can readily be adapted to other plan-of-care formats used by health care providers (e.g., critical paths, clinical practice guidelines). Each care plan is organized as follows:

INTRODUCTION

The introduction provides the reader with an overview of the condition including a basic definition and discussion of the pathophysiological mechanisms involved and/or a description of the surgical procedure or selected treatment modality. This overview is not intended to be a substitute for the information provided in medical-surgical nursing texts or other references but rather a quick refresher or a starting point for additional research. Within this section, the reader will also find the focus of the care plan (highlighted in bold print).

OUTCOME/DISCHARGE CRITERIA

This section includes criteria that serve as a guide for determining the client's readiness for discharge from the specific health care setting. Recognizing that client education is a vital aspect of health care, the authors use these criteria as the basis for the detailed teaching that is included at the end of each care plan.

NURSING AND COLLABORATIVE DIAGNOSES

The nursing and collaborative diagnoses describe the actual or potential health problems that a client with a particular condition may experience. The nursing diagnoses were selected from those approved by the North American Nursing Diagnosis Association (NANDA) through 2004. In a few instances the authors have included nursing diagnoses that have been modified or are not currently on the NANDA list. These diagnostic labels are usually noted in the text by an asterisk (*) and an explanatory footnote. Nursing diagnoses that are not unique to a particular condition but may be relevant for a client (e.g., spiritual distress) have not consistently been included but should be considered when individualizing each care plan. Collaborative diagnoses have been included to incorporate potential complications and electrolyte imbalances for which there are not established nursing diagnostic labels. Specific etiology statements that incorporate pathophysiological and psychosocial factors are identified for the majority of the nursing and collaborative diagnosis labels. As with other portions of the standardized care plans, these etiologies need to be individualized for each client. In most instances, the authors did not include etiologies for the nursing diagnosis labels that deal directly with client teaching (i.e., deficient knowledge, ineffective health maintenance, ineffective therapeutic regimen management) because of the numerous individual variables that may affect a client's ability to learn, maintain health, and manage his/her therapeutic regimen.

In order to provide consistency in the care plans, the nursing and collaborative diagnoses statements have usually been listed in the same order. No attempt has been made to prioritize the diagnoses. Priorities will need to be established by the student and practitioner based on the individual client's current needs.

DESIRED OUTCOMES

The desired outcomes for the nursing and collaborative diagnoses provide criteria for evaluating client progress and the effectiveness of care provided. The outcome criteria for the nursing diagnoses are based on the defining characteristics approved by NANDA. The student and practitioner should modify the goal and specific outcome criteria as needed to reflect what is realistic for each individual client. Target dates for the desired outcomes have not been included since these are determined by the client's current status.

NURSING ACTIONS AND SELECTED PURPOSES/RATIONALES

This column contains nursing actions that can assist the client to achieve the desired outcomes. The actions include detailed assessments that are based on the defining characteristics for the label as defined by NANDA. These assessments assist the user to determine if the nursing or collaborative diagnosis is an actual problem or if the client is at risk for developing it. The nursing interventions are specific and realistic yet global enough to allow for regional and multidisciplinary variations in standards of care. The selected purposes or rationales, which appear in italics, have been included to clarify actions that may not be fundamental nursing knowledge.

SUGGESTED NOC AND NIC LABELS

Suggested NOC outcomes and NIC interventions are listed for the nursing diagnoses in each care plan. These classification systems are included to demonstrate how they are linked to nursing diagnoses and to increase awareness and use of standardized outcome criteria and nursing interventions in the care planning process.

CLIENT TEACHING/CONTINUED CARE

Although client teaching is included throughout the care plans, the majority of the teaching is found in the actions for the nursing diagnoses of deficient knowledge, ineffective health maintenance, and ineffective therapeutic regimen management. The client teaching included uses terminology that most clients can understand.

* * *

An appendix of alphabetically arranged, NANDA-approved nursing diagnoses is included in this edition to facilitate the individualization of the care plans in this book. A bibliography is included after the Appendix. The page numbers for the general and unit-specific resources are listed at the end of each care plan. A comprehensive index assists the reader to locate specific care plans and nursing and collaborative diagnoses.

Ultimately, the value of a systematic approach to individualized client care is measured by its effect on the quality of care provided to the client. The authors hope that the sixth edition of this book will assist with the integration of the numerous aspects of client care, facilitate critical thinking and implementation of the nursing process, and provide both the student and the practitioner with a guide for planning and implementing high-quality client care.

ONLINE CARE PLANNER

The Online Care Planner allows users to access a web site that has many of these standardized care plans. The user can then customize and print the care plan. Care plans that are included on the web site have an EVOLVE icon next to the care plan title.

Acknowledgments

To our students who are a continual source of inspiration.

To our friends for their support and encouragement.

To Sharon Wendell for her participation in the first three editions of this book.

Most importantly to our families for their love, patience, and encouragement:
Curt, Shannon, and Chad Ulrich
Joe and Christopher Canale

Sue Ulrich
Suzanne Canale

Contents

UNIT I

Individualizing a Standardized Care Plan

STEPS IN INDIVIDUALIZING A STANDARDIZED CARE PLAN

Planning nursing care is an exciting challenge and a rewarding experience when one sees high quality client care provided as a result of the efforts. However, planning care that is individualized and comprehensive is often difficult to accomplish because of lack of time and adequate resources. This book is intended to facilitate the care planning process for adults with common recurring medical-surgical conditions. Within each care plan are nursing and collaborative diagnoses with etiological factors, desired outcomes with measurable behavioral criteria, and nursing actions with selected purposes or rationales. Safe, comprehensive care can be planned in a minimal amount of time using this book.

To be most effective, the standardized nursing care plan must be adapted to the client's individual needs. A process for planning individualized client care follows:

1. read the nurse's admission assessment/history information and the medication administration record of the assigned client
2. review the history, current diagnostic test results, nurses' notes for the last 48 hours, progress notes of health care providers (e.g., physician, dietitian, physical and occupational therapists, pain management specialist, social worker, discharge planner), and current consultation reports
3. interview the client and complete an assessment using the tool provided by your nursing school or health care facility
4. read about the client's diagnosis and nursing care in a current medical-surgical nursing text
5. select the appropriate standardized care plan(s) from this text and read the introductory information at the beginning of the care plan(s)
6. select the nursing and collaborative diagnoses that are appropriate for your client; choose the etiological factors that are relevant and modify them as appropriate
7. modify the desired outcomes so that they are measurable and realistic for your client; establish appropriate target dates
8. select the nursing actions that are relevant to the client's care; add to or modify the actions to meet the needs of your client; include specific medications and treatments as well as client preferences and other actions that will facilitate the achievement of the desired client outcomes.

The following situation is used to illustrate how these standardized nursing care plans can be used by the student and the practitioner in planning individualized client care:

> Mary G. is a 50-year-old woman who has been hospitalized in the terminal stages of cancer of the lung. She has been bedridden for the past 3 weeks because of severe bone pain due to metastatic lesions. She has four children ranging in age from 13 to 19 years. Both Mary and her husband have been trying to prepare the children for her death. They have no other family members living nearby.

1. **Read the nurse's admission assessment/history information and the medication administration record of the assigned client.**
   It is determined that Mary is a 50-year-old married woman. Her religious preference is Protestant. Her diagnosis is stage IV cancer of the lung. She is receiving morphine sulfate, 15 mg q2h; Dialose, 100 mg/day; and milk of magnesia, 30 ml p.o. every evening.
2. **Review the history, current diagnostic test results, nurses' notes for the last 48 hours, progress notes of health care providers (e.g., physician, dietitian, physical and occupational therapists, pain management specialist, social worker, discharge planner), and consultation reports.**
   From the history it is determined that Mary had a lobectomy 3 years ago and experienced disease recurrence 1 year ago. She was treated with chemotherapeutic drugs until 3 months ago when she elected to stop treatment. She has metastasis to the spine, ribs, and pelvis and has been bedridden for the last 3 weeks. The physician's progress notes indicate that Mary's physical condition is steadily deteriorating and the goal of care is to keep her comfortable.

Diagnostic test results reveal that Mary's RBC, Hgb, Hct, and serum protein levels are decreased.

The nurses' notes reveal that Mary needs assistance with all activities. She is able to feed herself but is only consuming 10% of her meals. She had a bowel movement this morning. Mary is voiding adequate amounts and her intake and output are balanced. She has been crying frequently and states that neither she nor her husband is ready for her death.

3. **Interview the client and complete an assessment using the tool provided by your nursing school or health care facility.**
   The interview and physical assessment reveal that Mary has persistent reddened areas on her left hip and coccyx; diminished breath sounds in the bases; shallow respirations of 24/minute; crackles (rales) in both lungs; and a cough that is productive of yellow, foul-smelling sputum. She has normal bowel sounds and states that she usually has a bowel movement every other day about 30 minutes after breakfast. Mary is alert and oriented and able to move all extremities. She complains of pain in her back, rib, and pelvic area.
4. **Read about the client's diagnosis and nursing care in a current medical-surgical nursing text.**
   Review cancer of the lung and care of the terminally ill client and the immobile client.
5. **Select the appropriate standardized care plan(s) from this text and read the introductory information at the beginning of the care plan(s).**
   Based on the physician's statement that Mary has been admitted for pain control and terminal care, it is determined that the appropriate care plans for Mary are Cancer of the Lung, Terminal Care, and Immobility.
6. **Select the nursing and collaborative diagnoses that are appropriate for your client. Choose the etiological factors that are relevant and modify them as appropriate.**
   It is determined that there are numerous diagnoses and etiological factors from the care plans on Cancer of the Lung, Terminal Care, and Immobility that are appropriate. Examples of some of these nursing diagnoses follow. The etiological factors have been modified to reflect Mary's situation.
   a. **Ineffective breathing pattern** related to:
      1. increased rate of respirations associated with fear, anxiety, and pain;
      2. decreased rate of respirations associated with depressant effect of morphine sulfate;
      3. decreased depth of respirations associated with compression of lung tissue by the tumor, recumbent positioning, weakness, fatigue, fear, anxiety, and reluctance to breathe deeply because of pain.
   b. **Ineffective airway clearance** related to:
      1. excessive mucus production associated with inflammation of lung tissue resulting from the disease process;
      2. stasis of secretions associated with decreased mobility, difficulty coughing up secretions, and impaired ciliary function;
      3. invasion of and/or pressure on airways by tumor.
   c. **Acute/Chronic pain: back, rib, and pelvic** related to bone metastasis.
   d. **Anticipatory grieving** related to loss of control over life and body functioning, changes in body image, loss of significant others, and imminent death.

The process for individualization of etiologies is demonstrated using the nursing diagnosis of **Risk for Constipation** as a prototype.

STANDARDIZED

Risk for Constipation related to:

(etiologies from Care Plan on Immobility)

a. diminished defecation reflex associated with:
   1. suppression of urge to defecate because of lack of privacy and reluctance to use bedpan
   2. decreased gravity filling of lower rectum resulting from horizontal positioning
b. weakened abdominal muscles associated with generalized loss of muscle tone resulting from prolonged immobility
c. decreased gastrointestinal motility associated with decreased activity and the increased sympathetic nervous system activity that occurs with anxiety.

(etiologies from Care Plan on Terminal Care)

a. diminished defecation reflex associated with decreased nervous system responses in terminal state, suppression of the urge to defecate because of reluctance to use bedpan, and decreased gravity filling of lower rectum resulting from horizontal positioning
b. decreased ability to respond to the urge to defecate associated with weakened abdominal muscles, impaired physical mobility, and decreased level of consciousness
c. decreased gastrointestinal motility associated with decreased activity, increased sympathetic nervous system activity that occurs with anxiety, and use of some medications (e.g., narcotic [opioid] analgesics, antacids containing aluminum or calcium)
d. decreased intake of fluid and foods high in fiber.

INDIVIDUALIZED

Risk for Constipation related to:

a. diminished defecation reflex associated with:
   1. suppression of urge to defecate because of increased back and pelvic pain when attempting to use bedpan
   2. decreased gravity filling of lower rectum resulting from horizontal positioning
b. weakened abdominal muscles associated with generalized loss of muscle tone resulting from prolonged immobility
c. decreased gastrointestinal motility associated with decreased activity and increased sympathetic nervous system activity that occurs with anxiety and pain.

a. diminished defecation reflex associated with decreased nervous system responses in terminal state, suppression of the urge to defecate because of increased back and pelvic pain when attempting to use bedpan, and decreased gravity filling of lower rectum resulting from horizontal positioning
b. decreased ability to respond to the urge to defecate associated with weakened abdominal muscles and impaired physical mobility
c. decreased gastrointestinal motility associated with decreased activity, use of morphine sulfate, and increased sympathetic nervous system activity that occurs with anxiety and pain
d. decreased intake of fluid and foods high in fiber.

7. **Modify the desired outcomes so that they are measurable and realistic for your client. Establish appropriate target dates.**
   The process for individualization of a desired outcome is demonstrated using the nursing diagnosis of **Risk for Constipation** as a prototype.

STANDARDIZED

(outcome from Care Plan on Immobility)

The client will not experience constipation as evidenced by:

a. usual frequency of bowel movements
b. passage of soft, formed stool
c. absence of abdominal distention and pain, feeling of rectal fullness or pressure, and straining during defecation.

INDIVIDUALIZED

Mary will not experience constipation as evidenced by:

a. passing soft, formed stool at least every other day
b. absence of abdominal distention, abdominal pain, feeling of rectal fullness or pressure, and straining during defecation.

STANDARDIZED

(outcome from Care Plan on Terminal Care)

The client will maintain a bowel routine that provides optimal comfort.

INDIVIDUALIZED

Same as previous example.

8. **Select the nursing actions that are relevant to the client's care. Add to or modify the actions to meet the needs of your client. Include specific medications and treatments as well as client preferences and other actions that will facilitate the achievement of the desired client outcomes.**
The process for individualization of nursing actions is demonstrated below using the nursing diagnosis of **Risk for Constipation** as a prototype.

STANDARDIZED

(actions from Care Plan on Immobility)

a. Assess for signs and symptoms of constipation (e.g., decrease in frequency of bowel movements; passage of hard, formed stools; anorexia; abdominal distention and pain; feeling of fullness or pressure in rectum; straining during defecation).
b. Assess bowel sounds. Report a pattern of decreasing bowel sounds.
c. Implement measures to prevent constipation:
   1. encourage client to defecate whenever the urge is felt
   2. place client in high Fowler's position for bowel movements unless contraindicated
   3. encourage client to relax, provide privacy, and have call signal within reach during attempts to defecate *(measures to promote relaxation enable client to relax the levator ani muscle and external anal sphincter, which facilitates evacuation of stool)*
   4. encourage client to establish a regular time for defecation, preferably within an hour after a meal
   5. instruct client to increase intake of foods high in fiber (e.g., bran, whole-grain breads and cereals, fresh fruits and vegetables) unless contraindicated
   6. instruct client to maintain a minimum fluid intake of 2500 ml/day unless contraindicated
   7. encourage client to drink hot liquids upon arising in the morning *in order to stimulate peristalsis*
   8. encourage client to perform isometric abdominal strengthening exercises unless contraindicated
   9. if client is taking analgesics for pain management, encourage the use of nonnarcotic rather than narcotic (opioid) analgesics when appropriate
   10. increase activity as allowed
   11. administer laxatives or cathartics and/or enemas if ordered.
d. Consult physician about checking for an impaction and digitally removing stool if client has not had a bowel movement in 3 days, if he/she is passing liquid stool, or if other signs and symptoms of constipation are present.
e. Consult appropriate health care provider if signs and symptoms of constipation persist and appear to be an ongoing problem.

INDIVIDUALIZED*

a. Assess Mary every shift for signs and symptoms of constipation (e.g., no bowel movement for 3 days; passage of hard, formed stool; increased anorexia; abdominal distention; abdominal pain; feeling of fullness or pressure in rectum; straining during defecation).
b. Assess bowel sounds. Report a pattern of decreasing bowel sounds.
c. Implement measures to prevent Mary's constipation:
   1. encourage Mary to defecate whenever she feels the urge
   2. place Mary on bedpan in high Fowler's position for bowel movements
   3. turn on soft music, provide privacy, and have call signal within reach during attempts to defecate
   4. encourage Mary to attempt to defecate about 30 minutes after breakfast
   5. offer bran cereal and fresh fruit for breakfast; encourage Mary to select foods high in fiber for lunch and dinner
   6. encourage Mary to increase her fluid intake; offer 200 ml of apple juice, orange juice, or water every hour while she is awake
   7. offer hot tea with breakfast
   8. omit—not appropriate for terminally ill client
   9. omit—Mary needs the narcotic analgesic for effective pain management
   10. omit—Mary is basically bedridden
   11. administer milk of magnesia, 30 ml p.o. each evening and Dialose, 100 mg p.o. each morning.
d. Consult physician about checking for an impaction and digitally removing stool if Mary has not had a bowel movement for 4 days and other signs and symptoms of constipation are present.
e. Consult appropriate health care provider if signs and symptoms of constipation occur and appear to be an ongoing problem.

*The italicized information from the standardized actions is purposes or rationales and is omitted in this column. The information would be included in the rationale column of an individualized care plan.

STANDARDIZED	INDIVIDUALIZED
(actions from Care Plan on Terminal Care)	
a. Refer to Care Plan on Immobility, Diagnosis 9 (p. 151), for measures related to assessment, prevention, and management of constipation.	a. Omit—individualization of these actions from the Care Plan on Immobility has already been completed above.
b. Assist client to toilet or bedside commode or place in high Fowler's position on bedpan for bowel movements unless contraindicated.	b. Omit—Mary is not able to get to the bathroom or sit on bedside commode.
c. If client is taking antacids containing aluminum or calcium, consult appropriate health care provider (e.g., physician, hospice nurse, palliative care nurse) about alternating them with antacids containing magnesium.	c. Omit—Mary is not currently taking antacids.

See next page for individualized care plan for Mary.

Individualized care plan for Mary for the nursing diagnosis of Risk for Constipation:

DATA	NURSING DIAGNOSIS	DESIRED OUTCOME	NURSING ACTIONS
States had a bowel movement this morning Normal bowel sounds Physician's orders: milk of magnesia, 30 ml p.o. each evening; Dialose, 100 mg p.o. every morning Bedridden for 3 weeks Consuming only 10% of meals States usually has bowel movement q.o.d. about 30 minutes after breakfast Activity: bed rest; requires assistance with all activities Receiving morphine sulfate every 2 hours	Risk for Constipation related to: a. diminished defecation reflex associated with decreased nervous system responses in terminal state, suppression of urge to defecate because of increased back and pelvic pain when attempting to use bedpan, and decreased gravity filling of lower rectum resulting from horizontal positioning; b. decreased ability to respond to urge to defecate associated with weakened abdominal muscles and impaired physical mobility; c. decreased gastrointestinal motility associated with decreased activity, use of morphine sulfate, and increased sympathetic nervous system activity that occurs with anxiety and pain; d. decreased intake of fluids and foods high in fiber.	Mary will not experience constipation as evidenced by: a. passing a soft, formed stool at least every other day b. absence of abdominal distention, abdominal pain, feeling of rectal fullness or pressure, and straining during defecation.	1. Assess Mary every shift for signs and symptoms of constipation (e.g., no bowel movement for 3 days; passage of hard, formed stool; increased anorexia; abdominal distention; abdominal pain; feeling of fullness or pressure in rectum; straining during defecation). 2. Assess bowel sounds. Report a pattern of decreasing bowel sounds. 3. Implement measures to prevent Mary's constipation: a. encourage Mary to defecate whenever she feels the urge b. place Mary on bedpan in high Fowler's position for bowel movements c. turn on soft music, provide privacy, and have call signal within reach during attempts to defecate d. encourage Mary to attempt to defecate about 30 minutes after breakfast e. offer bran cereal and fresh fruit for breakfast; encourage Mary to select foods high in fiber for lunch and dinner f. encourage Mary to increase her fluid intake; offer 200 ml of apple juice, orange juice, or water every hour while she is awake g. offer hot tea with breakfast h. administer milk of magnesia, 30 ml p.o. each evening and Dialose, 100 mg p.o. each morning. 4. Consult physician about checking for an impaction and digitally removing stool if Mary has not had a bowel movement for 4 days and other signs and symptoms of constipation are present. 5. Consult appropriate health care provider if signs and symptoms occur and appear to be an ongoing problem.

UNIT II

Actions, Rationales, and Documentation for Selected Nursing Diagnoses

NURSING DIAGNOSIS: ACTIVITY INTOLERANCE

Definition Insufficient physiological or psychological energy to endure or complete required or desired daily activities

Defining Characteristics Verbal report of fatigue or weakness; abnormal heart rate or blood pressure response to activity; exertional discomfort or dyspnea; electrocardiographic changes reflecting arrhythmias or ischemia

Related Factors Bedrest or immobility; generalized weakness; sedentary lifestyle; imbalance between oxygen supply/demand

Desired Outcome The client will demonstrate an increased tolerance for activity as evidenced by:

a. verbalization of feeling less fatigued and weak
b. ability to perform activities of daily living without exertional dyspnea, chest pain, diaphoresis, dizziness, and significant change in vital signs.

Documentation

a. Activity level
b. Statements of weakness and fatigue
c. Exertional dyspnea, chest pain, diaphoresis, or dizziness
d. Vital signs before, during, and after activity
e. Therapeutic interventions
f. Client teaching

Suggested NIC Interventions: Activity therapy; Energy management; Oxygen therapy; Nutrition management; Sleep enhancement; Cardiac care: rehabilitation; Teaching: prescribed activity

NURSING ACTIONS	RATIONALES
Assessments	
1. Assess for signs and symptoms of activity intolerance: a. statements of fatigue or weakness b. exertional dyspnea, chest pain, diaphoresis, or dizziness c. abnormal heart rate response to activity (e.g., increase in rate of 20 beats/minute above resting rate, rate not returning to preactivity level within 3 minutes after stopping activity, change from regular to irregular rate) d. a significant change (15 to 20 mm Hg) in blood pressure with activity.	1. Early recognition of signs and symptoms of activity intolerance allows for prompt intervention.
Prevention/Treatment	
2. Implement measures to promote rest and/or conserve energy (e.g., maintain prescribed activity restrictions, minimize environmental activity and noise, provide uninterrupted rest periods, assist with care, limit the number of visitors).	2. Cells utilize oxygen and fat, protein, and carbohydrate to produce the energy needed for all body activities. Rest and activities that conserve energy result in a lower metabolic rate, which preserves nutrients and oxygen for necessary activities.
3. Implement measures to increase cardiac output (e.g., administer positive inotropic agents, vasodilators, or antiarrhythmics as ordered; elevate head of bed) if decreased cardiac output is contributing to client's activity intolerance.	3. Sufficient cardiac output is necessary to maintain an adequate blood flow and oxygen supply to the tissues. Adequate tissue oxygenation promotes more efficient energy production, which subsequently improves the client's activity tolerance.
4. Implement measures to reduce fever if present (e.g., administer tepid sponge bath, administer antipyretics as ordered).	4. An elevated temperature increases the metabolic rate with subsequent depletion of available energy and a decrease in ability to tolerate activity.

NURSING ACTIONS *Prevention/Treatment*	RATIONALES
5. Discourage smoking and excessive intake of beverages high in caffeine such as coffee, tea, and colas.	5. Both nicotine and excessive caffeine intake can increase cardiac workload and myocardial oxygen utilization, thereby decreasing the amount of oxygen available for energy production.
6. Maintain oxygen therapy as ordered.	6. An oxygen deficiency results in anaerobic metabolism, which is less efficient than the aerobic mechanism of energy supply. Supplemental oxygen helps to alleviate hypoxia and restore the more efficient aerobic metabolism, thereby improving energy levels and activity tolerance.
7. Implement measures to improve respiratory status (e.g., encourage use of incentive spirometer; elevate head of bed; assist with turning, coughing, and deep breathing) if ineffective breathing pattern, ineffective airway clearance, or impaired gas exchange is contributing to client's activity intolerance.	7. Altered respiratory function can lead to inadequate tissue oxygenation, which results in less efficient energy production and a reduced ability to tolerate activity. Improving respiratory status increases the amount of oxygen available for energy production. It also eases the work of breathing, which reduces energy expenditure.
8. Implement measures to maintain an adequate nutritional status (e.g., provide a diet high in essential nutrients, provide dietary supplements as indicated, administer vitamins and minerals as ordered).	8. Metabolism is the process by which nutrients are transformed into energy. If nutrition is inadequate, energy production is decreased, which subsequently reduces one's ability to tolerate activity.
9. Implement measures to treat anemia if present (e.g., administer prescribed iron, folic acid, and/or vitamin B_{12}; administer packed red blood cells as ordered).	9. Anemia reduces the oxygen-carrying capacity of the blood. Resolution of anemia increases oxygen availability to the cells, which increases the efficiency of energy production and subsequently improves activity tolerance.
10. Increase client's activity gradually as allowed and tolerated.	10. A gradual increase in activity helps prevent a sudden increase in cardiac workload and myocardial oxygen consumption and the subsequent imbalance between oxygen supply and demand. Progressive activity also helps strengthen the myocardium, which enhances cardiac output and subsequently improves activity tolerance.
11. Instruct client to report a decreased tolerance for activity and to stop any activity that causes chest pain, shortness of breath, dizziness, or extreme fatigue or weakness.	11. These symptoms indicate that insufficient oxygen is reaching the tissues and that activity has been increased beyond a therapeutic level.
12. Consult physician if signs and symptoms of activity intolerance persist or worsen.	12. Notifying the physician allows for modification of treatment plan.

Nursing Diagnosis: Airway Clearance, Ineffective

Definition

Inability to clear secretions or obstructions from the respiratory tract to maintain a clear airway

Defining Characteristics

Dyspnea; orthopnea; diminished breath sounds; adventitious breath sounds (crackles, rhonchi, wheezes); cough, ineffective or absent; sputum production; difficulty vocalizing; wide-eyed; restlessness; changes in respiratory rate and rhythm; cyanosis

Related Factors

Environmental: Smoking; smoke inhalation; second-hand smoke

Obstructed airway: airway spasm; retained secretions; excessive mucus; presence of artificial airway; foreign body in airway; secretions in the bronchi; exudate in the alveoli

Physiological: Neuromuscular dysfunction; hyperplasia of the bronchial walls; chronic obstructive pulmonary disease; infection; asthma; allergic airways

Desired Outcome

The client will maintain clear, open airways as evidenced by:
a. normal breath sounds
b. normal rate and depth of respirations
c. absence of dyspnea.

Documentation

a. Breath sounds
b. Rate, depth, and ease of respirations
c. Characteristics of cough
d. Description of sputum
e. Therapeutic interventions
f. Client teaching

Suggested NIC Interventions: Respiratory monitoring; Airway management; Airway suctioning; Chest physiotherapy; Cough enhancement

NURSING ACTIONS	RATIONALES
Assessments	
1. Assess for and report signs and symptoms of ineffective airway clearance (e.g., abnormal breath sounds; rapid, shallow respirations; dyspnea; cough).	1. Early recognition and reporting of signs and symptoms of ineffective airway clearance allow for prompt intervention.
Prevention/Treatment	
2. Implement measures to decrease pain if present (e.g., splint chest or abdominal incision with pillow when coughing and deep breathing, administer prescribed analgesics before planned activity).	2. Pain often interferes with a client's willingness to move, cough, and deep breathe. Pain reduction enables the client to increase activity and cough and deep breathe more effectively, all of which promote effective airway clearance.
3. Instruct and assist client to change position, deep breathe, and cough or "huff" every 1 to 2 hours.	3. Repositioning helps mobilize secretions. Deep breathing helps clear the airways by loosening secretions and promoting a more effective cough. Coughing or "huffing" (a forced expiration technique) accelerates airflow through the airways, which helps mobilize and clear mucus and foreign matter from the respiratory tract.
4. Increase activity as allowed and tolerated.	4. Activity helps mobilize secretions and promotes deeper breathing. Deep breathing can help loosen secretions and enhance the effectiveness of coughing.
5. Implement measures to thin secretions and maintain adequate moisture of the respiratory mucous membranes (e.g., maintain a fluid intake of 2500 ml/day, humidify inspired air).	5. Adequate hydration and humidified inspired air help thin secretions, which facilitates the mobilization and expectoration of secretions. These actions also reduce dryness of the respiratory mucous membrane, which helps enhance mucociliary clearance.
6. Assist with administration of mucolytics (e.g., acetylcysteine) and diluent or hydrating agents (e.g., water, saline) via nebulizer as ordered.	6. Mucolytics and diluent or hydrating agents are mucokinetic substances that reduce the viscosity of mucus, thus making it easier for the client to mobilize and clear secretions from the respiratory tract.
7. Assist with or perform postural drainage therapy (PDT) if ordered.	7. Postural drainage therapy techniques (e.g., vibration, percussion, postural drainage) utilize the forces of motion and gravity to mobilize secretions from the periphery of the lungs to the larger central airways where they can be removed by coughing or suctioning.
8. Perform suctioning if needed.	8. Suctioning removes secretions from the large airways. It also stimulates coughing, which helps clear airways of mucus and foreign matter.

NURSING ACTIONS	RATIONALES
Prevention/Treatment	
9. Administer expectorants (e.g., guaifenesin, dornase alfa) if ordered.	9. Expectorants reduce the viscosity of sputum, making it easier to be removed by coughing or suctioning.
10. Discourage smoking.	10. Irritants present in smoke increase mucus production, impair ciliary function, and can cause inflammation and damage to the bronchial walls. This results in narrowed airways and stasis of pulmonary secretions.
11. Administer the following medications if ordered: a. bronchodilators: 1. methylxanthines (e.g., theophylline, aminophylline, oxtriphylline) 2. sympathomimetic (adrenergic) agents (e.g., albuterol, terbutaline, metaproterenol, salmeterol) 3. anticholinergic agents (e.g., ipratropium) b. corticosteroids (e.g., prednisone, methylprednisolone, beclomethasone, flunisolide, triamcinolone, budesonide) c. leukotriene modifiers (e.g., montelukast, zafirlukast).	11. These medications increase the patency of the airways and enhance bronchial airflow. Methylxanthines and sympathomimetics produce bronchodilation by relaxing the bronchial smooth muscle. Anticholinergic agents block cholinergic reflex constriction of the bronchioles and decrease mucus production. Corticosteroids and leukotriene modifiers reduce inflammation in the airways, which results in decreased bronchial hyperreactivity and constriction and mucus production.
12. Administer central nervous system depressants judiciously.	12. Central nervous system depressants depress the cough reflex, which can result in stasis of secretions.
13. Consult appropriate health care provider (e.g., physician, respiratory therapist) if signs and symptoms of ineffective airway clearance persist.	13. Notifying the appropriate health care provider allows for modification of the treatment plan.

Nursing Diagnosis: Anxiety

Definition

Vague uneasy feeling of discomfort or dread accompanied by an autonomic response (the source is often nonspecific or unknown to the individual); a feeling of apprehension caused by anticipation of danger. It is an altering signal that warns of impending danger and enables the individual to take measures to deal with threat

Defining Characteristics

Behavioral: diminished productivity; scanning and vigilance; poor eye contact; restlessness; glancing about; extraneous movement (e.g., foot shuffling, hand/arm movements); expressed concerns due to change in life events; insomnia; fidgeting
Affective: regretful; irritability; anguish; scared; jittery; overexcited; painful and persistent increased helplessness; rattled; uncertainty; increased wariness; focus on self; feelings of inadequacy; fearful; distressed; worried, apprehensive; anxious
Physiological: voice quivering; trembling/hand tremors; shakiness; increased respiration; urinary urgency; increased pulse; pupil dilation; increased reflexes; abdominal pain; sleep disturbance; tingling in extremities; cardiovascular excitation; increased perspiration; facial tension; anorexia; heart pounding; diarrhea; urinary hesitancy; fatigue; dry mouth; weakness; decreased pulse; facial flushing; superficial vasoconstriction; twitching; decreased blood pressure; nausea; urinary frequency; faintness; respiratory difficulties; increased blood pressure
Cognitive: blocking of thought; confusion; preoccupation; forgetfulness; rumination; impaired attention; decreased perceptual field; fear of unspecific consequences; tendency to blame others; difficulty concentrating; diminished ability to problem solve; diminished ability to learn; awareness of physiological symptoms

Related Factors

Exposure to toxins; threat to or change in role status; unconscious conflict about essential values/goals of life; familial association/heredity; unmet needs; interpersonal transmission/contagion; situational/maturational crises; threat of death; threat to or change in health status; threat to or change in interaction patterns; threat to or change in role function; threat to self-concept; threat to or change in environment; stress; threat to or change in economic status; substance abuse

Desired Outcome

The client will experience a reduction in anxiety as evidenced by:
a. verbalization of feeling less anxious
b. usual sleep pattern
c. relaxed facial expression and body movements
d. stable vital signs
e. usual perceptual ability and interactions with others.

Documentation

a. Verbalization of feeling anxious
b. Sleep pattern
c. Facial expression and body movement
d. Vital signs
e. Focus on self
f. Client's perception of precipitating factors
g. Therapeutic interventions
h. Client/family teaching

Suggested NIC Interventions: Anxiety reduction; Calming technique; Emotional support; Presence

NURSING ACTIONS	RATIONALES
Assessments	
1. Assess client for signs and symptoms of anxiety (e.g., verbalization of feeling anxious, insomnia, tenseness, shakiness, restlessness, diaphoresis, tachycardia, elevated B/P, self-focused behaviors).	1. Early recognition of signs and symptoms of anxiety allows for prompt intervention
Prevention/Treatment	
2. Encourage verbalization of feelings and concerns and assist client to identify specific stressors that may be causing anxiety. Provide feedback.	2. Verbalization of feelings and concerns helps the client identify factors that are causing anxiety. Providing feedback helps the client clarify and validate feelings and concerns and identify techniques that can reduce anxiety.
3. Orient client to environment, equipment, and routines.	3. Familiarity with the environment and usual routines reduces the client's anxiety about the unknown, provides a sense of security, and increases his/her sense of control, all of which help decrease anxiety.
4. Introduce staff who will be participating in the client's care. If possible, maintain consistency in staff assigned to his/her care.	4. Introduction of the staff familiarizes the client with those individuals who will be working with him/her, which provides a sense of comfort with the environment. Consistency in staff assignment provides the client with a feeling of stability, which reduces the anxiety that typically occurs with change.
5. Assure client that staff members are nearby. Respond to call signal as soon as possible.	5. Close contact and a prompt response to requests provide a sense of security and facilitate the development of trust, thus reducing the client's anxiety.
6. Maintain a calm, supportive, confident manner when interacting with the client.	6. A sense of calmness and confidence conveys to the client that someone is in control of the situation, which helps reduce anxiety.
7. Reinforce physician's explanations and clarify misconceptions the client has about the diagnostic tests, disease condition, treatment plan, surgical procedure, and/or prognosis.	7. Factual information and an awareness of what to expect help decrease the anxiety that arises from uncertainty.
8. Implement measures to reduce respiratory distress if present (e.g., elevate head of bed, encourage client to breathe deeply and more slowly, administer oxygen as ordered).	8. Improvement of respiratory status helps relieve anxiety associated with the feeling of not being able to breathe.

NURSING ACTIONS	RATIONALES
Prevention/Treatment	
9. Implement measures to reduce pain if present (e.g., administer prescribed analgesics, instruct and assist with relaxation techniques).	9. Pain can create or increase anxiety because it is often perceived as a threat to well-being. Pain also causes sympathetic nervous system stimulation with subsequent feelings of tenseness and increased anxiety.
10. Provide a calm, restful environment.	10. A calm, restful environment facilitates relaxation and promotes a sense of security, which reduces anxiety.
11. Instruct client in relaxation techniques and encourage participation in diversional activities.	11. Relaxation techniques reduce muscle tension and other physiological effects of anxiety. Activities that the client enjoys provide distraction, which may reduce anxiety.
12. When appropriate, assist client to meet spiritual needs (e.g., arrange for a visit from clergy).	12. Spiritual support is a source of comfort and security for many people and can help reduce the client's anxiety.
13. Initiate a social service referral and/or assist client to identify and contact appropriate community resources if indicated.	13. Concerns about factors such as finances, follow-up medical care, and home maintenance can be a source of great anxiety. Facilitating contact with the appropriate resource(s) can help reduce the client's anxiety and provide ongoing support.
14. Encourage significant others to project a caring, concerned attitude without obvious anxiousness.	14. Anxiety is easily transferable from one person to another. If significant others convey empathy, provide reassurance, and do not appear anxious, they can help reduce the client's anxiety.
15. Administer prescribed antianxiety agents if indicated.	15. Medications are sometimes prescribed to help reduce the client's anxiety. Benzodiazepines (e.g., lorazepam, diazepam, alprazolam, chlordiazepoxide) are the drugs of choice for management of short-term anxiety. These drugs augment the inhibitory effect of gamma-aminobutyric acid (GABA) on cell membrane responses to excitatory neurotransmitters.
16. Include significant others in orientation and teaching sessions and encourage their continued support of the client.	16. Significant others can help reduce the client's anxiety by reinforcing information that he/she has difficulty understanding or recalling. In addition, the presence of significant others often provides the client with a sense of support and security, which helps to reduce anxiety.
17. Provide information based on current needs of client at a level he/she can understand. Encourage client to ask questions and to seek clarification of information provided.	17. Providing the client with information that he/she is not ready to process or cannot understand tends to increase anxiety. Making the client feel comfortable enough to ask questions or clarify information helps to reduce anxiety.
18. Consult appropriate health care provider (e.g., psychiatric nurse clinician, physician) if above actions fail to control anxiety.	18. Notifying the appropriate health care provider allows for modification of the treatment plan.

Nursing Diagnosis: Aspiration, Risk For

Definition

At risk for entry of gastrointestinal secretions, oropharyngeal secretions, solids, or fluids into tracheobronchial passages

Risk Factors

Reduced level of consciousness; depressed cough and gag reflexes; presence of tracheostomy or endotracheal tube; incompetent lower esophageal sphincter; gastrointestinal tubes; tube feedings; medication administration; situations hindering elevation of upper body; increased intragastric pressure; increased gastric residual; decreased gastrointestinal motility; delayed gastric emptying; impaired swallowing; facial, oral, neck surgery or trauma; wired jaws

Desired Outcome

The client will not aspirate secretions or foods/fluids as evidenced by:
a. clear breath sounds
b. resonant percussion note over lungs
c. absence of cough, tachypnea, and dyspnea.

Documentation

a. Breath sounds
b. Percussion note over lungs
c. Respiratory rate and effort
d. Presence of cough
e. Pulse rate
f. Color of tracheal aspirate
g. Therapeutic interventions
h. Client/family teaching

Suggested NIC Interventions: Aspiration precautions; Respiratory monitoring; Swallowing therapy; Airway suctioning

NURSING ACTIONS / RATIONALES

Assessments

1. Assess for and report signs and symptoms of aspiration of secretions or foods/fluids (e.g., rhonchi, dull percussion note over affected lung area, cough, tachypnea, dyspnea, tachycardia, presence of tube feeding in tracheal aspirate).
   - *Rationale:* 1. Early recognition and reporting of signs and symptoms of aspiration allow for prompt intervention.
2. Assist with diagnostic studies to determine if aspiration is occurring during swallowing (e.g., videofluoroscopy).
   - *Rationale:* 2. Aspiration of foods/fluids during the swallowing process is evident on studies such as videofluoroscopy. Knowing when aspiration occurs during the swallowing process aids in the development of an individualized plan of care to prevent further aspiration.
3. Monitor chest x-ray results. Report findings of pulmonary infiltrate.
   - *Rationale:* 3. Evidence of pulmonary infiltrate on chest x-ray results can indicate that aspiration has occurred.

Prevention

4. Implement the following measures to prevent aspiration if client has a depressed or absent gag reflex, severe dysphagia, and/or decreased level of consciousness:
   - *Rationale:* 4. The risk for aspiration is high when mechanisms to protect the client's airway (e.g., gag reflex, swallowing reflex) are impaired or the client has a decreased level of consciousness.
   a. withhold oral foods/fluids
      - *Rationale:* a. Withholding oral foods/fluids eliminates the possibility of aspiration of same.
   b. place client in a side-lying position unless contraindicated
      - *Rationale:* b. Placing the client in a side-lying position allows oral secretions to accumulate in the mouth where they can be expectorated or removed by suctioning rather than flow into the pharynx where they can enter the larynx and be aspirated.
   c. perform oral hygiene and/or oropharyngeal suctioning as often as needed to remove excess secretions.
      - *Rationale:* c. Removing excess secretions from the mouth and pharynx prevents them from entering the larynx and being aspirated.
5. Implement measures to prevent vomiting (e.g., eliminate noxious sights and odors, administer antiemetics as ordered).
   - *Rationale:* 5. When the client vomits, gastric contents move up the esophagus, through the pharynx, and into the mouth. While vomitus is in the pharynx, it can spill into the larynx resulting in aspiration.
6. If client is receiving tube feedings, check tube placement before each feeding or on a routine basis if tube feeding is continuous.
   - *Rationale:* 6. Verification of feeding tube placement ensures that the tube feeding solution goes into the alimentary tract rather than the lungs.

NURSING ACTIONS / **RATIONALES**

Prevention

7. Implement measures to reduce the risk of regurgitation (e.g., maintain gastric decompression as ordered, provide small meals rather than large ones, do not administer tube feedings if the residual exceeds specified amount [usually 75 to 100 ml], maintain client in high Fowler's position for at least 30 minutes after meals and tube feedings, administer upper gastrointestinal stimulants as ordered).

   Rationale: 7. As gastric secretions or foods/fluids accumulate in the stomach, upward pressure is placed on the lower esophageal sphincter (LES). If the pressure increases significantly and/or the client has an incompetent LES, regurgitation can occur. Contents that move up through the esophagus into the pharynx can spill into the larynx, resulting in aspiration.

8. Implement measures to prevent aspiration when client is eating and drinking:

   Rationale: 8. When the client is eating and drinking, there is a high risk for aspiration before the swallowing reflex is triggered (the larynx and pharynx are at rest and the airway is open at this time), during swallowing if the larynx does not close completely, and after swallowing when the larynx opens again.

   a. perform actions to improve swallowing if indicated (e.g., select foods/fluids appropriate to client's swallowing ability, reinforce exercises to strengthen and develop muscles used in swallowing)

      Rationale: a. Improving the ability to swallow helps ensure that foods/fluids do not enter the larynx when the client is eating and drinking.

   b. place client in high Fowler's position unless contraindicated

      Rationale: b. This position uses gravity to facilitate movement of foods/fluids through the pharynx into the esophagus where the risk for aspiration is greatly reduced.

   c. instruct client to avoid laughing or talking when swallowing

      Rationale: c. Normally, when the swallowing reflex is triggered, the folds of the larynx that form its three valves contract so that aspiration does not occur as foods/fluids pass from the back of the mouth through the pharynx. When the client talks and laughs, air is forced through the trachea and the larynx opens. Instructing the client to avoid talking and laughing when swallowing reduces the risk of the airway being open when food/fluid is in the pharynx.

   d. encourage client to concentrate on eating and drinking and allow ample time for meals and snacks

      Rationale: d. If the client becomes distracted and/or is rushed during meals or snacks, swallowing and breathing attempts can become uncoordinated. This results in the larynx being open when the food/fluid is in the pharynx, which greatly increases the risk for aspiration.

   e. instruct client to dry swallow, cough twice, or clear his or her throat after swallowing if indicated.

      Rationale: e. If the client has a swallowing impairment such as decreased pharyngeal peristalsis, food/fluid can remain in the pharyngeal recesses after the swallowing reflex has occurred. Dry swallowing, coughing, or clearing the throat helps ensure that the pharynx is clear after swallowing, which reduces the risk for aspiration.

9. Instruct and assist the client to perform oral hygiene after meals.

   Rationale: 9. Good oral hygiene after meals results in removal of remaining food particles that could enter the larynx and be aspirated into the lungs.

NURSING DIAGNOSIS: BREATHING PATTERN, INEFFECTIVE

Definition Inspiration and/or expiration that does not provide adequate ventilation

Defining Characteristics Dyspnea; shortness of breath; orthopnea; respiratory rate (adults [ages 14 or greater] < 11 or > 24, infants < 25 or > 60, ages 1 to 4 < 20 or > 30, ages 5–14 < 14 or > 25); depth of breathing (tidal volume: adults 500 ml at rest, infants 6 to 8 ml/kg); decreased inspiratory/expiratory pressure; decreased minute ventilation; decreased vital capacity; nasal flaring; use of accessory muscles to breathe; assumption of three-point position; altered chest excursion; pursed-lip breathing; prolonged expiration phases; increased anterior-posterior diameter

Related Factors

Hyperventilation; hypoventilation syndrome; bony deformity; pain; chest wall deformity; anxiety; decreased energy/fatigue; neuromuscular dysfunction; musculoskeletal impairment; perception/cognitive impairment; obesity; spinal cord injury; body position; neurological immaturity; respiratory muscle fatigue

Desired Outcome

The client will maintain an effective breathing pattern as evidenced by:
a. normal rate and depth of respirations
b. symmetrical chest excursion
c. absence of dyspnea.

Documentation

a. Rate, depth, and ease of respirations
b. Chest excursion
c. Oximetry results
d. Therapeutic interventions
e. Client teaching

Suggested NIC Interventions: Respiratory monitoring; Ventilation assistance; Anxiety reduction

NURSING ACTIONS	RATIONALES
Assessments	
1. Assess for signs and symptoms of an ineffective breathing pattern (e.g., shallow respirations, tachypnea, limited chest excursion, dyspnea, use of accessory muscles when breathing).	1. Early recognition of signs and symptoms of an ineffective breathing pattern allows for prompt intervention.
2. Monitor for and report a significant decrease in oximetry results.	2. Oximetry is a noninvasive method of measuring arterial oxygen saturation. The results assist in evaluating respiratory status.
Prevention/Treatment	
3. Implement measures to reduce chest or abdominal pain if present (e.g., splint incision with pillow during coughing and deep breathing, administer prescribed analgesics before planned activity).	3. A client with chest or upper abdominal pain often guards respiratory efforts and breathes shallowly in an attempt to prevent additional discomfort. Pain reduction enables the client to breathe more deeply.
4. Implement measures to decrease fear and anxiety (e.g., assure client that breathing deeply will not dislodge tubes or cause incision to break open, interact with client in a confident manner).	4. Fear and anxiety may cause a client to breathe shallowly or to hyperventilate. Decreasing fear and anxiety allows the client to focus on breathing more slowly and taking deeper breaths.
5. Implement measures to increase strength and activity tolerance if client is weak and fatigued (e.g., provide uninterrupted rest periods, maintain optimal nutrition).	5. An increase in strength and activity tolerance enables the client to breathe more deeply and participate in activities to improve breathing pattern.
6. Place client in a semi- to high Fowler's position unless contraindicated. Position with pillows to prevent slumping.	6. A semi- to high Fowler's position allows for maximal diaphragmatic excursion and lung expansion. Prevention of slumping is essential because slumping causes the abdominal contents to be pushed up against the diaphragm and restrict lung expansion.
7. If client must remain flat in bed, assist with position change at least every 2 hours.	7. Compression of the thorax and subsequent limited chest wall and lung expansion occur when the client lies in one position. Frequent repositioning promotes maximal chest wall and lung expansion.
8. Instruct client to deep breathe or use incentive spirometer every 1–2 hours.	8. Deep breathing and use of an incentive spirometer promote maximal inhalation and lung expansion. Deep inhalation also stimulates surfactant production, which lowers alveolar surface tension and subsequently increases lung compliance and ease of inflation.

NURSING ACTIONS / **RATIONALES**

Prevention/Treatment

9. Assist with positive airway pressure techniques (e.g., continuous positive airway pressure [CPAP], bilevel positive airway pressure [BiPAP], flutter/positive expiratory pressure [PEP] device) if ordered.

   Rationale: 9. Positive airway pressure techniques increase intrapulmonary (alveolar) pressure, which helps reexpand collapsed alveoli and prevent further alveolar collapse.

10. Instruct client in and assist with diaphragmatic and pursed-lip breathing techniques if appropriate. NOTE: Diaphragmatic breathing is most often indicated for clients who have had thoracic surgery or clients who have chronic airflow limitation (e.g., emphysema) or neuromuscular conditions that cause fixation or weakening of the diaphragm.

    Rationale: 10. Diaphragmatic breathing promotes greater movement of the diaphragm and decreases the use of accessory muscles for inspiration. Use of this technique eases the work of breathing and ultimately promotes an increased efficiency of alveolar ventilation. Pursed-lip breathing causes a mild resistance to exhalation, which creates positive pressure in the airways. This pressure helps prevent airway collapse and subsequently promotes more complete alveolar emptying.

11. Instruct client to breathe slowly if hyperventilating.

    Rationale: 11. Hyperventilation is an ineffective breathing pattern that can eventually lead to respiratory alkalosis. The client can often slow breathing rate if he/she concentrates on doing so.

12. Instruct client in and assist with segmental or localized breathing exercises if appropriate (may be indicated for clients with painful respiratory conditions or clients who have had thoracic or abdominal surgery).

    Rationale: 12. Segmental or localized breathing exercises improve expansion of apical and/or basal areas of the lung by having the client focus on selectively expanding these areas of the chest.

13. Increase activity as allowed and tolerated.

    Rationale: 13. During activity, especially ambulation, the client usually takes deeper breaths, thus increasing lung expansion.

14. Administer central nervous system depressants judiciously. Hold medication and consult physician if respiratory rate is less than 12/minute.

    Rationale: 14. Central nervous system depressants cause depression of the respiratory center in the brainstem, which can result in a decreased rate and depth of respiration.

15. Consult appropriate health care provider (e.g., physician, respiratory therapist) if ineffective breathing pattern continues.

    Rationale: 15. Notifying the appropriate health care provider allows for modification of treatment plan.

Nursing Diagnosis: Cardiac Output, Decreased

Definition

Inadequate blood pumped by the heart to meet metabolic demands of the body

Defining Characteristics

Altered Heart Rate/Rhythm: arrhythmias; palpitations; EKG changes
Altered Preload: jugular vein distention; fatigue; edema; murmurs; increased/decreased central venous pressure (CVP); increased/decreased pulmonary artery wedge pressure (PAWP); weight gain
Altered Afterload: cold/clammy skin; shortness of breath/dyspnea; oliguria; prolonged capillary refill; decreased peripheral pulses; variations in blood pressure readings; increased/decreased systemic vascular resistance (SVR); increased/decreased pulmonary vascular resistance (PVR); skin color changes
Altered Contractility: crackles; cough; orthopnea/paroxysmal nocturnal dyspnea; cardiac output < 4 L/min; cardiac index < 2.5 L/min; decreased ejection fraction, Stroke Volume Index (SVI), Left Ventricular Stroke Work Index (LVSWI); S_3 or S_4 sounds
Behavioral/Emotional: anxiety; restlessness

Related Factors

Altered heart rate/rhythm
Altered stroke volume: altered preload; altered afterload; altered contractility

Desired Outcome

The client will maintain adequate cardiac output as evidenced by:

a. B/P within normal range for client
b. apical pulse regular and 60–100 beats/minute
c. absence of gallop rhythms
d. absence of fatigue and weakness

e. unlabored respirations at 12–20/minute
f. clear, audible breath sounds
g. usual mental status
h. absence of dizziness and syncope
i. palpable peripheral pulses
j. skin warm and usual color
k. capillary refill time less than 2–3 seconds
l. urine output at least 30 ml/hr
m. absence of edema and jugular vein distention
n. hemodynamic measurements such as cardiac output (CO), pulmonary artery pressure (PAP), pulmonary capillary wedge pressure (PCWP), and central venous pressure (CVP) within normal range.

Documentation

a. Vital signs
b. Heart sounds
c. Activity tolerance
d. Breath sounds
e. Ease of respirations
f. Mental status
g. Peripheral pulses
h. Capillary refill time
i. Skin color and temperature
j. Urine output
k. Presence of edema
l. Presence of jugular vein distention
m. Hemodynamic measurements (e.g., CO, PAP, PCWP, CVP)
n. Therapeutic interventions
o. Client teaching

Suggested NIC Interventions: Cardiac care: acute; Invasive hemodynamic monitoring; Hemodynamic regulation; Cardiac precautions; Dysrhythmia management; Oxygen therapy; Hypovolemia management; Hypervolemia management; Electrolyte management: hypomagnesemia; Electrolyte management: hypokalemia; Cardiac care: rehabilitative

NURSING ACTIONS

Assessments

1. Assess for and report signs and symptoms of decreased cardiac output:
   a. variations in B/P (may be increased because of compensatory vasoconstriction; may be decreased when compensatory mechanisms and pump fail)
   b. tachycardia
   c. presence of gallop rhythm
   d. fatigue and weakness
   e. dyspnea, tachypnea
   f. crackles (rales)
   g. restlessness, change in mental status
   h. dizziness, syncope
   i. diminished or absent peripheral pulses
   j. cool extremities
   k. pallor or cyanosis of skin
   l. capillary refill time greater than 2–3 seconds
   m. oliguria
   n. edema
   o. jugular vein distention (JVD)
   p. hemodynamic abnormalities such as decreased CO and increased PAP, PCWP, and CVP.

RATIONALES

1. Early recognition and reporting of signs and symptoms of decreased cardiac output allow for prompt intervention.

NURSING ACTIONS	RATIONALES
Assessments	
2. Monitor ECG readings and report significant abnormalities.	2. ECG readings provide data regarding functioning of the heart's electrical conduction system. Altered generation or transmission of electrical impulses often causes an abnormal heart rate or rhythm that can lead to decreased cardiac output.
3. Monitor chest x-ray results. Report findings of cardiomegaly, pulmonary vascular congestion, pleural effusion, or pulmonary edema.	3. Chest x-ray films provide data regarding the size of the heart, volume of blood in the pulmonary vessels, and fluid accumulation in the pleural space, pulmonary interstitium, and alveoli. Cardiomegaly often results in decreased cardiac output whereas pulmonary vascular congestion, pleural effusion, and pulmonary edema are often a result of decreased cardiac output.
Prevention/Treatment	
4. Implement measures to prevent hypovolemia (e.g., maintain a minimal fluid intake of 1000 ml/day unless ordered otherwise, consult physician before giving diuretics if excessive weight loss has occurred or client develops postural hypotension, administer blood and/or colloid or crystalloid solutions as ordered).	4. Hypovolemia reduces venous return to the heart, which subsequently decreases the amount of blood in the ventricles at the end of diastole (preload). This results in a decrease in stroke volume and cardiac output.
5. Implement measures to reduce cardiac workload:	5. Cardiac workload is the effort the heart expends to pump blood. The work of the heart is determined largely by the volume of blood distending the ventricles at the end of diastole (preload) and the amount of tension the ventricle must pump against to eject blood (afterload). Decreasing cardiac workload reduces the work that the compromised heart must perform in order to pump an adequate amount of blood. This results in increased cardiac output.
a. place client in a semi- to high Fowler's position	a. Elevation of client's upper body reduces cardiac workload by decreasing venous return from the periphery and subsequently reducing preload.
b. instruct client to avoid activities that create a Valsalva response (e.g., straining to have a bowel movement, holding breath while moving up in bed)	b. When a client exhales following the Valsalva maneuver, the intrathoracic pressure falls, causing a sudden increase in venous return and a subsequent increase in preload and cardiac workload. The rebound increase in heart rate and blood pressure that occurs following the Valsalva maneuver also causes an increase in cardiac workload.
c. perform actions to promote physical and emotional rest (e.g., maintain a calm, quiet environment; limit the number of visitors; maintain activity restrictions)	c. Physical rest reduces cardiac workload by lowering the body's energy requirements and subsequent need for oxygen. Promoting emotional rest reduces cardiac workload by preventing the increase in heart rate and blood pressure that accompanies stress-induced sympathetic nervous system stimulation.
d. perform actions to promote adequate tissue oxygenation (e.g., maintain oxygen therapy as ordered, encourage deep breathing exercises and use of incentive spirometer)	d. When tissue oxygenation is adequate, the heart does not need to work as hard to supply oxygen to the tissues; thus, more oxygen is available for myocardial use.
e. discourage smoking	e. Nicotine stimulates catecholamine output, which increases heart rate and causes vasoconstriction and subsequently increases cardiac workload. Smoking also reduces oxygen availability because hemoglobin has a greater affinity for the carbon monoxide in smoke than for oxygen. This increases cardiac workload as the heart tries to compensate for the reduced oxygen levels.

f. discourage excessive intake of beverages high in caffeine such as coffee, tea, and colas

f. Excessive caffeine can increase cardiac workload because caffeine is a myocardial stimulant and can increase the rate and force of myocardial contractions.

g. provide small meals rather than large ones

g. Large meals can increase cardiac workload because they require a greater increase in blood supply to the gastrointestinal tract to aid digestion.

h. perform actions to prevent or treat fluid volume excess (e.g., maintain prescribed fluid and dietary sodium restrictions, administer diuretics as ordered)

h. Preventing or treating excess fluid volume reduces vascular volume, which decreases preload and afterload and subsequently reduces cardiac workload.

i. increase activity gradually as allowed and tolerated.

i. A gradual increase in activity prevents a sudden increase in cardiac workload. A graded activity program also helps strengthen and tone the myocardium, which ultimately increases cardiac output.

6. Administer the following medications if ordered:

6.

a. positive inotropic agents (e.g., digitalis preparations, dobutamine, dopamine, inamrinone, milrinone)

a. Positive inotropic agents increase cardiac output by improving myocardial contractility.

b. nitrates (e.g., nitroglycerin, isosorbide dinitrate)

b. Nitrates decrease cardiac workload and myocardial oxygen demands by relaxing peripheral veins and, to a lesser extent, arterioles. This reduces venous return to the heart (preload) and peripheral vascular resistance (afterload). Nitrates also dilate nonsclerosed coronary arteries, which improves coronary blood flow and myocardial oxygen supply.

c. direct-acting vasodilators (e.g., sodium nitroprusside, hydralazine) or centrally acting or alpha-adrenergic inhibitors (e.g., clonidine, prazosin, doxazosin)

c. Vasodilators reduce cardiac workload by dilating the arterioles and subsequently decreasing peripheral vascular resistance (afterload). Certain vasodilators also dilate the veins, which decreases venous return and lowers diastolic ventricular filling pressure (preload).

d. angiotensin-converting enzyme (ACE) inhibitors (e.g., captopril, enalapril, lisinopril, benazepril, fosinopril, quinapril) or angiotensin II receptor antagonists (e.g., losartan, valsartan)

d. ACE inhibitors/angiotensin II receptor antagonists block the formation/effect of angiotensin II (a potent vasoconstrictor), which subsequently also causes a decrease in aldosterone output. The reduction in angiotensin II and aldosterone results in a decrease in total peripheral vascular resistance and reduced sodium and water retention, which leads to decreased cardiac workload.

e. beta-adrenergic blocking agents (e.g., propranolol, metoprolol, atenolol, nadolol, sotalol)

e. Beta-adrenergic blockers reduce cardiac workload by blocking sympathetic nervous system stimulation of beta receptors in the heart.

f. anticholinergic agents (e.g., atropine)

f. Cardiac output is dependent on stroke volume and heart rate. Anticholinergics increase the heart rate (have a positive chronotropic effect) and are used to increase cardiac output in clients with bradyarrhythmias.

g. antidysrhythmics (e.g., flecainide, lidocaine, disopyramide, procainamide, amiodarone, esmolol, sotalol, adenosine)

g. Antidysrhythmics improve cardiac output by correcting automaticity and/or conduction abnormalities in the heart. By slowing the heart rate and/or decreasing irregularity of the heart rate, the diastolic filling time is prolonged, resulting in an increased preload and stroke volume.

h. calcium channel blocking agents (e.g., nifedipine, verapamil, diltiazem, nicardipine, amlodipine).

h. Calcium channel blockers dilate the coronary arteries, thus improving coronary blood flow and myocardial oxygen supply. They also reduce cardiac workload by dilating peripheral arteries and subsequently reducing afterload. Certain calcium channel blockers (e.g., diltiazem, verapamil) also have an antidysrhythmic effect, which subsequently increases cardiac output by helping restore normal heart rate and rhythm.

NURSING ACTIONS	RATIONALES
Prevention/Treatment	
7. Consult physician if signs and symptoms of decreased cardiac output persist or worsen.	7. Notifying the physician allows for modification of treatment plan.

Nursing Diagnosis: Constipation

Definition

A decrease in normal frequency of defecation accompanied by difficult or incomplete passage of stool and/or passage of excessively hard, dry stool

Defining Characteristics

Change in bowel pattern; bright red blood with stool; presence of soft, pastelike stool in rectum; distended abdomen; dark, black, or tarry stool; increased abdominal pressure; percussed abdominal dullness; pain with defecation; decreased volume of stool; straining with defecation; decreased frequency; dry, hard, formed stool; palpable rectal mass; feeling of rectal fullness or pressure; abdominal pain; unable to pass stool; anorexia; headache; change in abdominal growling (borborygmi); indigestion; atypical presentations in older adults (e.g., change in mental status, urinary incontinence, unexplained falls, elevated body temperature); severe flatus; generalized fatigue; hypoactive or hyperactive bowel sounds; palpable abdominal mass; abdominal tenderness with or without palpable muscle resistance; nausea and/or vomiting; oozing liquid stool

Related Factors

Functional: recent environmental changes; habitual denying/ignoring of urge to defecate; insufficient physical activity; irregular defecation habits; inadequate toileting (e.g., timeliness, positioning for defecation, privacy); abdominal muscle weakness

Psychological: depression; emotional stress; mental confusion

Pharmacological: anticonvulsants; antilipemic agents; laxative overdose; calcium carbonate; aluminum-containing antacids; nonsteroidal anti-inflammatory agents; opiates; anticholinergics; diuretics; iron salts; phenothiazines; sedatives; sympathomimetics; bismuth salts; antidepressants; calcium channel blockers

Mechanical: rectal abscess or ulcer; pregnancy; rectal anal fissures; tumors; megacolon (Hirschsprung's disease); electrolyte imbalance; rectal prolapse; prostate enlargement; neurological impairment; rectal anal stricture; rectocele; postsurgical obstruction; hemorrhoids; obesity

Physiological: poor eating habits; decreased motility of gastrointestinal tract; inadequate dentition or oral hygiene; insufficient fiber intake; insufficient fluid intake; change in usual foods and eating pattern; dehydration

Desired Outcome

The client will maintain usual bowel elimination pattern as evidenced by:

a. usual frequency of bowel movements
b. passage of soft, formed stool
c. absence of abdominal distention and pain, feeling of rectal fullness or pressure, and straining during defecation.

Documentation

a. Occurrence of last bowel movement
b. Characteristics of stool
c. Abdominal distention or pain
d. Reports of fullness or pressure in rectum
e. Reports of straining at stool
f. Bowel sounds
g. Therapeutic interventions
h. Client teaching

Suggested NIC Intervention: Constipation/Impaction management

NURSING ACTIONS	RATIONALES
Assessments	
1. Ascertain client's usual bowel elimination habits.	1. Knowledge of the client's usual bowel elimination habits is essential in determining if constipation is present because the frequency of defecation varies among individuals.
2. Assess for signs and symptoms of constipation (e.g., decrease in frequency of bowel movements; passage of hard, formed stools; anorexia; abdominal distention and pain; feeling of fullness or pressure in rectum; straining during defecation).	2. Early recognition of signs and symptoms of constipation allows for prompt intervention.
3. Assess bowel sounds. Report a pattern of decreasing bowel sounds.	3. Bowel sounds are produced by peristaltic activity. A pattern of decreasing bowel sounds indicates a decrease in bowel motility, which can lead to and be present with constipation.
Prevention/Treatment	
4. Encourage client to defecate whenever the urge is felt.	4. If the client feels the urge to defecate but suppresses it by contracting the external anal sphincter, the defecation reflex will subside after a few minutes and not recur for several hours or until additional feces enters the rectum. Repeated inhibition of the defecation reflex results in progressive weakening of the reflex. In addition, when the defecation reflex is inhibited, feces remain in the colon longer and water continues to be absorbed from the feces, making the stool drier, harder, and subsequently more difficult to evacuate.
5. Assist client to toilet or bedside commode or place in high Fowler's position on bedpan for bowel movements unless contraindicated.	5. A sitting position aids in the expulsion of stool by taking advantage of gravity. This position also enhances the client's ability to perform the Valsalva maneuver, which increases intra-abdominal pressure and forces the fecal contents downward and into the rectum where the defecation reflex is then elicited.
6. Encourage client to relax, provide privacy, and have call signal within reach during attempts to defecate.	6. If the client is able to relax during attempts to defecate, he/she will be able to relax the levator ani muscle and external anal sphincter, thus facilitating the passage of stool.
7. Encourage the client to establish a regular time for defecation, preferably within an hour after a meal.	7. Attempting to have a bowel movement within an hour after a meal, particularly breakfast, takes advantage of mass peristalsis, which occurs only a few times a day and is strongest after meals. Mass peristalsis is stimulated by the gastrocolic reflex, which is initiated by the presence of foods/fluids in the stomach and duodenum.
8. Instruct client to increase intake of foods high in fiber (e.g., bran, whole-grain breads and cereals, fresh fruits and vegetables) unless contraindicated.	8. Foods high in fiber provide bulk to the fecal mass and keep the stool soft because of the ability of fiber to absorb water. The increased bulkiness (mass) of the stools stimulates peristalsis, which promotes more rapid movement of stool through the colon. Also, the shorter the time that feces remains in the intestine, the less water is absorbed from it, which helps prevent the formation of hard, dry stools that are difficult to expel.
9. Instruct client to maintain a minimal fluid intake of 2500 ml/day unless contraindicated.	9. Inadequate fluid intake reduces the water content of feces, which results in hard, dry stool that is difficult to evacuate.
10. Encourage client to drink hot liquids (e.g., coffee, tea) upon arising in the morning.	10. Ingestion of hot fluids can stimulate peristalsis.
11. Increase activity as allowed and tolerated.	11. Ambulation stimulates peristalsis, which promotes the passage of stool through the intestines.

NURSING ACTIONS	RATIONALES
Prevention/Treatment	
12. When appropriate, encourage the use of nonnarcotic rather than narcotic (opioid) analgesics for pain management.	12. Narcotic analgesics slow peristalsis, which delays transit of intestinal contents. This delay also results in increased absorption of fluid from the fecal mass with the subsequent formation of hard, dry stool.
13. Administer laxatives or cathartics (e.g., stool softeners, bulk-forming agents, irritants/stimulants, lubricants, saline/osmotic agents) as ordered.	13. Laxatives/cathartics act in a variety of ways to soften the stool, increase stool bulk, stimulate bowel motility, and/or lubricate the fecal mass and thereby promote the evacuation of stool.
14. Administer cleansing and/or oil retention enemas if ordered.	14. A cleansing enema stimulates peristalsis and evacuation of stool by distending the colon with a large volume of solution and/or by irritating the colonic mucosa. An oil retention enema facilitates the passage of stool by softening the fecal mass and lubricating the rectum and anal canal.
15. Consult physician about checking for an impaction and digitally removing stool if the client has not had a bowel movement in 3 days, if he/she is passing liquid stool, or if other signs and symptoms of constipation are present.	15. An impaction prohibits the normal passage of feces. Digital removal of an impacted fecal mass may be necessary before normal passage of stool can occur.
16. Consult appropriate health care provider if signs and symptoms of constipation persist and appear to be an ongoing problem.	16. Notifying the appropriate health care provider allows for modification of treatment plan.

Nursing Diagnosis: Coping, Ineffective

Definition

Inability to form a valid appraisal of the stressors, inadequate choices of practiced responses, and/or inability to use available resources

Defining Characteristics

Lack of goal-directed behavior/resolution of problem including inability to attend to and difficulty organizing information; sleep disturbance; abuse of chemical agents; decreased use of social support; use of forms of coping that impede adaptive behavior; poor concentration; inadequate problem solving; verbalization of inability to cope or inability to ask for help; inability to meet basic needs; destructive behavior toward self or others; inability to meet role expectations; high illness rate; change in usual communication patterns; fatigue; risk taking

Related Factors

Gender differences in coping strategies; inadequate level of confidence in ability to cope; uncertainty; inadequate social support created by characteristics of relationships; inadequate level of perception of control; inadequate resources available; high degree of threat; situational or maturational crisis; disturbance in pattern of tension release; inadequate opportunity to prepare for stressor; inability to conserve adaptive energies; disturbance in pattern of appraisal of threat

Desired Outcome

The client will demonstrate effective coping as evidenced by:

a. verbalization of ability to cope
b. use of appropriate problem-solving techniques
c. willingness to participate in treatment plan and meet basic needs
d. absence of destructive behavior toward self and others
e. appropriate use of defense mechanisms
f. use of available support systems.

Documentation

a. Client statements related to coping ability
b. Ability to meet basic needs and problem solve
c. Factors inhibiting successful coping
d. Current coping strategies used
e. Sleep pattern
f. Interactions with others
g. Support systems used
h. Therapeutic interventions
i. Client/family teaching

Suggested NIC Interventions: Coping enhancement; Decision-making support; Emotional support; Counseling; Support system enhancement; Crisis intervention

NURSING ACTIONS	RATIONALES
Assessments	
1. Assess for and report signs and symptoms of ineffective coping (e.g., verbalization of inability to cope or ask for help; inability to meet role expectations, problem solve, or meet basic needs; insomnia; withdrawal; destructive behavior toward self or others; inappropriate use of defense mechanisms).	1. Early recognition and reporting of signs and symptoms of ineffective coping allow for prompt intervention.
2. Assess client's perception of current situation.	2. The client's perception of the situation is the major determinant of his/her response. An awareness of the situation from the client's point of view helps the nurse develop interventions that will facilitate coping.
Prevention/Treatment	
3. Allow time for client to begin to adjust to his/her situation. Recognize that the amount of time needed will vary from client to client.	3. Time is necessary for cognitive appraisal of the situation and development of effective coping strategies.
4. Assist client to recognize and manage inappropriate denial if it is present.	4. Denial is a major defense mechanism used to deal with stressors such as illness, particularly when the client is having difficulty facing the reality of his/her situation or is grieving. If denial persists or is inappropriate, it inhibits the client's ability to cope.
5. Implement measures to reduce fear and anxiety (e.g., encourage verbalization about the situation, instruct in relaxation techniques, administer antianxiety agents as ordered).	5. Fear and anxiety inhibit clarity of thought and problem solving and the subsequent development and use of effective coping techniques.
6. Implement measures to reduce discomfort (e.g., administer prescribed analgesics, encourage use of relaxation techniques).	6. The presence of discomfort, particularly if it continues, can reduce the client's ability to effectively identify and use coping strategies.
7. Encourage verbalization about current situation and ways comparable situations have been handled in the past.	7. Verbalization assists the client to reflect on the situation with which he/she is dealing and to develop coping strategies based on previous successful experiences.
8. Assist client to identify personal strengths and resources that can be used to facilitate coping with the current situation.	8. The development of effective coping strategies is dependent on the client's ability to recognize and use personal strengths and resources.
9. Demonstrate acceptance of client and create an atmosphere of trust and support.	9. An environment of acceptance, trust, and support helps the client feel free to express feelings and concerns and subsequently begin to cope with the situation.
10. If acceptable to client, arrange for a visit with another individual who has successfully adjusted to a similar situation.	10. Contact with another individual who has experienced and successfully adjusted to a similar situation provides the client with support and insight into ways to effectively cope with his/her situation.
11. Include client in planning of care, encourage maximum participation in treatment plan, and allow choices when possible.	11. Active participation in the planning of care allows the client to maintain a sense of control. This enhances self-esteem and subsequently the ability to cope.
12. Instruct client in effective problem-solving techniques (e.g., accurate identification of stressors, determination of various options to solve problem).	12. Effective problem-solving skills are essential to the development of useful coping strategies because they enable the client to identify the problem clearly and select and implement viable options for dealing with it.

NURSING ACTIONS	RATIONALES
Prevention/Treatment	
13. Assist client to identify priorities and attainable goals as he/she starts to plan for necessary lifestyle and role changes.	13. The setting of appropriate priorities and realistic goals is necessary if the client is to cope effectively with the changes being experienced.
14. Assist client and significant others to identify ways that personal and family goals can be adjusted rather than abandoned.	14. Adjustment rather than abandonment of personal and family goals reduces the feeling of loss and increases the probability of positive adaptation to the situation being experienced.
15. Assist client through methods such as role playing to practice coping strategies.	15. Practicing coping strategies in a safe environment helps the client to integrate these skills so that they are more easily implemented when the need arises.
16. When appropriate, assist client to meet spiritual needs (e.g., arrange for a visit from clergy).	16. Spiritual support is a source of comfort, security, and strength for many people and can enhance the client's ability to cope.
17. Assist client to identify and use available support systems. Provide information about available community resources that can assist client and significant others in coping with the situation at hand.	17. Social support provides a sense of acceptance and reduces the feelings of aloneness, which are often experienced in a crisis situation. Various community resources can provide information and psychological support for the client and significant others and subsequently facilitate the development and success of coping strategies.
18. Encourage client to share with significant others the kind of support that would be most beneficial (e.g., listening, inspiring hope, providing reassurance and accurate information).	18. Techniques or behaviors that facilitate one's coping ability vary from person to person and need to be clearly communicated to significant others in order to maximize their support.
19. Support behaviors indicative of effective coping (e.g., participation in treatment plan and self-care activities, communication of the ability to cope, use of effective problem-solving strategies).	19. Positive reinforcement of effective coping strategies increases the likelihood of continued use of these strategies.
20. Consult appropriate health care provider (e.g., psychiatric nurse clinician, physician) if client continues to have difficulty coping with his/her situation.	20. If client continues to have difficulty coping with the situation, additional counseling, support, or training may be needed.

Nursing Diagnosis: Diarrhea

Definition Passage of loose, unformed stools

Defining Characteristics Hyperactive bowel sounds; at least three loose liquid stools per day; urgency; abdominal pain; cramping

Related Factors

Psychological: high stress levels and anxiety
Situational: alcohol abuse; toxins; laxative abuse; radiation; tube feedings; adverse effects of medications; contaminants; travel
Physiological: inflammation; malabsorption; infectious processes; irritation; parasites

Desired Outcome The client will have fewer bowel movements and more formed stool.

Documentation

a. Frequency of defecation
b. Characteristics of stool
c. Complaints of abdominal cramping
d. Bowel sounds
e. Therapeutic interventions
f. Client teaching

Suggested NIC Intervention: Diarrhea management

NURSING ACTIONS	RATIONALES
Assessments	
1. Ascertain client's usual bowel elimination habits.	1. Knowledge of the client's usual bowel elimination habits helps determine the severity of the diarrhea.
2. Assess for and report signs and symptoms of diarrhea (e.g., frequent, loose stools; urgency; abdominal cramping; hyperactive bowel sounds).	2. Early recognition and reporting of signs and symptoms of diarrhea allow for prompt intervention.
3. Assess for factors that may be causing diarrhea (e.g., antimicrobial agents, laxative use, tube feedings, gastrointestinal disorder, change in dietary intake, intestinal infection).	3. Knowing the cause of the diarrhea is a critical component in identifying the appropriate treatment.
Prevention/Treatment	
4. Limit oral intake to clear liquids and oral replacement solutions (e.g., Pedialyte, Resol, Rehydrate) as ordered.	4. Peristalsis is stimulated by the presence of foods/fluids in the stomach and duodenum. Restricting oral intake to clear liquids and/or replacement solutions during the acute phase of diarrhea allows the bowel to rest but also helps prevent malnutrition and fluid and electrolyte imbalances.
5. As diet advances, gradually progress from fluids to small meals.	5. Gradual introduction of small amounts of fluid and then food helps prevent a sudden increase in peristalsis and diarrhea.
6. Instruct client to avoid the following foods/fluids:	6.
a. those known to aggravate diarrhea (e.g., spicy foods, alcohol, coffee, fatty foods)	a. These substances are thought to increase intestinal motility and may also cause excessive mucus secretion, which increases the liquidity of the intestinal contents.
b. those that are extremely hot or cold	b. Extremes in temperature of ingested foods/fluids often stimulates peristalsis.
c. those high in lactose (e.g., milk, milk products)	c. Diarrhea may temporarily deplete the gastrointestinal enzyme lactase, which is essential for the hydrolysis and subsequent absorption of lactose. The nonabsorbed lactose has an osmotic effect and draws water into the colon, which results in more liquid stool. The lactose also serves as a base for bacterial fermentation in the colon. The lactic and fatty acids produced by this fermentation process irritate the colon with a subsequent increase in bowel motility and diarrhea.
d. those high in fiber (e.g., whole-grain cereals, raw fruits and vegetables)	d. Fiber increases bulk of the stool because of its ability to absorb water. The increased mass (bulk) of the stools stimulates peristalsis. Limiting fiber intake decreases the water content of the stool, which results in drier, firmer, and less bulky stools. The decrease in bulk (mass) results in less stimulation of peristalsis and the dryness of the stools slows intestinal transit time.
e. those made with synthetic, nonabsorbable sugars (e.g., sorbitol) that are found in many dietetic foods.	e. Synthetic, nonabsorbable sugars are not well absorbed from the gastrointestinal tract and tend to draw water into the intestine by osmosis. This excess water in the intestine increases the fluidity and volume of stool.
7. Implement measures to reduce fear and anxiety (e.g., provide client teaching, interact with client in a calm manner, administer prescribed antianxiety agents).	7. Parasympathetic activity may dominate in some stressful situations and cause increased gastrointestinal motility and diarrhea.
8. Encourage client to rest.	8. Physical activity stimulates peristalsis.

NURSING ACTIONS	RATIONALES
Prevention/Treatment	
9. If the client is receiving tube feeding, administer the solution at room temperature. Consult physician about reducing the rate of administration and/or the concentration of the tube feeding solution if diarrhea occurs.	9. Tube feedings can increase peristalsis if the solution is given while cold or if large amounts are given too quickly. Full-strength tube feeding solution has relatively high osmolality, which subsequently draws water into the intestine and causes an osmotic diarrhea. Reducing the concentration of the feeding solution lessens the risk for osmotic diarrhea.
10. Consult physician regarding measures to remove fecal impaction if present (e.g., digital removal of stool, oil retention enema).	10. When a fecal impaction is present, the secretory activity of the bowel increases in an attempt to lubricate and promote evacuation of the impacted feces. The liquid portion of the feces above the mass then leaks around the impaction, resulting in a continuous oozing of diarrheal stool.
11. Administer the following antidiarrheal agents if ordered:	11.
a. opioids (e.g., paregoric) or synthetic opioids (e.g., loperamide, diphenoxylate hydrochloride)	a. Opioids and synthetic opioids decrease gastrointestinal motility, which delays the passage of intestinal contents and subsequently allows more time for water to be absorbed from the feces. This results in fewer bowel movements and more formed stool.
b. bulk-forming agents (e.g., methylcellulose, psyllium hydrophilic mucilloid, polycarbophil)	b. Bulk-forming agents absorb water in the bowel, resulting in a more formed stool.
c. adsorbents/protectants (e.g., attapulgite [Kaopectate], bismuth subsalicylate [Pepto-Bismol]).	c. Adsorbents/protectants act locally to coat the walls of the gastrointestinal tract and absorb toxins that are stimulating gut motility and/or secretions.
12. Consult appropriate health care provider if diarrhea persists.	12. Notifying the appropriate health care provider allows for modification of the treatment plan.

Nursing Diagnosis: Fluid Volume, Deficient

NANDA International's definition of this diagnostic label has been altered slightly to reflect information in current resources.

Definition Decreased intravascular, interstitial and/or intracellular fluid

Defining Characteristics Decreased urine output; increased urine concentration; weakness; sudden weight loss (except in third-spacing); decreased venous filling; increased body temperature; decreased pulse volume/pressure; change in mental state; elevated hematocrit (Hct); decreased skin/tongue turgor; dry skin/mucus membranes; thirst; increased pulse rate; decreased blood pressure

Related Factors Active fluid volume loss; failure of regulatory mechanisms

Desired Outcome The client will not experience a deficient fluid volume as evidenced by:

a. normal skin turgor
b. moist mucous membranes
c. stable weight
d. B/P and pulse within normal range for client and stable with position change
e. capillary refill time less than 2–3 seconds
f. usual mental status
g. BUN and Hct within normal range
h. balanced intake and output.

Documentation

a. Vital signs
b. Condition of skin and mucous membranes
c. Weight

d. Capillary refill time
e. Appearance of neck veins when client is supine
f. Mental status
g. Intake and output
h. Presence of nausea, vomiting, or other contributing factors
i. Intravenous fluid therapy
j. Client teaching

Suggested NIC Interventions: Fluid monitoring; Fluid management; Hypovolemia management; Intravenous therapy (IV); Fever treatment

NURSING ACTIONS	RATIONALES
Assessments	
1. Assess for and report signs and symptoms of deficient fluid volume: a. decreased skin turgor b. dry mucous membranes, thirst c. weight loss of 2% or greater over a short period d. postural hypotension and/or low B/P e. weak, rapid pulse f. capillary refill time greater than 2–3 seconds g. neck veins flat when client is supine h. change in mental status i. elevated BUN and Hct j. decreased urine output.	1. Early recognition and reporting of signs and symptoms of deficient fluid volume allow for prompt intervention.
Prevention/Treatment	
2. Implement measures to reduce nausea and vomiting if present (e.g., administer antiemetics as ordered, instruct client to ingest foods/fluids slowly, eliminate noxious sights and odors).	2. Nausea often causes the client to have decreased fluid intake. Persistent vomiting results in excessive loss of fluid.
3. Implement measures to control diarrhea if present (e.g., administer antidiarrheal agents as ordered; discourage intake of spicy foods and foods high in fiber or lactose).	3. Persistent or severe diarrhea results in excessive loss of gastrointestinal fluid.
4. Implement measures to reduce fever if present (e.g., administer antipyretics as ordered, sponge client with tepid water, remove excessive clothing or bedcovers).	4. Fever may be accompanied by diaphoresis, which can result in excessive loss of fluid.
5. Carefully measure drainage (e.g., wound, nasogastric) and administer replacement fluids as ordered.	5. Replacing fluid that is lost helps prevent/treat deficient fluid volume.
6. Maintain a fluid intake of at least 2500 ml/day unless contraindicated. If oral intake is inadequate, maintain intravenous and/or enteral fluid therapy as ordered.	6. Adequate fluid intake needs to be provided in order to ensure adequate hydration.
7. Consult physician if signs and symptoms of deficient fluid volume persist or worsen.	7. Notifying the physician allows for modification of treatment plan.

Nursing Diagnosis: Fluid Volume, Excess

Definition Increased isotonic fluid retention

Defining Characteristics Jugular vein distention; decreased hemoglobin and hematocrit; weight gain over short period of time; dyspnea or shortness of breath; intake exceeds output; pleural effusion; orthopnea; S_3 heart sound; pulmonary congestion; change in respiratory pattern; change in mental status; blood pressure changes; pulmonary artery pressure changes; oliguria; specific gravity changes; azotemia; altered electrolytes; restlessness; anxiety; abnormal breath sounds (crackles); edema, may progress to anasarca; increased central venous pressure; positive hepatojugular reflex

Related Factors

Compromised regulatory mechanism; excess fluid intake; excess sodium intake

Desired Outcome

The client will not experience excess fluid volume as evidenced by:
a. stable weight
b. B/P within normal range for client
c. absence of S_3 heart sound
d. normal pulse volume
e. balanced intake and output
f. usual mental status
g. normal breath sounds
h. BUN and Hct within normal range
i. absence of dyspnea, orthopnea, peripheral edema, and distended neck veins
j. CVP within normal range.

Documentation

a. Blood pressure
b. Weight
c. Heart sounds
d. Pulse volume
e. Intake and output
f. Mental status
g. Breath sounds, ease of respirations
h. Presence of edema and neck vein distention
i. CVP readings
j. Therapeutic interventions
k. Client teaching

Suggested NIC Interventions: Fluid monitoring; Fluid management; Hypervolemia management

NURSING ACTIONS	RATIONALES
Assessments	
1. Assess for and report signs and symptoms of excess fluid volume: a. weight gain of 2% or greater in a short period b. elevated B/P (B/P may not be elevated if fluid has shifted out of vascular space) c. presence of an S_3 heart sound d. bounding pulse e. intake greater than output f. change in mental status g. crackles (rales), diminished or absent breath sounds h. decreased BUN and Hct i. dyspnea, orthopnea j. peripheral edema k. distended neck veins l. elevated CVP.	1. Early recognition and reporting of signs and symptoms of excess fluid volume allow for prompt intervention.
2. Monitor chest x-ray results. Report findings of pulmonary vascular congestion, pleural effusion, or pulmonary edema.	2. Chest x-ray films provide data about pulmonary vascular status and fluid accumulation in the pleural space, pulmonary interstitium, and alveoli.
Prevention/Treatment	
3. Maintain fluid restrictions as ordered.	3. Fluid restriction helps to reduce total body water and prevent the accumulation of excess fluid.
4. Restrict sodium intake as ordered.	4. Excess fluid volume is an isotonic retention of both sodium and water. Restricting sodium intake will result in less sodium and subsequently less water being reabsorbed by the kidneys.

5. Encourage client to rest periodically in a recumbent position if tolerated.

5. Lying flat promotes venous return, which leads to increased cardiac output and renal blood flow. This increases the glomerular filtration rate and promotes diuresis.

6. If client is receiving intravenous fluids that contain sizable amounts of sodium (e.g., 0.9% NaCl, lactated Ringer's), consult physician about a change in the solution or rate of infusion.

6. Excess fluid volume can result from overzealous or prolonged intravenous administration of sodium-containing fluids, particularly ones that contain sizable amounts of sodium.

7. If client is receiving numerous and/or large volume intravenous medications, consult pharmacist about ways to prevent excessive fluid administration (e.g., stop primary infusion during administration of intravenous medications, dilute medications in the minimum amount of solution).

7. Limiting the amount of IV solution infused at any one time and maximizing the concentration of intravenous medications helps prevent an additional fluid burden in the person who has or is at risk for excess fluid.

8. Administer diuretics if ordered.

8. Most diuretics inhibit sodium reabsorption in the renal tubules. This results in decreased water reabsorption and subsequent excretion of excess fluid.

9. Consult physician if signs and symptoms of excess fluid volume persist or worsen.

9. Notifying the physician allows for modification of treatment plan.

NURSING DIAGNOSIS: GAS EXCHANGE, IMPAIRED

Definition

Excess or deficit in oxygenation and/or carbon dioxide elimination at the alveolar-capillary membrane

Defining Characteristics

Visual disturbances; decreased carbon dioxide; tachycardia; hypercapnia; restlessness; somnolence; irritability; hypoxia; confusion; dyspnea; abnormal arterial blood gases; cyanosis (in neonates only); abnormal skin color (pale, dusky); hypoxemia; headache upon awakening; abnormal rate, rhythm, depth of breathing; diaphoresis; nasal flaring; abnormal arterial pH

Related Factors

Ventilation/perfusion imbalance; alveolar-capillary membrane changes

Desired Outcome

The client will experience adequate gas (O_2/CO_2) exchange as evidenced by:

a. usual mental status
b. unlabored respirations at 12–20/minute
c. oximetry results within normal range
d. blood gases within normal range.

Documentation

a. Respiratory rate
b. Difficulty breathing
c. Mental status
d. Oximetry results
e. Route and rate of oxygen administration
f. Therapeutic interventions
g. Client teaching

Suggested NIC Interventions: Respiratory monitoring; Oxygen therapy; Airway management; Chest physiotherapy; Cough enhancement; Acid-base management

NURSING ACTIONS

Assessments

1. Assess for and report signs and symptoms of impaired gas (O_2/CO_2) exchange:
   a. restlessness, irritability
   b. confusion, somnolence

RATIONALES

1. Early recognition and reporting of signs and symptoms of impaired gas exchange allow for prompt intervention.

NURSING ACTIONS	RATIONALES
Assessments	
c. tachypnea, dyspnea d. decreased PaO_2 and/or increased $PaCO_2$.	
2. Monitor for and report a significant decrease in oximetry results.	2. Oximetry is a noninvasive method of measuring arterial oxygen saturation. The results assist in evaluating respiratory status.
Prevention/Treatment	
3. Place client in a semi- to high Fowler's position unless contraindicated. Position with pillows to prevent slumping. If client is experiencing dyspnea or orthopnea, position overbed table so he/she can lean on it if desired.	3. These positions allow for increased diaphragmatic excursion and maximum lung expansion, which promotes optimal alveolar ventilation and O_2/CO_2 exchange.
4. Instruct and assist client to change position, deep breathe, and cough or "huff" every 1–2 hours.	4. Frequent repositioning helps mobilize secretions and aids lung expansion. Deep breathing helps loosen secretions and promotes a more effective cough. It also promotes maximum lung expansion and stimulates surfactant production. Coughing or "huffing" (a forced expiration technique) mobilizes secretions and facilitates removal of these secretions from the respiratory tract. These actions promote optimal alveolar ventilation and O_2/CO_2 exchange.
5. Reinforce correct use of incentive spirometer every 1–2 hours.	5. Incentive spirometer use promotes slow, deep inhalation, which improves lung expansion and helps clear airways by loosening secretions and promoting a more effective cough. These actions enhance alveolar ventilation and the exchange of O_2/CO_2.
6. Implement measures to reduce chest or abdominal pain if present (e.g., splint incision with pillow during coughing and deep breathing, administer prescribed analgesics before planned activity).	6. A client with chest or abdominal pain often guards respiratory efforts and breathes shallowly in an attempt to prevent additional discomfort. Pain reduction enables the client to breathe more deeply, which enhances alveolar ventilation and O_2/CO_2 exchange.
7. Implement measures to decrease fear and anxiety (e.g., assure client that breathing deeply will not dislodge tubes or cause incision to break open, interact with client in a confident manner).	7. Fear and anxiety may cause a client to breathe shallowly or to hyperventilate. Decreasing fear and anxiety allows the client to focus on breathing more slowly and taking deeper breaths, which subsequently enhances alveolar ventilation and the exchange of O_2/CO_2.
8. Implement measures to facilitate removal of pulmonary secretions (e.g., suction, postural drainage, percussion, vibration) if ordered.	8. Excessive secretions and/or client's inability to clear secretions from the respiratory tract lead to stasis of secretions, which can impair O_2/CO_2 exchange. Suction and chest physiotherapy techniques may be necessary to facilitate removal of pulmonary secretions and thereby promote adequate gas exchange.
9. Assist with positive airway pressure techniques (e.g., continuous positive airway pressure [CPAP], bilevel positive airway pressure [BiPAP], flutter/positive expiratory pressure [PEP] device) if ordered.	9. Positive airway pressure techniques increase intrapulmonary (alveolar) pressure, which helps re-expand collapsed alveoli and prevent further alveolar collapse so that gas exchange can take place.
10. Maintain oxygen therapy as ordered.	10. Supplemental oxygen increases the concentration of oxygen in the alveoli, which increases the diffusion of oxygen across the alveolar-capillary membrane.
11. Maintain activity restrictions as ordered. Increase activity gradually as allowed and tolerated.	11. Restricting activity lowers the body's oxygen requirements and thus increases the amount of oxygen available for gas exchange. A gradual increase in activity conserves energy and thereby lessens oxygen utilization, yet promotes mobilization of secretions and deeper breathing.

12. Instruct client in and assist with diaphragmatic breathing and pursed-lip breathing techniques if appropriate. NOTE: Diaphragmatic breathing is most often indicated for clients who have had thoracic surgery or clients who have chronic airflow limitation (e.g., emphysema) or neuromuscular conditions that cause fixation or weakening of the diaphragm.

12. Diaphragmatic breathing promotes greater movement of the diaphragm and decreases the use of the accessory muscles for inspiration. Use of this technique eases the work of breathing and ultimately promotes an increased efficiency of alveolar ventilation. Pursed-lip breathing causes a mild resistance to exhalation, which creates positive pressure in the airways. This pressure helps prevent airway collapse and subsequently promotes more complete alveolar emptying.

13. Discourage smoking.

13. Smoking impairs gas exchange because it:
    a. reduces effective airway clearance by increasing mucus production and impairing ciliary function
    b. decreases oxygen availability (hemoglobin binds with the carbon monoxide in smoke rather than with oxygen)
    c. causes damage to the bronchial and alveolar walls
    d. causes vasoconstriction and subsequently reduces pulmonary blood flow.

14. Administer medications that may be ordered to improve client's respiratory status (e.g., bronchodilators, analgesics, antibiotics, corticosteroids, anticoagulants, diuretics).

14. Medication therapy is an integral part of treating many respiratory conditions that impair alveolar gas exchange (e.g., bronchodilators improve bronchial airflow and subsequently increase O_2/CO_2 exchange; analgesics can reduce pain and promote deeper breathing and increased activity; antibiotics help resolve certain respiratory infections; corticosteroids reduce inflammation in the lungs and improve bronchial airflow; anticoagulants treat thromboemboli of the pulmonary vessels and subsequently improve pulmonary perfusion; diuretics reduce fluid accumulation in the pulmonary interstitium and alveoli, which subsequently improves gas exchange).

15. Administer central nervous system depressants judiciously. Hold medication and consult physician if respiratory rate is less than 12/minute.

15. Central nervous system depressants cause depression of the respiratory center and cough reflex. This can result in hypoventilation and stasis of secretions with subsequent impaired gas exchange.

16. Consult appropriate health care provider (e.g., physician, respiratory therapist) if signs and symptoms of impaired gas exchange persist or worsen.

16. Notifying the appropriate health care provider allows for modification of treatment plan.

NURSING DIAGNOSIS: GRIEVING

This diagnostic label includes anticipatory grieving and grieving following the actual loss.

Definition

Intellectual and emotional responses and behaviors by which individuals, families, and communities work through or attempt to work through the process of modifying self-concept based on the perception of potential or actual loss

Defining Characteristics

Anticipatory grieving: expression of distress at potential loss; sorrow; guilt; denial of potential loss; anger; altered communication patterns; potential loss of significant object (e.g., people, possessions, job, status, home, ideals, parts and processes of the body); denial of the significance of the loss; bargaining; alteration in eating habits, sleep patterns, dream patterns, activity level, libido; difficulty taking on new or different roles; resolution of grief prior to the reality of loss

Dysfunctional grieving: crying; sadness; reliving of past experiences with little or no reduction (diminishment) of intensity of the grief; labile affect; expression of unresolved issues; interference with life functioning; verbal expression of distress at loss; idealization of lost object (e.g., people, possessions, job, status, home, ideals, parts and processes of the body); difficulty in expressing loss; denial of loss; anger; alterations in: eating habits, sleep patterns, dream patterns, activity level, libido, concentration and/or pursuit of tasks; developmental regression; expression of guilt; repetitive use of ineffectual behaviors associated with attempts to reinvest in relationships; prolonged interference with life functioning; onset or exacerbation of somatic or psychosomatic responses

Related Factors

Anticipatory grieving: to be developed
Dysfunctional grieving: actual or perceived object loss (e.g., people, possessions, job, status, home, ideals, parts and processes of the body)

Desired Outcome

The client will demonstrate beginning progression through the grieving process as evidenced by:

a. verbalization of feelings about the loss
b. usual sleep pattern
c. participation in treatment plan and self-care activities
d. use of available support systems.

Documentation

a. Verbalization of feelings about the loss
b. Participation in activities
c. Eating pattern
d. Sleep pattern
e. Interaction with others
f. Measures used to adapt to loss
g. Client/family teaching

Suggested NIC Interventions: Grief work facilitation; Emotional support; Presence; Support system enhancement

NURSING ACTIONS	RATIONALES
Assessments	
1. Assess for signs and symptoms of grieving (e.g., expression of distress about the loss, change in eating habits, inability to concentrate, insomnia, anger, sadness, withdrawal from significant others, denial of loss).	1. Assessment of signs and symptoms of grieving helps the nurse determine the phase of grieving the client is experiencing. This knowledge aids in the development of effective strategies that can assist the client to progress through the phases of grieving.
2. Assess for factors that may hinder and facilitate client's acknowledgment of the loss.	2. In order for grief work to begin, the client needs to acknowledge the loss. An awareness of factors that may hinder and facilitate this acknowledgment assists in the development of effective strategies to accomplish this goal.
Prevention/Treatment	
3. Assist client to acknowledge the loss (e.g., encourage conversation about the loss including how or why it occurred and its impact on his/her future).	3. The client needs to acknowledge the loss in order for grief work to begin.
4. Discuss the grieving process and assist client to accept the phases of grieving as an expected response to an actual and/or anticipated loss.	4. An awareness of the feelings and behaviors commonly associated with each phase of the grieving process assists the client to accept his/her responses to the loss.
5. Allow time for client to progress through the phases of grieving (phases vary among theorists but progress from shock and alarm to acceptance).	5. Grieving is a process that occurs in phases or stages that progress over time. Some phases may not be experienced by the client and some may overlap or recur. The amount of time necessary to reach resolution of grief is very individual, may take months to years, and must be allowed to occur in order to reduce the risk for dysfunctional grieving.

6. Provide an atmosphere of care and concern (e.g., provide privacy, be available and nonjudgmental, display empathy and respect).

6. A supportive, nonthreatening environment provides the basis for a constructive, therapeutic relationship between the client and nurse. This allows the client to express feelings of grief and work toward its resolution.

7. Implement measures to promote trust (e.g., answer questions honestly, provide requested information).

7. A feeling of trust in the caregiver promotes the development of a therapeutic relationship in which the client can feel free to verbalize feelings. This facilitates the progression of grief work.

8. Encourage the verbal expression of anger and sadness about the loss experienced. Recognize displacement of anger and assist client to see the actual cause of angry feelings and resentment. Establish limits on abusive behavior if demonstrated.

8. The verbal expression of feelings of anger and sadness facilitates movement toward resolution of grief. Displacement of angry feelings needs to be acknowledged so that grieving can progress but should not be allowed to interfere with the therapeutic process.

9. Encourage client to express feelings in whatever ways are comfortable (e.g., writing, drawing, conversation).

9. Expression of feelings helps the client integrate both positive and negative aspects of the loss and move toward its acceptance.

10. Assist client to use techniques that have helped him/her cope in previous situations of loss.

10. Techniques that have previously facilitated the client's adjustment to situations of loss are often effective when used to help him/her cope with the current loss.

11. Support behaviors suggesting successful grief work (e.g., verbalizing feelings about loss, focusing on ways to adapt to loss, learning needed skills, developing or renewing relationships).

11. Positive feedback about behaviors that suggest successful grief work reinforces those behaviors and promotes positive adaptation to loss.

12. Explain the phases of the grieving process to significant others. Encourage their support and understanding.

12. When significant others are knowledgeable about the phases of the grieving process, they are more likely to understand and accept the client's behavior and assist him/her to move toward resolution of grief.

13. Facilitate communication between the client and significant others. Be aware that they may be in different phases of the grieving process.

13. Effective communication between the client and significant others enhances the client's ability to express feelings and successfully move through the phases of grieving.

14. Provide information about counseling services and support groups that might assist client in working through grief.

14. Counseling and support groups can assist the client in working through grief by:
    a. providing insight into his/her responses to the loss
    b. decreasing the feelings of aloneness and isolation that frequently accompany a loss
    c. helping identify methods or skills that can be used to help cope with the loss.

15. When appropriate, assist client to meet spiritual needs (e.g., arrange for a visit from clergy).

15. Spiritual support can be a source of strength and solace to the client and can facilitate resolution of grief.

16. Consult appropriate health care provider (e.g., psychiatric nurse clinician, physician) if signs of dysfunctional grieving (e.g., persistent denial of losses, excessive anger or sadness, emotional lability) occur.

16. Notifying the appropriate health care provider allows for modification of the treatment plan.

NURSING DIAGNOSIS: INFECTION, RISK FOR

Definition At increased risk for being invaded by pathogenic organisms

Risk Factors Inadequate primary defenses (broken skin, traumatized tissue, decrease in ciliary action, stasis of body fluids, change in pH of secretions, altered peristalsis); inadequate secondary defenses (decreased hemoglobin, leukopenia, suppressed inflammatory response); immunosuppression; inadequate acquired immunity; trauma; tissue destruction and increased environmental exposure; chronic disease; malnutrition; invasive procedures; pharmaceutical agents (e.g., immunosuppressants); rupture of amniotic membranes; insufficient knowledge to avoid exposure to pathogens

Desired Outcome

The client will remain free of infection as evidenced by:
a. absence of fever and chills
b. pulse within normal limits
c. usual mental status
d. normal breath sounds
e. cough productive of clear mucus only
f. voiding clear urine without reports of frequency, urgency, and burning
g. absence of heat, pain, redness, swelling, and unusual drainage in any area
h. WBC and differential counts within normal range for client
i. negative results of cultured specimens.

Documentation

a. Temperature
b. Pulse rate
c. Presence of chills
d. Mental status
e. Breath sounds
f. Characteristics of urine, sputum, and wound drainage
g. Evidence of inflammation in any area
h. Evidence of unusual drainage from any area
i. Therapeutic interventions
j. Client/family teaching

Suggested NIC Interventions: Infection control; Infection protection; Incision site care; Tube care; Wound care

NURSING ACTIONS	RATIONALES
Assessments	
1. Assess for and report signs and symptoms of infection (be aware that some signs and symptoms vary depending on the site of infection, the causative agent, and the age and immune status of the client): a. elevated temperature b. chills c. increased pulse d. malaise, lethargy, acute confusion e. loss of appetite f. abnormal breath sounds g. productive cough of purulent, green, or rust-colored sputum h. cloudy urine i. reports of frequency, urgency, or burning when urinating j. urinalysis showing a WBC count greater than 5, positive leukocyte esterase or nitrites, or presence of bacteria k. heat, pain, redness, swelling, or unusual drainage in any area l. elevated WBC count and/or significant change in differential.	1. Early recognition and reporting of signs and symptoms of infection allow for prompt intervention.
2. Obtain specimens (e.g., urine, wound drainage, vaginal drainage, sputum, blood) for culture as ordered. Report positive results.	2. Cultures are done to identify the specific organism(s) causing the infection. Culture results provide information that helps determine the most effective treatment.

Prevention

3. Maintain a fluid intake of at least 2500 ml/day unless contraindicated.

3. Adequate hydration helps prevent infection by:
   a. helping maintain adequate blood flow and nutrient supply to the tissues
   b. promoting urine formation and subsequent voiding, which flushes pathogens from the bladder and urethra
   c. thinning respiratory secretions so that they can more easily be removed by coughing or suctioning (respiratory secretions provide a good medium for growth and colonization of microorganisms).

4. Use good hand hygiene and encourage client to do the same.

4. Good hand hygiene removes transient flora, which reduces the risk of transmission of pathogens. Use of products such as an antibacterial soap, a chlorhexidine solution, or an alcohol-based handrub agent can actually inhibit the growth of or kill microorganisms, which further reduces infection risk.

5. Adhere to the appropriate precautions established to prevent transmission of infection to the client (standard precautions, transmission-based precautions on other clients, neutropenic precautions).

5. Adhering to the appropriate precautions that have been established to help prevent the transmission of microorganisms reduces the client's risk of infection.

6. Use sterile technique during invasive procedures (e.g., urinary catheterizations, venous and arterial punctures, injections, tracheal suctioning, wound care) and dressing changes.

6. Use of sterile technique reduces the possibility of introducing pathogens into the body.

7. Anchor catheters/tubings (e.g., urinary, intravenous, wound drainage) securely.

7. Catheters/tubings that are not securely anchored have some degree of in-and-out movement. This movement increases the risk of infection because it allows for the introduction of pathogens into the body. It can also cause tissue trauma, which can result in colonization of microorganisms.

8. Change equipment, tubings, and solutions used for treatments such as intravenous infusions, respiratory care, irrigations, and enteral feedings according to hospital policy.

8. The longer that equipment, tubings, and solutions are in use, the greater the chance of colonization of microorganisms, which can then be introduced into the body.

9. Maintain a closed system for drains (e.g., wounds, chest tubes, urinary catheters) and intravenous infusions whenever possible.

9. Each time a drainage or infusion system is opened, pathogens from the environment have an opportunity to enter the body. Maintaining a closed system decreases this risk, which reduces the possibility of infection.

10. Change peripheral intravenous line sites according to hospital policy.

10. Peripheral intravenous line sites are changed routinely to reduce persistent irritation of one area of a vein wall and the resultant colonization of microorganisms at that site.

11. Provide appropriate wound care (e.g., use dressing materials that maintain a moist wound surface, assist with debridement of necrotic tissue, use dressing materials that absorb excess exudate, protect granulating tissue from trauma and contamination, maintain patency of wound drains).

11. Proper wound care facilitates wound healing and reduces the number of pathogens that enter or are present in the wound, which reduce the risk of the wound becoming infected.

12. Protect client from others with infections.

12. Protecting the client from others with infections reduces his/her risk of exposure to pathogens.

13. Implement measures to maintain healthy, intact skin (e.g., keep skin lubricated, clean, and dry; instruct or assist client to turn every 2 hours; keep bed linens dry and wrinkle-free).

13. Healthy, intact skin reduces the risk for infection by:
    a. providing a physical barrier against the introduction of pathogens into the body
    b. removing many of the microorganisms on the surface of the skin by means of the constant shedding of the epidermis
    c. inhibiting the growth of some bacteria on the surface of the skin (sebum contains fatty acids, which create a slightly acidic environment that inhibits the growth of some bacteria).

NURSING ACTIONS	RATIONALES
Prevention	
14. Implement measures to reduce stress (e.g., reduce fear, anxiety, and pain; help client identify and use effective coping mechanisms).	14. Stress causes an increased secretion of cortisol. Cortisol interferes with some immune responses, which subsequently increases the client's susceptibility to infection.
15. Maintain an optimal nutritional status. Administer vitamins and minerals as ordered.	15. Adequate nutrition is needed to maintain normal function of the immune system.
16. Instruct and assist client to perform good perineal care routinely and after each bowel movement.	16. The perineal area contains a large number of organisms. Routine cleansing of the area reduces the risk of colonization of organisms and subsequent perineal, urinary tract, and/or vaginal infection.
17. Instruct and assist client to perform good oral hygiene as often as needed.	17. Frequent oral hygiene helps prevent infection by removing most of the food, debris, and many of the microorganisms that are present in the mouth. It also helps maintain the integrity of the oral mucosa, which provides a physical and chemical barrier to pathogens.
18. Implement measures to prevent urinary retention (e.g., instruct client to urinate when the urge is felt, promote relaxation during voiding attempts, administer bethanechol as ordered).	18. A client experiencing urinary retention is at increased risk for urinary tract infection because: a. the urine that accumulates in the bladder creates an environment conducive to the growth and colonization of microorganisms b. voiding does not occur so microorganisms are not flushed from the mucous lining of the urethra; these microorganisms can colonize and ascend into the bladder.
19. Implement measures to prevent stasis of respiratory secretions (e.g., assist client to turn, cough, and deep breathe; increase activity as allowed and tolerated; perform tracheal suctioning if indicated).	19. Respiratory secretions provide a good medium for growth of microorganisms. By preventing stasis, there is less chance of colonization of the microorganisms and a decreased risk for development of respiratory tract infection.
20. Instruct client to receive immunizations (e.g., influenza vaccine, pneumococcal vaccine) if appropriate.	20. Immunizations are often recommended to reduce the possibility of some infections in high-risk clients (e.g., those clients who are immunosuppressed, elderly, or have a chronic disease).
21. Consult appropriate health care provider regarding initiation of antimicrobial therapy if indicated. Question orders that do not seem appropriate (e.g., prolonged use of antimicrobials, excessively high dose of an antimicrobial, unnecessary use of broad-spectrum or multiple antimicrobials).	21. Most antimicrobials disrupt cell wall synthesis, which halts the growth of or kills microorganisms. This can effectively reduce the client's risk for infection. Antimicrobial orders that seem inappropriate should be questioned because they can result in the elimination of normal flora and/or the development of drug-resistant microorganisms, which actually increase the client's risk for infection.

Nursing Diagnosis: Nutrition, Imbalanced: Less Than Body Requirements

The defining characteristics listed by NANDA International that focus on related factors (causes) of imbalanced nutrition have been omitted.

Definition Intake of nutrients insufficient to meet metabolic needs

Defining Characteristics Loss of weight with adequate food intake; body weight 20% or more under ideal; sore, inflamed buccal cavity; capillary fragility; pale conjunctiva and mucous membranes; poor muscle tone; excessive loss of hair

Related Factors

Inability to ingest or digest food or absorb nutrients due to biological, psychological, or economic factors

Desired Outcome

The client will maintain an adequate nutritional status as evidenced by:
a. weight within normal range for client
b. normal BUN and serum albumin, prealbumin, Hct, Hgb, and lymphocyte levels
c. usual strength and activity tolerance
d. healthy oral mucous membrane.

Documentation

a. Weight
b. Activity tolerance
c. Condition of oral mucous membrane
d. Type of diet and amount consumed
e. Therapeutic interventions
f. Client/family teaching

Suggested NIC Interventions: Nutritional monitoring; Nutritional counseling; Nutrition management; Nutrition therapy; Weight gain assistance; Weight management

NURSING ACTIONS / RATIONALES

Assessments

1. Assess for and report signs and symptoms of malnutrition:
   a. weight significantly below client's usual weight or below normal for client's age, height, and body frame
   b. abnormal BUN and low serum albumin, prealbumin, Hct, Hgb, and lymphocyte levels
   c. weakness and fatigue
   d. sore, inflamed oral mucous membrane
   e. pale conjunctiva.

   Rationale: 1. Early recognition and reporting of signs and symptoms of malnutrition allow for prompt intervention.

2. Monitor percentage of meals and snacks client consumes. Report a pattern of inadequate intake.

   Rationale: 2. An awareness of the amount of foods/fluids the client consumes alerts the nurse to deficits in nutritional intake. Reporting an inadequate intake allows for prompt intervention.

3. Perform or assist with anthropometric measurements such as skinfold thickness, body circumferences (e.g., hip, waist, mid-upper arm), and bioelectrical impedance analysis if indicated. Report results that are lower than normal.

   Rationale: 3. Anthropometric measurements provide information about the amount of muscle mass, body fat, and protein reserves the client has. These assessments assist in evaluating the client's nutritional status.

Prevention/Treatment

4. Implement measures to prevent vomiting if indicated (e.g., administer antiemetics as ordered, eliminate noxious sights and odors).

   Rationale: 4. Vomiting results in an actual loss of nutrients.

5. Implement measures to control diarrhea if present (e.g., administer antidiarrheal agents as ordered, discourage intake of spicy foods and foods high in fiber or lactose).

   Rationale: 5. The increased intestinal motility that occurs with or causes diarrhea results in a decreased absorption of nutrients in the bowel. In addition, diarrhea causes an actual loss of nutrients.

6. Implement measures to improve oral intake:

   Rationale: 6. The client is more likely to achieve or maintain a good nutritional status if he/she has a good oral intake.

   a. perform actions to reduce nausea, pain, fear, and anxiety if present

      Rationale: a. Nausea, pain, fear, and/or anxiety can decrease the client's appetite and result in a decreased oral intake.

   b. perform actions to relieve gastrointestinal distention if present (e.g., encourage and assist client with frequent ambulation unless contraindicated, administer gastrointestinal stimulants as ordered)

      Rationale: b. Distention of the gastrointestinal tract (especially the stomach and duodenum) can result in stimulation of the satiety center and subsequent inhibition of the feeding center in the hypothalamus. This effect, along with the discomfort that occurs with distention, decreases appetite.

NURSING ACTIONS	RATIONALES
Prevention/Treatment	
c. increase activity as allowed and tolerated	c. Activity usually promotes a general feeling of well-being, which can result in improved appetite.
d. maintain a clean environment and a relaxed, pleasant atmosphere	d. Noxious sights and odors can inhibit the feeding center in the hypothalamus. Maintaining a clean environment helps prevent this from occurring. In addition, maintaining a relaxed, pleasant atmosphere can help reduce the client's stress and promote a feeling of well-being, which tends to improve appetite and oral intake.
e. encourage a rest period before meals if indicated	e. The physical activity of eating requires some expenditure of energy. Fatigue can reduce the client's desire and ability to eat.
f. provide oral hygiene before meals	f. Oral hygiene moistens the oral mucous membrane, which may make it easier to chew and swallow. It also freshens the mouth and removes unpleasant tastes. This can improve the taste of foods/fluids, which helps stimulate appetite and increase oral intake.
g. serve foods/fluids that are appealing to the client and adhere to personal and cultural (e.g., religious, ethnic) preferences whenever possible	g. Foods/fluids that appeal to the client's senses (especially sight and smell) and are in accordance with personal and cultural preferences are most likely to stimulate appetite and promote interest in eating.
h. serve frequent, small meals rather than large ones if client is weak, fatigues easily, and/or has a poor appetite	h. Providing small rather than large meals can enable a client who is weak or fatigues easily to finish a meal. Also, a client who has a poor appetite is often more willing to attempt to eat smaller meals because they seem less overwhelming than larger ones. If smaller meals are served, the number of meals per day should be increased to help ensure adequate nutrition.
i. encourage significant others to bring in client's favorite foods unless contraindicated and eat with him/her if client desires	i. A client's favorite foods/fluids tend to stimulate his/her appetite more than institutional foods/fluids. The presence of significant others during meals helps create a familiar social environment that can stimulate appetite and improve oral intake.
j. if client is experiencing dyspnea, place him/her in a high Fowler's position and provide supplemental oxygen therapy during meals if indicated	j. Because a person cannot swallow and breathe at the same time, relief of dyspnea increases the likelihood of maintaining a good oral intake. In addition, relieving dyspnea decreases the client's anxiety about and preoccupation with breathing efforts and increases the ability to focus on eating and drinking.
k. perform actions to compensate for taste alterations if present (e.g., add extra sweeteners to foods unless contraindicated, encourage client to experiment with different flavorings and seasonings, provide alternative sources of protein if meats such as beef or pork taste bitter or rancid)	k. Enhancing the taste of foods/fluids and providing nutritious alternatives to those that taste unpleasant to the client help to stimulate appetite and improve oral intake.
l. allow adequate time for meals; reheat foods/fluids if necessary	l. A client who feels rushed during meals tends to become anxious, lose his/her appetite, and stop eating. Appetite is also suppressed if foods/fluids normally served hot or warm become cold and do not appeal to the client.
m. limit fluid intake with meals unless the fluid has a high nutritional value.	m. When the stomach becomes distended, its volume receptors stimulate the satiety center in the hypothalamus and the client reduces his/her oral intake. Drinking liquids with meals distends the stomach and may cause satiety before an adequate amount of food is consumed.

7. Ensure that meals are well balanced and high in essential nutrients. Offer dietary supplements if indicated.

7. The client must consume a diet that is well balanced and high in essential nutrients in order to meet his/her nutritional needs. Dietary supplements are often needed to help accomplish this.

8. Administer vitamins and minerals if ordered.

8. Vitamins and minerals are needed to maintain metabolic functioning. If the client's dietary intake does not provide adequate amounts of them, oral and/or parenteral supplements may be necessary.

9. Allow the client to assist in the selection of foods/fluids that meet nutritional needs. Obtain a dietary consult if necessary.

9. The client who is actively involved in menu planning is more likely to adhere to the diet plan. In addition, the involvement increases his/her sense of control, which promotes a feeling of well-being and can lead to an increased oral intake. A dietitian is best able to evaluate whether the foods/fluids selected will meet the client's nutritional needs.

10. Perform a calorie count if ordered. Report information to dietitian and physician.

10. A calorie count provides information about the caloric and nutritional value of the foods/fluids the client consumes. The information obtained helps the dietitian and physician determine if an alternative method of nutritional support is needed.

11. Consult physician about an alternative method of providing nutrition (e.g., parenteral nutrition, tube feedings) if client does not consume enough food or fluids to meet nutritional needs.

11. If the client's oral intake is inadequate, an alternative method of providing nutrients needs to be implemented.

Nursing Diagnosis: Oral Mucous Membrane, Impaired

Definition

Disruption of the lips and soft tissue of the oral cavity

Defining Characteristics

Purulent drainage or exudates; gingival recession, pockets deeper than 4 mm; enlarged tonsils beyond what is developmentally appropriate; smooth atrophic, sensitive tongue; geographic tongue; mucosal denudation; presence of pathogens; difficult speech; self-report of bad taste; gingival or mucosal pallor; oral pain/discomfort; xerostomia (dry mouth); vesicles, nodules, or papules; white patches/plaques, spongy patches, or white curd-like exudate; oral lesions or ulcers; halitosis; edema; hyperemia; desquamation; coated tongue; stomatitis; self-report of difficulty eating or swallowing; self-report of diminished or absent taste; bleeding; macroplasia; gingival hyperplasia; fissures, chelitis; red or bluish masses (e.g., hemangiomas)

Related Factors

Chemotherapy; chemical (e.g., alcohol, tobacco, acidic foods, drugs, regular use of inhalers or other noxious agents); depression; immunosuppression; aging-related loss of connective, adipose, or bone tissue; barriers to professional care; cleft lip or palate; medication side effects; lack of or decreased salivation; trauma; pathological conditions: oral cavity (radiation to head or neck); NPO for more than 24 hours; mouth breathing; malnutrition or vitamin deficiency; dehydration; infection; ineffective oral hygiene; mechanical (e.g., ill-fitting dentures, braces, tubes [endotracheal/nasogastric], surgery in oral cavity); decreased platelets; immunocompromised; radiation therapy; barriers to oral self-care; diminished hormone levels (women); stress; loss of supportive structures

Desired Outcome

The client will maintain a healthy oral cavity as evidenced by:
a. absence of inflammation and discomfort
b. pink, moist, intact mucosa.

Documentation

a. Client reports of oral dryness and/or discomfort
b. Condition of oral mucous membrane
c. Therapeutic interventions
d. Client teaching

Suggested NIC Interventions: Oral health maintenance; Oral health restoration; Oral health promotion

NURSING ACTIONS	RATIONALES
Assessments	
1. Assess client for signs and symptoms of impaired oral mucous membrane (e.g., reports of oral dryness and discomfort, coated tongue, inflamed and/or ulcerated oral mucosa).	1. Early recognition of signs and symptoms of impaired oral mucous membrane allows for prompt intervention.
2. Culture oral lesions as ordered. Report positive results.	2. A positive culture reveals the organisms present in a lesion, which provides direction for the treatment plan.
Prevention/Treatment	
3. Instruct and assist client to perform oral hygiene as often as needed (e.g., after meals and at bedtime, at least every 2 hours if NPO).	3. Good oral hygiene helps maintain health of the oral mucous membrane by removing food particles and debris that harbor or promote the growth of pathogenic organisms that can cause inflammation and infection. Brushing the teeth also stimulates circulation to the gums.
4. Instruct and assist client to perform oral hygiene using a soft bristle toothbrush or sponge-tipped swab and to floss teeth gently.	4. Use of appropriate oral hygiene devices and techniques helps to effectively remove food particles and debris from client's mouth without causing trauma to the oral mucous membrane.
5. Avoid use of mouthwashes containing alcohol and oral care products that contain lemon and glycerin.	5. Mouthwashes containing alcohol and oral care products containing lemon and glycerin have a drying and irritating effect on the oral mucous membrane. Excessive use of the lemon-glycerin products also increases acidity in the mouth, which results in further irritation of the oral mucosa.
6. Encourage client to rinse mouth frequently with water.	6. Frequent rinsing of the mouth helps alleviate dryness, which reduces the risk for cracking and breakdown of the oral mucosa. Rinsing also helps prevent inflammation and infection in the mouth by removing food particles and debris that can harbor or promote the growth of pathogenic organisms.
7. Lubricate client's lips frequently.	7. Lubricating the client's lips helps keep them moist, which helps prevent drying and cracking of the lips.
8. Encourage client to breathe through nose rather than mouth.	8. Air inspired through the nose is humidified by the layer of mucus that coats the lining of the nasal cavity. Air inspired through the mouth lacks this moisture and is drying to the oral mucous membrane.
9. Encourage client not to smoke or chew tobacco.	9. Smoking dries the oral mucous membrane. Irritation and subsequent inflammation can occur when tobacco is in contact with the oral mucosa.
10. Encourage a fluid intake of at least 2500 ml/day unless contraindicated.	10. Adequate hydration helps keep the oral mucosa moist, which reduces the risk of cracking and breakdown.
11. Encourage client to suck on hard candy if allowed.	11. Sucking on hard candy stimulates salivation, which helps alleviate dryness of the oral mucosa and the subsequent risk of cracking and breakdown. Saliva also helps maintain oral mucosal health by washing away food particles and debris that harbor or promote the growth of pathogenic organisms and by directly destroying some of the bacteria present in the mouth.
12. Encourage client to use a saliva substitute such as Salivart if indicated.	12. A saliva substitute lubricates the oral mucous membrane in the absence of normal salivary flow. This helps reduce dryness and the subsequent risk of cracking and breakdown.
13. Assist client to select foods of moderate temperature and those that are soft and bland.	13. Foods that are extremely hot or cold; hard, crusty, or rough; spicy; and/or acidic may cause thermal, mechanical, or chemical trauma to the oral mucosa.

14. Encourage client to maintain an optimal nutritional status.

14. Adequate nutrition is needed to maintain the high cellular turnover of the oral mucous membrane. Good nutrition also promotes optimal function of the immune system, which reduces the client's risk of oral cavity infection.

15. Inspect client's dentures. Obtain a dental consult if dentures are rough, cracked, or ill-fitting.

15. Rough, cracked, or ill-fitting dentures can cause mechanical trauma and subsequent inflammation and breakdown of the oral mucosa. The discomfort in the affected area(s) can result in a decreased oral intake, which further compromises the health of the oral mucosa.

16. Administer topical anesthetics, oral protective agents, analgesics, and antimicrobials if ordered.

16. Topical anesthetics, oral protective agents, and analgesics promote comfort if the oral mucous membrane is inflamed or if breakdown is present. The increased comfort can result in an improved oral intake, which helps maintain health of the oral mucosa. Antimicrobials prevent or treat infection of the oral mucosa.

17. Consult appropriate health care provider if dryness, irritation, discomfort, and/or breakdown of the oral cavity persist or worsen.

17. Notifying the appropriate health care provider allows for modification of the treatment plan.

NURSING DIAGNOSIS: PAIN, ACUTE

Definition

Unpleasant sensory and emotional experience arising from actual or potential tissue damage or described in terms of such damage (International Association for the Study of Pain); sudden or slow onset of any intensity from mild to severe with an anticipated or predictable end and a duration of less than 6 months

Defining Characteristics

Verbal or coded report of pain; observed evidence; protective gestures; guarding behavior; facial mask; sleep disturbance (eyes lack luster, fixed or scattered movement, beaten look, grimace); self-focus; narrowed focus (altered time perception, impaired thought processes, reduced interaction with people and environment); distraction behavior (e.g., pacing, seeking out other people and/or activities, repetitive activities); autonomic change in muscle tone (may span from listless to rigid); autonomic responses (e.g., diaphoresis; changes in blood pressure, respiration, pulse; pupillary dilatation); expressive behavior (e.g., restlessness, moaning, crying, vigilance, irritability, sighing); changes in appetite and eating

Related Factors

Injury agents (biological, chemical, physical, psychological)

Desired Outcome

The client will experience diminished pain as evidenced by:
a. verbalization of decrease in or absence of pain
b. relaxed facial expression and body positioning
c. increased participation in activities
d. stable vital signs.

Documentation

a. Verbal description of pain
b. Rating of pain intensity
c. Facial expression
d. Body movement and position
e. Vital signs
f. Participation in activities
g. Factors that precipitate, aggravate, and alleviate pain
h. Therapeutic interventions
i. Client/family teaching

Suggested NIC Interventions: Pain management; Environmental management: comfort; Analgesic administration

NURSING ACTIONS	RATIONALES
Assessments	
1. Assess for signs and symptoms of pain (e.g., verbalization of pain, grimacing, reluctance to move, restlessness, diaphoresis, increased B/P, tachycardia).	1. Early recognition of signs and symptoms of pain allows for prompt intervention and improved pain control.
2. Assess client's perception of the severity of pain using a pain intensity rating scale.	2. An awareness of the severity of pain being experienced helps determine the most appropriate intervention(s) for pain management. Use of a pain intensity rating scale gives the nurse a clearer understanding of the pain being experienced and promotes consistency when communicating with others about the client's pain experience.
3. Assess the client's pain pattern (e.g., location, quality, onset, duration, precipitating factors, aggravating factors, alleviating factors).	3. Knowledge of the client's pain pattern assists in the identification of effective pain management interventions.
4. Ask the client to describe previous pain experiences and methods used to manage pain effectively.	4. Many variables affect a client's response to pain (e.g., age, sex, coping style, previous experience with pain, culture, cause of pain). Knowledge of the client's usual response to pain and methods previously used to manage pain effectively enables the nurse to evaluate the client's pain more accurately and facilitates the identification of effective strategies for pain management.
Prevention/Treatment	
5. Implement measures to reduce fear and anxiety (e.g., assure client that his/her need for pain relief is understood, plan methods for achieving pain control with client, provide a calm environment).	5. Fear and anxiety can decrease the client's threshold and tolerance for pain and thereby heighten the perception of pain. In addition, pain management methods are not as effective if the client is tense and unable to relax.
6. Implement measures to promote rest (e.g., minimize environmental activity and noise).	6. Fatigue can decrease the client's threshold and tolerance for pain and thereby heighten the perception of pain. If the client is well rested, he/she often experiences decreased pain and increased effectiveness of pain management measures.
7. Administer analgesics before activities and procedures that can cause pain and before pain becomes severe.	7. The administration of analgesics before a pain-producing event helps minimize the pain that will be experienced. Analgesics are also more effective if given before pain becomes severe because mild to moderate pain is controlled more quickly and effectively than severe pain.
8. Provide or assist with nonpharmacologic methods for pain relief. Examples include: a. cutaneous stimulation measures (e.g., pressure, massage, heat and cold applications, transcutaneous electrical nerve stimulation [TENS], acupuncture) b. relaxation techniques (e.g., progressive relaxation exercises, meditation, guided imagery) c. distraction measures (e.g., listening to music, conversing, watching television, playing cards, reading) d. position change.	8. Nonpharmacologic pain management includes a variety of interventions. It is believed that most of these are effective because they stimulate closure of the gating mechanism in the spinal cord and subsequently block the transmission of pain impulses. In addition, some interventions are thought to stimulate the release of endogenous analgesics (e.g., endorphins) that inhibit the transmission of pain impulses and/or alter the client's perception of pain. Many of the nonpharmacologic interventions also help decrease pain by promoting relaxation.
9. Administer the following medications as ordered:	9. Pharmacologic therapy is an effective method of reducing or relieving pain.
a. opioid (narcotic) analgesics	a. Opioid analgesics act mainly by altering the client's perception of pain and emotional response to the pain experience.
b. nonopioid (nonnarcotic) analgesics such as acetaminophen and salicylates and other nonsteroidal anti-inflammatory agents (e.g., ketorolac, ibuprofen, naproxen)	b. Nonopioid analgesics are thought to interfere with the transmission of pain impulses by inhibiting prostaglandin synthesis.
c. anesthetic agents (e.g., bupivacaine, etidocaine).	c. Anesthetics help control pain by inhibiting the initiation and conduction of pain impulses along the sensory pathways at and near the infusion site.

10. Consult physician about an order for patient-controlled analgesia (PCA) if indicated.

10. The use of PCA allows the client to self-administer analgesics within parameters established by the physician. This method facilitates pain management by ensuring prompt administration of the drug when needed, providing more continuous pain relief, and increasing the client's control over the pain.

11. Consult appropriate health care provider (e.g., physician, pharmacist, pain management specialist) if above measures fail to provide adequate pain relief.

11. Notifying the appropriate health care provider allows for modification of the treatment plan.

NURSING DIAGNOSIS: DISTURBED SELF-CONCEPT

This diagnostic label includes the nursing diagnoses of disturbed body image and situational low self-esteem

Definitions

Disturbed body image: Confusion in mental picture of one's physical self
Situational low self-esteem: Development of a negative perception of self-worth in response to a current situation (specify)

Defining Characteristics

Disturbed body image: Nonverbal response to actual or perceived change in body structure and/or function; verbalization of feelings or perceptions that reflect an altered view of one's body in appearance, structure, or function; behaviors of avoidance, monitoring, or acknowledgment of one's body; trauma to nonfunctioning part; missing body part; not touching body part; hiding or overexposing body part (intentional or unintentional); actual change in structure and/or function; change in social involvement; change in ability to estimate spatial relationship of body to environment; extension of body boundary to incorporate environmental objects; not looking at body part; refusal to verify actual change; preoccupation with change or loss; personalization of part or loss by name; depersonalization of part or loss by impersonal pronouns; negative feelings about body (e.g., feelings of helplessness, hopelessness, or powerlessness); verbalization of change in lifestyle; focus on past strength, function, or appearance; fear of rejection or reaction by others; emphasis on remaining strengths, heightened achievement
Situational low self-esteem: Verbally reports current situational challenge to self-worth; self-negating verbalizations; indecisive, nonassertive behavior; evaluation of self as unable to deal with situations or events; expressions of helplessness and uselessness

Related Factors

Disturbed body image: Psychosocial; biophysical; cognitive/perceptual; cultural or spiritual; developmental changes; illness; trauma or injury; surgery; illness treatment
Situational low self-esteem: Development changes; disturbed body image; functional impairment; loss; social role changes; lack of recognition/rewards; behavior inconsistent with values; failures/rejections

Desired Outcome

The client will demonstrate beginning adaptation to changes in appearance, level of independence, body functioning, lifestyle, and roles as evidenced by:
a. verbalization of feelings of self-worth
b. maintenance of relationships with significant others
c. active participation in activities of daily living
d. verbalization of a beginning plan for adapting lifestyle to changes resulting from the injury or disease and/or its treatment.

Documentation

a. Verbalization about changes that have occurred
b. Interactions with significant others
c. Reaction of significant others to changes in client's body functioning and/or appearance
d. Participation in activities of daily living
e. Client/family teaching
f. Referrals to community agencies

Suggested NIC Interventions: Body image enhancement; Self-esteem enhancement; Role enhancement; Counseling; Emotional support; Support system enhancement

NURSING ACTIONS	RATIONALES
Assessments	
1. Assess for signs and symptoms of a disturbed self-concept (e.g., verbalization of negative feelings about self, refusal to look at or touch a body part, withdrawal from significant others, lack of participation in activities of daily living, lack of plan for adapting to necessary changes in lifestyle).	1. Early recognition of signs and symptoms of a disturbed self-concept allows for prompt intervention.
2. Determine the meaning of the change in body image and/or functioning to the client by encouraging the verbalization of feelings and by noting nonverbal responses to changes experienced.	2. An understanding of what the change means to the client provides a basis for planning care.
Prevention/Treatment	
3. Implement measures to assist client through the beginning phases of grieving (e.g., shock, disbelief, denial, anger, sadness, depression).	3. A change in appearance, body functioning, and/or role can initiate a grieving response. Successful resolution of grief assists the client to accept changes experienced and integrate the changes into self-concept.
4. Discuss with client improvements in appearance and/or body functioning that can realistically be expected.	4. Realistic expectations about appearance and/or body functioning facilitate goal setting and are essential for positive adaptation to the changes experienced and integration of these changes into self-concept.
5. Implement measures to assist client to increase self-esteem (e.g., limit negative self-assessment, encourage positive comments about self, assist to identify strengths, give positive feedback about accomplishments and behaviors that are indicative of high self-esteem).	5. Self-esteem is a major component of one's view of self. It is a product of self-evaluation, reflected appraisals, social expectations, and perceptions of personal competence. An increase in self-esteem has a positive effect on the client's self-concept.
6. Assist client to identify and use coping techniques that have been helpful in the past.	6. Coping techniques help the client to manage or reduce the anxiety and stress that result when changes in appearance, body functioning, and/or role occur. This reduction in anxiety and stress facilitates adaptation to these changes and development of a positive self-concept.
7. Implement measures to assist client to adjust to alteration(s) in sexual functioning if appropriate (e.g., encourage questions and discussion about changes experienced, facilitate communication between client and his/her partner, discuss ways to be creative in expressing sexuality).	7. Sexual functioning is an important component of one's sense of self. Assistance may be necessary to help the client adjust to changes experienced and/or identify alternative ways of sexual expression.
8. Implement measures to assist client to adapt to changes in body functioning and/or appearance (e.g., instruct in use of assistive devices, assist with clothing selection that minimizes changes in body contour).	8. Measures that help minimize changes in appearance and/or body functioning reduce the impact of these changes on self-concept.
9. Assist client with usual grooming and makeup habits if necessary.	9. Appearance is an essential component of self-esteem and one's concept of self. Maintaining an appearance he/she is comfortable with has a positive effect on the client's self-concept.
10. Encourage client's participation in activities that can assist him/her to integrate physical changes that have occurred (e.g., exercise, grooming, bathing).	10. Activities that help the client acknowledge and deal with the changes that have occurred in his/her body facilitate the incorporation of the changes into the brain's schemata of the body.

11. Demonstrate acceptance of client with techniques such as touch and frequent visits. Encourage significant others to do the same.

11. Frequent visits and the use of touch convey a feeling of acceptance to the client. This enhances feelings of self-worth and assists in the development of a positive self-concept.

12. Support behaviors suggesting positive adaptation to changes that have occurred (e.g., willingness to care for wounds, compliance with treatment plan, verbalization of feelings of self-worth, maintenance of relationships with significant others).

12. Supporting behaviors indicative of positive adaptation to changes encourages the client to repeat these behaviors. Repetition of positive adaptive behaviors facilitates the development of a positive self-concept.

13. Encourage significant others to allow client to do what he/she is able.

13. Allowing the client to do as much as he/she is able facilitates the re-establishment of independence, which enhances feelings of self-esteem.

14. Encourage client contact with others if a change in appearance and body functioning has occurred.

14. Feedback from others is often a critical factor in the development of one's self-image. When a change in appearance and/or body functioning has occurred, contact with others provides the client with the opportunity to obtain feedback, test and establish a new self-image, and begin to adapt to the changes that have occurred.

15. Assist client's and significant others' adjustment by listening, facilitating communication, and providing information.

15. Listening, facilitating communication, and providing information assist the client and significant others to cope with the present situation. Effective coping facilitates the integration of changes that have occurred.

16. Assist client and significant others to have similar expectations and understanding of future lifestyle and to identify ways that personal and family goals can be adjusted rather than abandoned.

16. Congruent expectations of client and significant others facilitates their working together to meet common goals. Adjustment rather than abandonment of personal and family goals reduces the feeling of loss and increases the probability of positive adaptation to the changes that have occurred.

17. Teach client the rationale for treatments, encourage maximum participation in treatment regimen, and allow choices whenever possible.

17. An understanding of the reasons for treatments, active participation in treatment regimen, and the opportunity to make choices on one's behalf enable the client to maintain a sense of control, which enhances self-esteem.

18. Encourage client to pursue usual roles and interests and to continue involvement in social activities. If previous roles, interests, and hobbies cannot be pursued, encourage development of new ones.

18. The ability to pursue usual roles and activities has a positive effect on the client's self-esteem. The same effect can be achieved if the client is successful in new roles and activities that he/she chooses.

19. Provide information about and encourage use of community agencies and support groups (e.g., vocational rehabilitation; sexual, family, individual, and/or financial counseling).

19. Community agencies and support groups provide the opportunity for the client to see that he/she is not experiencing a unique problem, to share feelings and concerns, to profit from the experience of others with similar difficulties, and to learn new skills necessary to rebuild self-esteem. All of these factors help the client to establish a positive self-concept.

20. Consult appropriate health care provider (e.g., psychiatric nurse clinician, physician) if client seems unwilling or unable to adapt to changes resulting from the disease process and/or its treatment.

20. Additional counseling may be necessary to facilitate positive adaptation to the changes in appearance and/or body functioning that have occurred.

NURSING DIAGNOSIS: SKIN INTEGRITY, IMPAIRED, RISK FOR

Definition

At risk for skin being adversely altered

Risk Factors

External: radiation; physical immobilization; hypothermia or hyperthermia; chemical substance; mechanical factors (e.g., shearing forces, pressure, restraint); humidity; excretions and/or secretions; moisture; extremes of age

Internal: medication; skeletal prominence; immunologic factors; developmental factors; altered sensation; altered pigmentation; altered metabolic state; altered circulation;

alterations in skin turgor (changes in elasticity); alterations in nutritional state (e.g., obesity, emaciation); psychogenetic

Desired Outcome

The client will maintain skin integrity as evidenced by:
a. absence of redness and irritation
b. no skin breakdown.

Documentation

a. Appearance of skin
b. Therapeutic interventions
c. Client/family teaching

Suggested NIC Interventions: Pressure ulcer prevention; Skin surveillance; Bathing; Pressure management; Skin care: topical treatments; Positioning; Bed rest care

NURSING ACTIONS	RATIONALES
Assessments	
1. Determine client's risk for skin breakdown using a risk assessment tool (e.g., Norton Scale, Braden Scale, Gosnell Scale).	1. Prompt identification of the client's risk for skin breakdown leads to earlier implementation of actions to maintain skin integrity. Use of a risk assessment tool aids in the identification of factors that could cause skin breakdown.
2. Inspect the skin (especially bony prominences, dependent areas, pruritic areas, perineum, and areas of decreased sensation and/or edema) for pallor, redness, and breakdown.	2. Early recognition of signs of impaired skin integrity allows for prompt intervention.
Prevention	
3. Implement measures to prevent prolonged and/or excessive pressure on any area of the skin: a. assist client to turn at least every 2 hours unless contraindicated b. instruct or assist client to shift weight at least every 30 minutes c. position client properly using supportive devices such as pillows and pads as needed d. keep bed linens wrinkle-free e. ensure that external devices such as braces, casts, and restraints are applied properly f. ensure that client is not lying on tubings g. use pressure-reducing or pressure-relieving devices (e.g., gel or foam cushions, alternating pressure mattress, air-fluidized bed) if indicated.	3. Prolonged and/or excessive pressure on the skin obstructs capillary blood flow to that area. The resultant hypoxia, impaired flow of nutrients, and accumulation of waste products in the area of obstructed blood flow make that tissue more susceptible to breakdown. Measures that prevent the excessive pressure or ensure that pressure is relieved often enough to avoid obstruction of capillary blood flow help maintain skin integrity.
4. Gently massage around reddened areas at least every 2 hours.	4. Massage stimulates circulation to the skin and underlying tissues. The improved blood flow helps maintain skin integrity by increasing the supply of oxygen and nutrients available to the cells and by removing waste products of metabolism. To avoid damaging the capillaries, massage should be gentle rather than deep and massage over reddened areas should be avoided.
5. Implement measures to prevent shearing (e.g., keep head of bed as flat as possible, gatch knees slightly when head of bed is elevated 30° or higher, limit length of time client is in semi-Fowler's position to 30-minute intervals).	5. When one tissue layer slides past another in an opposite direction (shearing), the capillaries in the affected area are kinked, stretched, or severed. This compromises the area's blood supply and increases the risk of tissue breakdown. A client in a semi-Fowler's position is likely to slide down in the bed. When this occurs, his/her skin tends to remain stationary while the underlying tissues and skeletal structures shift position resulting in shearing.

6. Implement measures to reduce friction between the skin and another surface (e.g., apply a protective covering such as a hydrocolloid or transparent membrane dressing to susceptible areas of the skin, apply thin layer of a dry lubricant such as powder or cornstarch to bottom sheet or client's skin, lift and move client carefully using turn sheet and adequate assistance, adequately secure restraints and tubings, pat skin dry rather than rub).

6. The outermost layers of skin can be damaged when dragged along or rubbed against another surface. Reducing friction helps prevent skin surface irritation and abrasion.

7. Keep client's skin clean.

7. Keeping the skin clean removes many of the surface microorganisms, which, if allowed to accumulate, increase the risk of irritation or infection and subsequent skin breakdown.

8. Use a mild soap when bathing client.

8. Sebum, which is secreted by the skin, helps maintain skin integrity by preventing excess evaporation of moisture, keeping the skin soft and pliable, and destroying some of the bacteria on the skin's surface. Using a mild rather than a harsh, alkaline soap helps ensure that some sebum remains on the skin after bathing.

9. Implement measures to keep skin free of excessive moisture:
   a. thoroughly dry skin after bathing and as often as needed, paying special attention to skin folds and opposing skin surfaces (e.g., axillae, perineum, beneath breasts)
   b. keep bed linens dry
   c. protect skin surrounding wound from drainage (e.g., change dressing when damp, apply a drainage collection device if needed)
   d. if use of absorbent products such as pads or undergarments is necessary, select those that effectively absorb moisture and keep it away from the skin.

9. Excessive moisture on the skin or prolonged exposure of the skin to moisture softens the epidermal cells and makes them less resistant to damage. Moisture also harbors microorganisms that can cause irritation or infection and it increases the possibility of friction between the skin and the surface it is against. Removing excessive moisture and protecting the skin from prolonged contact with moisture reduces the risk of skin irritation and subsequent breakdown.

10. Increase activity as allowed and tolerated.

10. Activity stimulates circulation, which helps maintain skin integrity by increasing the flow of oxygen and nutrients to the skin and underlying tissues. In addition, increasing activity reduces the risk of prolonged pressure occurring on any area as a result of decreased mobility.

11. Maintain an optimal nutritional status.

11. An inadequate nutritional status results in muscle atrophy, a decrease in the amount of subcutaneous tissue, and skin that is thin and less elastic. Subsequently, the skin and tissue are more vulnerable to injury because they are less able to withstand minor trauma. In addition, a malnourished client is more susceptible to the effects of pressure because there is less padding between the skin and underlying bone.

12. Implement measures to prevent drying of the skin:
   a. encourage a fluid intake of 2500 ml/day unless contraindicated
   b. apply a moisturizing lotion and/or emollient to skin at least once a day.

12. Dry skin is more prone to cracking and has decreased elasticity, which make it susceptible to damage.
   a. An adequate fluid intake helps ensure that the skin remains well hydrated.
   b. Moisturizing lotion and some emollients provide a source of moisture to the skin. Emollients also form a protective barrier on the epidermis, which reduces the evaporation of moisture.

13. Protect skin from contact with urine and feces (e.g., perform actions to prevent incontinence and/or diarrhea, keep perineal area clean and dry, apply a protective ointment or cream to perineal area).

13. Urine and feces are irritants that can cause inflammation and breakdown of the skin. In addition, the moisture in urine and feces softens epidermal cells and increases friction between opposing skin surfaces and between the skin and bed linen.

NURSING ACTIONS	RATIONALES
Prevention	
14. If edema is present, handle edematous areas carefully and implement measures to reduce fluid accumulation in dependent areas (e.g., instruct client in and assist with range of motion exercises, elevate affected extremities whenever possible).	14. Edematous areas have an increased risk for skin breakdown because the oxygen and nutrient supply to the skin is compromised by the increased distance that exists between the capillaries and the cells. Handling edematous areas carefully and implementing measures to reduce edema decrease the risk for skin breakdown.
15. If the client is experiencing pruritus, implement measures to reduce the itching sensation (e.g., apply cool compress to pruritic area, administer prescribed antihistamines), keep his/her nails trimmed, and apply mittens if necessary.	15. The client experiencing pruritus is likely to scratch the affected areas, which irritates the skin and can cause excoriation. Implementing measures to reduce the itching sensation helps prevent scratching. Trimming the client's nails and applying mittens if necessary reduces the risk of trauma to the skin if he/she does scratch the pruritic areas.
16. Notify appropriate health care provider (e.g., physician, enterostomal therapist, wound care specialist) if skin breakdown occurs.	16. Notifying the appropriate health care provider allows for modification of treatment plan.

Nursing Diagnosis: Sleep Pattern, Disturbed

Definition

Time-limited disruption of sleep (natural, periodic suspension of consciousness) amount and quality

Defining Characteristics

Prolonged awakenings; sleep maintenance insomnia; self-induced impairment of normal pattern; sleep onset greater than 30 minutes; early morning insomnia; awakening earlier or later than desired; verbal complaints of difficulty falling asleep; verbal complaints of not feeling well-rested; increased proportion of Stage 1 sleep; dissatisfaction with sleep; less than age-normed total sleep time; three or more nighttime awakenings; decreased proportion of Stages 3 and 4 sleep (e.g., hyporesponsiveness, excess sleepiness, decreased motivation); decreased proportion of rapid eye movement (REM) sleep (e.g., REM rebound, hyperactivity, emotional lability, agitation and impulsivity, atypical polysomnographic features); decreased ability to function

Related Factors

Psychological: ruminative pre-sleep thoughts; daytime activity pattern; thinking about home; body temperature; temperament; dietary; childhood onset; inadequate sleep hygiene; sustained use of anti-sleep agents; circadian asynchrony; frequently changing sleep-wake schedule; depression; loneliness; frequent travel across time zones; daylight/darkness exposure; grief; anticipation; shift work; delayed or advanced sleep phase syndrome; loss of sleep partner, life change; preoccupation with trying to sleep; periodic gender-related hormonal shifts; biochemical agents; fear; separation from significant others; social schedule inconsistent with chronotype; aging-related sleep shifts; anxiety; medications; fear of insomnia; maladaptive conditioned wakefulness; fatigue; boredom

Environmental: noise; unfamiliar sleep furnishings; ambient temperature, humidity; lighting; other-generated awakening; excessive stimulation; physical restraint; lack of sleep privacy/control; interruptions for therapeutics, monitoring, lab tests; sleep partner; noxious odors

Parental: mother's sleep-wake pattern; parent-infant interaction; mother's emotional support

Physiological: urinary urgency, incontinence; fever; nausea; stasis of secretions; shortness of breath; position; gastroesophageal reflux

Desired Outcome

The client will attain optimal amounts of sleep as evidenced by statements of feeling well rested.

Documentation

a. Statements of difficulty falling asleep, interruptions in sleep, and/or not feeling well rested
b. Therapeutic interventions
c. Client teaching

Suggested NIC Intervention: Sleep enhancement

NURSING ACTIONS	RATIONALES
Assessments	
1. Assess for signs and symptoms of a disturbed sleep pattern (e.g., statements of difficulty falling asleep, sleep interruptions, or not feeling well rested).	1. Early recognition of signs and symptoms of a disturbed sleep pattern allows for prompt intervention.
2. Determine client's usual sleep habits.	2. Knowledge of the client's usual sleep-wake cycle and routines that help induce and maintain sleep helps the nurse plan interventions aimed at preventing a sleep pattern disturbance.
Prevention/Treatment	
3. Discourage long periods of sleep during the day unless signs and symptoms of sleep deprivation exist or daytime sleep is usual for client.	3. Long periods of sleep during the day are often a change in the client's usual sleep-wake cycle and cause desynchronization of his/her circadian rhythm. This can result in a poorer quality of sleep.
4. Implement measures to reduce fear and anxiety (e.g., maintain a calm, confident manner when working with client; assist client to identify specific stressors and ways to cope with them).	4. Fear and anxiety stimulate the sympathetic nervous system, which increases alertness and makes it difficult for the client to fall asleep. Sympathetic nervous system stimulation is also believed to shorten the duration of nonrapid eye movement (NREM) and REM sleep, which results in a poorer quality of sleep.
5. Encourage participation in relaxing diversional activities during the evening.	5. Involvement in relaxing activities in the evening helps the client fall asleep more easily.
6. Discourage intake of foods/fluids high in caffeine (e.g., chocolate, coffee, tea, colas) in the evening.	6. Caffeine acts as a central nervous system stimulant and can interfere with relaxation and subsequent sleep induction. Caffeine also acts as a diuretic, which can cause an interruption in sleep if the client awakens in response to the urge to urinate.
7. Offer client an evening snack that includes milk unless contraindicated.	7. Milk contains the amino acid L-tryptophan, which is believed to help induce and maintain sleep.
8. Allow client to continue usual sleep practices (e.g., position; time; presleep routines such as reading, watching television, listening to music, and meditating) whenever possible.	8. Adherence to usual sleep practices promotes mental and physical relaxation that assists the client to maintain his/her usual sleep-wake cycle.
9. Satisfy basic needs such as comfort and warmth before sleep.	9. When basic needs are met, the client is usually more comfortable and better able to relax. This facilitates sleep induction and reduces the probability of frequent awakenings.
10. Encourage client to urinate just before bedtime.	10. A full bladder stimulates an urge to urinate, which can interrupt sleep. Emptying the bladder just before bedtime reduces the risk of the client awakening more frequently and/or earlier than desired.
11. Reduce environmental distractions (e.g., close door to client's room; use night light rather than overhead light whenever possible; lower volume of paging system; keep staff conversations at a low level and away from client's room; close curtains between clients in a semi-private room or ward; keep beepers and alarms on low volume; provide client with "white noise" such as a fan, soft music, or tape-recorded sounds of the ocean or rain; have sleep mask and earplugs available for client if needed).	11. Environmental activity, noise, and light can interfere with the client's ability to fall asleep and stay asleep. Reducing stimuli helps prevent a sleep pattern disturbance.

NURSING ACTIONS	RATIONALES
Prevention/Treatment	
12. If client has orthopnea, assist him/her to assume a position that facilitates breathing (e.g., head of bed elevated with arms supported on pillows, resting forward on overbed table with good pillow support, sitting in a chair) and maintain oxygen therapy during sleep.	12. Hypoxemia stimulates the client's arousal system making it difficult to fall asleep and stay asleep. Proper positioning and administration of supplemental oxygen help ease breathing efforts and reduce hypoxemia, which makes it easier for the client to fall asleep and reduces the number of awakenings.
13. Encourage client to avoid drinking alcohol in the evening.	13. Although alcohol can induce drowsiness, which promotes sleep induction, it is known to interfere with REM sleep. Alcohol also inhibits the release of antidiuretic hormone (ADH), which can cause an interruption in sleep if the client awakens in response to the urge to urinate.
14. Encourage client to avoid smoking before bedtime.	14. Nicotine is a stimulant that can interfere with sleep by making it difficult for the client to relax and fall asleep and to stay asleep.
15. If possible, administer medications that can interfere with sleep (e.g., steroids, diuretics) early in the day rather than late afternoon or evening.	15. Administering these medications as early as possible during the day helps prevent nighttime insomnia and/or frequent awakenings.
16. Administer prescribed sedative-hypnotics if indicated.	16. Sedative-hypnotics are central nervous system depressants that promote sleep by reducing anxiety, shortening sleep induction, and/or reducing arousal level (wakefulness). These medications should be used for only a short time because they interfere with the length of REM sleep and can actually create a disturbance in the client's sleep-wake cycle.
17. Implement measures to reduce interruptions during sleep (e.g., restrict visitors, group care whenever possible) so that client is able to sleep undisturbed for 70 to 100 minute intervals.	17. One sleep cycle takes about 70–100 minutes to complete. Each time the cycle is interrupted, it begins again with NREM Stage 1 sleep so the client loses portions of NREM and/or REM sleep. When the client is deprived of NREM sleep, lethargy and depression occur. Loss of REM sleep results in irritability and anxiety. Reducing the frequency of sleep interruptions helps ensure that the client progresses through all of the sleep stages and does not experience a sleep pattern disturbance.
18. Consult appropriate health care provider if signs and symptoms of sleep deprivation (e.g., irritability, lethargy, agitation, inability to concentrate) occur and persist or worsen.	18. Notifying the appropriate health care provider allows for modification of treatment plan.

Nursing Diagnosis: Swallowing, Impaired

Definition

Abnormal functioning of the swallowing mechanism associated with deficits in oral, pharyngeal, or esophageal structure or function

Defining Characteristics

Pharyngeal phase impairment: altered head positions; inadequate laryngeal elevation; food refusal; unexplained fevers; delayed swallow; recurrent pulmonary infections; gurgly voice quality; nasal reflux; choking, coughing, or gagging; multiple swallows; abnormality in pharyngeal phase by swallow study

Esophageal phase impairment: heartburn or epigastric pain; acidic smelling breath; unexplained irritability surrounding mealtime; vomitus on pillow; repetitive swallowing or ruminating; regurgitation of gastric contents or wet burps; bruxism; nighttime coughing or awakening; observed evidence of difficulty in swallowing (e.g., stasis of food in oral cavity, coughing or choking); hyperextension of head, arching during or after meals; abnormality in esophageal phase by swallow study; odynophagia; food refusal or volume limiting; complaints of "something stuck"; hematemesis; vomiting

Oral phase impairment: lack of tongue action to form bolus; weak suck resulting in inefficient nippling; incomplete lip closure; food pushed out of mouth; slow bolus formation; premature entry of bolus; piecemeal deglutition; lack of chewing; food falls from mouth; nasal reflux; inability to clear oral cavity; long meals with little consumption; coughing, choking, gagging before a swallow; abnormality in oral phase of swallow study; pooling in lateral sulci; sialorrhea or drooling

Related Factors

Congenital deficits: upper airway anomalies; failure to thrive or protein energy malnutrition; conditions with significant hypotonia; respiratory disorders; history of tube feeding; behavioral feeding problems; self-injurious behavior; neuromuscular impairment (e.g., decreased or absent gag reflex, decreased strength or excursion of muscles involved in mastication, perceptual impairment, facial paralysis); mechanical obstruction (e.g., edema, tracheostomy tube, tumor); congenital heart disease; cranial nerve involvement

Neurological problems: upper airway anomalies; laryngeal abnormalities; achalasia; gastroesophageal reflux disease; acquired anatomic defects; cerebral palsy; internal traumas; tracheal, laryngeal, esophageal defects; traumatic head injury; developmental delay; external traumas; nasal or nasopharyngeal cavity defects; oral cavity or oropharynx abnormalities; premature infants

Desired Outcome

The client will experience an improvement in swallowing as evidenced by:
a. verbalization of same
b. absence of food in oral cavity after swallowing
c. absence of coughing and choking when eating and drinking.

Documentation

a. Verbalization of difficulty swallowing
b. Stasis of food in oral cavity
c. Coughing or choking when eating or drinking
d. Consistency of foods/fluids client is able to swallow without difficulty
e. Therapeutic interventions
f. Client/family teaching

Suggested NIC Interventions: Swallowing therapy; Aspiration precautions

NURSING ACTIONS	RATIONALES
Assessments	
1. Assess for signs and symptoms of impaired swallowing (e.g., statements of difficulty swallowing, stasis of food in oral cavity, coughing or choking when eating or drinking).	1. Early recognition of signs and symptoms of impaired swallowing allows for prompt intervention.
2. Assist with studies to evaluate client's swallowing (e.g., videofluoroscopy) if ordered.	2. Swallowing is a complex act that consists of voluntary and involuntary neuromotor components. Studies that evaluate the client's ability to swallow help identify the specific physiological dysfunction, which aids in planning effective interventions.
Prevention/Treatment	
3. Implement measures to reduce oral and pharyngeal discomfort if indicated (e.g., administer topical and/or systemic analgesics as ordered).	3. Oral and pharyngeal discomfort can interfere with the client's ability and willingness to adequately chew food and swallow effectively.
4. If client has viscous oral secretions, implement measures to liquefy these secretions (e.g., encourage a fluid intake of 2500 ml/day unless contraindicated, administer a papain product before meals as ordered).	4. Thick oral secretions interfere with movement of food in the mouth. Liquefying these secretions makes it easier for a bolus of food to be formed and moved to the back of the mouth. Liquefying the secretions also helps ensure that the bolus formed is moist so that it stays intact and triggers an effective swallowing reflex.
5. If client's mouth is dry, implement measures to moisten mouth prior to meals and snacks (e.g., provide good oral care, stimulate salivation by having client suck on hard candy unless contraindicated, encourage use of a saliva substitute such as Salivart).	5. A moist mouth helps lubricate food, which makes it easier to chew, form into a bolus, and manipulate toward the back of the mouth. A formed, moist bolus more effectively triggers the swallowing reflex and moves more easily through the esophagus.

NURSING ACTIONS	RATIONALES
Prevention/Treatment	
6. Consult speech pathologist about methods for dealing with client's specific swallowing impairment.	6. Consulting with persons who are knowledgeable about the management of swallowing difficulties aids in the development of an individualized plan of care to improve the client's swallowing.
7. Instruct and assist client to select foods/fluids that are appropriate for his/her swallowing ability. Some general guidelines include:	7. Impaired swallowing can result from structural or neurological problems. The types of foods/fluids a client can swallow effectively vary depending on the particular swallowing difficulty.
a. avoiding foods that tend to fall apart in mouth (e.g., applesauce, cake, muffins) and those that consist of small food particles (e.g., rice, peas, corn, nuts) if client has impaired tongue control	a. Clients with impaired tongue movement have difficulty keeping foods that tend to fall apart in the mouth or consist of small pieces in a bolus that can be transferred to the back of the mouth. Some small pieces of food may fall to the back of the mouth, but because the food is not in a bolus, it will not trigger a strong swallowing reflex.
b. avoiding foods that are sticky (e.g., peanut butter, soft bread, honey)	b. Sticky foods are difficult to move through the mouth because they tend to adhere to various structures, especially the hard palate. It is also difficult to form these foods into the distinct bolus needed to trigger the swallowing reflex.
c. moistening dry foods with gravy or sauces (e.g., catsup, sour cream, salad dressing)	c. Moist foods are more easily formed into a bolus and moved through the mouth and esophagus.
d. selecting thick rather than thin fluids or adding a thickening agent (e.g., "Thick-It," gelatin, baby cereal) if client has a delayed swallowing reflex and/or poor tongue control.	d. Thin fluids pass rapidly through the mouth and can pour over the back of the tongue without triggering an effective swallow. Thick fluids remain more cohesive and are able to stimulate the swallowing reflex more effectively.
8. Place client in a high Fowler's position for meals and snacks unless contraindicated.	8. A high Fowler's position uses gravity to aid in the flow of foods/fluids through the esophagus.
9. If client has difficulty chewing and maneuvering a bolus of food to the back of the mouth, instruct him/her to tilt head down when chewing and forming a bolus, then raise chin slightly when ready to swallow.	9. Tilting the head down allows client more time to chew and form a bolus because the food is in the front of the mouth where it does not trigger the swallowing reflex. Raising the chin facilitates movement of the bolus to the back of the mouth so that the swallowing reflex can be triggered. NOTE: Caution client to avoid tilting head back when swallowing since this position increases the risk for aspiration.
10. Serve foods/fluids that are hot or cold instead of room temperature.	10. Foods/fluids that are hot or cold trigger a more effective swallowing reflex because they have a greater stimulatory effect on the sensory receptors in the mouth.
11. If client has motor and sensory dysfunction of one side of the mouth or face, instruct and assist him/her to tilt head toward the unaffected side when eating and drinking and to place food in the unaffected side of the mouth.	11. When foods/fluids are directed toward the unaffected side of the mouth, the client is able to more effectively chew and use his/her tongue to form a bolus and move it to the back of the mouth. The unaffected side of the mouth also has more tension in the buccal musculature so foods/fluids are more likely to get to the back of the mouth rather than collect between the cheek and the mandible. Sensory receptors on the unaffected side also trigger a stronger swallowing reflex than those on the affected side.
12. Encourage client to concentrate on the act of swallowing. Provide verbal cueing as needed.	12. The client can achieve a more effective swallow by focusing on chewing and moving foods/fluids to the back of the mouth where the swallowing reflex is triggered.
13. Instruct client to avoid putting too much food/fluid in mouth at one time.	13. Overfilling the mouth makes it difficult for the client to form a distinct bolus and effectively move it to the back of the mouth where it triggers the swallowing reflex.

14. Encourage client to perform exercises to strengthen tongue and facial muscles if indicated (e.g., drinking through a straw; opening mouth and moving tongue anteriorly, posteriorly, and laterally; pushing tongue upward against resistance using an object such as a tongue blade, Popsicle, or sucker).

14. Strong tongue and facial muscles increase the client's ability to chew food, form a bolus, and direct the bolus to the back of the mouth where it triggers the swallowing reflex.

15. Consult appropriate health care provider (e.g., physician, speech pathologist) if swallowing difficulties persist or worsen.

15. Notifying the appropriate health care provider allows for modification of treatment plan.

Nursing Diagnosis: Tissue Perfusion, Ineffective

NANDA International identifies five types of ineffective tissue perfusion (renal, cerebral, cardiopulmonary, gastrointestinal, peripheral). A client can experience more than one type of ineffective tissue perfusion and the actions for the various types are often similar. The information presented here focuses on ineffective tissue perfusion in general rather than a specific type.

Definition

Decrease in oxygen resulting in failure to nourish the tissues at the capillary level

Defining Characteristics

Renal: altered blood pressure outside of acceptable parameters; hematuria; oliguria or anuria; elevation in BUN/creatinine ratio

Gastrointestinal: hypoactive or absent bowel sounds; nausea; abdominal distention; abdominal pain or tenderness

Peripheral: edema; positive Homans' sign; altered skin characteristics (hair, nails, moisture); weak or absent pulses; skin temperature changes; altered sensations; skin discolorations; diminished arterial pulsations; skin color pale on elevation, color does not return on lowering of leg; delayed healing; claudication; blood pressure changes in extremities; bruits

Cerebral: speech abnormalities; changes in pupillary reactions; extremity weakness or paralysis; altered mental status; difficulty in swallowing; changes in motor response; behavioral changes

Cardiopulmonary: altered respiratory rate outside of acceptable parameters; use of accessory muscles; capillary refill greater than 3 seconds; abnormal arterial blood gases; chest pain; sense of "impending doom"; bronchospasm; dyspnea; arrhythmias; nasal flaring; chest retraction

Related Factors

Hypovolemia; interruption of arterial flow; hypervolemia; exchange problems; interruption of venous flow; mechanical reduction of venous and/or arterial blood flow; hypoventilation; impaired transport of the oxygen across alveolar and/or capillary membrane; mismatch of ventilation with blood flow; decreased hemoglobin concentration in blood; enzyme poisoning; altered affinity of hemoglobin for oxygen

Desired Outcome

The client will maintain adequate systemic tissue perfusion as evidenced by:

a. B/P within normal range
b. usual mental status
c. extremities warm with absence of pallor and cyanosis
d. palpable peripheral pulses
e. capillary refill time less than 2–3 seconds
f. absence of edema
g. absence of exercise-induced pain
h. urine output at least 30 ml/hour.

Documentation

a. Blood pressure
b. Mental status
c. Skin color and temperature
d. Peripheral pulses
e. Capillary refill time
f. Presence of edema
g. Exercise-induced pain

h. Urine output
i. Therapeutic interventions
j. Client teaching

Suggested NIC Interventions: Circulatory care: arterial insufficiency; Circulatory care: venous insufficiency; Cardiac care: acute; Hypovolemia management

NURSING ACTIONS	RATIONALES
Assessments	
1. Assess for and report signs and symptoms of diminished tissue perfusion (e.g., decreased blood pressure, restlessness, confusion, cool extremities, pallor or cyanosis of extremities, diminished or absent peripheral pulses, slow capillary refill, edema, claudication, angina, oliguria).	1. Early recognition and reporting of signs and symptoms of diminished tissue perfusion allow for prompt intervention.
Prevention/Treatment	
2. Administer intravenous fluids and/or blood if ordered.	2. Intravenous fluids and/or blood help maintain vascular volume, which is essential for adequate tissue perfusion.
3. Maintain a minimum fluid intake of 2500 ml/day unless contraindicated.	3. Adequate hydration is essential for maintenance of a vascular volume sufficient to maintain adequate tissue perfusion.
4. Instruct client to change from a supine to an upright position slowly if he/she has postural hypotension.	4. Changing from a supine to a sitting or standing position slowly allows time for the baroreceptors to adjust to the change in the distribution of blood associated with an upright position; this helps keep the blood pressure at a level sufficient to maintain adequate tissue perfusion.
5. Discourage positions such as crossing legs, pillows under knees, and use of knee gatch.	5. These positions exert pressure on vessels in the lower extremities, which compromises blood flow.
6. Encourage client to avoid sitting or standing for prolonged periods.	6. Prolonged sitting or standing causes venous stasis.
7. If client is on bed rest, instruct and assist with range of motion exercises at least 3 times/day and active foot and leg exercises every 1–2 hours.	7. When a client is on bed rest, blood pools in the extremities as a result of decreased muscle activity. Range of motion exercises help reduce venous stasis. The rhythmic muscle contractions that occur during active foot and leg exercises cause intermittent compression of the veins, which improves venous return.
8. If client's activity is limited and/or venous insufficiency is a problem, consult physician about an order for antiembolism stockings or an intermittent pneumatic compression device.	8. Antiembolism stockings and intermittent pneumatic compression devices promote venous return by exerting either constant pressure or intermittent pressure on the vessels in the lower extremities.
9. Encourage and assist client with ambulation as soon as allowed and tolerated.	9. Ambulation causes rhythmic contractions of the leg muscles. This creates a pumping effect on the leg veins, which subsequently increases venous return.
10. Implement measures to improve cardiac output (e.g., administer positive inotropic agents, vasodilators, and/or antiarrhythmics if ordered; promote rest) if decreased cardiac output is contributing to inadequate tissue perfusion.	10. Improved cardiac output enhances tissue perfusion by increasing arterial and venous blood flow.
11. Implement measures to prevent vasoconstriction:	11. Vasoconstriction narrows vessel lumens, which results in diminished blood flow through the affected vessels. Vasoconstriction may also increase afterload, which can decrease cardiac output and systemic tissue perfusion.
a. perform actions to reduce stress	a. Stress stimulates the sympathetic nervous system, which results in vasoconstriction.

b. discourage smoking

b. Nicotine increases catecholamine output, which subsequently causes vasoconstriction.

c. perform actions to keep client from getting cold (e.g., maintain a comfortable room temperature, provide adequate clothing and blankets).

c. When the body is cold, peripheral vasoconstriction occurs in an attempt to contain body heat.

12. Administer the following medications if ordered:
   a. antiplatelet agents and/or anticoagulants
   b. hemorrheologic agents (e.g., pentoxifylline)
   c. peripheral vasodilators (e.g., isoxsuprine, cilostazol)
   d. antihypertensives.

12.
   a. Antiplatelet agents and anticoagulants may be used to prevent or treat clots that may obstruct blood flow.
   b. Pentoxifylline is a hemorrheologic agent that improves microcirculation by decreasing blood viscosity and improving RBC flexibility.
   c. These medications dilate cerebral and peripheral blood vessels making them useful in treatment of cerebral vascular insufficiency and peripheral vascular disease.
   d. Antihypertensives reduce systemic vascular resistance, which subsequently improves systemic tissue perfusion.

13. Consult appropriate health care provider if signs and symptoms of diminished tissue perfusion persist or worsen.

13. Notifying the appropriate health care provider allows for modification of treatment plan.

NURSING DIAGNOSIS: URINARY INCONTINENCE

NANDA International identifies five types of urinary incontinence (stress, reflex, urge, functional, and total). A client can experience a combination of types of incontinence and the actions for various types often are similar. The information presented here focuses on incontinence in general rather than a specific type.

Definition
Involuntary loss or passage of urine

Defining Characteristics
See NANDA International resource for defining characteristics for each type of urinary incontinence.

Related Factors
See NANDA International resource for related or risk factors for each type of urinary incontinence.

Desired Outcome
The client will experience urinary continence.

Documentation
a. Episodes of urinary incontinence
b. Statements of being unable to control urinary elimination
c. Therapeutic interventions
d. Client teaching

Suggested NIC Interventions: Urinary incontinence care; Urinary habit training; Urinary bladder training; Pelvic muscle exercise

NURSING ACTIONS	RATIONALES
1. Assess for and report urinary incontinence.	1. Early recognition and reporting of urinary incontinence allow for prompt intervention.
2. Monitor client's pattern of fluid intake and urination (e.g., times and amounts of fluid intake, types of fluids consumed, times and amounts of voluntary and involuntary voiding, reports of sensation of need to void, activities preceding incontinence).	2. Knowledge of the client's fluid intake and urination pattern assists in the identification of factors that may be causing urinary incontinence. This information helps the nurse plan individualized interventions that promote urinary continence.

NURSING ACTIONS	RATIONALES
Assessments	
3. Assist with urodynamic studies (e.g., urethral pressure profile, uroflowmetry, cystometrogram) if ordered.	3. Urodynamic studies may be done to determine the cause(s) of urinary incontinence. The studies provide information about the motor and sensory function of the bladder and urethra.
Prevention/Treatment	
4. Offer bedpan or urinal or assist client to bedside commode or bathroom every 2–4 hours if indicated.	4. Urinary incontinence occurs when the pressure in the bladder becomes greater than the pressure exerted by the urinary sphincters. Emptying the bladder before the pressure becomes too great reduces the risk of incontinence.
5. Allow client to assume a normal position for voiding (usually sitting for females and standing for males) unless contraindicated.	5. A sitting or standing position uses gravity to facilitate bladder emptying. The more completely the bladder is emptied, the less risk there is of incontinence.
6. Implement measures to reduce delays in toileting (e.g., have call signal within client's reach and respond promptly to requests for assistance; have bedpan, urinal, or bedside commode readily available to client; provide easy access to bathroom; provide client with easy-to-remove clothing such as pajamas with Velcro closures or an elastic waistband).	6. If client is having difficulty controlling urination, any delay in toileting increases the risk of incontinence. Measures that enable the client to use a bedpan, urinal, bedside commode, or toilet in a timely manner help reduce the risk of incontinence.
7. Instruct client to perform pelvic floor muscle exercises (e.g., stopping and starting stream during voiding; squeezing buttocks together, then relaxing the muscles) if appropriate.	7. Pelvic floor muscle exercises help strengthen the pelvic floor muscles and improve the tone of the external urinary sphincter. As this is achieved, the risk for incontinence decreases.
8. Instruct client to space fluids evenly throughout the day rather than drinking a large quantity at one time.	8. Drinking a large amount of fluid at one time results in rapid filling of the bladder, which increases pressure in the bladder and the subsequent risk of incontinence.
9. Limit oral fluid intake in the evening.	9. As the client's bladder fills and pressure in the bladder increases during sleep, he/she is less likely to be aware of and/or able to respond to the urge to urinate. By limiting fluid intake in the evening, bladder filling during the night is decreased, which reduces the risk of incontinence.
10. Instruct client to avoid drinking alcohol and beverages containing caffeine such as colas, coffee, and tea.	10. Alcohol and caffeinated beverages increase urine formation because of their mild diuretic effect. With increased urine formation, bladder filling increases, causing a rise in pressure in the bladder, which subsequently increases the risk of incontinence. Alcohol and caffeine also act as chemical irritants to the bladder and contribute to urge incontinence.
11. Administer the following medications if ordered:	11.
a. cholinergic (parasympathomimetic) agents (e.g., bethanechol)	a. If incontinence results from incomplete bladder emptying, cholinergic (parasympathomimetic) drugs may be prescribed to stimulate contraction of the detrusor muscle (smooth muscle of the bladder). This enhances bladder emptying and reduces the risk of incontinence.
b. anticholinergics (e.g., tolterodine, oxybutynin).	b. Hyperactivity of the bladder detrusor muscle can cause a sudden increase in pressure in the bladder and result in incontinence, especially if there is decreased bladder outlet resistance. Anticholinergics may be prescribed to reduce bladder detrusor muscle activity and thereby reduce the risk of incontinence.
12. Consult appropriate health care provider if urinary incontinence persists.	12. Notifying the appropriate health care provider allows for modification of treatment plan.

Nursing Diagnosis: Urinary Retention

Definition
Incomplete emptying of the bladder

Defining Characteristics
Bladder distention; small, frequent voiding or absence of urine output; sensation of bladder fullness; dysuria; dribbling of urine; residual urine; overflow incontinence

Related Factors
High urethral pressure caused by weak detrusor; inhibition of reflex arc; strong urinary sphincter; blockage of urine

Desired Outcome
The client will not experience urinary retention as evidenced by:
a. voiding at normal intervals
b. no reports of bladder fullness and suprapubic discomfort
c. absence of bladder distention and dribbling of urine
d. balanced intake and output.

Documentation
a. Frequency of urination and amount voided each time
b. Reports of bladder fullness and/or suprapubic discomfort
c. Bladder distention
d. Evidence or statements of dribbling of urine
e. Patency of urinary catheter if present
f. Intake and output
g. Therapeutic interventions
h. Client teaching

Suggested NIC Intervention: Urinary retention care

NURSING ACTIONS	RATIONALES
Assessments	
1. Assess for signs and symptoms of urinary retention: a. frequent voiding of small amounts (25–60 ml) of urine b. reports of bladder fullness or suprapubic discomfort c. bladder distention d. dribbling of urine e. output less than intake.	1. Early recognition of signs and symptoms of urinary retention allows for prompt intervention.
2. Assist with urodynamic studies (e.g., urethral pressure profile, uroflowmetry, cystometry) if ordered.	2. Urodynamic studies may be indicated when neurogenic dysfunction is the suspected cause of urinary retention. The studies provide information about the motor and sensory function of the bladder and urethra.
Prevention/Treatment	
3. Instruct client to urinate when the urge is first felt.	3. If the client feels the urge to urinate but suppresses it by contracting the external urinary sphincter, the urge will subside and not recur until the bladder fills more. If the client repeatedly suppresses the urge to urinate and the bladder fills too much or is chronically distended, the micturition reflex becomes less sensitive and does not effectively stimulate urination when the bladder fills.
4. Implement measures to promote relaxation during voiding attempts (e.g., provide privacy, hold a warm blanket against abdomen, administer prescribed analgesic if client is painful, encourage client to read).	4. If the client is relaxed when trying to urinate, he/she is better able to relax the pelvic floor muscles and external urinary sphincter and allow voiding to occur.
5. If client is having difficulty voiding, run water, place his/her hands in warm water, and/or pour warm water over perineum unless contraindicated.	5. These measures have been found to trigger the micturition reflex and thereby promote voiding. They also promote a sense of relaxation, which facilitates voiding.

NURSING ACTIONS	RATIONALES
Prevention/Treatment	
6. Allow client to assume a normal position for voiding (usually sitting for females and standing for males) unless contraindicated.	6. A sitting or standing position uses gravity to facilitate bladder emptying. Allowing the client to assume a normal voiding position also promotes relaxation, which facilitates voiding.
7. Instruct client to lean upper body forward and/or gently press downward on the lower abdomen when attempting to void unless contraindicated.	7. Leaning forward or gently pressing downward on the lower abdomen increases pressure on the bladder. This pressure helps create a sensation of bladder fullness, which stimulates the micturition reflex.
8. Administer cholinergic (parasympathomimetic) drugs (e.g., bethanechol) if ordered.	8. Cholinergic (parasympathomimetic) drugs promote urination by stimulating contraction of the bladder detrusor muscle.
9. If an indwelling urinary catheter is present, implement measures to ensure its patency (e.g., keep tubing free of kinks, keep collection bag below bladder level, irrigate catheter if indicated).	9. Maintaining patency of the indwelling catheter prevents urinary retention.
10. Consult appropriate health care provider if signs and symptoms of urinary retention persist.	10. Notifying the appropriate health care provider allows for modification of treatment plan.

UNIT III

Nursing Care of the Elderly Client

The Elderly Client

Persons who are 65 and older are the fastest growing segment of the population, making the elderly a major portion of the health care consumer population. Older persons are in the final stage of development during which many adaptations need to be made by the client because of the physiological changes that occur with aging. The extent or degree of the changes that take place depends on genetic and environmental factors as well as on the client's previous attention to health maintenance. As a client reaches old age, there may also be many changes in roles, relationships, and ability to maintain his/her usual lifestyle. These factors create psychosocial concerns that need to be addressed.

This care plan focuses on the elderly client needing health care. It includes the nursing diagnoses that reflect the biopsychosocial changes that commonly occur with old age and are intensified with the stressors of illness. **This care plan can be used in conjunction with the care plans in this text that are appropriate to the client's specific medical diagnosis(es) or surgery and is intended for use in an acute or extended care facility or in a home setting.**

NURSING DIAGNOSES

See p. 94 for additional diagnoses.

1. Nursing Diagnosis: INEFFECTIVE TISSUE PERFUSION

related to:
a. decreased cardiac output associated with:
   1. impaired relaxation and contractility of the heart associated with stiffening of the ventricular walls
   2. increased cardiac workload resulting from an increase in vascular resistance, thickened and rigid cardiac valves, and stress of current illness;
b. increased vascular resistance associated with decreased elasticity and increased rigidity of the arterial vessels associated with changes in the proportion of elastin and collagen in the vessel walls and accumulation of substances such as calcium and lipids;
c. decrease in baroreceptor sensitivity;
d. peripheral pooling of blood associated with loss of muscle tone in extremities, decreased competency of venous valves, and venous dilation (results from loss of vascular elasticity).

Suggested NOC Outcomes: Circulation status; Cardiac pump effectiveness

Suggested NIC Interventions: Circulatory care: arterial insufficiency; Circulatory care: venous insufficiency; Cardiac precautions

Desired Outcome

1. The client will maintain adequate tissue perfusion as evidenced by:
   a. B/P within normal range for client
   b. usual mental status
   c. absence of dizziness or lightheadedness and syncope
   d. extremities warm with absence of pallor and cyanosis
   e. palpable peripheral pulses
   f. capillary refill time less than 2–3 seconds
   g. absence of edema
   h. BUN and serum creatinine within normal limits for an elderly client
   i. urine output at least 30 ml/hour
   j. absence of exercise-induced pain.

Nursing Actions *and Selected Purposes/Rationales*

(see pp. 57–59 for additional rationales)

1.a. Assess for and report signs and symptoms of:
   1. decreased cardiac output (can lead to diminished tissue perfusion):
      a. variations in B/P (may be increased because of compensatory vasoconstriction; may be decreased when compensatory mechanisms and pump fail)
      b. irregular, rapid, or slow pulse (the incidence of dysrhythmias increases with age and is of concern *because of the coexisting decrease in cardiac reserve*)
      c. increase in loudness of existing systolic murmurs or presence of diastolic murmur (soft systolic murmurs are often present in elderly clients *because of sclerosed valves*)
      d. development of or an increase in loudness of S_3 and/or S_4 gallop rhythm (an S_4 can be present in a healthy elderly client)
      e. development of or increase in fatigue and weakness
      f. development of or increase in dyspnea
      g. new finding of or increased crackles (crackles in the morning are a common finding in an elderly client)
      h. edema
      i. jugular vein distention (JVD)
      j. abnormal ECG readings (expected age-related changes include left axis deviation and some prolongation of the PR and QT intervals)
      k. chest x-ray results showing pleural effusion or pulmonary edema
   2. diminished tissue perfusion:
      a. significant decrease in B/P (elevated systolic blood pressure is often present in elderly clients *because of the age-related stiffening of the arteries and impaired baroreceptor function*)
      b. decline in systolic B/P of greater than 20 mm Hg when client changes from a lying to sitting or standing position (in an elderly client, there is often a decline in systolic B/P of 15–20 mm Hg with this position change *because of a decrease in baroreceptor sensitivity and vasomotor responsiveness*)
      c. restlessness, confusion, or other change in mental status
      d. reports of dizziness or lightheadedness or occurrence of syncopal episodes

e. cool, pale, or cyanotic skin
f. diminished or absent peripheral pulses
g. capillary refill time greater than 2–3 seconds
h. edema
i. elevated BUN and serum creatinine (BUN and serum creatinine tend to be slightly elevated *because of the age-related decline in renal function*)
j. oliguria
k. claudication
l. angina.

b. Implement measures *to maintain adequate tissue perfusion:*
   1. perform actions *to reduce cardiac workload and help maintain an adequate cardiac output*
      a. place client in a semi- to high Fowler's position whenever possible
      b. instruct client to avoid activities that create a Valsalva response (e.g., straining to have a bowel movement, holding breath while moving up in bed)
      c. implement measures to promote rest and conserve energy (see Diagnosis 9, action b.1).
      d. implement measures to maintain an adequate respiratory status (see Diagnosis 2, action b) *in order to promote adequate tissue oxygenation*
      e. discourage smoking (*nicotine has a cardiostimulatory effect and causes vasoconstriction; the carbon monoxide in smoke reduces oxygen availability*)
      f. discourage excessive intake of beverages high in caffeine such as coffee, tea, and colas (*caffeine is a myocardial stimulant and can increase myocardial oxygen consumption*)
      g. provide small meals rather than large ones (*large meals can increase cardiac workload because they require an increase in blood supply to the gastrointestinal tract to aid digestion*)
      h. increase activity gradually as allowed and tolerated
   2. maintain a fluid intake of 1500–2000 ml/day unless contraindicated; if oral intake is inadequate or contraindicated, maintain intravenous and/or enteral fluid therapy as ordered (be alert to the greater risk for fluid overload in the elderly client *because of the age-related decline in the kidney's ability to excrete large volumes of water in response to sudden volume excess*)
   3. perform actions *to reduce peripheral pooling of blood and increase venous return:*
      a. instruct client in and assist with active foot and leg exercises every 1–2 hours during periods of decreased activity
      b. consult physician about an order for antiembolism stockings
      c. encourage and assist client with ambulation as allowed and tolerated
   4. instruct and assist client to change from a supine to an upright position slowly *in order to allow time for autoregulatory mechanisms to adjust to the change in the distribution of blood associated with an upright position*
   5. discourage positions that compromise blood flow in lower extremities (e.g., crossing legs, pillow under knees, use of knee gatch, sitting for long periods, prolonged standing)
   6. maintain a comfortable room temperature and provide client with adequate clothing and blankets (*exposure to cold causes generalized vasoconstriction*).

c. Consult appropriate health care provider if signs and symptoms of diminished tissue perfusion persist or worsen.

2. NURSING DIAGNOSIS: IMPAIRED RESPIRATORY FUNCTION*

a. ineffective breathing pattern related to:
   1. loss of alveolar elasticity (results in reduced efficiency of air expulsion)
   2. decreased chest expansion associated with calcification of costal cartilage and weakened respiratory muscles

*This diagnostic label includes the following nursing diagnoses: ineffective breathing pattern, ineffective airway clearance, and impaired gas exchange.

3. decreased responsiveness of chemoreceptors to hypoxia and hypercapnia;

b. ineffective airway clearance related to stasis of secretions associated with decreased activity during illness and an age-related decrease in ciliary activity and cough effectiveness;

c. impaired gas exchange related to:
   1. loss of effective lung surface associated with a reduced number of alveoli, changes in the alveolar walls, and accumulation of secretions in the bronchioles and alveoli (can result from ineffective airway clearance)
   2. reduced airflow associated with loss of alveolar elasticity, restricted chest expansion, and premature closure of small airways
   3. decreased pulmonary blood flow associated with a decrease in the number of capillaries surrounding the alveoli, fibrosis of the pulmonary vessels, and a generalized decrease in tissue perfusion.

Suggested NOC Outcomes: Respiratory status: ventilation; Respiratory status: airway patency; Respiratory status: gas exchange

Suggested NIC Interventions: Respiratory monitoring; Airway management; Chest physiotherapy; Oxygen therapy; Cough enhancement

Desired Outcome

2. The client will experience adequate respiratory function as evidenced by:
   a. normal rate and depth of respirations
   b. absence of dyspnea
   c. symmetrical chest excursion
   d. usual or improved breath sounds
   e. usual mental status
   f. oximetry results within normal range for an elderly client
   g. blood gases within normal range for an elderly client.

Nursing Actions *and Selected Purposes/Rationales*

(see pp. 12–14, 18–20, and 33–35 for additional rationales)

2.a. Assess for and report signs and symptoms of impaired respiratory function:
   1. rapid, shallow, or slow respirations
   2. dyspnea, orthopnea
   3. use of accessory muscles when breathing
   4. asymmetrical chest excursion
   5. adventitious breath sounds (e.g., crackles [rales], rhonchi); crackles may be heard, especially on initial morning assessment, *as a result of some alveolar collapse associated with age-related hypoventilation and decreased activity*
   6. diminished or absent breath sounds (diminished sounds are often present in the elderly client *because of reduced airflow*)
   7. cough
   8. restlessness, irritability
   9. confusion, somnolence
   10. abnormal blood gases (Pao_2 is normally lower in the elderly client)
   11. significant decrease in oximetry results (oxygen saturation is normally lower in the elderly client)
   12. abnormal chest x-ray results.

b. Implement measures *to maintain an adequate respiratory status:*
   1. place client in a semi- to high Fowler's position unless contraindicated; position with pillows *to prevent slumping*
   2. if client must remain flat in bed, assist with position change at least every 2 hours
   3. instruct client to deep breathe or use incentive spirometer every 1–2 hours
   4. perform actions to decrease pain if present (e.g., splint/protect painful area during movement, administer prescribed analgesics before planned activity) *in order to increase client's willingness to move, cough, and deep breathe*
   5. perform actions to decrease fear and anxiety (e.g., explain procedures, provide a calm environment) *in order to prevent the shallow and/or rapid breathing that can occur with fear and anxiety*
   6. instruct client in and assist with diaphragmatic and pursed-lip breathing techniques if indicated

7. perform actions *to promote the removal of pulmonary secretions:*
   a. instruct and assist client to cough or "huff" every 1–2 hours
   b. implement measures *to thin tenacious secretions and reduce dryness of the respiratory mucous membrane:*
      1. maintain a fluid intake of 1500–2000 ml/day unless contraindicated
      2. humidify inspired air if ordered
   c. if client has difficulty mobilizing secretions:
      1. assist with or perform postural drainage therapy (PDT) if ordered
      2. consult physician about use of a mucolytic (e.g., acetylcysteine) or diluent or hydrating agent (e.g., water, saline) via nebulizer
      3. suction as needed
8. assist with positive airway pressure techniques (e.g., continuous positive airway pressure [CPAP], bilevel positive airway pressure [BiPAP], flutter/positive expiratory pressure [PEP] device) if ordered
9. discourage smoking *(the irritants in smoke increase mucus production, further impair ciliary function, and can damage the bronchial and alveolar walls; the carbon monoxide decreases oxygen availability)*
10. maintain oxygen therapy if ordered
11. instruct client to avoid intake of gas-forming foods (e.g., beans, cabbage, cauliflower, onions), carbonated beverages, and large meals *in order to prevent gastric distention and pressure on the diaphragm*
12. maintain activity restrictions as ordered; increase activity gradually as allowed and tolerated
13. administer central nervous system depressants judiciously *because of their respiratory depressant effect* (the possibility of respiratory depression is increased in elderly clients *because of their altered metabolism, distribution, and excretion of drugs and decreased responsiveness of chemoreceptors to hypoxia and hypercapnia);* hold medication and consult physician if respiratory rate is less than 12/minute.

c. Consult appropriate health care provider (e.g., physician, respiratory therapist) if signs and symptoms of impaired respiratory function persist or worsen.

3. NURSING DIAGNOSIS: *RISK FOR DEFICIENT FLUID VOLUME*

related to:
a. age-related decrease in total body water;
b. decreased fluid intake associated with:
   1. restrictions imposed by current illness and/or treatment plan
   2. diminished thirst sensation
   3. desire to avoid nocturia and/or urinary incontinence;
c. age-related decline in kidney's ability to conserve water when a deficit is caused by disease or environmental factors.

Suggested NOC Outcome: Fluid balance

Suggested NIC Interventions: Fluid monitoring; Fluid management; Hypovolemia management; Intravenous (IV) therapy

Desired Outcome	**Nursing Actions** *and Selected Purposes/Rationales* (see pp. 30–31 for additional rationales)
3. The client will not experience deficient fluid volume as evidenced by: a. normal skin and tongue turgor for client b. moist mucous membranes c. stable weight	3.a. Assess for and report signs and symptoms of deficient fluid volume: 1. decreased skin turgor (not always a reliable indicator *because decreased skin turgor is a normal age-related change;* turgor is best assessed over the forehead or sternum in an elderly client) 2. decreased tongue turgor (the tongue will be smaller than usual and have more than one longitudinal furrow) 3. dry mucous membranes, thirst (may not be reliable indicators *because saliva production and sensation of thirst are diminished in elderly clients)*

Desired Outcome

d. B/P and pulse within normal range for client with no further increase in postural hypotension
e. capillary refill time less than 2–3 seconds
f. BUN and Hct within normal range for age
g. usual mental status
h. balanced intake and output.

Nursing Actions *and Selected Purposes/Rationales*

4. weight loss of 2% or greater over a short period
5. low B/P and/or decline in systolic B/P of greater than 20 mm Hg when client sits up (be aware that a drop of 15–20 mm Hg is not unusual in elderly clients *because of decreased baroreceptor sensitivity and vasomotor responsiveness*)
6. weak, rapid pulse
7. capillary refill time greater than 2–3 seconds
8. neck veins flat when client is supine
9. elevated BUN and Hct
10. change in mental status (e.g., confusion)
11. decreased urine output (reflects an actual rather than potential fluid volume deficit).

b. Implement measures *to prevent deficient fluid volume:*
   1. maintain a fluid intake of 1500–2000 ml/day and instruct client to continue this regimen following discharge unless contraindicated
   2. maintain intravenous and/or enteral fluid therapy if ordered (administer intravenous fluids cautiously *because the elderly client is also at risk for fluid overload*).

4. Nursing Diagnosis: *IMBALANCED NUTRITION: LESS THAN BODY REQUIREMENTS*

related to:

a. decreased oral intake associated with:
   1. anorexia resulting from factors such as depression, loneliness, diminished sense of smell and/or taste, early satiety, and dyspepsia
   2. difficulty chewing and swallowing food resulting from poor dentition, a decreased amount of saliva, and weakened chewing and swallowing muscles
   3. decreased ability to purchase and/or prepare healthy foods;

b. decreased utilization of nutrients associated with impaired digestion resulting from:
   1. decreased ability to chew foods thoroughly
   2. reduced secretion of digestive enzymes (e.g., salivary ptyalin, hydrochloric acid, pepsin, lipase);

c. reduced absorption of nutrients associated with hypochlorhydria, decreased intestinal blood flow, and atrophy of the absorptive surface of the intestine.

Suggested NOC Outcome: Nutritional status

Suggested NIC Interventions: Nutritional monitoring; Appetite; Nutrition management; Nutrition therapy; Nutritional counseling

Desired Outcome

4. The client will maintain an adequate nutritional status as evidenced by:
   a. weight within normal range for client
   b. normal serum albumin, prealbumin, Hct, Hgb, and lymphocyte levels for client's age
   c. usual strength and activity tolerance
   d. healthy oral mucous membrane.

Nursing Actions *and Selected Purposes/Rationales*
(see pp. 40–43 for additional rationales)

4.a. Assess for and report signs and symptoms of malnutrition:
   1. weight significantly below client's usual weight or below normal for client's age, height, and body frame; when using height and weight charts, be aware that weight is expected to decline gradually with age
   2. low serum albumin, prealbumin, Hct, Hgb, and lymphocyte levels
   3. weakness and fatigue
   4. sore, inflamed oral mucous membrane
   5. pale conjunctiva
   6. lower than normal anthropometric measurements such as skinfold thickness, body circumferences (e.g., hip, waist, mid-upper arm), and bioelectrical impedance analysis.

b. Monitor percentage of meals and snacks client consumes. Report a pattern of inadequate intake.

c. Implement measures *to maintain an adequate nutritional status:*
   1. perform actions *to improve oral intake:*
      a. implement measures to relieve dyspepsia, gastric fullness, and gas pain (see Diagnosis 5, action b)

   b. increase activity as allowed and tolerated *(activity usually promotes a sense of well-being, which can improve appetite; it also promotes gastric emptying, which reduces feeling of gastric fullness)*
   c. obtain a dietary consult if necessary to assist client in selecting foods/fluids that meet nutritional needs as well as personal and cultural preferences whenever possible
   d. maintain a clean environment and a relaxed, pleasant atmosphere
   e. implement measures to decrease sense of isolation and aloneness (see Diagnosis 21, action b) *in order to promote a sense of well-being, which can improve appetite*
   f. encourage a rest period before meals if client is weak or fatigues easily *(fatigue can reduce the client's desire and ability to eat)*
   g. provide frequent, small meals rather than large ones if client is weak, fatigues easily, and/or has a poor appetite
   h. provide oral hygiene before meals *(oral hygiene moistens the mouth, which may make it easier to chew and swallow; it also removes unpleasant tastes, which often improves the taste of foods/fluids)*
   i. if client has dentures, assist him/her to put them in before meals; if dentures do not fit properly, obtain a dental consult
   j. serve foods/fluids that are appealing to client (visual appeal is especially important if sense of smell is diminished)
   k. encourage significant others to bring in client's favorite foods unless contraindicated and eat with him/her *to make eating more of a familiar social experience*
   l. provide a soft, ground, or pureed diet if client has difficulty chewing
   m. implement measures *to compensate for taste alterations and/or dislike of prescribed diet:*
      1. serve foods warm *to stimulate sense of smell*
      2. encourage client to experiment with different flavorings and seasonings
      3. instruct client to use salt substitutes and salt-free herbs and spices if he/she is on low-sodium diet
      4. encourage client to add extra sweeteners to foods unless contraindicated
      5. provide alternative sources of protein if meats such as beef or pork taste bitter or rancid
   n. limit fluid intake with meals (unless the fluid has high nutritional value) *to reduce early satiety and subsequent decreased food intake*
   o. allow adequate time for meals; reheat foods/fluids if necessary
2. ensure that meals are well balanced and high in essential nutrients; offer high-protein supplements if client is having difficulty maintaining an adequate caloric intake
3. administer vitamins and minerals if ordered.

d. Perform a calorie count if ordered. Report information to dietitian and physician.
e. Consult physician regarding an alternative method of providing nutrition (e.g., parenteral nutrition, tube feedings) if client does not consume enough food or fluids to meet nutritional needs.
f. If indicated, obtain a social service consult to assist client in arranging for services such as Meals on Wheels and home health aides for feeding assistance at home.

NURSING DIAGNOSIS

ALTERED COMFORT: DYSPEPSIA, GASTRIC FULLNESS, AND/OR GAS PAIN

related to:

a. increased gastroesophageal sensitivity to irritants associated with thinning of the esophageal and gastric mucosa;
b. gastroesophageal reflux associated with decreased tone of the lower esophageal sphincter;
c. impaired digestion of many foods associated with reduced secretion of digestive enzymes (e.g., hydrochloric acid, pepsin, lipase);

d. delayed esophageal and gastric emptying associated with decreased gastroesophageal motility;
e. accumulation of intestinal gas associated with decreased peristalsis.

Suggested NOC Outcome: Comfort level

Suggested NIC Intervention: Flatulence reduction

Desired Outcome	Nursing Actions *and Selected Purposes/Rationales*
5. The client will experience diminished dyspepsia, gastric fullness, and gas pain as evidenced by: a. verbalization of same b. relaxed facial expression and body positioning c. diminished eructation.	5.a. Assess for signs and symptoms of dyspepsia, gastric fullness, or gas pain (e.g., verbal reports of indigestion, fullness, or gas pain; grimacing; clutching and guarding of abdomen; rubbing epigastric area; restlessness; reluctance to move; frequent eructation; reluctance to eat). b. Implement measures *to reduce dyspepsia, gastric fullness, and gas pain:* 1. perform actions *to reduce gastroesophageal reflux:* a. provide small, frequent meals rather than 3 large ones b. instruct client to ingest foods and fluids slowly c. maintain client in high Fowler's position during and for at least 30 minutes after meals and snacks unless contraindicated 2. instruct client to avoid the following foods/fluids: a. those that may irritate the gastroesophageal mucosa (e.g., spicy foods; alcohol; caffeine-containing beverages such as coffee, tea, and colas) b. those that are hard to digest (e.g., fried foods) 3. perform actions *to reduce accumulation of gas and fluid in gastrointestinal tract:* a. encourage and assist client with frequent position changes and ambulation as allowed and tolerated *(activity stimulates peristalsis and expulsion of flatus)* b. instruct client to avoid activities such as gum-chewing and drinking through a straw *in order to reduce air swallowing* c. instruct client to avoid intake of carbonated beverages and gas-producing foods (e.g., cabbage, onions, beans) d. encourage client to eructate and expel flatus whenever the urge is felt 4. encourage client to quit smoking *(smoking increases gastric acid production, alters the tone of the lower esophageal sphincter, and causes air swallowing)* 5. administer the following medications if ordered: a. antacids and cytoprotective agents (e.g., sucralfate, misoprostol) *to protect the gastroesophageal mucosa* b. antiflatulents (e.g., simethicone) *to reduce gas accumulation* c. gastrointestinal stimulants (e.g., metoclopramide) *to promote gastric emptying.* c. Consult appropriate health care provider if signs and symptoms of dyspepsia, gastric fullness, or gas pain persist or worsen.

6. Nursing Diagnosis: DISTURBED SENSORY PERCEPTION

a. visual related to the lens becoming more opaque, losing elasticity, and yellowing; loss of ciliary muscle tone; decreased pupil size; and changes in the cornea, retina, macula, and vitreous humor;
b. auditory related to degenerative changes in the inner ear and eardrum and cerumen accumulation;
c. gustatory related to a diminished sense of smell and atrophy of the taste buds (there is usually only a modest, quality-specific loss of taste in healthy elderly clients);
d. olfactory related to a decreased number of sensory cells in the nasal lining and atrophy of the olfactory bulb at the base of the brain;

e. kinesthetic related to a decrease in vestibular sensitivity and ability to perceive movement;
f. tactile related to a decreased number of sensory receptors in the skin.

Suggested NOC Outcomes: Hearing compensation behavior; Sensory function: cutaneous; Sensory function: hearing; Sensory function: proprioception; Sensory function: taste and smell; Sensory function: vision

Suggested NIC Interventions: Communication enhancement: visual deficit; Communication enhancement: hearing deficit; Environmental management; Peripheral sensation management

Desired Outcome

6. The client will demonstrate adaptation to disturbed sensory perception as evidenced by:
   a. appropriate verbal and nonverbal responses
   b. expected level of participation in self-care activities and treatment plan
   c. safe responses to environmental stimuli.

Nursing Actions *and Selected Purposes/Rationales*

6.a. Assess client for the following:
   1. vision changes (e.g., statements of decreased visual acuity, altered depth perception, inability to adjust to changes in lighting, increased sensitivity to glare, or altered color perception; overreaching or underreaching for objects)
   2. decreased auditory ability (e.g., statements of not being able to hear or understand what others are saying, inappropriate responses to auditory stimuli, irritability, increased volume of speech, not speaking when spoken to, increased volume of radio and television)
   3. altered sense of taste and smell (e.g., statements of same, decreased food intake, heavy use of sugar or seasonings)
   4. diminished kinesthetic sense (e.g., unsteadiness on feet, swaying, lack of coordination)
   5. diminished tactile sensation (e.g., statements of diminished feeling in extremities, holding or touching very hot objects, use of heating pad at higher than expected temperatures).

b. If client's vision is impaired:
   1. ensure that lighting is adequate but not too bright *(elderly persons have increased sensitivity to glare)*
   2. avoid sudden changes in light intensity *(elderly clients often adjust more slowly to changes in lighting)*
   3. reduce the glare from windows by partially closing blinds or curtains
   4. provide a night light *to facilitate adaptation to a darkened environment and improve night vision*
   5. provide large-print reading material if available
   6. keep frequently used items within the visual field *(the visual field narrows with aging)*
   7. encourage client to wear his/her glasses; make sure glasses are clean
   8. provide auditory rather than visual diversionary activities if indicated
   9. inform client of resources available if he/she desires additional information about visual aids (e.g., American Foundation for the Blind)
   10. assist with activities such as filling out menus and reading mail and legal documents as needed.

c. If client's hearing is impaired:
   1. assess auditory canal for excessive cerumen accumulation; if present, consult appropriate health care provider about removal of ear wax
   2. implement measures *to facilitate communication:*
      a. provide adequate lighting in room *so client can read lips and see facial expressions and gestures*
      b. reduce environmental noise
      c. get client's attention (e.g., touch his/her shoulder, stand within visual field) before beginning conversation
      d. remind client to use hearing aid; ensure that it is functioning well, positioned correctly, and free of cerumen

Desired Outcome | **Nursing Actions** *and Selected Purposes/Rationales*

e. face client and stay within 3–6 feet of him/her while speaking
f. avoid chewing gum, eating, and covering mouth while talking to client
g. lower tone of voice, speak slightly louder than usual, and avoid talking rapidly
h. avoid lowering voice at end of sentences
i. use simple sentences
j. articulate clearly but avoid overenunciation of words
k. rephrase sentences if client does not understand what is being said
l. employ related nonverbal cues such as gestures when appropriate
m. use alternative forms of communication (e.g., word cards, paper and pencil, Magic Slate) if indicated
n. respond to client's call signal in person rather than over intercommunication system

3. encourage client to have an audiometric examination if indicated
4. provide client and significant others with information about available resources that can assist with recommendations about hearing aids and assisted listening devices (e.g., amplifiers for the telephone and television, lighted rather than sound-producing smoke alarms).

d. Implement measures to compensate for taste alterations if present (see Diagnosis 4, action c.1.m).
e. Implement measures to prevent burns (see Diagnosis 18, action a.1) if client has diminished tactile sensation.
f. Implement measures to reduce the risk for falls (see Diagnosis 16, action a) if client's vision and/or sense of position or balance seems impaired.
g. Instruct client and significant others in above methods of adapting to disturbed sensory perceptions.
h. Consult appropriate health care provider if disturbed sensory perceptions worsen.

7. Nursing Diagnosis: RISK FOR IMPAIRED SKIN INTEGRITY

related to:
a. increased fragility of the skin associated with decreased nutritional status and age-related dryness, loss of elasticity, and thinning of skin;
b. frequent contact with irritants if urinary incontinence is present;
c. accumulation of waste products and decreased oxygen and nutrient supply to the skin and subcutaneous tissue associated with decreased blood flow to the skin resulting from:
   1. an age-related decrease in dermal vascularity
   2. prolonged pressure on the tissues if mobility is decreased.

Suggested NOC Outcome: Tissue integrity: skin and mucous membrane

Suggested NIC Interventions: Skin surveillance; Positioning; Skin care: topical treatments; Pressure ulcer prevention

Desired Outcome | **Nursing Actions** *and Selected Purposes/Rationales* (see pp. 49–52 for additional rationales)

7. The client will maintain skin integrity as evidenced by:
   a. absence of redness and irritation
   b. no skin breakdown.

7.a. Determine client's risk for skin breakdown using a risk assessment tool (e.g., Norton Scale, Braden Scale, Gosnell Scale).
b. Inspect the skin (especially bony prominences, dependent areas, perineum, and areas of decreased sensation and/or edema) for pallor, redness, and breakdown.
c. Implement measures *to prevent skin breakdown:*
   1. assist client to turn at least every 2 hours (elderly clients may require more frequent position change *because of decreased blood flow to the skin, reduced amounts of protective subcutaneous fat, and a decreased ability to sense pressure and discomfort)*

2. position client properly; use pressure-reducing or pressure-relieving devices (e.g., pillows, gel or foam cushions, alternating pressure mattress, air-fluidized bed) if indicated
3. gently massage around reddened areas at least every 2 hours
4. apply a thin layer of a dry lubricant such as powder or cornstarch to bottom sheet or skin and to opposing skin surfaces (e.g., axillae, beneath breasts) if indicated *to reduce friction*
5. lift and move client carefully using a turn sheet and adequate assistance
6. perform actions to keep client from sliding down in bed (e.g., gatch knees slightly when head of bed is elevated 30° or higher, limit length of time client is in a semi-Fowler's position to 30-minute intervals) *in order to reduce the risk of skin surface abrasion and shearing*
7. instruct or assist client to shift weight at least every 30 minutes
8. keep client's skin clean
9. keep bed linens dry and wrinkle-free
10. thoroughly dry skin after bathing and as often as needed, paying special attention to skin folds and opposing skin surfaces (e.g., axillae, perineum, beneath breasts); pat skin dry rather than rub
11. ensure that external devices such as braces, casts, and restraints are applied properly
12. provide elbow and heel protectors if indicated
13. encourage client to wear socks while in bed *(helps reduce friction on heels)*
14. increase activity as allowed and tolerated
15. perform actions *to reduce dryness of the skin:*
    a. avoid use of harsh soaps and hot water; use a mild soap and tepid water for bathing
    b. apply moisturizing lotion and/or emollient to skin at least once a day
    c. assist client with total bath or shower every other day rather than daily
    d. encourage a fluid intake of 1500–2000 ml/day unless contraindicated
16. perform actions *to prevent skin irritation resulting from urinary incontinence if present:*
    a. implement measures to reduce episodes of urinary incontinence (see Diagnosis 12, action e.2)
    b. assist client to thoroughly cleanse and dry perineal area with soft tissue or cloth after each episode of incontinence; apply a protective ointment or cream
    c. if use of absorbent products such as pads or undergarments is necessary, select those that effectively absorb moisture and keep it away from the skin
17. apply a protective covering such as a hydrocolloid or transparent membrane dressing to areas of the skin susceptible to breakdown (e.g., coccyx, elbows, heels)
18. use caution with application of heat or cold to areas of decreased sensation or circulatory impairment
19. perform actions to maintain an adequate nutritional status (see Diagnosis 4, action c)
20. perform actions to maintain adequate tissue perfusion (see Diagnosis 1, action b) *in order to improve blood flow to the skin.*

d. If skin breakdown occurs:
   1. notify appropriate health care provider (e.g., physician, wound care specialist)
   2. perform care of involved area(s) as ordered or per standard hospital procedure.

IMPAIRED ORAL MUCOUS MEMBRANE

a. dryness related to decreased saliva production associated with a gradual decline in salivary gland activity;

b. irritation and breakdown related to dryness and thinning of the oral mucosa.

Suggested NOC Outcome: Oral hygiene

Suggested NIC Interventions: Oral health maintenance; Oral health restoration; Oral health promotion

Desired Outcome	Nursing Actions *and Selected Purposes/Rationales* (see pp. 43–45 for additional rationales)
8. The client will maintain a moist, intact oral mucous membrane.	8.a. Assess client for dryness, irritation, and breakdown of the oral mucosa. b. Implement measures *to decrease dryness and irritation of the oral mucous membrane:* 1. instruct and assist client to perform oral hygiene as often as needed; avoid products that contain lemon and glycerin and mouthwashes containing alcohol *(these products have a drying and irritating effect on the oral mucous membrane)* 2. instruct and assist client to perform oral hygiene using a soft bristle toothbrush or sponge-tipped swab and to floss teeth gently 3. encourage client to rinse mouth frequently with water 4. lubricate client's lips frequently 5. encourage client to breathe through nose rather than mouth 6. encourage client not to smoke or chew tobacco *(smoking dries the mucosa; tobacco acts as an irritant to the oral mucosa)* 7. encourage a fluid intake of 1500–2000 ml/day unless contraindicated 8. encourage client to chew sugarless gum or suck on sugarless hard candy *in order to stimulate salivation* 9. encourage client to use artificial saliva *to lubricate the mucous membrane* 10. inspect client's dentures; obtain a dental consult if dentures are rough, cracked, or ill-fitting. c. If oral mucosa is irritated or cracked, implement measures *to relieve discomfort and promote healing:* 1. assist client to select soft, bland foods 2. instruct client to avoid foods/fluids that are extremely hot 3. if client has dentures, remove and replace only for meals 4. administer topical anesthetics, oral protective agents, and analgesics if ordered. d. Consult appropriate health care provider if dryness, irritation, breakdown, or discomfort persists.

9. Nursing Diagnosis: RISK FOR ACTIVITY INTOLERANCE

related to:

a. decreased tissue oxygenation associated with diminished functional reserve capacity of the respiratory and cardiac systems during stress/illness;
b. decrease in strength and endurance associated with the loss of muscle mass that occurs with aging;
c. inadequate nutritional status;
d. inadequate rest and sleep associated with age-related changes in sleep pattern and effects of current illness and hospitalization on sleep pattern.

Suggested NOC Outcomes: Activity tolerance; Energy conservation; Self-care: activities of daily living; Self-care status

Suggested NIC Interventions: Energy management; Nutrition management; Sleep enhancement

Desired Outcome	Nursing Actions *and Selected Purposes/Rationales* (see pp. 11–12 for additional rationales)
9. The client will not experience activity intolerance as evidenced by: a. no reports of fatigue and weakness b. ability to perform activities of daily living without exertional dyspnea, chest pain, diaphoresis, dizziness, and a significant change in vital signs.	9.a. Assess for signs and symptoms of activity intolerance: 1. statements of fatigue or weakness 2. exertional dyspnea, chest pain, diaphoresis, or dizziness 3. abnormal heart rate response to activity (e.g., increase in rate of 20 beats/minute above resting rate, rate not returning to preactivity level within 10 minutes after stopping activity, change from regular to irregular rate); be aware that the pulse rate increases only slightly with activity and returns to preactivity level slowly in an elderly client 4. a significant change (15–20 mm Hg) in blood pressure with activity. b. Implement measures *to maintain adequate activity tolerance:* 1. perform actions *to promote rest and/or conserve energy:* a. maintain activity restrictions as ordered b. minimize environmental activity and noise c. organize nursing care to allow for periods of uninterrupted rest d. limit the number of visitors and their length of stay e. assist client with self-care activities as needed f. keep supplies and personal articles within easy reach g. instruct client in energy-saving techniques (e.g., using shower chair when showering, sitting to brush teeth or comb hair) h. implement measures to promote sleep (see Diagnosis 14, action b) 2. perform actions to maintain adequate cardiac output and tissue perfusion (see Diagnosis 1, action b) 3. perform actions to maintain an adequate respiratory status (see Diagnosis 2, action b) 4. perform actions to maintain an adequate nutritional status (see Diagnosis 4, action c) 5. increase client's activity gradually as allowed and tolerated; periods of activity should be short, frequent, and interspersed with rest periods. c. Instruct client to: 1. report a decreased tolerance for activity; caution client that tolerance for vigorous activity may be diminished *because of age-related changes in thermoregulatory mechanisms and sympathetic nervous system responses* 2. stop any activity that causes chest pain, shortness of breath, dizziness, or extreme fatigue or weakness 3. continue with a regular exercise program following discharge to improve activity tolerance. d. Consult physician if signs and symptoms of activity intolerance develop and persist or worsen.

10. Nursing Diagnosis: *IMPAIRED PHYSICAL MOBILITY*

related to:

a. decreased muscle strength associated with the loss of muscle mass that occurs with aging;
b. weakness and fatigue associated with decreased functional reserve capacity of the respiratory and cardiac systems during stress and illness, inadequate nutritional status, and difficulty resting and sleeping;
c. joint aching and stiffness that may be present as a result of degenerative changes in the joints;
d. fear of falling;
e. physical limitations/activity restrictions associated with current diagnosis and/or treatment plan.

Suggested NOC Outcomes: Mobility; Ambulation: balance

Suggested NIC Interventions: Exercise therapy: joint mobility; Exercise therapy: ambulation; Exercise promotion

Desired Outcome	**Nursing Actions** *and Selected Purposes/Rationales*
10. The client will maintain an optimal level of physical mobility within prescribed activity restrictions.	10.a. Implement measures *to maintain an optimal level of physical mobility:* 1. perform actions to maintain adequate strength and activity tolerance (see Diagnosis 9, action b) 2. perform actions to prevent falls (see Diagnosis 16, action a) *in order to reduce client's fear of injury* 3. instruct client in and assist with use of mobility aids (e.g., cane, walker) if indicated 4. instruct client in and assist with range of motion exercises at least 3 times/day unless contraindicated 5. if client complains of joint aching or stiffness: a. encourage him/her to perform mild exercise of affected joint(s) upon awakening in the morning *in order to reduce stiffness* b. consult physician regarding application of heat to affected joint(s) c. administer analgesics (e.g., nonsteroidal anti-inflammatories) if ordered 6. encourage activity and participation in self-care as allowed and tolerated 7. encourage client to continue a regular exercise program following discharge. b. Encourage the support of significant others. Allow them to assist with range of motion exercises, positioning, and activity unless contraindicated. c. Consult appropriate health care provider if client is unable to achieve expected level of mobility or if range of motion becomes more restricted.

11. Nursing Diagnosis:

SELF-CARE DEFICIT

related to:
a. impaired physical mobility;
b. weakness and fatigue;
c. lack of motivation and/or presence of cognitive impairments that result in the elderly client attaching less importance to or forgetting usual grooming and hygiene practices.

Suggested NOC Outcome:
Self-care: activities of daily living

Suggested NIC Intervention: Self-care assistance

Desired Outcome	**Nursing Actions** *and Selected Purposes/Rationales*
11. The client will perform self-care activities within physical limitations and activity restrictions imposed by the treatment plan.	11.a. With client, develop a realistic plan for meeting daily physical needs. b. Implement measures *to facilitate client's ability to perform self-care activities:* 1. schedule care at a time when client is most likely to be able to participate (e.g., after rest periods, not immediately after meals or treatments) 2. keep needed objects within easy reach 3. consult occupational therapist about assistive devices available (e.g., long-handled hairbrush and shoehorn) if indicated 4. allow adequate time for the accomplishment of self-care activities, remembering that elderly clients tend to be slower in reacting to stimuli and in moving 5. perform actions to maintain an optimal level of mobility (see Diagnosis 10, action a) 6. perform actions to maintain adequate strength and activity tolerance (see Diagnosis 9, action b). c. Encourage maximum independence within physical limitations and prescribed activity restrictions. d. Assist the client with activities he/she is unable to perform independently.

e. Inform significant others of client's abilities to perform own care. Explain the importance of encouraging and allowing client to maintain an optimal level of independence and allowing client to complete activities at his/her own pace.

12. NURSING DIAGNOSIS:

IMPAIRED URINARY ELIMINATION

a. frequency and urgency related to incomplete bladder emptying, decrease in bladder capacity, and uninhibited bladder contractions in response to small volumes of urine (bladder detrusor muscle hyperactivity or instability);
b. retention related to:
   1. decrease in bladder muscle tone
   2. obstruction of the bladder outlet by an enlarged prostate or fecal impaction
   3. decreased attention to the urge to urinate
   4. difficulty urinating associated with anxiety about a lack of privacy and possibly having to use a bedpan or urinal
   5. the effect of some medications (e.g., sedatives, narcotic [opioid] analgesics, anticholinergics);
c. incontinence (stress, urge, functional) related to:
   1. decreased tone of the external urinary sphincter and an incompetent bladder outlet (a result of lessening of the urethrovesical junction angle in women) associated with degenerative changes in the urethra and pelvic floor muscles and structural supports of the bladder (occurs more in women as a result of childbearing and estrogen deficiency)
   2. decreased bladder capacity and an increase in uninhibited bladder contractions in response to small volumes of urine (bladder detrusor muscle hyperactivity or instability)
   3. overflow of urine associated with overdistention of the bladder if urinary retention is present
   4. delays in toileting associated with:
      a. inability to get to the toilet in time to urinate resulting from unfamiliar environment and impaired physical mobility
      b. difficulty removing clothing in a timely manner when needing to urinate resulting from reduced manual dexterity.

Suggested NOC Outcomes: Urinary continence; Urinary elimination

Suggested NIC Interventions: Urinary incontinence care; Urinary retention care; Urinary habit training; Urinary bladder training; Pelvic muscle exercise

Desired Outcome	**Nursing Actions** *and Selected Purposes/Rationales* (see pp. 59–62 for additional rationales)
12. The client will maintain or regain optimal urinary elimination as evidenced by: a. voiding at normal intervals b. no reports of urgency, frequency, bladder fullness, and suprapubic discomfort c. absence of bladder distention d. absence of incontinence e. balanced intake and output.	12.a. Assess for signs and symptoms of impaired urinary elimination: 1. frequent voiding of small amounts (25–60 ml) of urine 2. nocturia 3. reports of urgency, frequency, bladder fullness, or suprapubic discomfort 4. bladder distention 5. incontinence 6. output less than intake. b. Monitor client's pattern of fluid intake and urination (e.g., times and amounts of fluid intake, types of fluids consumed, times and amounts of voluntary and involuntary voiding, reports of sensation of need to void, activities preceding incontinence). c. Catheterize client if ordered *to determine the amount of residual urine.* d. Assist with urodynamic studies (e.g., urethral pressure profile, uroflowmetry, cystometrogram) if performed *to determine cause of altered urinary elimination.*

Desired Outcome	Nursing Actions *and Selected Purposes/Rationales*

e. Implement measures *to promote optimal urinary elimination:*
   1. perform actions *to prevent or treat urinary retention:*
      a. offer bedpan or urinal or assist client to bedside commode or bathroom every 2–4 hours if indicated
      b. instruct client to urinate when the urge is first felt
      c. implement measures *to promote relaxation during voiding attempts* (e.g., provide privacy, encourage client to read)
      d. implement measures *that may help trigger the micturition reflex and promote a sense of relaxation during voiding attempts* (e.g., run water, place client's hands in warm water, pour warm water over perineum)
      e. allow client to assume a normal position for voiding unless contraindicated
      f. instruct client to lean upper body forward and/or gently press downward on lower abdomen during voiding attempts unless contraindicated *in order to put pressure on the bladder (pressure helps create a sensation of bladder fullness, which stimulates the micturition reflex)*
      g. implement measures to prevent or treat constipation (see Diagnosis 13, actions c and d) *in order to prevent increased pressure on bladder outlet*
      h. administer parasympathomimetic (cholinergic) drugs (e.g., bethanechol) if ordered *to stimulate bladder contraction*
      i. consult physician about intermittent catheterization or insertion of an indwelling catheter if signs and symptoms of urinary retention persist
   2. perform actions *to prevent or treat urinary incontinence:*
      a. offer bedpan or urinal or assist client to bedside commode or bathroom every 2–4 hours or more frequently depending on the client's usual urinary elimination pattern
      b. allow client to assume a normal position for voiding unless contraindicated *in order to promote complete bladder emptying*
      c. implement measures *to reduce delays in toileting* (e.g., have call signal within client's reach and respond promptly to requests for assistance; have bedpan, urinal, or bedside commode readily available to client; provide easy access to bathroom; provide client with easy-to-remove clothing such as pajamas with Velcro closures or an elastic waistband)
      d. instruct client to perform pelvic floor muscle exercises (e.g., stopping and starting stream during voiding; squeezing buttocks together, then relaxing the muscles) several times a day if appropriate *in order to strengthen pelvic floor muscles and improve tone of the external urinary sphincter;* instruct client to continue these exercises following discharge, emphasizing that it will take several weeks of exercise before improvement may be noted
      e. instruct client to space fluids evenly throughout the day rather than drinking a large quantity at one time *(rapid filling of bladder can result in incontinence if client has decreased urinary sphincter control)*
      f. limit oral fluid intake in the evening *to decrease the possibility of nighttime incontinence*
      g. instruct client to avoid drinking alcohol and beverages containing caffeine *(alcohol and caffeine have a mild diuretic effect and act as irritants to the bladder; both factors may make urinary control more difficult)*
      h. administer the following medications if ordered:
         1. cholinergic (parasympathomimetic) agents (e.g., bethanechol) *to stimulate bladder contractions and promote complete bladder emptying if incontinence is associated with overflow resulting from urinary retention*
         2. estrogen preparations (may be used to treat stress incontinence in postmenopausal women)
         3. anticholinergics (e.g., oxybutynin, tolterodine) *to decrease bladder detrusor muscle hyperactivity and reduce episodes of urge incontinence*

4. sympathomimetic agents (e.g., ephedrine) *to increase urethral sphincter tone and reduce episodes of stress incontinence*

i. if urinary incontinence persists:
   1. utilize biofeedback techniques if appropriate *to assist client to regain control over the pelvic floor muscles and external urinary sphincter*
   2. instruct and assist client with bladder retraining program if appropriate
   3. consult physician regarding intermittent catheterization, insertion of an indwelling catheter, or use of an external collection device (e.g., condom catheter).

13. Nursing Diagnosis: RISK FOR CONSTIPATION

related to:

a. decreased gastrointestinal motility associated with age and exacerbated by decreased activity and anxiety during illness;
b. failure to respond to the urge to defecate associated with dulling of the impulses that sense the signal to defecate, inability to get to the toilet independently, and/or reluctance to use a bedpan or bedside commode;
c. difficulty evacuating stool associated with weakened abdominal muscles and decreased lubrication of stools (a result of diminished intestinal mucus production);
d. decreased intake of fiber and fluids;
e. possible chronic laxative use.

Suggested NOC Outcomes: Bowel elimination; Symptom control

Suggested NIC Intervention: Constipation/Impaction management

Desired Outcome	Nursing Actions *and Selected Purposes/Rationales* (see pp. 24–26 for additional rationales)
13. The client will not experience constipation as evidenced by: a. usual frequency of bowel movements b. passage of soft, formed stool c. absence of abdominal distention and pain, feeling of rectal fullness or pressure, and straining during defecation.	13.a. Assess for signs and symptoms of constipation (e.g., decrease in frequency of bowel movements; passage of hard, formed stools; anorexia; abdominal distention and pain; feeling of fullness or pressure in rectum; straining during defecation). b. Assess bowel sounds. Report a pattern of decreasing bowel sounds. c. Implement measures *to prevent constipation:* 1. encourage client to defecate whenever the urge is felt 2. assist client to toilet or bedside commode or place in high Fowler's position on bedpan for bowel movements unless contraindicated 3. encourage client to relax, provide privacy, and have call signal within reach during attempts to defecate *(measures to promote relaxation enable client to relax the levator ani muscle and external anal sphincter, which facilitates evacuation of stool)* 4. encourage client to establish a regular time for defecation, preferably within an hour after a meal 5. instruct client to increase intake of foods high in fiber (e.g., bran, whole-grain breads and cereals, fresh fruits and vegetables) unless contraindicated 6. instruct client to maintain a minimum fluid intake of 1500–2000 ml/day unless contraindicated 7. encourage client to drink hot liquids (e.g., tea) upon arising in the morning 8. increase activity as allowed and tolerated 9. encourage client to perform isometric abdominal strengthening exercises unless contraindicated 10. perform actions to reduce fear and anxiety (e.g., explain procedures, provide care in a confident manner)

Desired Outcome	Nursing Actions and Selected Purposes/Rationales

11. if client is taking analgesics for pain management, encourage the use of nonnarcotic rather than narcotic (opioid) analgesics when appropriate
12. administer laxatives or cathartics and/or enemas if ordered
13. instruct client to continue with actions to promote regular bowel function following discharge (e.g., maintain a fluid intake of at least 6–8 glasses/day, increase intake of foods high in fiber, participate in regular exercise program).

d. Consult physician about checking for an impaction and digitally removing stool if client has not had a bowel movement in 3 days, if he/she is passing liquid stool, or if other signs and symptoms of constipation are present.
e. Consult appropriate health care provider if signs and symptoms of constipation persist and appear to be an ongoing problem.

14. Nursing Diagnosis: DISTURBED SLEEP PATTERN

related to:
a. fear, anxiety, change in environment if in hospital or extended care facility, and discomfort associated with present illness;
b. age-related nocturia;
c. age-related changes in the stages of sleep resulting in frequent awakenings and less deep restorative sleep.

Suggested NOC Outcome: Sleep

Suggested NIC Intervention: Sleep enhancement

Desired Outcome	Nursing Actions and Selected Purposes/Rationales (see pp. 52–54 for additional rationales)

14. The client will attain optimal amounts of sleep as evidenced by statements of feeling well rested.

14.a. Assess for signs and symptoms of a disturbed sleep pattern (e.g., statements of difficulty falling asleep, frequent awakenings, or not feeling well rested).

b. Implement measures *to promote sleep:*
1. discourage excessive napping during the day unless signs and symptoms of sleep deprivation exist
2. perform actions to reduce fear and anxiety (e.g., explain procedures, provide care in a confident manner)
3. perform actions to reduce dyspepsia, gastric fullness, and gas pain if present (see Diagnosis 5, action b) and discomfort associated with client's diagnosis and treatment
4. inform client of normal changes in sleep pattern that occur with aging *in order to reduce concerns about quantity of sleep necessary to maintain health*
5. encourage participation in relaxing diversional activities during the evening
6. discourage intake of foods and fluids high in caffeine (e.g., chocolate, coffee, tea, colas) in the evening
7. offer client an evening snack that includes milk unless contraindicated *(milk contains L-tryptophan, which is believed to help induce and maintain sleep)*
8. allow client to continue usual sleep practices (e.g., position; time; presleep routines such as reading, watching television, and listening to music) whenever possible
9. satisfy basic needs such as comfort and warmth before sleep
10. instruct client to limit intake of fluids in the evening and urinate just before bedtime *in order to reduce nocturia*

11. encourage client to avoid drinking alcohol in the evening *(alcohol interferes with REM sleep)*
12. encourage client to avoid smoking before bedtime *(nicotine is a stimulant)*
13. review medications that client takes with pharmacist or physician and identify those that can interfere with sleep (e.g., nicotine transdermal systems, theophylline, corticosteroids, diuretics, diphenhydramine or other over-the-counter sleep aids, some antidepressants); if possible, administer medications such as steroids and diuretics early in the day rather than late afternoon or evening and encourage client to continue this schedule for these medications at home
14. reduce environmental distractions (e.g., close door to client's room; use night light rather than overhead light whenever possible; lower volume of paging system; keep staff conversations at a low level and away from client's room; close curtains between clients in a semi-private room or ward; keep beepers and alarms on low volume; have earplugs available for client if needed)
15. administer prescribed sedative-hypnotic only if indicated; administer these agents cautiously *because the metabolism, distribution, and excretion of drugs are often altered in the elderly client;* inform client that over-the-counter sleep aids (e.g., diphenhydramine) can interfere with the quality of sleep and daytime functioning and should not be taken on a regular basis
16. perform actions *to reduce interruptions during sleep (70–100 minutes of uninterrupted sleep is usually needed to complete one sleep cycle):*
    a. restrict visitors
    b. group care (e.g., medications, treatments, physical care, assessments) whenever possible.

c. Consult appropriate health care provider if signs and symptoms of sleep deprivation (e.g., irritability, lethargy, agitation, inability to concentrate) occur and persist or worsen.

15. NURSING DIAGNOSIS: ***RISK FOR INFECTION***

related to:

a. stasis of respiratory secretions associated with decreased activity during illness and age-related decrease in ciliary activity and cough effectiveness;
b. decrease in immunity associated with:
    1. an age-related decline in T-cell and B-cell function and the number of functional macrophages in the skin and alveoli
    2. an inadequate nutritional status (if present);
c. decrease in effectiveness of the body's physical barriers associated with changes in the skin and mucous membranes;
d. urinary stasis associated with decreased activity during illness and the urinary retention that can result from a decrease in bladder muscle tone, the effect of certain medications, an enlarged prostate, and difficulty urinating in a new environment;
e. favorable environment for growth of pathogens in vagina associated with an increase in the pH of vaginal secretions.

Suggested NOC Outcomes: Immune status; Infection severity

Suggested NIC Interventions: Infection protection; Infection control; Incision site care; Tube care; Wound care

Desired Outcome	**Nursing Actions** *and Selected Purposes/Rationales* (see pp. 37–40 for additional rationales)
15. The client will remain free of infection as evidenced by: a. absence of fever and chills b. pulse within normal limits c. normal breath sounds d. cough productive of clear mucus only e. voiding clear urine without reports of burning and increased frequency and urgency f. absence of heat, pain, redness, swelling, and unusual drainage in any area g. usual mental status h. WBC and differential counts within normal range for elderly client i. negative results of cultured specimens.	15.a. Assess for and report signs and symptoms of infection (be aware that some signs and symptoms vary *because of an age-related decline in thermoregulatory, immune, and sympathetic nervous system responses;* some signs and symptoms also vary depending on the site of infection and causative organism): 1. increase in temperature above client's usual level (be aware that normal temperature in the elderly client may be less than 37° C) 2. chills (may not be present in the elderly *because they may have a diminished shivering reflex)* 3. increased pulse (the elderly client may not demonstrate the classic elevation in pulse rate that occurs with infection *because of his/her decreased sympathetic nervous system responses)* 4. abnormal breath sounds 5. cough productive of purulent, green, or rust-colored sputum 6. loss of appetite 7. cloudy urine 8. reports of burning when urinating 9. reports of increased urinary frequency or urgency 10. urinalysis showing a WBC count greater than 5, positive leukocyte esterase or nitrites, or the presence of bacteria 11. heat, pain, redness, swelling, or unusual drainage in any area 12. malaise, lethargy, acute confusion 13. increase in WBC count and/or significant change in differential 14. positive results of cultured specimens (e.g., urine, vaginal drainage, wound drainage, sputum, blood). b. Implement measures *to prevent infection:* 1. maintain a fluid intake of at least 1500–2000 ml/day unless contraindicated 2. use good hand hygiene and encourage client to do the same 3. adhere to the appropriate precautions established to prevent transmission of infection to the client (standard precautions, transmission-based precautions on other clients, neutropenic precautions) 4. use sterile technique during invasive procedures (e.g., urinary catheterizations, venous and arterial punctures, injections, wound care) and dressing changes 5. anchor catheters/tubings (e.g., urinary, intravenous, wound drainage) securely *in order to reduce the risk for trauma to the tissues and the risk for introduction of pathogens associated with in-and-out movement of the tubing* 6. change equipment, tubings, and solutions used for treatments such as intravenous infusions, respiratory care, irrigations, and enteral feedings according to hospital policy 7. change peripheral intravenous line sites according to hospital policy 8. maintain a closed system for drains (e.g., wound, chest tube, urinary catheter) and intravenous infusions whenever possible 9. protect client from others with infections and instruct him/her to continue this after discharge 10. perform actions to maintain an adequate nutritional status (see Diagnosis 4, action c) 11. perform actions to prevent and treat irritation and breakdown of the oral mucous membrane (see Diagnosis 8, actions b and c) 12. instruct and assist client to perform good perineal care routinely and after each bowel movement 13. perform actions to maintain an adequate respiratory status (see Diagnosis 2, action b) *in order to reduce the risk of respiratory tract infection* 14. perform actions to prevent or treat urinary retention (see Diagnosis 12, action e.1) *in order to prevent urinary stasis*

15. perform actions to prevent skin breakdown (see Diagnosis 7, action c)
16. if client has a wound, provide appropriate wound care (e.g., use dressing materials that maintain a moist wound surface, assist with debridement of necrotic tissue, use dressing materials that absorb excess exudate, maintain patency of wound drains) *to facilitate wound healing and reduce the number of pathogens that enter or are present in the wound*
17. perform actions *to reduce stress* (e.g., reduce fear, anxiety, and pain; help client identify and use effective coping mechanisms) *in order to prevent an increase in cortisol secretion (cortisol interferes with some immune responses)*
18. instruct client to receive vaccinations (e.g., pneumococcal pneumonia, tetanus, influenza) at recommended intervals if appropriate
19. consult appropriate health care provider regarding:
    a. initiation of antimicrobial therapy if indicated
    b. antimicrobial orders that do not seem appropriate (e.g., prolonged use of antimicrobials, excessively high doses of an antimicrobial, unnecessary use of broad-spectrum or multiple antimicrobials) *in order to reduce the risk of elimination of the client's natural flora and/or the development of drug-resistant microorganisms.*

16. NURSING DIAGNOSIS: ***RISK FOR FALLS***

related to:

a. dizziness or syncope associated with decreased cerebral tissue perfusion that can result from certain medications (e.g., antihypertensive agents) and from age-related vascular changes, decrease in cardiac output, and postural hypotension;
b. loss of balance associated with the effect of certain medications (e.g., sedatives, narcotic [opioid] analgesics) and the changes in posture, reduced coordination, delayed reaction time, and impaired proprioception that can occur with aging;
c. tripping associated with age-related gait abnormalities (e.g., decreased step height and length) and impaired vision;
d. weakness associated with an age-related decrease in muscle strength and the general deconditioning that can occur with reduced physical activity.

Suggested NOC Outcomes: Fall prevention behavior; Knowledge: fall prevention

Suggested NIC Interventions: Fall prevention; Environmental management: safety

Desired Outcome	**Nursing Actions** *and Selected Purposes/Rationales*
16. The client will not experience falls.	16.a. Implement measures *to reduce the risk for falls:* 1. keep bed in low position with side rails up when client is in bed 2. keep needed items within easy reach and assist client to identify their location 3. encourage client to request assistance whenever needed; have call signal within easy reach 4. use lap belt when client is in chair if indicated 5. instruct client to wear well-fitting slippers/shoes with nonslip soles and low heels when ambulating 6. keep floor free of clutter and wipe up spills promptly 7. instruct and assist client to get out of bed slowly *in order to reduce dizziness associated with postural hypotension* 8. carefully position tubings and equipment so that they will not interfere with ambulation 9. accompany client during ambulation and use a transfer safety belt if he/she is weak or dizzy 10. provide ambulatory aids (e.g., walker, cane) if client is weak or unsteady on feet

Desired Outcome	Nursing Actions *and Selected Purposes/Rationales*

11. reinforce instructions from physical therapist on correct ambulation and transfer techniques
12. if vision is impaired, orient client to surroundings, room, and arrangement of furniture and identify obstacles during ambulation
13. instruct client to move slowly, use wider stance when ambulating, and avoid rapidly turning head or body *in order to prevent loss of balance*
14. instruct client to ambulate in well-lit areas and to use handrails if needed
15. do not rush client; allow adequate time for ambulation to the bathroom and in hallway
16. make sure that shower has a nonslip bottom surface and that shower chair, secure bath mat, call signal, grab bars, and adequate lighting are present
17. implement measures to maintain adequate strength and activity tolerance (see Diagnosis 9, action b) and an optimal level of physical mobility (see Diagnosis 10, action a)
18. if client is at high risk for falls and gets up without assistance despite reminders to request assistance:
    a. attach an alarm device to bed or chair
    b. consult physician about the temporary use of jacket or wrist restraints
19. administer central nervous system depressants judiciously.

b. Include client and significant others in planning and implementing measures to prevent falls. Discuss:
   1. the need to evaluate living environment for hazards (e.g., thick or loose carpets, inadequate or loose railings, insufficient lighting) and make necessary modifications
   2. the importance of participating in a regular exercise program for conditioning and muscle strengthening and continuing with therapy for gait and balance training if needed
   3. the importance of continuing appropriate safety precautions after discharge.

c. If falls occur, initiate appropriate first aid and notify physician.

17. Nursing Diagnosis: RISK FOR ASPIRATION

related to a diminished gag reflex and the gastroesophageal reflux that can occur as a result of decreased tone of the lower esophageal sphincter.

Suggested NOC Outcome: Aspiration prevention

Suggested NIC Intervention: Aspiration precautions

Desired Outcome	Nursing Actions *and Selected Purposes/Rationales*

Desired Outcome

17. The client will not aspirate secretions or foods/fluids as evidenced by:
    a. clear breath sounds
    b. resonant percussion note over lungs
    c. absence of cough, tachypnea, and dyspnea.

Nursing Actions

17.a. Assess for and report signs and symptoms of aspiration of secretions or foods/fluids (e.g., rhonchi, dull percussion note over affected lung area, cough, tachypnea, dyspnea, tachycardia, presence of tube feeding in tracheal aspirate, chest x-ray results showing pulmonary infiltrate).

b. Implement measures *to reduce the risk for aspiration:*
   1. perform actions to reduce gastroesophageal reflux (see Diagnosis 5, action b.1)
   2. instruct client to avoid laughing and talking while eating and drinking
   3. encourage client to concentrate on eating and drinking and allow ample time for meals and snacks
   4. instruct and assist client to perform oral hygiene after meals *to ensure that food particles do not remain in mouth*
   5. if client is receiving tube feedings, check tube placement before each feeding or on a routine basis if tube feeding is continuous, and do not administer tube feeding if the residual exceeds specified amount (usually 75–100 ml).

c. If signs and symptoms of aspiration occur:
   1. perform tracheal suctioning
   2. withhold oral intake
   3. prepare client for chest x-ray.

18. NURSING DIAGNOSIS: RISK FOR INJURY

a. burns related to age-related decrease in tactile sensation;
b. pathologic fractures related to osteoporosis associated with an imbalance between bone resorption and bone formation resulting from decreased estrogen levels in women, calcium deficiency (results from decreased dietary intake and decreased absorption due to vitamin D deficiency), and decreased activity;
c. drug toxicity related to:
   1. an increase in cell receptor sensitivity to some drugs
   2. changes in the usual distribution of drugs associated with factors such as a decrease in total body water, a decrease in lean body mass, an increase in total body fat, and a decrease in serum albumin
   3. impaired metabolism and excretion of drugs associated with diminished liver and kidney function
   4. synergistic effect that occurs with some combinations of medications (elderly clients are often taking a number of medications).

Suggested NOC Outcomes:
Knowledge: personal safety;
Knowledge: medication

Suggested NIC Interventions: Environmental management: safety; Medication management

Desired Outcomes	Nursing Actions *and Selected Purposes/Rationales*
18.a. The client will not experience burns.	18.a.1. Implement measures *to prevent burns:* a. let hot foods and fluids cool slightly before serving b. supervise client while smoking if indicated c. assess temperature of bath water and direct heat application (e.g., heating pad, warm compress) before and during use. 2. If burns occur, initiate appropriate first aid and notify physician.
18.b. The client will not experience pathologic fractures as evidenced by: 1. usual mobility and range of motion 2. absence of unusual motion, abnormal joint position, and obvious deformity of any body part 3. absence of pain and swelling over skeletal structures 4. x-ray reports showing absence of fractures.	18.b.1. Assess for and report signs and symptoms of pathologic fractures (e.g., decrease in mobility or range of motion, motion at site where motion does not usually occur, abnormal joint position or obvious deformity, pain or swelling over skeletal structures, x-ray reports showing pathologic fracture). 2. Implement measures *to prevent pathologic fractures:* a. move client carefully; obtain adequate assistance as needed b. when turning client, logroll and support all extremities c. use smooth movements when moving client; avoid pulling or pushing on body parts d. correctly apply back brace or corset if ordered e. perform actions to prevent falls (see Diagnosis 16, action a) f. perform actions *to prevent or delay bone demineralization:* 1. assist client to maintain maximum mobility *(weight bearing reduces bone breakdown)* 2. consult physician about use of a tilt table to facilitate weight bearing if client is immobile 3. administer calcium preparations, vitamin D, and medications that inhibit bone resorption (e.g., calcitonin, alendronate) if ordered 4. discourage smoking and excessive caffeine and alcohol intake 5. encourage client to consume a diet that has adequate amounts of protein, vitamins, and calcium 6. emphasize need for client to follow a regular exercise program after discharge.

Desired Outcomes	Nursing Actions *and Selected Purposes/Rationales*

3. If fractures occur:
   a. maintain activity restrictions if ordered
   b. apply external stabilization device (e.g., cervical collar, brace, splint, sling) if ordered
   c. prepare client for surgery (e.g., internal fixation) if planned
   d. administer analgesics and/or muscle relaxants if ordered *to control pain.*

18.c. The client will not develop drug toxicity as evidenced by absence of signs and symptoms commonly associated with drug toxicity such as:
1. ataxia, agitation, confusion, and blurred vision
2. anorexia, nausea, vomiting, and diarrhea
3. dizziness, dysrhythmias, and postural hypotension
4. dyspnea and stridor
5. rash and urticaria
6. elevated BUN, creatinine, and transaminase levels.

18.c.1. Assess client for signs and symptoms that might be indicative of drug toxicity (e.g., ataxia, agitation, confusion, blurred vision, anorexia, nausea, vomiting, diarrhea, dizziness, dysrhythmias, postural hypotension, dyspnea, stridor, rash, urticaria, elevated BUN and creatinine, elevated transaminase levels). Be aware that the signs and symptoms will vary depending on drugs being taken.

2. Implement measures *to prevent drug toxicity:*
   a. consult appropriate resource (e.g., pharmacist, physician, drug book, geriatrician) for:
      1. information about possible drug interactions of the medications client is taking
      2. appropriate dosages of medications for elderly clients (the smallest effective dose of a medication should be ordered for elderly persons *to reduce the risk of adverse effects*)
      3. schedule for and order of administration of medications *(the absorption, distribution, metabolism, and excretion of many medications may be altered by other medications as well as the age-related changes in body function and the client's current illness)*
   b. administer central nervous system depressants judiciously
   c. inform client of common adverse effects of drugs being taken and ways to avoid toxicity; encourage him/her to report adverse effects or any other unusual symptoms immediately
   d. obtain baseline vital signs and results of laboratory studies indicative of renal and hepatic function *to facilitate assessment of the effects of medications on these systems*
   e. monitor blood levels (e.g., peak, trough) of drugs as ordered and report results to physician; be aware that the elderly client may experience toxic effects when drug levels are within the "normal" therapeutic range
   f. prior to discharge:
      1. provide client and family members with clear, simple, written instructions for taking medications prescribed; include drug name, dose, schedule, route of administration, special precautions such as incompatible foods or drugs, and adverse reactions to observe for
      2. assist client to set up a system for remembering to take medication as prescribed (e.g., divided pill container, use of timer)
      3. emphasize the importance of taking only those medications that are prescribed, following the directions carefully, and keeping the physician informed of adverse effects experienced
      4. provide client with a written schedule for any laboratory tests that are to be done to monitor the therapeutic effect or side effects of medications being taken
      5. encourage client to get all of medications from one pharmacy and to provide them with a complete medical history and list of medications being taken.

3. If signs and symptoms of drug toxicity occur, withhold dose and notify appropriate health care provider (e.g., physician, practitioner, pharmacist).

19. NURSING DIAGNOSIS: *INEFFECTIVE SEXUALITY PATTERNS*

related to:
a. fear of rejection associated with feelings of loss of physical attractiveness;
b. inadequate opportunities for sexual expression associated with lack of available partner;
c. misconceptions about sexual functioning in old age;
d. fear of urinary incontinence;
e. dyspareunia associated with vaginal changes (e.g., decreased vaginal lubrication, thinning and loss of elasticity of the vaginal wall, shortening and narrowing of the vagina) resulting from decreased estrogen levels;
f. embarrassment associated with possible impotence (erections are usually less intense and slower in the elderly male and may be further affected by certain disease processes [e.g., diabetes, vascular disorders, chronic renal failure] and medications [e.g., thiazide diuretics, tricyclic antidepressants, certain antihypertensive agents]).

Suggested NOC Outcomes: Psychosocial adjustment: life change; Sexual identity

Suggested NIC Interventions: Body image enhancement; Sexual counseling

Desired Outcome

19. The client will demonstrate beginning adaptation to changes in sexuality patterns as evidenced by:
    a. verbalization of a perception of self as sexually acceptable and adequate
    b. statements reflecting ways to adjust to effects of aging on sexual functioning.

Nursing Actions *and Selected Purposes/Rationales*

19.a. Assess for symptoms of altered sexuality patterns (e.g., verbalization of sexual concerns, limitations, or difficulties; reports of changes in sexual activities or behaviors).

b. Determine client's perception of desired sexuality, usual pattern of sexual expression, recent changes in sexuality patterns, and knowledge of age-related changes in sexual functioning. Be aware that the client may be reluctant to express concerns *because of the common stereotype that elderly are not sexually active.*

c. Implement measures *to promote an optimal sexuality pattern:*
   1. inform client of age-related changes in sexual functioning (e.g., sexual responses are slower and less intense, vaginal secretions are diminished, erections take longer to achieve, seminal fluid volume is reduced, erection is rapidly lost after orgasm, refractory time between orgasms is longer); encourage questions and clarify misconceptions
   2. facilitate communication between client and partner; focus on feelings shared by the couple and assist them to identify changes that may affect their sexual relationship
   3. discuss ways to be creative in expressing sexuality (e.g., massage, fantasies, cuddling)
   4. arrange for uninterrupted privacy if desired by couple
   5. perform actions to improve client's self-concept (see Diagnosis 20, actions c–p)
   6. if dyspareunia is a problem:
      a. encourage female client to use a water-soluble lubricant before sexual intercourse *to reduce vaginal dryness*
      b. suggest experimentation with different positions during intercourse *to reduce the depth of penetration*
      c. administer estrogen if ordered or provide client with information about estrogen therapy as a way *to reduce vaginal dryness and thinning of vaginal epithelium*
   7. if impotence is a problem:
      a. encourage client to discuss it with physician *(impotence may be due to reversible factors such as medication therapy, alcohol, or poorly controlled chronic disease conditions)*
      b. assure client that occasional episodes of impotence are normal
      c. suggest alternative methods of sexual gratification if appropriate

Desired Outcome	Nursing Actions *and Selected Purposes/Rationales*

d. encourage client to discuss various treatment options (e.g., penile prosthesis, sildenafil, vardenafil, intraurethral alprostadil pellet placement, external vacuum device) with physician if appropriate
8. reinforce the importance of rest before sexual activity
9. if incontinence of urine is a problem, encourage client to void just before intercourse and other sexual activity
10. include partner in above discussions and encourage continued support of the client.

d. Consult appropriate health care provider if counseling appears indicated.

20. Nursing Diagnosis: *DISTURBED SELF-CONCEPT**

related to:
a. changes in appearance and body functioning (e.g., graying and thinning of hair; sagginess of eyelids, earlobes, and breasts; dry, wrinkled skin; reduced height; increase in and change in distribution of body fat; reduction in lean body mass; decreased bladder control; diminished visual acuity and hearing);
b. increased dependence on others to meet basic needs;
c. feelings of powerlessness;
d. changes in usual lifestyle and roles associated with decreased strength and endurance and disturbed sensory perception.

*This diagnostic label includes the nursing diagnoses of disturbed body image, low self-esteem, and ineffective role performance.

Suggested NOC Outcomes: Body image; Self-esteem; Personal autonomy; Psychosocial adjustment: life change; Quality of life

Suggested NIC Interventions: Body image enhancement; Self-esteem enhancement; Role enhancement; Hope instillation; Emotional support; Support system enhancement

Desired Outcome	Nursing Actions *and Selected Purposes/Rationales* (see pp. 47–49 for additional rationales)
20. The client will demonstrate beginning adaptation to changes in appearance, body functioning, level of independence, lifestyle, and roles as evidenced by: a. verbalization of feelings of self-worth and sexual adequacy b. maintenance of relationships with significant others c. active participation in activities of daily living d. verbalization of a beginning plan for adapting lifestyle to changes associated with the aging process and current diagnosis.	20.a. Assess for signs and symptoms of a disturbed self-concept (e.g., verbalization of negative feelings about self, withdrawal from significant others, lack of participation in activities of daily living, lack of plan for adapting to necessary changes in lifestyle). b. Determine the meaning of changes in appearance, body functioning, lifestyle, and roles to the client by encouraging the verbalization of feelings and by noting nonverbal responses to the changes experienced. c. Implement measures *to assist client to increase self-esteem* (e.g., limit negative self-assessment, encourage positive comments about self, assist to identify strengths, give positive feedback about accomplishments and behaviors that are indicative of high self-esteem). d. Assist client to identify and use coping techniques that have been helpful in the past. e. Reinforce measures to promote an optimal sexuality pattern (see Diagnosis 19, action c). f. Implement measures to assist client to adapt to impaired sensory perceptions (see Diagnosis 6, actions b–f). g. If client is incontinent, instruct in ways to minimize the problem *so that socialization is possible* (e.g., placing disposable liners in underwear, wearing absorbent undergarments such as Attends). h. Assist client with usual grooming and makeup habits if necessary. i. Implement measures *to assist the client to maintain a sense of dignity and feeling of well-being about appearance* (e.g., do not expose client unnecessarily during assessments, procedures, and care; do not discuss incontinence episodes in front of client's visitors; assist client with bathing, makeup, hair-styling, and shaving before visitors arrive).

j. Implement measures to reduce client's feelings of powerlessness (e.g., discuss the purpose and benefits of having advanced directives for health care; encourage client to ask questions and participate in decision making about treatment regimen and future living situation; encourage client to do as much for self as possible).
k. Demonstrate acceptance of client using techniques such as touch and frequent visits. Encourage significant others to do the same.
l. Support behaviors suggesting positive adaptation to changes that have occurred (e.g., interest in personal appearance, verbalization of feelings of self-worth, maintenance of relationships with significant others).
m. Encourage visits and support from significant others.
n. Encourage client to pursue usual roles and interests and continue involvement in social activities. If previous roles, interests, and hobbies cannot be pursued, encourage development of new ones.
o. Instruct client in ways to promote and maintain optimal body functioning after discharge (e.g., maintain good nutritional status, participate in an active exercise program).
p. Provide information about and encourage use of community agencies and support groups (e.g., senior centers; family, individual, and/or financial counseling).
q. Consult appropriate health care provider about psychological counseling if client desires or seems unwilling or unable to adapt to changes resulting from the aging process.

21. NURSING DIAGNOSIS: ***RISK FOR LONELINESS***

related to:

a. reduced opportunities for socialization associated with inadequate financial resources, death or disability of friends and family members, reluctance of others to include the elderly in activities, reluctance to establish new relationships and try new activities, and/or a move to a different location (e.g., family member's home, foster home, extended care facility);
b. decreased desire to communicate with others associated with an imbalance between the effort required to interact with others and the anticipated rewards of the interaction;
c. decreased participation in usual activities associated with changes in sensory and motor function and fear of falls;
d. withdrawal from others associated with fear of embarrassment resulting from functional changes such as incontinence or hearing loss.

Suggested NOC Outcomes: Social support; Psychosocial adjustment: life change; Quality of life

Suggested NIC Interventions: Socialization enhancement; Visitation facilitation; Support system enhancement

Desired Outcome	**Nursing Actions** *and Selected Purposes/Rationales*
21. The client will not experience a sense of isolation and loneliness as evidenced by: a. maintenance of relationships with significant others b. no expression of feelings of isolation and loneliness.	21.a. Assess for indications of isolation and loneliness (e.g., absence of supportive significant others; uncommunicative and withdrawn; expression of feelings of rejection, being different from others, or being lonely; hostility; sad, dull affect). b. Implement measures *to decrease isolation and reduce the risk for loneliness:* 1. assist client to identify reasons for feeling isolated and alone; aid him/her in developing a plan of action to reduce these feelings 2. use touch to demonstrate acceptance of client 3. encourage significant others to visit 4. encourage client to maintain telephone contact with others 5. schedule time each day to sit and talk with client 6. assist client to identify a few persons he/she feels comfortable with and encourage interactions with them

Desired Outcome	Nursing Actions *and Selected Purposes/Rationales*

7. make objects such as telephone, TV, radio, newspapers, and greeting cards accessible to client
8. have significant others bring client's favorite objects from home and place in room
9. change room assignments as feasible *to provide client with roommate with similar interests;* encourage their interaction
10. emphasize the importance of maintaining active friendships and seeking out new relationships; encourage participation in support groups if appropriate
11. encourage client to participate in structured activity programs following discharge; provide information about community senior centers and the programs they offer.

22. Nursing Diagnosis: *INEFFECTIVE THERAPEUTIC REGIMEN MANAGEMENT*

related to:
a. lack of motivation, inadequate support and supervision, and insufficient financial resources;
b. confusion about appropriate health care practices and a decreased level of trust associated with conflicting advice from multiple health care providers;
c. conflicting values between client and health care providers;
d. knowledge deficit regarding current diagnosis, medications and treatments prescribed, and consequences of failure to comply with treatment plan.

Suggested NOC Outcomes: Knowledge: treatment regimen; Knowledge: disease process; Participation in health care decisions; Compliance behavior; Health beliefs: perceived resources

Suggested NIC Interventions: Discharge planning; Health system guidance; Self-modification assistance; Teaching: disease process; Teaching: procedure/treatment; Support group; Values clarification; Financial resource assistance

Desired Outcome	Nursing Actions *and Selected Purposes/Rationales*
22. The client will demonstrate the probability of effective management of therapeutic regimen as evidenced by: a. willingness to learn about and participate in treatments and care b. statements reflecting ways to modify personal habits and integrate treatments into lifestyle c. statements reflecting an understanding of the implications of not following the prescribed treatment plan.	22.a. Assess for indications that the client may be unable to effectively manage the therapeutic regimen: 1. statements reflecting inability to manage care at home 2. failure to adhere to treatment plan (e.g., not adhering to dietary modifications, refusing medications, refusing to ambulate) 3. statements reflecting a lack of understanding of the factors that will cause further progression of current illness and/or accelerate aging process 4. statements reflecting an unwillingness or inability to modify personal habits and integrate necessary treatments into lifestyle 5. statements reflecting view that situation is hopeless and that efforts to comply are useless. b. Implement measures *to promote effective management of the therapeutic regimen:* 1. discuss with client the specific factors that may interfere with management of care (e.g., inadequate financial resources, religious or cultural conflicts, lack of support systems) 2. explain the aging process and current diagnosis in terms the client can understand; stress the fact that adherence to the treatment plan is necessary in order to delay and/or prevent complications associated with the diagnosis and minimize some of the changes that occur with aging 3. assist client to clarify values and to identify ways to incorporate the therapeutic goals and priorities into value system 4. encourage questions and clarify misconceptions the client has about aging and his/her diagnosis and effects of each 5. perform actions to promote trust in caregivers (e.g., validate conflicting advice, explain reasons for treatment plan) 6. encourage client to participate in treatment plan (e.g., take medications as prescribed, perform recommended exercises)

7. provide instruction regarding medications and treatments prescribed; allow time for return demonstration of procedures; determine areas of difficulty and misunderstanding and reinforce teaching as necessary
8. provide client with written instructions about medications and treatments
9. assist client to identify ways to incorporate treatments into lifestyle; focus on modifications of lifestyle rather than complete change if possible
10. encourage client to discuss financial concerns; obtain a social service consult to assist client with financial planning and to obtain financial aid if indicated
11. provide information about and encourage use of community resources that can assist client to make necessary lifestyle changes if appropriate
12. encourage client to attend follow-up educational classes if appropriate
13. reinforce behaviors suggesting future compliance with the therapeutic regimen (e.g., statements reflecting plans for integrating treatments into lifestyle, active participation in exercise program, changes in personal habits)
14. include significant others in explanations and teaching sessions and encourage their support; reinforce the need for client to assume responsibility for managing as much of care as possible.

c. Consult appropriate health care provider about referrals to community health agencies if continued instruction, support, or supervision is needed.

23. NURSING DIAGNOSIS: *INTERRUPTED FAMILY PROCESSES*

related to:

a. financial, physical, and psychological stresses associated with family member's illness and/or progressive disability;
b. inadequate knowledge about the normal aging process, client's current diagnosis, and necessary care;
c. inadequate support services;
d. decreased ability of client to fulfill usual family roles;
e. guilt associated with need to change client's living situation resulting from family's inability to provide necessary care.

Suggested NOC Outcomes: Family coping; Family functioning; Family involvement promotion; Family normalization; Family resiliency

Suggested NIC Interventions: Family integrity promotion; Family process maintenance; Family support

Desired Outcome

23. The family members* will demonstrate beginning adjustment to changes in functioning of family member and family roles and structure as evidenced by:
    a. meeting client's needs
    b. verbalization of ways to adapt to required role and lifestyle changes
    c. active participation in decision making and client's rehabilitation
    d. positive interactions with one another.

*The term *family members* is being used here to include client's significant others.

Nursing Actions *and Selected Purposes/Rationales*

23.a. Assess for signs and symptoms of interrupted family processes (e.g., inability to meet client's needs, statements of not being able to accept client's disabilities or make necessary role and lifestyle changes, inability to make decisions, inability or refusal to participate in client's care and/or rehabilitation, negative family interactions).

b. Identify components of the family and their patterns of communication and role expectations.

c. Implement measures *to facilitate family members' adjustment to age- or diagnosis-related changes in client and resultant changes in family roles and structure:*
1. encourage family members to verbalize feelings about changes in client and the effect of these changes on family structure; actively listen to each family member and maintain a nonjudgmental attitude about feelings shared
2. instruct client and family about normal aging processes (e.g., sensory deficits, decreased muscle strength, reduced coordination)
3. reinforce physician's explanation of the effects of the current diagnosis and planned treatment and rehabilitation
4. assist family members to gain a realistic perspective of client's situation, conveying as much hope as appropriate

Desired Outcome	Nursing Actions *and Selected Purposes/Rationales*

5. provide privacy *so that family members and client can share their feelings with one another;* stress the importance of and facilitate the use of good communication techniques
6. assist family members to progress through their own grieving processes; explain that they may encounter times when they need to focus on meeting their own rather than the client's needs
7. emphasize the need for family members to obtain adequate rest and nutrition and to identify and utilize stress management techniques *so they are better able to emotionally and physically deal with changes experienced*
8. encourage and assist family members to identify coping strategies for dealing with client's age-related changes and changes in health status and their effect on the family
9. assist family members to identify realistic goals and ways of reaching these goals
10. include family members in decision making about client's care; convey appreciation for their input and continued support of client
11. encourage and allow family members to participate in client's care and rehabilitation; instruct family in any special procedures and allow them to practice with supervision prior to discharge of the client
12. assist family members to identify resources that could assist them in coping with their feelings and meeting their immediate and long-term needs (e.g., counseling and social services; pastoral care; service, church, and support groups); initiate a referral if indicated.

d. Consult appropriate health care provider if family members continue to demonstrate difficulty adapting to changes in client's functioning, roles, and family structure.

ADDITIONAL NURSING DIAGNOSES

*FEAR/ANXIETY**

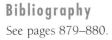

related to unfamiliar environment; signs and symptoms of current diagnosis; lack of understanding of diagnostic tests, diagnosis, and treatment plan; financial concerns; and effects of diagnosis on health status, usual roles, and ability to live independently.

RISK FOR POWERLESSNESS

related to:

a. increased dependence on others to meet basic needs;
b. inability to pursue usual life activities and roles associated with age-related changes in body functioning, current diagnosis and its treatment, and inadequate financial resources;
c. inability to control many of the changes that occur with aging.

*See Unit II for outcomes, actions, and rationales.

Bibliography

See pages 879–880.

UNIT IV

Nursing Care of the Client Having Surgery

Preoperative Care

The preoperative phase begins when the client decides to have surgery and ends when the client enters the operating room area. Although surgical procedures are performed in a variety of settings (e.g., hospitals, day surgery centers, physicians' offices), the basic preoperative client care is similar. The goals of preoperative care are to prepare the client physically and psychologically for the surgery and the postoperative period. Thorough preoperative preparation reduces the client's postoperative fear and anxiety and the risk of postoperative complications. In order to individualize this care plan, the client's psychological and physiological status, the surgical setting, the length of time before the surgical procedure, the type of anesthesia to be used, and the planned surgical procedure must be considered.

This care plan focuses on the adult client who is scheduled for a surgical procedure. It should be used in conjunction with each surgical care plan.

PREOPERATIVE GOALS

THE CLIENT WILL:

- share thoughts and feelings about the impending surgery and its anticipated effects
- verbalize an understanding of the surgical procedure, preoperative care, and postoperative sensations and care
- demonstrate the ability to perform activities designed to prevent postoperative complications.

NURSING DIAGNOSES

CLIENT TEACHING

1. Nursing Diagnosis: *FEAR/ANXIETY*

related to:

a. unfamiliar environment and separation from significant others;
b. anticipated loss of control associated with effects of anesthesia;
c. lack of understanding of diagnostic tests and planned surgical procedure;
d. financial concerns associated with the surgery and recovery period;
e. potential embarrassment or loss of dignity associated with body exposure;
f. risk of disease if blood transfusions are necessary;
g. anticipated pain; surgical findings; and changes in appearance, body functioning, and usual lifestyle and roles;
h. possibility of death.

Suggested NOC Outcomes: Anxiety level; Anxiety self-control; Fear level; Fear self-control

Suggested NIC Interventions: Anxiety reduction; Calming technique; Emotional support; Presence; Teaching: preoperative

Desired Outcome	**Nursing Actions** *and Selected Purposes/Rationales* (see pp. 14–16 for additional rationales)
1. The client will experience a reduction in fear and anxiety as evidenced by: a. verbalization of feeling less anxious b. usual sleep pattern	1.a. Gather the following data from the client during the preoperative period: 1. level of understanding of planned surgical procedure 2. perceptions about the surgery and its anticipated results 3. significance of the surgical procedure and hospitalization 4. previous surgical and hospital experiences 5. availability of adequate support systems

Desired Outcome	Nursing Actions *and Selected Purposes/Rationales*
c. relaxed facial expression and body movements d. stable vital signs e. usual perceptual ability and interactions with others.	6. arrangements made for responsibilities such as job, child care, meal preparation, and home maintenance if needed during the recovery period. b. Assess client for signs and symptoms of fear and anxiety (e.g., verbalization of feeling anxious, insomnia, tenseness, shakiness, restlessness, diaphoresis, tachycardia, elevated blood pressure, self-focused behaviors). c. Implement measures *to reduce fear and anxiety:* 1. orient client to environment, equipment, and routines 2. introduce client to staff who will be participating in care; if possible maintain consistency in staff assigned to his/her care 3. assure client that staff members are nearby; respond to call signal as soon as possible 4. maintain a calm, supportive, confident manner when interacting with client 5. encourage verbalization of fear and anxiety; provide feedback 6. reinforce physician's explanations and clarify misconceptions the client has about the surgical procedure (e.g., purpose, size and location of incision, anticipated outcome) 7. explain all presurgical diagnostic tests 8. provide information about preoperative routines and anticipated postoperative care (see Diagnosis 4, actions a.1–4 and b.1) 9. enable client *to maintain a sense of control by:* a. including him/her in planning of preoperative care and allowing choices whenever possible b. explaining purpose of the written consent form (e.g., indicates voluntary and informed consent, protects against unsanctioned surgery) c. discussing the purpose and benefits of an advanced directive for health care and providing assistance as needed to complete the necessary documents 10. provide a calm, restful environment 11. instruct client in relaxation techniques and encourage participation in diversional activities 12. assist client to identify specific stressors and ways to cope with them 13. provide information based on current needs of client at a level he/she can understand; encourage questions and clarification of information provided 14. perform actions *to help client maintain a sense of dignity* (e.g., provide privacy when appropriate; avoid unnecessary body exposure during preoperative procedures; allow client to wear dentures, glasses, wig, etc. into the operating room suite if possible) 15. assure client that pain relief needs will be met postoperatively 16. assure client that blood is screened carefully and that the risk for contracting blood-borne disease is minimal 17. initiate a social service referral if indicated 18. encourage significant others to project a caring, concerned attitude without obvious anxiousness 19. include significant others in orientation and teaching sessions and encourage their continued support of client 20. when appropriate, assist client to meet spiritual needs (e.g., arrange for a visit from clergy) 21. administer prescribed antianxiety agents if indicated. d. Consult appropriate health care provider (e.g., psychiatric nurse clinician, physician) if above actions fail to control fear and anxiety.

2. Nursing Diagnosis: ***DISTURBED SLEEP PATTERN***

related to fear, anxiety, presurgical treatments and procedures, and unfamiliar environment.

Suggested NOC Outcome: Sleep

Suggested NIC Intervention: Sleep enhancement

Desired Outcome	Nursing Actions *and Selected Purposes/Rationales* (see pp. 52–54 for additional rationales)
2. The client will attain optimal amounts of sleep as evidenced by statements of feeling well rested.	2.a. Assess for signs and symptoms of a disturbed sleep pattern (e.g., statements of difficulty falling asleep, interrupted sleep, or not feeling well rested). b. Implement measures *to promote sleep:* 1. perform actions to reduce fear and anxiety (see Diagnosis 1, action c) 2. encourage participation in relaxing diversional activities during the evening 3. discourage intake of foods/fluids high in caffeine (e.g., chocolate, coffee, tea, colas) in the evening 4. offer client an evening snack that includes milk unless contraindicated *(milk contains L-tryptophan, which is believed to help induce and maintain sleep)* 5. allow client to continue usual sleep practices (e.g., position; time; presleep routines such as reading, watching television, listening to music, and meditating) whenever possible 6. satisfy basic needs such as comfort and warmth before sleep 7. encourage client to urinate just before bedtime 8. reduce environmental distractions (e.g., close door to client's room, use night light rather than overhead light whenever possible, lower volume of paging system, keep staff conversations at a low level and away from client's room, close curtains between clients in a semi-private room or ward, keep beepers and alarms on low volume, have earplugs available for client if needed) 9. encourage client to avoid drinking alcohol in the evening *(alcohol interferes with REM sleep)* 10. encourage client to avoid smoking before bedtime *(nicotine is a stimulant)* 11. administer prescribed sedative-hypnotics if indicated 12. perform actions *to reduce interruptions during sleep (70–100 minutes of uninterrupted sleep is usually needed to complete one sleep cycle):* a. restrict visitors b. group care (e.g., medications, treatments, physical care, assessments) whenever possible.

3. NURSING DIAGNOSIS: ***ANTICIPATORY GRIEVING***

related to potential loss of or change in a body part and/or usual body functioning, appearance, lifestyle, and roles.

Suggested NOC Outcome: Grief resolution

Suggested NIC Interventions: Grief work facilitation; Emotional support

Desired Outcome	Nursing Actions *and Selected Purposes/Rationales* (see pp. 35–37 for additional rationales)
3. The client will demonstrate beginning progression through the grieving process as evidenced by: a. verbalization of feelings about anticipated losses and changes following surgery b. usual sleep pattern	3.a. Assess for signs and symptoms of anticipatory grieving (e.g., expression of distress about the losses or changes that may occur as a result of the surgery, change in eating habits, inability to concentrate, insomnia, anger, sadness, withdrawal from significant others). b. Implement measures *to facilitate the grieving process:* 1. assist client to acknowledge the anticipated losses *so grief work can begin;* assess for factors that may hinder and facilitate acknowledgment

Desired Outcome	Nursing Actions *and Selected Purposes/Rationales*
c. participation in preoperative care and self-care activities d. use of available support systems.	2. discuss the grieving process and assist client to accept the phases of grieving (phases vary among theorists but progress from shock and alarm to acceptance) as an expected response to the anticipated losses 3. provide an atmosphere of care and concern (e.g., provide privacy, be available and nonjudgmental, display empathy and respect) *so client will feel free to express feelings* 4. perform actions *to promote trust* (e.g., answer questions honestly, provide requested information) 5. encourage the verbal expression of anger and sadness about the anticipated losses; recognize displacement of anger and assist client to see the actual cause of angry feelings and resentment 6. encourage client to express feelings in whatever ways are comfortable (e.g., writing, drawing, conversation) 7. assist client to identify and use techniques that have helped him/her cope in previous situations of loss 8. support realistic hope about changes that may result from the surgery 9. support behaviors suggesting successful grief work (e.g., verbalizing feelings about anticipated losses, expressing sorrow, focusing on ways to adapt to anticipated losses) 10. explain the phases of the grieving process to significant others; encourage their support and understanding 11. provide information about counseling services and support groups that might assist client in working through grief 12. when appropriate, assist client to meet spiritual needs (e.g., arrange for a visit from clergy). c. Consult appropriate health care provider regarding a referral for counseling if signs of dysfunctional grieving (e.g., persistent denial of the anticipated loss, excessive anger or sadness, emotional lability) occur.

Client Teaching

4. Nursing Diagnosis: ***DEFICIENT KNOWLEDGE***

regarding the surgical procedure, routines associated with surgery, physical preparation for the surgical procedure, sensations that normally occur following surgery and anesthesia, and postoperative care.

Suggested NOC Outcomes: Knowledge: disease process; Knowledge: treatment regimen

Suggested NIC Interventions: Teaching: preoperative; Teaching: individual

Desired Outcomes	Nursing Actions *and Selected Purposes/Rationales*
4.a. The client will verbalize an understanding of the surgical procedure, preoperative care, and postoperative sensations and care.	4.a.1. Provide information about usual preoperative routines for the surgery to be performed (e.g., blood work, ECG, urinalysis, chest x-ray, insertion of urinary catheter and/or nasogastric tube, bowel and skin preparation, removal of prosthetic devices). 2. Provide information about: a. scheduled time and estimated length of surgery b. food and fluid restrictions before surgery c. preoperative medications and planned anesthesia d. body position during surgical procedure e. purpose for and estimated length of stay in preoperative holding area and postanesthesia care unit (PACU) f. sensations that can occur after surgery (e.g., dryness of mouth, sore throat following endotracheal intubation, pain at surgical site).

3. Reinforce information provided by the anesthesiologist and surgeon about the surgery.
4. Inform client of the anticipated postoperative care:
   a. equipment (e.g., dressings, intravenous lines, drainage tubes, traction devices, antiembolism stockings, intermittent pneumatic compression device)
   b. activity limitations and expectations
   c. dietary modifications
   d. treatments (e.g., respiratory care, circulatory management, wound care) and expected frequency
   e. assessments (e.g., intake and output, lung sounds, vital signs, neurological checks, bowel sounds) and expected frequency
   f. medications (e.g., antiemetics, analgesics, antimicrobials)
   g. pain management measures (e.g., oral, parenteral, and/or intravenous medications; epidural analgesia; patient-controlled analgesia [PCA]; positioning; relaxation techniques).
5. Allow time for questions and clarification. Provide feedback.

4.b. The client will demonstrate the ability to perform activities designed to prevent postoperative complications.

4.b.1. Provide instructions about activities the client will be expected to perform postoperatively. These may include:
   a. effective coughing and deep breathing techniques
   b. correct use of incentive spirometer
   c. active foot and leg exercises
   d. correct methods for moving in bed, getting out of bed, and ambulating.
2. Allow time for questions, clarification, and return demonstration.

Bibliography

See pages 879 and 880.

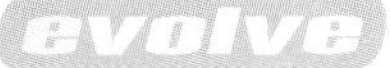

Postoperative Care

The postoperative phase begins when the client is transferred from surgery to a postanesthesia care unit (PACU) and ends when he/she has recovered from the surgical intervention. The length of the postoperative phase varies depending on factors such as the client's age and preoperative health status, type of anesthesia used, length and type of surgery, and the client's physiological and psychological responses postoperatively.

This care plan focuses on postoperative care of an adult client who has received general anesthesia and has been transferred from the recovery area to the clinical care unit. Much of the information is applicable to clients having surgery in an outpatient setting (e.g., physician's office, surgical care center) and to those receiving follow-up care in an extended care facility or home setting. This care plan should be used in conjunction with all surgical care plans.

OUTCOME/DISCHARGE CRITERIA

THE CLIENT WILL:

- tolerate prescribed diet
- tolerate expected level of activity
- have surgical pain controlled
- have clear, audible breath sounds throughout lungs
- have evidence of normal wound healing
- have no signs and symptoms of infection or postoperative complications
- identify ways to prevent postoperative infection
- demonstrate the ability to perform wound care
- state signs and symptoms to report to the health care provider
- share thoughts and feelings about the surgery, diagnosis, prognosis, and treatment plan
- verbalize an understanding of and a plan for adhering to recommended follow-up care including future appointments with health care provider, dietary modifications, activity level, treatments, and medications prescribed.

NURSING/COLLABORATIVE DIAGNOSES

c. thromboembolism
d. paralytic ileus
e. dehiscence

21. Fear/Anxiety p. 124

DISCHARGE TEACHING

22. Deficient knowledge, Ineffective therapeutic regimen management, or Ineffective health maintenance p. 125

1. NURSING DIAGNOSIS: *INEFFECTIVE TISSUE PERFUSION*

related to:

a. hypovolemia associated with fluid loss and decreased fluid intake;
b. peripheral pooling of blood associated with decreased activity and diminished vasomotor responses resulting from the effects of anesthesia and some medications (e.g., narcotic [opioid] analgesics).

Suggested NOC Outcome: Circulation status

Suggested NIC Interventions: Circulatory care: venous insufficiency; Circulatory care: arterial insufficiency; Hypovolemia management

Desired Outcome	Nursing Actions *and Selected Purposes/Rationales* (see pp. 57–59 for additional rationales)
1. The client will maintain adequate tissue perfusion as evidenced by: a. B/P within normal range for client and stable with position change b. usual mental status c. extremities warm with absence of pallor and cyanosis d. palpable peripheral pulses e. capillary refill time less than 2–3 seconds f. urine output at least 30 ml/hour.	1.a. Assess for and report signs and symptoms of diminished tissue perfusion (e.g., significant decrease in B/P, postural hypotension, dizziness or lightheadedness when changing to an upright position, restlessness, confusion, cool extremities, pallor or cyanosis of extremities, diminished or absent peripheral pulses, slow capillary refill, oliguria). b. Implement measures *to maintain adequate tissue perfusion:* 1. maintain a minimum fluid intake of 2500 ml/day unless contraindicated; if oral intake is inadequate or contraindicated, maintain intravenous fluid therapy as ordered 2. administer blood and blood products as ordered 3. instruct client to change from a supine to an upright position slowly *in order to allow time for autoregulatory mechanisms to adjust to the change in the distribution of blood associated with an upright position* 4. perform actions *to prevent peripheral pooling of blood and increase venous return:* a. instruct and assist client to perform active foot and leg exercises every 1–2 hours while awake b. encourage and assist with ambulation as soon as allowed and tolerated (client should be instructed to pick up feet instead of shuffling *in order to promote contractions of the leg muscles*) c. discourage positions that compromise blood flow in lower extremities (e.g., crossing legs, pillows under knees, sitting for long periods) d. consult physician about an order for antiembolism stockings or an intermittent pneumatic compression device during period of reduced activity 5. perform actions *to prevent vasoconstriction:* a. implement measures *to reduce stress* (e.g., explain procedures, reduce discomfort, maintain calm environment) b. discourage smoking c. implement measures *to keep client from getting cold* (e.g., maintain a comfortable room temperature, provide adequate clothing and blankets). c. Consult physician if signs and symptoms of diminished tissue perfusion persist or worsen.

2. Nursing Diagnosis: *INEFFECTIVE BREATHING PATTERN*

related to:

a. increased rate of respirations associated with fear and anxiety;
b. decreased rate of respirations associated with the depressant effect of anesthesia and some medications (e.g., narcotic [opioid] analgesics, some antiemetics);
c. decreased depth of respirations associated with:
    1. depressant effect of anesthesia and some medications (e.g., narcotic [opioid] analgesics, some antiemetics)
    2. reluctance to breathe deeply because of pain
    3. fear, anxiety, weakness, and fatigue
    4. restricted chest expansion resulting from positioning and elevation of the diaphragm if abdominal distention is present.

Suggested NOC Outcome: Respiratory status: ventilation

Suggested NIC Interventions: Respiratory monitoring; Ventilation assistance

Desired Outcome	Nursing Actions *and Selected Purposes/Rationales* (see pp. 18–20 for additional rationales)
2. The client will maintain an effective breathing pattern as evidenced by: a. normal rate and depth of respirations b. absence of dyspnea.	2.a. Assess for signs and symptoms of an ineffective breathing pattern (e.g., shallow or slow respirations, limited chest excursion, tachypnea, dyspnea, use of accessory muscles when breathing). b. Implement measures *to improve breathing pattern:* 1. perform actions to reduce fear and anxiety (see Diagnosis 21, action b) *in order to prevent the shallow and/or rapid breathing that can occur with fear and anxiety* 2. perform actions to reduce pain (see Diagnosis 6, action d) *in order to increase the client's willingness to move and breathe more deeply* 3. perform actions to reduce the accumulation of gas and fluid in the gastrointestinal tract (see Diagnosis 7, action b) *in order to decrease pressure on the diaphragm* 4. perform actions to increase strength and improve activity tolerance (see Diagnosis 11, action b) *in order to enable the client to breathe more deeply and participate in activities to improve breathing pattern* 5. instruct client to deep breathe or use incentive spirometer every 1–2 hours 6. assist with positive airway pressure techniques (e.g., continuous positive airway pressure [CPAP], bilevel positive airway pressure [BiPAP], flutter/positive expiratory pressure [PEP] device) if ordered 7. instruct client to breathe slowly if hyperventilating 8. place client in a semi- to high Fowler's position unless contraindicated; position with pillows *to prevent slumping* 9. if client must remain flat in bed, assist with position change at least every 2 hours 10. increase activity as allowed and tolerated 11. administer central nervous system depressants judiciously; hold medication and consult physician if respiratory rate is less than 12/minute. c. Consult appropriate health care provider (e.g., physician, respiratory therapist) if: 1. ineffective breathing pattern continues 2. signs and symptoms of impaired gas exchange (e.g., restlessness, irritability, confusion, significant decrease in oximetry results, decreased Pa_{O_2} and increased Pa_{CO_2} levels) are present.

3. NURSING DIAGNOSIS: **INEFFECTIVE AIRWAY CLEARANCE**

related to:
a. occlusion of the pharynx in the immediate postoperative period associated with relaxation of the tongue resulting from effect of anesthesia and some medications (e.g., narcotic [opioid] analgesics);
b. stasis of secretions associated with:
 1. decreased activity
 2. depressed ciliary function resulting from effects of anesthesia
 3. difficulty coughing up secretions resulting from the depressant effect of anesthesia and some medications (e.g., narcotic [opioid] analgesics, some antiemetics), pain, weakness, fatigue, and presence of tenacious secretions (can occur as a result of deficient fluid volume);
c. increased secretions associated with irritation of the respiratory tract (can result from inhalation anesthetics and endotracheal intubation).

Suggested NOC Outcomes: Respiratory status: ventilation; Respiratory status: airway patency

Suggested NIC Interventions: Respiratory monitoring; Airway management; Cough enhancement

Desired Outcome	Nursing Actions *and Selected Purposes/Rationales* (see pp. 12–14 for additional rationales)

3. The client will maintain clear, open airways as evidenced by:
 a. normal breath sounds
 b. normal rate and depth of respirations
 c. absence of dyspnea.

3.a. Assess for signs and symptoms of ineffective airway clearance (e.g., abnormal breath sounds; rapid, shallow respirations; dyspnea; cough).
 b. Implement measures *to promote effective airway clearance:*
  1. position client on side and/or insert an artificial airway if necessary *to prevent obstruction of airway by tongue*
  2. perform actions to reduce pain (see Diagnosis 6, action d) *in order to increase the client's willingness to move, cough, and deep breathe*
  3. instruct and assist client to change position at least every 2 hours while in bed
  4. increase activity as allowed and tolerated
  5. perform actions *to promote the removal of secretions:*
   a. instruct and assist client to deep breathe and cough or "huff" every 1–2 hours
   b. implement measures *to thin tenacious secretions and reduce drying of the respiratory mucous membrane:*
    1. maintain a fluid intake of at least 2500 ml/day unless contraindicated
    2. humidify inspired air as ordered
   c. assist with administration of mucolytics (e.g., acetylcysteine) and diluent or hydrating agents (e.g., water, saline) via nebulizer if ordered
   d. perform suctioning if needed
  6. discourage smoking *(the irritants in smoke increase mucus production, impair ciliary function, and can cause inflammation and damage to the bronchial walls)*
  7. administer central nervous system depressants judiciously.
 c. Consult appropriate health care provider (e.g., physician, respiratory therapist) if:
  1. signs and symptoms of ineffective airway clearance persist
  2. signs and symptoms of impaired gas exchange (e.g., restlessness, irritability, confusion, significant decrease in oximetry results, decreased $Pa{O_2}$ and increased $Pa{CO_2}$ levels) are present.

4. Nursing/Collaborative Diagnosis: RISK FOR IMBALANCED FLUID AND ELECTROLYTES

a. **deficient fluid volume** related to restricted oral fluid intake before, during, and after surgery; blood loss; and loss of fluid associated with vomiting, nasogastric tube drainage, and/or profuse wound drainage;
b. **hypokalemia, hypochloremia, and metabolic alkalosis** related to loss of electrolytes and hydrochloric acid associated with vomiting and nasogastric tube drainage;
c. **excess fluid volume** related to vigorous fluid therapy during and immediately following surgery and an increased secretion of antidiuretic hormone (output of ADH is stimulated by trauma, pain, and anesthetic agents).

Suggested NOC Outcomes: Fluid balance; Electrolyte and acid-base balance

Suggested NIC Interventions: Fluid monitoring; Fluid management; Electrolyte management: hypokalemia; Fluid/Electrolyte management; Acid-base monitoring; Acid-base management: metabolic alkalosis

Desired Outcomes

4.a. The client will not experience deficient fluid volume, hypokalemia, hypochloremia, or metabolic alkalosis as evidenced by:
1. normal skin turgor
2. moist mucous membranes
3. stable weight
4. B/P and pulse within normal range for client and stable with position change
5. capillary refill time less than 2–3 seconds
6. usual mental status
7. balanced intake and output within 48 hours after surgery
8. urine specific gravity within normal range
9. return of peristalsis within expected time
10. absence of cardiac dysrhythmias, muscle weakness, paresthesias, twitching, spasms, and dizziness
11. BUN, serum electrolytes, and blood gases within normal range.

Nursing Actions *and Selected Purposes/Rationales*

(see pp. 30–33 for additional rationales)

4.a.1. Assess for and report signs and symptoms of:
- a. deficient fluid volume:
  1. decreased skin turgor, dry mucous membranes, thirst
  2. weight loss of 2% or greater over a short period
  3. postural hypotension and/or low B/P
  4. weak, rapid pulse
  5. capillary refill time greater than 2–3 seconds
  6. neck veins flat when client is supine
  7. change in mental status
  8. continued low urine output 48 hours after surgery with a change in specific gravity (the specific gravity will usually increase with an actual fluid volume deficit but may be decreased depending on the cause of the deficit)
  9. elevated BUN
- b. hypokalemia (e.g., cardiac dysrhythmias, postural hypotension, muscle weakness, nausea and vomiting, continued abdominal distention and hypoactive or absent bowel sounds, low serum potassium)
- c. hypochloremia and metabolic alkalosis (e.g., dizziness, paresthesias, muscle twitching or spasms, hypoventilation, low serum chloride, elevated pH and TCO_2).

2. Implement measures *to prevent or treat deficient fluid volume, hypokalemia, hypochloremia, and metabolic alkalosis:*
- a. perform actions to prevent nausea and vomiting (see Diagnosis 8, action b)
- b. if a nasogastric tube is present and needs to be irrigated frequently and/or with large volumes of solution, irrigate it with normal saline rather than water
- c. perform actions to reduce fever if present (e.g., administer antipyretics as ordered, sponge client with tepid water, remove excessive clothing or bedcovers) *in order to prevent diaphoresis and subsequent loss of fluid*
- d. carefully measure drainage (e.g., wound, nasogastric) and administer replacement fluids as ordered
- e. administer fluid and electrolyte replacements if ordered
- f. maintain a fluid intake of at least 2500 ml/day unless contraindicated
- g. when oral intake is allowed and tolerated, assist client to select foods/fluids high in potassium (e.g., bananas, orange juice, potatoes, raisins, cantaloupe, tomato juice).

3. Consult physician if signs and symptoms of deficient fluid volume and electrolyte imbalances persist or worsen.

4.b. The client will not experience excess fluid volume as evidenced by:
1. stable weight
2. stable B/P
3. absence of an S_3 heart sound
4. normal pulse volume
5. balanced intake and output within 48 hours following surgery
6. usual mental status
7. normal breath sounds
8. BUN, Hct, and serum sodium and osmolality levels within normal range
9. absence of dyspnea, orthopnea, edema, and distended neck veins.

4.b.1. Assess for and report signs and symptoms of excess fluid volume:
- a. weight gain of 2% or greater over a short period
- b. elevated B/P (B/P may not be elevated if fluid has shifted out of vascular space)
- c. presence of an S_3 heart sound
- d. bounding pulse
- e. intake that continues to be greater than output 48 hours postoperatively (for the first 48 hours after surgery, output is expected to be less than intake *due to increased secretion of ADH*)
- f. change in mental status
- g. crackles (rales), diminished or absent breath sounds
- h. low serum sodium and osmolality (indicates hypoosmolar overhydration [water intoxication])
- i. decreased BUN and Hct (low Hct could also indicate blood loss)
- j. dyspnea, orthopnea
- k. edema
- l. distended neck veins
- m. chest x-ray results showing pulmonary vascular congestion, pleural effusion, or pulmonary edema.

2. Implement measures *to prevent or treat excess fluid volume:*
   - a. administer fluid replacement therapy judiciously, especially within first 48 hours after surgery
   - b. maintain fluid restrictions if ordered
   - c. if client is receiving intravenous fluids that contain sizable amounts of sodium (e.g., 0.9% NaCl, lactated Ringer's), consult physician about a change in the solution or a decrease in the rate of infusion
   - d. if client is receiving numerous and/or large volume intravenous medications, consult pharmacist about ways to prevent excessive fluid administration (e.g., stop primary infusion during administration of intravenous medications, dilute medication in the minimum amount of solution)
   - e. administer diuretics if ordered *to increase excretion of water.*
3. Consult physician if signs and symptoms of excess fluid volume persist or worsen.

5. NURSING DIAGNOSIS: *IMBALANCED NUTRITION: LESS THAN BODY REQUIREMENTS*

related to:
- a. decreased oral intake associated with prescribed dietary modifications, pain, weakness, fatigue, nausea, dislike of prescribed diet, and feeling of fullness (can occur as a result of abdominal distention);
- b. inadequate nutritional replacement therapy;
- c. loss of nutrients associated with vomiting;
- d. increased nutritional needs associated with the increased metabolic rate that occurs during wound healing.

Suggested NOC Outcome: Nutritional status

Suggested NIC Interventions: Nutritional monitoring; Nutrition management; Nutrition therapy; Diet staging

Desired Outcome

Nursing Actions *and Selected Purposes/Rationales*

(see pp. 40–43 for additional rationales)

5. The client will maintain an adequate nutritional status as evidenced by:
   a. weight within normal range for client

5.a. Assess for and report signs and symptoms of malnutrition:
1. weight significantly below client's usual weight or below normal for client's age, height, and body frame
2. abnormal BUN and low serum albumin, Hct, Hgb, and lymphocyte levels (decreased Hct and Hgb may also result from blood loss)
3. weakness and fatigue

Desired Outcome	Nursing Actions *and Selected Purposes/Rationales*

b. normal BUN and serum albumin, Hct, Hgb, and lymphocyte levels
c. usual strength and activity tolerance
d. healthy oral mucous membrane.

4. sore, inflamed oral mucous membrane
5. pale conjunctiva.

b. Assess for return of bowel function every 2–4 hours. Notify physician when client has bowel sounds and is expelling flatus *so that oral intake can be resumed as soon as possible.*
c. When oral intake is allowed, monitor percentage of meals and snacks client consumes. Report pattern of inadequate intake.
d. Implement measures *to maintain an adequate nutritional status:*
   1. when food or oral fluids are allowed, perform actions *to improve oral intake:*
      a. implement measures to prevent nausea and vomiting (see Diagnosis 8, action b)
      b. implement measures to reduce pain (see Diagnosis 6, action d)
      c. implement measures to reduce the accumulation of gas and fluid in the gastrointestinal tract and prevent constipation (see Diagnoses 7, action b and 15, action c) *in order to reduce the risk of gastrointestinal distention and subsequent feeling of fullness and early satiety*
      d. increase activity as allowed and tolerated *(activity promotes gastric emptying, which reduces feeling of gastric fullness; it also usually promotes a sense of well-being, which can improve appetite)*
      e. encourage a rest period before meals *to minimize fatigue*
      f. obtain a dietary consult if necessary to assist client in selecting foods/fluids that meet nutritional needs, are appealing, and adhere to personal and cultural preferences as well as the prescribed dietary modifications
      g. maintain a clean environment and a relaxed, pleasant atmosphere
      h. provide oral hygiene before meals *(oral hygiene moistens the mouth, which may make it easier to chew and swallow; it also removes unpleasant tastes, which often improves the taste of foods/fluids)*
      i. serve frequent, small meals rather than large ones if client is weak, fatigues easily, and/or has a poor appetite
      j. encourage significant others to bring in client's favorite foods unless contraindicated
      k. allow adequate time for meals; reheat foods/fluids if necessary
      l. limit fluid intake with meals (unless the fluid has high nutritional value) *to reduce early satiety and subsequent decreased food intake*
   2. ensure that meals are well balanced and high in essential nutrients; offer dietary supplements if indicated
   3. administer vitamins and minerals if ordered.
e. Perform a calorie count if ordered. Report information to dietitian and physician.
f. Consult physician about an alternative method of providing nutrition (e.g., parenteral nutrition, tube feedings) if client does not consume enough food or fluids to meet nutritional needs.

6. Nursing Diagnosis: ACUTE PAIN

related to tissue trauma and reflex muscle spasms associated with the surgery; irritation from drainage tubes; and stress on surgical area associated with deep breathing, coughing, and/or movement.

Suggested NOC Outcomes: Pain control; Pain: adverse psychological response; Comfort level

Suggested NIC Interventions: Pain management; Analgesic administration

Desired Outcome	Nursing Actions *and Selected Purposes/Rationales* (see pp. 45–47 for additional rationales)
6. The client will experience diminished pain as evidenced by: a. verbalization of a decrease in or absence of pain b. relaxed facial expression and body positioning c. increased participation in activities d. stable vital signs.	6.a. Assess for signs and symptoms of pain (e.g., verbalization of pain, grimacing, reluctance to move, restlessness, diaphoresis, increased B/P, tachycardia). b. Assess client's perception of the severity of pain using a pain intensity rating scale. c. Assess the client's pain pattern (e.g., location, quality, onset, duration, precipitating factors, aggravating factors, alleviating factors). d. Implement measures *to reduce pain:* 1. perform actions *to reduce fear and anxiety about the pain experience* (e.g., assure client that his/her need for pain relief is understood, plan methods for achieving pain control with client) 2. perform actions to reduce fear and anxiety (see Diagnosis 21, action b) *in order to promote relaxation and subsequently increase the client's threshold and tolerance for pain* 3. administer analgesics before activities and procedures that can cause pain and before pain becomes severe 4. perform actions to promote rest (e.g., minimize environmental activity and noise) *in order to reduce fatigue and subsequently increase the client's threshold and tolerance for pain* 5. provide or assist with nonpharmacologic methods for pain relief (e.g., massage; position change; progressive relaxation exercises; restful environment; diversional activities such as watching television, reading, or conversing) 6. instruct and assist client to support abdominal or chest incision with a pillow or hands when turning, coughing, and deep breathing 7. if client has an abdominal incision, instruct him/her to bend knees while coughing and deep breathing *in order to reduce tension on abdominal muscles and incision* 8. securely anchor drainage tubes *to decrease tissue irritation resulting from movement of tubes* 9. encourage client to use patient-controlled analgesia (PCA) device as instructed 10. maintain integrity of analgesia delivery system (e.g., epidural, intravenous, subcutaneous, transdermal) 11. administer the following medications as ordered: a. narcotic (opioid) analgesics b. nonnarcotic analgesics such as acetaminophen and salicylates and other nonsteroidal anti-inflammatory agents c. local anesthetics (e.g., bupivacaine, etidocaine) d. muscle relaxants. e. Consult appropriate health care provider (e.g., physician, pharmacist, pain management specialist) if above measures fail to provide adequate pain relief.

7. NURSING DIAGNOSIS: ALTERED COMFORT: ABDOMINAL DISTENTION AND GAS PAIN

related to accumulation of gas and fluid in the gastrointestinal tract associated with:

a. decreased peristalsis resulting from manipulation of the bowel during abdominal surgery and depressant effect of anesthesia and some medications (e.g., narcotic [opioid] analgesics);
b. decreased activity.

Suggested NOC Outcomes: Comfort level; Symptom control

Suggested NIC Intervention: Flatulence reduction

Desired Outcome	Nursing Actions *and Selected Purposes/Rationales*
7. The client will experience diminished abdominal distention and gas pain as evidenced by: a. verbalization of decreased abdominal fullness and pain b. relaxed facial expression and body positioning c. decrease in abdominal girth.	7.a. Assess for signs and symptoms of abdominal distention or gas pain (e.g., verbal reports of abdominal fullness or gas pain, clutching or guarding of abdomen, restlessness, reluctance to move, grimacing, increasing abdominal girth). b. Implement measures *to reduce the accumulation of gas and fluid in the gastrointestinal tract:* 1. encourage and assist client with frequent position changes and ambulation as soon as allowed and tolerated *(activity stimulates peristalsis and expulsion of flatus)* 2. instruct the client to avoid activities such as chewing gum, drinking through a straw, and smoking *in order to reduce air swallowing* 3. maintain patency of nasogastric, gastric, or intestinal tube if present 4. maintain food and oral fluid restrictions as ordered 5. when oral intake is allowed, instruct client to avoid intake of carbonated beverages and gas-producing foods (e.g., cabbage, onions, beans) 6. encourage client to expel flatus whenever the urge is felt 7. consult physician regarding insertion of a rectal tube or administration of a return flow enema if indicated 8. encourage use of nonnarcotic analgesics once the period of severe pain has subsided *(narcotic [opioid] analgesics depress gastrointestinal activity)* 9. administer gastrointestinal stimulants (e.g., metoclopramide, bisacodyl) if ordered *to increase gastrointestinal motility.* c. Consult physician if signs and symptoms of abdominal distention and gas pain persist or worsen.

8. NURSING DIAGNOSIS:

NAUSEA

related to stimulation of the vomiting center associated with:

a. stimulation of visceral afferent pathways resulting from abdominal distention and/or the irritating effect of some medications on the gastric mucosa;
b. stimulation of the cerebral cortex resulting from pain, stress, and/or noxious environmental stimuli;
c. stimulation of the chemoreceptor trigger zone resulting from rapid movement and the effect of some medications (e.g., morphine).

Suggested NOC Outcome: Nausea and vomiting severity

Suggested NIC Interventions: Nausea management; Vomiting management; Environmental management: comfort

Desired Outcome	Nursing Actions *and Selected Purposes/Rationales*
8. The client will experience relief of nausea and vomiting as evidenced by: a. verbalization of relief of nausea b. absence of vomiting.	8.a. Assess client for nausea and vomiting. b. Implement measures *to prevent nausea and vomiting:* 1. perform actions to reduce the accumulation of gas and fluid in the gastrointestinal tract (see Diagnosis 7, action b) 2. perform actions to reduce pain (see Diagnosis 6, action d) 3. perform actions to reduce fear and anxiety (see Diagnosis 21, action b) 4. eliminate noxious sights and odors from the environment *(noxious stimuli can cause stimulation of the vomiting center)* 5. encourage client to take deep, slow breaths when nauseated 6. instruct client to change positions slowly *(rapid movement can result in chemoreceptor trigger zone stimulation and subsequent excitation of the vomiting center)* 7. provide oral hygiene after each emesis 8. when oral intake is allowed: a. advance diet slowly (usually beginning with clear liquids and progressing to solid food)

b. avoid serving foods with an overpowering aroma; remove lids from hot foods before entering room
c. provide small, frequent meals rather than 3 large ones
d. instruct client to ingest foods and fluids slowly
e. instruct client to avoid foods/fluids that irritate the gastric mucosa (e.g., spicy foods; caffeine-containing beverages such as coffee, tea, and colas)
f. encourage client to eat dry foods (e.g., toast, crackers) and avoid drinking liquids with meals if nauseated
g. instruct client to avoid foods high in fat *(fat delays gastric emptying)*
h. instruct client to rest after eating with head of bed elevated
i. administer medications known to cause gastric irritation (e.g., aspirin and aspirin-containing products, corticosteroids, ibuprofen) with or immediately after meals unless contraindicated

9. administer antiemetics and gastrointestinal stimulants (e.g., metoclopramide) if ordered.

c. Consult physician if above measures fail to control nausea and vomiting.

9. NURSING DIAGNOSIS: IMPAIRED ORAL MUCOUS MEMBRANE: DRYNESS

related to:
a. deficient fluid volume associated with restricted oral intake and fluid loss;
b. decreased salivation associated with food and fluid restrictions and the effect of anesthesia and some medications (e.g., narcotic [opioid] analgesics).

Suggested NOC Outcome: Oral hygiene

Suggested NIC Interventions: Oral health maintenance; Oral health promotion

Desired Outcome	**Nursing Actions** *and Selected Purposes/Rationales* (see pp. 43–45 for additional rationales)
9. The client will maintain a moist, intact oral mucous membrane.	9.a. Assess client for dryness of the oral mucosa. b. Implement measures *to relieve dryness of the oral mucous membrane:* 1. instruct and assist client to perform oral hygiene as often as needed; avoid use of products that contain lemon and glycerin and use of mouthwashes containing alcohol *(these products have a drying and irritating effect on the oral mucous membrane)* 2. encourage client to rinse mouth frequently with water 3. lubricate client's lips frequently 4. encourage client to breathe through nose rather than mouth 5. encourage client not to smoke *(smoking dries the mucosa)* 6. maintain intravenous fluid therapy as ordered *to improve hydration* 7. encourage client to suck on hard candy unless contraindicated *in order to stimulate salivation* 8. increase oral fluid intake as soon as allowed and tolerated *to improve hydration and stimulate salivation.* c. Consult physician if signs and symptoms of parotitis (e.g., pain, tenderness, and swelling at the angle of the jaw; fever) occur.

10. NURSING DIAGNOSIS: ACTUAL/RISK FOR IMPAIRED TISSUE INTEGRITY

related to:
a. disruption of tissue associated with the surgical procedure;
b. delayed wound healing associated with factors such as decreased nutritional status and inadequate blood supply to wound area;
c. irritation of skin associated with contact with wound drainage, pressure from tubes, and use of tape.

Suggested NOC Outcomes: Wound healing: primary intention; Wound healing: secondary intention; Tissue integrity: skin and mucous membranes

Suggested NIC Interventions: Skin surveillance; Pressure management; Positioning; Wound care; Incision site care

Desired Outcomes	**Nursing Actions** *and Selected Purposes/Rationales* (see pp. 49–52 for additional rationales)
10.a. The client will experience normal healing of surgical wound(s) as evidenced by: 1. gradual reduction in periwound swelling and redness 2. presence of granulation tissue if healing is by secondary or tertiary intention 3. intact, approximated wound edges if healing is by primary intention.	10.a.1. Assess for and report signs and symptoms of impaired wound healing (e.g., increasing periwound swelling and redness, pale or necrotic tissue in wounds healing by secondary or tertiary intention, separation of wound edges in wounds healing by primary intention). 2. Implement measures *to promote wound healing:* a. perform actions to maintain an adequate nutritional status (see Diagnosis 5, action d) b. perform actions *to maintain adequate circulation to wound area:* 1. implement measures to maintain adequate tissue perfusion (see Diagnosis 1, action b) 2. do not apply dressings tightly unless ordered *(excessive pressure impairs circulation to the area)* c. perform actions *to protect the wound from mechanical injury:* 1. ensure that dressings are secure enough to keep them from rubbing and irritating wound 2. carefully remove tape and dressings when performing wound care 3. remind client to keep hands away from wound area 4. implement measures to prevent falls (see Diagnosis 18, action a) d. perform actions *to decrease stress on wound area:* 1. instruct and assist client to support the involved area when moving 2. instruct and assist client to splint abdominal and chest wounds when coughing 3. apply an abdominal binder during periods of activity if ordered *for additional support following abdominal surgery* 4. implement measures to reduce the accumulation of gas and fluid in the gastrointestinal tract (see Diagnosis 7, action b) in clients who have had abdominal surgery 5. implement measures to prevent nausea and vomiting (see Diagnosis 8, action b) in clients who have had chest, back, or abdominal surgery e. perform actions to prevent wound infection (see Diagnosis 17, action b.2). 3. If signs and symptoms of impaired wound healing occur: a. perform or assist with wound care (e.g., debridement, packing, irrigation) as ordered b. prepare client for surgical revision of the wound if planned.
10.b. The client will maintain tissue integrity in areas in contact with wound drainage, tape, and tubings as evidenced by: 1. absence of redness and irritation 2. no skin breakdown.	10.b.1. Inspect skin areas that are in contact with wound drainage, tape, and tubings for signs of irritation and breakdown. 2. Implement measures *to prevent tissue irritation and breakdown in areas in contact with wound drainage, tape, and tubings:* a. perform actions *to prevent wound drainage from contacting or remaining on skin:* 1. inspect dressings, wounds, and areas around drains and puncture sites; cleanse skin and change dressings when appropriate 2. maintain patency of drainage tubes *to decrease risk of leakage around the tubes* 3. apply a collection device over drains and incisions that are draining continuously and/or copiously

4. apply a protective barrier product to skin that is likely to be in frequent contact with drainage
b. when positioning client, ensure that he/she is not lying on tubings *(pressure on the skin can compromise circulation to that area; in addition, if a drainage tubing is occluded, there is an increased risk for leakage of drainage around the tube)*
c. anchor all tubings securely *to prevent excessive movement of tubes against tissues*
d. apply a water-soluble lubricant to external nares every 2–4 hours *to decrease irritation from nasogastric tube and nasal airway or cannula*
e. perform actions *to decrease skin irritation resulting from the use of tape:*
   1. use only necessary amount of tape
   2. use hypoallergenic tape whenever possible
   3. apply skin sealant or barrier before applying tape if indicated
   4. use Montgomery straps or tubular netting *to avoid repeated application and removal of tape if frequent dressing changes are anticipated*
   5. when removing tape, pull it in the direction of hair growth; use adhesive solvents if necessary.

3. If tissue breakdown occurs:
   a. notify appropriate health care provider (e.g., physician, wound care specialist)
   b. perform care of involved areas as ordered or per standard hospital procedure.

11. NURSING DIAGNOSIS: ACTIVITY INTOLERANCE

related to:
a. tissue hypoxia associated with anemia if present;
b. inadequate nutritional status;
c. difficulty resting and sleeping associated with discomfort, fear, and anxiety.

Suggested NOC Outcomes: Energy conservation; Rest; Self-care: activities of daily living; Activity tolerance

Suggested NIC Interventions: Energy management; Nutrition management; Sleep enhancement; Pain management

Desired Outcome	Nursing Actions *and Selected Purposes/Rationales* (see pp. 11–12 for additional rationales)
11. The client will demonstrate an increased tolerance for activity as evidenced by: a. verbalization of feeling less fatigued and weak b. ability to perform activities of daily living without exertional dyspnea, chest pain, diaphoresis, dizziness,.and a significant change in vital signs.	11.a. Assess for signs and symptoms of activity intolerance: 1. statements of fatigue or weakness 2. exertional dyspnea, chest pain, diaphoresis, or dizziness 3. abnormal heart rate response to activity (e.g., increase in rate of 20 beats/minute above resting rate, rate not returning to preactivity level within 3 minutes after stopping activity, change from regular to irregular rate) 4. a significant change (15–20 mm Hg) in blood pressure with activity. b. Implement measures *to improve activity tolerance:* 1. perform actions *to promote rest and/or conserve energy:* a. maintain activity restrictions as ordered b. minimize environmental activity and noise c. organize nursing care to allow for periods of uninterrupted rest d. limit number of visitors and their length of stay e. assist client with self-care activities as needed f. keep supplies and personal articles within easy reach g. instruct client in energy-saving techniques (e.g., using shower chair when showering, sitting to brush teeth or comb hair) h. implement measures to reduce fear and anxiety (see Diagnosis 21, action b) i. implement measures to promote sleep (see Diagnosis 16, action b) j. implement measures to reduce discomfort (see Diagnoses 6, action d; 7, action b; and 8, action b)

Desired Outcome	Nursing Actions *and Selected Purposes/Rationales*
	2. perform actions to improve breathing pattern and facilitate airway clearance (see Diagnoses 2, action b and 3, action b) *in order to promote maximum tissue oxygenation* 3. maintain oxygen therapy as ordered 4. perform actions to maintain an adequate nutritional status (see Diagnosis 5, action d) 5. administer packed red blood cells if ordered 6. increase client's activity gradually as allowed and tolerated. c. Instruct client to: 1. report a decreased tolerance for activity 2. stop any activity that causes chest pain, shortness of breath, dizziness, or extreme fatigue or weakness. d. Consult physician if signs and symptoms of activity intolerance persist or worsen.

12. Nursing Diagnosis: ***IMPAIRED PHYSICAL MOBILITY***

related to:
a. weakness and fatigue associated with tissue hypoxia, inadequate nutritional status, and difficulty resting and sleeping;
b. pain and nausea;
c. depressant effect of anesthesia and some medications (e.g., narcotic [opioid] analgesics, some antiemetics);
d. fear of falling, dislodging tubes, and compromising surgical wound;
e. activity restrictions imposed by the treatment plan.

Suggested NOC Outcome: Mobility

Suggested NIC Interventions: Exercise therapy: ambulation; Environmental management

Desired Outcome	Nursing Actions *and Selected Purposes/Rationales*
12. The client will achieve maximum physical mobility within the limitations imposed by the surgical procedure and postoperative treatment plan.	12.a. Implement measures *to increase mobility:* 1. perform actions to improve activity tolerance (see Diagnosis 11, action b) *in order to reduce weakness and fatigue* 2. perform actions to reduce pain (see Diagnosis 6, action d) 3. perform actions to prevent nausea and vomiting (see Diagnosis 8, action b) 4. schedule attempts to increase activity when analgesics and/or antiemetics are at peak effect 5. encourage use of nonnarcotic analgesics rather than narcotic (opioid) analgesics once severe pain has subsided 6. perform actions *to decrease client's fear of injury:* a. implement measures to prevent falls (see Diagnosis 18, action a) b. anchor all dressings and tubings securely *to decrease risk of inadvertent removal during activity* 7. assure client that level of activity ordered is expected to facilitate rather than compromise wound healing and postoperative recovery 8. encourage activity and participation in self-care as allowed and tolerated; put side rails up and provide overhead trapeze if appropriate *to promote independent movement.* b. Encourage the support of significant others. Allow them to assist client with activity unless contraindicated. c. Consult appropriate health care provider (e.g., physician, physical therapist) if client is unable to achieve expected level of mobility.

13. Nursing Diagnosis: ***SELF-CARE DEFICIT***

related to impaired physical mobility associated with weakness, fatigue, pain, nausea, depressant effect of some medications, fear of dislodging tubes and compromising surgical wound, and activity restrictions.

Suggested NOC Outcome: Self-care: activities of daily living

Suggested NIC Intervention: Self-care assistance

Desired Outcome	Nursing Actions *and Selected Purposes/Rationales*
13. The client will perform self-care activities within physical limitations and postoperative activity restrictions.	13.a. With client, develop a realistic plan for meeting daily physical needs. b. Implement measures *to facilitate the client's ability to perform self-care activities:* 1. schedule care at a time when client is most likely to be able to participate (e.g., when analgesics are at peak effect, after rest periods, not immediately after meals or treatments) 2. keep needed objects within easy reach 3. allow adequate time for accomplishment of self-care activities 4. perform actions to increase physical mobility (see Diagnosis 12, action a). c. Encourage maximum independence within physical limitations and postoperative activity restrictions. d. Assist the client with activities he/she is unable to perform independently. e. Inform significant others of client's abilities to perform own care. Explain the importance of encouraging and allowing client to maintain an optimal level of independence.

14. NURSING DIAGNOSIS: URINARY RETENTION

related to:

a. increased tone of the urinary sphincters associated with sympathetic nervous system stimulation resulting from pain, fear, and anxiety;
b. decreased perception of bladder fullness associated with depressant effect of anesthesia and some medications (e.g., narcotic [opioid] analgesics);
c. relaxation of the bladder muscle associated with depressant effect of anesthesia and some medications (e.g., narcotic [opioid] analgesics) and stimulation of the sympathetic nervous system (can result from pain, fear, and anxiety).

Suggested NOC Outcome: Urinary elimination

Suggested NIC Intervention: Urinary retention care

Desired Outcome	Nursing Actions *and Selected Purposes/Rationales* (see pp. 61–62 for additional rationales)
14. The client will not experience urinary retention as evidenced by: a. voiding at normal intervals b. no reports of bladder fullness and suprapubic discomfort c. absence of bladder distention and dribbling of urine d. balanced intake and output within 48 hours following surgery.	14.a. Assess for signs and symptoms of urinary retention: 1. frequent voiding of small amounts (25–60 ml) of urine 2. reports of bladder fullness or suprapubic discomfort 3. bladder distention 4. dribbling of urine. b. Monitor intake and output. Consult physician if there is no urine output within 6–8 hours after surgery or if output continues to be less than intake 48 hours after surgery (for first 48 hours postoperatively, urine output is expected to be less than intake *due to factors such as blood loss and increased secretion of ADH*). c. Implement measures *to prevent urinary retention:* 1. instruct client to urinate when the urge is first felt 2. perform actions *to promote relaxation during voiding attempts* (e.g., provide privacy, hold a warm blanket against abdomen, encourage client to read) 3. perform actions *that may help trigger the micturition reflex and promote a sense of relaxation during voiding attempts* (e.g., run water, place client's hands in warm water, pour warm water over perineum) 4. allow client to assume a normal position for voiding unless contraindicated

Desired Outcome	Nursing Actions *and Selected Purposes/Rationales*
	5. instruct client to lean upper body forward and/or gently press downward on lower abdomen during voiding attempts unless contraindicated *in order to put pressure on the bladder (pressure helps create a sensation of bladder fullness, which stimulates the micturition reflex)* 6. perform actions to reduce postoperative pain (see diagnosis 6, action d) 7. encourage use of nonnarcotic rather than narcotic (opioid) analgesics once period of severe pain has subsided 8. administer cholinergic (parasympathomimetic) drugs (e.g., bethanechol) if ordered *to stimulate bladder contraction.* d. Consult physician regarding intermittent catheterization or insertion of an indwelling catheter if above actions fail to alleviate urinary retention. e. If urinary catheter is present, prevent urinary retention by maintaining patency of the catheter (e.g., keep tubing free of kinks, irrigate as ordered).

15. Nursing Diagnosis: RISK FOR CONSTIPATION

related to:
a. decreased gastrointestinal motility associated with manipulation of bowel during abdominal surgery, depressant effect of anesthesia and narcotic (opioid) analgesics, and decreased activity;
b. decreased fluid intake;
c. decreased intake of foods high in fiber.

Suggested NOC Outcome: Bowel elimination

Suggested NIC Intervention: Constipation/Impaction management

Desired Outcome	Nursing Actions *and Selected Purposes/Rationales* (see pp. 24–26 for additional rationales)
15. The client will not experience constipation as evidenced by: a. usual frequency of bowel movements about two days after usual oral intake is resumed b. passage of soft, formed stool c. absence of increasing abdominal distention and pain, feeling of rectal fullness or pressure, and straining during defecation.	15.a. Assess for signs and symptoms of constipation (e.g., decrease in frequency of bowel movements; passage of hard, formed stools; anorexia; increasing abdominal distention and pain; feeling of fullness or pressure in rectum; straining during defecation). b. Assess bowel sounds. Report a pattern of diminishing sounds or sounds that do not return to normal when expected. c. Implement measures *to prevent constipation:* 1. increase activity as allowed and tolerated 2. encourage client to defecate whenever the urge is felt 3. assist client to the bathroom or bedside commode or place in high Fowler's position on bedpan for bowel movements unless contraindicated 4. encourage client to relax, provide privacy, and have call signal within reach during attempts to defecate *(measures to promote relaxation enable client to relax the levator ani muscle and external anal sphincter, which facilitates evacuation of stool)* 5. encourage client to establish a regular time for defecation, preferably an hour after a meal 6. encourage use of nonnarcotic rather than narcotic (opioid) analgesics once period of severe pain has subsided 7. when oral intake is allowed: a. instruct client to maintain a minimum fluid intake of 2500 ml/day unless contraindicated b. encourage client to drink hot liquids upon arising in the morning *in order to stimulate peristalsis* c. when diet advances, instruct client to increase intake of foods high in fiber (e.g., bran, whole-grain breads and cereals, fresh fruits and vegetables) unless contraindicated

8. administer laxatives or cathartics and/or enemas if ordered.

d. Consult appropriate health care provider if signs and symptoms of constipation persist.

16. NURSING DIAGNOSIS:

DISTURBED SLEEP PATTERN

related to fear, anxiety, discomfort, inability to assume usual sleep position, and frequent assessments and treatments.

Suggested NOC Outcome: Sleep

Suggested NIC Intervention: Sleep enhancement

Desired Outcome	Nursing Actions *and Selected Purposes/Rationales* (see pp. 52–54 for additional rationales)
16. The client will attain optimal amounts of sleep as evidenced by statements of feeling well rested.	16.a. Assess for signs and symptoms of a disturbed sleep pattern (e.g., statements of difficulty falling asleep, interrupted sleep, or not feeling well rested).

b. Implement measures *to promote sleep:*
   1. discourage long periods of sleep during the day unless signs and symptoms of sleep deprivation exist or daytime sleep is usual for client
   2. perform actions to reduce fear and anxiety (see Diagnosis 21, action b)
   3. perform actions to reduce discomfort (see Diagnoses 6, action d; 7, action b; and 8, action b)
   4. encourage participation in relaxing diversional activities during the evening
   5. when oral intake is allowed:
      a. discourage intake of foods and fluids high in caffeine (e.g., chocolate, coffee, tea, colas) in the evening
      b. offer client an evening snack that includes milk unless contraindicated *(milk contains L-tryptophan, which is believed to help induce and maintain sleep)*
   6. allow client to continue usual sleep practices (e.g., position; time; presleep routines such as reading, watching television, listening to music, and meditating) whenever possible
   7. satisfy basic needs such as comfort and warmth before sleep
   8. encourage client to urinate just before bedtime
   9. reduce environmental distractions (e.g., close door to client's room; use night light rather than overhead light whenever possible; lower volume of paging system; keep staff conversations at a low level and away from client's room; close curtains between clients in a semi-private room or ward; keep beepers and alarms on low volume; provide client with "white noise" such as fan, soft music, or tape-recorded sounds of the ocean or rain; have earplugs available for client if needed)
   10. encourage client to avoid smoking before bedtime *(nicotine is a stimulant)*
   11. if possible, administer medications that can interfere with sleep (e.g., steroids, diuretics) early in the day rather than late afternoon or evening
   12. administer prescribed sedative-hypnotics if indicated
   13. perform actions *to reduce interruptions during sleep (70–100 minutes of uninterrupted sleep is usually needed to complete one sleep cycle):*
      a. restrict visitors
      b. group care (e.g., medications, treatments, physical care, assessments) whenever possible.

c. Consult appropriate health care provider if signs and symptoms of sleep deprivation (e.g., irritability, lethargy, agitation, inability to concentrate) occur and persist or worsen.

17. Nursing Diagnosis: RISK FOR INFECTION

a. pneumonia related to stasis of pulmonary secretions and aspiration (if it occurs);
b. wound infection related to:
   1. wound contamination associated with introduction of pathogens during or following surgery
   2. decreased resistance to infection associated with factors such as diminished tissue perfusion of wound area and inadequate nutritional status;
c. urinary tract infection related to:
   1. increased growth and colonization of microorganisms associated with urinary stasis
   2. introduction of pathogens associated with an indwelling catheter if present.

Suggested NOC Outcomes: Immune status; Infection severity; Wound healing: primary intention; Wound healing: secondary intention

Suggested NIC Interventions: Infection protection; Infection control; Cough enhancement; Airway management; Tube care; Incision site care; Wound care; Urinary retention care

Desired Outcomes	Nursing Actions *and Selected Purposes/Rationales* (see pp. 37–40 for additional rationales)
17.a. The client will not develop pneumonia as evidenced by: 1. normal breath sounds 2. resonant percussion note over lungs 3. absence of tachypnea 4. cough productive of clear mucus only 5. afebrile status 6. absence of pleuritic pain 7. WBC count declining toward normal 8. blood gases within normal range for client 9. negative sputum culture.	17.a.1. Assess for and report signs and symptoms of pneumonia: a. abnormal breath sounds (e.g., crackles [rales], pleural friction rub, bronchial breath sounds, diminished or absent breath sounds) b. dull percussion note over affected lung area c. increase in respiratory rate d. cough productive of purulent, green, or rust-colored sputum e. chills and fever f. pleuritic pain g. persistent elevation of or increase in WBC count h. abnormal oximetry and blood gas results i. positive sputum culture results j. chest x-ray results indicative of pneumonia. 2. Implement measures *to prevent pneumonia:* a. perform actions to maintain an effective breathing pattern and airway clearance (see Diagnoses 2, action b and 3, action b) b. perform actions to reduce risk for aspiration (see Diagnosis 19, action b) c. encourage and assist client to perform frequent oral hygiene *in order to remove pathogens and secretions that could be aspirated* d. replace or cleanse equipment used for respiratory care as often as needed e. protect client from persons with respiratory tract infections. 3. If signs and symptoms of pneumonia occur: a. administer oxygen as ordered b. administer antimicrobials if ordered.
17.b. The client will remain free of wound infection as evidenced by: 1. absence of chills and fever 2. absence of redness, heat, swelling, and increased pain in wound area 3. usual drainage from wounds	17.b.1. Assess for and report signs and symptoms of wound infection (e.g., chills; fever; redness, heat, swelling, and increased pain in wound area; unusual wound drainage; foul odor from wound area; persistent elevation of WBC count and significant change in differential; positive results of wound drainage cultures). 2. Implement measures *to prevent wound infection:* a. perform actions to promote wound healing (see Diagnosis 10, actions a.2.a–d) b. perform actions *to reduce the introduction of pathogens into the wound:* 1. use good hand hygiene and encourage client to do the same

4. WBC and differential counts returning toward normal
5. negative cultures of wound drainage.

2. instruct client to avoid touching incisions, dressings, drainage tubings, and open wounds
3. use sterile technique during all dressing changes and wound care
4. replace equipment and solutions used for wound care according to hospital policy *in order to reduce the risk of colonization of microorganisms*
5. anchor wound drainage tubings securely *to reduce in-and-out movement of the tubes*
6. maintain a closed system for wound drains whenever possible
7. protect client from others with infections

c. administer antimicrobials if ordered.

3. Consult appropriate health care provider if signs and symptoms of infection are present.

17.c. The client will remain free of urinary tract infection as evidenced by:
1. clear urine
2. absence of frequency, urgency, and burning on urination
3. absence of chills and fever
4. urinalysis showing fewer than 5 WBCs, negative leukocyte esterase and nitrites, and absence of bacteria
5. negative urine culture.

17.c.1. Assess for and report signs and symptoms of urinary tract infection (e.g., cloudy urine; reports of frequency, urgency, or burning on urination; chills; elevated temperature; urinalysis showing a WBC count greater than 5, positive leukocyte esterase or nitrites, or presence of bacteria; positive urine culture).

2. Implement measures *to prevent urinary tract infection*:
   a. perform actions to prevent urinary retention (see Diagnosis 14, actions c–e)
   b. instruct female client to wipe from front to back after urinating or defecating
   c. assist client with perineal care routinely and after each bowel movement
   d. maintain fluid intake of at least 2500 ml/day unless contraindicated *to promote urine formation and subsequent voiding, which flushes pathogens from the bladder and urethra*
   e. increase activity as allowed and tolerated *to decrease urinary stasis*
   f. maintain sterile technique during urinary catheterizations and irrigations
   g. if an indwelling urinary catheter is present:
      1. secure the catheter tubing to lower abdomen or thigh on males or to thigh on females *to minimize risk of accidental traction on the catheter and subsequent trauma to the bladder and urethra*
      2. perform catheter care as often as needed *to prevent accumulation of mucus around the meatus*
      3. anchor tubing securely *to reduce the amount of in-and-out movement of the catheter (this movement can result in the introduction of pathogens into the urinary tract and can cause tissue trauma, which can result in colonization of microorganisms)*
      4. maintain a closed drainage system whenever possible *to reduce the risk of the introduction of pathogens into the urinary tract*
      5. keep urine collection container lower than level of the bladder at all times *to prevent reflux or stasis of urine*
      6. remove catheter as soon as allowed *(the risk for urinary tract infection increases the longer the catheter is in place)*.

3. If signs and symptoms of urinary tract infection are present, administer antimicrobials if ordered.

18. NURSING DIAGNOSIS: RISK FOR FALLS

related to:

a. weakness and fatigue;
b. dizziness or syncope associated with postural hypotension resulting from peripheral pooling of blood and blood loss during surgery;
c. central nervous system depressant effect of some medications (e.g., narcotic [opioid] analgesics, some antiemetics);
d. presence of tubings or equipment.

Suggested NOC Outcomes: Fall prevention behavior; Falls occurrence

Suggested NIC Interventions: Fall prevention, Environmental management

Desired Outcome	Nursing Actions *and Selected Purposes/Rationales*
18. The client will not experience falls.	18.a. Implement measures *to prevent falls:* 1. keep bed in low position with side rails up when client is in bed 2. keep needed items within easy reach 3. encourage client to request assistance whenever needed; have call signal within easy reach 4. use lap belt when client is in chair if indicated 5. instruct client to wear well-fitting slippers/shoes with nonslip soles and low heels when ambulating 6. keep floor free of clutter and wipe up spills promptly 7. instruct and assist client to rise and change positions slowly *in order to reduce dizziness or syncope associated with postural hypotension* 8. carefully position tubings and equipment so that they will not interfere with ambulation 9. provide ambulatory aids (e.g., walker, cane) if client is weak or unsteady on feet 10. accompany client during ambulation and use a transfer safety belt if he/she is weak or dizzy 11. instruct client to ambulate in well-lit areas and to utilize handrails if needed 12. do not rush client; allow adequate time for ambulation to the bathroom and in hallway 13. make sure that shower area has a nonslip bottom surface and that shower chair, secure bath mat, call signal, grab bars, and adequate lighting are present 14. perform actions to increase strength and improve activity tolerance (see Diagnosis 11, action b). b. Include client and significant others in planning and implementing measures to prevent falls. c. If client falls, initiate first aid measures if appropriate and notify physician.

19. Nursing Diagnosis: *RISK FOR ASPIRATION*

related to:

a. decreased level of consciousness and absent or diminished gag reflex associated with depressant effect of anesthesia and narcotic (opioid) analgesics;
b. supine positioning;
c. increased risk for gastroesophageal reflux associated with increased gastric pressure resulting from decreased gastrointestinal motility.

Suggested NOC Outcomes: Respiratory status: airway patency; Aspiration prevention; Respiratory status: gas exchange

Suggested NIC Interventions: Respiratory monitoring; Aspiration precautions; Airway suctioning

Desired Outcome	Nursing Actions *and Selected Purposes/Rationales* (see pp. 16–18 for additional rationales)
19. The client will not aspirate secretions, vomitus, or foods/fluids as evidenced by: a. clear breath sounds b. resonant percussion note over lungs c. absence of cough, tachypnea, and dyspnea.	19.a. Assess for and report signs and symptoms of aspiration of secretions, vomitus, or foods/fluids (e.g., rhonchi, dull percussion note over affected lung area, cough, tachypnea, dyspnea, tachycardia, chest x-ray results showing pulmonary infiltrate). b. Implement measures *to reduce the risk for aspiration:* 1. withhold oral foods/fluids and place client in a side-lying position unless contraindicated if gag reflex is absent or client is not alert 2. perform oropharyngeal suctioning and provide oral hygiene as often as needed *to remove secretions, vomitus, and/or food particles* 3. perform actions to prevent nausea and vomiting (see Diagnosis 8, action b) 4. perform actions to reduce accumulation of gas and fluid in the gastrointestinal tract (see Diagnosis 7, action b) *in order to prevent gastric distention and gastroesophageal reflux* 5. place client in high Fowler's position during and for at least 30 minutes after eating or drinking unless contraindicated. c. If signs and symptoms of aspiration occur: 1. perform tracheal suctioning 2. withhold oral intake 3. prepare client for chest x-ray.

20. COLLABORATIVE DIAGNOSES: ***POTENTIAL COMPLICATIONS FOLLOWING SURGERY***

a. hypovolemic shock related to:
   1. hemorrhage associated with opening of wound (can occur as a result of inadequate wound closure, stress on incision line, and/or poor wound healing), slippage of closures on ligated vessels, and/or disruption of clots at incision site
   2. deficient fluid volume associated with restricted oral intake and excessive fluid loss;

b. atelectasis related to shallow respirations, stasis of secretions in the alveoli and bronchioles, and decreased surfactant production (results from inadequate deep breathing and changes in regional blood flow in the lungs);

c. thromboembolism related to:
   1. venous stasis associated with decreased activity, positioning during and following surgery, increased blood viscosity (can result from deficient fluid volume), and abdominal distention (the distended intestine may put pressure on the abdominal vessels)
   2. hypercoagulability associated with increased release of tissue thromboplastin into the blood (occurs as a result of surgical trauma) and hemoconcentration and increased blood viscosity (can occur as a result of deficient fluid volume)
   3. trauma to vein walls during surgery;

d. paralytic ileus related to manipulation of intestines during abdominal surgery, depressant effect of anesthesia and some medications (e.g., narcotic [opioid] analgesics, some antiemetics) on bowel motility, hypokalemia, and hypovolemia (can cause decreased blood supply to the intestine);

e. dehiscence related to:
   1. inadequate wound closure
   2. stress on incision line associated with persistent coughing, distention, or vomiting
   3. poor wound healing associated with decreased tissue perfusion of wound area, inadequate nutritional status, and infection.

Desired Outcomes	Nursing Actions *and Selected Purposes/Rationales*

20.a. The client will not develop hypovolemic shock as evidenced by:
1. usual mental status
2. stable vital signs
3. skin warm and usual color
4. palpable peripheral pulses
5. urine output at least 30 ml/hour.

20.a.1. Assess for and report signs and symptoms of hypovolemic shock:
- a. restlessness, agitation, confusion, or other change in mental status
- b. significant decrease in B/P
- c. postural hypotension
- d. rapid, weak pulse
- e. rapid respirations
- f. cool skin
- g. pallor, cyanosis
- h. diminished or absent peripheral pulses
- i. urine output less than 30 ml/hour.

2. Implement measures *to prevent hypovolemic shock:*
- a. if bleeding occurs, apply firm, prolonged pressure to area if possible
- b. perform actions to prevent deficient fluid volume (see Diagnosis 4, actions a.2.a–f).

3. If signs and symptoms of hypovolemic shock occur:
- a. place client flat in bed with legs elevated unless contraindicated
- b. monitor vital signs frequently
- c. administer oxygen as ordered
- d. administer blood and/or volume expanders if ordered
- e. prepare client for insertion of hemodynamic monitoring devices (e.g., central venous catheter, intra-arterial catheter) if indicated.

20.b. The client will not develop atelectasis as evidenced by:
1. clear, audible breath sounds
2. resonant percussion note over lungs
3. unlabored respirations at 12–20/minute
4. pulse rate within normal range for client
5. afebrile status.

20.b.1. Assess for and report signs and symptoms of atelectasis (e.g., diminished or absent breath sounds, dull percussion note over affected area, increased respiratory rate, dyspnea, tachycardia, elevated temperature, chest x-ray results showing atelectasis).

2. Implement measures *to prevent atelectasis:*
- a. perform actions to improve breathing pattern (see Diagnosis 2, action b)
- b. perform actions to promote effective airway clearance (see Diagnosis 3, action b).

3. If signs and symptoms of atelectasis occur:
- a. increase frequency of position change, coughing or "huffing," deep breathing, and use of incentive spirometer
- b. consult physician if signs and symptoms of atelectasis persist or worsen.

20.c.1. The client will not develop a deep vein thrombus as evidenced by:
- a. absence of pain, tenderness, swelling, and distended superficial vessels in extremities
- b. usual temperature of extremities
- c. negative Homans' sign.

20.c.1.a. Assess for and report signs and symptoms of a deep vein thrombus:
1. pain or tenderness in extremity
2. increase in circumference of extremity
3. distention of superficial vessels in extremity
4. unusual warmth of extremity
5. positive Homans' sign (not always a reliable indicator).

b. Implement measures *to prevent thrombus formation*:
1. perform actions to prevent peripheral pooling of blood (see Diagnosis 1, action b.4)
2. maintain a minimum fluid intake of 2500 ml/day (unless contraindicated) *to prevent increased blood viscosity*
3. administer anticoagulants (e.g., low- or adjusted-dose heparin, fondaparinux, warfarin, low-molecular-weight heparin) if ordered.

c. If signs and symptoms of a deep vein thrombus occur:
1. maintain client on bed rest until activity orders received
2. elevate foot of bed 15–20° above heart level if ordered
3. discourage positions that compromise blood flow (e.g., pillows under knees, crossing legs, sitting for long periods)
4. prepare client for diagnostic studies (e.g., venography, duplex ultrasound, impedance plethysmography) if indicated
5. administer anticoagulants (e.g., heparin, fondaparinux, warfarin) if ordered.

20.c.2. The client will not experience a pulmonary embolism as evidenced by:
- a. absence of sudden chest pain
- b. unlabored respirations at 12–20/minute
- c. pulse 60–100 beats/minute
- d. blood gases within normal range.

20.c.2.a. Assess for and report signs and symptoms of a pulmonary embolism (e.g., sudden chest pain, dyspnea, tachypnea, tachycardia, apprehension, low PaO_2).

b. Implement measures *to prevent a pulmonary embolism:*
   1. perform actions to prevent and treat a deep vein thrombus (see actions c.1.b and c.1.c in this diagnosis)
   2. do not exercise, check for Homans' sign in, or massage any extremity known to have a thrombus
   3. caution client to avoid activities that create a Valsalva response (e.g., straining to have bowel movement, holding breath while moving up in bed) *in order to prevent dislodgment of existing thrombi*
   4. prepare client for a vena caval interruption (e.g., insertion of an intracaval filtering device) if planned.

c. If signs and symptoms of a pulmonary embolism occur:
   1. maintain client on strict bed rest in a semi- to high Fowler's position
   2. maintain oxygen therapy as ordered
   3. prepare client for diagnostic tests (e.g., blood gases, D-dimer level, ventilation-perfusion lung scan, pulmonary angiography)
   4. administer anticoagulants (e.g., heparin, warfarin) if ordered
   5. prepare client for the following if planned:
      - a. vena caval interruption (e.g., insertion of an intracaval filtering device) *to prevent further pulmonary emboli*
      - b. embolectomy.

20.d. The client will not develop a paralytic ileus as evidenced by:
1. absence or resolution of abdominal pain and cramping
2. soft, nondistended abdomen
3. gradual return of bowel sounds
4. passage of flatus.

20.d.1. Assess for and report signs and symptoms of paralytic ileus (e.g., development of or persistent abdominal pain and cramping; firm, distended abdomen; absent bowel sounds; failure to pass flatus; abdominal x-ray showing distended bowel).

2. Implement measures *to prevent paralytic ileus:*
   - a. increase activity as soon as allowed and tolerated
   - b. perform actions to prevent hypokalemia (see Diagnosis 4, action a.2) *in order to prevent the resultant decrease in peristalsis*
   - c. perform actions to maintain adequate tissue perfusion (see Diagnosis 1, action b) *in order to maintain adequate blood supply to the bowel*
   - d. administer gastrointestinal stimulants (e.g., metoclopramide) if ordered.

3. If signs and symptoms of paralytic ileus occur:
   - a. withhold all oral intake
   - b. insert nasogastric tube and maintain suction as ordered.

20.e. The client will not experience dehiscence as evidenced by intact, approximated wound edges.

20.e.1. Assess for and report evidence of dehiscence (separation of edges of the wound).

2. Implement measures to promote wound healing (see Diagnosis 10, action a.2) *in order to decrease the risk of dehiscence.*

3. If dehiscence occurs:
   - a. implement measures *to reduce stress on the wound* (e.g., limit movement of affected area; if client has a chest or abdominal incision, instruct him/her to avoid coughing; if client has an abdominal incision, place him/her on bed rest in a semi-Fowler's position with knees slightly flexed)
   - b. apply skin closures (e.g., butterfly tape, Steri-Strips) to the incision line if appropriate
   - c. cover wound with a sterile, nonadherent dressing
   - d. assist with resuturing the wound if indicated
   - e. if client has an abdominal incision, assess for and immediately report signs and symptoms of evisceration (e.g., client statements that "something popped" or "gave way," sudden profuse drainage of serosanguineous fluid from wound; protrusion of intestinal contents).

21. Nursing Diagnosis: FEAR/ANXIETY

related to unfamiliar environment; pain; lack of understanding of surgical procedure performed, diagnosis, and postoperative treatment plan; possible change in body image and roles; and financial concerns.

Suggested NOC Outcomes:
Anxiety level; Fear level; Anxiety self-control; Fear self-control

Suggested NIC Interventions: Anxiety reduction; Calming technique; Emotional support; Presence; Pain management

Desired Outcome

21. The client will experience a reduction in fear and anxiety as evidenced by:
    a. verbalization of feeling less anxious
    b. usual sleep pattern
    c. relaxed facial expression and body movements
    d. stable vital signs
    e. usual perceptual ability and interactions with others.

Nursing Actions *and Selected Purposes/Rationales*

(see pp. 14–16 for additional rationales)

21.a. Assess client for signs and symptoms of fear and anxiety (e.g., verbalization of feeling anxious, insomnia, tenseness, shakiness, restlessness, diaphoresis, tachycardia, elevated blood pressure, self-focused behaviors). Validate perceptions carefully, remembering that some behavior may result from factors such as pain, fluid and electrolyte imbalances, and infection.

b. Implement measures *to reduce fear and anxiety:*
   1. orient client to environment, equipment, and routines
   2. introduce client to staff who will be participating in care; if possible, maintain consistency in staff assigned to his/her care
   3. assure client that staff members are nearby; respond to call signal as soon as possible
   4. maintain a calm, supportive, confident manner when interacting with client
   5. encourage verbalization of fear and anxiety; provide feedback
   6. reinforce the physician's explanations and clarify any misconceptions the client has about the diagnosis, surgical procedure performed, treatment plan, and prognosis
   7. perform actions to reduce pain (see Diagnosis 6, action d)
   8. provide a calm, restful environment
   9. instruct client in relaxation techniques and encourage participation in diversional activities
   10. assist client to identify specific stressors and ways to cope with them
   11. provide information based on current needs of client at a level he/she can understand; encourage questions and clarification of information provided
   12. when appropriate, assist client to meet spiritual needs (e.g., arrange for a visit from clergy)
   13. initiate social service referral and/or assist client to identify and contact appropriate community agencies if indicated
   14. encourage significant others to project a caring, concerned attitude without obvious anxiousness
   15. include significant others in orientation and teaching sessions and encourage their continued support of the client
   16. administer prescribed antianxiety agents if indicated.

c. Consult appropriate health care provider if above actions fail to control fear and anxiety.

Discharge Teaching/Continued Care

22. NURSING DIAGNOSIS: DEFICIENT KNOWLEDGE, INEFFECTIVE THERAPEUTIC REGIMEN MANAGEMENT, OR INEFFECTIVE HEALTH MAINTENANCE*

*The nurse should select the diagnostic label that is most appropriate for the client's discharge teaching needs.

Suggested NOC Outcome: Knowledge: treatment regimen

Suggested NIC Interventions: Teaching: individual; Teaching: prescribed activity/exercise; Teaching: prescribed medication; Health system guidance

Desired Outcomes	Nursing Actions *and Selected Purposes/Rationales*
22.a. The client will identify ways to prevent postoperative infection.	22.a. Instruct client in ways to prevent postoperative infection: 1. continue with coughing (unless contraindicated) and deep breathing every 2 hours while awake 2. continue to use incentive spirometer if activity is limited 3. increase activity as ordered 4. avoid contact with persons who have infections 5. avoid crowds during flu and cold seasons 6. decrease or stop smoking 7. drink at least 10 glasses of liquid/day unless contraindicated 8. maintain a balanced nutritional intake 9. maintain proper balance of rest and activity 10. maintain good personal hygiene (especially oral care, hand washing, and perineal care) 11. avoid touching any wound unless it is completely healed 12. maintain sterile or clean technique as ordered during wound care.
22.b. The client will demonstrate the ability to perform wound care.	22.b. 1. Discuss the rationale for, frequency of, and equipment necessary for the prescribed wound care. 2. Provide client with the necessary supplies (e.g., dressings, irrigating solution, tape) for wound care and with names and addresses of places where additional supplies can be obtained. 3. Demonstrate wound care and proper cleansing of any reusable equipment. Allow time for questions, clarification, and return demonstration.
22.c. The client will state signs and symptoms to report to the health care provider.	22.c. Instruct the client to report the following signs and symptoms: 1. persistent low-grade or significantly elevated (38.3° C [101° F]) temperature 2. difficulty breathing 3. chest pain 4. cough productive of purulent, green, or rust-colored sputum 5. increasing weakness or inability to tolerate prescribed activity level 6. increasing discomfort or discomfort not controlled by prescribed medications and treatments 7. continued nausea or vomiting 8. increasing abdominal distention and/or discomfort 9. separation of wound edges 10. increasing redness, warmth, pain, or swelling around wound 11. unusual or excessive drainage from any wound site 12. pain or swelling in calf of one or both legs 13. urine retention 14. frequency, urgency, or burning on urination 15. cloudy or foul-smelling urine.

Desired Outcomes	Nursing Actions *and Selected Purposes/Rationales*
22.d. The client will verbalize an understanding of and a plan for adhering to recommended follow-up care including future appointments with health care provider, dietary modifications, activity level, treatments, and medications prescribed.	22.d.1. Reinforce importance of keeping scheduled follow-up appointments with the health care provider. 2. Reinforce physician's instructions about dietary modifications. Obtain a dietary consult for client if needed. 3. Reinforce physician's instructions on suggested activity level and treatment plan. 4. Explain the rationale for, side effects of, and importance of taking medications prescribed. Inform client of pertinent food and drug interactions. 5. Implement measures to improve client compliance: a. include significant others in teaching sessions if possible b. encourage questions and allow time for reinforcement and clarification of information provided c. provide written instructions on scheduled appointments with health care provider, dietary modifications, activity level, treatment plan, medications prescribed, and signs and symptoms to report.

Bibliography

See pages 879 and 880.

UNIT V

Nursing Care of the Immobile Client

IMMOBILITY

Immobility refers to a limitation of physical activity as a result of a disease process, trauma, or therapeutic intervention. Immobility or complete bed rest for periods greater than 48 to 72 hours will result in changes in all body systems.

This care plan focuses on the adult client who is on complete bed rest for a prolonged period. Many of the actions included in the care plan will help prevent disuse syndrome, which is a deterioration of body systems as a result of prescribed or unavoidable musculoskeletal inactivity. The information provided is applicable to clients receiving care in an acute or extended care facility or in a home setting.

OUTCOME/DISCHARGE CRITERIA

THE CLIENT WILL:

- have no signs or symptoms of complications of immobility
- have no evidence of tissue irritation or breakdown
- have clear, audible breath sounds throughout lungs
- have an adequate nutritional status
- verbalize an understanding of ways to prevent problems associated with continued decreased mobility
- demonstrate techniques for meeting self-care needs
- state signs and symptoms to report to the health care provider
- identify community agencies that can provide assistance with home care and transportation
- verbalize an understanding of and a plan for adhering to recommended follow-up care including future appointments with health care provider and physical therapist, exercise regimen, and medications prescribed.

NURSING/COLLABORATIVE DIAGNOSES

DISCHARGE TEACHING

1. Nursing Diagnosis: ***INEFFECTIVE BREATHING PATTERN***

related to:

a. decreased rate of respirations associated with the depressant effect of some medications (e.g., narcotic [opioid] analgesics, sedatives, centrally acting muscle relaxants) that may be given for treatment of current diagnosis;

b. decreased depth of respirations associated with:
   1. recumbent positioning (in this position, full expansion of the lungs is restricted by the bed surface and by the abdominal contents pushing up against the diaphragm)
   2. weakness, fear, and anxiety.

Suggested NOC Outcome: Respiratory status: ventilation

Suggested NIC Interventions: Respiratory monitoring; Ventilation assistance

Desired Outcome	**Nursing Actions** *and Suggested Purposes/Rationales* (see pp. 18–20 for additional rationales)
1. The client will maintain an effective breathing pattern as evidenced by normal rate and depth of respirations.	1.a. Assess for signs and symptoms of an ineffective breathing pattern (e.g., shallow or slow respirations). b. Implement measures *to improve breathing pattern:* 1. place client in a semi- to high Fowler's position unless contraindicated; position client with pillows *to prevent slumping* 2. if client must remain flat in bed, assist with position change at least every 2 hours unless contraindicated 3. instruct client to deep breathe or use incentive spirometer every 1–2 hours 4. perform actions to reduce chest or abdominal pain if present (e.g., splint chest/abdomen with a pillow when positioning, coughing, and deep breathing; administer prescribed analgesics) *in order to increase the client's willingness to move and breathe more deeply* 5. perform actions to decrease fear and anxiety (see Diagnosis 13, action b) *in order to prevent the shallow and/or rapid breathing that can occur with fear and anxiety* 6. assist with positive airway pressure techniques (e.g., continuous positive airway pressure [CPAP], bilevel positive airway pressure [BiPAP], flutter/positive expiratory pressure [PEP] device) if ordered 7. instruct client to avoid intake of gas-forming foods (e.g., beans, cauliflower, cabbage, onions), carbonated beverages, and large meals *in order to prevent gastric distention and additional pressure on the diaphragm* 8. increase activity as allowed 9. administer central nervous system depressants judiciously; hold medication and consult physician if respiratory rate is less than 12/minute. c. Consult appropriate health care provider (e.g., physician, respiratory therapist) if: 1. ineffective breathing pattern continues 2. signs and symptoms of impaired gas exchange (e.g., restlessness, irritability, confusion, significant decrease in oximetry results, decreased Pao_2 and increased $Paco_2$ levels) are present.

2. Nursing Diagnosis: ***INEFFECTIVE AIRWAY CLEARANCE***

related to stasis of secretions associated with:

a. decreased mobility;

b. decreased effectiveness of cough resulting from diminished lung/chest wall expansion, depressant effect of certain medications (e.g., narcotic [opioid] analgesics, centrally acting muscle relaxants, sedatives), and possible tenacious secretions if fluid intake is inadequate.

Suggested NOC Outcome:
Respiratory status: airway patency

Suggested NIC Interventions: Respiratory monitoring; Airway management; Cough enhancement; Chest physiotherapy

Desired Outcome	**Nursing Actions** *and Suggested Purposes/Rationales* (see pp. 12–14 for additional rationales)

2. The client will maintain clear, open airways as evidenced by:
   a. normal breath sounds
   b. normal rate and depth of respirations
   c. absence of dyspnea.

2.a. Assess for signs and symptoms of ineffective airway clearance (e.g., abnormal breath sounds; rapid, shallow respirations; dyspnea; cough).

b. Implement measures *to promote effective airway clearance:*
   1. perform actions to decrease pain if present (e.g., splint/protect painful area during movement, administer prescribed analgesics) *in order to increase the client's willingness to move, cough, and deep breathe*
   2. instruct and assist client to change position at least every 2 hours
   3. perform actions *to promote the removal of secretions:*
      a. instruct and assist client to deep breathe and cough or "huff" every 1–2 hours
      b. implement measures *to thin tenacious secretions and reduce drying of the respiratory mucous membrane:*
         1. maintain a fluid intake of at least 2500 ml/day unless contraindicated
         2. humidify inspired air as ordered
      c. assist with administration of mucolytics (e.g., acetylcysteine) and diluent or hydrating agents (e.g., water, saline) via nebulizer if ordered
      d. assist with or perform postural drainage therapy (PDT) if ordered
      e. perform suctioning if needed
   4. discourage smoking *(the irritants in smoke increase mucus production, impair ciliary function, and can cause inflammation and damage to the bronchial walls)*
   5. administer central nervous system depressants judiciously
   6. increase activity as allowed.

c. Consult appropriate health care provider (e.g., physician, respiratory therapist) if:
   1. signs and symptoms of ineffective airway clearance persist
   2. signs and symptoms of impaired gas exchange (e.g., restlessness, irritability, confusion, significant decrease in oximetry results, decreased PaO_2 and increased $PaCO_2$ levels) are present.

3. NURSING DIAGNOSIS: *IMBALANCED NUTRITION: LESS THAN BODY REQUIREMENTS*

related to:

a. decreased oral intake associated with:
   1. anorexia resulting from decreased activity, depression and social isolation, the effect of negative nitrogen balance, and early satiety that occurs with decreased gastrointestinal motility
   2. difficulty feeding self as a result of impaired or limited physical mobility;

b. increased nutritional needs associated with an imbalance in the rate of catabolism and anabolism (in the immobilized person, catabolic processes occur at a faster rate than anabolic processes).

Suggested NOC Outcome:
Nutritional status

Suggested NIC Interventions: Nutritional monitoring; Nutrition management; Nutrition therapy

Desired Outcome	**Nursing Actions** *and Suggested Purposes/Rationales* (see pp. 40–43 for additional rationales)

3. The client will maintain an adequate nutritional status as evidenced by:
   a. weight within normal range for client
   b. normal BUN and serum albumin, prealbumin, Hct, Hgb, and lymphocyte levels
   c. no further decline in strength and activity tolerance
   d. healthy oral mucous membrane.

3.a. Assess for and report signs and symptoms of malnutrition:
   1. weight below client's usual weight or below normal for client's age, height, and body frame
   2. abnormal BUN and low serum albumin, prealbumin, Hct, Hgb, and lymphocyte levels
   3. weakness and fatigue
   4. sore, inflamed oral mucous membrane
   5. pale conjunctiva.

b. Monitor percentage of meals and snacks client consumes. Report a pattern of inadequate intake.

c. Implement measures *to maintain an adequate nutritional status:*
   1. perform actions *to improve oral intake:*
      a. obtain a dietary consult if necessary to assist client in selecting foods/fluids that meet nutritional needs, are appealing, and adhere to personal and cultural preferences
      b. encourage a rest period before meals *to minimize fatigue*
      c. maintain a clean environment and relaxed, pleasant atmosphere
      d. provide oral hygiene before meals *(removes unpleasant tastes, which often improves the taste of foods/fluids)*
      e. serve frequent, small meals rather than large ones if client is weak, fatigues easily, and/or has a poor appetite
      f. implement measures to prevent gastrointestinal distention (e.g., perform actions to prevent constipation, administer prescribed gastrointestinal stimulants) *in order to prevent feeling of fullness and early satiety*
      g. encourage significant others to bring in client's favorite foods unless contraindicated and eat with him/her *to make eating more of a familiar social experience*
      h. encourage significant others to be present to assist client with meals if needed
      i. allow adequate time for meals; reheat foods/fluids if necessary
      j. limit fluid intake with meals (unless the fluid has high nutritional value) *to reduce early satiety and subsequent decreased food intake*
      k. enable client to feed self if possible; if client needs to be fed, offer foods/fluids in the order he/she prefers
      l. increase activity as allowed *(activity usually promotes a sense of well-being, which can improve appetite; it also promotes gastric emptying, which reduces feeling of fullness)*
   2. ensure that meals are well balanced and high in essential nutrients; offer high-protein, high-calorie dietary supplements if indicated
   3. administer vitamins and minerals if ordered.

d. Perform a calorie count if ordered. Report information to dietitian and physician.

e. Consult physician about an alternative method of providing nutrition (e.g., parenteral nutrition, tube feedings) if client does not consume enough food or fluids to meet nutritional needs.

4. Nursing Diagnosis: *RISK FOR IMPAIRED TISSUE INTEGRITY*

related to:

a accumulation of waste products and decreased oxygen and nutrient supply to the skin and subcutaneous tissue associated with reduced blood flow resulting from prolonged pressure on the tissues;

b damage to the skin and/or subcutaneous tissue associated with friction or shearing;

c increased fragility of the skin associated with dependent edema and inadequate nutritional status.

Suggested NOC Outcome:
Tissue integrity: skin and mucous membranes

Suggested NIC Interventions:
Skin surveillance; Pressure management; Positioning; Bed rest care; Skin care: topical treatments; Pressure ulcer prevention

Desired Outcome	Nursing Actions *and Suggested Purposes/Rationales* (see pp. 49–52 for additional rationales)

4. The client will maintain tissue integrity as evidenced by:
   a. absence of redness and irritation
   b. no skin breakdown.

4.a. Determine client's risk for skin breakdown using a risk assessment tool (e.g., Norton Scale, Braden Scale, Gosnell Scale).

b. Inspect the skin, especially bony prominences and dependent areas, for pallor, redness, and breakdown.

c. Implement measures *to prevent tissue breakdown:*
   1. assist client to turn at least every 2 hours unless contraindicated
   2. position client properly; use pressure-reducing or pressure-relieving devices (e.g., pillows, gel or foam cushions, alternating pressure mattress, air-fluidized bed, kinetic bed) if indicated
   3. gently massage around reddened areas at least every 2 hours
   4. apply a thin layer of a dry lubricant such as powder or cornstarch to bottom sheet or skin and to opposing skin surfaces (e.g., axillae, beneath breasts) if indicated *to reduce friction*
   5. lift and move client carefully using a turn sheet and adequate assistance
   6. perform actions to keep client from sliding down in bed (e.g., gatch knees slightly when head of bed is elevated 30° or higher) *in order to reduce the risk of skin surface abrasion and shearing*
   7. instruct or assist client to shift weight at least every 30 minutes
   8. keep client's skin clean
   9. thoroughly dry skin after bathing and as often as needed, paying special attention to skin folds and opposing skin surfaces (e.g., axillae, perineum, beneath breasts); pat skin dry rather than rub
   10. keep bed linens dry and wrinkle-free
   11. ensure that external devices such as braces, casts, and restraints are applied properly
   12. protect the skin from contact with urine and feces (e.g., keep perineal area clean and dry, apply a protective ointment or cream to perineal area)
   13. perform actions *to prevent drying of the skin:*
       a. encourage a fluid intake of 2500 ml/day unless contraindicated
       b. provide a mild soap for bathing
       c. apply moisturizing lotion and/or emollient to skin at least once a day
   14. apply a protective covering such as a hydrocolloid or transparent membrane dressing to areas of the skin susceptible to breakdown (e.g., coccyx, heels, elbows)
   15. perform actions to maintain an adequate nutritional status (see Diagnosis 3, action c)
   16. if edema is present:
       a. perform actions *to reduce fluid accumulation in dependent areas:*
          1. instruct client in and assist with range of motion exercises
          2. elevate affected extremities whenever possible
       b. handle edematous areas carefully
   17. increase activity as allowed.

d. If tissue breakdown occurs:
   1. notify appropriate health care provider (e.g., physician, wound care specialist)
   2. perform care of involved areas as ordered or per standard hospital procedure.

5. NURSING DIAGNOSIS: *RISK FOR ACTIVITY INTOLERANCE*

related to:

a. decrease in available energy associated with an inadequate nutritional status and a slowed metabolic rate when inactive;
b. loss of muscle mass, tone, and strength associated with disuse and inadequate nutritional status;

c. eventual decrease in cardiac reserve associated with:
   1. increased cardiac workload resulting from the increased venous return in a recumbent position
   2. decreased coronary blood flow resulting from a shortened diastolic filling time (a result of the progressive increase in heart rate that occurs when a person is immobile)
   3. weakening of the myocardium (not usually a factor until client has been immobilized for 3 weeks or longer);

d. difficulty resting and sleeping associated with inability to assume usual sleep position, frequent assessments and treatments, fear, anxiety, unfamiliar environment, and discomfort resulting from current illness/injury.

Suggested NOC Outcomes: Activity tolerance; Energy conservation

Suggested NIC Interventions: Energy management; Nutrition management; Sleep enhancement; Exercise therapy: muscle control

Desired Outcome	**Nursing Actions** *and Suggested Purposes/Rationales* (see pp. 11–12 for additional rationales)
5. The client will not experience activity intolerance as evidenced by: a. no reports of fatigue and weakness b. ability to perform activities of daily living within physical limitations/restrictions without exertional dyspnea, chest pain, diaphoresis, dizziness, and a significant change in vital signs.	5.a. Assess for signs and symptoms of activity intolerance: 1. statements of fatigue or weakness 2. exertional dyspnea, chest pain, diaphoresis, or dizziness 3. abnormal heart rate response to activity (e.g., increase in rate of 20 beats/minute above resting rate, rate not returning to preactivity level within 3 minutes after stopping activity, change from regular to irregular rate) 4. a significant change (15–20 mm Hg) in blood pressure with activity. b. Implement measures *to prevent activity intolerance:* 1. perform actions *to promote rest and/or conserve energy:* a. minimize environmental activity and noise b. organize nursing care to allow for periods of uninterrupted rest c. limit the number of visitors and their length of stay d. assist client with self-care activities as needed e. keep supplies and personal articles within easy reach f. implement measures to reduce fear and anxiety (see Diagnosis 13, action b) g. implement measures to promote sleep (see Diagnosis 10, action c) 2. perform additional actions *to reduce cardiac workload and help maintain adequate cardiac reserve:* a. place client in a semi- to high Fowler's position periodically if allowed b. instruct client to avoid activities that create a Valsalva response (e.g., straining to have a bowel movement, holding breath while moving up in bed) c. implement measures to improve breathing pattern and airway clearance (see Diagnoses 1, action b, and 2, action b) *in order to promote adequate tissue oxygenation* d. discourage smoking and excessive intake of beverages high in caffeine such as coffee, tea, and colas 3. perform actions to help maintain muscle strength (see Diagnosis 6, actions a.1–4) 4. perform actions to maintain an adequate nutritional status (see Diagnosis 3, action c) 5. when activity can be increased: a. increase activity gradually b. instruct client in energy-saving techniques (e.g., using shower chair when showering, sitting to brush teeth or comb hair). c. Instruct client to: 1. report a decreased tolerance for activity 2. stop any activity that causes chest pain, shortness of breath, dizziness, or extreme fatigue or weakness.

d. Consult physician if signs and symptoms of activity intolerance develop and persist or worsen.

6. NURSING DIAGNOSIS

IMPAIRED PHYSICAL MOBILITY

related to:
a. activity limitations imposed by current diagnosis and/or treatment plan;
b. loss of muscle mass, tone, and strength associated with prolonged disuse and inadequate nutritional status.

Suggested NOC Outcomes:
Joint movement;
Coordinated movement

Suggested NIC Interventions: Bed rest care; Exercise therapy: joint mobility; Exercise therapy: muscle control; Self-care assistance: IADL

Desired Outcome	Nursing Actions *and Suggested Purposes/Rationales*
6. The client will maintain maximum physical mobility within limitations imposed by the disease or injury and treatment plan.	6.a. Implement measures *to maintain optimal joint mobility and muscle function during period of immobility:* 1. instruct client in and assist with range of motion exercises at least 3 times/day unless contraindicated 2. reinforce instructions, activities, and exercise plan recommended by physical and occupational therapists 3. assist with use of electrical stimulation devices that promote muscle strengthening if ordered 4. encourage participation in self-care as allowed; put side rails up and provide overhead trapeze unless contraindicated *to promote independent movement* 5. perform actions to reduce the risk of contractures (see Diagnosis 12, actions d.2–6) 6. perform actions to maintain an adequate nutritional status (see Diagnosis 3, action c) *in order to help maintain muscle mass, tone, and strength.* b. Encourage the support of significant others. Allow them to assist with range of motion exercises and positioning unless contraindicated. c. Consult appropriate health care provider (e.g., physician, physical therapist) if client's mobility and range of motion are more limited than expected.

7. NURSING DIAGNOSIS

SELF-CARE DEFICIT

related to:
a. activity limitations imposed by current diagnosis and/or treatment plan;
b. weakness and fatigue associated with factors such as inadequate nutritional status, cardiac deconditioning, loss of muscle strength, and difficulty resting and sleeping.

Suggested NOC Outcome:
Self-care: activities of daily living

Suggested NIC Intervention: Self-care assistance

Desired Outcome	Nursing Actions *and Suggested Purposes/Rationales*
7. The client will perform self-care activities within physical limitations and activity restrictions imposed by current diagnosis and treatment plan.	7.a. With client, develop a realistic plan for meeting daily physical needs. b. Implement measures *to facilitate client's ability to perform self-care activities:* 1. schedule care at a time when client is most likely to be able to participate (e.g., when analgesics are at peak effect, after rest periods, not immediately after meals or treatments) 2. keep needed objects within easy reach 3. perform actions to prevent activity intolerance (see Diagnosis 5, action b) *in order to help maintain client's strength and prevent weakness and fatigue*

Desired Outcome	Nursing Actions *and Suggested Purposes/Rationales*
	4. perform actions to maintain optimal joint mobility and muscle function (see Diagnosis 6, action a) 5. consult occupational therapist about assistive devices available if indicated 6. allow adequate time for accomplishment of self-care activities. c. Encourage client to perform as much of self-care as possible within physical limitations and activity restrictions imposed by the current diagnosis and treatment plan. d. Assist the client with activities he/she is unable to perform independently. e. Inform significant others of client's abilities to perform own care. Explain importance of encouraging and allowing client to maintain an optimal level of independence within prescribed activity restrictions and physical capabilities.

8. NURSING DIAGNOSIS:

URINARY RETENTION

related to:

a. stasis of urine in the kidney and bladder associated with prolonged horizontal positioning;
b. difficulty urinating associated with anxiety regarding use of bedpan or urinal;
c. incomplete bladder emptying associated with:
   1. horizontal positioning (the gravity needed for complete bladder emptying is lost)
   2. decreased bladder muscle tone resulting from the generalized loss of muscle tone that occurs with prolonged immobility.

Suggested NOC Outcome: Urinary elimination

Suggested NIC Intervention: Urinary retention care

Desired Outcome	Nursing Actions *and Suggested Purposes/Rationales* (see pp. 61–62 for additional rationales)
8. The client will not experience urinary retention as evidenced by: a. voiding at normal intervals b. no reports of bladder fullness and suprapubic discomfort c. absence of bladder distention and dribbling of urine d. balanced intake and output.	8.a. Assess for signs and symptoms of urinary retention: 1. frequent voiding of small amounts (25–60 ml) of urine 2. reports of bladder fullness or suprapubic discomfort 3. bladder distention 4. dribbling of urine 5. output less than intake. b. Catheterize client if ordered *to determine the amount of residual urine.* c. Implement measures *to prevent urinary retention:* 1. instruct client to urinate when the urge is first felt 2. perform actions *to promote relaxation during voiding attempts* (e.g., provide privacy, hold a warm blanket against abdomen, encourage client to read) 3. perform actions *that may help trigger the micturition reflex and promote a sense of relaxation during voiding attempts* (e.g., run water, place client's hands in warm water, pour warm water over perineum) 4. allow client to assume a normal position for voiding unless contraindicated 5. instruct and/or assist client to lean upper body forward and/or gently press downward on lower abdomen during voiding attempts unless contraindicated *in order to put pressure on the bladder (pressure helps create a sensation of bladder fullness, which stimulates the micturition reflex)* 6. administer cholinergic (parasympathomimetic) drugs (e.g., bethanechol) if ordered *to stimulate bladder contraction.* d. Consult physician about intermittent catheterization or insertion of an indwelling catheter if above actions fail to alleviate urinary retention.

9. NURSING DIAGNOSIS:

RISK FOR CONSTIPATION

related to:
a. diminished defecation reflex associated with:
   1. suppression of urge to defecate because of lack of privacy and reluctance to use bedpan
   2. decreased gravity filling of lower rectum resulting from horizontal positioning;
b. weakened abdominal muscles associated with generalized loss of muscle tone resulting from prolonged immobility;
c. decreased gastrointestinal motility associated with decreased activity and the increased sympathetic nervous system activity that occurs with anxiety.

Suggested NOC Outcome:
Bowel elimination

Suggested NIC Intervention: Constipation/Impaction management

Desired Outcome	**Nursing Actions** *and Suggested Purposes/Rationales* (see pp. 24–26 for additional rationales)
9. The client will not experience constipation as evidenced by: a. usual frequency of bowel movements b. passage of soft, formed stool c. absence of abdominal distention and pain, feeling of rectal fullness or pressure, and straining during defecation.	9.a. Assess for signs and symptoms of constipation (e.g., decrease in frequency of bowel movements; passage of hard, formed stools; anorexia; abdominal distention and pain; feeling of fullness or pressure in rectum; straining during defecation). b. Assess bowel sounds. Report a pattern of decreasing bowel sounds. c. Implement measures *to prevent constipation:* 1. encourage client to defecate whenever the urge is felt 2. place client in high Fowler's position for bowel movements unless contraindicated 3. encourage client to relax, provide privacy, and have call signal within reach during attempts to defecate *(measures to promote relaxation enable client to relax the levator ani muscle and external anal sphincter, which facilitates evacuation of stool)* 4. encourage client to establish a regular time for defecation, preferably within an hour after a meal 5. instruct client to increase intake of foods high in fiber (e.g., bran, whole-grain breads and cereals, fresh fruits and vegetables) unless contraindicated 6. instruct client to maintain a minimum fluid intake of 2500 ml/day unless contraindicated 7. encourage client to drink hot liquids upon arising in the morning *in order to stimulate peristalsis* 8. encourage client to perform isometric abdominal strengthening exercises unless contraindicated 9. if client is taking analgesics for pain management, encourage the use of nonnarcotic rather than narcotic (opioid) analgesics when appropriate 10. increase activity as allowed 11. administer laxatives or cathartics and/or enemas if ordered. d. Consult physician about checking for an impaction and digitally removing stool if client has not had a bowel movement in 3 days, if he/she is passing liquid stool, or if other signs and symptoms of constipation are present. e. Consult appropriate health care provider if signs and symptoms of constipation persist and appear to be an ongoing problem.

10. NURSING DIAGNOSIS:

DISTURBED SLEEP PATTERN

related to decreased physical activity, fear, anxiety, inability to assume usual sleep position, frequent assessments or treatments, unfamiliar environment, and discomfort resulting from current illness/injury.

Suggested NOC Outcome: Sleep

Suggested NIC Intervention: Sleep enhancement

Desired Outcome	**Nursing Actions** *and Suggested Purposes/Rationales* (see pp. 52–54 for additional rationales)
10. The client will attain optimal amounts of sleep as evidenced by statements of feeling well rested.	10.a. Assess for signs and symptoms of a disturbed sleep pattern (e.g., statements of difficulty falling asleep, not feeling well rested, or interrupted sleep). b. Determine the client's usual sleep habits. c. Implement measures *to promote sleep:* 1. perform actions to reduce fear and anxiety (see Diagnosis 13, action b) 2. discourage long periods of sleep during the day unless signs and symptoms of sleep deprivation exist or daytime sleep is usual for client 3. perform actions to relieve discomfort if present (e.g., reposition client; administer prescribed analgesics, antiemetics, or muscle relaxants) 4. encourage participation in relaxing diversional activities during the evening 5. discourage intake of foods and fluids high in caffeine (e.g., chocolate, coffee, tea, colas) in the evening 6. offer client an evening snack that includes milk unless contraindicated *(milk contains L-tryptophan, which is believed to help induce and maintain sleep)* 7. allow client to continue usual sleep practices (e.g., position; time; presleep routines such as reading, watching television, listening to music, and meditating) whenever possible 8. satisfy basic needs such as comfort and warmth before sleep 9. encourage client to urinate just before bedtime 10. reduce environmental distractions (e.g., close door to client's room; use night light rather than overhead light whenever possible; lower volume of paging system; keep staff conversations at a low level and away from client's room; close curtains between clients in a semi-private room or ward; keep beepers and alarms on low volume; provide client with "white noise" such as a fan, soft music, or tape-recorded sounds of the ocean or rain; have sleep mask and earplugs available for client if needed) 11. ensure good room ventilation 12. encourage client to avoid drinking alcohol in the evening *(alcohol interferes with REM sleep)* 13. encourage client to avoid smoking before bedtime *(nicotine is a stimulant)* 14. if possible, administer medications that can interfere with sleep (e.g., steroids, diuretics) early in the day rather than late afternoon or evening 15. administer prescribed sedative-hypnotics if indicated 16. perform actions *to reduce interruptions during sleep (70–100 minutes of uninterrupted sleep is usually needed to complete one sleep cycle)* a. restrict visitors b. group care (e.g., medications, treatments, physical care, assessments) whenever possible. d. Consult appropriate health care provider if signs and symptoms of sleep deprivation (e.g., irritability, lethargy, agitation, inability to concentrate) occur and persist or worsen.

11. Nursing Diagnosis: *RISK FOR INFECTION*

a. **pneumonia** related to stasis of secretions in the lungs (secretions provide a good medium for bacterial growth);

b. **urinary tract infection** related to:

1. increased growth and colonization of microorganisms associated with urinary stasis

2. introduction of pathogens into the urinary tract associated with the presence of an indwelling catheter and/or difficulty maintaining good perineal hygiene during period of immobility.

Suggested NOC Outcomes: Immune status; Infection severity

Suggested NIC Interventions: Infection protection; Infection control; Cough enhancement; Airway management; Perineal care; Tube care: urinary; Urinary retention care

Desired Outcomes	**Nursing Actions** *and Suggested Purposes/Rationales* (see pp. 37–40 for additional rationales)
11.a. The client will not develop pneumonia as evidenced by: 1. normal breath sounds 2. resonant percussion note over lungs 3. absence of tachypnea 4. cough productive of clear mucus only 5. afebrile status 6. absence of pleuritic pain 7. blood gases and WBC count within normal range for client 8. negative sputum culture.	11.a.1. Assess for and report signs and symptoms of pneumonia: a. abnormal breath sounds (e.g., crackles [rales], pleural friction rub, bronchial breath sounds, diminished or absent breath sounds) b. dull percussion note over affected lung area c. tachypnea d. cough productive of purulent, green, or rust-colored sputum e. chills and fever f. pleuritic pain g. elevated WBC count h. abnormal oximetry and blood gas results i. positive sputum culture results j. chest x-ray results indicative of pneumonia. 2. Implement measures *to prevent pneumonia:* a. perform actions to promote effective airway clearance (see Diagnosis 2, action b) b. protect client from persons with respiratory tract infections c. encourage and assist client to perform frequent oral hygiene *in order to remove pathogens and secretions that could be aspirated.* 3. If signs and symptoms of pneumonia occur: a. administer oxygen as ordered b. administer antimicrobials if ordered.
11.b. The client will remain free of urinary tract infection as evidenced by: 1. clear urine 2. absence of frequency, urgency, and burning on urination 3. absence of chills and fever 4. urinalysis showing fewer than 5 WBCs, negative leukocyte esterase and nitrites, and absence of bacteria 5. negative urine culture.	11.b.1. Assess for and report signs and symptoms of urinary tract infection (e.g., cloudy urine; reports of frequency, urgency, or burning on urination; chills; elevated temperature; urinalysis showing a WBC count greater than 5, positive leukocyte esterase or nitrites, or the presence of bacteria; positive urine culture). 2. Implement measures *to prevent urinary tract infection:* a. perform actions to prevent urinary stasis (see Diagnosis 12, action c.2.a) b. maintain a fluid intake of at least 2500 ml/day unless contraindicated *to promote urine formation and subsequent voiding, which flushes pathogens from the urethra and bladder* c. instruct female client to wipe from front to back after urinating or defecating d. assist client with perineal care routinely and after each bowel movement e. maintain sterile technique during urinary catheterization and irrigations f. if an indwelling urinary catheter is present: 1. secure the catheter tubing to lower abdomen or thigh on males or to thigh on females *to minimize risk of accidental traction on the catheter and subsequent trauma to the bladder and urethra;* anchor tubing securely *to reduce the amount of in-and-out movement of the catheter (this movement can result in introduction of pathogens into the urinary tract and cause tissue trauma, which can result in colonization of microorganisms)* 2. perform catheter care as often as needed *to prevent accumulation of mucus around the meatus*

Desired Outcomes	Nursing Actions *and Suggested Purposes/Rationales*
	3. maintain a closed drainage system whenever possible *to reduce the risk of introducing pathogens into the urinary tract* 4. keep urine collection container below bladder level at all times *to prevent reflux or stasis of urine* 5. change catheter according to hospital policy. 3. If signs and symptoms of urinary tract infection occur, administer antimicrobials if ordered.

12. Collaborative Diagnoses: POTENTIAL COMPLICATIONS OF IMMOBILITY

a. thromboembolism related to:
   1. venous stasis associated with decreased mobility and increased blood viscosity if fluid intake is inadequate
   2. injury to the vessel wall associated with external pressure on the calf vessels from the mattress, pillows, or knee gatch when in a recumbent position
   3. hypercoagulability associated with increased blood viscosity (if fluid intake is inadequate) and increased levels of calcium in the blood from bone demineralization;

b. atelectasis related to shallow respirations and stasis of secretions in the alveoli and bronchioles associated with prolonged recumbent positioning;

c. renal calculi related to crystallization of calcium salts in the urine associated with:
   1. urinary stasis that occurs in a recumbent position
   2. oversaturation of the urine with calcium resulting from:
      a. increased urinary excretion of calcium that occurs with bone demineralization
      b. decreased urine formation if fluid intake is inadequate
   3. decreased solubility of calcium in the urine resulting from an increased urinary calcium level in proportion to the citrate level (citrate is an inhibitor of calcium stone formation);

d. contractures related to muscle atrophy and lack of joint movement associated with prolonged immobility;

e. pathologic fractures related to increased bone fragility associated with the osteoporosis that can develop with prolonged immobility.

Desired Outcomes	Nursing Actions *and Suggested Purposes/Rationales*
12.a.1. The client will not develop a deep vein thrombus as evidenced by: a. absence of pain, tenderness, swelling, and distended superficial vessels in extremities b. usual temperature of extremities c. negative Homans' sign.	12.a.1.a. Assess for and report signs and symptoms of a deep vein thrombus: 1. pain or tenderness in extremity 2. increase in circumference of extremity 3. distention of superficial vessels in extremity 4. unusual warmth of extremity 5. positive Homans' sign (not always a reliable indicator). b. Implement measures *to prevent thrombus formation:* 1. encourage and assist client to perform active foot and leg exercises every 1–2 hours while awake 2. instruct client to avoid positions that compromise blood flow (e.g., pillows under knees, crossing legs, sitting for long periods) 3. elevate foot of bed for 20-minute intervals several times a shift unless contraindicated 4. consult physician about an order for antiembolism stockings or an intermittent pneumatic compression device 5. maintain a minimum fluid intake of 2500 ml/day unless contraindicated *to prevent increased blood viscosity* 6. administer anticoagulants (e.g., low- or adjusted-dose heparin, fondaparinux, warfarin, low-molecular-weight heparin) if ordered 7. progress activity as allowed. c. If signs and symptoms of a deep vein thrombus occur: 1. maintain client on bed rest until activity orders are received 2. elevate foot of bed 15–20° above heart level if ordered

3. discourage positions that compromise blood flow (e.g., pillows under knees, crossing legs, sitting for long periods)
4. prepare client for diagnostic studies (e.g., venography, duplex ultrasound, impedance plethysmography) if indicated
5. administer anticoagulants (e.g., continuous intravenous heparin, low-molecular-weight heparin, fondaparinux, warfarin) as ordered
6. prepare client for intravenous injection of a thrombolytic agent (e.g., streptokinase, tissue plasminogen activator [tPA]) or catheter-directed fibrinolysis (infusion of a fibrinolytic agent into the thrombus) if planned.

12.a.2. The client will not experience a pulmonary embolism as evidenced by:
a. absence of sudden chest pain
b. unlabored respirations at 12–20/minute
c. pulse 60–100 beats/minute
d. blood gases within normal range.

12.a.2.a. Assess for and report signs and symptoms of pulmonary embolism (e.g., sudden chest pain, dyspnea, tachypnea, tachycardia, apprehension, low PaO_2).
b. Implement measures *to prevent a pulmonary embolism:*
   1. perform actions to prevent and treat a deep vein thrombus (see actions a.1.b and c in this diagnosis)
   2. do not exercise, check for Homans' sign in, or massage any extremity known to have a thrombus
   3. caution client to avoid activities that create a Valsalva response (e.g., straining to have a bowel movement, holding breath while moving up in bed) *in order to prevent dislodgment of existing thrombi*
   4. prepare client for a vena caval interruption (e.g., insertion of an intracaval filtering device) if planned.
c. If signs and symptoms of a pulmonary embolism occur:
   1. maintain client on strict bed rest in a semi- to high Fowler's position
   2. maintain oxygen therapy as ordered
   3. prepare client for diagnostic tests (e.g., blood gases, D-dimer level, ventilation-perfusion lung scan, pulmonary angiography)
   4. administer anticoagulants (e.g., heparin, warfarin) as ordered
   5. prepare client for the following if planned:
      a. injection of a thrombolytic agent (e.g., streptokinase, urokinase, tissue plasminogen activator [tPA])
      b. vena caval interruption (e.g., insertion of an intracaval filtering device) *to prevent further pulmonary emboli*
      c. embolectomy.

12.b. The client will not develop atelectasis as evidenced by:
1. clear, audible breath sounds
2. resonant percussion note over lungs
3. unlabored respirations at 12–20/minute
4. pulse rate within normal range for client
5. afebrile status.

12.b.1. Assess for and report signs and symptoms of atelectasis (e.g., diminished or absent breath sounds, dull percussion note over affected area, increased respiratory rate, dyspnea, tachycardia, elevated temperature, chest x-ray results showing atelectasis).
2. Implement measures *to prevent atelectasis:*
   a. perform actions to maintain an effective breathing pattern (see Diagnosis 1, action b)
   b. perform actions to maintain effective airway clearance (see Diagnosis 2, action b).
3. If signs and symptoms of atelectasis occur:
   a. increase frequency of position change, coughing or "huffing," deep breathing, and use of incentive spirometer
   b. consult physician if signs and symptoms of atelectasis persist or worsen.

12.c. The client will not develop renal calculi as evidenced by:
1. absence of flank pain, hematuria, nausea, and vomiting
2. clear urine without calculi.

12.c.1. Assess for and report signs and symptoms of renal calculi (e.g., dull, aching or severe, colicky flank pain; hematuria; nausea; vomiting).
2. Implement measures *to prevent calcium stone formation:*
   a. perform actions *to prevent urinary stasis:*
      1. assist client to change position at least every 2 hours; elevate head of bed periodically unless contraindicated
      2. progress activity as allowed
      3. implement measures to prevent urinary retention (see Diagnosis 8, action c)
      4. maintain patency of urinary catheter if present

Desired Outcomes	Nursing Actions *and Suggested Purposes/Rationales*
	b. encourage a minimum fluid intake of 2500 ml/day unless contraindicated *to promote adequate urine formation and subsequently reduce the concentration of calcium in the urine* (some physicians encourage clients to increase intake of citrus fruit juices, in particular lemonade, *to increase urinary citrate*) c. perform actions to prevent or delay bone demineralization (see action e.2.a in this diagnosis) *in order to reduce the amount of calcium present in the urine* d. instruct client to avoid excessive intake of foods/fluids high in calcium (e.g., dairy products) e. perform actions to prevent urinary tract infection (see Diagnosis 11, action b.2); *infections caused by urea-splitting organisms increase urine alkalinity, which promotes a favorable environment for the formation of struvite and calcium phosphate stones* f. instruct client to reduce intake of foods/fluids high in oxalate (e.g., tea, instant coffee, peanuts, chocolate, spinach) *in order to help prevent precipitation of calcium oxalate stones* g. maintain dietary sodium and protein restrictions if ordered *(sodium increases the urinary excretion of calcium and decreases citrate excretion; protein can increase urinary calcium excretion)* h. administer thiazide diuretic if ordered *to reduce urinary calcium excretion.* 3. If signs and symptoms of renal calculi occur: a. strain all urine carefully and save any calculi for analysis; report finding to physician b. encourage maximum fluid intake allowed c. administer analgesics and antispasmodic agents (e.g., oxybutynin) as ordered d. prepare client for removal of calculi (e.g., extracorporeal shock wave lithotripsy [ESWL], percutaneous nephrolithotomy, ureteroscopy with lithotripsy and stone extraction) if planned.
12.d. The client will not develop contractures as evidenced by normal or expected range of motion.	12.d.1. Assess for reports of joint stiffness and limitations in range of motion. 2. Implement general measures *to prevent contractures:* a. maintain proper body alignment at all times b. perform actions to maintain optimal joint mobility and muscle function during period of immobility (see Diagnosis 6, actions a.1–4). 3. Implement measures *to prevent hip and knee contractures:* a. place client in a flat, supine position at least every 4 hours unless contraindicated b. limit length of time client is in high Fowler's position (usually no longer than 1 hour at a time) c. avoid use of knee gatch and pillows under knees d. instruct client to do quadriceps- and gluteal-setting exercises if able *in order to maintain muscle strength and tone and improve ability to perform range of motion exercises of hips and knees* e. when client is in a supine or Fowler's position, place trochanter roll or sandbag along outer aspect of each thigh *to prevent external rotation of the hips.* 4. Implement measures *to prevent footdrop:* a. instruct and assist client to perform active foot exercises every 1–2 hours while awake b. if necessary, use devices to keep feet in a neutral or slightly dorsiflexed position (e.g., high-topped tennis shoes, foam boots) c. keep bed linen from exerting excessive pressure on toes and feet d. if extremity is in traction or a suspension device, be certain that pressure is not being exerted on the lateral aspect of the knee *(pressure on the peroneal nerve may result in footdrop).* 5. Implement measures *to prevent contractures in upper extremities:* a. encourage client to use upper extremities to perform self-care and assist in moving unless contraindicated

b. reposition upper extremities at least every 2 hours
c. use handroll and wrist splints if indicated.
6. Use a small rather than large pillow to support client's head and shoulders *in order to prevent a neck flexion contracture.*
7. Consult appropriate health care provider (e.g., physician, physical therapist) if range of motion becomes restricted.

12.e. The client will not experience pathologic fractures as evidenced by:
1. usual mobility and range of motion
2. absence of unusual motion, abnormal joint position, and obvious deformity of any body part
3. absence of pain and swelling over skeletal structures
4. x-ray reports showing absence of fractures.

12.e.1. Assess for and report signs and symptoms of pathologic fractures (e.g., further decrease in mobility or range of motion, motion at site where motion does not usually occur, abnormal joint position or obvious deformity, pain or swelling over skeletal structures, x-ray reports showing pathologic fracture).
2. Implement measures *to prevent pathologic fractures:*
a. perform actions *to prevent or delay bone demineralization:*
1. consult physician about the use of a tilt table while client is immobile
2. assist client with weight-bearing activities as soon as allowed *(weight bearing reduces bone breakdown)*
3. administer medications *that inhibit bone resorption* (e.g., alendronate, calcitonin) if ordered
4. encourage client to consume a diet that has adequate amounts of protein, vitamins, and calcium
5. discourage smoking and excessive caffeine and alcohol intake
b. if evidence of osteoporosis exists:
1. move client carefully; obtain adequate assistance as needed
2. when turning client, logroll and support all extremities
3. use smooth movements when moving client; avoid pulling or pushing on body parts
4. correctly apply back brace or corset if ordered.
3. If fractures occur:
a. apply external stabilization device (e.g., cervical collar, brace, splint, sling) if ordered
b. administer analgesics and/or muscle relaxants if ordered *to control pain*
c. prepare client for surgery (e.g., internal fixation) if planned.

13. Nursing Diagnosis: FEAR/ANXIETY

related to unfamiliar environment; lack of understanding of diagnosis, diagnostic tests, and treatments; financial concerns; and feelings of confinement.

Suggested NOC Outcomes:
Anxiety self-control; Anxiety level; Fear level; Fear self-control

Suggested NIC Interventions: Anxiety reduction; Calming technique; Emotional support; Presence; Financial resource assistance

Desired Outcome	Nursing Actions *and Suggested Purposes/Rationales* (see pp. 14–16 for additional rationales)

13. The client will experience a reduction in fear and anxiety as evidenced by:
a. verbalization of feeling less anxious
b. usual sleep pattern
c. relaxed facial expression and body movements
d. stable vital signs
e. usual perceptual ability and interactions with others.

13.a. Assess client for signs and symptoms of fear and anxiety (e.g., verbalization of feeling anxious, insomnia, tenseness, shakiness, restlessness, diaphoresis, tachycardia, elevated blood pressure, self-focused behaviors).
b. Implement measures *to reduce fear and anxiety:*
1. orient client to environment, equipment, and routines; explain the purpose for and operation of a kinetic bed if indicated
2. introduce client to staff who will be participating in care; if possible, maintain consistency in staff assigned to his/her care
3. assure client that staff members are nearby; respond to call signal as soon as possible
4. keep door and curtains open as much as possible *to reduce feeling of confinement*

Desired Outcome	Nursing Actions *and Suggested Purposes/Rationales*
	5. maintain a calm, supportive, confident manner when interacting with client 6. encourage verbalization of fear and anxiety; provide feedback 7. reinforce physician's explanations and clarify misconceptions client has about the diagnosis, treatment plan, and prognosis 8. explain all diagnostic tests 9. provide a calm, restful environment 10. instruct client in relaxation techniques and encourage participation in diversional activities 11. assist client to identify specific stressors and ways to cope with them 12. initiate social service referral and/or assist client to identify and contact appropriate community resources if indicated 13. provide information based on current needs of client at a level he/she can understand; encourage questions and clarification of information provided 14. encourage significant others to project a caring, concerned attitude without obvious anxiousness 15. include significant others in orientation and teaching sessions and encourage their continued support of the client 16. administer prescribed antianxiety agents if indicated. c. Consult appropriate health care provider if above actions fail to control fear and anxiety.

14. Nursing Diagnosis: ***DISTURBED SELF-CONCEPT****

related to dependence on others to meet basic needs, feelings of powerlessness, and change in body functioning and usual roles and lifestyle associated with physical limitations and/or prescribed activity restrictions.

*This diagnostic label includes the nursing diagnoses of disturbed body image, low self-esteem, and ineffective role performance.

Suggested NOC Outcomes: Body image; Self-esteem; Psychosocial adjustment: life change

Suggested NIC Interventions: Body image enhancement; Self-esteem enhancement; Emotional support; Support system enhancement; Role enhancement; Counseling

Desired Outcome	Nursing Actions *and Suggested Purposes/Rationales* (see pp. 47–49 for additional rationales)
14. The client will demonstrate beginning adaptation to changes in body functioning, lifestyle, roles, and level of independence as evidenced by: a. verbalization of feelings of self-worth b. maintenance of relationships with significant others c. active participation in activities of daily living d. verbalization of a beginning plan for adapting lifestyle to changes resulting from the injury or disease and/or its treatment.	14.a. Assess for signs and symptoms of a disturbed self-concept (e.g., verbalization of negative feelings about self, withdrawal from significant others, lack of participation in activities of daily living, lack of plan for adapting to necessary changes in lifestyle). b. Determine the meaning of feelings of dependency and changes in body functioning, lifestyle, and roles to the client by encouraging the verbalization of feelings and by noting nonverbal responses to the changes experienced. c. Discuss with client improvements in body functioning and ability to resume usual roles and lifestyle that can realistically be expected. d. Implement measures *to assist client to increase self-esteem* (e.g., limit negative self-assessment, encourage positive comments about self, assist to identify strengths, give positive feedback about accomplishments). e. Assist client to identify and use coping techniques that have been helpful in the past. f. Assist client with usual grooming and makeup habits if necessary.

g. Implement measures to reduce client's feelings of powerlessness (see Diagnosis 15, actions c–n).
h. Support behaviors suggesting positive adaptation to changes that have occurred (e.g., verbalization of feelings of self-worth, maintenance of relationships with significant others).
i. Assist client's and significant others' adjustment by listening, facilitating communication, and providing information.
j. Encourage visits and support from significant others.
k. Encourage client to continue involvement in interests and hobbies if possible. If previous interests and hobbies cannot be pursued, encourage development of new ones.
l. Provide information about and encourage use of community agencies and support groups (e.g., vocational rehabilitation; family, individual, and/or financial counseling).
m. Consult appropriate health care provider about psychological counseling if client desires or seems unwilling or unable to adapt to changes that have occurred as a result of the disease or injury and its treatment.

15. NURSING DIAGNOSIS: *RISK FOR POWERLESSNESS*

related to:
a. physical limitations and/or prescribed activity restrictions;
b. dependence on others to meet basic needs;
c. alterations in roles, relationships, and future plans.

Suggested NOC Outcomes: Health beliefs: perceived control; Participation in health care decisions; Personal autonomy

Suggested NIC Interventions: Self-esteem enhancement; Emotional support; Self-responsibility facilitation

Desired Outcome

15. The client will demonstrate a feeling of control over his/her situation as evidenced by:
a. verbalization of same
b. active participation in planning of care
c. participation in self-care activities within physical limitations and prescribed activity restrictions.

Nursing Actions *and Suggested Purposes/Rationales*

15.a. Assess for behaviors that may indicate feelings of powerlessness (e.g., verbalization of lack of control over self-care or current situation, anger, irritability, passivity, lack of participation in self-care or care planning).
b. Obtain information from client and significant others regarding client's usual response to situations in which he/she has had limited control (e.g., loss of job, financial stress).
c. Evaluate client's perception of current situation, strengths, weaknesses, expectations, and parts of current situation that are under his/her control. Correct misinformation and inaccurate perceptions and encourage discussion of feelings about areas in which there is a perceived lack of control.
d. Reinforce physician's explanations about the disease or injury and treatment plan. Clarify misconceptions.
e. Support realistic hope about probability of future independence and ability to resume usual roles and lifestyle.
f. Assist client to meet spiritual needs (e.g., arrange for a visit from clergy if desired by client).
g. Remind client of the right to ask questions about condition and treatment regimen.
h. Support client's efforts to increase knowledge of and control over condition. Provide relevant pamphlets and audiovisual materials.
i. Include client in the planning of care, encourage maximum participation in the treatment plan, and allow choices whenever possible *to promote a sense of control.*
j. Consult physical and/or occupational therapists if indicated about assistive devices and environmental modifications that would allow client more independence in performing activities of daily living.

Desired Outcome	Nursing Actions *and Suggested Purposes/Rationales*
	k. Inform client of scheduled procedures and tests *so that he/she knows what to expect, which promotes a sense of control.* l. Encourage significant others to allow client to do as much as he/she is able *so that a feeling of independence can be maintained.* m. Assist client to establish realistic short- and long-term goals. n. Encourage client's participation in support groups if indicated.

16. Nursing Diagnosis: ***RISK FOR LONELINESS***

related to inability to participate in usual activities, limited contact with significant others, and decreased exposure to events in the outside world associated with prolonged immobility.

Suggested NOC Outcomes: Psychosocial adjustment: life change; Social involvement

Suggested NIC Interventions: Socialization enhancement; Visitation facilitation; Support system enhancement

Desired Outcome	Nursing Actions *and Suggested Purposes/Rationales*
16. The client will not experience a sense of isolation and loneliness as evidenced by: a. maintenance of relationships with significant others b. no expression of feelings of isolation and loneliness.	16.a. Assess for indications of isolation and loneliness (e.g., absence of supportive significant others; uncommunicative and withdrawn; expression of feelings of rejection or being lonely; sad, dull affect). b. Implement measures *to decrease isolation and reduce the risk for loneliness:* 1. assist client to identify reasons for feeling isolated and alone; aid him/her in developing a plan of action to reduce these feelings 2. encourage significant others to visit 3. encourage client to maintain telephone contact with others 4. schedule time each day to sit and talk with client 5. make objects such as clock, TV, radio, newspapers, and greeting cards accessible to client 6. have significant others bring client's favorite objects from home and place in room 7. move client periodically to a more stimulating environment (e.g., hall, lounge, garden) when condition allows 8. change room assignments as feasible *to provide client with roommate with similar interests.*

Discharge Teaching/Continued Care

17. Nursing Diagnosis: ***DEFICIENT KNOWLEDGE, INEFFECTIVE THERAPEUTIC REGIMEN MANAGEMENT, OR INEFFECTIVE HEALTH MAINTENANCE****

*The nurse should select the diagnostic label that is most appropriate for the client's discharge teaching needs.

Suggested NOC Outcome: Knowledge: treatment regimen

Suggested NIC Interventions: Teaching: individual; Teaching: prescribed activity/exercise; Health system guidance; Self-care assistance: IADL

Desired Outcomes	Nursing Actions *and Suggested Purposes/Rationales*
17.a. The client will verbalize an understanding of ways to prevent problems associated with continued decreased mobility.	17.a.1. Provide instructions regarding ways to prevent respiratory tract infection: a. avoid contact with persons having respiratory tract infections b. drink at least 10 glasses of liquid/day unless contraindicated c. continue with respiratory care (e.g., incentive spirometer, coughing and deep breathing) as long as mobility is impaired d. avoid smoking.

2. Provide instructions regarding ways to prevent urinary tract infection:
   a. drink at least 10 glasses of liquid/day unless contraindicated
   b. void whenever the urge is felt
   c. wipe from front to back after urinating or defecating (if female) and keep perineal area clean.
3. Provide instructions regarding ways to prevent urinary calcium stone formation:
   a. drink at least 10 glasses of liquid/day unless contraindicated
   b. void whenever the urge is felt
   c. avoid excessive intake of foods/fluids high in calcium (e.g., dairy products) and oxalate (e.g., tea, instant coffee, peanuts, chocolate, rhubarb, spinach).
4. Provide instructions regarding ways to prevent a thromboembolism:
   a. drink at least 10 glasses of liquid/day unless contraindicated
   b. avoid placing pillows under knees, crossing legs, and prolonged sitting
   c. perform active foot and leg exercises every 1–2 hours during periods of inactivity
   d. wear elastic stockings as prescribed
   e. do not massage extremities.
5. Provide instructions regarding ways to prevent fainting spells associated with position change:
   a. wear elastic stockings as prescribed
   b. change from a lying to sitting or standing position slowly.
6. Provide instructions regarding ways to prevent skin breakdown:
   a. change position at least every 2 hours
   b. avoid pressure on any reddened or irritated area
   c. keep skin clean and dry
   d. place an alternating pressure pad or foam or gel cushion on bed and chair if prone to skin breakdown or if activity is severely limited.
7. Provide instructions regarding ways to prevent contractures:
   a. continue with recommended exercises to increase muscle tone and joint mobility
   b. avoid sitting for prolonged periods
   c. use devices to keep feet in a neutral or slightly dorsiflexed position (e.g., high-topped tennis shoes, foam boots) if in bed for prolonged periods.
8. Provide instructions regarding ways to reduce the risk for pathologic fractures:
   a. continue recommended weight-bearing activities
   b. take prescribed medications that inhibit bone resorption (e.g., alendronate, calcitonin)
   c. avoid smoking and excessive intake of caffeine and alcohol
   d. maintain an adequate dietary intake of protein, vitamins, and calcium
   e. take precautions to reduce the risk for falls.
9. Provide instructions regarding ways to prevent constipation:
   a. drink at least 10 glasses of liquid/day unless contraindicated
   b. increase intake of foods high in fiber (e.g., bran, whole-grain breads and cereals, fresh fruits and vegetables)
   c. defecate whenever the urge is felt
   d. assume a sitting position for defecation if possible.

17.b. The client will demonstrate techniques for meeting self-care needs.

17.b.1. Assist the client to identify techniques that will allow him/her to perform as much self-care as possible.
2. Reinforce physical/occupational therapist's instructions about use of assistive devices.
3. Allow time for return demonstration of self-care techniques and use of assistive devices.

Desired Outcomes	**Nursing Actions** *and Suggested Purposes/Rationales*
17.c. The client will state signs and symptoms to report to the health care provider.	17.c. Instruct client to report the following signs and symptoms: 1. temperature elevation lasting longer than 2 days 2. skin breakdown 3. cough productive of purulent, green, or rust-colored sputum 4. pain or swelling in any extremity 5. chest pain 6. flank pain 7. nausea and vomiting 8. frequency, urgency, or burning on urination 9. cloudy or foul-smelling urine 10. increased restriction of any joint motion.
17.d. The client will identify community agencies that can provide assistance with home care and transportation.	17.d.1. Provide information about community agencies that can provide assistance to client with home care or transportation (e.g., home health agencies, Meals on Wheels, church groups, transportation agencies). 2. Initiate a referral if indicated.
17.e. The client will verbalize an understanding of and a plan for adhering to recommended follow-up care including future appointments with health care provider and physical therapist, exercise regimen, and medications prescribed.	17.e.1. Reinforce the importance of keeping follow-up appointments with health care provider and physical therapist. 2. Reinforce physician's instructions regarding exercises and activity limitations. 3. Explain the rationale for, side effects of, and importance of taking medications prescribed. 4. Implement measures to improve client compliance: a. include significant others in teaching sessions if possible b. encourage questions and allow time for reinforcement and clarification of information provided c. provide written instructions regarding scheduled appointments with health care provider and physical therapist, medications prescribed, and signs and symptoms to report.

Bibliography

See pages 879 and 880.

UNIT VI

Nursing Care of the Client Who Is Dying

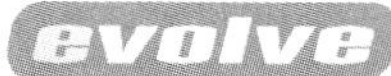

TERMINAL CARE

This care plan focuses on care of the adult client who is expected to die soon. The information included is appropriate for clients in acute or extended care settings or in the home. The major goals of nursing care are to prevent or control physiological problems that could reduce the quality of the client's remaining life; facilitate the client's psychological adjustment to his/her imminent death; and assist the client to experience a peaceful, dignified death. The nurse also assists the significant others to understand the dying process, support the dying person, meet their own physical and emotional needs, and adjust to their loss of the client.

This care plan does not deal with any particular medical diagnosis. The nursing diagnoses included are those that are relatively common to all persons facing death. Care plans that pertain to the client's specific medical diagnosis will provide additional guidelines for nursing care during the terminal stages of that illness.

Use in conjunction with the Care Plan on Immobility and care plans that pertain to the client's medical diagnosis.

NURSING DIAGNOSES

Refer to p. 165, Care Plan on Immobility (pp. 129–148), and care plans that pertain to the client's medical diagnosis for additional diagnoses.

1. NURSING DIAGNOSIS: ***IMPAIRED RESPIRATORY FUNCTION****

a. ineffective breathing pattern related to:
   1. increased rate of respirations associated with fear, anxiety, and pain
   2. decreased rate of respirations associated with the depressant effect of some medications (e.g., narcotic [opioid] analgesics, some antiemetics and antianxiety agents)
   3. decreased depth of respirations associated with recumbent positioning (in this position, full expansion of the lungs is restricted by the bed surface and by the abdominal contents pushing up against the diaphragm), fear, anxiety, weakness, fatigue, and/or abdominal distention

*This diagnostic label includes the following nursing diagnoses: ineffective breathing pattern, ineffective airway clearance, and impaired gas exchange.

4. altered function of the respiratory center (can occur as a result of the underlying disease process);

b. ineffective airway clearance related to:
   1. stasis of secretions associated with:
      a. decreased mobility
      b. difficulty coughing up secretions resulting from diminished lung/chest wall expansion and presence of tenacious secretions if fluid intake is inadequate
   2. fluid accumulation in the alveoli and bronchioles associated with pulmonary edema if present
   3. airway obstruction associated with the underlying disease process and/or relaxation of the tongue (can occur with decreased level of consciousness and as a result of administration of central nervous system depressants);

c. impaired gas exchange related to:
   1. loss of effective lung tissue (can occur as a result of the underlying disease process)
   2. a thickened alveolar-capillary membrane associated with stasis of pulmonary secretions and pulmonary edema if present
   3. decreased oxygen availability associated with anemia (can result from decreased nutritional status and/or the underlying disease process).

Suggested NOC Outcomes: Respiratory status: ventilation; Respiratory status: airway patency; Respiratory status: gas exchange; Comfortable death; Comfort level

Suggested NIC Interventions: Respiratory monitoring; Airway management; Oxygen therapy; Anxiety reduction

Desired Outcome	**Nursing Actions** *and Selected Purposes/Rationales* (see pp. 12–14, 18–20, and 33–35 for additional rationales)
1. The client will not experience respiratory distress as evidenced by: a. unlabored respirations b. absence of restlessness and agitation c. absence of gurgling or rattling respirations d. no reports of feeling of suffocation or drowning.	1.a. Assess for signs and symptoms of impaired respiratory function: 1. rapid, shallow, slow, or irregular respirations 2. dyspnea, orthopnea 3. use of accessory muscles when breathing 4. adventitious breath sounds (e.g., crackles [rales], rhonchi) 5. diminished or absent breath sounds 6. restlessness, agitation 7. cough, gurgling or rattling respirations 8. confusion, somnolence 9. reports of feeling of suffocation or drowning 10. significant decrease in oximetry results. b. Implement measures *to maintain an adequate respiratory status and prevent respiratory distress:* 1. perform actions to reduce pain (see Diagnosis 3, action e) *in order to prevent any change in the depth or rate of respirations that can occur in response to pain* 2. perform actions to decrease accumulation of gastrointestinal gas and fluid (see Diagnosis 5, action b) *in order to decrease pressure on the diaphragm* 3. perform actions to decrease fear and anxiety (see Diagnosis 12) *in order to prevent the shallow and/or rapid breathing that can occur with fear and anxiety* 4. perform actions to reduce the risk for aspiration (see Diagnosis 2, action c) 5. place client in a semi- to high Fowler's position unless contraindicated; position client with pillows *to prevent slumping* 6. instruct client to breathe slowly if hyperventilating 7. assist client with position change at least every 2 hours

8. perform actions *to promote removal of secretions:*
   a. instruct and assist client to deep breathe and cough or "huff" every 1–2 hours
   b. implement measures *to thin tenacious secretions and reduce dryness of the respiratory mucous membrane:*
      1. encourage maximum fluid intake allowed and tolerated
      2. humidify inspired air as ordered
   c. perform oral, pharyngeal, and/or tracheal suctioning if necessary (tracheal suctioning should be avoided during the final stage of dying)
9. maintain oxygen therapy as ordered
10. encourage activity as tolerated
11. administer the following medications if ordered:
    a. diuretics *to decrease fluid accumulation in the lungs*
    b. morphine sulfate *to reduce dyspnea*
    c. bronchodilators (e.g., theophylline)
    d. anticholinergics (e.g., scopolamine, hyoscyamine [Levsin], atropine) *to reduce bronchial secretions if frequent suctioning is necessary or the sound of excessive secretions is disturbing to significant others.*

c. Consult appropriate health care provider (e.g., respiratory therapist, palliative care nurse, hospice nurse, physician) if the client is experiencing respiratory distress.

2. NURSING DIAGNOSIS: *RISK FOR ASPIRATION*

related to:

a. decreased level of consciousness;
b. absent or diminished gag reflex associated with the underlying disease process and/or the depressant effect of some medications (e.g., narcotic [opioid]analgesics, some antiemetics and antianxiety agents);
c. supine positioning;
d. increased risk for gastroesophageal reflux associated with increased gastric pressure resulting from decreased gastrointestinal motility;
e. impaired swallowing associated with dry mouth and absent or diminished swallowing reflex (can occur as a result of the underlying disease process).

Suggested NOC Outcomes: Aspiration prevention; Respiratory status: gas exchange

Suggested NIC Interventions: Respiratory monitoring; Aspiration precautions; Airway precautions

Desired Outcome	**Nursing Actions** *and Selected Purposes/Rationales* (see pp. 16–18 for additional rationales)
2. The client will not aspirate secretions or foods/fluids as evidenced by: a. clear or usual breath sounds b. resonant percussion note over lungs c. absence of cough and tachypnea d. absence of or no increase in dyspnea.	2.a. Assess for and report signs and symptoms of aspiration of secretions, vomitus, or foods/fluids (e.g., rhonchi, dull percussion note over affected lung area, cough, tachypnea, tachycardia, development of or increase in dyspnea, presence of tube feeding in tracheal aspirate, chest x-ray results showing pulmonary infiltrate). b. Implement measures *to reduce the risk for aspiration:* 1. position client in side-lying or semi- to high Fowler's position at all times 2. perform oropharyngeal suctioning and oral hygiene as often as needed *to remove excess secretions, vomitus, and food particles* 3. perform actions to prevent nausea and vomiting (see Diagnosis 4, action b) 4. perform actions to reduce the accumulation of gastrointestinal gas and fluid (see Diagnosis 5, action b) *in order to reduce the risk of gastric distention and gastroesophageal reflux* 5. withhold oral food/fluids if gag reflex is depressed or absent, client is not alert, or he/she is experiencing severe dysphagia

Desired Outcome	**Nursing Actions** *and Selected Purposes/Rationales*

6. if client is receiving tube feedings:
   a. check tube placement before each feeding or on a routine basis if continuous feeding
   b. do not increase rate of continuous tube feeding unless allowed and tolerated; administer intermittent tube feedings slowly
   c. maintain client in a high Fowler's position during and for at least 30 minutes after feeding unless contraindicated
   d. stop tube feeding and notify physician if residuals exceed established parameters
7. if client is taking foods/fluids orally:
   a. offer foods/fluids that promote an effective swallow (e.g., thick rather than thin fluids, moist rather than dry foods)
   b. encourage client to concentrate on eating and drinking and allow ample time for meals
   c. instruct client to avoid talking or laughing when swallowing
   d. maintain client in high Fowler's position during and for at least 30 minutes after meals and snacks unless contraindicated
   e. assist client with oral hygiene after eating *to ensure that food particles do not remain in mouth.*

c. If signs and symptoms of aspiration occur:
   1. perform tracheal suctioning
   2. withhold oral intake
   3. prepare client for chest x-ray if ordered.

3. Nursing Diagnosis: ***ACUTE/CHRONIC PAIN***

related to:
a. the underlying disease process;
b. muscle spasms or stiff joints associated with decreased mobility;
c. reluctance to take pain medication associated with fear of loss of control and/or oversedation, feeling that taking medication is a sign of weakness or that pain has redemptive qualities, and/or need to be stoic.

Suggested NOC Outcomes: Comfort level; Pain control

Suggested NIC Interventions: Analgesic administration; Pain management; Patient-controlled analgesia (PCA) assistance; Environmental management: comfort; Dying care

Desired Outcome	**Nursing Actions** *and Selected Purposes/Rationales* (see pp. 45–47 for additional rationales)
3. The client will experience diminished pain as evidenced by: a. verbalization of decrease in or absence of pain b. relaxed facial expression and body positioning c. stable vital signs.	3.a. Assess for signs and symptoms of pain (e.g., verbalization of pain, grimacing, reluctance to move, restlessness, diaphoresis, increased B/P, tachycardia). b. Assess client's perception of the severity of pain using a pain intensity rating scale. c. Assess the client's pain pattern (e.g., location, quality, onset, duration, precipitating factors, aggravating factors, alleviating factors). d. Ask the client to describe previous pain experiences and methods used to manage pain effectively. e. Implement measures *to reduce pain:* 1. perform actions *to reduce fear and anxiety about the pain experience* (e.g., assure client that his/her need for pain relief is understood, plan methods for achieving pain control with client) 2. perform actions to reduce fear and anxiety (see Diagnosis 12) *in order to promote relaxation and subsequently increase the client's threshold and tolerance for pain* 3. administer analgesics before activities and procedures that can cause pain and before pain becomes severe

4. perform actions to promote rest (e.g., minimize environmental activity and noise) *in order to reduce fatigue and subsequently increase the client's threshold and tolerance for pain*
5. plan methods for achieving pain control with client *in order to assist him/her to maintain a sense of control over the pain experience*
6. provide or assist with nonpharmacologic methods for pain relief (e.g., massage; position change; progressive relaxation exercise; restful environment; diversional activities such as watching television, reading, or conversing)
7. if client has a patient-controlled analgesia (PCA) device, encourage him/her to use it as instructed
8. maintain integrity of analgesia delivery system (e.g., epidural, intravenous, subcutaneous, transdermal)
9. administer the following medications as ordered *to provide maximum pain relief with minimal side effects:*
   a. narcotic (opioid) analgesics
   b. nonnarcotic (nonopioid) analgesics such as salicylates or other nonsteroidal anti-inflammatory agents or acetaminophen
   c. local anesthetics (e.g., bupivacaine, etidocaine)
   d. muscle relaxants.

f. Consult appropriate health care provider (e.g., hospice nurse, palliative care nurse, pharmacist, physician, pain management specialist) if above measures fail to provide adequate pain relief.

4. NURSING DIAGNOSIS: NAUSEA

related to stimulation of the vomiting center associated with:
a. stimulation of the visceral afferent pathways resulting from abdominal distention if present;
b. stimulation of the cerebral cortex resulting from pain and stress;
c. stimulation of the chemoreceptor trigger zone by some medications (e.g., morphine sulfate).

Suggested NOC Outcome: Nausea and vomiting severity

Suggested NIC Interventions: Nausea management; Vomiting management

Desired Outcome	Nursing Actions *and Selected Purposes/Rationales*
4. The client will experience relief of nausea and vomiting as evidenced by: a. verbalization of relief of nausea b. absence of vomiting.	4.a. Assess client for nausea and vomiting. b. Implement measures *to prevent nausea and vomiting:* 1. perform actions to reduce accumulation of gastrointestinal gas and fluid (see Diagnosis 5, action b) 2. perform actions to reduce pain (see Diagnosis 3, action e) 3. perform actions to reduce fear and anxiety (see Diagnosis 12) 4. eliminate noxious sights and odors from the environment *(noxious stimuli can cause stimulation of the vomiting center)* 5. encourage client to take deep, slow breaths when nauseated 6. instruct client to change positions slowly *(rapid movement can result in stimulation of the chemoreceptor trigger zone and subsequent excitation of the vomiting center)* 7. provide oral hygiene after each emesis 8. if oral intake is allowed and tolerated: a. avoid serving foods with an overpowering aroma; remove lids from hot foods before entering room b. provide small, frequent meals; instruct client to ingest foods and fluids slowly c. encourage client to eat dry foods (e.g., toast, crackers) and avoid drinking liquids with meals if nauseated d. instruct client to avoid foods/fluids that irritate the gastric mucosa (e.g., spicy foods; caffeine-containing beverages such as coffee, tea, and colas)

Desired Outcome	Nursing Actions *and Selected Purposes/Rationales*
	e. instruct client to avoid foods high in fat *(fat delays gastric emptying)* f. instruct client to rest after eating with head of bed elevated g. administer medications known to cause gastric irritation (e.g., aspirin and aspirin-containing products, corticosteroids, ibuprofen) with or immediately after meals or snacks unless contraindicated 9. administer medications ordered to control nausea and vomiting (e.g., ondansetron, metoclopramide, lorazepam, ABR [Ativan, Benadryl, and Reglan] suppository). c. If above measures fail to control nausea and vomiting: 1. consult physician 2. be prepared to insert a nasogastric tube and maintain suction as ordered.

5. Nursing Diagnosis: ***ALTERED COMFORT: ABDOMINAL DISTENTION AND GAS PAIN***

related to an accumulation of gas and fluid in the gastrointestinal tract associated with decreased gastrointestinal motility resulting from depressant effect of some medications (e.g., narcotic [opioid] analgesics) and decreased activity.

Suggested NOC Outcome: Comfort level

Suggested NIC Intervention: Flatulence reduction

Desired Outcome	Nursing Actions *and Selected Purposes/Rationales*
5. The client will experience diminished abdominal distention and gas pain as evidenced by: a. verbalization of decreased abdominal fullness and pain b. relaxed facial expression and body positioning c. decrease in abdominal girth.	5.a. Assess for signs and symptoms of abdominal distention and gas pain (e.g., verbal reports of abdominal fullness or gas pain, grimacing, clutching or guarding of abdomen, restlessness, reluctance to move, increasing abdominal girth). b. Implement measures *to reduce the accumulation of gastrointestinal gas and fluid:* 1. encourage and assist client with frequent position changes and ambulation as tolerated *(activity stimulates peristalsis and expulsion of flatus)* 2. instruct client to avoid activities such as chewing gum and smoking *in order to reduce air swallowing* 3. maintain patency of nasogastric tube if present 4. maintain food and oral fluid restrictions if ordered 5. instruct client to avoid intake of carbonated beverages and gas-producing foods (e.g., cabbage, onions, beans) 6. encourage client to eructate and expel flatus whenever the urge is felt 7. consult physician about insertion of a rectal tube or administration of a return flow enema if indicated 8. if appropriate, encourage the use of nonnarcotic analgesics rather than narcotic (opioid) analgesics for pain management 9. administer the following medications if ordered: a. antiflatulents (e.g., simethicone) *to reduce gas accumulation* b. gastrointestinal stimulants (e.g., metoclopramide, bisacodyl) *to increase gastrointestinal motility.* c. Consult appropriate health care provider (e.g., hospice nurse, palliative care nurse, physician) if signs and symptoms of abdominal distention or gas pain persist or worsen.

6. Nursing Diagnosis: ***RISK FOR IMPAIRED TISSUE INTEGRITY***

related to:

a. accumulation of waste products and decreased oxygen and nutrient supply to the skin and subcutaneous tissue associated with reduced blood flow from prolonged pressure on the tissues resulting from decreased mobility;
b. damage to the skin and/or subcutaneous tissue associated with friction or shearing;
c. frequent contact with irritants associated with incontinence of urine or stool;

d. increased fragility of skin associated with inadequate nutritional status, dryness, and dependent edema.

Suggested NOC Outcome: Tissue integrity: skin and mucous membrane

Suggested NIC Interventions: Skin surveillance; Skin care: topical treatments; Pressure ulcer prevention; Positioning

Desired Outcome	**Nursing Actions** *and Selected Purposes/Rationales* (see pp. 49–52 for additional rationales)
6. The client will maintain tissue integrity as evidenced by: a. absence of redness and irritation b. no skin breakdown.	6.a. Determine client's risk for skin breakdown using a risk assessment tool (e.g., Norton Scale, Braden Scale, Gosnell Scale). b. Inspect the skin (especially bony prominences; dependent, edematous, and pruritic areas; and perianal area) for pallor, redness, and breakdown. c. Refer to Care Plan on Immobility, Diagnosis 4, action c (p. 133), for measures to prevent tissue breakdown. d. Implement measures *to prevent skin irritation resulting from incontinence of urine or stool in order to help prevent tissue breakdown:* 1. perform actions to reduce the episodes of urinary and bowel incontinence (see Diagnoses 8, actions b and c.1 and 10, action b) 2. assist client to thoroughly cleanse and dry perineal area with soft tissue or cloth after each episode of incontinence; apply a protective ointment or cream 3. apply a fecal incontinence pouch if bowel incontinence is a persistent problem 4. if use of absorbent products such as pads or undergarments is necessary, select those that effectively absorb moisture and keep it away from the skin. e. If tissue breakdown occurs: 1. notify appropriate health care provider (e.g., wound care specialist, physician) 2. perform pressure ulcer care as ordered or per standard hospital procedure (extensiveness of treatment is usually limited to that necessary to maintain comfort).

7. NURSING DIAGNOSIS: ***IMPAIRED ORAL MUCOUS MEMBRANE: DRYNESS AND IRRITATION***

related to:

a. decreased salivation associated with decreased oral intake and some medications (e.g., tricyclic antidepressants, anticholinergics, narcotic [opioid] analgesics, phenothiazines);
b. deficient fluid volume associated with decreased fluid intake and increased fluid loss;
c. prolonged oxygen therapy (especially if administered by mask);
d. mouth breathing;
e. inadequate nutritional status.

Suggested NOC Outcome: Oral hygiene

Suggested NIC Interventions: Oral health maintenance; Oral health restoration

Desired Outcome	**Nursing Actions** *and Selected Purposes/Rationales* (see pp. 43–45 for additional rationales)
7. The client will maintain a healthy oral cavity as evidenced by: a. absence of inflammation and discomfort b. moist, intact mucosa.	7.a. Assess client for signs and symptoms of impaired oral mucous membrane (e.g., reports of oral dryness and discomfort, coated tongue, inflamed and/or ulcerated oral mucosa). b. Implement measures *to reduce dryness of the oral mucous membrane:* 1. assist client to perform oral hygiene as often as needed; avoid use of products that contain lemon and glycerin and mouthwashes containing alcohol *(these have a drying and irritating effect on the oral mucous membrane)*

Desired Outcome	Nursing Actions *and Selected Purposes/Rationales*

2. assist client to rinse mouth frequently with water
3. lubricate client's lips frequently
4. encourage client to breathe through nose rather than mouth
5. encourage client not to smoke or chew tobacco *(smoking dries the mucosa; tobacco acts as an irritant to the oral mucosa)*
6. perform actions *to prevent further fluid loss:*
   a. implement measures to prevent nausea and vomiting if present (see Diagnosis 4, action b)
   b. implement measures *to reduce fever if present* (e.g., administer antipyretics if ordered, sponge client with tepid water, remove excessive clothing or bedcovers)
7. encourage fluid intake as allowed and tolerated; if client has difficulty drinking from a glass or through a straw:
   a. give frequent sips of water or juice using a syringe
   b. use a spoon to provide small amounts of ice chips
   c. provide frozen juice bars if client desires
8. encourage client to suck on hard candy unless contraindicated *in order to stimulate salivation*
9. encourage client to use a saliva substitute such as Salivart if needed *to lubricate the mucous membrane.*

c. If oral mucosa is irritated or cracked, implement measures *to relieve discomfort and promote healing:*
   1. if client is alert and able to take nourishment by mouth, assist him/her to select soft, bland foods
   2. instruct client to avoid foods/fluids that are extremely hot
   3. use a soft bristle brush, gauze-wrapped tongue blade, sponge-tipped applicator, or low-pressure power spray for oral hygiene
   4. administer topical anesthetics, oral protective agents, and analgesics if ordered.

d. Consult appropriate health care provider (e.g., hospice nurse, palliative care nurse, physician) if dryness, irritation, and/or discomfort persist.

8. Nursing Diagnosis: *URINARY INCONTINENCE*

related to:

a. decreased ability to respond to the urge to urinate associated with decreased level of consciousness and impaired physical mobility;
b. decreased awareness of full bladder and poor urinary sphincter control associated with decreased level of consciousness and/or the underlying disease process.

Suggested NOC Outcome: Urinary continence	**Suggested NIC Interventions:** Urinary incontinence care; Self-care assistance: toileting; Urinary catheterization

Desired Outcome	Nursing Actions *and Selected Purposes/Rationales* (see pp. 59–60 for additional rationales)
8. The client will experience urinary continence.	8.a. Assess for urinary incontinence.

b. Implement measures *to maintain or regain urinary continence:*
   1. offer bedpan or urinal or assist client to bedside commode or bathroom every 2–4 hours if indicated
   2. allow client to assume a normal position for voiding unless contraindicated *in order to promote complete bladder emptying*
   3. perform actions *to reduce delays in toileting* (e.g., have call signal within client's reach and respond promptly to requests for assistance; have bedpan, urinal, or bedside commode readily available to client;

provide client with easy-to-remove clothing such as pajamas with Velcro closures or an elastic waistband)
4. if client has a good fluid intake, encourage him/her to space fluids evenly throughout the day rather than drinking a large quantity at one time *(rapid filling of bladder can result in incontinence if client has decreased urinary sphincter control)*
5. encourage client to avoid drinking alcohol and beverages containing caffeine *(alcohol and caffeine have a mild diuretic effect and act as irritants; these factors may make urinary control more difficult).*

c. If urinary incontinence persists:
1. consult physician about intermittent catheterization, insertion of indwelling catheter, or use of external collection device (e.g., condom catheter)
2. provide client with or apply disposable undergarments (e.g., Depends, Attends) if indicated.

9. NURSING DIAGNOSIS:

RISK FOR CONSTIPATION

related to:
a. diminished defecation reflex associated with decreased nervous system responses in terminal state, suppression of the urge to defecate because of reluctance to use bedpan, and decreased gravity filling of lower rectum resulting from horizontal positioning;
b. decreased ability to respond to the urge to defecate associated with weakened abdominal muscles, impaired physical mobility, and decreased level of consciousness;
c. decreased gastrointestinal motility associated with decreased activity, increased sympathetic nervous system activity that occurs with anxiety, and use of some medications (e.g., narcotic [opioid] analgesics, antacids containing aluminum or calcium);
d. decreased intake of fluids and foods high in fiber.

Suggested NOC Outcome:
Bowel elimination

Suggested NIC Intervention: Constipation/Impaction management

Desired Outcome	Nursing Actions *and Selected Purposes/Rationales* (see pp. 24–26 for additional rationales)
9. The client will maintain a bowel routine that provides optimal comfort.	9.a. Refer to Care Plan on Immobility, Diagnosis 9 (p. 137), for measures related to assessment, prevention, and management of constipation. b. Implement additional measures *to prevent constipation:* 1. assist client to toilet or place in high Fowler's position or on bedside commode for bowel movements unless contraindicated 2. if client is taking antacids containing aluminum or calcium, consult appropriate health care provider (e.g., physician, hospice nurse, palliative care nurse) about alternating them with antacids containing magnesium.

10. NURSING DIAGNOSIS:

BOWEL INCONTINENCE

related to:
a. decreased ability to respond to the urge to defecate associated with decreased level of consciousness and impaired physical mobility;
b. decreased awareness of urge to defecate and poor anal sphincter control associated with decreased level of consciousness;
c. fecal impaction if present (continuous stimulation of the defecation reflex by the fecal mass inhibits the internal anal sphincter and results in loss of ability to retain the mucus and fluid that collect proximal to and leak around the fecal mass).

Suggested NOC Outcome: Bowel continence

Suggested NIC Interventions: Bowel incontinence care; Self-care assistance: toileting

Desired Outcome	Nursing Actions *and Selected Purposes/Rationales*
10. The client will maintain optimal bowel control as evidenced by absence of or decrease in episodes of incontinence.	10.a. Monitor for episodes of bowel incontinence. b. Implement measures *to reduce the risk of bowel incontinence:* 1. perform bowel care routinely *to promote emptying of the lower colon* 2. perform actions *to reduce delays in toileting* (e.g., have call signal within client's reach and respond promptly to requests for assistance; have bedpan or bedside commode readily available to client; provide client with easy-to-remove clothing such as pajamas with Velcro closures or an elastic waistband) 3. consult physician regarding measures to remove fecal impaction if present (e.g., digital removal of stool, oil retention enema). c. If bowel incontinence persists: 1. consult appropriate health care provider (e.g., hospice nurse, palliative care nurse, physician) about use of a fecal incontinence pouch 2. provide client with disposable liners for underwear or disposable undergarments such as Attends or Depends.

11. Nursing Diagnosis: *DISTURBED THOUGHT PROCESSES**

related to:

a. drug toxicity associated with organ failure;
b. deficient fluid volume and imbalanced electrolytes associated with decreased oral intake, and the underlying disease process;
c. cerebral hypoxia, cerebral tissue damage, and/or metabolic changes associated with the underlying disease process;
d. uncontrolled pain.

*The diagnostic label of acute or chronic confusion may be more appropriate depending on the client's symptoms.

Suggested NOC Outcomes: Cognitive orientation; Communication

Suggested NIC Interventions: Reality orientation; Hallucination management

Desired Outcome	Nursing Actions *and Selected Purposes/Rationales*
11. The client will maintain optimal thought processes.	11.a. Assess client for disturbed thought processes (e.g., impaired memory, shortened attention span, slowed verbal response time, confusion). b. Ascertain from significant others client's usual level of cognitive functioning. c. If client shows evidence of disturbed thought processes: 1. assess for possible causes (e.g., drug toxicity, pain, hypoxia, imbalanced fluid and electrolytes) and implement measures to treat them if appropriate 2. reorient client to person, place, time, and others as necessary 3. address client by name 4. encourage significant others to bring in client's favorite items and place them within client's view 5. approach client in a slow, calm manner; allow adequate time for communication 6. repeat instructions as necessary using clear, simple language and short sentences 7. keep environmental stimuli to a minimum 8. have client perform only one activity at a time and allow adequate time for performance of activities

9. if client is having vision-like experiences (e.g., hearing and talking to persons not in the room), affirm, rather than deny or argue about, the experience
10. encourage significant others to spend time with and to be supportive of client; instruct them in methods of dealing with client's disturbed thought processes
11. leave light on at night *to facilitate client's orientation to surroundings.*

12. Nursing Diagnosis:

DEATH ANXIETY

related to:

a. concern about the well-being of caregivers and the impact of death on significant others;
b. fear of loss of physical and mental capabilities during dying process;
c. anticipated discomfort (e.g., pain, nausea, difficulty breathing) during dying process;
d. feeling of powerlessness over issues related to death;
e. feeling of doubt about existence of a god or higher being;
f. unfinished business and unresolved conflicts;
g. fear of abandonment and dying alone.

Suggested NOC Outcomes: Anxiety self-control; Fear self-control; Dignified life closure; Spiritual health

Suggested NIC Interventions: Anxiety reduction; Presence; Emotional support; Spiritual support; Decision-making support; Self-esteem enhancement

Desired Outcome

Nursing Actions *and Selected Purposes/Rationales*
(see pp. 14–16 for additional rationales)

12. The client will experience a reduction in death anxiety as evidenced by:
    a. verbalization of feeling less anxious
    b. usual sleep pattern
    c. relaxed facial expression and body movements
    d. stable vital signs
    e. statements reflecting resolution of unfinished business, conflicts, and concerns.

12.a. Refer to Care Plan on Immobility, Diagnosis 13 (pp. 143–144), for measures related to assessment and reduction of fear and anxiety.
b. Implement additional measures *to reduce fear and anxiety about dying:*
   1. perform actions to reduce discomfort (see Diagnoses 3, action e; 4, action b; 5, action b; and 7, action b)
   2. perform actions to improve respiratory status (see Diagnosis 1, action b) *in order to relieve dyspnea if present*
   3. spend time with client *to reduce feelings of abandonment and aloneness*
   4. assist client to formulate plans for completing unfinished business and providing for care of significant others if appropriate
   5. if appropriate, encourage and assist client to record (e.g., write, audiotape, videotape) information he/she would like others to know at the present time and after his/her death
   6. encourage significant others to stay with client and participate in care if their presence seems to relieve the client's fear and anxiety
   7. perform actions to promote resolution of spiritual distress and a sense of spiritual well-being (see Diagnosis 14, action c)
   8. perform actions *to reduce feelings of powerlessness* (e.g., provide information about advance directives, encourage participation in decisions about care and after-death arrangements, involve client in as much of self-care as possible).

13. Nursing Diagnosis:

ANTICIPATORY GRIEVING

related to loss of control over life and body functioning, changes in body image, loss of significant others, and imminent death.

Suggested NOC Outcome: Grief resolution

Suggested NIC Interventions: Grief work facilitation; Emotional support; Presence; Support system enhancement; Dying care

Desired Outcome	Nursing Actions *and Selected Purposes/Rationales* (see pp. 35–37 for additional rationales)
13. The client will demonstrate progression through the grieving process as evidenced by: a. verbalization of feelings about dying b. usual sleep pattern c. use of available support systems.	13.a. Assess for signs and symptoms of grieving (e.g., expression of distress about terminal illness and dying, change in eating habits, inability to concentrate, insomnia, anger, sadness, withdrawal from significant others, denial of impending death).

b. Implement measures *to facilitate the grieving process:*

1. assist client to acknowledge that death is imminent *so that grief work can progress;* assess for factors that may hinder and facilitate acknowledgment
2. discuss the grieving process and assist client to accept the phases of grieving as an expected response to anticipated losses and impending death
3. allow time for client to progress through the phases of grieving (phases vary among theorists, but progress from shock and alarm to acceptance); be aware that not every phase is expressed by all individuals, that phases do not necessarily occur in sequential order, and that recurrence of phases is common during the course of an illness and the dying process
4. provide an atmosphere of care and concern (e.g., provide privacy, be available and nonjudgmental, display empathy and respect) *so client will feel free to express feelings*
5. perform actions *to promote trust* (e.g., answer questions honestly, provide requested information)
6. encourage the verbal expression of anger and sadness about anticipated losses; recognize displacement of anger and assist client to see the actual cause of angry feelings and resentment; establish limits on abusive behavior if demonstrated
7. encourage client to express feelings in whatever ways are comfortable (e.g., writing, drawing, conversation)
8. assist client to identify and utilize techniques that have helped him/her cope in previous situations of loss
9. if desired by client, assist with after-death arrangements (e.g., funeral, religious service, who should be called)
10. perform actions *to assist the client to maintain a positive self-concept and feel good about the life he/she has experienced:*
    a. visit frequently and encourage verbalization about past events, life accomplishments, interests, and feelings
    b. help client to focus on positive rather than negative aspects of his/her life experience
    c. maintain a nonjudgmental attitude about the kind of life client has led and his/her beliefs
    d. encourage participation in decisions about care
    e. encourage and assist client with good physical hygiene and grooming; suggest use of personal rather than hospital clothing *to assist client to maintain his/her identity*
11. support behaviors suggesting successful grief work (e.g., verbalizing feelings about dying, statements reflecting that dying is difficult but a part of life, comfortable and realistic remembrances about significant relationships, use of available support systems)
12. explain the phases of the grieving process to significant others; encourage their support and understanding
13. facilitate communication between the client and significant others; be aware that they may be in different phases of the grieving process
14. provide information about counseling services and support groups that might assist client and significant others in working through grief
15. perform actions to promote a sense of spiritual well-being (see Diagnosis 14, action c).

c. Consult appropriate health care provider (e.g., hospice nurse, palliative care nurse, psychiatric nurse clinician, physician) regarding a referral for counseling if signs of dysfunctional grieving (e.g., persistent denial of terminal state, excessive anger or sadness, emotional lability) occur.

14. NURSING DIAGNOSIS: RISK FOR SPIRITUAL DISTRESS

related to:
a. challenged belief and value system as a result of intense or prolonged suffering and imminent death;
b. separation from religious/cultural ties;
c. overwhelming grief and sense of hopelessness.

Suggested NOC Outcomes: Hope; Spiritual health; Dignified life closure

Suggested NIC Interventions: Spiritual support; Grief work facilitation; Spiritual growth facilitation

Desired Outcome

14. The client will not experience spiritual distress as evidenced by:
    a. expression of a sense of spiritual well-being
    b. participation in usual religious/spiritual practices when possible
    c. maintaining connectedness with significant others.

Nursing Actions *and Selected Purposes/Rationales*

14.a. Assess client's religious/spiritual beliefs and practices.

b. Assess for signs and symptoms of spiritual distress (e.g., verbalization of conflict about beliefs and relationship with deity, reports of anger toward God, questioning the purpose for suffering, verbalizing that illness and imminent death are a punishment, refusal to participate in usual religious practices or to have visits from clergy, apathy, hostility, withdrawal).

c. Implement measures *to promote a sense of spiritual well-being:*
   1. give client permission to express feelings and concerns about his/her religious/spiritual beliefs
   2. maintain a nonjudgmental attitude about client's beliefs and any inner conflicts client is experiencing
   3. encourage client to use available spiritual resources (e.g., clergy, prayer, religious rituals) for support
   4. perform actions to facilitate the grieving process (see Diagnosis 13, action b)
   5. perform actions to reduce feelings of hopelessness (see Diagnosis 15, action b).

d. Consult appropriate resource (e.g., clergy, psychiatric nurse clinician, physician, palliative care nurse, hospice nurse) if signs and symptoms of spiritual distress occur and client's response is inappropriate and/or destructive.

15. NURSING DIAGNOSIS: HOPELESSNESS

related to deteriorating physical condition, feelings of abandonment, loss of belief in religious/cultural values, and inability to reach self-fulfillment associated with terminal state.

Suggested NOC Outcomes: Hope; Decision making; Quality of life; Dignified life closure; Spiritual well-being

Suggested NIC Interventions: Decision-making support; Presence; Grief work facilitation; Hope instillation

Desired Outcome

15. The client will maintain hope as evidenced by:
    a. verbal expression of same
    b. maintenance of satisfying relationships with others
    c. participation in self-care and decision making as able
    d. identification of realistic goals.

Nursing Actions *and Selected Purposes/Rationales*

15.a. Assess client for signs and symptoms of hopelessness (e.g., statements of feeling hopeless, decreased response to significant others, decreased participation in self-care and decision making, decreased verbalization, flat affect).

b. Implement measures *to assist client to reduce feelings of hopelessness:*
   1. perform actions to facilitate the grieving process (see Diagnosis 13, action b)
   2. perform actions to promote a sense of spiritual well-being (see Diagnosis 14, action c)
   3. allow client to retain as much control as possible over activities of daily living; involve him/her in as much self-care and decision making as feasible

Desired Outcome	Nursing Actions *and Selected Purposes/Rationales*

4. assist client to identify goals that are achievable in the time that he/she has left, ways to continue working toward goals previously set even if not possible to achieve them totally, and the purpose remaining in his/her life such as role model or advisor to significant others.

c. Consult appropriate health care provider (e.g., palliative care nurse, hospice nurse, psychiatric nurse clinician, physician) if client demonstrates increased feelings of hopelessness.

16. NURSING DIAGNOSIS: *INTERRUPTED FAMILY PROCESSES*

related to excessive anxiety, grief, disorganization and role changes within the family unit, inadequate support systems, and fatigue.

Suggested NOC Outcomes: Family coping; Family functioning; Family resiliency; Family normalization

Suggested NIC Interventions: Family involvement promotion; Family integrity promotion; Family process maintenance; Family support; Caregiver support; Support system enhancement

Desired Outcome	Nursing Actions *and Selected Purposes/Rationales*

16. The family members* will demonstrate beginning adjustment to loss of client and changes in family roles and structure as evidenced by:
   a. verbalization of ways to adapt to required role and lifestyle changes
   b. active participation in decision making and client's care
   c. positive interactions with one another

16.a. Assess for signs and symptoms of interrupted family processes (e.g., statements of not being able to accept client's imminent death or to make necessary role and lifestyle changes, inability to make decisions, infrequent visits, inappropriate response to client's situation, verbalization of guilt, preoccupation with other aspects of life, negative family interactions).

b. Identify components of the family and their patterns of communication and role expectations.

c. Implement measures *to facilitate family members' adjustment to imminent loss of client and altered family roles and structure:*
   1. encourage and assist family members to verbalize feelings about the death of the client and the effect of it on their lifestyle and family structure; actively listen to each family member and maintain a nonjudgmental attitude about feelings shared
   2. assist family members to confront the reality of the client's imminent death when they are ready; encourage them to imagine life after death of the client and to set some personal goals if appropriate
   3. provide privacy *so that family members can share their feelings and grief with one another;* stress the importance of and facilitate the use of good communication techniques
   4. explain the phases of grieving and assist family members to progress through their own grieving process; explain that they may encounter times when they need to focus on meeting their own rather than the client's needs
   5. emphasize the need for family members to obtain adequate rest and nutrition and to identify and use stress management techniques *so that they are better able to emotionally and physically deal with the death of the client;* assure them that the client will be well cared for in their absence
   6. encourage and assist family members to identify coping strategies for dealing with the client's death and its effect on those left behind
   7. include family members in decision making about client and his/her care; convey appreciation of their input and continued support of the client
   8. encourage and allow family members to participate in client's care if desired by both client and family members
   9. assist family members to make necessary postmortem arrangements for or with the client (e.g., funeral home, burial place, clergy visitation)

*The term "family members" is being used here to include client's significant others.

10. provide information to family members about:
    a. the current status of client
    b. behaviors to expect as the client progresses through terminal stages of disease and his/her own grieving
    c. physical signs and symptoms of approaching death (e.g., decrease in appetite and thirst; lack of interest in environment; withdrawal from relationships; disorientation; restlessness; agitation; vision-like experiences; "out-of-character" statements or requests; increased sleeping; incontinence; decreased level of consciousness; reduced urine output; cool, mottled extremities; respiratory sounds such as gurgling or rattling, labored breathing, or periods of no breathing)
    d. ways they can best assist in meeting client's needs
11. when appropriate, help and encourage family members to "let go" of client and say goodbye
12. assist family members to identify resources that can assist them in coping with their feelings and in meeting their immediate and long-term needs (e.g., counseling and social services; pastoral care; service, bereavement, and church groups; Hospice); initiate a referral if indicated
13. assist family members to contact appropriate persons (e.g., funeral home director, clergy) when death occurs.

d. Consult appropriate health care provider (e.g., hospice nurse, palliative care nurse, physician) if family members continue to demonstrate difficulty adjusting to the loss of the client and role changes within the family unit.

ADDITIONAL NURSING DIAGNOSES

*RISK FOR DEFICIENT FLUID VOLUME**

related to decreased oral intake and increased fluid loss associated with vomiting and/or diaphoresis if client has a fever.

IMPAIRED PHYSICAL MOBILITY

related to:
a. weakness and fatigue;
b. dyspnea and/or sensory and motor deficits (can occur as a result of the underlying disease process);
c. reluctance to move associated with pain and nausea if present;
d. decreased level of consciousness.

SELF-CARE DEFICIT

related to:
a. weakness and fatigue;
b. activity limitations associated with the underlying disease process;
c. pain, nausea, dyspnea, and/or disturbed thought processes if present;
d. decreased level of consciousness.

*DISTURBED SLEEP PATTERN**

related to decreased physical activity, fear, anxiety, unfamiliar environment, discomfort, and inability to assume usual sleep position associated with orthopnea if present.

RISK FOR FALLS

related to weakness, fatigue, and attempting activity unassisted because of agitation or confusion.

*See Unit II for outcomes, actions, and rationales.

Bibliography

See pages 879 and 880.

UNIT VII

Nursing Care of the Client Receiving Treatment for Neoplastic Disorders

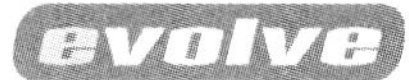

Chemotherapy

This care plan focuses on the use of cytotoxic drugs (chemotherapeutic agents) in the treatment of cancer. Chemotherapy is used alone or in combination with radiation therapy, surgery, and/or biotherapy to achieve a cure, control tumor growth, or provide relief of symptoms associated with advanced disease (palliation). Success of the therapy depends on the size, type, and location of the tumor in addition to the client's physiological and psychological condition.

Cytotoxic drugs are classified according to chemical structure (e.g., antimetabolites, mitotic inhibitors [vinca alkaloids, plant alkaloids], alkylating agents), primary mode of action (e.g., interfere with folic acid synthesis, produce cross-links of DNA strands), or effect on the cell life cycle. Some drugs are more effective during a specific phase of the cell cycle and are referred to as cell cycle phase-specific or cell cycle-specific (e.g., mitotic inhibitors, antimetabolites). The cytotoxic agents that interrupt the cell replication process without regard to the phase of the cell cycle are classified as cell cycle phase-nonspecific or cell cycle-nonspecific (e.g., alkylating agents, antitumor antibiotics).

The primary effect of cytotoxic drugs is to interrupt cell replication. It is believed that cytotoxic drugs kill a fixed percentage, rather than a specific number, of tumor cells with each dose and that tumors with a large percentage of growing cells will experience greater cell death than tumors with a smaller percentage of growing cells. Cells in the resting phase are less responsive to chemotherapeutic agents and are better able to repair themselves if damaged during treatment.

The finding that tumor cells may develop resistance to chemotherapeutic agents has resulted in the development of multiple drug protocols in which a combination of drugs are given simultaneously or in a particular sequence. The additive and sometimes synergistic effects that occur when drugs are used together allow an increased percentage of tumor cell kill without a concomitant increase in drug-induced toxicities. The dose, combination, and treatment schedule for the drugs are determined by factors such as the physiologic status of the client and the drug's action on the cell cycle, metabolism, toxic effects, and nadir. Cytotoxic agents are most frequently given intravenously, but routes such as oral, subcutaneous, topical, and direct instillation into the target area (e.g., peritoneum, bladder, cerebral spinal fluid) are used when appropriate.

Cytotoxic drugs do not discriminate between the normal and the cancerous cell and, as a result, the client may experience certain side effects and/or toxic effects following their administration. The drugs have the greatest effect on rapidly dividing cancerous and normal cells (e.g., bone marrow, skin, hair follicles, lining of the gastrointestinal tract). Because of this lack of selectivity between the cancerous and the normal cell, nursing care of the recipient of the drugs is indeed a challenge.

This care plan focuses on the adult client hospitalized for an initial or subsequent cycle of chemotherapy and/or management of side effects of treatment with cytotoxic agents. Much of the information is applicable to clients receiving chemotherapy and/or follow-up care in an outpatient facility or home setting.

OUTCOME/DISCHARGE CRITERIA

THE CLIENT WILL:

- have no signs and symptoms of toxic effects of cytotoxic agents
- have side effects of cytotoxic agents under control
- have fatigue at a manageable level
- have an adequate or improved nutritional status
- identify ways to prevent infection during periods of lowered immunity
- demonstrate appropriate oral hygiene techniques
- identify techniques to control nausea and vomiting
- verbalize ways to improve appetite and nutritional status
- verbalize ways to manage and cope with persistent fatigue
- verbalize ways to prevent bleeding when platelet counts are low
- verbalize ways to adjust to alterations in reproductive and sexual functioning
- verbalize ways to promote independence and prevent injury if neuropathies are present
- demonstrate the ability to care for a central venous catheter, a peritoneal catheter, or an implanted infusion device if in place
- verbalize an understanding of the care and precautions necessary if an Ommaya reservoir is in place
- verbalize an understanding of an implanted infusion pump and precautions necessary if one is in place
- state signs and symptoms to report to the health care provider
- share thoughts and feelings about changes in body image resulting from chemotherapy

- identify community resources that can assist with home management and adjustment to the diagnosis of cancer and chemotherapy and its effects
- verbalize an understanding of and a plan for adhering to recommended follow-up care including medications prescribed and schedule for chemotherapy, laboratory studies, and future appointments with health care provider.

NURSING/COLLABORATIVE DIAGNOSES

DISCHARGE TEACHING

See pp. 194–195 for additional diagnoses.

1. Nursing Diagnosis: *FEAR/ANXIETY*

related to:

a. unfamiliar environment;
b. lack of knowledge about chemotherapy including administration procedure, expected side effects, and impact on usual lifestyle and roles if admitted for chemotherapy;
c. need for hospitalization to manage current side effects and/or toxic effects of chemotherapy and possibility of additional untoward effects with a subsequent cycle of chemotherapy;
d. financial concerns;
e. diagnosis of cancer with potential for premature death.

Suggested NOC Outcomes: Anxiety self-control; Anxiety level; Fear self-control; Fear level

Suggested NIC Interventions: Anxiety reduction; Calming technique; Emotional support; Presence; Teaching: procedure/treatment; Financial resource assistance

Desired Outcome	Nursing Actions *and Selected Purposes/Rationales* (see pp. 14–16 for additional rationales)
1. The client will experience a reduction in fear and anxiety as evidenced by: a. verbalization of feeling less anxious or fearful b. usual sleep pattern c. relaxed facial expression and body movements d. stable vital signs e. usual perceptual ability and interactions with others.	1.a. Assess client on admission for: 1. fears, misconceptions, and level of understanding of chemotherapy and its effects on body functioning, lifestyle, and roles 2. perception of anticipated results of planned chemotherapeutic regimen 3. feelings about past experiences with chemotherapy or other treatments for cancer 4. availability of an adequate support system 5. signs and symptoms of fear and anxiety (e.g., verbalization of feeling anxious, insomnia, tenseness, shakiness, restlessness, diaphoresis, tachycardia, elevated blood pressure, self-focused behaviors). b. Implement measures *to reduce fear and anxiety:* 1. orient client to environment, equipment, and routines 2. introduce client to staff who will be participating in care; if possible, maintain consistency in staff assigned to his/her care 3. assure client that staff members are nearby; respond to call signal as soon as possible 4. maintain a calm, supportive, confident manner when interacting with client 5. encourage verbalization of fear and anxiety; provide feedback 6. explain all tests that may be done before the initiation of chemotherapy (e.g., blood and urine studies, ECG, pulmonary function studies) 7. reinforce physician's explanations and clarify misconceptions the client has about how prescribed drugs work, expected side effects, and potential drug toxicities 8. provide a calm, restful environment 9. instruct client in relaxation techniques (e.g., listening to music, exercise, yoga, guided imagery) and encourage participation in diversional activities 10. assist client to identify specific stressors and ways to cope with them 11. initiate a social service referral and/or assist client to identify and contact appropriate community resources if indicated 12. provide information based on current needs of client at a level he/she can understand; encourage questions and clarification of information provided 13. provide client with a note pad and pencil, printed information, and/or a tape recorder so he/she can review the information presented as often as desired 14. encourage significant others to project a caring, concerned attitude without obvious anxiousness 15. include significant others in orientation and teaching sessions and encourage their continued support of the client 16. initiate preoperative teaching if placement of a peritoneal or central venous catheter, Ommaya reservoir, or implanted infusion device is planned 17. administer prescribed antianxiety agents if indicated. c. Consult appropriate health care provider (e.g., psychiatric nurse clinician, oncology nurse specialist, physician) if above actions fail to control fear and anxiety.

2. NURSING DIAGNOSIS: *IMBALANCED NUTRITION: LESS THAN BODY REQUIREMENTS*

related to:

a. decreased oral intake associated with:
   1. oral, pharyngeal, and esophageal pain and difficulty swallowing resulting from mucositis if it has developed

2. anorexia resulting from factors such as depression, fear, anxiety, fatigue, discomfort, early satiety, altered sense of taste and smell, and increased levels of certain cytokines that depress appetite (e.g., interleukin-1, tumor necrosis factor)
3. altered mental status (can result from fluid and electrolyte imbalances, hypoxia, or tumor involvement of the brain);

b. loss of nutrients associated with vomiting and diarrhea if present;

c. impaired utilization of nutrients associated with:
1. accelerated and inefficient metabolism of proteins, carbohydrates, and/or fats resulting from factors such as increased levels of cortisol, glucagon, and certain cytokines (e.g., tumor necrosis factor, interleukin-1)
2. decreased absorption of nutrients resulting from loss of intestinal absorptive surface if mucositis has developed;

d. utilization of available nutrients by the malignant cells rather than the host.

Suggested NOC Outcomes: Nutritional status; Appetite

Suggested NIC Interventions: Nutritional monitoring; Nutrition management; Nutrition therapy; Nausea management; Pain management

Desired Outcome	**Nursing Actions** *and Selected Purposes/Rationales* (see pp. 40–43 for additional rationales)
2. The client will have or attain an adequate nutritional status as evidenced by: a. weight within or returning toward normal range for client b. normal BUN and serum prealbumin, albumin, and transferrin levels c. usual strength and activity tolerance d. healthy oral mucous membrane.	2.a. Assess for and report signs and symptoms of malnutrition: 1. significant weight loss 2. abnormal BUN and low serum prealbumin, albumin, and transferrin levels 3. weakness and fatigue 4. sore, inflamed oral mucous membrane 5. pale conjunctiva. b. Monitor percentage of meals and snacks client consumes. Report a pattern of inadequate intake. c. Implement measures *to maintain or promote an adequate nutritional status:* 1. perform actions *to improve oral intake:* a. implement measures to reduce nausea and vomiting (see Diagnosis 4, action c) b. implement measures to reduce oral, pharyngeal, esophageal, and abdominal pain (see Diagnosis 3, action d.4) c. implement measures to assist client to adjust psychologically to the diagnosis of cancer and treatment with chemotherapy (see Diagnoses 10, actions c–j and 11, action b) d. implement measures *to compensate for taste alterations that might be present:* 1. encourage client to select mild-tasting fish, cold chicken or turkey, eggs, and cheese as protein sources if beef or pork tastes bitter or rancid 2. provide meat for breakfast if aversion to meat tends to increase as day progresses 3. marinate meats in red wine or sweet and sour sauce 4. add extra sweeteners to foods if acceptable to client 5. experiment with different flavorings, seasonings, and textures 6. serve food cold or at room temperature *(can decrease some peculiar tastes)* 7. provide client with plastic rather than metal eating utensils if metallic taste is present e. if client is having difficulty swallowing: 1. implement measures to reduce the severity of stomatitis and/or relieve dryness of the oral mucous membrane (see Diagnosis 5, actions b and c) 2. assist client to select foods that require little or no chewing and are easily swallowed (e.g., custard, eggs, canned fruit, mashed potatoes)

3. avoid serving foods that are sticky (e.g., peanut butter, soft bread, honey)
4. moisten dry foods with gravy or sauces

f. serve food warm if indicated *(can stimulate sense of smell and subsequent appeal of certain foods)*
g. increase activity as tolerated *(activity usually promotes a sense of well-being, which can improve appetite)*
h. obtain a dietary consult if necessary to assist client in selecting foods/fluids that are appealing and adhere to personal and cultural preferences
i. encourage a rest period before meals *to minimize fatigue*
j. maintain a clean environment and a relaxed, pleasant atmosphere
k. provide oral hygiene before meals *(oral hygiene moistens the mouth, which makes it easier to chew and swallow; it also removes unpleasant tastes, which often improves the taste of foods/fluids)*
l. provide largest amount of calories and protein when appetite is the best (usually at breakfast)
m. serve frequent, small meals rather than large ones if client is weak, fatigues easily, and/or has a poor appetite
n. encourage significant others to bring in client's favorite foods and eat with him/her *to make eating more of a familiar social experience*
o. limit fluid intake with meals (unless the fluid has high nutritional value) *to reduce early satiety and subsequent decreased food intake*
p. allow adequate time for meals; reheat foods/fluids if necessary
q. administer appetite stimulants (e.g., megestrol acetate, dronabinol) if ordered

2. ensure that meals are well balanced and high in essential nutrients; offer high-calorie, high-protein dietary supplements (e.g., milk shakes, puddings, or eggnog made with cream or powdered milk reconstituted with whole milk; commercially-prepared dietary supplements) if indicated
3. perform actions to control diarrhea (see Diagnosis 7, action b)
4. administer vitamins and minerals if ordered.

d. Perform a calorie count if ordered. Report information to dietitian and physician.
e. Consult physician regarding an alternative method of providing nutrition (e.g., parenteral nutrition, tube feedings) if client does not consume enough food or fluids to meet nutritional needs.

3. NURSING DIAGNOSIS: ***ACUTE/CHRONIC PAIN***

a. oral, pharyngeal, esophageal, and/or abdominal pain related to mucositis associated with the effects of cytotoxic drugs on the rapidly dividing cells of the gastrointestinal mucosa;
b. muscle and bone pain (the cause is not known but it sometimes occurs in persons receiving paclitaxel and high doses of vinblastine or etoposide);
c. neuropathic pain related to the effects of some cytotoxic drugs (e.g., paclitaxel, cisplatin, vinca alkaloids) on the peripheral nerves.

Suggested NOC Outcomes: Pain control; Comfort level

Suggested NIC Interventions: Pain management; Environmental management: comfort; Analgesic administration; Oral health restoration

Desired Outcome	**Nursing Actions** *and Selected Purposes/Rationales* (see pp. 45–47 for additional rationales)
3. The client will experience diminished pain as evidenced by: a. verbalization of a decrease in or absence of pain	3.a. Assess client for: 1. reports of oral, pharyngeal, esophageal, and/or abdominal pain 2. statements of painful swallowing 3. reports of gastric pain induced by spicy or acidic foods 4. reports of achiness (usually in lower extremities) 5. reports of numbness, tingling, burning, or shooting pain in extremity(ies)

Desired Outcome	**Nursing Actions** *and Selected Purposes/Rationales*
b. relaxed facial expression and body positioning c. increased participation in activities.	6. grimacing, reluctance to move, clutching abdomen, or restlessness.

b. Assess client's perception of the severity of pain using a pain intensity rating scale.

c. Assess the client's pain pattern (e.g., location, quality, onset, duration, precipitating factors, alleviating factors).

d. Implement measures *to reduce pain:*
   1. perform actions to reduce fatigue (see Diagnosis 6, action d) *in order to increase the client's threshold and tolerance for pain*
   2. perform actions to reduce fear and anxiety (see Diagnosis 1, action b) *in order to promote relaxation and subsequently increase the client's threshold and tolerance for pain*
   3. provide or assist with nonpharmacologic methods for pain relief (e.g., massage; position change; progressive relaxation exercises; guided imagery; restful environment; diversional activities such as watching television, reading, or conversing)
   4. if client has oral, pharyngeal, esophageal, or abdominal pain:
      a. perform actions to reduce the severity of stomatitis (see Diagnosis 5, actions b and c)
      b. instruct client to avoid substances that might further irritate the gastrointestinal mucosa (e.g., extremely hot, spicy, or acidic foods/fluids; dry or hard foods; raw vegetables)
      c. offer cool, soothing liquids such as nonacidic juices and ices
      d. instruct client to gargle with a saline solution every 2 hours or spray mouth with a solution containing diphenhydramine and water (1 oz diphenhydramine and 1 qt water) if ordered *to soothe the oral mucous membrane*
      e. administer topical anesthetics/analgesics and oral protective agents (e.g., mixture of diphenhydramine, antacid, and Xylocaine Viscous; sucralfate oral suspension) if ordered
   5. administer the following medications if ordered *to manage pain:*
      a. nonopioid (nonnarcotic) analgesics (e.g., acetaminophen, tramadol, nonsteroidal anti-inflammatory agents)
      b. skeletal muscle relaxants *to reduce pain resulting from muscle spasms*
      c. antidepressants (e.g., amitriptyline) or anticonvulsants such as phenytoin, clonazepam, carbamazepine, or gabapentin *(used to treat neuropathic pain)*
      d. opioid (narcotic) analgesics or opioid analgesics combined with *N*-methyl-D-aspartate (NMDA) receptor antagonists (e.g., Morphidex)
      e. corticosteroids
   6. apply a cooling pad or ice pack to painful extremity unless contraindicated *(may help reduce mild neuropathic pain).*

e. Consult appropriate health care provider (e.g., pharmacist, physician, pain management specialist) if pain persists or worsens.

4. Nursing Diagnosis: *NAUSEA*

related to stimulation of the vomiting center associated with:

a. the effect of some cytotoxic drugs (those with a high emetic potential include carboplatin, cisplatin, dacarbazine, mechlorethamine, streptozocin, and carmustine), the by-products of cellular destruction, and the foul taste created by some cytotoxic agents;

b. stimulation of the visceral afferent pathways resulting from inflammation of the gastrointestinal mucosa if mucositis is present;

c. stimulation of the cerebral cortex resulting from stress and a conditioned response to previous experience with nausea and vomiting after the administration of cytotoxic drugs.

Suggested NOC Outcome:
Nausea and vomiting severity

Suggested NIC Interventions: Nausea management; Vomiting management

Desired Outcome	***Nursing Actions** and Selected Purposes/Rationales*
4. The client will experience a reduction in nausea and vomiting as evidenced by: a. verbalization of decreased nausea b. reduction in the number of episodes of vomiting.	4.a. Assess client for nausea and vomiting. Determine whether nausea and vomiting are acute, delayed, or anticipatory; the frequency of occurrence; what factors improve or worsen it; and if the nausea and vomiting interfere with activities. b. Assess client's perception of the severity of nausea using a scale of 1–10 or the terms mild, moderate, or severe. c. Implement measures *to reduce nausea and vomiting:* 1. perform actions to reduce fear and anxiety and promote psychological adjustment to the diagnosis of cancer and treatment with chemotherapy (see Diagnoses 1, action b; 10, actions c–j; and 11, action b) *in order to reduce stress* 2. convey an attitude that nausea and vomiting might not occur *(not every client experiences nausea and vomiting every time)* 3. administer the following medications as ordered 1–24 hours before initiating chemotherapy and routinely for the expected period of nausea and vomiting for the specific chemotherapeutic agents being administered: a. serotonin antagonists (e.g., dolasetron, granisetron, ondansetron) b. phenothiazines (e.g., thiethylperazine, prochlorperazine) c. butyrophenones (e.g., droperidol) d. gastrointestinal stimulants (e.g., metoclopramide) e. benzodiazepines (e.g., lorazepam, diazepam) *to decrease anxiety and/or induce amnesia in order to lessen the possibility of client's developing a conditioned response to chemotherapy* f. corticosteroids (e.g., dexamethasone) g. neurokinin receptor antagoniosts (e.g., aprepitant) h. synthetic cannabinoids such as dronabinol (may be prescribed as primary treatment or if severe nausea and vomiting has not been controlled by other medications) 4. administer intravenous cytotoxic drugs slowly unless contraindicated *to decrease stimulation of the vomiting center* 5. if feasible, administer the cytotoxic drugs at night *so client will sleep and experience less nausea* 6. provide mints or sour hard candy for client to suck on if he/she can taste the drug 7. eliminate noxious sights and odors from the environment *(noxious stimuli can cause stimulation of the vomiting center)* 8. encourage client to take deep, slow breaths when nauseated 9. encourage client to change positions slowly *(rapid movement can result in chemoreceptor trigger zone stimulation and subsequent excitation of the vomiting center)* 10. provide oral hygiene after each emesis and before meals 11. provide carbonated beverages for client to sip if nauseated 12. delay meals until 3–4 hours after chemotherapy administration 13. avoid serving foods with an overpowering aroma; remove lids from hot foods before entering room 14. provide small, frequent meals; instruct client to ingest foods and fluids slowly 15. encourage client to eat dry foods (e.g., toast, crackers) and avoid drinking liquids with meals if nauseated 16. instruct client to avoid foods/fluids that irritate the gastric mucosa (e.g., spicy foods; caffeine-containing beverages such as coffee, tea, and colas) 17. encourage the use of nonpharmacologic measures (e.g., self-hypnosis, relaxation, biofeedback, imagery, acupressure, music therapy) to control nausea.

Desired Outcome	**Nursing Actions** *and Selected Purposes/Rationales*
	d. Consult appropriate health care provider (e.g., oncology nurse specialist, physician) if above measures fail to control nausea and vomiting.

5. NURSING DIAGNOSIS:

IMPAIRED ORAL MUCOUS MEMBRANE

a. dryness related to reduced oral intake;
b. stomatitis related to:
   1. malnutrition and inadequate oral hygiene
   2. disruption in the renewal process of mucosal epithelial cells associated with toxic effects of cytotoxic drugs (particularly antimetabolites, antitumor antibiotics, mitotic inhibitors, and taxanes)
   3. infection, particularly gingival, during the period of myelosuppression.

Suggested NOC Outcome: Oral hygiene

Suggested NIC Interventions: Oral health maintenance; Oral health restoration

Desired Outcome	**Nursing Actions** *and Selected Purposes/Rationales* (see pp. 43–45 for additional rationales)
5. The client will maintain a healthy oral cavity as evidenced by: a. absence of inflammation b. pink, moist, intact mucosa c. no reports of oral dryness and burning d. ability to swallow without discomfort.	5.a. Assess client for dryness of the oral mucosa and signs and symptoms of stomatitis (e.g., inflamed and/or ulcerated oral mucosa; reports of burning pain in mouth, difficulty swallowing, or taste changes; viscous saliva; positive results of cultured specimens from oral lesions). b. Implement measures *to prevent or reduce the severity of stomatitis and/or relieve dryness of the oral mucous membrane:* 1. encourage client to chew on ice during chemotherapy infusion, especially if receiving 5-fluorouracil 2. reinforce importance of and assist client with oral hygiene after meals and snacks; avoid use of products that contain lemon and glycerin and mouthwashes containing alcohol *(these products have a drying and irritating effect on the oral mucous membrane)* 3. instruct and assist client to perform oral hygiene using a soft bristle toothbrush or sponge-tipped swab and to floss teeth gently 4. have client rinse mouth frequently with warm saline solution, baking soda and warm water, or chlorhexidene gluconate (Peridex) or mist oral cavity frequently using a spray bottle 5. lubricate client's lips frequently 6. encourage client to suck on sugarless candy or chew sugarless gum *to stimulate salivation* 7. encourage a fluid intake of at least 2500 ml/day unless contraindicated 8. encourage client not to smoke or chew tobacco *(smoking dries the mucosa; tobacco acts as an irritant to the oral mucosa)* 9. encourage client to use a saliva substitute such as Salivart if indicated 10. instruct client to avoid substances that might further irritate the oral mucosa (e.g., hot, spicy, or acidic foods/fluids) 11. perform actions to promote an adequate nutritional status (see Diagnosis 2, action c) 12. provide client with a prophylactic antifungal oral suspension or lozenge (e.g., nystatin) if ordered. c. If stomatitis is not controlled: 1. increase frequency of oral hygiene 2. if client has dentures, remove and replace only for meals. d. Consult appropriate health care provider (e.g., oncology nurse specialist, physician) if signs and symptoms of dryness and stomatitis persist or worsen.

6. NURSING DIAGNOSIS: FATIGUE

related to*:
a. a build up of cellular waste products associated with rapid lysis of cancerous and normal cells exposed to cytotoxic drugs;
b. difficulty resting and sleeping associated with fear, anxiety, and discomfort;
c. tissue hypoxia associated with anemia (a result of malnutrition and chemotherapy-induced bone marrow suppression);
d. overwhelming emotional demands associated with the diagnosis of cancer and treatment with chemotherapy;
e. increased energy expenditure associated with an increase in the metabolic rate resulting from continuous, active tumor growth and increased levels of certain cytokines (e.g., tumor necrosis factor, interleukin-1);
f. malnutrition;
g. side effects of other medications client may be receiving (e.g., narcotic [opioid] analgesics, antiemetics, antianxiety agents, biotherapy agents such as interferons and interleukins).

*Some of the etiological factors presented here are under investigation.

Suggested NOC Outcomes: Endurance; Energy conservation; Rest; Psychomotor energy

Suggested NIC Interventions: Energy management; Nutrition management; Sleep enhancement; Mood management

Desired Outcome

6. The client will experience a reduction in fatigue as evidenced by:
   a. verbalization of feelings of increased energy
   b. ability to perform usual activities of daily living
   c. increased interest in surroundings and ability to concentrate.

Nursing Actions *and Selected Purposes/Rationales*

6.a. Assess for:
   1. signs and symptoms of fatigue (e.g., verbalization of lack of energy and inability to maintain usual routines, lack of interest in surroundings, decreased ability to concentrate, lethargy)
   2. client's perception of the severity of fatigue using a fatigue rating scale; have client try to determine the severity of fatigue currently and an average for each week since last treatment.

b. Inform client that a feeling of persistent fatigue is not unusual and is a result of the disease itself as well as a side effect of chemotherapy and other medications he/she may be taking.

c. Assist client to identify personal patterns of fatigue (e.g., time of day, after certain activities) and to plan activities so that times of greatest fatigue are avoided.

d. Implement measures *to reduce fatigue:*
   1. perform actions *to promote rest and/or conserve energy:*
      a. schedule several short rest periods during the day
      b. minimize environmental activity and noise
      c. limit the number of visitors and their length of stay
      d. assist client with self-care activities as needed
      e. keep supplies and personal articles within easy reach
      f. implement measures to reduce fear and anxiety (see Diagnosis 1, action b)
      g. implement measures *to promote sleep* (e.g., encourage relaxing diversional activities in the evening, allow client to continue usual sleep practices unless contraindicated, reduce environmental stimuli, administer prescribed sedative-hypnotics)
      h. implement measures to reduce discomfort (see Diagnoses 3, action d and 4, action c)
      i. instruct client in energy-saving techniques (e.g., using shower chair when showering, sitting to brush teeth or comb hair, prioritizing activities and eliminating those that are optional)
   2. perform actions to promote an adequate nutritional status (see Diagnosis 2, action c)

Desired Outcome	Nursing Actions *and Selected Purposes/Rationales*

3. encourage client to maintain a fluid intake of at least 2500 ml/day unless contraindicated *to promote elimination of the by-products of cellular breakdown*
4. administer the following if ordered for treatment of anemia:
   a. iron preparations (e.g., ferrous gluconate, ferrous sulfate)
   b. folic acid (e.g., folate)
   c. erythropoiesis stimulating growth factor such as epoetin alfa (e.g., Epogen, EPO, Procrit) or darbepoetin alfa (e.g., Aranesp)
   d. blood transfusions (e.g., packed red blood cells)
   e. peripheral blood stem cell transplantation
5. increase activity gradually as tolerated
6. perform actions to facilitate client's psychological adjustment to the diagnosis of cancer and the treatment regimen and its effects (see Diagnoses 10, actions c–j and 11, action b).

e. Consult appropriate health care provider (e.g., oncology nurse specialist, physician) if signs and symptoms of fatigue worsen.

7. Nursing Diagnosis: *DIARRHEA*

related to increased peristalsis and disorders of intestinal secretion and absorption associated with inflammation and ulceration of the gastrointestinal mucosa resulting from effects of cytotoxic drugs (particularly many of the antimetabolites, topoisomerase-1 inhibitors, and antitumor antibiotics) on the rapidly dividing epithelial cells in the intestine.

Suggested NOC Outcome: Bowel elimination

Suggested NIC Intervention: Diarrhea management

Desired Outcome	Nursing Actions *and Selected Purposes/Rationales* (see pp. 28–30 for additional rationales)

7. The client will have fewer bowel movements and more formed stool if diarrhea occurs.

7.a. Assess for signs and symptoms of diarrhea (e.g., frequent, loose stools [more than 3 stools/day]; urgency; abdominal cramping; hyperactive bowel sounds).

b. Implement measures *to control diarrhea:*
1. restrict oral intake if ordered and progress diet gradually (elemental formulas may be ordered to minimize stimulation of the bowel)
2. instruct client to avoid the following foods/fluids that may stimulate or irritate the bowel or cause the stool to be more liquid:
   a. those high in fiber (e.g., whole-grain cereals, raw fruits and vegetables)
   b. coffee, alcohol, or foods that are spicy or fatty
   c. extremely hot or cold foods/fluids
   d. those high in lactose (e.g., milk, milk products)
   e. those made with synthetic, nonabsorbable sugars (e.g., sorbitol) that are found in dietetic foods
3. encourage intake of foods/fluids high in pectin (e.g., peeled apples, pear or apple juice, avocados, bananas)
4. administer the following medications if ordered *to control diarrhea:*
   a. opioids (e.g., paregoric) or synthetic opioids (e.g., loperamide, diphenoxylate hydrochloride) *to decrease gastrointestinal motility*
   b. adsorbents/protectants (e.g., attapulgite [Kaopectate], bismuth subsalicylate [Pepto-Bismol])
   c. antisecretory agents (e.g., octreotide acetate [Sandostatin]) *to suppress the output of gastroenterohepatic peptides and slow intestinal motility.*

c. Consult appropriate health care provider (e.g., oncology nurse specialist, physician) if diarrhea persists or worsens.

8. NURSING DIAGNOSIS: RISK FOR INFECTION

related to:
a. lowered natural resistance associated with:
   1. malnutrition
   2. chemotherapy-induced bone marrow suppression
   3. long-term treatment with corticosteroids (may be used in treatment of certain types of cancer)
   4. disruption in normal, endogenous microbial flora resulting from antimicrobial therapy
   5. impaired immune system functioning resulting from certain malignancies (e.g., Hodgkin's disease, lymphoma, multiple myeloma, leukemia);
b. break in mucosal surfaces associated with delayed cellular renewal resulting from effects of cytotoxic agents;
c. break in integrity of the skin associated with placement of a central venous catheter (e.g., Groshong), implanted infusion device (e.g., Port-a-Cath), or peritoneal catheter (e.g., Tenckhoff);
d. stasis of secretions in lungs and urinary stasis if mobility is decreased.

Suggested NOC Outcomes: Immune status; Infection severity

Suggested NIC Interventions: Infection control; Infection protection; Wound care

Desired Outcome

8. The client will remain free of infection as evidenced by:
   a. absence of fever and chills
   b. pulse within normal limits
   c. normal breath sounds
   d. usual mental status
   e. cough productive of clear mucus only
   f. voiding clear urine without reports of frequency, urgency, and burning
   g. absence of heat, pain, redness, swelling, and unusual drainage in any area
   h. no reports of increased weakness and fatigue
   i. WBC and differential counts within normal range for client
   j. negative results of cultured specimens.

Nursing Actions *and Selected Purposes/Rationales* (see pp. 37–40 for additional rationales)

8.a. Assess for and report:
   1. absolute neutrophil count (WBC count multiplied by the percentage of neutrophils) below 1000/mm^3 (indicative of severely impaired immune function)
   2. signs and symptoms of infection (be alert to subtle changes in the client since the signs of infection may be minimal as a result of immunosuppression; also be aware that some signs and symptoms vary depending on the site of the infection, the causative organism, and the age of the client):
      a. increase in client's usual temperature
      b. chills
      c. increased pulse
      d. abnormal breath sounds
      e. development of or increased malaise
      f. lethargy, acute confusion
      g. further loss of appetite
      h. cough productive of purulent, green, or rust-colored sputum
      i. cloudy urine
      j. reports of frequency, urgency, or burning when urinating
      k. urinalysis showing a WBC count greater than 5, positive leukocyte esterase or nitrites, or presence of bacteria
      l. heat, pain, redness, swelling, or unusual drainage in any area
      m. reports of increased weakness or fatigue
      n. increase in WBC count and/or significant change in differential
      o. positive results of cultured specimens (e.g., urine, vaginal drainage, mouth, sputum, stool, blood).

b. Implement measures *to reduce the risk for infection:*
   1. protect client from others with infections and those who have recently been vaccinated *(a person may have a subclinical infection after a vaccination)*
   2. use good hand hygiene and encourage client to do the same
   3. adhere to the appropriate precautions established to prevent transmission of infection to the client (standard precautions, neutropenic precautions)

Desired Outcome	Nursing Actions *and Selected Purposes/Rationales*

4. maintain a fluid intake of at least 2500 ml/day unless contraindicated
5. perform actions to promote an adequate nutritional status (see Diagnosis 2, action c)
6. provide a low-microbial diet (e.g., cooked foods, fresh fruits and vegetables that have been washed thoroughly) if the client is likely to be immunosuppressed
7. perform actions to prevent or reduce severity of stomatitis and relieve dryness of the oral mucous membrane (see Diagnosis 5, actions b and c); clean or replace oral hygiene items (e.g., denture cup, toothbrush) regularly
8. avoid invasive procedures (e.g., urinary catheterizations, arterial and venous punctures, injections) whenever possible; if such procedures are necessary, perform them using sterile technique
9. change intravenous insertion sites according to hospital policy
10. anchor catheters/tubings (e.g., urinary, intravenous) securely *in order to reduce trauma to the tissues and the risk for introduction of pathogens associated with the in-and-out movement of the tubing*
11. maintain a closed system for drains (e.g., urinary catheter) and intravenous infusions whenever possible
12. change equipment, tubings, and solutions used for treatments such as intravenous infusions, respiratory care, irrigations, and enteral feedings according to hospital policy
13. initiate measures to prevent constipation (e.g., offer client a daily fiber supplement such as a mixture of bran, applesauce, and prune juice; encourage a minimum fluid intake of 2500 ml/day; encourage increased intake of foods high in fiber; administer laxatives as ordered) *in order to prevent damage to the bowel mucosa from hard stool*
14. avoid unnecessary rectal invasion (e.g., temperature taking, enemas, suppositories, rectal tube) *to prevent trauma to rectal mucosa and possible abscess formation*
15. perform actions to reduce stress and discomfort (see Diagnoses 1, action b; 3, action d; 4, action c; and 5, actions b and c) *in order to prevent an increase in the secretion of cortisol (cortisol interferes with some immune responses)*
16. perform actions *to prevent stasis of respiratory secretions* (e.g., assist client to turn, cough, and deep breathe; increase activity as tolerated)
17. perform actions to prevent urinary retention (e.g., instruct client to void when the urge is first felt, promote relaxation during voiding attempts) *in order to prevent urinary stasis*
18. instruct and assist client to perform good perineal care routinely and after every bowel movement
19. instruct and assist client in proper care of the exit site of a central venous catheter or insertion site of an implanted infusion device or peritoneal catheter (see Diagnosis 12, actions i.1–3)
20. administer the following as ordered:
    a. antimicrobial agents
    b. colony-stimulating factors (e.g., filgrastim, pegfilgrastim, sargramostim) *to accelerate WBC recovery.*

9. COLLABORATIVE DIAGNOSES: POTENTIAL COMPLICATIONS OF CHEMOTHERAPY

a. **bleeding** related to thrombocytopenia associated with chemotherapy-induced bone marrow suppression;
b. **impaired renal function** related to:
   1. direct toxic effects of some cytotoxic agents (e.g., cisplatin, high doses of methotrexate, streptozocin) on renal cells
   2. nephropathy associated with:
      a. excessive uric acid accumulation resulting from the rapid lysis of large numbers of tumor cells

b. precipitation of certain drugs (e.g., high doses of methotrexate) in the renal tubules and collecting ducts as a result of low urinary pH and inadequate hydration before, during, and after drug administration;

c. hemorrhagic cystitis related to irritation and ulceration of the bladder mucosa by toxic metabolites of certain cytotoxic agents, particularly cyclophosphamide and ifosfamide;

d. local tissue irritation and sloughing related to extravasation of vesicant drugs (e.g., most antitumor antibiotics, teniposide, vinblastine, vincristine, paclitaxel);

e. cardiac dysrhythmias related to cardiotoxic effects of certain cytotoxic drugs (e.g., cyclophosphamide, high doses of ifosfamide, doxorubicin, daunorubicin, paclitaxel);

f. inflammation and fibrosis of lung tissue related to toxic effects of some cytotoxic agents on the lung (e.g., busulfan, bleomycin, carmustine, mitomycin);

g. neurotoxicity related to the toxic effects of certain cytotoxic agents (e.g., vincristine, vinblastine, cisplatin, ifosfamide, etoposide, high doses of methotrexate or cytarabine) on the nerves;

h. anaphylactic reaction related to a hypersensitivity response to a cytotoxic drug (e.g., cyclophosphamide, cisplatin, L-asparaginase, teniposide, paclitaxel).

Desired Outcomes	**Nursing Actions** *and Selected Purposes/Rationales*
9.a. The client will not experience unusual bleeding as evidenced by: 1. skin and mucous membranes free of petechiae, purpura, ecchymoses, and active bleeding 2. absence of unusual joint pain 3. absence of frank and occult blood in stool, urine, and vomitus 4. no increase in abdominal girth 5. usual menstrual flow 6. usual mental status 7. vital signs within normal range for client 8. stable or improved Hct and Hgb.	9.a.1. Assess client for and report signs and symptoms of unusual bleeding: a. petechiae, purpura, or ecchymoses b. gingival bleeding c. prolonged bleeding from puncture sites d. epistaxis, hemoptysis e. unusual joint pain f. frank or occult blood in stool, urine, or vomitus g. increase in abdominal girth h. menorrhagia i. restlessness, confusion j. decreasing B/P and increased pulse rate k. decrease in Hct and Hgb levels. 2. Monitor platelet count and coagulation test results (e.g., bleeding time). Report significant worsening of values. 3. If platelet count is low, coagulation test results are abnormal, or Hct and Hgb levels decrease, test all stools, urine, and vomitus for occult blood. Report positive results. 4. Implement measures *to prevent bleeding:* a. avoid giving injections whenever possible; consult physician about prescribing an alternative route for medications ordered to be given intramuscularly or subcutaneously b. when giving injections or performing venous and arterial punctures, use the smallest gauge needle possible c. apply gentle, prolonged pressure to puncture sites after injections, venous and arterial punctures, and diagnostic tests such as bone marrow aspiration d. take B/P only when necessary and avoid overinflating the cuff e. caution client to avoid activities that increase the risk for trauma (e.g., shaving with a straight-edge razor, using stiff bristle toothbrush or dental floss) f. whenever possible, avoid intubations (e.g., nasogastric) and procedures that can cause injury to rectal mucosa (e.g., taking temperatures rectally, inserting a rectal suppository or tube, administering an enema) g. pad side rails if client is confused or restless h. perform actions *to reduce the risk for falls* (e.g., keep bed in low position with side rails up when client is in bed, avoid unnecessary clutter in room, instruct client to wear slippers/shoes with nonslip soles when ambulating)

Desired Outcomes	Nursing Actions *and Selected Purposes/Rationales*
	i. instruct client to avoid blowing nose forcefully or straining to have a bowel movement; consult physician about an order for a decongestant and/or laxative if indicated j. administer the following if ordered: 1. platelet-stimulating factor (oprelvekin [Neumega]) 2. estrogen-progestin preparations *to suppress menses* 3. platelets. 5. If bleeding occurs and does not subside spontaneously: a. apply firm, prolonged pressure to bleeding area(s) if possible b. if epistaxis occurs, place client in high Fowler's position and apply pressure and ice pack to nasal area c. maintain oxygen therapy as ordered d. administer whole blood or blood products (e.g., platelets) as ordered.
9.b. The client will maintain adequate renal function as evidenced by: 1. urine output at least 30 ml/hour 2. BUN, serum creatinine, and creatinine clearance within normal range.	9.b.1. Assess for and report a urine output below 100 ml/hour during and for 24 hours after administration of nephrotoxic drugs (consult physician about insertion of a urinary catheter if output cannot be monitored accurately). 2. Assess for and report signs and symptoms of impaired renal function (e.g., urine output less than 30 ml/hour, urine specific gravity fixed at or less than 1.010, elevated BUN and serum creatinine levels, decreased creatinine clearance). 3. Implement measures *to maintain adequate renal function:* a. hydrate client with at least 150 ml fluid/hour unless contraindicated for 6–24 hours before administration of drugs known to be nephrotoxic (e.g., cisplatin, high doses of methotrexate, streptozocin) b. administer intravenous fluids as ordered during administration of nephrotoxic drugs and for 24 hours after therapy *to maintain a high rate of glomerular blood flow* c. administer the following medications as ordered: 1. diuretics (e.g., furosemide, mannitol) *to promote more rapid plasma clearance of the cytotoxic agent* 2. xanthine oxidase inhibitor (e.g., allopurinol) *to decrease the formation of uric acid* 3. sodium bicarbonate *to alkalinize the urine and subsequently increase the solubility of uric acid in the urine and prevent the precipitation of methotrexate in renal tubules and collecting ducts* 4. leucovorin calcium (e.g., folinic acid) *to diminish the toxic effects of cytotoxic agents such as methotrexate on the renal cells* 5. chemoprotectant agent (e.g., amifostine) *to protect the renal cells against toxicity from some cytotoxic agents (e.g., cisplatin).* 4. If signs and symptoms of impaired renal function occur: a. assess for and report signs of acute renal failure (e.g., oliguria or anuria; weight gain of 2% or greater over a short time; edema; elevated B/P; lethargy and confusion; increasing BUN and serum creatinine, phosphorus, and potassium levels) b. prepare client for dialysis if indicated.
9.c. The client will not develop hemorrhagic cystitis as evidenced by absence of dysuria, urinary frequency and urgency, suprapubic pain, and hematuria.	9.c.1. Assess for and report signs and symptoms of hemorrhagic cystitis (e.g., dysuria, urinary frequency and/or urgency, suprapubic pain, frank or occult blood in urine). 2. Implement measures *to prevent hemorrhagic cystitis:* a. ensure that client is vigorously hydrated; maintain intravenous fluids at the rate ordered (often as high as 200 ml/hr during chemotherapy) *in order to reduce the concentration of toxic drug metabolites in the bladder* b. administer cyclophosphamide early in the day and encourage client to void at least every 4 hours, before going to bed, and at least once during the night *in order to prevent stasis of toxic drug metabolites in the bladder*

c. administer mesna (Mesnex) if ordered *to interact with and inactivate the toxic drug metabolites of ifosfamide*
d. maintain continuous bladder irrigation before and after administration of cyclophosphamide or ifosfamide if ordered.

3. If signs and symptoms of hemorrhagic cystitis occur:
   a. discontinue cytotoxic drug administration and notify physician
   b. continue with fluid administration as ordered
   c. administer diuretics as ordered *to increase urine output and thereby decrease the concentration of toxic drug metabolites in the urine*
   d. assist with or perform bladder irrigations as ordered *to facilitate removal of drug metabolites and flush clots from the bladder*
   e. maintain continuous bladder irrigation with silver nitrate or alum (potassium aluminum sulfate) solution if ordered *to stop bleeding*
   f. prepare client for the following if planned:
      1. cystoscopy *to cauterize bleeding vessels*
      2. intravesical instillation of formalin *to control persisent, severe bleeding.*

9.d. The client will not experience drug extravasation as evidenced by:
1. absence of swelling, blanching, and coolness of skin around infusion site
2. no reports of stinging or burning pain at infusion site or along the vein.

9.d.1. Assess for signs and symptoms of drug extravasation (e.g., swelling, blanching, or coolness of skin around infusion site; reports of stinging or burning pain at infusion site or along vein). Ensure that infusion site and surrounding tissue are visible at all times.

2. Implement measures *to prevent drug extravasation:*
   a. select the best vein possible for vesicant drug administration:
      1. do not use a vein that has been previously used for vesicant agents
      2. use a large vein in forearm if possible; avoid the antecubital fossa and small veins in the hand *(extravasation in these areas can destroy nerves and tendons)*
      3. do not use an existing peripheral intravenous catheter that is more than 24 hours old
      4. avoid extremities with compromised circulation
      5. consult physician about insertion of a central venous catheter if large and/or frequent doses of a vesicant are planned
   b. do not perform multiple punctures in the same vein *in order to prevent leakage from the vessel after infusion has begun*
   c. tape intravenous catheter securely, but not too tight
   d. do not irrigate catheter forcefully or use a high pressure setting on infusion device
   e. perform actions *to ensure that the drug is infusing into the vein:*
      1. test patency of vein before administration of cytotoxic drug
      2. stay with client while a vesicant drug is infusing; check site every 2–3 minutes
   f. perform actions *to prevent increased irritation of the vein:*
      1. dilute drug according to manufacturer's recommendations
      2. administer drug at recommended rate of infusion
   g. stop infusion if there is any indication that the drug is not infusing properly
   h. when the drug infusion is complete, flush intravenous catheter with a minimum of 30 ml of normal saline; apply pressure to site for at least 4 minutes after catheter removal *to minimize oozing.*
3. If signs and symptoms of drug extravasation occur:
   a. stop infusion immediately
   b. treat area of extravasation as ordered (treatment varies depending on drug used) or per standard hospital procedure
   c. assess the site frequently for signs of increased inflammation, blistering, and necrosis
   d. administer analgesics as ordered *(severe pain is common following extravasation).*

Desired Outcomes	**Nursing Actions** *and Selected Purposes/Rationales*
9.e. The client will experience resolution of cardiac dysrhythmias if they occur as evidenced by: 1. regular apical pulse at 60–100 beats/minute 2. equal apical and radial pulse rates 3. absence of syncope and palpitations 4. ECG reading showing normal sinus rhythm.	9.e.1. Assess for and report signs and symptoms of cardiac dysrhythmias (e.g., irregular apical pulse; pulse rate below 60 or above 100 beats/minute; apical-radial pulse deficit; syncope; palpitations; abnormal rate, rhythm, or configurations on ECG). 2. Monitor liver and kidney function studies and report abnormal results *(cardiotoxicity can result from delayed metabolism or excretion of cytotoxic drugs by the liver or kidneys).* 3. Administer a cardioprotectant agent (e.g., dexrazoxane) if ordered *to reduce the risk of anthracycline-induced cardiac damage.* 4. If cardiac dysrhythmias occur: a. initiate cardiac monitoring and prepare client for an ECG if ordered b. administer antidysrhythmic agents (e.g., lidocaine, digoxin, diltiazem, esmolol, amiodarone, atropine) if ordered c. restrict client's activity based on his/her tolerance and severity of the dysrhythmia d. maintain oxygen therapy as ordered e. assess cardiovascular status frequently and report signs and symptoms of inadequate tissue perfusion (e.g., decrease in B/P, cool skin, cyanosis, diminished peripheral pulses, declining urine output, restlessness and agitation, shortness of breath) f. have emergency cart readily available for defibrillation, cardioversion, or cardiopulmonary resuscitation.
9.f. The client will experience decreased signs and symptoms of pulmonary inflammation and fibrosis if they occur as evidenced by: 1. decreased coughing 2. afebrile status 3. decreased dyspnea 4. improved breath sounds.	9.f.1. Assess for and report signs and symptoms of pulmonary inflammation and fibrosis (e.g., dry, hacking, persistent cough; fever; tachypnea; dyspnea on exertion; wheezing; crackles) particularly if client is reaching total allowable cumulative dose of cytotoxic agent(s) known to cause pulmonary toxicity. 2. If signs and symptoms of pulmonary inflammation and fibrosis occur: a. discontinue infusion of cytotoxic agent as ordered b. prepare client for diagnostic studies (e.g., chest x-ray, pulmonary function studies, CT or gallium scan, fiberoptic bronchoscopy) if planned c. maintain oxygen therapy as ordered d. administer the following medications if ordered: 1. corticosteroids *to reduce inflammatory response* 2. bronchodilators.
9.g. The client will adapt to the signs and symptoms of neurotoxicity if it occurs and not experience injury associated with those signs and symptoms.	9.g.1. Assess for and report signs and symptoms of neurotoxicity (e.g., constipation, ataxia, numbness and tingling of extremities, burning pain in extremity, unusual muscle weakness, gait disturbances, difficulty with fine motor movements, footdrop or wristdrop, hearing loss, blurred vision, nystagmus, memory loss, confusion, expressive aphasia, seizures). 2. Assure client that most changes in neurological function may be reversible if reported immediately and the neurotoxic drug is discontinued. 3. If signs and symptoms of neurotoxicity occur: a. implement measures *to prevent falls* (e.g., keep bed in low position with side rails up when client is in bed, avoid unnecessary clutter in room, instruct client to wear slippers/shoes with nonslip soles when ambulating) b. implement measures *to prevent burns* (e.g., let hot foods/fluids cool slightly before serving, assess temperature of bath water before bathing) *and cuts* (e.g., assist with shaving) c. institute seizure precautions if indicated d. implement measures *to assist client to adapt to the following if present:* 1. constipation (e.g., encourage a fluid intake of 2500 ml/day, increase fiber intake, administer prescribed laxatives)

2. pain in extremities (e.g., assist with nonpharmacologic methods such as distraction, position change, and guided imagery; administer anticonvulsants [clonazepam, gabapentin, phenytoin] or antidepressants [e.g., amitriptyline] if prescribed)
3. footdrop (e.g., instruct client to perform active foot exercises every 1–2 hours while awake, use high-topped tennis shoes or foam boots to keep feet in a neutral or slightly dorsiflexed position)
4. wristdrop (e.g., instruct client to perform active wrist exercises every 1–2 hours while awake, provide a wrist splint if necessary)
5. impaired hearing (e.g., face client when speaking, use gestures, respond to client's call signal in person rather than over the intercommunication system)
6. memory loss (e.g., assist to make lists, repeat information as needed)
7. confusion (e.g., decrease environmental stimuli, keep daily routines consistent and simple if possible, maintain consistency in staff assigned to care for client)
8. expressive aphasia (e.g., encourage client to use short words or phrases, provide an alphabet or word board, encourage client to use gestures)

e. consult physician if signs and symptoms of neurotoxicity persist or worsen.

9.h. The client will not develop an anaphylactic reaction as evidenced by:
1. usual mental status
2. usual skin color
3. absence of urticaria and pruritus
4. no reports of abdominal cramps, tightness in throat, ringing in ears, and numbness
5. absence of dyspnea, wheezing, and stridor
6. stable vital signs
7. absence of edema.

9.h.1. Assess for and report signs and symptoms of an anaphylactic reaction (usually some or all of the signs and symptoms will occur within minutes of drug administration):
a. anxiety, agitation
b. flushing of skin
c. generalized urticaria and pruritus
d. reports of abdominal cramps, tightness in throat, ringing in ears, or numbness
e. dyspnea, wheezing, stridor
f. irregular and/or increased pulse rate, decline in B/P
g. edema (particularly common in face, hands, and feet).

2. Implement measures *to prevent an anaphylactic reaction:*
a. consult physician before giving any drug that is the same as or similar to one the client has reacted to previously
b. administer a test dose before giving drug if appropriate
c. administer the following medications if ordered *to reduce sensitivity to the cytotoxic agent:*
1. corticosteroids (e.g., dexamethasone)
2. $histamine_1$ receptor antagonists (e.g., diphenhydramine) alone or in combination with $histamine_2$ receptor antagonists (e.g., famotidine, cimetidine, ranitidine).

3. If signs and symptoms of an anaphylactic reaction occur:
a. discontinue the cytotoxic drug but keep intravenous line open with a normal saline solution
b. administer oxygen as ordered
c. administer the following medications if ordered:
1. sympathomimetics such as epinephrine *(relieves bronchospasm and stimulates peripheral vasoconstriction)* or dopamine *(maintains blood pressure and organ perfusion)*
2. antihistamines (e.g., diphenhydramine) *to reduce the sensitivity reaction and control pruritus and urticaria*
3. bronchodilators (e.g., theophylline) *to relieve bronchospasm*
4. corticosteroids *to reduce the allergic response and maintain usual vascular wall permeability*

d. assess for and report signs and symptoms of anaphylactic shock (e.g., increased restlessness; significant decrease in B/P; rapid, weak pulse; increased dyspnea; cool, pale skin).

10. Nursing Diagnosis: *DISTURBED SELF-CONCEPT**

related to:

a. changes in appearance associated with the side effects of chemotherapy (e.g., alopecia, excessive weight loss, skin and nail changes) and external drug infusion catheter if present;
b. possible alteration in usual sexual activities associated with weakness, fatigue, reduced levels of testosterone (can occur with chemotherapy for prostate or testicular cancer or lymphoma), psychological factors, and vaginal discomfort (may result from mucositis and premature menopause if ovarian failure occurs);
c. possible temporary or permanent infertility associated with gonadal dysfunction resulting from extensive therapy with some cytotoxic drugs (e.g., some alkylating agents);
d. increased dependence on others to meet self-care needs;
e. changes in lifestyle and roles associated with effects of the disease process and its treatment.

*This diagnostic label includes the nursing diagnoses of disturbed body image, low self-esteem, and ineffective role performance.

Suggested NOC Outcomes: Self-esteem; Personal autonomy; Psychosocial adjustment: life change; Body image

Suggested NIC Interventions: Body image enhancement; Self-esteem enhancement; Role enhancement; Emotional support; Support system enhancement

Desired Outcome

10. The client will demonstrate beginning adaptation to changes in appearance, body functioning, lifestyle, and roles as evidenced by:
    a. verbalization of feelings of self-worth and sexual adequacy
    b. maintenance of relationships with significant others
    c. active participation in activities of daily living
    d. verbalization of a beginning plan for adapting lifestyle to changes resulting from the disease process and residual effects of chemotherapy.

Nursing Actions *and Selected Purposes/Rationales*

(see pp. 47–49 for additional rationales)

10.a. Assess for signs and symptoms of a disturbed self-concept (e.g., verbalization of negative feelings about self, withdrawal from significant others, lack of participation in activities of daily living, lack of a plan for adapting to necessary changes in lifestyle).

b. Implement measures to facilitate the grieving process (see Diagnosis 11, action b).

c. Discuss with client improvements in appearance and functioning that can realistically be expected.

d. Implement measures *to assist client to adapt to the following changes in body functioning and appearance if appropriate:*
   1. alopecia:
      a. inform client that hair loss can be expected approximately 2 weeks after initiation of chemotherapy; may be sudden, gradual, partial, or complete; and can include scalp hair, pubic hair, beard, eyebrows, and eyelashes
      b. reassure client that hair loss is temporary (regrowth sometimes occurs before cessation of treatment but usually occurs 2–3 months after it)
      c. inform client that hair regrowth may be a different color, texture, and consistency
      d. encourage client to cut hair very short *to decrease the anxiety related to seeing large quantities of hair fall out*
      e. inform client that he/she can reduce rate of scalp hair loss by:
         1. brushing hair gently using a soft bristle brush
         2. shampooing hair only once or twice a week and using a gentle shampoo and lukewarm water
         3. avoiding use of equipment/products that dry hair (e.g., hot rollers, hair dryers, curling iron, dyes)
         4. avoiding hair styles that create tension on hair (e.g., ponytails, braids)

f. encourage client to wear a wig, scarf, hat, false eyelashes, or makeup if desired *to camouflage hair loss*
g. inform client of community resources that can provide information and assistance with ways to facilitate adjustment to changes in appearance (e.g., American Cancer Society, Look Good-Feel Better Program)

2. skin changes (e.g., redness, rashes, peeling, increased sensitivity to sun, acne, darkening along the vein used for cytotoxic drug administration):
   a. inform client that skin and vein hyperpigmentation may occur if he/she is receiving cytotoxic drugs such as bleomycin, busulfan, methotrexate, and fluorouracil
   b. inform client that skin and vein discoloration is usually temporary
   c. instruct client to avoid exposure to sunlight and to use sun screen to prevent an increase in photosensitivity reactions
   d. assist client to identify types of clothing that can be worn to camouflage skin changes
3. nail changes:
   a. inform client that his/her nails may thicken and stop growing, develop ridges, darken, and detach from nail bed during treatment with certain cytotoxic drugs (e.g., cyclophosphamide, doxorubicin, bleomycin, fluorouracil)
   b. reassure client that normal nail growth will resume when chemotherapy is completed
4. infertility:
   a. clarify physician's explanation that infertility is a possible permanent effect of chemotherapy
   b. discuss alternative methods of becoming a parent (e.g., artificial insemination, adoption) if of concern to client
5. impotence:
   a. encourage client to discuss it with physician (impotence usually resolves after cessation of therapy)
   b. suggest alternative methods of sexual gratification if appropriate
   c. discuss ways to be creative in expressing sexuality (e.g., massage, fantasies, cuddling).

e. Assist client with usual grooming and makeup habits if necessary.
f. Support behaviors suggesting positive adaptation to changes that have occurred (e.g., interest in personal appearance, maintenance of relationships with significant others).
g. Assist client's and significant others' adjustment to changes by listening, facilitating communication, and providing information.
h. Encourage significant others to allow client to do what he/she is able *so that independence can be re-established and/or self-esteem redeveloped.*
i. Encourage client contact with others *so that he/she can test and establish a new self-image.*
j. Encourage visits and support from significant others.
k. Consult appropriate health care provider (e.g., psychiatric nurse clinician, physician) if client seems unwilling or unable to adapt to changes that have occurred as a result of cancer and its treatment.

11. NURSING DIAGNOSIS: GRIEVING*

related to:
a. changes in body image and usual roles and lifestyle;
b. diagnosis of cancer with potential for premature death.

*This diagnostic label includes anticipatory grieving and grieving following the actual losses.

Suggested NOC Outcomes:
Grief resolution;
Psychosocial adjustment: life change

Suggested NIC Interventions: Grief work facilitation; Emotional support; Support system enhancement; Spiritual growth facilitation

Desired Outcome	**Nursing Actions** *and Selected Purposes/Rationales* (see pp. 35–37 for additional rationales)
11. The client will demonstrate beginning progression through the grieving process as evidenced by: a. verbalization of feelings about the diagnosis of cancer and chemotherapy b. usual sleep pattern c. participation in the treatment plan and self-care activities d. use of available support systems e. verbalization of a plan for integrating prescribed follow-up care into lifestyle.	11.a. Assess for signs and symptoms of grieving (e.g., expression of distress about having cancer, change in eating habits, inability to concentrate, insomnia, anger, sadness, withdrawal from significant others, denial of losses). b. Implement measures *to facilitate the grieving process:* 1. assist client to acknowledge the losses *so grief work can begin;* assess for factors that may hinder and facilitate acknowledgment 2. discuss the grieving process and assist client to accept the phases of grieving as an expected response to actual and/or anticipated losses 3. allow time for client to progress through the phases of grieving (phases vary among theorists but progress from shock and alarm to acceptance); be aware that not every phase is expressed by all individuals, phases may overlap or recur, the amount of time needed to reach resolution of grief is very individual, and the grieving process may take months to years 4. provide an atmosphere of care and concern (e.g., provide privacy, be available and nonjudgmental, display empathy and respect) *so client will feel free to express feelings* 5. perform actions *to promote trust* (e.g., answer questions honestly, provide requested information) 6. encourage the verbal expression of anger and sadness about the diagnosis and losses; recognize displacement of anger and assist client to see the actual cause of angry feelings and resentment 7. encourage client to express feelings in whatever ways are comfortable (e.g., writing, drawing, conversation) 8. assist client to identify and use techniques that have helped him/her cope in previous situations of loss 9. support realistic hope about the prognosis and the temporary nature of most of the physical changes 10. if acceptable to client, arrange for a visit with a person who has been successfully treated for cancer with cytotoxic drugs 11. support behaviors suggesting successful grief work (e.g., verbalizing feelings about the diagnosis and losses, focusing on ways to adapt to losses) 12. explain the phases of the grieving process to significant others; encourage their support and understanding 13. facilitate communication between the client and significant others; be aware that they may be in different phases of the grieving process 14. provide information regarding counseling services and support groups that might assist client in working through grief 15. when appropriate, assist client to meet spiritual needs (e.g., arrange for visit from clergy) 16. administer antidepressant agents if ordered 17. assist client to identify and use available support systems; provide information about available community resources that can assist client and significant others in coping with the effects of chemotherapy and the diagnosis of cancer (e.g., American Cancer Society; support groups; individual, family, and financial counselors). c. Consult appropriate health care provider (e.g., psychiatric nurse clinician, physician) if signs of dysfunctional grieving (e.g., persistent denial of diagnosis or losses, excessive anger or sadness, emotional lability) occur.

Discharge Teaching/Continued Care

12. NURSING DIAGNOSIS: DEFICIENT KNOWLEDGE, INEFFECTIVE THERAPEUTIC REGIMEN MANAGEMENT, OR INEFFECTIVE HEALTH MAINTENANCE*

*The nurse should select the diagnostic label that is most appropriate for the client's discharge teaching needs.

Suggested NOC Outcomes: Knowledge: disease process; Knowledge: treatment regimen; Knowledge: energy conservation; Knowledge: treatment procedure(s)

Suggested NIC Interventions: Health system guidance; Teaching: disease process; Teaching: prescribed medication; Teaching: prescribed activity/exercise; Teaching: procedure/treatment; Nutrition management

Desired Outcomes	**Nursing Actions** *and Selected Purposes/Rationales*
12.a. The client will identify ways to prevent infection during periods of lowered immunity.	12.a.1. Explain to client that his/her resistance to infection is reduced when WBC counts are low. Emphasize need to adhere closely to recommended techniques to prevent infection. 2. Instruct the client in ways to prevent infection: a. avoid crowds, persons with any sign of infection, and persons who have recently been vaccinated b. utilize good hand hygiene (e.g., wash hands using an antibacterial soap, use an alcohol-base hand rub) c. wear gloves to protect hands during activities such as cleaning and gardening d. take axillary rather than oral temperature if stomatitis is present e. lubricate skin frequently to prevent dryness and subsequent cracking f. maintain sterile technique when caring for a central venous or peritoneal catheter, Ommaya reservoir, or implanted infusion device (e.g., MediPort) if in place g. avoid unnecessary rectal invasion (e.g., temperature taking, enemas, suppositories, sexual activity) to prevent rectal trauma h. avoid constipation to prevent damage to the bowel mucosa from hard or impacted stool i. wash perianal area thoroughly with soap and water after each bowel movement and after sexual activity; instruct female client to always wipe from front to back after urination and defecation j. drink at least 10 glasses of liquid/day unless contraindicated k. cough and deep breathe or use incentive spirometer every 2 hours until usual activity is resumed l. stop smoking m. perform meticulous oral hygiene after meals and at bedtime, change denture care solution daily, and replace toothbrush routinely n. avoid douching unless ordered (douching disturbs normal vaginal flora and may cause trauma to the vaginal mucosa) o. maintain an optimal nutritional status (e.g., diet high in protein, calories, vitamins, and minerals) p. avoid sharing eating utensils q. maintain an adequate balance between activity and rest r. cleanse respiratory equipment as instructed; change water in humidifiers daily s. decrease risk of food-borne illness 1. avoid intake of foods with a high microorganism content (e.g., unwashed fruits and vegetables; undercooked eggs, meat, poultry, and seafood) 2. be sure that juices and ciders are pasteurized or processed and that milk and cheese are pasteurized

Desired Outcomes	Nursing Actions *and Selected Purposes/Rationales*
	3. thoroughly wash hands and food preparation items and surfaces (e.g., knives, cutting board, countertop) before and after cooking, especially when working with raw meat, poultry, and fish 4. thaw food items in the refrigerator rather than on kitchen counter t. avoid picking up animal waste or cleaning animal litter boxes and bird cages u. avoid elective surgery and dental work v. reinforce the importance of taking prescribed medications such as colony-stimulating factors and prophylactic antimicrobial agents.
12.b. The client will demonstrate appropriate oral hygiene techniques.	12.b.1. Explain the rationale for and importance of frequent oral hygiene. 2. Provide instructions regarding oral hygiene techniques: a. cleanse mouth after eating and at bedtime; increase frequency to every 2 hours if stomatitis is present b. use a soft bristle toothbrush to prevent trauma to fragile mucous membranes c. rinse mouth with the following solutions as prescribed: 1. salt or baking soda and warm water 2. chlorhexidine gluconate (Peridex) d. mist oral cavity frequently using a spray bottle and/or take sips of water frequently to reduce mouth dryness e. avoid commercial mouthwashes that have an alcohol base (these are drying to oral mucosa).
12.c. The client will identify techniques to control nausea and vomiting.	12.c. Instruct client in methods to control nausea and vomiting: 1. eat foods that are cool or room temperature (hot foods frequently have an overpowering aroma that stimulates nausea) 2. eat dry foods (e.g., toast, crackers) or sip cold carbonated beverages if nausea is present 3. eat several small meals per day instead of 3 large ones 4. avoid drinking liquids with meals 5. select bland foods (e.g., mashed potatoes, cottage cheese) rather than fatty, spicy foods 6. rest after eating 7. if feasible, have someone else prepare the food 8. avoid offensive odors and sights 9. cleanse mouth frequently 10. take deep, slow breaths when nauseated 11. take antiemetics on a regular basis for prescribed length of time and if nausea is persistent.
12.d. The client will verbalize ways to improve appetite and nutritional status.	12.d. Instruct client in ways to improve appetite and maintain an adequate nutritional status: 1. try fish, cheese, chicken, and eggs as protein sources instead of beef and pork if taste distortion is a problem 2. increase amount of sugar or sweeteners and seasonings usually used in foods and beverages 3. use plastic utensils and cook food in glass or plastic containers if metallic taste is present 4. eat in a pleasant environment with company if possible 5. perform frequent meticulous oral hygiene to eliminate unpleasant tastes in mouth 6. try recommended methods of controlling nausea (see action c in this diagnosis) 7. eat several high-calorie, high-protein, nutritious small meals/day rather than 3 large ones; use nutritional supplements if needed to maintain an adequate caloric intake 8. plan ahead for low-energy days (e.g., have some prepared meals available; maintain an ample supply of nutritious, minimal

preparation foods such as eggs, tuna fish, cheese, peanut butter, and yogurt; keep nutritious snacks and beverages within easy reach)
9. take vitamins, minerals, and appetite stimulants (e.g., megestrol acetate, dronabinol) as prescribed.

12.e. The client will verbalize ways to manage and cope with persistent fatigue.

12.e. Instruct client in ways to manage and cope with persistent fatigue:
1. view fatigue as a protective mechanism rather than a problematic limitation
2. determine ways in which daily patterns of activity can be modified to conserve energy and prevent excessive fatigue (e.g., spread light and heavy tasks throughout the day, take short rests during an activity whenever possible, sit during an activity whenever possible, take several short rest periods during the day instead of one long one)
3. determine if life demands are realistic in light of physical state and adjust short- and long-term goals accordingly
4. avoid situations that are particularly fatiguing such as those that are boring, frustrating, or require prolonged or strenuous physical activity
5. participate in a moderate exercise program (e.g., walking or bicycling 20–30 minutes 3–4 times/week)
6. participate in "attention-restoring" activities (e.g., walking outside, gardening).

12.f. The client will verbalize ways to prevent bleeding when platelet counts are low.

12.f.1. Instruct client in ways to minimize risk of bleeding:
a. avoid taking aspirin and other nonsteroidal anti-inflammatory agents (e.g., ibuprofen)
b. consult health care provider before routinely taking herbs that can increase the risk of bleeding (e.g., ginkgo, arnica, chamomile)
c. brush teeth gently using a soft bristle toothbrush; do not use dental floss or put sharp objects (e.g., toothpicks) in mouth
d. use an electric rather than a straight-edge razor
e. cut nails and cuticles carefully
f. use caution when ambulating to prevent falls or bumps and do not walk barefoot
g. be attentive when using scissors, knives, and tools to reduce the risk of cuts
h. avoid contact sports and other activities that could result in injury
i. avoid straining to have a bowel movement
j. avoid blowing nose forcefully
k. avoid wearing constrictive clothing (e.g., garters, knee-high stockings)
l. use an ample amount of water-soluble lubricant prior to sexual intercourse and avoid anal sexual activity, douching, use of rectal suppositories, and enemas in order to prevent trauma to the vaginal and rectal mucosa
m. avoid heavy lifting.

2. Instruct client to control any bleeding by applying firm, prolonged pressure to the area if possible.

12.g. The client will verbalize ways to adjust to alterations in reproductive and sexual functioning.

12.g.1. Assure client that many of the side effects of chemotherapy (e.g., decreased libido, impotence) are temporary or can be treated.
2. Explain to the female client that ovarian failure during chemotherapy may result in irritability, hot flashes, and other symptoms of premature menopause.
3. Instruct client in the childbearing years to use contraception during chemotherapy and for at least 2 years after completion of chemotherapy (many cytotoxic drugs cause genetic abnormalities in the developing fetus).
4. Encourage client to rest before sexual activity if fatigue is a problem.
5. Instruct client in measures to decrease discomfort associated with decreased vaginal secretions and mucositis:
a. use an ample amount of water-soluble lubricant prior to intercourse

Desired Outcomes	**Nursing Actions** *and Selected Purposes/Rationales*
	b. use vaginal steroid cream if prescribed to ease dryness and inflammation if present c. take a sitz bath 2–3 times a day d. avoid intercourse until mucositis of the vaginal canal resolves. 6. Instruct client to take hormone replacements (e.g., estrogen, testosterone) as prescribed.
12.h. The client will verbalize ways to promote independence and prevent injury if neuropathies are present.	12.h. Instruct client in measures to promote independence and prevent injury if neuropathies are present: 1. use adaptive devices to facilitate performance of activities of daily living (e.g., zipper pulls; buttoners; molded sock aids; elastic shoe laces or Velcro straps; special pens, pencils, or utensils that are easy to grasp) 2. take extra precautions to prevent falls (e.g., have handrails in hallways and tubs and showers, avoid unnecessary clutter in pathways, wear shoes/slippers with nonskid soles, secure all carpets/rugs) 3. adhere to precautions to prevent burns (e.g., check temperature of bath water [should be less than 110° F], wear mitts when handling hot items) and cuts (e.g., shield fingers when using a sharp knife, avoid the use of motorized tools such as lawnmowers and saws, use adapted nail clippers).
12.i. The client will demonstrate the ability to care for a central venous catheter, a peritoneal catheter, or an implanted infusion device if in place.	12.i.1. Provide instructions related to care of a central venous catheter (e.g., Groshong) if appropriate: a. change dressing if present according to protocol using aseptic technique b. observe exit site for changes in appearance, redness, swelling, and unusual drainage c. flush catheter according to protocol to maintain patency d. replace injection cap as directed e. tape catheter securely to the chest wall to prevent accidental dislodgment f. notify physician if unable to flush catheter, if signs and symptoms of infection occur at exit site, or if catheter appears to be leaking. 2. Provide instructions related to care of a peritoneal catheter if in place: a. change dressing according to protocol utilizing aseptic technique b. keep catheter capped between treatments c. keep water below the level of the catheter when taking a tub bath (a tub bath may be taken 7–10 days after catheter insertion) d. observe for and notify physician if any of the following occur: 1. redness, swelling, or change in appearance of insertion site 2. unusual drainage from exit site 3. increasing abdominal pain 4. chills or fever 5. increased abdominal distention between treatments 6. persistent nausea or vomiting 7. dyspnea. 3. Provide instructions related to care of an implanted infusion device (e.g., MediPort, Port-a-Cath) if in place: a. keep appointment to have device flushed or flush as instructed b. avoid trauma to insertion site c. notify physician if area around infusion device becomes reddened or painful. 4. Allow time for questions, clarification, and return demonstration of procedures.

12.j. The client will verbalize an understanding of the care and precautions necessary if an Ommaya reservoir is in place.

12.j. Provide instructions related to care and precautions necessary if an Ommaya reservoir is in place:
1. wash site daily with soap and water
2. observe for and report redness, drainage, or discomfort at insertion site; stiff neck; persistent headache; or persistent nausea and vomiting
3. avoid activities that could result in trauma to the head and damage to the reservoir (e.g., contact sports).

12.k. The client will verbalize an understanding of an implanted infusion pump and precautions necessary if one is in place.

12.k.1. Reinforce physician's explanation about the purpose of the pump and how it works.
2. Instruct client to avoid activities that could result in abdominal trauma and dislodgment of pump.
3. Caution client to notify physician if:
   a. air travel is planned (client should carry an explanatory letter since pump may trigger airport weapon security devices; flow rate of pump may also need to be adjusted if the flight time is lengthy)
   b. body temperature is elevated more than 2° F for more than 24 hours (an increase in vapor pressure in the pump can increase flow rate)
   c. he/she plans to move to an area of greater or lesser altitude (alterations in the pump's flow rate may need to be made)
   d. redness, swelling, or drainage occurs at incisional or refilling site.
4. Emphasize importance of keeping appointments to have pump refilled (permanent blockage of the catheter can occur if pump is allowed to empty completely).

12.l. The client will state signs and symptoms to report to the health care provider.

12.l.1. Instruct client to observe for and report the following:
   a. signs and symptoms of infection (stress that usual signs of infection are diminished in people with altered bone marrow function and/or a suppressed immune system and that it is necessary to monitor closely for the following signs and symptoms):
      1. temperature above 38° C (100.4° F)
      2. changes in odor, color, or consistency of urine or pain with urination
      3. white patches in mouth
      4. crusted ulcerations around or in oral cavity
      5. swollen, reddened, coated tongue
      6. painful rectal or vaginal area
      7. unusual vaginal drainage
      8. changes in the appearance or temperature of skin, particularly around puncture sites
      9. persistent productive or nonproductive cough
   b. signs and symptoms of bleeding (e.g., excessive bruising, black stools, persistent nosebleeds or bleeding from gums, sudden swelling in joints, red or smoke-colored urine, blood in vomitus)
   c. signs and symptoms of hemorrhagic cystitis (e.g., blood in urine, pain on urination, urinary frequency or urgency)
   d. signs and symptoms of extravasation (e.g., coolness, pain, swelling, and/or skin changes at infusion site)
   e. signs and symptoms of pulmonary dysfunction (e.g., shortness of breath; persistent, dry, hacking cough; fever)
   f. signs and symptoms of dehydration (e.g., dry mouth, significant weight loss, concentrated urine, lightheadedness)
   g. signs and symptoms of cardiotoxicity (e.g., irregular or rapid heart rate, increased weakness and fatigue, shortness of breath, unexplained weight gain, swelling of extremities); emphasize that cardiotoxicity can occur several days to months after administration of drugs known to cause it
   h. new or increased signs and symptoms of neurotoxicity (e.g., numbness and tingling of extremities, change in hearing acuity, blurred vision, constipation, change in motor function and coordination, burning pain in extremity, impaired memory or ability to communicate)

Desired Outcomes	Nursing Actions and Selected Purposes/Rationales
	i. persistent diarrhea, nausea, vomiting, and/or decreased oral intake j. significant weight loss k. inability to cope with the effects of the diagnosis and treatment. 2. Instruct client to keep a record of signs and symptoms, activities at the time the symptoms occur, measures taken to achieve relief, and the effect of the measures taken. Instruct client to take the information to each appointment with the health care provider.
12.m. The client will identify community resources that can assist with home management and adjustment to the diagnosis of cancer and chemotherapy and its effects.	12.m.1. Provide information about and encourage use of community resources that can assist client and significant others with home management and adjustment to diagnosis of cancer and chemotherapy and its effects (e.g., American Cancer Society, counselors, social service agencies, Meals on Wheels, Make Today Count, Look Good-Feel Better Program, hospice, community support groups). 2. Initiate a referral if indicated.
12.n. The client will verbalize an understanding of and a plan for adhering to recommended follow-up care including medications prescribed and schedule for chemotherapy, laboratory studies, and future appointments with health care provider.	12.n.1. Thoroughly explain rationale for, side effects of, and importance of taking medications prescribed. Inform client of pertinent food and drug interactions. 2. Reinforce physician's explanation of planned chemotherapy schedule. 3. Discuss with client any difficulties he/she might have adhering to the schedule and assist in planning ways to overcome these. 4. Reinforce importance of keeping appointments for chemotherapy and laboratory studies. 5. Reinforce importance of keeping follow-up appointments with health care provider. 6. Implement measures to improve client compliance: a. include significant others in teaching sessions b. encourage questions and allow time for reinforcement and clarification of information provided c. provide written instructions regarding ways to maintain nutritional status, future appointments with health care provider and laboratory, medications prescribed, and signs and symptoms to report.

Additional Nursing Diagnoses

RISK FOR IMPAIRED SKIN INTEGRITY*

related to:

a. increased skin fragility associated with malnutrition and dryness (a result of the effects of cytotoxic drugs on sebaceous and sweat glands);
b. frequent contact of the skin with irritants associated with diarrhea if present;
c. damage to the skin and/or subcutaneous tissue associated with prolonged pressure on tissues, friction, or shearing if mobility is decreased.

RISK FOR CONSTIPATION*

related to decreased gastrointestinal motility associated with:

a. autonomic neuropathy resulting from some cytotoxic drugs (e.g., vinblastine, teniposide, vindesine, vinorelbine);
b. depressant effect of medications administered to control symptoms such as pain, nausea, and vomiting (e.g., narcotic [opioid] analgesics, some antiemetics);
c. decreased activity;
d. increased sympathetic nervous system activity resulting from anxiety;
e. decreased intake of fiber and fluids.

*See Unit II for outcomes, actions, and rationales.

SELF-CARE DEFICIT

related to:
a. fatigue, weakness, and discomfort;
b. sedation associated with the effects of some medications administered to control pain, anxiety, nausea, and vomiting;
c. tactile and proprioceptive impairments associated with the neurotoxic effects of some cytotoxic agents (particularly platinum, procarbazine, paclitaxel, or etoposide).

*DISTURBED SLEEP PATTERN**

related to:
a. nausea, vomiting, and pain;
b. anxiety, fear, and grief;
c. frequent need to defecate associated with diarrhea if present.

INEFFECTIVE COPING/IMPAIRED ADJUSTMENT*

related to persistent discomfort associated with the side effects of chemotherapy, fear, anxiety, chronic fatigue, feeling of powerlessness, and uncertainty of prognosis.

RISK FOR POWERLESSNESS

related to:
a. the possibility of disease progression and death despite treatment;
b. dependence on others to assist with basic needs as a result of fatigue, weakness, and discomfort;
c. possible alterations in roles, relationships, and future plans associated with changes that occur as a result of the cancer and the side effects/toxic effects of the cytotoxic drugs.

---

*See Unit II for outcomes, actions, and rationales.

Bibliography

See pages 879–881.

External Radiation Therapy (Teletherapy)

Radiation therapy is one of the four major modes of treatment for cancer. It can be either external (teletherapy) or internal (brachytherapy) and is a local treatment in which cellular destruction occurs only at the treatment site. It is most effective on well-oxygenated tumors with a high growth fraction. Unfortunately, radiation therapy is not a selective process and changes in cellular structure and function occur in both cancerous and normal cells within the treatment field. The normal cells, however, have a greater capacity for self-repair.

The effect of radiation therapy on the cell begins immediately and continues through several reproductive cycles of the cell. The time of cellular death and the side effects experienced by the client depend on the number of grays (Gy) or centigrays (cGy) received, the volume of tissue irradiated, whether or not both strands of DNA are broken, the extent of the damage to the cell's reproductive abilities, and the cell's ability to repair damage. The side effects that most clients receiving external radiation experience are a skin reaction at the radiation treatment site, fatigue, malaise, and anorexia. Other side effects experienced depend on the anatomic site being radiated, the mitotic rate of the cells within the treatment field, fractionation of the dose, total dose delivered, and the general condition of the client.

Although it may be used alone, radiation therapy is increasingly being used in combination with surgery, chemotherapy, and/or biotherapy to achieve palliation, control, or cure of cancer. External radiation is also used with brachytherapy to treat certain cancers (e.g., prostate, endometrial) more effectively. Radiation therapy in combination with surgical treatment of some cancers has resulted in the need for less extensive surgery.

Minimization of damage to normal tissue with maximum tumor kill is a primary goal of radiation therapy. This goal is being accomplished more frequently as a result of advances in technology and techniques. Computerized three-dimensional treatment planning provides more accurate targeting of tumor tissue and the use of equipment that contains multiple, computer-operated shields results in preservation of a greater amount of the normal tissue surrounding the tumor. Radiosensitizers that increase the sensitivity of tumor cells to radiation and radioprotectants that help protect normal cells from radiation damage may be used during teletherapy for some clients to achieve this same goal. In addition, changes in standard radiation protocols (e.g., more frequent, smaller doses of radiation) are being made in some instances to increase tumor cell kill and decrease damage to normal cells.

This care plan focuses on the adult client hospitalized for initiation of external radiation therapy or for management of side effects associated with radiation therapy. Much of the information is applicable to the client undergoing treatment on an outpatient basis.

OUTCOME/DISCHARGE CRITERIA

THE CLIENT WILL:

- have an adequate or improved nutritional status
- have fatigue at a manageable level
- have evidence of normal healing of skin at site of irradiation
- have no signs and symptoms of complications of radiation therapy
- verbalize an understanding of appropriate skin care for site of irradiation
- identify techniques to control nausea and vomiting
- verbalize ways to improve appetite and nutritional status
- identify ways to reduce the risk of dental caries and periodontal disease and manage stomatitis if present
- identify ways to prevent bleeding if platelet counts are low
- identify ways to prevent infection if WBC counts are low
- verbalize an understanding of and ways to manage the effects of radiation therapy on sexual and reproductive functioning
- verbalize ways to manage and cope with persistent fatigue
- verbalize an understanding of the signs and symptoms of lymphedema and ways to manage it if it occurs
- state signs and symptoms to report to the health care provider
- share feelings and thoughts about the diagnosis of cancer and the effects of radiation therapy on body image
- identify community resources that can assist with home management and adjustment to the diagnosis of cancer and radiation therapy and its effects
- verbalize an understanding of and a plan for adhering to recommended follow-up care including medications prescribed and future appointments with health care provider, radiation department, and laboratory.

NURSING/COLLABORATIVE DIAGNOSES

Client Teaching

1. NURSING DIAGNOSIS: *DEFICIENT KNOWLEDGE: PRE-RADIATION*

regarding how radiation works, pre- and post-radiation routines, what to expect during actual radiation treatment, and expected side effects of radiation.

Suggested NOC Outcomes: Knowledge: treatment regimen; Knowledge: treatment procedure(s)

Suggested NIC Interventions: Teaching: treatment/procedure; Teaching: individual

Desired Outcome	Nursing Actions *and Selected Purposes/Rationales*
1. The client will verbalize an understanding of radiation therapy and what to expect before, during, and after radiation treatments.	1.a. Provide the client with the following information about radiation therapy including: 1. how radiation therapy works and why the total radiation dose prescribed is fractionated 2. that he/she will be alone in the room during the few minutes of therapy but will be observed continuously via a television monitor and that communication will be possible by means of an intercommunication system 3. that the machine may click or make a whirring noise but no discomfort will be felt during the treatment 4. the possible general side effects of radiation therapy (e.g., fatigue; anorexia; itchy, dry, reddened skin; moist desquamation and increase in skin pigmentation at radiation site), anticipated side effects for the particular site being irradiated, and when the side effects can be expected to occur and resolve 5. the treatment simulation process that occurs before initiation of therapy (the simulation process is done to accurately determine the treatment field and design devices such as plastic or plaster molds or lead blocks that will be used to ensure proper positioning and/or shield vital body organs within the treatment field)

Desired Outcome	Nursing Actions *and Selected Purposes/Rationales*

6. that vital organs within the radiation treatment field are shielded during treatment to prevent unnecessary exposure to radiation, that the treatment field will include the smallest amount of normal tissue possible, and the field may be changed or reduced as the tumor shrinks in size
7. how the treatment field will be outlined (e.g., skin markings with an indelible dye, ink, or felt tip marker) and that the markings will be replaced by pinpoint tattoos once the reproducibility of the field is ensured.

b. Arrange for client and significant others to visit the radiation department and meet those individuals responsible for his/her care.
c. Prepare client for waiting room experiences with others receiving radiation therapy. Emphasize that each individual has a different treatment plan, response, and prognosis and that comparison should be avoided.
d. Allow adequate time for questions and clarification of information provided.

2. Nursing Diagnosis: FEAR/ANXIETY

related to:
a. unfamiliar environment;
b. lack of knowledge about radiation therapy if admitted to initiate therapy;
c. need for hospitalization to manage existing side effects of radiation therapy and concern that additional untoward effects will occur with subsequent radiation treatments;
d. financial concerns;
e. diagnosis of cancer with potential for premature death.

Suggested NOC Outcomes: Anxiety level; Fear level; Anxiety self-control; Fear self-control

Suggested NIC Interventions: Anxiety reduction; Calming technique; Emotional support; Presence; Teaching: procedure/treatment; Financial resource assistance

Desired Outcome	Nursing Actions *and Selected Purposes/Rationales* (see pp. 14–16 for additional rationales)

2. The client will experience a reduction in fear and anxiety as evidenced by:
   a. verbalization of feeling less anxious
   b. usual sleep pattern
   c. relaxed facial expression and body movements
   d. stable vital signs
   e. usual perceptual ability and interactions with others.

2.a. Assess client on admission for:
1. fears, misconceptions, and level of understanding of radiation therapy and its therapeutic and nontherapeutic effects
2. significance to client of the site to be irradiated
3. perception of the impact of the radiation therapy treatment schedule on usual lifestyle, roles, and personal relationships
4. availability of an adequate support system
5. past experience with radiation therapy or other treatments for cancer
6. signs and symptoms of fear and anxiety (e.g., verbalization of feeling anxious, insomnia, tenseness, shakiness, restlessness, diaphoresis, tachycardia, elevated blood pressure, self-focused behaviors).

b. Implement measures *to reduce fear and anxiety:*
1. orient client to hospital environment, equipment, and routines
2. introduce client to staff who will be participating in care; if possible, maintain consistency in staff assigned to his/her care
3. assure client that staff members are nearby; respond to call signal as soon as possible
4. maintain a calm, supportive, confident manner when interacting with client
5. encourage verbalization of fear and anxiety; provide feedback
6. provide information about radiation therapy (see Diagnosis 1, actions a–c)

7. reinforce physician's explanations and clarify misconceptions client has about the diagnosis of cancer, treatment plan and its effects, and prognosis
8. provide a calm, restful environment
9. instruct client in relaxation techniques (e.g., listening to music, exercise, yoga, guided imagery) and encourage participation in diversional activities
10. assist client to identify specific stressors and ways to cope with them
11. initiate a social service referral and/or assist client to identify and contact appropriate community resources if indicated
12. provide information based on current needs of client at a level he/she can understand; encourage questions and clarification of information provided
13. provide client with a note pad and pencil, printed information, and/or a tape recorder so he/she can review the information presented as often as desired
14. encourage significant others to project a caring, concerned attitude without obvious anxiousness
15. include significant others in orientation and teaching sessions and encourage their continued support of client
16. administer prescribed antianxiety agents if indicated.

c. Consult appropriate health care provider (e.g., psychiatric nurse clinician, oncology nurse specialist, physician) if above actions fail to control fear and anxiety.

3. NURSING DIAGNOSIS: *IMBALANCED NUTRITION: LESS THAN BODY REQUIREMENTS*

related to:

a. decreased oral intake associated with:
   1. anorexia resulting from factors such as depression, fear, anxiety, fatigue, discomfort, early satiety, an altered sense of taste (often reported by persons with cancer; can also result from damage to the taste buds and salivary glands with radiation to the head and neck), and increased levels of certain cytokines that depress appetite (e.g., interleukin-1, tumor necrosis factor)
   2. impaired swallowing resulting from pharyngitis, esophagitis, dry mouth, and/or viscous oral secretions if present as a result of radiation treatment to the head, neck, or mediastinum;
b. loss of nutrients associated with vomiting and diarrhea if present;
c. impaired utilization of nutrients associated with:
   1. accelerated and inefficient metabolism of proteins, carbohydrates, and/or fats resulting from factors such as increased levels of cortisol, glucagon, and certain cytokines (e.g., tumor necrosis factor, interleukin-1)
   2. decreased absorption of nutrients resulting from loss of intestinal absorptive surface if mucositis has developed (can occur with radiation to the abdomen or lower back);
d. utilization of available nutrients by the malignant cells rather than the host.

Suggested NOC Outcomes: Nutritional status; Appetite

Suggested NIC Interventions: Nutritional monitoring; Nutrition management; Nutrition therapy; Pain management; Nausea management

Desired Outcome	**Nursing Actions** *and Selected Purposes/Rationales* (see pp. 40–43 for additional rationales)
3. The client will have or attain an adequate nutritional status as evidenced by: a. weight within or returning toward normal range for client	3.a. Assess for and report signs and symptoms of malnutrition: 1. significant weight loss (a loss of 1–2 pounds during each week of radiation therapy is often expected) 2. abnormal BUN and low serum prealbumin, albumin, Hct, Hgb, and transferrin levels 3. weakness and fatigue 4. sore, inflamed oral mucous membrane

Desired Outcome	**Nursing Actions** *and Selected Purposes/Rationales*
b. normal BUN and serum prealbumin, albumin, Hct, Hgb, and transferrin levels c. usual strength and activity tolerance d. healthy oral mucous membrane.	5. pale conjunctiva.

b. Monitor percentage of meals and snacks client consumes. Report a pattern of inadequate intake.

c. Implement measures *to maintain or promote an adequate nutritional status:*
   1. perform actions *to improve oral intake:*
      a. implement measures to control nausea and vomiting (see Diagnosis 6, action b)
      b. implement measures to reduce pain (see Diagnosis 5, action d)
      c. implement measures to assist client to adjust psychologically to the diagnosis of cancer and treatment with radiation therapy (see Diagnoses 14, actions c–j and 15, action b)
      d. implement measures to improve client's ability to swallow (see Diagnosis 4, action b)
      e. implement measures *to compensate for taste alterations* if present (loss of sense of taste often occurs within 2 weeks of initiation of radiation treatment to head and neck, may persist for 4–6 weeks after completion of therapy, and usually is not permanent):
         1. encourage client to select mild-tasting fish, cold turkey or chicken, eggs, and cheese as protein sources if beef or pork tastes bitter or rancid
         2. provide meat for breakfast if aversion to meat tends to increase during day
         3. marinate meats in red wine or sweet and sour sauce
         4. add extra sweeteners to foods if acceptable to client
         5. experiment with different flavorings, seasonings, and textures
         6. serve food cold or at room temperature *(can decrease some peculiar tastes)*
      f. increase activity as tolerated *(activity usually promotes a sense of well-being, which can improve appetite)*
      g. obtain a dietary consult if necessary to assist client in selecting foods/fluids that meet nutritional needs, are appealing, and adhere to personal and cultural preferences
      h. encourage a rest period before meals *to minimize fatigue*
      i. maintain a clean environment and a relaxed, pleasant atmosphere
      j. provide oral hygiene before meals *(oral hygiene moistens the mouth, which makes it easier to chew and swallow; it also removes unpleasant tastes, which often improves the taste of foods/fluids)*
      k. provide largest amount of calories and protein when appetite is best (usually at breakfast)
      l. serve frequent, small meals rather than large ones if client is weak, fatigues easily, and/or has a poor appetite
      m. encourage significant others to bring in client's favorite foods and eat with him/her *to make eating more of a familiar social experience*
      n. limit fluid intake with meals (unless the fluid has high nutritional value) *to reduce early satiety and subsequent decreased food intake*
      o. allow adequate time for meals; reheat foods/fluids if necessary
      p. administer appetite stimulants (e.g., megestrol acetate, dronabinol) if ordered
   2. ensure that meals are well balanced and high in essential nutrients; offer high-protein, high-calorie dietary supplements (e.g., milk shakes, puddings, or eggnog made with cream or powdered milk reconstituted with whole milk; commercially prepared dietary supplements) if indicated
   3. perform actions to control diarrhea (see Diagnosis 11, action b)
   4. administer vitamins and minerals if ordered.

d. Perform a calorie count if ordered. Report information to dietitian and physician.

e. Consult physician about an alternative method of providing nutrition (e.g., parenteral nutrition, tube feedings) if client does not consume enough food or fluids to meet nutritional needs.

4. Nursing Diagnosis:

IMPAIRED SWALLOWING

related to:

a. oral, pharyngeal, or esophageal pain associated with inflammation and/or ulceration of the mucosa if the treatment field includes the head, neck, or mediastinum;
b. dry mouth and viscous oral secretions associated with:
   1. destruction of the salivary glands (particularly the parotids) if the treatment field includes the head and neck
   2. decreased oral intake.

Suggested NOC Outcome: Swallowing status

Suggested NIC Interventions: Swallowing therapy; Pain management; Oral health restoration

Desired Outcome

Nursing Actions *and Selected Purposes/Rationales* (see pp. 54–57 for additional rationales)

4. The client will experience an improvement in swallowing as evidenced by:
   a. verbalization of same
   b. absence of food in oral cavity after swallowing
   c. absence of coughing and choking when eating and drinking.

4.a. Assess for signs and symptoms of impaired swallowing (e.g., statements of difficulty swallowing, stasis of food in oral cavity, coughing or choking when eating or drinking).

b. Implement measures *to improve ability to swallow:*
   1. perform actions to reduce oral, pharyngeal, and esophageal pain (see Diagnosis 5, action d.7)
   2. perform actions to reduce the severity of stomatitis and/or relieve dryness of the oral mucous membrane (see Diagnosis 9, action b)
   3. assist client to select foods that require little or no chewing and are easily swallowed (e.g., custard, eggs, canned fruit, mashed potatoes)
   4. avoid serving foods that are sticky (e.g., peanut butter, soft bread, honey)
   5. moisten dry foods with gravy or sauces (e.g., sour cream, salad dressing)
   6. perform actions *to stimulate salivation at meal time:*
      a. provide oral hygiene before meals
      b. provide a piece of hard candy for client to suck on just before meals unless contraindicated
      c. serve foods that are visually pleasing
   7. perform actions *to reduce and/or liquefy viscous oral secretions:*
      a. encourage a fluid intake of 2500 ml/day unless contraindicated
      b. encourage client to avoid milk, milk products, and chocolate *(when combined with saliva, they produce very thick secretions).*

c. Consult appropriate health care provider (e.g., oncology nurse specialist, physician) if swallowing difficulties persist or worsen.

5. Nursing Diagnosis:

ACUTE PAIN

related to inflammation and/or moist desquamation (if it occurs) in irradiated area.

Suggested NOC Outcomes: Pain control; Comfort level

Suggested NIC Interventions: Pain management; Analgesic administration; Environmental management: comfort; Wound care; Oral health restoration

Desired Outcome

Nursing Actions *and Selected Purposes/Rationales* (see pp. 45–47 for additional rationales)

5. The client will experience diminished pain as evidenced by:
   a. verbalization of decreased pain
   b. relaxed facial expression and body positioning

5.a. Assess for signs and symptoms of pain (e.g., verbalization of pain, grimacing, reluctance to move, restlessness, diaphoresis, increased B/P, tachycardia).

b. Assess client's perception of the severity of pain using a pain intensity rating scale.

c. Assess the client's pain pattern (e.g., location, quality, onset, duration, precipitating factors, aggravating factors, alleviating factors).

Desired Outcome	**Nursing Actions** *and Selected Purposes/Rationales*
c. increased participation in activities d. stable vital signs.	d. Implement measures *to reduce pain:* 1. perform actions *to reduce fear and anxiety about the pain experience* (e.g., assure client that his/her need for pain relief is understood, plan methods of achieving pain control with client) 2. perform actions to reduce fear and anxiety (see Diagnosis 2, action b) *in order to promote relaxation and subsequently increase the client's threshold and tolerance for pain* 3. administer analgesics before activities and procedures that can cause pain and before pain becomes severe 4. perform actions to reduce fatigue (see Diagnosis 10, action d) *in order to increase the client's threshold and tolerance for pain* 5. perform actions *to reduce pain associated with moist desquamation:* a. implement measures identified in Diagnosis 8, action b.1.i to treat a moist desquamation reaction b. if open method of treatment is being used, position a covered bed cradle over affected area *to reduce airflow over exposed nerve endings* 6. perform actions *to reduce perianal pain* (can occur if the perineum is in the treatment field or if diarrhea is present): a. provide a foam pad for client to sit on b. consult physician about an order for sitz baths unless contraindicated c. implement measures to decrease skin irritation and prevent breakdown associated with diarrhea (see Diagnosis 8, action b.2) d. avoid taking temperature rectally or administering rectal suppositories e. apply a topical anesthetic/corticosteroid cream (e.g., Corticaine) if ordered 7. perform actions *to reduce oral, pharyngeal, and esophageal pain* (can occur with radiation to the head, neck, and mediastinum): a. implement measures to reduce severity of stomatitis (see Diagnosis 9, actions b and c) b. offer cool, soothing liquids such as nonacidic juices and ices c. instruct client to gargle with a saline solution every 2 hours or spray mouth with a solution containing diphenhydramine and water (1 oz diphenhydramine and 1 qt water) if ordered *to soothe the oral mucous membrane* d. administer oral protective agents and topical anesthetics or analgesics (e.g., mixture of diphenhydramine, antacid, and Xylocaine Viscous; sucralfate oral suspension) if ordered 8. provide or assist with nonpharmacologic measures for pain relief (e.g., relaxation exercises; guided imagery; restful environment; diversional activities such as watching television, reading, or conversing) 9. administer analgesics if ordered. e. Consult appropriate health care provider (e.g., oncology nurse specialist, physician) if above measures fail to provide adequate pain relief.

6. NURSING DIAGNOSIS: *NAUSEA*

related to stimulation of the vomiting center associated with:

a. presence of by-products of cellular destruction if client is receiving a large daily fraction of radiation or daily treatments over a period of several weeks;
b. stimulation of the visceral afferent pathways resulting from inflammation of the gastrointestinal mucosa (occurs when areas of the chest, back, abdomen, or pelvis are irradiated);
c. stimulation of the cerebral cortex resulting from cerebral inflammation (if client is receiving whole brain irradiation) and stress.

Suggested NOC Outcome:
Nausea and vomiting severity

Suggested NIC Interventions: Nausea management; Vomiting management

Desired Outcome	Nursing Actions *and Selected Purposes/Rationales*
6. The client will experience relief of nausea and vomiting as evidenced by: a. verbalization of relief of nausea b. absence of vomiting.	6.a. Assess client for nausea and vomiting (tends to occur within 1–3 hours after treatment). b. Implement measures *to control nausea and vomiting:* 1. perform actions to reduce fear and anxiety and promote psychological adjustment to the diagnosis of cancer and treatment with external radiation (see Diagnoses 2, action b; 14, actions c–j; and 15, action b) 2. eliminate noxious sights and odors from the environment *(noxious stimuli can cause stimulation of the vomiting center)* 3. encourage client to take deep, slow breaths when nauseated 4. encourage client to change positions slowly *(rapid movement can result in stimulation of the chemoreceptor trigger zone and subsequent excitation of the vomiting center)* 5. provide oral hygiene after each emesis and before meals 6. maintain food and fluid restrictions if ordered (client may be placed on a clear liquid or bland diet for short periods if nausea is severe) 7. provide carbonated beverages for client to sip if nauseated 8. avoid serving foods with an overpowering aroma; remove lids from hot foods before entering room 9. provide small, frequent meals; instruct client to ingest foods and fluids slowly 10. if nausea tends to peak after each treatment, instruct client to eat his/her major meal of the day at least 3 hours before treatment if possible and to eat lightly for 3–4 hours after the treatment 11. encourage client to eat dry foods (e.g., toast, crackers) and avoid drinking liquids with meals if nauseated 12. instruct client to avoid foods/fluids that irritate the gastric mucosa (e.g., spicy foods; caffeine-containing beverages such as coffee, tea, and colas) 13. instruct client to rest after eating 14. administer antiemetics as ordered (these are often given on a regular schedule 1–2 hours before radiation therapy and every 4–6 hours for 12 hours after treatment). c. Consult appropriate health care provider (e.g., oncology nurse specialist, physician) if above measures fail to control nausea and vomiting.

7. NURSING DIAGNOSIS:

ALTERED COMFORT: PRURITUS

related to dry skin associated with decreased function of sebaceous and sweat glands within the treatment field.

Suggested NOC Outcomes:
Comfort level; Symptom control

Suggested NIC Intervention: Pruritus management

Desired Outcome	Nursing Actions *and Selected Purposes/Rationales*
7. The client will experience relief of pruritus as evidenced by: a. verbalization of same b. no scratching and rubbing of skin.	7.a. Assess for the following: 1. reports of itchiness 2. persistent scratching or rubbing of skin 3. dryness and redness or excoriation of skin within the treatment field. b. Instruct client in and/or implement measures *to relieve pruritus in the treatment area:* 1. apply cool, moist compresses to pruritic areas 2. maintain a cool environment

Desired Outcome	Nursing Actions *and Selected Purposes/Rationales*

3. perform actions *to reduce skin dryness:*
   a. use tepid water and mild soaps for bathing, being careful not to remove temporary skin markings
   b. apply water-based lubricant lotions (e.g., Lubriderm, Eucerin) 2–3 times daily and after bath (avoid lotions that contain lanolin or petrolatum *because they must be removed before treatments)*
   c. limit bathing to every other day
   d. encourage a fluid intake of 2500 ml/day unless contraindicated
   e. utilize a room humidifier *to increase moisture in the air*
4. add emollients, cornstarch, baking soda, or colloidal-based bath products to bath water
5. apply a light dusting of cornstarch to areas of dry desquamation (cornstarch should not be used if moist desquamation is present)
6. make an oatmeal paste, apply to pruritic areas, let dry for 3–5 minutes, and then rinse with cool water
7. pat skin dry after bathing, making sure to dry thoroughly
8. encourage participation in diversional activities and use of relaxation techniques (e.g., music, imagery)
9. use cutaneous stimulation techniques (e.g., stroking with a soft brush, light massage, pressure) at sites of itching or acupressure points (skin within the treatment field should never be rubbed or deeply massaged)
10. encourage client to wear loose cotton garments
11. administer antihistamines and/or apply topical anesthetic cream (e.g., Lanacane) if ordered.

c. Consult appropriate health care provider (e.g., oncology nurse specialist, physician) if above measures fail to relieve pruritus or if the skin becomes more excoriated.

8. Nursing Diagnosis: ACTUAL/RISK FOR IMPAIRED SKIN INTEGRITY

related to:

a. dry desquamation of irradiated site associated with increased sensitivity of skin in certain areas (e.g., opposing skin surfaces, face, perineum) and destruction of rapidly dividing epithelial cells of the skin;
b. moist desquamation of irradiated area associated with damage to the basal cells of the skin;
c. increased skin fragility associated with:
   1. tissue edema resulting from vascular changes in irradiated area
   2. malnutrition;
d. excessive scratching associated with pruritus;
e. frequent contact of the skin with irritants associated with diarrhea if present.

Suggested NOC Outcomes: Tissue integrity: skin and mucous membranes; Wound healing: secondary intention

Suggested NIC Interventions: Skin surveillance; Skin care: topical treatments; Wound care

Desired Outcome	Nursing Actions *and Selected Purposes/Rationales* (see pp. 49–52 for additional rationales)
8. The client will maintain or regain skin integrity as evidenced by: a. minimal redness and irritation within the treatment field	8.a. Inspect the following areas for pallor, redness, and breakdown: 1. treatment field and area on the body surface opposite to it (should be assessed before treatment, every week during treatment, and on every subsequent visit) 2. opposing skin surfaces 3. bony prominences 4. dependent, pruritic, and edematous areas 5. perineum.

b. absence of redness and irritation in body areas not in treatment field
c. no skin breakdown.

b. Implement measures *to maintain or regain skin integrity:*
   1. perform actions *to prevent or treat skin irritation or breakdown within the treatment field:*
      a. cleanse irradiated area gently each shift with tepid water and mild soap (may be contraindicated initially when temporary skin markings rather than tattoos are used)
      b. pat skin dry using soft materials, paying particular attention to opposing skin surfaces within the treatment field
      c. expose irradiated area to the air as much as possible, avoiding extremes in temperature
      d. apply a skin sealant to the area to be irradiated if ordered
      e. avoid use of tape within irradiated area
      f. instruct client to:
         1. wear loose cotton clothing
         2. avoid use of perfumed lotions or soaps, cosmetics, and deodorants *to prevent chemical irritation (many of these products contain heavy metals that will augment effects of radiation on the skin)*
         3. apply a light dusting of cornstarch to areas of dry desquamation *to reduce friction*
         4. apply a mild, water-based lubricant lotion (e.g., Lubriderm, Eucerin) *to reduce skin dryness and subsequent cracking*
         5. avoid use of hydrophobic products (e.g., Vaseline) *because they are difficult to remove*
         6. use an electric rather than a straight-edge razor if it is absolutely necessary to shave in irradiated area
      g. avoid applications of heat and cold to irradiated area
      h. implement measures *to prevent skin breakdown associated with scratching:*
         1. perform actions to relieve pruritus (see Diagnosis 7, action b)
         2. keep nails trimmed and/or apply mittens if necessary
         3. instruct client to apply firm pressure to pruritic areas rather than scratching
      i. implement measures *to treat a moist desquamation reaction if it has occurred*
         1. cleanse area well with a saline solution, water, or a dilute solution of chlorhexidine 3 times/day; apply an astringent soak if ordered
         2. keep involved area exposed to the air as much as possible
         3. apply a metal-free gel (e.g., RadiaCare) to involved area if ordered
         4. apply a topical antimicrobial agent as ordered if signs and symptoms of a localized infection occur
   2. perform actions *to decrease skin irritation and prevent breakdown associated with diarrhea:*
      a. implement measures to control diarrhea (see Diagnosis 11, action b)
      b. assist client to thoroughly cleanse and dry perineal area with soft tissue or cloth after each bowel movement; apply a protective ointment or cream, being sure to remove it before treatments if rectal area is within treatment field
      c. if use of absorbent products such as pads or undergarments is necessary, select those that effectively absorb moisture and keep it away from the skin
   3. if edema is present:
      a. perform actions *to reduce fluid accumulation in dependent areas:*
         1. instruct client in and assist with range of motion exercises
         2. elevate affected extremities whenever possible
      b. handle edematous areas carefully
   4. perform actions to promote an adequate nutritional status (see Diagnosis 3, action c).

Desired Outcome	Nursing Actions *and Selected Purposes/Rationales*
	c. If unexpected skin irritation or breakdown occurs: 1. notify appropriate health care provider (e.g., oncology nurse specialist, wound care specialist, physician) 2. perform care of involved areas as ordered or per standard hospital procedure.

9. Nursing Diagnosis:

IMPAIRED ORAL MUCOUS MEMBRANE

a. dryness related to decreased oral intake and destruction of salivary glands if the treatment field includes the head and neck;
b. stomatitis related to malnutrition, inadequate oral hygiene, and disruption in the renewal process of mucosal epithelial cells if the oral cavity is irradiated.

Suggested NOC Outcome: Oral hygiene

Suggested NIC Interventions: Oral health maintenance; Oral health restoration

Desired Outcome	Nursing Actions *and Selected Purposes/Rationales* (see pp. 43–45 for additional rationales)
9. The client will maintain a healthy oral cavity as evidenced by: a. no reports of oral dryness and burning b. pink, moist, intact mucosa c. absence of inflammation d. ability to swallow without discomfort.	9.a. Assess client for: 1. dryness of the oral mucosa and presence of thick, ropey saliva (reduction in salivary flow may occur after a cumulative dose of as little as 1000 cGy to the head and neck and may persist for many months after treatment; dryness will be permanent after a radiation exposure of over 6000 cGy) 2. signs and symptoms of stomatitis (e.g., inflamed and/or ulcerated oral mucosa; reports of burning pain in mouth, difficulty swallowing, or taste changes; positive results of cultured specimens from oral lesions). b. Implement measures *to prevent or reduce the severity of stomatitis and/or relieve dryness of the oral mucous membrane:* 1. administer amifostine 15–30 minutes prior to radiation treatment that includes the parotid glands in client with head and neck cancer *(amifostine is used as a protectant agent to reduce the incidence of xerostomia)* 2. instruct and assist client to perform oral hygiene after eating and as often as needed; avoid use of products that contain lemon and glycerin and mouthwashes containing alcohol *(these products have a drying and irritating effect on the oral mucous membrane)* 3. instruct and assist client to perform oral hygiene using a soft bristle toothbrush or a sponge-tipped swab and to floss teeth gently 4. have client rinse mouth frequently with warm saline solution, baking soda and warm water, or chlorhexidene gluconate (Peridex) or mist oral cavity frequently using a spray bottle 5. lubricate client's lips frequently 6. encourage a fluid intake of 2500 ml/day unless contraindicated 7. encourage client not to smoke or chew tobacco *(smoking dries the mucosa; tobacco acts as an irritant to the oral mucosa)* 8. perform actions *to stimulate salivation:* a. encourage client to suck on sugarless candy or chew sugarless gum b. administer silagogues (e.g., oral pilocarpine [Salagen]) if ordered 9. instruct client to avoid substances that might further irritate the oral mucosa (e.g., hot, spicy, or acidic foods/fluids) 10. perform actions to promote an adequate nutritional status (see Diagnosis 3, action c) 11. encourage client to use a saliva substitute such as Salivart if indicated 12. provide client with a prophylactic antifungal oral suspension or lozenge (e.g., nystatin) if ordered.

c. If stomatitis is not controlled:
   1. increase frequency of oral hygiene
   2. if client has dentures, remove them and replace only for meals.

d. Consult appropriate health care provider (e.g., oncology nurse specialist, physician) if oral dryness and signs and symptoms of stomatitis persist or worsen.

10. Nursing Diagnosis: FATIGUE

related to*:

a. a build up of cellular waste products associated with rapid lysis of cancerous and normal cells exposed to radiation;
b. tissue hypoxia associated with anemia (can result from malnutrition or depression of bone marrow activity if large amounts of active bone marrow are included in the treatment field);
c. difficulty resting and sleeping associated with fear, anxiety, and discomfort;
d. overwhelming emotional demands associated with the diagnosis of cancer and treatment with radiation;
e. increased energy expenditure associated with an increase in the metabolic rate resulting from continuous active tumor growth and increased levels of certain cytokines (e.g., tumor necrosis factor, interleukin-1);
f. malnutrition;
g. side effects of medications client may be receiving (e.g., narcotic [opioid] analgesics, antiemetics, antianxiety agents).

*Some of the etiological factors presented here are under investigation.

Suggested NOC Outcomes: Endurance; Energy conservation; Rest; Psychomotor energy

Suggested NIC Interventions: Energy management; Nutrition management; Sleep enhancement; Mood management

Desired Outcome	**Nursing Actions** *and Selected Purposes/Rationales*
10. The client will experience a reduction in fatigue as evidenced by: a. verbalization of feelings of increased energy b. ability to perform usual activities of daily living c. increased interest in surroundings and ability to concentrate.	10.a. Assess for: 1. signs and symptoms of fatigue (e.g., verbalization of lack of energy and inability to maintain usual routines, lack of interest in surroundings, decreased ability to concentrate, lethargy) 2. client's perception of the severity of fatigue using a fatigue rating scale; have client try to determine the severity of fatigue currently and an average for each week since last treatment. b. Inform client that a feeling of persistent fatigue is not unusual and can result from the disease itself, cell breakdown that occurs with radiation therapy, and side effects of some medications he/she may be taking. c. Assist client to identify personal patterns of fatigue (e.g., time of day, after treatments or certain activities) and to plan activities so that times of greatest fatigue are avoided. d. Implement measures *to reduce fatigue:* 1. perform actions *to promote rest and/or conserve energy:* a. schedule several short rest periods during the day b. minimize environmental activity and noise c. limit the number of visitors and their length of stay d. assist client with self-care activities as needed e. keep supplies and personal articles within easy reach f. implement measures to reduce fear and anxiety (see Diagnosis 2, action b) g. implement measures *to promote sleep* (e.g., encourage relaxing diversional activities in the evening, allow client to continue usual sleep practices unless contraindicated, reduce environmental stimuli, administer prescribed sedative-hypnotics)

Desired Outcome	Nursing Actions *and Selected Purposes/Rationales*
	h. implement measures to reduce discomfort (see Diagnoses 5, action d; 6, action b; and 7, action b) i. instruct client in energy-saving techniques (e.g., using shower chair when showering, sitting to brush teeth or comb hair, prioritizing activities and eliminating those that are optional) 2. perform actions to promote an adequate nutritional status (see Diagnosis 3, action c) 3. encourage client to maintain a fluid intake of at least 2500 ml/day unless contraindicated *to promote elimination of the by-products of cellular breakdown* 4. administer the following if ordered *to treat anemia:* a. iron preparations (e.g., ferrous gluconate, ferrous sulfate) b. folic acid (e.g., folate) c. erythropoiesis stimulating growth factor such as epoetin alfa (e.g., Epogen, EPO, Procrit) or darbepoetin alfa (e.g., Aranesp) d. blood transfusions (e.g., packed red blood cells) 5. increase activity gradually as tolerated 6. perform actions to facilitate client's psychological adjustment to the diagnosis of cancer and the treatment regimen and its effects (see Diagnoses 14, actions c–j and 15, action b). e. Consult appropriate health care provider (e.g., oncology nurse specialist, physician) if signs and symptoms of fatigue worsen.

11. Nursing Diagnosis: DIARRHEA

related to increased peristalsis and disorders of intestinal secretion and absorption associated with damage to the intestinal mucosa if the treatment field includes the pelvis, abdomen, or lower back.

Suggested NOC Outcome:
Bowel elimination

Suggested NIC Intervention: Diarrhea management

Desired Outcome	Nursing Actions *and Selected Purposes/Rationales* (see pp. 28–30 for additional rationales)
11. The client will have fewer bowel movements and more formed stool if diarrhea occurs.	11.a. Assess for signs and symptoms of diarrhea (e.g., frequent, loose stools [more than 3 stools/day]; urgency; abdominal cramping; hyperactive bowel sounds). Diarrhea will usually begin after 1500–3000 cGy have been received and end 2–3 weeks after cessation of treatment. b. Implement measures *to control diarrhea:* 1. restrict oral intake if ordered and progress diet gradually (elemental formulas may be ordered to minimize stimulation of the bowel) 2. instruct client to avoid the following foods/fluids that may stimulate or irritate the inflamed bowel or cause the stool to be more liquid: a. those high in fiber (e.g., whole-grain cereals, raw fruits and vegetables) b. extremely hot or cold foods/fluids c. those high in lactose (e.g., milk, milk products) d. coffee, alcohol, or foods that are spicy or fatty e. those made with synthetic, nonabsorbable sugars (e.g., sorbitol) that are found in dietetic foods 3. encourage intake of foods/fluids high in pectin (e.g., pear or apple juice, peeled apples, avocados, bananas) 4. administer the following medications if ordered *to control diarrhea:* a. opioids (e.g., paregoric) or synthetic opioids (e.g., loperamide, diphenoxylate hydrochloride) *to decrease gastrointestinal motility* b. adsorbents/protectants (e.g., attapulgite [Kaopectate], bismuth subsalicylate [Pepto-Bismol])

c. antisecretory agents (e.g., octreotide acetate [Sandostatin]) *to suppress the output of gastroenterohepatic peptides and slow intestinal motility.*

c. Consult appropriate health care provider (e.g., oncology nurse specialist, physician) if diarrhea persists.

12. Nursing Diagnosis: RISK FOR INFECTION

related to:
a. break in the integrity of the skin associated with dry or moist desquamation;
b. lowered natural resistance associated with:
   1. malnutrition
   2. neutropenia resulting from bone marrow suppression if large amounts of active bone marrow are included in the treatment field
   3. impaired immune system functioning resulting from certain malignancies (e.g., Hodgkin's disease, lymphoma);
c. stasis of respiratory secretions and urinary stasis if mobility is decreased.

Suggested NOC Outcomes: Immune status; Infection severity

Suggested NIC Interventions: Infection protection; Infection control; Wound care

Desired Outcome

12. The client will remain free of infection as evidenced by:
   a. absence of fever and chills
   b. pulse within normal limits
   c. normal breath sounds
   d. usual mental status
   e. cough productive of clear mucus only
   f. voiding clear urine without reports of frequency, urgency, and burning
   g. absence of redness, heat, pain, swelling, and unusual drainage in any area
   h. no reports of increased weakness and fatigue
   i. WBC and differential counts within normal range for client
   j. negative results of cultured specimens.

Nursing Actions *and Selected Purposes/Rationales*

(see pp. 37–40 for additional rationales)

12.a. Assess for and report signs and symptoms of infection (be alert to subtle changes in the client since the signs of infection may be minimal as a result of immunosuppression; also be aware that some signs and symptoms vary depending on the site of the infection, the causative organism, and the age of the client):
   1. elevated temperature
   2. chills
   3. increased pulse
   4. abnormal breath sounds
   5. development of or increased malaise
   6. lethargy, acute confusion
   7. further loss of appetite
   8. cough productive of purulent, green, or rust-colored sputum
   9. cloudy urine
   10. reports of frequency, urgency, or burning when urinating
   11. urinalysis showing a WBC count greater than 5, positive leukocyte esterase or nitrites, or presence of bacteria
   12. redness, heat, pain, swelling, or unusual drainage in any area
   13. reports of increased weakness or fatigue
   14. elevated WBC count and/or significant change in differential
   15. positive results of cultured specimens (e.g., urine, vaginal drainage, mouth, sputum, blood, moist desquamation sites).

b. Implement measures *to reduce the risk for infection:*
   1. protect client from others with infections and those who have recently been vaccinated *(a person may have a subclinical infection after a vaccination)*
   2. use good hand hygiene and encourage client to do the same
   3. adhere to the appropriate precautions established to prevent transmission of infection to the client (e.g., standard precautions, neutropenic precautions)
   4. maintain a fluid intake of at least 2500 ml/day unless contraindicated
   5. perform actions to promote an adequate nutritional status (see Diagnosis 3, action c)
   6. provide a low-microbial diet (e.g., cooked foods, fresh fruits and vegetables that have been washed thoroughly) if client is immunosuppressed

Desired Outcome	Nursing Actions *and Selected Purposes/Rationales*

7. perform actions to prevent or reduce the severity of stomatitis (see Diagnosis 9, actions b and c)
8. clean or replace oral hygiene items (e.g., denture cup, toothbrush) regularly
9. perform actions to maintain or regain skin integrity (see Diagnosis 8, actions b and c)
10. avoid invasive procedures (e.g., urinary catheterizations, arterial and venous punctures, injections) whenever possible; if such procedures are necessary, perform them using sterile technique
11. change intravenous insertion sites according to hospital policy
12. anchor catheters/tubings (e.g., urinary, intravenous) securely *in order to reduce trauma to the tissues and the risk for introduction of pathogens associated with the in-and-out movement of the tubing*
13. maintain a closed system for drains (e.g., urinary catheter) and intravenous infusions whenever possible
14. change equipment, tubings, and solutions used for treatments such as intravenous infusions, respiratory care, irrigations, and enteral feedings according to hospital policy
15. initiate measures to prevent constipation (e.g., offer client a daily fiber supplement such as a mixture of bran, applesauce, and prune juice; encourage a minimum fluid intake of 2500 ml/day; administer laxatives as ordered) *in order to prevent damage to the bowel mucosa from hard stool*
16. avoid unnecessary rectal invasion (e.g., temperature taking, enemas, suppositories, rectal tube) *to prevent trauma to rectal mucosa and possible abscess formation*
17. perform actions to reduce stress and discomfort (see Diagnoses 2, action b; 5, action d; 6, action b; 7, action b; and 9, actions b and c) *in order to prevent an increase in the secretion of cortisol (cortisol interferes with some immune responses)*
18. perform actions *to prevent stasis of respiratory secretions* (e.g., assist client to turn, cough, and deep breathe; increase activity as tolerated)
19. perform actions to prevent urinary retention (e.g., instruct client to urinate when the urge is first felt, promote relaxation during voiding attempts) *in order to prevent urinary stasis*
20. instruct and assist client to perform good perineal care routinely and after each bowel movement
21. administer the following as ordered:
    a. antimicrobial agents
    b. colony-stimulating factors (e.g., filgrastim, pegfilgrastim, sargramostim) *to accelerate WBC recovery.*

13. Collaborative Diagnoses: POTENTIAL COMPLICATIONS OF EXTERNAL RADIATION THERAPY

a. bleeding related to thrombocytopenia associated with bone marrow suppression if large amounts of active bone marrow are included in the treatment field;
b. radiation cystitis related to irritation of the bladder mucosa if the bladder is in the treatment field;
c. radiation pneumonitis related to inflammation of lung tissue resulting from radiation to the chest;
d. lymphedema related to damage to and subsequent obstruction of lymphatic vessels in the area being irradiated (seen most frequently in persons having radiation for breast cancer, melanoma in an upper or lower extremity, gynecologic cancer, or prostate cancer).

Desired Outcomes | **Nursing Actions** *and Selected Purposes/Rationales*

13.a. The client will not experience unusual bleeding as evidenced by:
1. skin and mucous membranes free of petechiae, purpura, ecchymoses, and active bleeding
2. absence of unusual joint pain
3. no increase in abdominal girth
4. absence of frank and occult blood in stool, urine, and vomitus
5. usual menstrual flow
6. usual mental status
7. vital signs within normal range for client
8. stable or improved Hct and Hgb.

13.a.1. Assess client for and report signs and symptoms of unusual bleeding:
   a. petechiae, purpura, or ecchymoses
   b. gingival bleeding
   c. prolonged bleeding from puncture sites
   d. epistaxis, hemoptysis
   e. unusual joint pain
   f. increase in abdominal girth
   g. frank or occult blood in stool, urine, or vomitus
   h. menorrhagia
   i. restlessness, confusion
   j. decreasing B/P and increased pulse rate
   k. decrease in Hct and Hgb levels.
2. Monitor platelet count and coagulation test results (e.g., bleeding time). Report significant worsening of values.
3. If platelet count is low, coagulation test results are abnormal, or Hct and Hgb levels decrease, test all stools, urine, and vomitus for occult blood. Report positive results.
4. Implement measures *to prevent bleeding:*
   a. avoid giving injections whenever possible; consult physician about prescribing an alternative route for medications ordered to be given intramuscularly or subcutaneously
   b. when giving injections or performing venous or arterial punctures, use the smallest gauge needle possible and apply gentle, prolonged pressure to the site after the needle is removed
   c. take B/P only when necessary and avoid overinflating the cuff
   d. caution client to avoid activities that increase the risk for trauma (e.g., shaving with a straight-edge razor, using stiff bristle toothbrush or dental floss)
   e. whenever possible, avoid intubations (e.g., nasogastric) and procedures that can cause injury to rectal mucosa (e.g., taking temperature rectally, inserting a rectal suppository, administering an enema)
   f. pad side rails if client is confused or restless
   g. perform actions *to reduce the risk for falls* (e.g., keep bed in low position with side rails up when client is in bed, avoid unnecessary clutter in room, instruct client to wear slippers/shoes with nonslip soles when ambulating)
   h. instruct client to avoid blowing nose forcefully or straining to have a bowel movement; consult physician regarding an order for a decongestant and/or laxative if indicated
   i. administer the following if ordered:
      1. platelet-stimulating factor (oprelvekin [Neumega])
      2. estrogen-progestin preparations *to suppress menses*
      3. platelets.
5. If bleeding occurs and does not subside spontaneously:
   a. apply firm, prolonged pressure to bleeding area(s) if possible
   b. if epistaxis occurs, place client in a high Fowler's position and apply pressure and ice pack to nasal area
   c. maintain oxygen therapy as ordered
   d. administer whole blood or blood products (e.g., platelets) as ordered.

13.b. The client will experience resolution of radiation cystitis if it occurs as evidenced by:
1. reports of decreasing dysuria, urinary frequency and urgency, and suprapubic discomfort
2. absence of hematuria.

13.b.1. Assess for and report signs and symptoms of radiation cystitis (e.g., reports of dysuria, urinary frequency and/or urgency, or suprapubic discomfort; frank or occult blood in the urine). Symptoms of acute cystitis may appear 2–3 weeks after radiation therapy is initiated and persist for 1 month following the completion of treatment.
2. If signs and symptoms of radiation cystitis occur:
   a. implement measures *to reduce discomfort associated with cystitis:*
      1. encourage a minimum fluid intake of 2500 ml/day unless contraindicated *to keep urine dilute and thereby reduce further irritation of the bladder lining*

Desired Outcomes	Nursing Actions *and Selected Purposes/Rationales*
	2. instruct client to avoid substances that can cause bladder irritation (e.g., caffeinated beverages, alcohol, tobacco, spicy foods) 3. administer urinary tract analgesic/anesthetic agents (e.g., phenazopyridine) and bladder smooth muscle relaxants (e.g., tolterodine, oxybutynin) if ordered b. assist with measures *to control bleeding* (e.g., continuous bladder irrigation with silver nitrate, cystoscopy to cauterize bleeding vessels, instillation of formalin into the bladder) if bleeding occurs and is persistent or severe.
13.c. The client will have improvement of radiation pneumonitis if it occurs as evidenced by: 1. decreased dyspnea and coughing 2. temperature declining toward normal 3. fewer reports of night sweats.	13.c.1. Assess for and report signs and symptoms of radiation pneumonitis (e.g., dyspnea, cough, fever, night sweats, finding of infiltrates on chest x-ray results). 2. If signs and symptoms of radiation pneumonitis occur: a. implement measures *to improve respiratory function:* 1. instruct and assist client to turn, cough, and deep breathe every 1–2 hours 2. reinforce correct use of incentive spirometer every 1–2 hours 3. maintain oxygen therapy if ordered b. administer the following medications if ordered: 1. corticosteroids *to reduce pulmonary inflammation* 2. bronchodilators c. consult physician if signs and symptoms of pneumonitis worsen or signs and symptoms of impaired gas exchange (e.g., restlessness, irritability, confusion, decreased PaO_2 and increased $PaCO_2$) develop.
13.d. The client will have decreasing signs and symptoms of lymphedema if it occurs as evidenced by: 1. decreased pain and feeling of heaviness and tightness in involved extremity 2. reduction in size of involved extremity 3. improved motor and sensory function in involved extremity.	13.d.1. Assess extremities in or near the treatment field for signs and symptoms of lymphedema (e.g., pain or feeling of heaviness, fullness, or tightness in extremity; increase in size of extremity [determined by daily measurement of limb circumference]; sensory or motor deficits in extremity). 2. If signs and symptoms of lymphedema occur: a. elevate the involved extremity b. avoid use of involved extremity for B/P measurements, injections, and venipunctures c. apply a graded-pressure or sequential compression device to involved extremity if ordered d. administer the following medications if ordered: 1. antimicrobial agents *to prevent or treat cellulitis and lymphangitis* 2. analgesics e. consult physician if signs and symptoms of lymphedema persist or worsen or if signs and symptoms of infection (e.g., redness or unusual warmth in extremity, fever) develop.

14. Nursing Diagnosis: ***DISTURBED SELF-CONCEPT****

related to:

a. changes in appearance (e.g., temporary or permanent hair loss within the treatment field; skin changes such as erythema, uneven skin texture, or hyperpigmentation within the treatment field; excessive weight loss);

b. possible alteration in usual sexual activities associated with:
   1. fatigue, decreased levels of testosterone (if testes are in the treatment field), psychological factors, and vaginal and/or urethral discomfort (if the lower abdomen, pelvis, or perineal area is irradiated)
   2. temporary or permanent impotence resulting from psychological factors, decreased levels of testosterone (if testes are in the treatment field), and/or injury to pelvic nerves and blood vessels if included within the treatment field;

*This diagnostic label includes the nursing diagnoses of disturbed body image, low self-esteem, and ineffective role performance.

c. altered reproductive function:
   1. sterility associated with exposure of testes or ovaries to radiation
   2. potential for genetic mutations associated with sperm or ova chromosomal damage resulting from irradiation of the gonads;

d. increased dependence on others to meet self-care needs;

e. changes in lifestyle and roles associated with the effects of the disease process and its treatment.

Suggested NOC Outcomes: Self-esteem; Psychosocial adjustment: life change; Personal autonomy; Body image

Suggested NIC Interventions: Body image enhancement; Self-esteem enhancement; Role enhancement; Emotional support; Support system enhancement

Desired Outcome	**Nursing Actions** *and Selected Purposes/Rationales* (see pp. 47–49 for additional rationales)
14. The client will demonstrate beginning adaptation to changes in appearance, body functioning, lifestyle, and roles as evidenced by: a. verbalization of feelings of self-worth and sexual adequacy b. maintenance of relationships with significant others c. active participation in activities of daily living d. verbalization of a beginning plan for adapting lifestyle to changes resulting from the disease process and the residual effects of radiation therapy.	14.a. Assess for signs and symptoms of a disturbed self-concept (e.g., verbalization of negative feelings about self, withdrawal from significant others, lack of participation in activities of daily living, lack of a plan for adapting to necessary changes in lifestyle). b. Implement measures to facilitate the grieving process (see Diagnosis 15, action b). c. Discuss with client improvements in appearance and functioning that can realistically be expected. d. Implement measures *to assist client to adapt to the following changes in appearance and body functioning if appropriate:* 1. alopecia: a. inform client that hair loss in the treatment field usually begins 2–3 weeks after initiation of therapy b. reassure client that regrowth of hair within the treatment field will occur within 2–3 months after cessation of therapy if the loss is temporary (temporary or patchy loss will usually occur with a radiation dose of 2000–3000 cGy; delayed hair growth or complete, permanent hair loss within the treatment field may result from a radiation exposure above 4000 cGy); explain that regrowth may be a different color, texture, and thickness c. instruct the client in ways *to minimize scalp hair loss if thinning or partial hair loss is anticipated:* 1. brush and comb hair gently 2. wash hair only when necessary and avoid harsh shampoo, cream rinse, and other hair care products 3. do not use hair dryer, curling iron, curlers, or constrictive decorations (e.g., clips, rubber bands) on hair 4. avoid hairstyles that create tension on hair (e.g., ponytails, braids) d. encourage the client to wear a wig, scarf, hat, or turban if desired to conceal hair loss; contact the American Cancer Society for a wig if client is unable to obtain one but desires to do so e. encourage use of the wig before hair loss *to facilitate adjustment to wig and its integration into body image;* caution client to remove wig several times/day to allow for exposure of treatment area to the air 2. skin changes within the treatment field: a. reinforce physician's explanation about skin changes that will occur and when they can be expected b. suggest possible clothing styles that will make changes in skin texture and pigmentation less obvious 3. sterility or chromosomal damage: a. clarify physician's explanation about probable effects of radiation therapy on the gonads if they are in the treatment field b. discuss alternative methods of becoming a parent (e.g., artificial insemination, adoption) if of concern to client

Desired Outcome	Nursing Actions *and Selected Purposes/Rationales*

4. impotence:
   a. reinforce physician's explanation about the temporary or permanent nature of impotence; if it will be permanent, encourage client to discuss various treatment options (e.g., vacuum erection aids, penile prosthesis) with physician
   b. suggest alternative methods of sexual gratification if appropriate
   c. discuss ways to be creative in expressing sexuality (e.g., massage, fantasies, cuddling).

e. Assist client with usual grooming and makeup habits if necessary.
f. Support behaviors suggesting positive adaptation to changes that have occurred (e.g., interest in personal appearance, maintenance of relationships with significant others).
g. Encourage significant others to allow client to do what he/she is able *so that independence can be re-established and/or self-esteem redeveloped.*
h. Assist client's and significant others' adjustment by listening, facilitating communication, and providing information.
i. Encourage visits and support from significant others.
j. Provide information about and encourage use of community agencies and support groups (e.g., vocational rehabilitation; sexual, family, individual, and/or financial counseling).
k. Consult appropriate health care provider (e.g., psychiatric nurse clinician, oncology nurse specialist, physician) if client seems unwilling or unable to adapt to changes resulting from cancer and radiation therapy.

15. Nursing Diagnosis: GRIEVING*

related to:
a. changes in body image and usual lifestyle and roles;
b. diagnosis of cancer with potential for premature death.

*This diagnostic label includes anticipatory grieving and grieving following the actual losses.

Suggested NOC Outcomes:
Grief resolution;
Psychosocial adjustment: life change

Suggested NIC Interventions: Grief work facilitation; Emotional support; Support system enhancement; Spiritual growth facilitation

Desired Outcome	Nursing Actions *and Selected Purposes/Rationales* (see pp. 35–37 for additional rationales)

15. The client will demonstrate beginning progression through the grieving process as evidenced by:
    a. verbalization of feelings about the diagnosis of cancer and radiation therapy and its effects
    b. usual sleep pattern
    c. participation in treatment plan and self-care activities
    d. use of available support systems
    e. verbalization of a plan for integrating prescribed follow-up care into lifestyle.

15.a. Assess for signs and symptoms of grieving (e.g., expression of distress about having cancer, change in eating habits, inability to concentrate, insomnia, anger, sadness, withdrawal from significant others, denial of losses).

b. Implement measures *to facilitate the grieving process:*
   1. assist client to acknowledge the losses *so grief work can begin;* assess for factors that may hinder and facilitate acknowledgment
   2. discuss the grieving process and assist client to accept the phases of grieving as an expected response to actual and/or anticipated losses
   3. allow time for client to progress through the phases of grieving (phases vary among theorists but progress from shock and alarm to acceptance); be aware that not every phase is expressed by all individuals, phases may overlap or recur, the amount of time needed to reach resolution of grief is very individual, and the grieving process may take months to years
   4. provide an atmosphere of care and concern (e.g., provide privacy, be available and nonjudgmental, display empathy and respect) *so client will feel free to express feelings*

5. perform actions *to promote trust* (e.g., answer questions honestly, provide requested information)
6. encourage the verbal expression of anger and sadness about the diagnosis and losses experienced; recognize displacement of anger and assist client to see the actual cause of angry feelings and resentment
7. encourage client to express feelings in whatever ways are comfortable (e.g., writing, drawing, conversation)
8. assist client to identify and use techniques that have helped him/her cope in previous situations of loss
9. support realistic hope about the prognosis and the temporary nature of most of the changes in appearance
10. if acceptable to client, arrange for a visit from a person who has been successfully treated for cancer with radiation therapy
11. support behaviors suggesting successful grief work (e.g., verbalizing feelings about the diagnosis, expressing sorrow, focusing on ways to adapt to losses)
12. explain the phases of the grieving process to significant others; encourage their support and understanding
13. facilitate communication between the client and significant others; be aware that they may be in different phases of the grieving process
14. provide information regarding counseling services and support groups that might assist client in working through grief
15. when appropriate, assist client to meet spiritual needs (e.g., arrange for visit from clergy)
16. administer antidepressant agents if ordered
17. assist client to identify and use available support systems; provide information about available community resources that can assist client and significant others in coping with the effects of radiation therapy and the diagnosis of cancer (e.g., American Cancer Society; support groups; individual, family, and financial counselors).

c. Consult appropriate health care provider (e.g., psychiatric nurse clinician, physician) if signs of dysfunctional grieving (e.g., persistent denial of losses, excessive anger or sadness, emotional lability) occur.

Discharge Teaching/Continued Care

16. NURSING DIAGNOSIS: ***DEFICIENT KNOWLEDGE, INEFFECTIVE THERAPEUTIC REGIMEN MANAGEMENT, OR INEFFECTIVE HEALTH MAINTENANCE****

*The nurse should select the diagnostic label that is most appropriate for the client's discharge teaching needs.

Suggested NOC Outcomes: Knowledge: disease process; Knowledge: treatment regimen; Knowledge: energy conservation; Knowledge: treatment procedure(s)

Suggested NIC Interventions: Teaching: disease process; Health system guidance; Teaching: prescribed activity/exercise; Teaching: procedure/treatment; Nutrition management

Desired Outcomes	**Nursing Actions** *and Selected Purposes/Rationales*
16.a. The client will verbalize an understanding of appropriate skin care for site of irradiation.	16.a.1. Reinforce teaching about the expected skin reaction at the site of irradiation (e.g., redness, tanned appearance, peeling, itching, loss of hair, decreased perspiration). 2. Instruct the client to: a. cleanse irradiated area gently using a mild soap and tepid water, being careful not to wash off temporary skin markings b. pat skin dry with a soft cotton towel c. avoid rubbing, scratching, and massaging irradiated skin

Desired Outcomes	Nursing Actions *and Selected Purposes/Rationales*
	d. relieve itching by: 1. applying a light dusting of cornstarch to area of dry desquamation 2. adding emollients, colloidal-based bath products, cornstarch, or baking soda to bath water e. relieve dryness by applying a water-based lubricant lotion (e.g., Lubriderm, Eucerin) f. avoid use of deodorant if treatment field includes axilla g. check with physician before using cosmetics or perfumed lotions or creams in treatment area h. protect irradiated skin from exposure to temperature extremes and wind i. avoid exposure of treated area to direct sunlight or tanning beds during treatment period and for at least 1 month after therapy is complete (burns can occur easily because melanin production in new epidermal cells is slowed) and always use sunscreen with SPF of 15 or greater j. wear soft cotton garments next to treatment area; use a gentle detergent to launder clothing k. avoid wearing tight or constrictive clothing over irradiated area in order to reduce mechanical irritation l. avoid shaving and using tape within treatment field; use an electric razor if shaving is absolutely necessary m. care for a moist desquamation reaction by: 1. performing wound care and applying sterile dressings as prescribed (stretchable netting should be used instead of tape to hold dressings in place) 2. exposing area to the air as much as possible. 3. Demonstrate care of treatment site. 4. Allow time for questions, clarification, and return demonstration of skin and wound care.
16.b. The client will identify techniques to control nausea and vomiting.	16.b. Instruct client in the following techniques to control nausea and vomiting: 1. cleanse mouth frequently 2. avoid offensive odors and sights 3. eat several small meals/day instead of 3 large ones 4. eat the largest meal 3–4 hours before treatments and eat lightly for at least 3–4 hours after a treatment 5. eat foods that are cool or at room temperature (hot foods frequently have an overpowering aroma that stimulates nausea) 6. eat dry foods (e.g., toast, crackers) or sip cold carbonated beverages if nausea is present 7. select bland foods (e.g., mashed potatoes, cottage cheese) rather than fatty, spicy foods 8. if feasible, have someone else prepare the food 9. avoid drinking liquids with meals 10. rest after eating 11. take deep, slow breaths when nauseated 12. follow prescribed antiemetic regimen.
16.c. The client will verbalize ways to improve appetite and nutritional status.	16.c. Instruct client in ways to improve appetite and maintain an adequate nutritional status: 1. try chicken, fish, cheese, and eggs as protein sources instead of beef and pork if taste distortion is a problem 2. increase the amount of sweeteners and seasonings usually used in foods or beverages 3. use plastic eating utensils and cook foods in glass or plastic containers rather than metal ones if metallic taste is experienced

4. moisten dry foods with sauces, salad dressing, or sour cream if mouth is dry or sore
5. eat in a pleasant environment with company if possible
6. perform frequent oral hygiene to eliminate unpleasant tastes in mouth
7. try recommended methods of controlling nausea (see action b in this diagnosis)
8. eat several high-calorie, high-protein, nutritious small meals/day rather than 3 large ones; use nutritional supplements if needed to maintain an adequate calorie intake
9. plan ahead for low-energy days (e.g., have some prepared meals available; maintain an ample supply of nutritious, minimal preparation foods such as eggs, tuna fish, cheese, peanut butter, and yogurt; keep nutritious snacks and beverages within easy reach)
10. take vitamins and minerals as prescribed.

16.d. The client will identify ways to reduce the risk of dental caries and periodontal disease and manage stomatitis if present.

16.d.1. Inform client that dental caries and periodontal disease can occur months to years after irradiation of the jaw, neck, or oral cavity. Emphasize that a meticulous daily oral hygiene program is essential, particularly if salivary flow is permanently reduced.

2. Instruct client in ways to reduce the risk of dental caries and periodontal disease:
   a. use appropriate technique for cleansing teeth
   b. brush teeth with a fluoride toothpaste several times a day, particularly after eating
   c. use a small, soft, flexible toothbrush to brush teeth
   d. rinse mouth with a fluoride solution after brushing.
3. If stomatitis is present, instruct client to:
   a. rinse mouth with the following solutions as prescribed:
      1. salt or baking soda and warm water
      2. chlorhexidine gluconate (Peridex)
   b. consult physician about use of preparations to soothe the oral mucous membrane (e.g., diphenhydramine and water mixture) if mouth is painful
   c. wear dentures only at mealtime
   d. eat soft, bland foods and avoid substances that might further irritate the mouth (e.g., extremely hot, spicy, or acidic foods/fluids).
4. Allow time for questions, clarification, and practice of oral hygiene techniques.
5. Instruct client to discuss any planned dental care with the radiologist and to inform the dentist that he/she is receiving or has had radiation to the oral cavity.

16.e. The client will identify ways to prevent bleeding if platelet counts are low.

16.e.1. Instruct client in ways to minimize the risk of bleeding:
   a. avoid taking aspirin and other nonsteroidal anti-inflammatory agents (e.g., ibuprofen)
   b. consult health care provider before routinely taking herbs that can increase the risk of bleeding (e.g., ginkgo, arnica, chamomile)
   c. brush teeth gently using a soft bristle toothbrush; do not use dental floss or put sharp objects (e.g., toothpicks) in mouth
   d. be attentive when using scissors, knives, and tools to reduce the risk of cuts
   e. use an electric rather than a straight-edge razor
   f. cut nails and cuticles carefully
   g. use caution when ambulating to prevent falls or bumps and do not walk barefoot
   h. avoid blowing nose forcefully
   i. avoid contact sports and other activities that could result in injury
   j. avoid straining to have a bowel movement
   k. avoid wearing constrictive clothing (e.g., garters, knee-high stockings)

Desired Outcomes	Nursing Actions *and Selected Purposes/Rationales*
	l. use an ample amount of water-soluble lubricant prior to sexual intercourse and avoid anal sexual activity, douching, use of rectal suppositories, and enemas in order to prevent trauma to the vaginal and rectal mucosa m. avoid heavy lifting. 2. Instruct client to control any bleeding by applying firm, prolonged pressure to the area(s) if possible.
16.f. The client will identify ways to prevent infection if WBC counts are low.	16.f.1. Explain to client that his/her resistance to infection is reduced when WBC counts are low. Emphasize the need to adhere closely to recommended techniques to prevent infection. 2. Instruct client in ways to prevent infection: a. avoid crowds, persons with any sign of infection, and persons who have recently been vaccinated b. utilize good hand hygiene (e.g., wash hands using an antibacterial soap, use an alcohol-base hand rub) c. wear gloves to protect hands during activities such as cleaning and gardening d. take an axillary rather than an oral temperature if stomatitis is present e. lubricate the skin outside irradiated area frequently to prevent dryness and subsequent cracking f. cleanse and care for skin within treatment field as recommended (see action a.2 in this diagnosis) g. avoid unnecessary rectal invasion (e.g., temperature taking, enemas, suppositories, sexual activity) to prevent trauma to the rectal mucosa h. avoid constipation to prevent trauma to the bowel mucosa from hard or impacted stool i. wash perianal area thoroughly with soap and water after each bowel movement; inform female client to always wipe from front to back after defecating and urinating j. avoid douching unless ordered (douching disturbs the normal vaginal flora and may cause trauma to the vaginal mucosa) k. drink at least 10 glasses of liquid/day unless contraindicated l. cough and deep breathe or use incentive spirometer every 2 hours until usual activity level is resumed m. stop smoking n. perform meticulous oral hygiene after meals and at bedtime or more often if directed, change denture care solution daily, and replace toothbrush routinely o. maintain an optimal nutritional status (e.g., diet high in protein, calories, vitamins, and minerals) p. avoid sharing eating utensils q. maintain an adequate balance between activity and rest r. cleanse respiratory equipment as instructed; change water in humidifiers daily s. decrease risk of food-borne illness: 1. avoid intake of foods with a high microorganism content (e.g., unwashed fruits and vegetables; undercooked eggs, meat, poultry, and seafood) 2. be sure that juices and ciders are pasteurized or processed and that milk and cheese are pasteurized 3. thoroughly wash hands and food preparation items and surfaces (e.g., knives, cutting boards, countertop) before and after cooking, especially when working with raw meat, poultry, and fish 4. thaw food items in the refrigerator rather than on kitchen counter

t. avoid picking up animal waste or cleaning animal litter boxes and bird cages
u. avoid elective surgery and dental work
v. reinforce the importance of taking prescribed medications such as colony-stimulating factors and prophylactic antimicrobial agents.

16.g. The client will verbalize an understanding of and ways to manage the effects of radiation therapy on sexual and reproductive functioning.

16.g.1. Clarify physician's explanation about the possible effects of irradiation on the gonads if included in the treatment field.
2. Explain that a temporary decrease in libido may occur as a result of radiation treatment.
3. Encourage client to rest before sexual activity if fatigue is a problem.
4. Instruct client in measures to reduce discomfort associated with decreased vaginal secretions and mucositis:
   a. use an ample amount of water-soluble lubricant to prevent trauma to the vaginal mucosa and increase lubrication during intercourse
   b. use a vaginal steroid cream, if prescribed, to ease dryness and inflammation
   c. avoid intercourse until mucositis of the vaginal canal and/or urethra resolves
   d. have male partner use a condom during intercourse to prevent contact of vaginal area with semen (semen can cause a burning sensation in the early months after vaginal irradiation).
5. Emphasize the need for frequent intercourse or vaginal dilatation once mucositis has resolved to prevent stenosis of the vaginal canal (stenosis may develop several weeks or months after cessation of treatment that includes the vaginal area).
6. Explain to the female client that ovarian failure during therapy may result in decreased libido, irritability, hot flashes, and other symptoms of premature menopause.
7. Inform the female client that her usual menstrual cycle will resume within 6 months to 1 year after treatment if sterility is temporary.
8. Emphasize the need for both male and female clients to practice birth control during treatment and for at least 2 years after it. Encourage both male and female clients to seek genetic counseling before attempting conception to ascertain the risk of chromosomal anomalies.
9. Instruct client to take hormone replacements (e.g., estrogen, testosterone) as prescribed.

16.h. The client will verbalize ways to manage and cope with persistent fatigue.

16.h. Instruct client in ways to manage and cope with persistent fatigue:
1. view fatigue as a protective mechanism rather than a problematic limitation
2. determine ways that daily patterns of activity can be modified to conserve energy and prevent excessive fatigue (e.g., spread light and heavy tasks throughout the day, take short rests during an activity whenever possible, take several short rest periods during the day instead of one long one)
3. determine whether life demands are realistic in light of physical state and adjust short- and long-term goals accordingly
4. avoid situations that are particularly fatiguing such as those that are boring, frustrating, or require prolonged or strenuous physical activity
5. participate in a moderate exercise program (e.g., walking or bicycling 20–30 minutes 3–4 times/week)
6. participate in "attention-restoring" activities (e.g., walking outside, gardening).

16.i. The client will verbalize an understanding of the signs and symptoms of lymphedema and ways to manage it if it occurs.

16.i.1. Instruct the client at risk for lymphedema (e.g., person receiving radiation for breast cancer, melanoma in an extremity, gynecologic cancer or prostate cancer) to:
   a. monitor for and report signs and symptoms of lymphedema (e.g., pain or a feeling of heaviness or tightness in involved extremity)

Desired Outcomes	**Nursing Actions** *and Selected Purposes/Rationales*

b. measure the circumference of involved arm or leg daily if the extremity appears swollen and report a sudden increase in size to the physician.

2. Provide the following instructions about ways to manage and prevent complications associated with lymphedema if it occurs:
   a. keep pressure off the involved extremity (e.g., avoid wearing tight jewelry, clothes with constricting bands, and elastic stockings with constricting bands; carry bags on unaffected arm; do not cross legs)
   b. keep involved extremity elevated as much as possible
   c. perform prescribed exercises
   d. gently clean and apply oil or skin cream to involved extremity daily
   e. avoid injury to the involved extremity (e.g., do not allow finger sticks or venipunctures in involved extremity, use an electric rather than straight-edge razor when shaving involved extremity, wear gardening and cooking gloves and use a thimble for sewing if upper extremity is affected, do not walk barefoot if lower extremity is affected, avoid extreme hot or cold on affected extremity, do not cut cuticles on hand or foot of involved extremity).

16.j. The client will state signs and symptoms to report to the health care provider.

16.j.1. Instruct the client to observe for and report the following:
   a. signs and symptoms of infection (stress that the usual signs of infection are diminished in people with a suppressed immune system and that it is necessary to monitor closely for the following signs and symptoms):
      1. temperature above 38° C (100.4° F)
      2. changes in odor, color, or consistency of urine or pain on urination
      3. white patches in mouth
      4. crusted ulcerations around or in oral cavity
      5. swollen, reddened, coated tongue
      6. painful rectal or vaginal area
      7. unusual vaginal drainage
      8. persistent or productive cough
      9. redness, heat, swelling, or unusual drainage in any area, particularly site being irradiated or venipuncture sites
   b. signs and symptoms of bleeding (e.g., excessive bruising, black stools, persistent nosebleeds or bleeding from gums, sudden swelling in joints, red or smoke-colored urine, blood in vomitus)
   c. signs and symptoms of radiation cystitis (e.g., blood in the urine, pain on urination, urinary frequency or urgency)
   d. signs and symptoms of radiation pneumonitis (e.g., shortness of breath, persistent cough, night sweats, fever); radiation pneumonitis can occur 2–3 months after cessation of treatment depending on total dose of radiation received, fractionation of dose, and volume of lung tissue within the treatment field
   e. signs and symptoms of tissue fibrosis within treatment field (e.g., LUNG: increasing shortness of breath, cough; BOWEL: inability to move bowels, distended abdomen, loss of appetite, alternating diarrhea and constipation; ESOPHAGUS: difficulty swallowing; VAGINA: pain during intercourse)
   f. excessive tooth decay
   g. persistent nausea, vomiting, or decreased oral intake
   h. significant weight loss (weight loss of 1–2 pounds/week during radiation therapy is not unusual)
   i. persistent diarrhea
   j. excessive depression or difficulty coping with the effects of the diagnosis and treatment.

2. Instruct client to keep a record of signs and symptoms, activities at the time the symptoms occur, measures to achieve relief, and the effect of the measures taken. Instruct client to take the information to each appointment with the health care provider.

16.k. The client will identify community resources that can assist with home management and adjustment to the diagnosis of cancer and radiation therapy and its effects.

16.k.1. Provide information about and encourage use of community resources that can assist the client and significant others with home management and adjustment to cancer and the effects of radiation therapy (e.g., local support groups, American Cancer Society, home health agencies, counselors, social service agencies, Meals on Wheels, Make Today Count, hospice).

2. Initiate a referral if indicated.

16.l. The client will verbalize an understanding of and a plan for adhering to recommended follow-up care including medications prescribed and future appointments with health care provider, radiation department, and laboratory.

16.l.1. Explain the rationale for, side effects of, and importance of taking medications prescribed. Inform client of pertinent food and drug interactions.

2. Reinforce physician's explanation of planned radiation therapy schedule.
3. Discuss with client any difficulties he/she might have adhering to the schedule and assist in planning ways to overcome these.
4. Reinforce the importance of keeping appointments for radiation treatments and follow-up laboratory studies.
5. Reinforce the importance of keeping follow-up appointments with health care provider.
6. Implement measures to improve client compliance:
   a. include significant others in teaching sessions
   b. encourage questions and allow time for reinforcement and clarification of information provided
   c. provide written instructions regarding future appointments with health care provider, radiation department, and laboratory; medications prescribed; and signs and symptoms to report.

Bibliography

See pages 879–881.

UNIT VIII

Nursing Care of the Client with Disturbances of Neurological Function

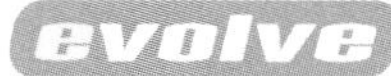

Cerebrovascular Accident

A cerebrovascular accident (CVA, stroke, brain attack) is the result of an interruption in the blood flow in areas of the brain and is characterized by the sudden development of neurological deficits that last for at least 24 hours. These deficits range from mild symptoms such as tingling, weakness, and slight speech impairment to more severe symptoms such as hemiplegia, aphasia, dysphagia, loss of portions of visual field, spatial-perceptual changes, altered cognitive function, and loss of consciousness. Clinical manifestations depend on factors such as the area(s) of the brain affected, the adequacy of collateral cerebral circulation, and the extensiveness of subsequent cerebral edema.

Cerebrovascular accidents are classified according to etiology. The major classifications are ischemic and hemorrhagic. Ischemic CVAs are most frequently the result of a thrombosis (which is usually associated with atherosclerosis) or an embolus. Conditions most often associated with a hemorrhagic CVA are extreme hypertension, cerebral aneurysm, or arteriovenous malformation. Treatment following a CVA is determined by the etiology and the neurological deficits that are present.

This care plan focuses on the adult client hospitalized with signs and symptoms of a CVA. Much of the information is also applicable to clients receiving follow-up care in an extended care or rehabilitation facility or home setting. This care plan focuses on the more common problems that occur as a result of a CVA. The reader should refer to neurological texts for additional information about specific speech, motor, and sensory deficits that can occur.

OUTCOME/DISCHARGE CRITERIA

THE CLIENT WILL:

- have improved cerebral tissue perfusion
- have improved or stable neurological function
- experience optimal control of urinary elimination
- have no signs or symptoms of complications
- communicate an awareness of ways to decrease the risk of a recurrent CVA
- identify ways to manage sensory and speech impairments and disturbed thought processes
- identify ways to improve ability to swallow
- identify ways to manage urinary incontinence
- demonstrate measures to facilitate the performance of activities of daily living and increase physical mobility
- communicate an awareness of signs and symptoms to report to the health care provider share thoughts and feelings about the effects of the CVA on lifestyle, roles, and self-concept
- communicate knowledge of community resources that can assist with home management and adjustment to changes resulting from the CVA
- communicate an understanding of and a plan for adhering to recommended follow-up care including future appointments with health care provider and therapists and medications prescribed.

Use in Conjunction with the Care Plan on Immobility.

NURSING/COLLABORATIVE DIAGNOSES

NURSING/COLLABORATIVE DIAGNOSES

DISCHARGE TEACHING

See pp. 242–243 and Care Plan on Immobility (pp. 129–148) for additional diagnoses.

1. Nursing Diagnosis: *INEFFECTIVE TISSUE PERFUSION: CEREBRAL*

related to decreased cerebral blood flow associated with thrombus, embolus, cerebral hemorrhage, hypotension, and/or subsequent spasm or compression of cerebral vessel(s).

Suggested NOC Outcomes: Neurological status; Tissue perfusion: cerebral

Suggested NIC Interventions: Cerebral edema management; Cerebral perfusion promotion; Intracranial pressure (ICP) monitoring

Desired Outcome

1. The client will experience improved cerebral tissue perfusion as evidenced by:
   a. absence of or reduction in dizziness, visual disturbances, and speech impairments
   b. improved mental status
   c. improved sensory and motor function.

Nursing Actions *and Selected Purposes/Rationales*

1.a. Assess the client for signs and symptoms of decreased cerebral tissue perfusion:
   1. dizziness
   2. visual disturbances (e.g., blurred or dimmed vision, diplopia, change in visual field)
   3. aphasia
   4. irritability and restlessness
   5. decreased level of consciousness
   6. paresthesias, weakness, paralysis.

b. Implement measures *to improve cerebral tissue perfusion:*
   1. if a thrombus or embolus is present:
      a. assist with administration of a thrombolytic agent (e.g., tenecteplase, alteplase [tPA]) if ordered
      b. administer anticoagulants (e.g., heparin, warfarin) or platelet aggregation inhibitors (e.g., aspirin, clopidogrel) if ordered
   2. if intracerebral hemorrhage occurred as a result of cerebral aneurysm rupture, administer a hemostatic agent (e.g., aminocaproic acid) if ordered *to prevent the lysis of formed clots and subsequent rebleeding*
   3. if intracerebral hemorrhage occurred as a result of extreme hypertension, perform actions *to control high blood pressure* (e.g., administer prescribed antihypertensive agents, reduce stress)
   4. if client is hypotensive, perform actions *to improve cerebral blood flow* (e.g., administer prescribed sympathomimetic agents, maintain intravenous fluid therapy as ordered)
   5. administer calcium-channel blockers (e.g., nimodipine) if ordered *to reduce cerebral vasospasm (the calcium that is released by the injured neural cells can cause vasospasm)*
   6. perform actions to prevent and treat increased intracranial pressure (see Diagnosis 12, actions a.2 and 3)
   7. prepare client for surgery (e.g., evacuation of hematoma, repair of ruptured aneurysm) if planned.

c. Consult physician if signs and symptoms of decreased cerebral tissue perfusion worsen.

2. NURSING DIAGNOSIS:

IMPAIRED SWALLOWING

related to weakness or paralysis of the swallowing muscles on the affected side and diminished or absent swallowing reflex.

Suggested NOC Outcomes: Swallowing status: oral phase; Swallowing status: pharyngeal phase

Suggested NIC Intervention: Swallowing therapy

Desired Outcome	Nursing Actions *and Selected Purposes/Rationales* (see pp. 54–57 for additional rationales)

2. The client will experience an improvement in swallowing as evidenced by:
   a. communication of same
   b. absence of food in oral cavity after swallowing
   c. absence of coughing and choking when eating and drinking.

2.a. Assess for signs and symptoms of impaired swallowing (e.g., communication of difficulty swallowing, stasis of food in oral cavity, coughing or choking when eating or drinking, abnormal results of swallow study).

b. Implement measures *to improve ability to swallow:*
   1. place client in high Fowler's position for meals and snacks; head and neck should be tilted forward slightly *to facilitate elevation of the larynx and posterior movement of the tongue*
   2. provide oral care before meals and snacks *(oral care stimulates sensory awareness and salivation, which facilitates swallowing)*
   3. assist client to select foods that require little or no chewing and are easily swallowed (e.g., custard, eggs, canned fruit, mashed potatoes)
   4. instruct client to avoid mixing foods of different texture in his/her mouth at the same time
   5. avoid serving foods that are sticky (e.g., peanut butter, soft bread, honey)
   6. avoid foods that tend to fall apart in mouth (e.g., cake, muffins) and those that consist of small food particles (e.g., rice, peas, corn) if client has impaired tongue control
   7. serve foods/fluids that are hot or cold instead of room temperature *(the more extreme temperatures stimulate the sensory receptors and swallowing reflex)*
   8. serve thick rather than thin fluids or add a thickening agent (e.g., "Thick-It," gelatin, baby cereal) to thin fluids
   9. moisten dry foods with gravy or sauces (e.g., catsup, salad dressing, sour cream)
   10. utilize assistive devices (e.g., long-handled spoon) to place food that does not need to be chewed (e.g., gelatin, mashed potatoes, custard) in the back of mouth on unaffected side if tongue movement is impaired
   11. instruct client to avoid putting too much food/fluid in mouth at one time
   12. encourage client to concentrate on the act of swallowing; provide verbal cueing as needed
   13. if client has decreased lip control, instruct him/her to gently hold lips closed with fingers after putting food in mouth
   14. gently stroke client's throat when he/she is swallowing if indicated
   15. consult speech pathologist or therapist about methods for dealing with impaired swallowing; reinforce recommended exercises and techniques.

c. Consult appropriate health care provider (e.g., speech pathologist, physician) if swallowing difficulties persist or worsen.

3. NURSING DIAGNOSIS:

DISTURBED SENSORY PERCEPTION

a. visual related to ischemia of portions of the visual pathways in the occipital lobe and the parieto-occipitotemporal interpretative (association) area;

b. kinesthetic related to visual deficits and ischemia of portions of the parietal lobe (primarily of the nondominant hemisphere) and the cerebellum.

Suggested NOC Outcomes: Sensory function: proprioception; Sensory function: vision

Suggested NIC Interventions: Environmental management; Cerebral perfusion promotion

Desired Outcome	Nursing Actions *and Selected Purposes/Rationales*
3. The client will experience a reduction in and/or demonstrate beginning adaptation to disturbed sensory perception as evidenced by: a. communication of same b. increased participation in activities.	3.a. Assess for signs and symptoms of: 1. visual impairments such as homonymous hemianopsia and/or diplopia (e.g., lack of response to visual stimuli on side of hemiplegia, reports of double vision, decreased participation in activities) 2. kinesthetic impairment (e.g., difficulty maintaining balance, determining body position, buttoning clothing, or locating mouth when trying to feed self; decreased participation in activities). b. Implement measures to improve cerebral tissue perfusion (see Diagnosis 1, action b) *in order to reduce cerebral ischemia.* c. Implement measures *to assist client to adapt to changes in visual and/or kinesthetic functioning:* 1. provide an eyepatch or opaque lens for client to wear if diplopia is present 2. if client is experiencing homonymous hemianopsia: a. perform actions *to decrease the risk of startling client* (e.g., approach client from unaffected side whenever possible, verbally acknowledge client before touching him/her if approaching on affected side) b. perform actions *to ensure client receives visual stimuli* (e.g., position client's bed and chair so that window or door to hall rather than blank wall is within visual field, instruct visitors to sit or stand on client's unaffected side) c. after condition has stabilized, place some items (e.g., television, clock, calendar, pictures) on affected side *to promote environmental scanning* 3. if client is experiencing kinesthetic impairments, place him/her in front of a full-length mirror during activities when possible after condition has stabilized *(viewing his/her reflection may help the client to identify body position and vertical and horizontal planes)* 4. perform actions to facilitate performance of self-care activities (see Diagnosis 7, actions b.3 and 4) 5. consult physical and occupational therapists about additional ways to facilitate client's adaptation to disturbed sensory perceptions 6. inform significant others and health care personnel of approaches being used to increase client's awareness of affected side; encourage their use of these techniques. d. Consult appropriate health care provider (e.g., physical therapist, occupational therapist, physician) if disturbed sensory perceptions worsen or client is unable to adapt to the ones he/she is experiencing.

4. Nursing Diagnosis: ***UNILATERAL NEGLECT***

related to ischemia of portions of the brain (primarily the parietal lobe of the non-dominant cerebral hemisphere).

Suggested NOC Outcomes: Body image; Body positioning: self-initiated

Suggested NIC Interventions: Unilateral neglect management; Sensory function: proprioception; Sensory function: vision; Vision compensation behavior

Desired Outcome	Nursing Actions *and Selected Purposes/Rationales*
4. The client will experience a gradual reduction in and/or demonstrate beginning adaptation to unilateral neglect as evidenced by: a. awareness of stimuli on affected side b. awareness of the affected side of body.	4.a. Assess client for presence of unilateral neglect (e.g., not looking toward affected side, no response to stimuli on affected side, lack of awareness of affected extremities). b. Implement measures to improve cerebral tissue perfusion (see Diagnosis 1, action b) *in order to reduce cerebral ischemia.* c. If unilateral neglect is present: 1. ensure that affected extremities are positioned properly at all times 2. protect affected extremities from injury 3. touch and move affected extremities routinely *(provides sensory stimulation and can help client experience normal movement patterns)* 4. after client's condition stabilizes, implement measures *to increase client's awareness of affected side:* a. encourage client to handle affected extremities when bathing, dressing, and repositioning self b. assist client to participate in activities that bring affected extremities across midline of body (e.g., range of motion exercises, some recreational activities) c. place some items (e.g., television, clock, calendar, pictures) on affected side *to increase the likelihood of the client viewing the affected extremities* d. place familiar items (e.g., favorite bracelet or watch, frequently worn shoe or slipper) on affected extremities *to assist client to recognize that the extremities are a part of his/her body* 5. consult physical and occupational therapists about additional ways to facilitate client's reintegration of neglected body parts 6. inform significant others and health care personnel of approaches being used to increase client's awareness of affected side; encourage their use of these techniques. 7. consult appropriate health care provider (e.g., physical therapist, occupational therapist, physician) if client is unable to begin to adapt to unilateral neglect.

5. NURSING DIAGNOSIS: ***IMPAIRED VERBAL COMMUNICATION***

related to:
a. impaired function of the muscles that are used to produce speech;
b. ischemia in the dominant cerebral hemisphere (ischemia of Wernicke's area in the temporoparietal cortex will result in receptive [fluent, sensory] aphasia; ischemia of Broca's area in the frontal cortex will result in expressive [nonfluent, motor] aphasia).

Suggested NOC Outcomes: Communication: receptive; Communication: expressive; Communication

Suggested NIC Interventions: Communication enhancement: speech deficit; Active listening

Desired Outcome	Nursing Actions *and Selected Purposes/Rationales*
5. The client will communicate needs and desires effectively.	5.a. Assess client for impaired verbal communication (e.g., inability to speak, difficulty forming words or sentences, difficulty expressing thoughts verbally, inappropriate verbalization). Validate verbal responses with an assessment of nonverbal behavior *in order to determine if client is experiencing receptive aphasia.* b. Implement measures *to facilitate communication:* 1. answer call signal in person rather than using the intercommunication system 2. maintain a patient, calm approach; listen attentively and allow ample time for communication

Desired Outcome	Nursing Actions *and Selected Purposes/Rationales*

3. maintain a calm, quiet environment *so that client can concentrate on communication efforts, does not have to speak loudly, and is able to hear others clearly*
4. ask questions that require short answers, eyeblinks, or nod of head if client is having difficulty speaking and/or is frustrated or fatigued
5. schedule rest periods before visiting hours and speech therapy sessions *to maximize communication ability during those times*
6. when speaking to client, face him/her; speak slowly; use direct, short statements; repeat key words; present only one idea or thought at a time; and avoid using unrelated gestures
7. provide materials such as Magic Slate, pad and pencil, computer, word cards, and/or picture board if appropriate; try to ensure that placement of intravenous line does not interfere with client's use of these communication aids
8. consult speech pathologist or therapist regarding methods for dealing with speech impairments; reinforce exercises and techniques recommended.

c. Inform significant others and health care personnel of techniques being used to facilitate client's ability to communicate. Stress the importance of consistent use of these techniques.
d. Encourage significant others and staff to talk to client even if he/she is unresponsive or unable to communicate.
e. Consult appropriate health care provider (e.g., speech pathologist, physician) if client experiences increasing impairment of verbal communication.

6. Nursing Diagnosis: ***IMPAIRED PHYSICAL MOBILITY***

related to:

a. activity limitations associated with decreased motor function and spatial-perceptual impairments;
b. loss of muscle tone during period of flaccidity of affected extremities (flaccid paralysis is usually present during the first few days following a CVA);
c. hypertonia of affected extremities (as muscle tone returns after period of flaccidity, it often progresses to spasticity within about 6–8 weeks);
d. reluctance to move associated with fear of injuring self (occurs mainly with ischemia of the dominant hemisphere);
e. loss of muscle mass, tone, and strength associated with prolonged disuse.

Suggested NOC Outcomes: Mobility; Coordinated movement; Joint movement; Transfer performance

Suggested NIC Interventions: Exercise therapy: joint mobility; Exercise therapy: balance; Exercise therapy: ambulation; Exercise therapy: muscle control; Positioning

Desired Outcome	Nursing Actions *and Selected Purposes/Rationales*
6. The client will achieve maximum physical mobility within limitations imposed by the CVA.	6.a. Refer to Care Plan on Immobility, Diagnosis 6 (p. 135), for measures related to ways to maintain optimal joint mobility and muscle function. b. Implement additional measures *to increase mobility:* 1. provide adequate rest periods before activity sessions 2. administer muscle relaxants (e.g., baclofen, dantrolene) if ordered *to relieve spasticity in affected extremities* 3. perform actions to prevent falls (see Diagnosis 10, action a.1) *in order to decrease client's fear of injury* 4. instruct client in and assist with use of mobility aids (e.g., cane, walker) if appropriate 5. after client's condition has stabilized, assist with and reinforce the following if appropriate: a. balance training (sitting, standing, walking)

b. neurodevelopmental treatment (e.g., Bobath approach) *to promote more normal movement of the affected extremities*
c. neuromuscular re-education techniques (e.g., electromyographic biofeedback) *to improve muscle strength and reduce spasticity of the affected extremities.*

c. Encourage the support of significant others. Allow them to assist with range of motion exercises, positioning, and activity if desired.
d. Consult appropriate health care provider (e.g., physical therapist, physician) if client is unable to achieve expected level of mobility or if range of motion becomes restricted.

7. NURSING DIAGNOSIS: *SELF-CARE DEFICIT*

related to impaired physical mobility, visual and spatial-perceptual impairments, apraxia, unilateral neglect, and disturbed thought processes.

Suggested NOC Outcome:
Self-care: activities of daily living

Suggested NIC Interventions: Self-care assistance; Self-care assistance: IADL; Exercise therapy: muscle control

Desired Outcome	Nursing Actions *and Selected Purposes/Rationales*
7. The client will perform self-care activities within cognitive and physical limitations.	7.a. Refer to Care Plan on Immobility, Diagnosis 7, action b (pp. 135–136), for measures to facilitate client's ability to perform self-care activities.

b. Implement additional measures *to facilitate client's ability to perform self-care activities:*
1. if apraxia is present, explain and demonstrate use of items such as toothbrush, comb, and washcloth as often as necessary
2. encourage client to wear eyepatch or opaque lens if diplopia is present
3. perform actions *to enable client to feed self:*
   a. place foods/fluids within client's visual field until he/she learns to effectively utilize scanning techniques
   b. place only a few items on the tray at one time if spatial-perceptual deficits are present
   c. identify where items are placed on the plate and tray and open containers, cut meat, and butter bread as indicated
   d. consult with occupational therapist about assistive devices available (e.g., broad-handled utensils, rocker knife, nonslip tray mat, plate guard); reinforce use of these devices
4. perform actions *to enable client to dress self:*
   a. encourage use of assistive devices such as button hooks, long-handled shoehorns, and pull loops for pants
   b. encourage client to select clothing that is easy to put on and remove (e.g., shirts with zippers or Velcro closures rather than buttons, loose-fitting clothing, pants with an elastic waistband or Velcro closures, shoes with Velcro fasteners or elastic laces)
   c. if client has difficulty distinguishing right from left, mark outer aspect of shoes with tape
5. perform actions to increase mobility (see Diagnosis 6) *in order to further facilitate the client's ability to perform self-care activities*
6. reinforce exercises and activities recommended by the occupational therapist to improve fine motor skills.

c. Assist the client with activities he/she is unable to perform independently.
d. Inform significant others of client's abilities to perform own care. Explain importance of encouraging and allowing client to maintain an optimal level of independence.

8. Nursing Diagnosis: *IMPAIRED URINARY ELIMINATION: INCONTINENCE*

related to:
a. increased reflex activity of the bladder and loss of voluntary control of urinary elimination associated with upper motor neuron involvement if it has occurred;
b. decreased ability to control urination associated with decreased level of consciousness or inability to recognize sensation of bladder fullness;
c. inability to get to bedside commode or bathroom in a timely manner associated with:
   1. delay in obtaining assistance resulting from inability to communicate the urge to urinate
   2. impaired physical mobility.

Suggested NOC Outcomes: Urinary continence; Self-care: toileting

Suggested NIC Interventions: Prompted voiding; Self-care assistance: toileting; Urinary habit training

Desired Outcome	**Nursing Actions** *and Selected Purposes/Rationales* (see pp. 59–60 for additional rationales)
8. The client will experience urinary continence.	8.a. Assess client's pattern of fluid intake and urination (e.g., times and amounts of fluid intake, types of fluids consumed, times and amounts of voluntary and involuntary voiding, reports of sensation of need to void, activities preceding incontinence). b. Implement measures *to reduce the risk of urinary incontinence:* 1. offer bedpan or urinal or assist client to bedside commode or bathroom every 2–4 hours if indicated 2. allow client to assume a normal position for voiding unless contraindicated *in order to promote complete bladder emptying* 3. perform actions *to reduce delays in toileting* (e.g., have call signal within client's reach and respond promptly to requests for assistance; have bedpan, urinal, or bedside commode readily available to client; provide client with easy-to-remove clothing such as pajamas with Velcro closures or an elastic waistband) 4. if client is aphasic, establish an effective method for him/her to communicate the urge to urinate 5. instruct client to space fluids evenly throughout the day rather than drinking a large quantity at one time *(rapid filling of bladder can result in incontinence if client has decreased urinary sphincter control)* 6. limit oral fluid intake in the evening *to decrease possibility of nighttime incontinence* 7. instruct client to avoid drinking alcohol and beverages containing caffeine *(alcohol and caffeine have a mild diuretic effect and act as irritants to the bladder; these factors may make urinary control more difficult).* c. If urinary incontinence persists, consult physician about intermittent catheterization, insertion of indwelling catheter, or use of external catheter.

9. Nursing Diagnosis: *DISTURBED THOUGHT PROCESSES**

related to damage to cerebral tissue associated with cerebral ischemia.

*The diagnostic label of acute or chronic confusion may be more appropriate depending on the client's symptoms.

Suggested NOC Outcomes: Information processing; Neurological status: consciousness; Cognition; Memory

Suggested NIC Interventions: Reality orientation; Cognitive stimulation; Cognitive restructuring; Cerebral perfusion promotion; Socialization enhancement

Desired Outcome	Nursing Actions *and Selected Purposes/Rationales*
9. The client will experience improvement in thought processes as evidenced by: a. improved attention span, memory, and problem-solving abilities b. improved level of orientation c. reduction in instances of inappropriate responses.	9.a. Assess client for disturbed thought processes (e.g., shortened attention span, impaired memory, decreased ability to problem solve, confusion, inappropriate responses). b. Ascertain from significant others client's usual level of cognitive and emotional functioning. c. Implement measures to improve cerebral tissue perfusion (see Diagnosis 1, action b) *in order to reduce cerebral ischemia and subsequently improve thought processes.* d. If client shows evidence of disturbed thought processes: 1. reorient to person, place, and time as necessary 2. address client by name 3. place familiar objects, clock, and calendar within client's view 4. face client when conversing with him/her 5. approach client in a slow, calm manner; allow adequate time for communication 6. repeat instructions as necessary using clear, simple language and short sentences 7. keep environmental stimuli to a minimum but avoid sensory deprivation 8. maintain a consistent and fairly structured routine 9. provide written or taped information whenever possible for client to review as often as necessary 10. have client perform only one activity at a time and allow adequate time for performance of activities 11. encourage client to make lists of planned activities, questions, and concerns 12. assist client to problem solve if necessary 13. implement measures *to stop emotional outbursts and inappropriate responses if they occur* (e.g., provide distraction by clapping hands, handing client an object to look at or hold, or turning on the radio or television) 14. maintain realistic expectations of client's ability to learn, comprehend, and remember information provided 15. encourage significant others to be supportive of client; instruct them in methods of dealing with client's disturbed thought processes 16. discuss physiological basis for disturbed thought processes with client and significant others; inform them that cognitive and emotional functioning may improve gradually during the next 6–12 months 17. consult physician if disturbed thought processes worsen.

10. NURSING DIAGNOSIS: ***RISK FOR INJURY: FALLS, BURNS, AND LACERATIONS***

related to:

a. motor, visual, and spatial-perceptual impairments;
b. spasticity if present;
c. quick, impulsive behavior (occurs primarily with ischemia of the nondominant cerebral hemisphere);
d. disturbed thought processes (e.g., impaired memory, shortened attention span, confusion).

Suggested NOC Outcomes: Fall prevention behavior; Balance

Suggested NIC Interventions: Fall prevention; Environmental management; Surveillance: safety; Peripheral sensation management

Desired Outcome	**Nursing Actions** *and Selected Purposes/Rationales*

10. The client will not experience falls, burns, or lacerations.

10.a. Implement measures *to reduce the risk for injury:*
  1. perform actions *to prevent falls:*
    a. keep bed in low position with side rails up when client is in bed
    b. keep needed items within easy reach and within client's visual field
    c. encourage client to request assistance whenever needed; have call signal within easy reach
    d. if vision is impaired:
      1. orient client to surroundings, room, and arrangement of furniture and identify obstacles during ambulation
      2. provide an eyepatch or opaque lens for client to wear if diplopia is present
      3. encourage visual scanning if homonymous hemianopsia is present
    e. use lap belt when client is in chair if indicated
    f. instruct client to wear well-fitting slippers/shoes with nonslip soles and low heels when ambulating
    g. keep floor free of clutter and wipe up spills promptly
    h. accompany client during ambulation utilizing a transfer safety belt
    i. provide ambulatory aids (e.g., walker, cane) if client is weak or unsteady on feet
    j. reinforce instructions from physical therapist on correct transfer and ambulation techniques
    k. instruct client to ambulate in well-lit areas and to utilize handrails if needed
    l. do not rush client; allow adequate time for ambulation to the bathroom and in hallway
    m. make sure that shower has a nonslip bottom surface and that shower chair, secure bath mat, call signal, grab bars, and adequate lighting are present
    n. stabilize client's affected arm with a sling when he/she is out of bed *in order to improve balance*
  2. perform actions *to prevent burns:*
    a. let hot foods/fluids cool slightly before serving
    b. supervise client while smoking if indicated
    c. assess temperature of bath water and direct heat application device (e.g., heating pad, warm compress) before and during use
  3. assist client with tasks that require fine motor skills (e.g., shaving) *in order to prevent lacerations*
  4. if client is confused or irrational:
    a. reorient frequently to surroundings and necessity of adhering to safety precautions
    b. provide appropriate level of supervision
    c. consult physician about the temporary use of a bed alarm or jacket or wrist restraints if necessary
    d. administer prescribed antianxiety and antipsychotic medications if indicated
  5. administer muscle relaxants if ordered *to reduce spasticity of affected muscles.*

b. Include client and significant others in planning and implementing measures to prevent injury.

c. If injury does occur, initiate appropriate first aid and notify physician.

11. Nursing Diagnosis: *RISK FOR ASPIRATION*

related to impaired swallowing, depressed cough and gag reflexes, and decreased level of consciousness.

Suggested NOC Outcomes: Respiratory status: airway patency; Aspiration prevention; Respiratory status: gas exchange

Suggested NIC Interventions: Respiratory monitoring; Aspiration precautions; Airway suctioning; Swallowing therapy

Desired Outcome	**Nursing Actions** *and Selected Purposes/Rationales* (see pp. 16–18 for additional rationales)
11. The client will not aspirate secretions or foods/fluids as evidenced by: a. clear breath sounds b. resonant percussion note over lungs c. absence of cough, tachypnea, and dyspnea.	11.a. Assess for and report signs and symptoms of aspiration of secretions or foods/fluids (e.g., rhonchi, dull percussion note over affected lung area, cough, tachypnea, tachycardia, dyspnea, presence of tube feeding in tracheal aspirate, chest x-ray results showing pulmonary infiltrate). b. Implement measures *to reduce the risk for aspiration:* 1. withhold oral foods/fluids and place client in side-lying position if he/she has a depressed or absent gag reflex, severe dysphagia, and/or is not alert 2. perform oropharyngeal suctioning, encourage client to use tonsil-tip suction, and provide oral hygiene as often as needed *to remove excess secretions* 3. if client is receiving tube feedings: a. check tube placement before each feeding or on a routine basis if feeding is continuous b. do not increase rate of continuous tube feeding infusion unless ordered; administer intermittent tube feedings slowly c. maintain client in a high Fowler's position during and for at least 30 minutes after feeding unless contraindicated d. stop tube feeding and notify physician if residuals exceed established parameters (usually 75–100 ml) 4. if oral intake is allowed: a. perform actions to improve ability to swallow (see Diagnosis 2, action b) b. allow ample time for meals c. instruct client to avoid laughing and talking while eating and drinking d. maintain client in high Fowler's position during and for at least 30 minutes after meals and snacks unless contraindicated e. assist client with oral hygiene after eating *to ensure that food particles do not remain in mouth.* c. If signs and symptoms of aspiration occur: 1. perform tracheal suctioning 2. withhold oral intake 3. prepare client for chest x-ray.

12. COLLABORATIVE DIAGNOSES: ***POTENTIAL COMPLICATIONS OF CEREBROVASCULAR ACCIDENT***

related to:

a. **increased intracranial pressure (IICP)**
   1. accumulation of blood in the cerebral tissue (can occur if CVA resulted from conditions such as ruptured cerebral aneurysm)
   2. cerebral edema associated with increased capillary permeability of cerebral vessels and disruption of the sodium pump within the cells (both occur as a result of cerebral hypoxia)
   3. increase in cerebral vascular volume associated with vasodilation of the cerebral vessels;

b. **corneal irritation and abrasion** related to inability to close eye on affected side if facial nerve paresis or paralysis has occurred;

c. **subluxation of shoulder** related to muscle weakness in affected upper arm and shoulder and gravity pull on affected arm.

Desired Outcomes	Nursing Actions *and Selected Purposes/Rationales*
12.a. The client will not develop IICP as evidenced by: 1. usual or improved level of consciousness 2. no reports of headache 3. stable or improved motor and sensory function 4. absence of vomiting, papilledema, and seizure activity 5. usual papillary size and reactivity 6. stable vital signs.	12.a.1. Assess for and report signs and symptoms of IICP: a. restlessness, agitation, confusion, lethargy b. reports of headache c. decreasing motor and sensory function d. abnormal posturing (e.g., extension [decerebrate], flexion [decorticate]) e. vomiting (usually without nausea) f. papilledema g. seizures h. change in pupil size or reactivity i. altered respiratory pattern (e.g., shallow, slow respirations; periods of apnea; central neurogenic hyperventilation) j. bounding, slow pulse k. rise in systolic B/P with widening pulse pressure. 2. Implement measures *to prevent IICP:* a. maintain fluid restrictions as ordered b. administer the following medications if ordered *to reduce cerebral edema:* 1. osmotic diuretics (e.g., mannitol) 2. loop diuretics (e.g., furosemide) 3. corticosteroids (e.g., dexamethasone) c. perform actions *to promote adequate cerebral venous drainage:* 1. elevate head of bed 30° unless contraindicated 2. keep client's head and neck in neutral, midline position; avoid flexion, extension, and rotation of head and neck 3. administer a laxative, antitussive, and antiemetic if ordered *to prevent straining to have a bowel movement, coughing, and vomiting (these conditions cause an increase in intrathoracic pressure that subsequently impedes venous return from the brain)* d. perform actions *to prevent further cerebral hypoxia and the subsequent vasodilation and cerebral edema:* 1. implement measures to improve cerebral tissue perfusion (see Diagnosis 1, action b) 2. implement measures *to maintain a patent airway* (e.g., position client on side, suction if necessary) 3. administer oxygen as ordered and before and after tracheal suctioning e. perform actions *to prevent an increase in blood pressure and subsequent dilation of the cerebral vessels:* 1. observe for and control conditions that can cause agitation (e.g., fear, anxiety, distended bladder) 2. instruct client to avoid activities that result in isometric muscle contractions (e.g., pushing feet against footboard, tightly gripping side rails) f. schedule care so activities that could raise intracranial pressure (e.g., suctioning, bathing, repositioning) are not grouped together. 3. If signs and symptoms of IICP are present: a. initiate seizure precautions b. prepare client for insertion of an intracranial pressure monitoring device or surgical intervention to treat the underlying cause (e.g., ligation of bleeding vessel, evacuation of expanding hematoma) if planned.
12.b. The client will not experience corneal irritation or abrasion as evidenced by: 1. absence of excessive tearing and eye redness 2. no reports of eye discomfort 3. usual visual acuity.	12.b.1. Assess for and report signs and symptoms of corneal irritation and abrasion (e.g., excessive tearing; reddened eye; reports of sensation of foreign body in eye, eye pain, itchy eye, or blurred vision). 2. Implement measures *to prevent corneal irritation and abrasion of eye on affected side:* a. reduce client's exposure to irritants such as powder, dust, and smoke b. have client wear his/her glasses *to protect eye* c. lubricate conjunctiva with isotonic eyedrops frequently d. tape eyelid shut if client is unable to close eye e. instruct client to avoid rubbing eye.

3. If signs and symptoms of corneal irritation or abrasion occur:
   a. assist with removal of any foreign body in the eye
   b. administer antimicrobial and anti-inflammatory ophthalmic ointments or solutions if ordered.

12.c. The client will not experience subluxation of shoulder as evidenced by:
1. absence of shoulder pain, tenderness, and swelling
2. maintenance of full range of motion of shoulder.

12.c.1. Assess for and report signs and symptoms of subluxation of the shoulder (e.g., shoulder pain, tenderness, or swelling; decreased range of motion of shoulder).
2. Implement measures *to prevent subluxation of the shoulder on the affected side:*
   a. perform actions *to improve muscle tone in affected shoulder and upper arm:*
      1. instruct client in and assist with range of motion exercises of affected shoulder and arm
      2. encourage client to use affected upper extremity to perform self-care and to assist in moving whenever possible
   b. when client is in bed or chair, position arm in correct alignment using pillows or lap board for support if necessary
   c. assist client with application of an arm support before sitting up in bed or getting out of bed
   d. use turn sheet or transfer belt when assisting client to move; never pull on shoulder or arm.
3. If signs and symptoms of shoulder subluxation occur:
   a. apply heat or cold to area as ordered
   b. administer anti-inflammatory medications and analgesics if ordered.

13. NURSING DIAGNOSIS: DISTURBED SELF-CONCEPT*

related to:
a. change in appearance (e.g., hemiplegia, facial droop, ptosis);
b. lifestyle and role changes associated with motor and spatial-perceptual impairments and disturbed thought processes;
c. impaired verbal communication;
d. loss of self-control (e.g., automatic speech, emotional lability, inappropriate behavior) or exaggerated emotional responses;
e. urinary incontinence;
f. dependence on others to meet basic needs.

*This diagnostic label includes the nursing diagnoses of disturbed body image, low self-esteem, and ineffective role performance.

Suggested NOC Outcomes: Body image; Self-esteem; Personal autonomy; Psychosocial adjustment: life change

Suggested NIC Interventions: Body image enhancement; Self-esteem enhancement; Emotional support; Support system enhancement; Role enhancement; Counseling

Desired Outcome

Nursing Actions *and Selected Purposes/Rationales* (see pp. 47–49 for additional rationales)

13. The client will demonstrate beginning adaptation to changes in appearance, physical and cognitive functioning, level of independence, lifestyle, and roles (see Care Plan on Immobility, Diagnosis 14 [p. 144], for outcome criteria).

13.a. Refer to Care Plan on Immobility, Diagnosis 14 (pp. 144–145), for measures related to assessment and promotion of a positive self-concept.
b. Implement additional measures *to assist client to adapt to changes in appearance, physical and cognitive functioning, level of independence, lifestyle, and roles:*
   1. reinforce measures to assist client to cope with effects of CVA (see Diagnosis 14, action c)
   2. discuss techniques the client can utilize *to adapt to disturbed thought processes:*
      a. encourage client to make lists and jot down messages and refer to these notes rather than relying on memory

Desired Outcome	**Nursing Actions** *and Selected Purposes/Rationales*

b. instruct client to place self in a calm environment when making decisions
c. encourage client to validate decisions, clarify information, and seek assistance with problem solving if indicated
3. instruct significant others in ways to manage client's emotional lability and inappropriate laughing, crying, or swearing (e.g., provide privacy; distract client by clapping hands, turning on television, or handing him/her an object)
4. provide privacy for the client when he/she is relearning skills such as feeding and dressing self *(helps to decrease the embarrassment that may be experienced initially)*
5. perform actions to reduce the risk of urinary incontinence (see Diagnosis 8, action b)
6. instruct and assist client to position self with affected extremities well supported and in proper alignment *(if extremities are positioned awkwardly, the impairment is more obvious)*
7. demonstrate acceptance of client using techniques such as touch and frequent visits; encourage significant others to do the same
8. perform actions to facilitate communication (see Diagnosis 5, action b)
9. reinforce use of assistive devices (e.g., plate guards, broad-handled utensils, universal cuff, button hook, long-handled shoehorn) and mobility aids (e.g., walker, cane) *to increase client's independence*
10. encourage significant others to allow client to do what he/she is able *so that independence can be re-established and/or self-esteem redeveloped*
11. use adjectives such as weak, affected, or right- or left-sided rather than "bad" when referring to side of hemiplegia.

14. Nursing Diagnosis: INEFFECTIVE COPING

related to fear; anxiety; depression; decreased ability to communicate verbally; changes in motor and sensory function, thought processes, and future lifestyle and roles; and need for lengthy rehabilitation.

Suggested NOC Outcomes: Coping; Adaptation to physical disability; Acceptance: health status; Psychosocial adjustment: life change

Suggested NIC Interventions: Coping enhancement; Counseling; Emotional support; Support system enhancement

Desired Outcome	**Nursing Actions** *and Selected Purposes/Rationales* (see pp. 26–28 for additional rationales)

14. The client will demonstrate effective coping as evidenced by:
   a. communication of ability to cope with the effects of the CVA
   b. utilization of appropriate problem-solving techniques
   c. willingness to participate in treatment plan and meet basic needs
   d. appropriate use of defense mechanisms
   e. utilization of available support systems.

14.a. Assess for and report signs and symptoms of ineffective coping (e.g., communication of inability to cope or ask for help; inability to meet role expectations, problem solve, or meet basic needs; insomnia; withdrawal; reluctance to participate in treatment plan; inappropriate use of defense mechanisms). Validate perceptions carefully, remembering that some behaviors may be a result of neurological changes.

b. Assess client's perception of current situation.

c. Implement measures *to promote effective coping:*
   1. allow time for client to begin to adjust to the diagnosis and planned treatment, residual effects of the CVA, and anticipated lifestyle and role changes
   2. perform actions to facilitate communication (see Diagnosis 5, action b)
   3. perform actions *to reduce fear and anxiety* (e.g., if speech or comprehension is impaired, establish an effective communication system as soon as possible; avoid startling client who is experiencing homonymous hemianopsia by approaching on unaffected side within his/her visual field; simplify client's environment as much as possible)

4. assist client to recognize and manage inappropriate denial if it is present
5. assist client to identify personal strengths and resources that can be utilized to facilitate coping with the current situation
6. perform actions *to support realistic hope about the effects of treatment on the residual impairments:*
   a. focus on what the client is able to accomplish independently and with the use of assistive devices
   b. reinforce knowledge that impairments may improve with time
   c. reinforce positive effects of speech, physical, and occupational therapies and control of underlying cause of the CVA (e.g., hypertension, diabetes)
7. if acceptable to client, arrange for a visit with another individual who has successfully adjusted to the effects of a CVA
8. instruct client in effective problem-solving techniques (e.g., accurate identification of stressors, determination of various options to solve problem)
9. assist client to maintain usual daily routines whenever possible
10. assist client to identify priorities and attainable goals as he/she starts to plan for necessary lifestyle and role changes
11. assist client through methods such as role playing to prepare for negative reactions of others to his/her altered appearance and other neurological impairments
12. if client is incontinent, instruct in ways to minimize the problem *so that socialization with others is possible* (e.g., placing disposable liners in underwear, wearing absorbent undergarments such as Depends)
13. set up a home evaluation appointment with occupational and physical therapists *so that changes in home environment (e.g., installation of ramps and handrails, widening doorways, altering kitchen facilities) can be completed by discharge*
14. assist client and significant others to identify ways that personal and family goals can be adjusted rather than abandoned
15. inform client that he/she may have times when impairments worsen; assure client that this is usually temporary and the result of physical and/or emotional stress or fatigue rather than an indication of deteriorating neurological status
16. administer antianxiety and/or antidepressant agents if ordered
17. if appropriate, assist client to meet spiritual needs (e.g., arrange for a visit from clergy)
18. assist client to identify and utilize available support systems; provide information regarding available community resources that can assist client and significant others in coping with effects of the CVA (e.g., stroke support groups, local chapter of the American Heart Association)
19. encourage the client to share with significant others the kind of support that would be most beneficial (e.g., listening, inspiring hope, providing reassurance and accurate information)
20. support behaviors indicative of effective coping (e.g., participation in treatment plan and self-care activities, communication of ability to cope, utilization of effective problem-solving strategies).

d. Consult appropriate health care provider (e.g., psychiatric nurse clinician, physician) if client continues to have difficulty coping with the effects of the CVA.

15. NURSING DIAGNOSIS: ***INTERRUPTED FAMILY PROCESSES***

related to change in family roles and structure associated with a family member's verbal, motor, and sensory impairments; disturbed thought processes; and need for lengthy rehabilitation.

Suggested NOC Outcomes:
Family coping; Family functioning; Family resiliency; Family normalization

Suggested NIC Interventions: Family involvement promotion; Family integrity promotion; Family process maintenance; Family support; Family mobilization; Support system enhancement

Desired Outcome	Nursing Actions *and Selected Purposes/Rationales*
15. The family members* will demonstrate beginning adjustment to changes in functioning of family member and family roles and structure as evidenced by: a. meeting client's needs b. verbalization of ways to adapt to required role and lifestyle changes c. active participation in decision making and client's rehabilitation d. positive interactions with one another.	15.a. Assess for signs and symptoms of interrupted family processes (e.g., inability to meet client's needs, statements of not being able to accept client's diagnosis of CVA and its effects or make necessary role and lifestyle changes, inability to make decisions, inability or refusal to participate in client's rehabilitation, negative family interactions). b. Identify components of the family and their patterns of communication and role expectations. c. Implement measures *to facilitate family members' adjustment to client's diagnosis, changes in client's functioning within the family system, and resultant changes in family roles and structure:* 1. encourage verbalization of feelings about the CVA and its effects on family structure; actively listen to each family member and maintain a nonjudgmental attitude about feelings shared 2. reinforce physician's explanation about the CVA and planned treatment and rehabilitation 3. assist family members to gain a realistic perspective of client's situation, conveying as much hope as appropriate 4. provide privacy *so that family members and client can share their feelings with one another;* stress the importance of and facilitate the use of good communication techniques 5. assist family members to progress through their own grieving process; explain that they may encounter times when they need to focus on meeting their own rather than the client's needs 6. emphasize the need for family members to obtain adequate rest and nutrition and to identify and utilize stress management techniques *so that they are better able to emotionally and physically deal with the changes and losses experienced and the physical care of the client* 7. encourage and assist family members to identify coping strategies for dealing with the client's impairments and their effects on the family 8. assist family members to identify realistic goals and ways of reaching these goals 9. include family members in decision making about client and his/her care; convey appreciation for their input and continued support of client 10. encourage and allow family members to participate in client's care and rehabilitation as appropriate 11. assist family members to identify resources that could assist them in coping with their feelings and meeting their immediate and long-term needs (e.g., counseling and social services; pastoral care; adult day care or respite program; service, church, and stroke support groups); initiate a referral if indicated. d. Consult appropriate health care provider (e.g., psychiatric nurse clinician, physician) if family members continue to demonstrate difficulty adapting to changes in client's functioning, roles, and family structure.

Discharge Teaching/Continued Care

16. NURSING DIAGNOSIS: ***DEFICIENT KNOWLEDGE, INEFFECTIVE THERAPEUTIC REGIMEN MANAGEMENT, OR INEFFECTIVE HEALTH MAINTENANCE****

*The nurse should select the diagnostic label that is most appropriate for the client's discharge teaching needs.

*The term "family members" is being used here to include client's significant others.

Suggested NOC Outcomes: Knowledge: disease process; Knowledge: treatment regimen; Knowledge: health behavior; Knowledge: health resources; Knowledge: fall prevention; Knowledge: treatment procedure(s)

Suggested NIC Interventions: Teaching: individual; Teaching: disease process; Teaching: prescribed activity/exercise; Teaching: psychomotor skills; Health system guidance

Desired Outcomes	**Nursing Actions** *and Selected Purposes/Rationales*
16.a. The client will communicate an awareness of ways to decrease the risk of a recurrent CVA.	16.a.1. Assist client to recognize factors that may have contributed to the CVA (e.g., hypertension, elevated serum lipids, diabetes, atrial fibrillation, use of oral contraceptives). 2. Identify appropriate actions client can take to decrease risk of a recurrent CVA (e.g., take medications as prescribed, decrease stress, stop smoking, modify diet, adhere to medical treatment plan to control hypertension and diabetes, use another form of birth control if taking oral contraceptives). 3. Provide information about resources that can help client to control risk factors (e.g., National Stroke Association, American Heart Association, smoking cessation and stress management programs). Initiate a referral if indicated.
16.b. The client will identify ways to manage sensory and speech impairments and disturbed thought processes.	16.b.1. Reinforce instructions regarding ways to adapt to visual impairments if present: a. utilize scanning techniques if visual field cut is present b. arrange home setting so that when in favorite chair or in bed, stimuli other than wall or furniture are within visual field c. wear eyepatch or opaque lens if double vision persists. 2. Reinforce use of established communication techniques and continuation with speech therapy if indicated. 3. If client is experiencing spatial-perceptual deficits and/or unilateral neglect, stress need for assistance with usual daily activities and strict adherence to safety measures to prevent injury. 4. Reinforce methods of adapting to impaired memory and shortened attention span (e.g., make lists of planned activities, review taped or written instructions frequently). 5. Instruct client to request assistance when problem solving and setting priorities and to seek validation of decisions if reasoning ability is impaired.
16.c. The client will identify ways to improve ability to swallow.	16.c.1. Reinforce instructions regarding appropriate swallowing techniques (e.g., sit upright for meals and snacks, tilt head and neck forward slightly when eating, place food in unaffected side of mouth, do not put a lot of food in mouth at one time). 2. Reinforce information about selecting or preparing foods/fluids that will promote more effective swallowing (e.g., avoid sticky foods; use "Thick-It," gelatin, or baby cereal to thicken liquids that are thin; moisten dry foods with gravy or sauces). 3. Allow time for questions and clarification of information provided.
16.d. The client will identify ways to manage urinary incontinence.	16.d.1. Reinforce instructions regarding client's bladder training program. Stress the importance of adhering to the program in order to reduce the risk of incontinence. 2. Demonstrate procedures that are included in client's bladder training program (e.g., intermittent catheterization, application of an external catheter). 3. Allow time for questions, clarification, and return demonstration.

Desired Outcomes	Nursing Actions *and Selected Purposes/Rationales*
16.e. The client will demonstrate measures to facilitate the performance of activities of daily living and increase physical mobility.	16.e.1. Reinforce measures that the client is using to improve his/her ability to perform activities of daily living and increase physical mobility (e.g., participation in exercise program; use of assistive devices and mobility aids; continued concentration on body positioning, balance, and movement). 2. Allow time for questions, clarification, and return demonstration.
16.f. The client will communicate an awareness of signs and symptoms to report to the health care provider.	16.f.1. Refer to Care Plan on Immobility, Diagnosis 17, action c (p. 148), for signs and symptoms to report to health care provider. 2. Instruct client to report development of or increase in these additional signs and symptoms: a. weakness or loss of sensation in extremities b. visual disturbances such as tunnel vision, blurred vision, or transient blindness c. lethargy, irritability, or confusion d. difficulty chewing or swallowing e. difficulty speaking or understanding verbal and nonverbal communication f. difficulty maintaining balance g. seizures (can begin to occur months after the CVA as scar tissue forms in the ischemic area).
16.g. The client will communicate knowledge of community resources that can assist with home management and adjustment to changes resulting from the CVA.	16.g.1. Provide information about community resources that can assist client and significant others with home management and adjustment to impairments in motor and sensory function and disturbed thought processes resulting from the CVA (e.g., home health agencies, stroke support groups, Meals on Wheels, social and financial services, local chapter of the American Heart Association, local service groups that can help obtain assistive devices, individual and family counselors). 2. Initiate a referral if indicated.
16.h. The client will communicate an understanding of and a plan for adhering to recommended follow-up care including future appointments with health care provider and therapists and medications prescribed	16.h.1. Reinforce the importance of keeping follow-up appointments with health care provider and physical, occupational, and speech therapists. 2. Teach client the rationale for, side effects of, and importance of taking prescribed medications (e.g., anticoagulants, platelet aggregation inhibitors, antihypertensives). Inform client of pertinent food and drug interactions. 3. Implement measures to improve client compliance: a. include significant others in teaching sessions if possible b. encourage questions and allow time for reinforcement and clarification of information provided c. provide written instructions on scheduled appointments with health care provider and occupational, physical, and speech therapists; medications prescribed; signs and symptoms to report; and exercise program.

Additional Nursing Diagnoses

*IMBALANCED NUTRITION: LESS THAN BODY REQUIREMENTS**

related to decreased oral intake associated with difficulty chewing, swallowing, and feeding self.

*RISK FOR CONSTIPATION**

related to:

a. decreased gastrointestinal motility associated with decreased activity;
b. decreased intake of fluids and foods high in fiber associated with difficulty chewing, swallowing, and feeding self;

---

*See Unit II for outcomes, actions, and rationales.

c. failure to respond to the urge to defecate associated with decreased level of consciousness or inability to recognize sensation of rectal fullness;
d. weakened abdominal muscles associated with generalized loss of muscle tone resulting from prolonged immobility.

SEXUAL DYSFUNCTION

related to:
a. alteration in usual sexual activities associated with impaired motor function;
b. decreased libido and/or impotence associated with impaired motor and sensory function, fear of urinary incontinence, depression, disturbed self-concept, and fear of rejection by partner.

*FEAR/ANXIETY**

related to impaired verbal communication and/or motor and sensory function; unfamiliar environment; lack of understanding of diagnosis, diagnostic tests, and treatments; uncertain prognosis; disturbed thought processes; financial concerns; and anticipated effect of the CVA on future lifestyle and roles.

*GRIEVING**

related to changes in motor and sensory function and thought processes and the effect of these changes on future lifestyle and roles.

---

*See Unit II for outcomes, actions, and rationales.

Bibliography

See pages 879 and 881.

Craniocerebral Trauma

The leading causes of craniocerebral trauma (head injury, traumatic brain injury) are motor vehicle accidents, falls, sports/recreational injuries, and assaults. Examples of skull and brain injury that can occur include skull fracture; dural tear; cerebral contusion, concussion, and laceration; diffuse axonal injury (DAI); brain stem damage; and intracranial hemorrhage. Brain damage can occur during the initial injury and as a result of subsequent cerebral damage resulting from factors such as cerebral hematoma, infection, and edema; seizure activity; and/or obstruction of the flow of cerebral spinal fluid (CSF).

Following craniocerebral trauma, a person may have a disturbance in consciousness ranging from a brief loss of contact with the environment to persistent coma. As the level of consciousness improves, clients often experience headache, dizziness, and alterations in thought processes. These signs and symptoms tend to subside gradually but can persist for weeks to years. Additional signs and symptoms following craniocerebral trauma vary depending on the area of the brain that has been affected. For example, tissue damage in the frontal lobe could result in loss of voluntary motor control, personality changes, and/or expressive aphasia; damage to the occipital lobe could cause visual disturbances; and damage to the temporal lobe could result in receptive aphasia and/or hearing impairment.

Craniocerebral trauma is classified according to location (e.g., skull, epidural area, brain stem), effect (e.g., concussion, diffuse axonal injury, depressed fracture of the skull, contusion, subdural hematoma), and/or severity. The severity of trauma ranges from minor (usually a concussion with no alteration in consciousness or a loss of consciousness lasting 5 minutes or less) to severe, in which extensive contusion and/or laceration of brain tissue and possible brain stem injury occurs. Severe craniocerebral trauma usually involves a period of prolonged unconsciousness and results in permanent neurological impairments that require extensive rehabilitation and long-term care.

This care plan focuses on the adult client hospitalized following craniocerebral trauma. It deals mainly with nursing and collaborative diagnoses appropriate for a client who has regained consciousness after sustaining a moderate brain injury. Much of the information is also applicable to clients receiving follow-up care in an extended care or rehabilitation facility or home setting. Nursing care and discharge teaching need to be individualized according to the areas of the brain affected and the extensiveness of the tissue damage. If the client has sustained more severe craniocerebral trauma, refer also to the Care Plans on Immobility and Cerebrovascular Accident.

OUTCOME/DISCHARGE CRITERIA

THE CLIENT WILL:

- have improved cerebral tissue perfusion
- have improved or stable neurological function
- have an adequate nutritional status
- have no signs or symptoms of complications
- identify ways to adapt to neurological deficits that may persist following craniocerebral trauma
- identify ways to reduce headache
- state signs and symptoms to report to the health care provider
- share thoughts and feelings about residual neurological impairments
- identify community resources that can assist with home management and adjustment to changes resulting from craniocerebral trauma
- verbalize an understanding of and a plan for adhering to recommended follow-up care including future appointments with health care provider and therapists and medications prescribed.

NURSING/COLLABORATIVE DIAGNOSES

1. Ineffective tissue perfusion: cerebral p. 245
2. Imbalanced nutrition: less than body requirements p. 245
3. Acute pain: headache p. 247
4. Disturbed thought processes p. 247
5. Risk for injury: falls, burns, and lacerations p. 248
6. Potential complications p. 249
   a. increased intracranial pressure (IICP)
   b. meningitis
   c. seizures
   d. cranial nerve damage
   e. diabetes insipidus

NURSING/COLLABORATIVE DIAGNOSES

f. syndrome of inappropriate antidiuretic hormone (SIADH)
g. gastrointestinal (GI) bleeding
7. Disturbed self-concept p. 255
8. Ineffective coping p. 256
9. Interrupted family processes p. 257

DISCHARGE TEACHING

10. Deficient knowledge, Ineffective therapeutic regimen management, or Ineffective health maintenance p. 259

See pp. 260–261 for additional diagnoses.

1. NURSING DIAGNOSIS:

INEFFECTIVE TISSUE PERFUSION: CEREBRAL

related to decreased cerebral blood flow associated with:
a. cerebral hemorrhage resulting from laceration of blood vessels at the time of injury;
b. pressure on cerebral vessels resulting from hematoma formation and/or edema;
c. spasm of cerebral vessels (can occur in response to damage to and stretching of cerebral vessels).

Suggested NOC Outcomes: Neurological status; Tissue perfusion: cerebral

Suggested NIC Interventions: Cerebral edema management; Cerebral perfusion promotion; Intracranial pressure (ICP) monitoring

Desired Outcome	**Nursing Actions** *and Selected Purposes/Rationales*
1. The client will experience improved cerebral tissue perfusion as evidenced by: a. decrease in or absence of dizziness, visual disturbances, and speech impairments b. improved mental status c. improved or usual sensory and motor function.	1.a. Assess client for signs and symptoms of decreased cerebral tissue perfusion: 1. dizziness 2. visual disturbances (e.g., blurred or dimmed vision, diplopia, change in visual field) 3. aphasia 4. irritability and restlessness 5. decreased level of consciousness 6. paresthesias, weakness, paralysis. b. Implement measures *to improve cerebral tissue perfusion:* 1. perform actions to prevent and treat increased intracranial pressure (see Diagnosis 6, actions a.2 and 3) 2. if client is hypotensive, perform actions *to improve cerebral blood flow* (e.g., administer prescribed sympathomimetic agents, maintain intravenous fluid therapy as ordered) 3. administer calcium-channel blockers (e.g., nimodipine) if ordered *to reduce cerebral vasospasm (the calcium that is released by the injured neural cells can cause vasospasm)* 4. prepare client for surgery (e.g., evacuation of hematoma, ligation of bleeding vessels) if planned. c. Consult physician if signs and symptoms of decreased cerebral tissue perfusion persist or worsen.

2. NURSING DIAGNOSIS:

IMBALANCED NUTRITION: LESS THAN BODY REQUIREMENTS

related to:
a. decreased oral intake associated with:
   1. anorexia resulting from headache and impaired sense of taste (can occur with damage to the facial nerves and/or as a result of loss of sense of smell [the olfactory nerves are often impaired because they are extremely sensitive to pressure])
   2. dysphagia if present

3. difficulty feeding self if visual disturbances are present or if motor function is impaired
4. prescribed dietary restrictions (may be necessary if client has a decreased level of consciousness or if damage to cranial nerves has resulted in a depressed or absent gag reflex or severe dysphagia)
5. restlessness, agitation, and/or shortened attention span;

b. the increased metabolic rate that occurs following craniocerebral trauma.

Suggested NOC Outcome: Nutritional status

Suggested NIC Interventions: Nutritional monitoring; Nutrition management; Nutrition therapy; Self-care assistance: feeding; Swallowing therapy

Desired Outcome	**Nursing Actions** *and Selected Purposes/Rationales* (see pp. 40–43 for additional rationales)
2. The client will maintain an adequate nutritional status as evidenced by: a. weight within normal range for client b. normal BUN and serum albumin, prealbumin, Hct, Hgb, and lymphocyte levels c. usual strength and activity tolerance d. healthy oral mucous membrane.	2.a. Assess the client for signs and symptoms of malnutrition: 1. weight significantly below client's usual weight or below normal for client's age, height, and body frame 2. abnormal BUN and low serum albumin, prealbumin, Hct, Hgb, and lymphocyte levels 3. weakness and fatigue 4. sore, inflamed oral mucous membrane 5. pale conjunctiva. b. Monitor percentage of meals and snacks client consumes. Report a pattern of inadequate intake. c. Implement measures *to maintain an adequate nutritional status:* 1. when food or oral fluids are allowed, perform actions *to improve oral intake:* a. implement measures to reduce headache (see Diagnosis 3, action d) b. implement measures to assist client to adapt to loss of or diminished sense of smell, visual impairments, impaired swallowing ability, and/or altered sense of taste if present (see Diagnosis 6, actions d.3.a and b; d.3.d.2.b; and d.3.e) c. increase activity as allowed and tolerated *(activity usually promotes a sense of well-being, which can improve appetite)* d. obtain a dietary consult if necessary to assist client in selecting foods/fluids that meet nutritional needs, are appealing, and adhere to personal and cultural preferences e. maintain a clean environment and a relaxed, quiet, pleasant atmosphere f. provide oral hygiene before meals *(oral hygiene moistens the mouth, which may make it easier to chew and swallow; it also removes unpleasant tastes, which often improves the taste of foods/fluids)* g. serve frequent, small meals rather than large ones if client is weak, quickly loses interest in eating, and/or has a poor appetite h. allow adequate time for meals; reheat foods/fluids if necessary i. implement measures *to enable client to feed self* (e.g., place only a few items on the tray at one time if spatial-perceptual deficits are present; reinforce use of assistive devices such as broad-handled utensils, rocker knives, and plate guards); if client needs to be fed, offer foods/fluids in the order he/she prefers 2. ensure that meals are well balanced and high in essential nutrients; offer dietary supplements if indicated 3. administer all vitamins and minerals if ordered. d. Perform a calorie count if ordered. Report information to dietitian and physician. e. Consult physician regarding an alternative method of providing nutrition (e.g., parenteral nutrition, tube feedings) if client does not consume enough food or fluids to meet nutritional needs.

3. NURSING DIAGNOSIS:

ACUTE PAIN: HEADACHE

related to:
a. trauma to the scalp, dura, and cerebral vessels and tissue;
b. stretching or compression of cerebral vessels and tissue associated with increased intracranial pressure if it occurs;
c. irritation of the meninges (occurs primarily if blood is present in the cerebrospinal fluid or meningitis develops).

Suggested NOC Outcomes: Comfort level; Pain control

Suggested NIC Interventions: Pain management; Analgesic administration

Desired Outcome

Nursing Actions *and Selected Purposes/Rationales*
(see pp. 45–47 for additional rationales)

3. The client will experience diminished headache as evidenced by:
   a. verbalization of same
   b. relaxed facial expression and body positioning
   c. increased participation in activities.

3.a. Assess for signs and symptoms of headache (e.g., statement of same, new or increased restlessness or irritability, grimacing, rubbing head, avoidance of bright lights and noises, reluctance to move).
b. Assess client's perception of the severity of the headache using a pain intensity rating scale.
c. Assess the client's pain pattern (e.g., location, quality, onset, duration, precipitating factors, aggravating factors, alleviating factors).
d. Implement measures *to reduce headache:*
   1. perform actions to reduce fear and anxiety (e.g., assure client that staff members are nearby, respond to call signal as soon as possible) *in order to promote relaxation and subsequently increase the client's threshold and tolerance for pain*
   2. administer analgesics before activities and procedures that can cause headache and before headache becomes severe
   3. perform actions *to minimize environmental stimuli* (e.g., provide a quiet environment, limit number of visitors and their length of stay, dim lights)
   4. avoid jarring bed or startling client *to minimize risk of sudden movements*
   5. perform actions to prevent and treat increased intracranial pressure and meningitis (see Diagnosis 6, actions a.2 and 3 and b.3 and 4)
   6. provide or assist with nonpharmacologic measures to reduce headache (e.g., cool cloth to forehead, progressive relaxation exercises)
   7. administer nonnarcotic analgesics or codeine if ordered (other narcotic [opioid] analgesics are usually contraindicated *because they have a greater depressant effect on the central nervous system*).
e. Consult physician if above actions fail to reduce headache.

4. NURSING DIAGNOSIS:

DISTURBED THOUGHT PROCESSES*

related to impaired cerebral functioning associated with cerebral tissue irritation and ischemia resulting from craniocerebral trauma.

*The diagnostic label of acute or chronic confusion may be more appropriate depending on the client's symptoms.

Suggested NOC Outcomes: Information processing; Neurological status: consciousness; Cognition; Memory

Suggested NIC Interventions: Reality orientation; Cognitive stimulation; Cognitive restructuring; Cerebral perfusion promotion; Socialization enhancement

Desired Outcome	Nursing Actions *and Selected Purposes/Rationales*
4. The client will experience improvement in thought processes as evidenced by: a. improved attention span, memory, reasoning ability, and judgment b. decreased irritability and instances of inappropriate responses c. improved level of orientation.	4.a. Assess client for disturbed thought processes (e.g., shortened attention span, impaired memory, decreased ability to concentrate, slow response time, poor reasoning ability or judgment, irritability, inappropriate responses, confusion). b. Ascertain from significant others client's usual level of cognitive and emotional functioning. c. Implement measures to improve cerebral tissue perfusion (see Diagnosis 1, action b) *in order to reduce cerebral ischemia and subsequently improve thought processes.* d. If client shows evidence of disturbed thought processes: 1. reorient client to person, place, and time as necessary 2. address client by name 3. place familiar objects, clock, and calendar within client's view 4. face client when conversing with him/her 5. approach client in a slow, calm manner; allow adequate time for communication 6. repeat instructions as necessary using clear, simple language and short sentences 7. keep environmental stimuli to a minimum but avoid sensory deprivation 8. maintain a consistent and fairly structured routine 9. provide written or taped information whenever possible for client to review as often as necessary 10. have client perform only one activity at a time and allow adequate time for performance of activities 11. encourage client to make lists of planned activities, questions, and concerns 12. assist client to problem solve if necessary 13. implement measures *to stop emotional outbursts and inappropriate responses if they occur* (e.g., provide distraction by taking client for a walk, decrease environmental stimuli by turning off television or radio and/or requesting that visitors leave for short while) 14. maintain realistic expectations of client's ability to learn, comprehend, and remember information provided 15. encourage significant others to be supportive of client; instruct them in methods of dealing with client's disturbed thought processes 16. discuss physiological basis for disturbed thought processes with client and significant others; inform them that cognitive and emotional functioning usually improve gradually but caution them that post-traumatic response (a postconcussion syndrome manifested in part by disturbed thought processes) can develop within weeks or months following the injury and persist for months to years 17. assist with neuropsychological testing if indicated 18. consult appropriate health care provider (e.g., psychiatric nurse clinician, physician) if disturbed thought processes worsen.

5. Nursing Diagnosis: RISK FOR INJURY: FALLS, BURNS, AND LACERATIONS

related to:
a. dizziness;
b. motor, visual, and/or spatial-perceptual impairments if present;
c. quick, impulsive behavior (can occur with injury involving the nondominant cerebral hemisphere);
d. ataxia (can occur with cerebellar injury);
e. disturbed thought processes (e.g., impaired memory, shortened attention span, confusion, slow response time).

Suggested NOC Outcomes: Fall prevention behavior; Balance

Suggested NIC Interventions: Fall prevention; Environmental management; Surveillance: safety; Peripheral sensation management

Desired Outcome	**Nursing Actions** *and Selected Purposes/Rationales*

5. The client will not experience falls, burns, or laceration.

5.a. Implement measures *to reduce the risk for injury:*
   1. perform actions *to prevent falls:*
      a. keep bed in low position with side rails up when client is in bed; consult physician about use of a floor bed or cubicle bed (large mattress on floor with surrounding "wall" of mattresses or padding) if indicated
      b. keep needed items within easy reach
      c. encourage client to request assistance whenever needed; have call signal within easy reach
      d. use lap belt when client is in chair if indicated
      e. instruct client to wear well-fitting slippers/shoes with nonslip soles and low heels when ambulating
      f. keep floor free of clutter and wipe up spills promptly
      g. accompany client during ambulation utilizing a transfer safety belt
      h. provide ambulatory aids (e.g., walker, cane) if client is weak or unsteady on feet
      i. reinforce instructions from physical therapist on correct transfer and ambulation techniques
      j. instruct client to ambulate in well-lit areas, utilize handrails if needed, and avoid sudden movements
      k. do not rush client; allow adequate time for ambulation to the bathroom and in hallway
      l. if vision is impaired:
         1. orient client to surroundings, room, and arrangement of furniture and identify obstacles during ambulation
         2. instruct client to wear an eyepatch or opaque lens if diplopia is present
         3. encourage visual scanning if a visual field cut is present
      m. make sure that shower has a nonslip bottom surface and that shower chair, secure bath mat, call signal, grab bars, and adequate lighting are present
   2. perform actions *to prevent burns* (e.g., let hot foods and fluids cool slightly before serving, supervise client while smoking if indicated)
   3. assist client with tasks that require fine motor skills (e.g., shaving) *in order to prevent lacerations*
   4. administer central nervous system depressants judiciously
   5. if client is confused or irrational:
      a. reorient frequently to surroundings and necessity of adhering to safety precautions
      b. provide appropriate level of supervision
      c. consult physician about the temporary use of a bed alarm or jacket or wrist restraints if necessary
      d. administer prescribed antianxiety and antipsychotic medications if indicated.

b. Include client and significant others in planning and implementing measures to prevent injury.

c. If injury does occur, initiate appropriate first aid and notify physician.

6. COLLABORATIVE DIAGNOSES: POTENTIAL COMPLICATIONS OF CRANIOCEREBRAL TRAUMA

a. increased intracranial pressure (IICP) related to:
   1. accumulation of blood in the cerebral tissue associated with trauma to the cerebral vessels
   2. cerebral edema associated with:
      a. increased capillary permeability of cerebral vessels (occurs with cerebral hypoxia)
      b. an increase in cellular volume resulting from disruption of the sodium pump within the cells (occurs as a result of cerebral hypoxia) and syndrome of inappropriate antidiuretic hormone (SIADH) if it occurs

3. hydrocephalus associated with obstruction of normal cerebrospinal fluid (CSF) flow resulting from edema, hematoma, and/or presence of blood in the subarachnoid space
4. increase in cerebral vascular volume associated with vasodilation of the cerebral vessels;

b. **meningitis** related to:
1. irritation of the meninges associated with trauma to the meningeal vessels or presence of blood in the CSF
2. introduction of pathogens into the meninges or CSF associated with a tear in the dura (more likely to occur with a compound fracture of the skull, a linear fracture of the frontal or temporal bone, and/or penetration of the skull by an object such as a bullet) and presence of an intracranial monitoring device and/or external ventricular drain;

c. **seizures** related to altered activity of the cerebral neurons associated with irritation of the brain tissue resulting from the initial injury and IICP and meningitis if they occur;

d. **cranial nerve damage** related to trauma to the nerves during the initial injury and/or compression of the nerves associated with the development of cerebral hematoma or edema;

e. **diabetes insipidus** related to decreased production and/or impaired release of antidiuretic hormone (ADH) associated with trauma to the hypothalamus and/or the posterior lobe of the pituitary gland;

f. **syndrome of inappropriate antidiuretic hormone (SIADH)** related to:
1. increased production and/or release of ADH associated with trauma to the hypothalamus and/or the posterior lobe of the pituitary gland
2. stimulation of ADH output associated with pain, trauma, and stress;

g. **gastrointestinal (GI) bleeding** related to the development of an ulcer (often referred to as stress-induced ulcer, stress-related mucosal damage [SRMD], or Cushing's ulcer) associated with:
1. gastric ischemia resulting from vasoconstriction (occurs with sympathetic nervous system stimulation that can result from cerebral injury)
2. hypersecretion of hydrochloric acid resulting from parasympathetic nervous system stimulation that can occur with cerebral injury and stress.

Desired Outcomes

6.a. The client will not develop IICP as evidenced by:
1. usual or improved level of consciousness
2. no reports of increased headache
3. stable or improved motor and sensory function
4. absence of vomiting, papilledema, and seizure activity
5. usual pupillary size and reactivity
6. stable vital signs.

Nursing Actions *and Selected Purposes/Rationales*

6.a.1. Assess for and report signs and symptoms of IICP:
- a. increased restlessness, agitation, confusion, or lethargy
- b. reports of increased headache
- c. decreasing motor and sensory function
- d. abnormal posturing (e.g., extension [decerebrate], flexion [decorticate])
- e. vomiting (usually without nausea)
- f. papilledema
- g. seizures
- h. change in pupil size or reactivity
- i. altered respiratory pattern (e.g., shallow, slow respirations; periods of apnea; central neurogenic hyperventilation)
- j. bounding, slow pulse
- k. rise in systolic B/P with widening pulse pressure.

2. Implement measures *to prevent IICP:*
- a. maintain fluid restrictions as ordered
- b. administer the following medications if ordered *to reduce cerebral edema:*
  1. osmotic diuretics (e.g., mannitol)
  2. loop diuretics (e.g., furosemide)
  3. corticosteroids (e.g., dexamethasone)
- c. perform actions *to promote adequate cerebral venous drainage:*
  1. elevate head of bed 30° unless contraindicated
  2. keep head and neck in neutral, midline position; avoid flexion, extension, and rotation of head and neck

3. administer a laxative, antitussive, and antiemetic if ordered *to prevent straining to have a bowel movement, coughing, and vomiting (these conditions cause an increase in intrathoracic pressure, which subsequently impedes venous return from the brain)*

d. perform actions *to prevent cerebral hypoxia and the subsequent vasodilation and cerebral edema:*
   1. implement measures to improve cerebral tissue perfusion (see Diagnosis 1, action b)
   2. implement measures *to maintain a patent airway* (e.g., position client on side, suction if necessary)
   3. administer central nervous system depressants judiciously; hold medication and consult physician if respiratory rate is less than 12/minute
   4. administer oxygen as ordered and before and after tracheal suctioning

e. perform actions to prevent and treat SIADH (see actions f.2 and 3 in this diagnosis) *in order to further reduce the risk for cerebral edema*

f. perform actions *to prevent excessive cerebral blood flow and/or dilation of cerebral vessels:*
   1. implement measures *to prevent an increase in blood pressure:*
      a. observe for and control conditions that can cause or increase restlessness and agitation (e.g., fear, anxiety, pain, distended bladder); administer an antianxiety agent (e.g., lorazepam) if ordered *to reduce persistent restlessness and agitation*
      b. instruct client to avoid activities that result in isometric muscle contractions (e.g., pushing feet against footboard, tightly gripping side rails)
   2. implement measures *to prevent an increase in metabolic rate:*
      a. administer anticonvulsants (e.g., phenytoin) if ordered *to prevent seizure activity*
      b. perform actions *to prevent and treat increased body temperature* (e.g., apply a hypothermia blanket if ordered, administer antipyretics if ordered)

g. perform actions to prevent and treat meningitis (see actions b.3 and 4 in this diagnosis) *in order to prevent obstruction of the flow of CSF and an increase in metabolic rate (infection causes an increase in metabolic rate and subsequent increase in cerebral blood flow, which results in cerebral vasodilation)*

h. schedule care so activities that could raise intracranial pressure (e.g., suctioning, bathing, repositioning) are not grouped together.

3. If signs and symptoms of IICP are present:
   a. initiate seizure precautions
   b. prepare client for the following if planned:
      1. insertion of an intracranial pressure monitoring device
      2. lumbar or ventricular puncture *to remove excess CSF*
      3. surgical intervention (e.g., ligation of bleeding vessel, aspiration of hematoma, elevation of depressed bone, removal of bone fragments).

6.b. The client will not develop meningitis as evidenced by:
   1. absence of fever and chills
   2. gradual resolution of headache
   3. absence of nuchal rigidity and photophobia
   4. negative Kernig's and Brudzinski's signs
   5. normal CSF analysis.

6.b.1. Assess for and report signs and symptoms of a CSF leak *(indicates a tear in the dura):*
   a. presence of glucose in clear drainage from nose, ear, or wound as shown by positive results on a glucose reagent strip
   b. yellowish ring ("halo") around bloody or serosanguineous drainage on dressing or pillowcase *(CSF dries in concentric rings)*
   c. reports of postnasal drip
   d. constant swallowing.

2. Assess for and report signs and symptoms of meningitis:
   a. fever, chills
   b. increasing or persistent headache
   c. nuchal rigidity

Desired Outcomes	**Nursing Actions** *and Selected Purposes/Rationales*

d. photophobia
e. positive Kernig's sign (inability to straighten knee when hip is flexed)
f. positive Brudzinski's sign (flexion of hip and knee in response to forward flexion of the neck)
g. CSF that is cloudy (can indicate elevated WBC and protein levels in the CSF)
h. elevated CSF pressure (pressure is often elevated with meningitis)
i. CSF analysis showing increased WBC and protein levels.

3. Implement measures *to prevent meningitis:*
   a. assist with thorough cleansing and debridement of head wound if indicated
   b. use sterile technique when changing dressings and working with intracranial pressure monitoring device and external ventricular drain
   c. instruct client to keep hands away from head wound, drainage tube(s), and dressing; apply wrist restraints or mittens if necessary
   d. if a CSF leak is present:
      1. instruct client to avoid excessive movement and activity (bed rest is usually ordered *to prevent further stress on the torn dura)*
      2. instruct client to avoid coughing, blowing nose, or straining to have a bowel movement *(these activities raise intracranial pressure and can cause extension of the dural tear);* consult physician regarding an order for an antitussive, decongestant, and laxative if indicated
      3. if CSF is leaking from nose:
         a. position client with head of bed elevated at least 20° unless contraindicated *to allow the fluid to drain*
         b. if client needs to sneeze, instruct him/her to do so with mouth open *(withholding the sneeze can force bacteria backward through the torn dura)*
         c. instruct client to avoid putting finger in nose
         d. do not perform nasal suctioning or insert a nasogastric tube
         e. do not attempt to clean nose unless ordered by physician
      4. if CSF is leaking from ear:
         a. position client on side of CSF leakage unless contraindicated *to allow the fluid to drain*
         b. instruct client to avoid putting finger in ear
         c. do not attempt to clean ear unless ordered by physician
      5. do not pack dressing into area of CSF leakage (nose, ear, or wound) *because it will interfere with the drainage of fluid;* place a sterile pad over area of CSF leakage to absorb drainage and change pad as soon as it becomes damp
      6. prepare client for surgical repair of the torn dura if the leak does not heal spontaneously
   e. administer antimicrobials if ordered.
4. If signs and symptoms of meningitis occur:
   a. initiate seizure precautions *(cerebral irritation can cause seizures)*
   b. provide a quiet environment with dim lighting *to reduce discomfort associated with headache and photophobia*
   c. administer antimicrobials as ordered.

6.c. The client will not experience seizure activity or injury if seizure occurs.

6.c.1. Assess for and report signs and symptoms of seizure activity (e.g., twitching [usually of face or hands], clonic-tonic movements).
2. Implement measures *to prevent seizures:*
   a. perform actions to prevent and treat IICP and meningitis (see actions a.2 and 3 and b.3 and 4 in this diagnosis)
   b. administer anticonvulsants (e.g., phenytoin, carbamazepine) if ordered.
3. Initiate and maintain seizure precautions:
   a. have oral airway and suction equipment readily available

b. pad side rails with blankets or soft pads
c. keep bed in low position with side rails up when client is in bed.

4. If seizures do occur:
   a. implement measures *to decrease risk of injury:*
      1. ease client to the floor if he/she is sitting in chair or ambulating at onset of seizure
      2. remain with but do not restrain client during seizure activity
      3. do not force any object between clenched teeth or try to pry mouth open
      4. clear area of objects that may cause injury
      5. place towel under client's head if he/she is on floor
      6. as seizure activity subsides, perform actions *to maintain a patent airway* (e.g., turn client on side, insert an oral airway, suction as needed)
   b. observe for and report characteristics of seizures (e.g., progression, time elapsed)
   c. administer intravenous anticonvulsants (e.g., phenytoin, phenobarbital) if ordered.

6.d. The client will not experience cranial nerve damage or will adapt to cranial nerve damage if it occurs.

6.d.1. Assess for and report signs and symptoms of damage to the following cranial nerves:
   a. olfactory (e.g., decreased or absent sense of smell)
   b. optic, oculomotor, trochlear, or abducens (e.g., diplopia, visual field cut, decreased visual acuity, abnormal extraocular movements)
   c. trigeminal (e.g., decreased or absent corneal reflex, difficulty chewing, pain when chewing)
   d. vagus or glossopharyngeal (e.g., loss of gag reflex, difficulty swallowing, hoarseness, inability to speak clearly)
   e. hypoglossal (e.g., difficulty chewing, swallowing, or speaking)
   f. facial (e.g., facial ptosis, impaired sense of taste).

2. Implement measures to prevent and treat IICP (see actions a.2 and 3 in this diagnosis) *in order to reduce the risk for compression of and subsequent damage to the cranial nerves.*

3. Implement measures *to help the client compensate for cranial nerve damage if it has occurred:*
   a. if the olfactory nerve is affected, provide meals that are visually appealing *to help stimulate appetite*
   b. if vision is impaired, provide an eyepatch or opaque lens *(helps reduce double vision)*, instruct client in visual scanning techniques (if experiencing visual field cut), and assist client with self-care and ambulation if indicated
   c. if the corneal reflex is absent or the client is unable to close his/her eye, perform actions *to protect the cornea from irritation and abrasion* (e.g., instruct client to avoid rubbing eye; reduce exposure to dust, powder, and smoke; instill isotonic eyedrops frequently)
   d. if the trigeminal, hypoglossal, vagus, and/or glossopharyngeal nerves are affected:
      1. withhold oral foods/fluids until gag reflex returns and client is better able to chew and swallow *in order to reduce the risk for aspiration;* provide parenteral nutrition or tube feedings if indicated
      2. when oral intake is allowed:
         a. perform actions *to prevent aspiration* (e.g., place client in high Fowler's position during and for at least 30 minutes after meals and snacks, assist client with oral hygiene after eating *to ensure that food particles do not remain in mouth,* instruct client to avoid laughing and talking while eating and drinking)
         b. perform actions *to improve client's ability to swallow* (e.g., avoid serving sticky foods such as peanut butter and bananas, assist client to select foods that require little or no chewing and are easily swallowed, serve thick fluids or thicken thin fluids with substances such as "Thick-It" or gelatin)

Desired Outcomes	**Nursing Actions** *and Selected Purposes/Rationales*

3. perform actions *to facilitate communication* (e.g., maintain quiet environment; provide pad and pencil, Magic Slate, computer, or word cards; listen carefully when client speaks)
4. consult speech pathologist about additional ways to facilitate swallowing and communication

e. if the sensory component of the facial nerve is affected, instruct client to add extra sweeteners or seasonings to food/fluids if desired *in order to compensate for impaired sense of taste.*

6.e. The client will not experience diabetes insipidus as evidenced by:
1. absence of polyuria
2. absence of intense thirst (polydipsia).

6.e.1. Assess for and report signs and symptoms of diabetes insipidus:
a. polyuria (urine output can range from 4–10 or more liters/day)
b. reports of intense thirst (if oral fluids are allowed and tolerated, the client's intake is often an amount that corresponds to the high volume of urine output)
c. a decrease in urine specific gravity (often 1.005 or less).

2. Administer osmotic diuretics (e.g., mannitol), loop diuretics (e.g., furosemide), and/or corticosteroids (e.g., dexamethasone) if ordered *to decrease edema of the hypothalamus, pituitary gland, and surrounding tissue and subsequently reduce the risk for the development of diabetes insipidus.*

3. If signs and symptoms of diabetes insipidus occur:
a. maintain fluid intake equal to output *in order to prevent water deficit*
b. administer an ADH replacement (e.g., vasopressin, desmopressin [DDAVP]) if ordered
c. assess for and report signs and symptoms of water deficit (e.g., decreased skin turgor; dry mucous membranes; weight loss of 2% or greater over a short period; postural hypotension and/or low B/P; weak, rapid pulse; elevated serum sodium and osmolality).

6.f. The client will not develop SIADH as evidenced by:
1. stable weight
2. balanced intake and output
3. stable or improved mental status
4. stable or improved muscle strength
5. decreased reports of headache
6. absence of cellular edema, abdominal cramping, nausea, vomiting, and seizure activity
7. urine and serum sodium and osmolality levels within normal limits.

6.f.1. Assess for and report signs and symptoms of SIADH:
a. weight gain of 2% or greater over a short period
b. intake greater than output
c. increased irritability or confusion
d. increasing muscle weakness
e. reports of persistent or increased headache
f. fingerprint edema over sternum (reflects cellular edema)
g. abdominal cramping, nausea, or vomiting
h. seizures
i. elevated urine sodium and osmolality levels
j. low serum sodium and osmolality levels.

2. Implement measures *to reduce the risk for the development of SIADH:*
a. perform actions to reduce pain (see Diagnosis 3, action d)
b. perform actions *to reduce fear and anxiety* (e.g., assure client that staff members are nearby, respond to call signal as soon as possible)
c. administer osmotic diuretics (e.g., mannitol), loop diuretics (e.g., furosemide), and/or corticosteroids (e.g., dexamethasone) if ordered *to decrease edema of the hypothalamus, pituitary gland, and surrounding tissue.*

3. If signs and symptoms of SIADH occur:
a. maintain fluid restrictions if ordered *to prevent further fluid retention* (typically, this is a restriction of free water)
b. encourage intake of foods/fluids high in sodium (e.g., tomato juice, cured meats, processed cheese, canned soups, catsup, canned vegetables, dill pickles, bouillon) if oral intake is allowed and tolerated
c. initiate seizure precautions
d. administer the following if ordered:
   1. diuretics (usually furosemide) *to promote water excretion*
   2. intravenous infusion of a hypertonic saline solution *to treat severe hyponatremia*

3. demeclocycline *to promote water excretion (inhibits the effect of ADH on the renal tubules).*

6.g. The client will not experience GI bleeding as evidenced by:
1. no reports of epigastric discomfort and fullness
2. absence of frank and occult blood in stool and gastric contents
3. B/P and pulse within normal range for client
4. RBC, Hct, and Hgb levels within normal range.

6.g.1. Assess for and report signs and symptoms of GI bleeding (e.g., reports of epigastric discomfort or fullness; frank or occult blood in stool or gastric contents; decreased B/P; increased pulse; decreasing RBC, Hct, and Hgb levels).
2. Implement measures *to prevent ulceration of the gastric and duodenal mucosa:*
   a. perform actions *to decrease fear and anxiety* (e.g., assure client that staff members are nearby, respond to call signal as soon as possible)
   b. when oral intake is allowed:
      1. administer ulcerogenic medications (e.g., corticosteroids, phenytoin) with meals or snacks *to decrease gastric irritation*
      2. instruct client to avoid foods/fluids that stimulate hydrochloric acid secretion or irritate the gastric mucosa (e.g., coffee; caffeine-containing tea and colas; spices such as black pepper, chili powder, and nutmeg)
   c. administer histamine$_2$ receptor antagonists (e.g., ranitidine, famotidine), proton-pump inhibitors (e.g., omeprazole, rabeprazole), antacids, and/or cytoprotective agents (e.g., sucralfate) if ordered.
3. If signs and symptoms of GI bleeding occur:
   a. insert nasogastric tube and maintain suction as ordered
   b. administer blood products and/or volume expanders if ordered
   c. assist with measures to control bleeding (e.g., gastric lavage, endoscopic electrocoagulation) if planned.

7. NURSING DIAGNOSIS: DISTURBED SELF-CONCEPT*

related to:
a. change in appearance (e.g., periocular edema and ecchymosis, loss of hair on head if an area was shaved to repair lacerations);
b. changes in motor and sensory function;
c. dependence on others to meet basic needs;
d. anticipated changes in lifestyle and roles associated with sensory and motor impairments and disturbed thought processes.

*This diagnostic label includes the nursing diagnoses of disturbed body image, low self-esteem, and ineffective role performance.

Suggested NOC Outcomes: Body image; Self-esteem; Psychosocial adjustment: life change

Suggested NIC Interventions: Body image enhancement; Self-esteem enhancement; Emotional support; Support system enhancement; Role enhancement; Counseling

Desired Outcome	**Nursing Actions** *and Selected Purposes/Rationales* (see pp. 47–49 for additional rationales)

7. The client will demonstrate beginning adaptation to changes in appearance, physical and cognitive functioning, lifestyle, roles, and level of independence as evidenced by:
   a. verbalization of feelings of self-worth
   b. maintenance of relationships with significant others

7.a. Assess for signs and symptoms of a disturbed self-concept (e.g., verbalization of negative feelings about self, withdrawal from significant others, lack of participation in activities of daily living, lack of plan for adapting to necessary changes in lifestyle).
b. Discuss with client improvements in appearance and neurological function that can realistically be expected.
c. Implement measures to assist the client to cope with the effects of craniocerebral trauma (see Diagnosis 8, action c).
d. If periocular edema and ecchymosis are present:
   1. reinforce that they are temporary (edema usually begins to subside 48–72 hours after the injury and ecchymosis usually disappears in 10–14 days)

Desired Outcome	Nursing Actions *and Selected Purposes/Rationales*
c. active participation in activities of daily living d. verbalization of a beginning plan for adapting lifestyle to changes resulting from craniocerebral trauma.	2. instruct and assist client with measures *to reduce swelling* (e.g., cold compresses to affected area, lying on unaffected side, keeping head of bed elevated 30° unless contraindicated). e. Implement measures *to reduce client's embarrassment about loss of hair* (e.g., assist with hair styling that makes shaved area less obvious; provide client with a turban, hat, scarf, surgical cap). Reinforce the fact that the hair will grow back. f. Discuss techniques the client can utilize *to adapt to disturbed thought processes:* 1. encourage client to make lists and write or record messages and to refer to these rather than relying on memory 2. instruct the client to place self in a calm environment when making decisions 3. encourage client to validate decisions, clarify information, and seek assistance to problem solve if indicated 4. encourage client to schedule adequate rest periods and reduce stressors *in order to decrease irritability.* g. Instruct significant others in ways to manage client's emotional lability and inappropriate behavior (e.g., provide privacy, reduce environmental stimuli, distract client by clapping hands). h. Reinforce use of assistive devices (e.g., plate guard, nonslip tray mat, broad-handled utensils, universal cuff, button hook, long-handled shoehorn) and mobility aids (e.g., walker, cane) *to increase client's independence.* i. Encourage significant others to allow client to do what he/she is able *so that independence can be re-established and/or self-esteem redeveloped.* j. Assist client's and significant others' adjustment by listening, facilitating communication, and providing information. k. Support behaviors suggesting positive adaptation to changes that have occurred (e.g., use of assistive devices to perform self-care, verbalization of feelings of self-worth, maintenance of relationships with significant others). l. Assist client and significant others to have similar expectations and understanding of future lifestyle. m. Encourage client to continue involvement in social activities and to pursue usual roles and interests. If previous roles, interests, and hobbies cannot be pursued, encourage development of new ones. n. Provide information about and encourage utilization of community agencies and support groups (e.g., brain injury support groups, vocational rehabilitation, family and individual counseling) if appropriate. o. Consult appropriate health care provider (e.g., psychiatric nurse clinician, physician) about psychological counseling if client desires or seems unwilling or unable to adapt to changes resulting from craniocerebral trauma.

8. Nursing Diagnosis: *INEFFECTIVE COPING*

related to persistent headache, changes in motor and sensory function and thought processes, and possibility of lengthy rehabilitation and changes in future lifestyle and roles.

Suggested NOC Outcomes: Coping; Psychosocial adjustment: life change

Suggested NIC Interventions: Coping enhancement; Counseling; Emotional support; Support system enhancement

Desired Outcome	**Nursing Actions** *and Selected Purposes/Rationales* (see pp. 26–28 for additional rationales)
8. The client will demonstrate effective coping as evidenced by: a. verbalization of ability to cope with the effects of craniocerebral trauma b. utilization of appropriate problem-solving techniques c. willingness to participate in treatment plan and meet basic needs d. absence of destructive behavior toward self and others e. appropriate use of defense mechanisms f. utilization of available support systems.	8.a. Assess for and report signs and symptoms of ineffective coping (e.g., verbalization of inability to cope or ask for help; inability to meet role expectations, problem solve, or meet basic needs; insomnia; withdrawal; reluctance to participate in treatment plan; destructive behavior toward self or others; inappropriate use of defense mechanisms). Validate perceptions carefully, remembering that some behaviors may be the result of neurological changes. b. Assess client's perception of current situation. c. Implement measures *to promote effective coping:* 1. allow time for client to begin to adjust to planned treatment, residual effects of craniocerebral trauma, and anticipated lifestyle and role changes 2. perform actions to reduce headache (see Diagnosis 3, action d) 3. assist client to identify personal strengths and resources that can be utilized to facilitate coping with the current situation 4. demonstrate acceptance of client but set limits on inappropriate behavior 5. if acceptable to client, arrange for a visit with another individual who has successfully recovered from craniocerebral trauma 6. instruct client in effective problem-solving techniques (e.g., accurate identification of stressors, determination of various options to solve problem) 7. assist client to maintain usual daily routines whenever possible 8. assist client to identify priorities and attainable goals as he/she starts to plan for necessary lifestyle and role changes 9. set up a home evaluation appointment with occupational and physical therapists if indicated *so that changes in the home environment (e.g., installation of ramps and handrails, widening doorways, altering kitchen facilities) can be completed by discharge* 10. assist client and significant others to identify ways that personal and family goals can be adjusted rather than abandoned 11. inform client that he/she may have days when impairments worsen; assure client that this is usually temporary and the result of physical and/or emotional stress or fatigue rather than an indication of deteriorating neurological status 12. administer antianxiety and/or antidepressant agents if ordered 13. assist client to identify and utilize available support systems; provide information regarding available community resources that can assist client and significant others in coping with effects of craniocerebral trauma (e.g., brain injury support groups; individual, family, and financial counseling services) 14. encourage client to share with significant others the kind of support that would be most beneficial (e.g., listening, inspiring hope, providing reassurance and accurate information) 15. support behaviors indicative of effective coping (e.g., participation in treatment plan and self-care activities, communication of ability to cope, utilization of effective problem-solving strategies). d. Consult appropriate health care provider (e.g., psychiatric nurse clinician, physician) if client continues to have difficulty coping with the effects of the craniocerebral trauma.

9. NURSING DIAGNOSIS: ***INTERRUPTED FAMILY PROCESSES***

related to change in family roles and structure associated with a family member's motor and sensory impairments, disturbed thought processes, and possible need for lengthy rehabilitation.

Suggested NOC Outcomes: Family coping; Family functioning; Family resiliency; Family normalization

Suggested NIC Interventions: Family involvement promotion; Family integrity promotion; Family process maintenance; Family support; Family mobilization; Support system enhancement

Desired Outcome	**Nursing Actions** *and Selected Purposes/Rationales*

9. The family members* will demonstrate beginning adjustment to changes in functioning of family member and family roles and structure as evidenced by:
   a. meeting client's needs
   b. verbalization of ways to adapt to required role and lifestyle changes
   c. active participation in decision making and client's rehabilitation
   d. positive interactions with one another.

9.a. Assess for signs and symptoms of interrupted family processes (e.g., inability to meet client's needs, statements of not being able to accept client's physical impairments and changes in thought processes or make necessary role and lifestyle changes, inability to make decisions, inability or refusal to participate in client's rehabilitation, negative family interactions).

b. Identify components of the family and their patterns of communication and role expectations.

c. Implement measures *to facilitate family members' adjustment to client's diagnosis, changes in client's functioning within the family system, and resultant changes in family roles and structure:*
   1. encourage verbalization of feelings about client's disabilities and the effect of these on their family structure; actively listen to each member and maintain a nonjudgmental attitude about feelings shared
   2. reinforce physician's explanation about the effects of craniocerebral trauma and planned treatment and rehabilitation
   3. assist family members to gain a realistic perspective of client's situation, conveying as much hope as appropriate
   4. provide privacy *so that family members and client can share their feelings with one another;* stress the importance of and facilitate the use of good communication techniques
   5. assist family members to progress through their own grieving process; explain that they may encounter times when they need to focus on meeting their own rather than the client's needs
   6. emphasize the need for family members to obtain adequate rest and nutrition and to identify and utilize stress management techniques *so that they are better able to emotionally and physically deal with the changes and losses experienced*
   7. encourage and assist family members to identify coping strategies for dealing with the client's disabilities and the effects on the family
   8. assist family members to identify realistic goals and ways of reaching these goals
   9. include family members in decision making about client and his/her care; convey appreciation for their input and continued support of client
   10. encourage and allow family members to participate in client's care and rehabilitation
   11. assist family members to identify resources that could assist them in coping with their feelings and meeting their immediate and long-term needs (e.g., counseling and social services; pastoral care; adult day care or respite program; service, church, and brain injury support groups); initiate a referral if indicated.

d. Consult appropriate health care provider (e.g., psychiatric nurse clinician, physician) if family members continue to demonstrate difficulty adapting to changes in client's functioning, roles, and family structure.

---

*The term "family members" is being used here to include client's significant others.

Discharge Teaching/Continued Care

10. NURSING DIAGNOSIS: ***DEFICIENT KNOWLEDGE, INEFFECTIVE THERAPEUTIC REGIMEN MANAGEMENT, OR INEFFECTIVE HEALTH MAINTENANCE****

*The nurse should select the diagnostic label that is most appropriate for the client's discharge teaching needs.

Suggested NOC Outcomes: Knowledge: treatment regimen; Knowledge: health behavior; Knowledge: health resources

Suggested NIC Interventions: Health system guidance; Teaching: individual; Teaching: prescribed activity/exercise; Teaching: prescribed medication

Desired Outcomes	**Nursing Actions** *and Selected Purposes/Rationales*
10.a. The client will identify ways to adapt to neurological deficits that may persist following craniocerebral trauma.	10.a.1. Instruct client in ways to adapt to neurological deficits* resulting from craniocerebral trauma: a. wear an eyepatch or opaque lens if double vision is a problem b. utilize scanning techniques if visual field cut is present c. utilize paper and pencil, Magic Slate, computer, pictures, and gestures to express self if verbal communication is impaired d. make lists, write or record messages and reminders, and refer to written instructions repeatedly if experiencing difficulty concentrating or remembering e. request assistance when problem solving and setting priorities and seek validation of decisions if reasoning ability is impaired f. continue with techniques and exercises to improve swallowing if indicated g. prepare meals that are visually appealing to help stimulate appetite if senses of smell and/or taste are impaired h. utilize assistive devices (e.g., broad-handled eating utensils, plate guard) and mobility aids (e.g., wheelchair, cane, walker) if motor function is impaired i. plan daily activities to allow for adequate rest periods in order to reduce irritability that often occurs after craniocerebral trauma. 2. Allow time for questions, clarification, and return demonstration of techniques.
10.b. The client will identify ways to reduce headache.	10.b. Instruct client in ways to reduce headache (headache may persist for months following injury): 1. dim environmental lighting if possible or wear sunglasses when light is bright 2. reduce environmental noise whenever possible (e.g., lower volume on TV and radio) 3. avoid situations that increase stress 4. take analgesics as prescribed.
10.c. The client will state signs and symptoms to report to the health care provider.	10.c. Instruct client to report the following signs and symptoms: 1. increased drowsiness unrelated to a significant increase in activity or decease in amount of sleep obtained 2. increased irritability or restlessness 3. changes in behavior, increased difficulty remembering or concentrating

*Neurological deficits can range from a temporary increase in irritability or a slight facial droop to hemiplegia, aphasia, or severely disturbed thought processes depending on the areas of the brain that have been affected. Ways of adapting to a few of the more common deficits are included here. For more specific rehabilitative measures and a more extensive discussion of deficits, refer to textbooks on neurological nursing and the Care Plan on Cerebrovascular Accident.

Desired Outcomes	Nursing Actions *and Selected Purposes/Rationales*
	4. new or increased weakness of extremities 5. decreased sensation in extremities 6. severe headache 7. difficulty speaking or understanding what others are saying 8. difficulty chewing or swallowing 9. changes in vision (e.g., double vision, blurred vision, visual field cut) 10. increased dizziness, difficulty maintaining balance 11. bloody, yellowish, or clear drainage from nose or ears 12. stiff neck 13. sudden weight gain or loss, excessive thirst, and/or unusual increase or decrease in amount of urination (indicative of SIADH or diabetes insipidus) 14. unexplained fever 15. seizures 16. exaggerated startle response; angry outbursts; diminished interest or participation in significant activities; feeling of detachment from others; and recurrent, intrusive, disturbing images and thoughts of the event that resulted in the craniocerebral trauma (these are signs and symptoms of post-traumatic stress disorder [PTSD] that can occur a few weeks to months following involvement in a traumatic event).
10.d. The client will identify community resources that can assist with home management and adjustment to changes resulting from craniocerebral trauma.	10.d.1. Inform client and significant others of community resources that can assist with home management and adjustment to changes resulting from craniocerebral trauma (e.g., home health agencies, Meals on Wheels, social and financial services, brain injury support groups, local service groups that can help obtain assistive devices, individual and family counseling services). 2. Initiate a referral if indicated.
10.e. The client will verbalize an understanding of and a plan for adhering to recommended follow-up care including future appointments with health care provider and therapists and medications prescribed.	10.e.1. Reinforce the importance of keeping follow-up appointments with health care provider and physical, occupational, and speech therapists. 2. Teach client the rationale for, side effects of, schedule for taking, and importance of taking medications prescribed (e.g., anticonvulsants, analgesics, antimicrobials). Inform client of pertinent food and drug interactions. 3. Implement measures to improve client compliance: a. include significant others in teaching sessions if possible b. encourage questions and allow time for reinforcement and clarification of information provided c. provide written instructions on scheduled appointments with health care provider and occupational, physical, and speech therapists; medications prescribed; and signs and symptoms to report.

Additional Nursing Diagnoses

RISK FOR IMBALANCED BODY TEMPERATURE: INCREASED

related to direct trauma to the hypothalamus and/or pressure on the hypothalamus associated with hematoma formation or edema of the surrounding tissue.

IMPAIRED PHYSICAL MOBILITY

related to motor and spacial-perceptual impairments if present, activity restrictions imposed by the treatment plan, and reluctance to move because of headache.

SELF-CARE DEFICIT

related to impaired physical mobility, disturbed thought processes, and/or visual impairments if present.

FEAR/ANXIETY*

related to impaired motor and/or sensory function; disturbed thought processes; uncertainty as to permanence of neurological deficits; unfamiliar environment; and lack of understanding of diagnostic tests, diagnosis, and treatments.

RISK FOR POST-TRAUMA SYNDROME

related to having experienced a situation that resulted in physical injury and involved intense feelings of fear and helplessness.

*See Unit II for outcomes, actions, and rationales.

Bibliography

See pages 879 and 881.

evolve

Craniotomy

A craniotomy is a surgical opening into the skull to gain access to the brain. Reasons for the surgery include removing a tumor, abscess, hematoma, bone fragments, or foreign object (e.g., bullet); controlling cerebral vascular bleeding; repairing a vascular abnormality (e.g., aneurysm, arteriovenous malformation); and improving ventricular drainage. A craniectomy (excision of a portion of the skull) is the usual method of entering the brain. If this portion of the skull is replaced (using the preserved bone or a synthetic substance), it can be done on completion of the surgery or sometime in the future after there are no longer concerns about increased intracranial pressure and/or cerebral infection.

A craniotomy is described in relation to the approach (i.e. supratentorial, infratentorial) and the location of the pathology (e.g., temporal, occipital, parietal). The neurological deficits that can occur following the surgical procedure depend primarily on the areas of the brain that are disrupted to gain access to the desired area (e.g., speech may be impaired following a temporal approach, ataxia is expected after a cerebellar approach) and the amount and location of the brain tissue that is excised or traumatized at the site of the pathology.

This care plan focuses on the adult client hospitalized for a craniotomy. Much of the information is also applicable to clients receiving follow-up care in an extended care or rehabilitation facility or home setting. Client care and discharge teaching need to be individualized based on the diagnosis and the neurological deficits he/she is experiencing. For more detailed coverage of nursing care measures for various neurological deficits, refer to the Care Plan on Cerebrovascular Accident.

OUTCOME/DISCHARGE CRITERIA

THE CLIENT WILL:

- have adequate cerebral tissue perfusion
- have improved or stable neurological function
- have no signs and symptoms of complications
- have surgical pain controlled
- have evidence of normal wound healing
- identify ways to adapt to neurological deficits resulting from the underlying disease condition and/or surgical procedure
- identify ways to protect the surgical site from injury
- state signs and symptoms to report to the health care provider
- share thoughts and feelings about the diagnosis and neurological deficits resulting from the underlying disease process and/or surgery
- identify community resources that can assist with home management and adjustment to changes resulting from the diagnosis and/or surgery
- verbalize an understanding of and a plan for adhering to recommended follow-up care including future appointments with health care provider, activity level, pain management, and medications prescribed.

NURSING/COLLABORATIVE DIAGNOSES

DISCHARGE TEACHING

See Standardized Preoperative and Postoperative Care Plans (pp. 97–126) for additional diagnoses.

PREOPERATIVE *Use in conjunction with the Standardized Preoperative Care Plan.*

1. NURSING DIAGNOSIS: FEAR/ANXIETY

related to:
a. unfamiliar environment and separation from significant others;
b. lack of understanding of diagnostic tests and planned surgical procedure;
c. anticipated loss of control associated with effects of anesthesia;
d. financial concerns associated with hospitalization and follow-up care;
e. possibility of continued and/or new neurological impairments;
f. anticipated pain, surgical findings, and changes in appearance (e.g., shaved head, skull indentation) and usual lifestyle and roles;
g. possibility of death.

Suggested NOC Outcomes: Anxiety level; Anxiety self-control; Fear level; Fear self-control

Suggested NIC Interventions: Anxiety reduction; Calming technique; Emotional support; Presence; Teaching: preoperative

Desired Outcome	**Nursing Actions** *and Selected Purposes/Rationales* (see pp. 14–16 for additional rationales)
1. The client will experience a reduction in fear and anxiety (see Standardized Preoperative Care Plan, Diagnosis 1 [pp. 97–98], for outcome criteria).	1.a. Refer to Standardized Preoperative Care Plan, Diagnosis 1 (pp. 97–98), for measures related to assessment and reduction of fear and anxiety. b. Implement additional measures *to reduce fear and anxiety:* 1. explain the necessity for intensive care monitoring after most craniotomies; orient client to the critical care unit if appropriate 2. describe and explain the rationale for equipment and tubes that may be present postoperatively (e.g., intracranial pressure monitoring device, ventilator, ventricular drain, wound drain, intravenous lines) 3. establish an effective method of communicating (e.g., Magic Slate, word cards, picture board, hand signals) if client is expected to be intubated or speech impairment is anticipated following surgery 4. perform actions *to reduce fear and anxiety about anticipated changes in physical appearance:* a. if the surgical site is shaved before anesthesia induction, cover client's head with a surgical cap, stockinette, or clean scarf *(helps keep the client warm and reduce embarrassment)* b. inform client that the incision line is usually made behind the hairline (with a supratentorial approach) or just above the nape of the neck (with an infratentorial approach) and should not be apparent when hair grows back c. assure client that when head dressing is removed, he/she can wear a surgical cap, turban, hat, or scarf if desired (most physicians advise clients to avoid wearing a wig or hairpiece until incision has healed) d. discuss alternative hair styles that might make incision, skull indentation, and/or shaved portion of scalp less apparent e. assure client that the swollen eyes and facial bruising that can occur after surgery are temporary (these are usually the result of prone positioning and/or pressure from devices used to immobilize the head during surgery) 5. if neurological impairments are anticipated following surgery, discuss resources that will be available to assist client to adapt to them (e.g., speech, occupational, and physical therapy).

POSTOPERATIVE

Use in conjunction with the Standardized Postoperative Care Plan.

1. Nursing Diagnosis: INEFFECTIVE TISSUE PERFUSION: CEREBRAL

related to decreased cerebral blood flow associated with:
a. cerebral hemorrhage resulting from the underlying disease process or loss of integrity of the ligated vessels;
b. compression of cerebral vessels (occurs mainly as a result of cerebral edema or accumulation of blood in cerebral tissue);
c. spasm of the cerebral vessels resulting from trauma to and stretching of the vessels during surgery;
d. hypotension (can occur as a result of factors such as hypovolemia and peripheral pooling of blood).

Suggested NOC Outcomes: Neurological status; Tissue perfusion: cerebral

Suggested NIC Interventions: Cerebral edema management; Cerebral perfusion promotion; Intracranial pressure (ICP) monitoring

Desired Outcome	**Nursing Actions** *and Selected Purposes/Rationales*
1. The client will maintain adequate cerebral tissue perfusion as evidenced by: a. absence of dizziness, visual disturbances, and speech impairments b. usual or improved mental status c. usual or improved sensory and motor function.	1.a. Assess for and report signs and symptoms of ineffective cerebral tissue perfusion: 1. dizziness 2. visual disturbances (e.g., blurred or dimmed vision, diplopia, change in visual field) 3. aphasia 4. irritability and restlessness 5. decreased level of consciousness 6. paresthesias, weakness, paralysis. b. Implement measures *to maintain adequate cerebral tissue perfusion:* 1. perform actions to prevent and treat increased intracranial pressure (see Postoperative Diagnosis 3, actions a.2 and 3) 2. if client is hypotensive, perform actions *to improve cerebral blood flow* (e.g., administer prescribed sympathomimetic agents, maintain intravenous fluid therapy as ordered) 3. administer calcium-channel blockers (e.g., nimodipine) if ordered *to reduce cerebral vasospasm (the calcium that is released by the injured neural cells can cause vasospasm)* 4. prepare client for surgical intervention (e.g., evacuation of hematoma, ligation of bleeding vessels) if planned. c. Consult physician if signs and symptoms of decreased cerebral tissue perfusion persist or worsen.

2. Nursing Diagnosis: ACUTE PAIN: HEADACHE

related to:
a. trauma to the cerebral tissue associated with the surgical procedure;
b. stretching or compression of cerebral vessels and tissue associated with increased intracranial pressure if it occurs;
c. irritation of the meninges associated with bleeding from meningeal vessels, leakage of blood into the cerebrospinal fluid (CSF), and/or inflammation of the meninges.

Suggested NOC Outcomes: Comfort level; Pain control

Suggested NIC Interventions: Pain management; Analgesic administration

Desired Outcome	**Nursing Actions** *and Selected Purposes/Rationales* (see pp. 45–47 for additional rationales)
2. The client will obtain relief from headache as evidenced by: a. verbalization of same b. relaxed facial expression and body positioning.	2.a. Assess for signs and symptoms of headache (e.g., statements of same, restlessness, irritability, grimacing, rubbing head, avoidance of bright lights and noises, reluctance to move). b. Assess client's perception of the severity of the headache using a pain intensity rating scale. c. Assess the client's pain pattern (e.g., location, quality, onset, duration, precipitating factors, aggravating factors, alleviating factors). d. Implement measures *to relieve headache:* 1. perform actions *to reduce fear and anxiety about the pain experience* (e.g., assure client that his/her need for headache relief is understood, plan methods for relieving headache with client) 2. perform actions to reduce fear and anxiety (e.g., assure client that staff members are nearby, respond to call signal as soon as possible) *in order to promote relaxation and subsequently increase the client's threshold and tolerance for pain* 3. administer analgesics before activities and procedures that can cause headache and before headache becomes severe 4. perform actions *to minimize environmental stimuli* (e.g., provide a quiet environment, limit number of visitors and their length of stay, dim lights) 5. avoid jarring bed or startling client *to minimize risk of sudden movements* 6. perform actions to prevent and treat increased intracranial pressure and meningitis (see Postoperative Diagnosis 3, actions a.2 and 3 and b.3 and 4) 7. provide or assist with nonpharmacologic measures for headache relief (e.g., cool cloth to forehead, progressive relaxation exercises) 8. administer nonnarcotic analgesics or codeine if ordered (other narcotic [opioid] analgesics are usually contraindicated *because they have a greater depressant effect on the central nervous system*). e. Consult physician if above actions fail to relieve headache.

3. COLLABORATIVE DIAGNOSES:

POTENTIAL COMPLICATIONS OF CRANIOTOMY

a. increased intracranial pressure (IICP) related to:
   1. accumulation of blood in the cerebral tissue associated with surgical trauma to the cerebral vessels
   2. cerebral edema associated with increased capillary permeability of cerebral vessels and an increase in cellular volume resulting from disruption of the sodium pump within the cells (both can occur as a result of cerebral hypoxia)
   3. hydrocephalus associated with obstruction of normal CSF flow resulting from edema, hematoma, presence of blood in the subarachnoid space, and/or occlusion of ventricular shunt if present
   4. increase in cerebral vascular volume associated with vasodilation of the cerebral vessels;

b. meningitis related to:
   1. irritation of the meninges associated with trauma to the meningeal vessels or presence of blood in the CSF
   2. introduction of pathogens into the meninges or CSF associated with surgical incision (interrupts the integrity of the dura) and presence of an intracranial monitoring device and/or external ventricular drain;

c. seizures related to altered activity of the cerebral neurons associated with irritation of the brain tissue during surgery (especially if a supratentorial approach was used) or IICP and meningitis if they occur;

d. diabetes insipidus related to decreased production and/or impaired release of antidiuretic hormone (ADH) associated with altered function of the hypothalamus or posterior lobe of the pituitary gland (can occur as a result of surgical trauma or postoperative edema or hematoma in that area);

e. syndrome of inappropriate antidiuretic hormone (SIADH) related to increased production and/or release of ADH associated with:
   1. altered function of the hypothalamus or the posterior lobe of the pituitary gland (can occur as a result of surgical trauma or postoperative edema or hematoma in that area)
   2. pain, fear, anxiety, and some anesthetic agents;

f. cranial nerve damage related to trauma to the nerves prior to or during surgery and/or compression of the nerves associated with postoperative cerebral hematoma or edema.

Desired Outcomes	**Nursing Actions** *and Selected Purposes/Rationales*
3.a. The client will not develop IICP as evidenced by: 1. usual or improved level of consciousness 2. no reports of increased headache 3. stable or improved motor and sensory function 4. absence of vomiting, papilledema, and seizure activity 5. usual pupillary size and reactivity 6. stable vital signs.	3.a.1. Assess for and report signs and symptoms of IICP: a. restlessness, agitation, confusion, lethargy b. reports of increased headache c. decreasing motor and sensory function d. abnormal posturing (e.g., extension [decerebrate], flexion [decorticate]) e. vomiting (usually without nausea) f. elevation of bone flap or bulging in area where bone was removed g. papilledema h. seizures i. change in pupil size or reactivity j. altered respiratory pattern (e.g., shallow, slow respirations; periods of apnea; central neurogenic hyperventilation) k. bounding, slow pulse l. rise in systolic B/P with widening pulse pressure. 2. Implement measures *to prevent IICP:* a. maintain fluid restrictions as ordered b. administer the following medications if ordered *to reduce cerebral edema:* 1. osmotic diuretics (e.g., mannitol) 2. loop diuretics (e.g., furosemide) 3. corticosteroids (e.g., dexamethasone) c. perform actions *to promote adequate cerebral venous drainage:* 1. elevate head of bed 30° unless contraindicated (if surgery was performed using the infratentorial approach, head of bed is usually kept flat postoperatively *to reduce pressure on the brain stem)* 2. keep head and neck in neutral, midline position; avoid flexion, extension, and rotation of head and neck 3. administer a laxative, antitussive, and antiemetic if ordered *to prevent straining to have a bowel movement, coughing, and vomiting (these conditions cause an increase in intrathoracic pressure, which subsequently impedes venous return from the brain)* d. perform actions *to prevent cerebral hypoxia and the subsequent vasodilation and cerebral edema:* 1. implement measures *to maintain a patent airway* (e.g., position client on side, suction if necessary) 2. administer central nervous system depressants judiciously; hold medication and consult physician if respiratory rate is less than 12/minute 3. administer oxygen as ordered and before and after tracheal suctioning e. perform actions *to prevent excessive cerebral blood flow and/or dilation of cerebral vessels:* 1. implement measures *to prevent an increase in blood pressure:* a. observe for and control conditions that can cause agitation (e.g., fear, anxiety, distended bladder) b. instruct client to avoid activities that result in isometric muscle contractions (e.g., pushing feet against footboard, tightly gripping side rails)

2. implement measures *to prevent an increase in metabolic rate:*
   a. administer anticonvulsants (e.g., phenytoin) if ordered *to prevent seizure activity*
   b. perform actions *to prevent and treat increased body temperature* (e.g., apply a hypothermia blanket if ordered, administer antipyretics if ordered)

f. perform actions to prevent and treat meningitis (see actions b.3 and 4 in this diagnosis) *in order to prevent obstruction of the flow of CSF and an increase in metabolic rate (infection causes an increase in metabolic rate and subsequent increase in cerebral blood flow, which results in cerebral vasodilation)*

g. schedule care so activities that could raise intracranial pressure (e.g., suctioning, bathing, repositioning) are not grouped together

h. position client on unoperative side if bone flap and/or large mass was removed *(helps prevent increased pressure and venous congestion in the operative area)*

i. if client has a wound drain, perform actions *to maintain its patency* (e.g., keep tubing free of kinks, empty drainage collection device when appropriate, maintain wound suction as ordered)

j. if client has an internal shunt, perform actions *to maintain its patency* (e.g., avoid pressure on the skin over the shunt, tubing, and reservoir site; pump shunt as ordered)

k. if client has an external shunt, perform actions *to maintain its patency* (e.g., avoid kinks in tubing, keep client's head and drainage collection device at the prescribed levels).

3. If signs and symptoms of IICP are present:
   a. initiate seizure precautions
   b. prepare client for the following if planned:
      1. insertion of an intracranial pressure monitoring device
      2. lumbar or ventricular puncture *to remove excess CSF*
      3. surgical intervention (e.g., ligation of bleeding vessel, repair of blocked shunt, removal of bone flap or hematoma).

3.b. The client will not develop meningitis as evidenced by:
1. absence of fever and chills
2. absence of nuchal rigidity and photophobia
3. gradual resolution of headache
4. negative Kernig's and Brudzinski's signs
5. normal CSF analysis.

3.b.1. Assess for and report signs and symptoms of a CSF leak *(indicates an opening in the dura):*
   a. presence of glucose in clear drainage from nose, ear, or wound as shown by positive results on a glucose reagent strip
   b. yellowish ring ("halo") around bloody or serosanguineous drainage on dressing or pillowcase *(CSF dries in concentric circles)*
   c. reports of postnasal drip
   d. constant swallowing.

2. Assess for and report signs and symptoms of meningitis:
   a. fever, chills
   b. nuchal rigidity
   c. photophobia
   d. increasing or persistent headache
   e. positive Kernig's sign (inability to straighten knee when hip is flexed)
   f. positive Brudzinski's sign (flexion of hip and knee in response to forward flexion of the neck)
   g. CSF that is cloudy (can indicate elevated WBC and protein levels in the CSF)
   h. elevated CSF pressure (pressure is often elevated with meningitis)
   i. CSF analysis showing increased WBC and protein levels.

3. Implement measures *to prevent meningitis:*
   a. use sterile technique when changing dressings and working with an external ventricular shunt and intracranial pressure monitoring device
   b. instruct client to keep hands away from drains and dressings; apply wrist restraints or mittens if necessary.
   c. if a CSF leak is present:
      1. instruct client to avoid excessive movement and activity (bed rest is usually ordered *to prevent further stress on the incised dura)*

Desired Outcomes	Nursing Actions *and Selected Purposes/Rationales*

2. instruct client to avoid coughing, blowing nose, and straining to have a bowel movement *(these activities raise intracranial pressure and can cause extension of the dural tear);* consult physician about an order for an antitussive, decongestant, and laxative if indicated
3. if CSF is leaking from nose:
   a. position client with head of bed elevated at least 20° unless contraindicated *to allow the fluid to drain*
   b. if client needs to sneeze, instruct him/her to do so with mouth open *(withholding the sneeze can force bacteria backward through the torn dura)*
   c. instruct client to avoid putting finger in nose
   d. do not perform nasal suctioning or insert a nasogastric tube
   e. do not attempt to clean nose unless ordered by physician
4. if CSF is leaking from ear:
   a. position client on side of CSF leakage unless contraindicated *to allow the fluid to drain*
   b. instruct client to avoid putting finger in ear
   c. do not attempt to clean ear unless ordered by physician
5. do not pack dressing into area of CSF leakage (nose, ear, or wound) *because it will interfere with the drainage of fluid;* place a sterile pad over area of CSF leakage to absorb drainage and change pad as soon as it becomes damp
6. prepare client for surgical repair of the dura if leak does not heal spontaneously (the area usually heals without surgical intervention within 7–10 days)

d. administer antimicrobials if ordered.

4. If signs and symptoms of meningitis occur:
   a. initiate seizure precautions *(cerebral irritation can cause seizures)*
   b. provide a quiet environment with dim lighting *to reduce discomfort associated with headache and photophobia*
   c. administer antimicrobials as ordered.

3.c. The client will not experience seizure activity or injury if seizure occurs.

3.c.1. Assess for and report signs and symptoms of seizure activity (e.g., twitching [usually of face or hands], clonic-tonic movements).

2. Implement measures *to prevent seizures:*
   a. perform actions to prevent and treat IICP and meningitis (see actions a.2 and 3 and b.3 and 4 in this diagnosis)
   b. administer anticonvulsants (e.g., phenytoin, carbamazepine) if ordered.
3. Initiate and maintain seizure precautions:
   a. have an oral airway and suction equipment readily available
   b. pad side rails with blankets or soft pads
   c. keep bed in low position with side rails up when client is in bed.
4. If seizures occur:
   a. implement measures *to decrease risk of injury:*
      1. ease client to the floor if he/she is sitting in chair or ambulating at onset of seizure
      2. remain with but do not restrain client during seizure activity
      3. do not force any object between clenched teeth or try to pry mouth open
      4. clear area of objects that may cause injury
      5. place towel under client's head if he/she is on the floor
      6. as seizure activity subsides, perform actions *to maintain a patent airway* (e.g., turn client on side, insert an oral airway, suction as needed)
   b. observe for and report characteristics of seizures (e.g., progression, time elapsed)
   c. administer intravenous anticonvulsants (e.g., phenytoin, phenobarbital) if ordered.

3.d. The client will not experience diabetes insipidus as evidenced by:
1. absence of polyuria
2. absence of intense thirst (polydipsia).

3.d.1. Assess for and report signs and symptoms of diabetes insipidus:
a. polyuria (urine output can range from 4–10 or more liters/day)
b. reports of intense thirst (if oral fluids are allowed and tolerated, the client's intake is often an amount that corresponds to the high volume of urine output)
c. low urine specific gravity (often 1.005 or less).
2. Administer osmotic diuretics (e.g., mannitol), loop diuretics (e.g., furosemide), and/or corticosteroids (e.g., dexamethasone) if ordered *to reduce edema of the hypothalamus, pituitary gland, and surrounding tissue and subsequently reduce the risk for the development of diabetes insipidus.*
3. If signs and symptoms of diabetes insipidus occur:
a. maintain fluid intake equal to output *in order to prevent water deficit*
b. administer an ADH replacement (e.g., vasopressin, desmopressin [DDAVP]) as ordered
c. assess for and report signs and symptoms of water deficit (e.g., decreased skin turgor; dry mucous membranes; weight loss of 2% or greater over a short period; postural hypotension and/or low B/P; weak, rapid pulse; elevated serum sodium and osmolality).

3.e. The client will not develop SIADH as evidenced by:
1. stable weight
2. balanced intake and output
3. usual or improved mental status
4. usual or improved muscle strength
5. decreased reports of headache
6. absence of cellular edema, abdominal cramping, nausea, vomiting, and seizure activity
7. urine and serum sodium and osmolality levels within normal limits.

3.e.1. Assess for and report signs and symptoms of SIADH:
a. weight gain of 2% or greater over a short period
b. intake significantly greater than output
c. development of or increase in irritability or confusion
d. development of or increase in muscle weakness
e. reports of persistent or increased headache
f. fingerprint edema over sternum (reflects cellular edema)
g. abdominal cramping, nausea, or vomiting
h. seizures
i. elevated urine sodium and osmolality levels
j. low serum sodium and osmolality levels.
2. Implement measures *to reduce the risk of SIADH:*
a. perform actions to reduce headache (see Postoperative Diagnosis 2, action d)
b. perform actions to reduce fear and anxiety (see Standardized Postoperative Care Plan, Diagnosis 21, action b [p. 124]).
c. administer osmotic diuretics (e.g., mannitol), loop diuretics (e.g., furosemide), and/or corticosteroids (e.g., dexamethasone) if ordered *to reduce edema of the hypothalamus, pituitary gland, and surrounding tissue.*
3. If signs and symptoms of SIADH occur:
a. maintain fluid restrictions if ordered *to prevent further fluid retention* (typically, this is a restriction of free water)
b. initiate seizure precautions
c. administer the following if ordered:
1. diuretics (usually furosemide) *to promote water excretion*
2. intravenous infusion of a hypertonic saline solution *to treat severe hyponatremia*
3. demeclocycline *to promote water excretion (inhibits the effect of ADH on the renal tubules).*

3.f. The client will not experience cranial nerve damage or will adapt to cranial nerve damage if it occurs.

3.f.1. Assess for and report signs and symptoms of damage to the following cranial nerves:
a. olfactory (e.g., decreased or absent sense of smell)
b. optic, oculomotor, trochlear, or abducens (e.g., diplopia, visual field cut, decreased visual acuity, abnormal extraocular movements)
c. trigeminal (e.g., decreased or absent corneal reflex, difficulty chewing, pain when chewing)
d. vagus or glossopharyngeal (e.g., loss of gag reflex, difficulty swallowing, hoarseness, inability to speak clearly)

Desired Outcomes	Nursing Actions *and Selected Purposes/Rationales*

e. hypoglossal (e.g., difficulty chewing, swallowing, or speaking)
f. facial (e.g., facial ptosis, impaired sense of taste).

2. Implement measures to prevent and treat IICP (see actions a.2 and 3 in this diagnosis) *in order to reduce the risk for compression of and subsequent damage to the cranial nerves.*
3. Implement measures *to assist the client to adapt to cranial nerve damage if it has occurred:*
   a. if the olfactory nerve is affected, provide meals that are visually appealing *to help stimulate appetite*
   b. if vision is affected, provide an eyepatch or opaque lens *(helps reduce double vision),* instruct client in visual scanning techniques if experiencing visual field cut, and assist client with self-care and ambulation if indicated
   c. if the corneal reflex is absent or the client is unable to close his/her eye, perform actions *to protect the cornea from irritation and abrasion* (e.g., instruct client to avoid rubbing eye; reduce exposure to dust, powder, and smoke; instill isotonic eyedrops frequently)
   d. if the trigeminal, hypoglossal, vagus, and/or glossopharyngeal nerves are affected:
      1. withhold oral foods/fluids until gag reflex returns and client is better able to chew and swallow *in order to reduce the risk for aspiration;* provide parenteral nutrition or tube feedings if indicated
      2. when oral intake is allowed:
         a. perform actions *to prevent aspiration* (e.g., place client in high Fowler's position during and for at least 30 minutes after meals and snacks unless contraindicated, assist client with oral hygiene after eating *to ensure that food particles do not remain in mouth,* instruct client to avoid laughing and talking while eating and drinking)
         b. perform actions *to improve client's ability to swallow* (e.g., avoid serving sticky foods such as peanut butter and bananas, assist client to select foods that require little or no chewing and are easily swallowed, serve thick fluids or thicken thin fluids with substances such as "Thick-It" or gelatin)
      3. perform actions *to facilitate communication* (e.g., maintain quiet environment; provide pad and pencil, Magic Slate, computer, or word cards; listen carefully when client speaks)
      4. consult speech pathologist about additional ways to facilitate swallowing and communication
   e. if the sensory component of the facial nerve is affected, instruct client to add extra sweeteners or seasonings to foods/fluids if desired *in order to compensate for impaired sense of taste.*

4. Nursing Diagnosis: ***DISTURBED SELF-CONCEPT****

related to:
a. changes in appearance (e.g., periocular edema and ecchymosis, skull indentation, loss of scalp hair);
b. dependence on others to meet basic needs;
c. anticipated changes in lifestyle and roles associated with changes that occur as a result of cerebral tissue damage (e.g., impaired motor and sensory function, disturbed thought processes).

*This diagnostic label includes the nursing diagnoses of disturbed body image, low self-esteem, and ineffective role performance.

Suggested NOC Outcomes: Body image; Self-esteem; Psychosocial adjustment: life changes

Suggested NIC Interventions: Body image enhancement; Self-esteem enhancement; Emotional support; Support system enhancement; Role enhancement; Counseling

Desired Outcome	**Nursing Actions** *and Selected Purposes/Rationales* (see pp. 47–49 for additional rationales)
4. The client will demonstrate beginning adaptation to changes in appearance, physical and cognitive functioning, lifestyle, and roles as evidenced by: a. verbalization of feelings of self-worth b. maintenance of relationships with significant others c. active participation in activities of daily living d. verbalization of a beginning plan for adapting lifestyle to changes resulting from the underlying disease process and/or residual effects of the surgery.	4.a. Assess for signs and symptoms of a disturbed self-concept (e.g., verbalization of negative feelings about self, withdrawal from significant others, lack of participation in activities of daily living, lack of plan for adapting to necessary changes in lifestyle). b. Be aware that client may recognize and grieve for the losses experienced. Provide support during the grieving process. c. Discuss with client improvements in appearance and neurological function that can realistically be expected. d. If periocular edema and ecchymosis are present: 1. reinforce that they are temporary (edema usually begins to subside 48–72 hours after surgery and ecchymosis usually disappears in 10–14 days) 2. instruct client in and assist with measures *to reduce swelling* (e.g., cold compresses to affected area, lying on unoperative side unless contraindicated, keeping head of bed elevated 30° unless contraindicated). e. Implement measures *to reduce client's embarrassment about partial or total loss of hair and misshapen skull if bone flap was not replaced* (e.g., provide client with a surgical cap, turban, hat, or scarf; assist client to obtain a wig or hairpiece to wear after the incision has healed). Reinforce the fact that the hair will grow back and encourage client to discuss with physician the possibility of a cranioplasty in the future to restore the original shape of the skull. f. Discuss techniques the client can utilize *to adapt to disturbed thought processes if present:* 1. encourage client to make lists and write or record messages and to refer to these rather than relying on memory 2. instruct the client to place self in a calm environment when making decisions 3. encourage client to validate decisions, clarify information, and seek assistance to problem solve if indicated 4. encourage client to schedule adequate rest periods and reduce stressors *in order to decrease irritability.* g. Support behaviors suggesting positive adaptation to changes that have occurred (e.g., scanning environment or wearing eyepatch if visual disturbances are present, utilizing alternative methods of communicating if speech is impaired, utilizing assistive devices to perform self-care activities). h. Encourage significant others to allow client to do what he/she is able *so that independence can be re-established and/or self-esteem redeveloped.* i. Assist client's and significant others' adjustment by listening, facilitating communication, and providing information. j. Assist client and significant others to have similar expectations and understanding of future lifestyle and to identify ways that personal and family goals can be adjusted rather than abandoned. k. Encourage client to continue involvement in social activities and to pursue usual roles and interests. If previous roles, interests, and hobbies cannot be pursued, encourage development of new ones. l. Provide information about and encourage utilization of community agencies and support groups (e.g., brain injury support groups; vocational rehabilitation; American Cancer Society; family, individual, and/or financial counseling) if appropriate. m. Consult appropriate health care provider (e.g., psychiatric nurse clinician, physician) about psychological counseling if client desires or seems unwilling or unable to adapt to changes resulting from the disease and/or the surgery.

Discharge Teaching/Continued Care

DEFICIENT KNOWLEDGE, INEFFECTIVE THERAPEUTIC REGIMEN MANAGEMENT, OR INEFFECTIVE HEALTH MAINTENANCE*

*The nurse should select the diagnostic label that is most appropriate for the client's discharge teaching needs.

Suggested NOC Outcomes: Knowledge: treatment regimen; Knowledge: health behavior; Knowledge: health resources

Suggested NIC Interventions: Health system guidance; Teaching: individual; Teaching: prescribed activity/exercise; Teaching: prescribed medications

Desired Outcomes	Nursing Actions and Selected Purposes/Rationales
5.a. The client will identify ways to adapt to neurological deficits resulting from the underlying disease condition and/or surgical procedure.	5.a.1. Instruct client in ways to adapt to neurological deficits* resulting from the underlying disease condition and/or surgical procedure: a. wear an eyepatch or opaque lens if double vision is a problem b. utilize scanning techniques if visual field cut is present c. utilize pencil and paper, Magic Slate, computer, pictures, and gestures to express self if verbal communication is impaired d. make lists, write or record messages and reminders, and refer to written instructions repeatedly if experiencing difficulty concentrating or memory is impaired e. request assistance when problem solving and setting priorities and seek validation of decisions if reasoning ability is impaired f. prepare meals that are visually appealing to help stimulate appetite if sense of smell and/or taste is diminished g. utilize assistive devices (e.g., broad-handled eating utensils, plate guard) and mobility aids (e.g., walker, wheelchair, cane) if motor function is impaired h. plan daily activities to allow for adequate rest periods in order to reduce the irritability that can occur after cerebral tissue trauma. 2. Allow time for questions, clarification, and return demonstration of techniques.
5.b. The client will identify ways to protect the surgical site from injury.	5.b. Instruct the client in ways to protect the surgical site from injury: 1. wear a scarf, turban, hat, or cap until hair has grown back 2. do not shampoo hair until the incision has healed (usually 7–10 days following surgery) 3. when shampooing hair, avoid vigorous scrubbing; pat surgical site dry rather than rubbing 4. avoid use of hair dryer on hot setting, curling iron, and hot curlers at or near surgical site until hair has grown back (the direct heat can burn the unprotected scalp) 5. avoid scratching the surgical site; if it itches as the incision heals and the hair grows back, apply light pressure to the surgical site or distract self with activities like taking a walk or watching television 6. if the bone flap was not replaced, avoid bumping or putting excessive pressure on the surgical site (if the skull depression is large, client may need to wear a protective helmet as level of activity increases).

*Neurological deficits can range from a temporary increase in irritability or a slight facial droop to hemiplegia, aphasia, or severely disturbed thought processes depending on the area(s) of the brain that have been affected. Ways of adapting to a few of the more common deficits are included here. For more specific rehabilitative measures and a more extensive discussion of deficits, refer to textbooks on neurological and neurosurgical nursing and the Care Plan on Cerebrovascular Accident.

5.c. The client will state signs and symptoms to report to the health care provider.

5.c.1. Refer to Standardized Postoperative Care Plan, Diagnosis 22, action c (p. 125), for signs and symptoms to report to the health care provider.
2. Instruct client to report these additional signs and symptoms:
a. increased drowsiness unrelated to a significant increase in activity or a decrease in amount of sleep obtained
b. increased irritability or restlessness
c. changes in behavior, decreased ability to concentrate
d. decreased sensation in extremities
e. new or increased weakness of extremities
f. difficulty speaking or understanding what others are saying
g. change in vision (e.g., double vision, blurred vision, visual field cut)
h. increased difficulty chewing or swallowing
i. dizziness, difficulty maintaining balance
j. increased swelling at wound site
k. bloody, yellowish, or clear drainage from ears, nose, or incision
l. stiff neck
m. excessive thirst and excessive urination (can indicate diabetes insipidus)
n. sudden weight gain and unusual decrease in amount of urination (can indicate SIADH)
o. severe or persistent headache
p. seizures.

5.d. The client will identify community resources that can assist with home management and adjustment to changes resulting from the diagnosis and/or surgery.

5.d.1. Inform client and significant others of community resources that can assist with home management and adjustment to neurological changes resulting from the diagnosis and/or surgery (e.g., physical, occupational, and speech therapists; Meals on Wheels; social services; home health agencies; American Cancer Society; brain injury support groups).
2. Initiate a referral if indicated.

5.e. The client will verbalize an understanding of and a plan for adhering to recommended follow-up care including future appointments with health care provider, activity level, pain management, and medications prescribed.

5.e.1. Refer to Standardized Postoperative Care Plan, Diagnosis 22 (pp. 125–126), for routine postoperative instructions and measures to improve client compliance.
2. Instruct client in ways to reduce headache if present (e.g., reduce environmental lighting and noise whenever possible, avoid situations that increase stress, take analgesics as prescribed).
3. Explain the rationale for, side effects of, schedule for taking, and importance of taking the prescribed medications (e.g., anticonvulsants, analgesics, antimicrobials). Inform client of pertinent food and drug interactions.

Bibliography

See pages 879 and 881.

Spinal Cord Injury

Spinal cord injury (spinal cord trauma) is most frequently the result of sudden, external trauma (e.g., motor vehicle accident, fall, sports or recreational injury, act of violence), although it can be caused by a tumor or conditions affecting the vertebrae (e.g., stenosis, pathologic fractures). Spinal cord injury is classified according to the cause of cord injury (e.g., contusion, compression, transection), direction of movement of the vertebrae or mechanism of injury (e.g., flexion, hyperextension, rotation), level of injury (e.g., cervical, sacral), stability of the vertebral column (i.e. stable, unstable), and/or degree of cord involvement (i.e. complete, incomplete).

Immediately following traumatic injury to the spinal cord, spinal shock (loss of motor, sensory, autonomic, and reflex activity below the level of the injury) occurs. Spinal shock usually lasts between 1 and 6 weeks but can persist for months. The neurological impairments that remain following the period of spinal shock depend upon the level of the cord injury (the higher the level, the greater the loss of body function) and the degree of cord involvement (if complete, there is total loss of sensory function and voluntary motor function below the level of the injury; if incomplete, some of the motor and/or sensory fibers below the level of injury are able to function).

This care plan focuses on the adult client hospitalized with a complete injury of the spinal cord at the level of the fifth cervical vertebra (C5). After the period of spinal shock, a client with a complete cord injury at the C5 level experiences loss of voluntary motor function below the clavicles; however, full neck, upper shoulder, and some bicep control and elbow flexion are retained. Sensory function is intact above the clavicles and in certain areas of the deltoids and forearms. With rehabilitation, the client may be able to do things such as operate an electric wheelchair and a manual wheelchair with hand rim projections (quad pegs), feed self using assistive devices, utilize reflex activity to achieve an erection and stimulate bowel and bladder elimination, accomplish some change in body position, and operate some equipment (e.g., typewriter, computer, telephone) using assistive devices.

Much of the information provided in this care plan is also applicable to spinal cord injured clients in extended care, rehabilitation, and home settings. Although the focus is on injury at the C5 level, the information can easily be individualized to plan nursing care for clients with injury to other segments of the spinal cord.

OUTCOME/DISCHARGE CRITERIA

THE CLIENT WILL:

- have clear, audible breath sounds throughout lungs
- have no evidence of tissue irritation or breakdown
- have an adequate nutritional status
- experience optimal control of urinary and bowel elimination
- direct own care and perform or participate in self-care when possible
- have adequate tissue perfusion and thermoregulation
- have no signs and symptoms of complications resulting from the spinal cord injury and decreased mobility
- identify ways to prevent complications associated with spinal cord injury and decreased mobility
- demonstrate the ability to correctly use and maintain assistive devices
- identify ways to manage altered bowel and bladder function
- state signs and symptoms to report to the health care provider
- identify resources that can assist with financial needs, home management, and adjustment to changes resulting from spinal cord injury
- share thoughts and feelings about the effects of spinal cord injury on self-concept, lifestyle, and roles
- verbalize an understanding of and a plan for adhering to recommended follow-up care including future appointments with health care provider and occupational and physical therapists and medications prescribed.

Use in Conjunction with the Care Plan on Immobility.

NURSING/COLLABORATIVE DIAGNOSES

DISCHARGE TEACHING

See pp. 298–299 and Care Plan on Immobility (pp. 129–148) for additional diagnoses.

1. Nursing Diagnosis: *FEAR/ANXIETY*

related to extensive loss of motor and sensory function; application of immobilization device to stabilize and align the cervical spine; lack of understanding of diagnostic tests, diagnosis, and treatment; unfamiliar environment; financial concerns; and anticipated effect of the spinal cord injury on lifestyle and roles.

Suggested NOC Outcomes: Anxiety level; Fear level; Stress level; Anxiety self-control; Fear self-control

Suggested NIC Interventions: Anxiety reduction; Calming technique; Emotional support; Presence; Teaching: procedure/treatment

Desired Outcome	**Nursing Actions** *and Selected Purposes/Rationales* (see pp. 14–16 for additional rationales)
1. The client will experience a reduction in fear and anxiety as evidenced by: a. verbalization of feeling less anxious b. usual sleep pattern c. relaxed facial expression d. usual perceptual ability and interactions with others.	1.a. Assess client for signs and symptoms of fear and anxiety (e.g., verbalization of feeling anxious, insomnia, tenseness, self-focused behaviors). b. Implement measures *to reduce fear and anxiety:* 1. remain with client while immobilization device is being applied 2. explain necessity of frequent neurological checks 3. provide information about the insertion of skull pins: a. assure client that the pins penetrate only the outer table of the skull, not the brain b. assure client that very little pain is associated with the insertion but that the procedure will be quite loud since bone is such a good sound conductor c. assure client that only a small amount of hair is clipped at each insertion site d. explain that tongs and traction, a halo ring and traction, or a halo ring and halo vest will be attached to the pins in order to keep the cervical spine immobilized and in correct alignment 4. explain the purpose and safety features of the kinetic bed if appropriate; assure client that measures have been taken to keep him/her from falling out of bed (e.g., side rails up) 5. if client is placed on a kinetic bed (e.g., Roto Rest bed), explain the sensations that may be experienced as the bed continually rotates from side-to-side (e.g., motion sickness, fear of falling); assure client that these sensations usually disappear after being on the bed for a day or two 6. once cervical spine immobilization is accomplished: a. orient client to environment, equipment, and routines b. assure client that staff members are nearby; provide call signal that has been adapted to meet client's needs (e.g., voice-activated call light) and respond to call signal as soon as possible c. introduce client to staff who will be participating in care; if possible, maintain consistency in staff assigned to his/her care d. maintain a calm, supportive, confident manner when interacting with client e. avoid startling client (e.g., speak client's name and identify yourself when entering room and before physical contact, place self in client's visual field whenever possible during care and conversation) f. provide prism glasses and/or position mirrors in strategic places to increase client's ability to view his/her surroundings during the time that head movement is limited because of the immobilization device and/or recumbent position g. reinforce physician's explanations and clarify misconceptions client has about spinal cord injury, treatment plan, and prognosis h. explain all diagnostic tests i. explain that the flaccid paralysis and lack of reflex activity below the level of the cord injury that occurs immediately following the injury is a result of spinal shock; emphasize that some reflex activity will return after spinal shock subsides j. provide a calm, restful environment; instruct client in relaxation techniques k. initiate a social service referral and/or assist client to identify and contact appropriate community resources if indicated l. provide information based on current needs of client at a level he/she can understand; encourage questions and clarification of information provided m. encourage significant others to project a caring, concerned attitude without obvious anxiousness n. if comfortable for nurse and client, reinforce verbal messages of caring by touching areas where client has sensation (e.g., shoulders, head, neck); encourage significant others to do the same.

c. Consult appropriate health care provider (e.g., psychiatric nurse clinician, physician) if above actions fail to control fear and anxiety.

2. NURSING DIAGNOSIS:

INEFFECTIVE TISSUE PERFUSION

related to:

a. decreased cardiac output associated with:
   1. bradycardia resulting from loss of sympathetic nervous system activity and subsequent unopposed action of the parasympathetic nervous system on the heart
   2. decreased venous return resulting from vasodilation below the level of the injury (the vasodilation occurs because of loss of sympathetic nervous system activity below the level of cord injury);
b. peripheral pooling of blood associated with vasodilation below the level of the injury and loss of muscle tone in extremities resulting from paralysis of extremities and decreased mobility.

Suggested NOC Outcome: Circulation status

Suggested NIC Interventions: Circulatory care: venous insufficiency; Circulatory care: arterial insufficiency

Desired Outcome	**Nursing Actions** *and Selected Purposes/Rationales* (see pp. 57–59 for additional rationales)

2. The client will maintain adequate tissue perfusion as evidenced by:
   a. B/P within normal range for client
   b. usual mental status
   c. extremities warm with absence of pallor and cyanosis
   d. palpable peripheral pulses
   e. capillary refill time less than 2–3 seconds
   f. absence of edema
   g. urine output at least 30 ml/hour.

2.a. Assess for and report signs and symptoms of diminished tissue perfusion (e.g., decreased blood pressure, restlessness, confusion, cool extremities, pallor or cyanosis of extremities, diminished or absent peripheral pulses, slow capillary refill, edema, oliguria).

b. Implement measures *to maintain adequate tissue perfusion:*
   1. avoid activities that cause vagal stimulation (e.g., suctioning) unless absolutely necessary *in order to prevent a further reduction in pulse rate*
   2. administer the following medications if ordered:
      a. anticholinergics (e.g., atropine) *to increase heart rate*
      b. sympathomimetics (e.g., dopamine) *to increase cardiac output and maintain arterial pressure*
   3. perform actions *to prevent peripheral pooling of blood and/or increase venous return:*
      a. perform passive range of motion exercises at least 3 times/day
      b. avoid positions that compromise blood flow in the lower extremities (e.g., crossing legs, pillows under knees, sitting for long periods)
      c. apply thigh-high elastic stockings as ordered
      d. apply/maintain a sequential compression device to lower extremities if ordered
      e. apply an abdominal binder if ordered before placing client in a sitting or upright position *(the binder reduces pooling of blood in the abdominal/pelvic vessels)*
   4. perform actions *to allow time for remaining autoregulatory mechanisms to adjust to position changes:*
      a. change client's position slowly
      b. gradually progress client to a sitting or upright position using a recliner wheelchair or tilt table when allowed and tolerated.

c. Consult physician if signs and symptoms of decreased tissue perfusion persist or worsen.

3. NURSING DIAGNOSIS:

INEFFECTIVE BREATHING PATTERN

related to:

a. decreased depth of respirations associated with:
   1. the depressant effect of some medications (e.g., narcotic [opioid] analgesics, centrally acting muscle relaxants)
   2. weakness, fatigue, and decreased activity

3. restricted chest expansion resulting from:
   a. loss of abdominal and intercostal muscle function (innervation of these muscles occurs at the thoracic level)
   b. impaired function of the diaphragm (the diaphragm is innervated by the phrenic nerve, which travels through segments 3–5 of the cervical spine)
   c. upward pressure on the diaphragm (can occur as a result of gastric distension if paralytic ileus develops during period of spinal shock)
   d. recumbent positioning (in this position, full expansion of the lungs is restricted by the bed surface and the abdominal contents pushing up against the diaphragm)
   e. improper fit or application of halo vest or abdominal binder;

b. decreased rate of respirations associated with the depressant effect of some medications (e.g., narcotic [opioid] analgesics, centrally acting muscle relaxants).

Suggested NOC Outcome: Respiratory status: ventilation

Suggested NIC Interventions: Respiratory monitoring; Ventilation assistance

Desired Outcome	**Nursing Actions** *and Selected Purposes/Rationales* (see pp. 18–20 for additional rationales)
3. The client will maintain an effective breathing pattern (see Care Plan on Immobility, Diagnosis 1 [p. 130], for outcome criteria).	3.a. Refer to Care Plan on Immobility, Diagnosis 1 (p. 130), for measures related to assessment and improvement of breathing pattern. b. Assist with pulmonary function studies (e.g., tidal volume, vital capacity, inspiratory force) if done to evaluate respiratory status and effectiveness of treatment measures. c. Implement additional measures *to promote lung/chest wall expansion in order to improve breathing pattern:* 1. perform actions to treat paralytic ileus (see Diagnosis 15, action b.2) *in order to reduce gastric distention and upward pressure on diaphragm* 2. if client needs an abdominal binder, make sure it is positioned below the rib cage 3. progress client to a sitting or upright position when allowed and tolerated 4. if client is wearing a halo vest, consult appropriate health care provider (e.g., physician, orthotist) about having it readjusted if it appears too tight 5. encourage and assist client to perform exercises that strengthen the accessory muscles used in breathing (e.g., shoulder shrugs to strengthen the trapezius muscles) when allowed and tolerated.

4. Nursing Diagnosis: *INEFFECTIVE AIRWAY CLEARANCE*

related to stasis of secretions associated with:

a. decreased mobility;
b. decreased effectiveness of cough resulting from diminished lung/chest wall expansion, depressant effect of certain medications (e.g., narcotic [opioid] analgesics, centrally acting muscle relaxants), and possible tenacious secretions if fluid intake is inadequate.

Suggested NOC Outcomes: Respiratory status: ventilation; Respiratory status: airway patency

Suggested NIC Interventions: Respiratory monitoring; Airway management; Cough enhancement; Chest physiotherapy

Desired Outcome	**Nursing Actions** *and Selected Purposes/Rationales* (see pp. 12–14 for additional rationales)
4. The client will maintain clear, open airways (see Care Plan on Immobility, Diagnosis 2 [p. 131], for outcome criteria).	4.a. Refer to Care Plan on Immobility, Diagnosis 2 (p. 131), for measures related to assessment and promotion of effective airway clearance. b. Implement measures *to facilitate the client's cough efforts in order to further promote effective airway clearance:* 1. place client in a horizontal position during cough efforts unless contraindicated *(this position promotes a more effective forced expiration by decreasing the effect of gravity on the diaphragm)* 2. use an assisted coughing technique (e.g., place palm of hand below diaphragm and push upward as client exhales).

5. NURSING DIAGNOSIS:

ACUTE/CHRONIC PAIN

a. headache related to contractions of the neck muscles (can occur in response to stress and/or neck pain);
b. neck pain related to nerve root irritation at the site of spinal cord injury, muscle stiffness while immobilization device is in place, and muscle strain associated with increased use of neck muscles following removal of immobilization device;
c. upper arm and shoulder pain related to muscle strain associated with increased use of biceps and shoulders as activity progresses.

Suggested NOC Outcomes: Pain control; Comfort level

Suggested NIC Interventions: Pain management; Analgesic administration

Desired Outcome	**Nursing Actions** *and Selected Purposes/Rationales* (see pp. 45–47 for additional rationales)
5. The client will experience diminished pain as evidenced by: a. verbalization of same b. relaxed facial expression c. increased participation in activities when allowed.	5.a. Assess for signs and symptoms of pain (e.g., verbalization of pain, grimacing or tense facial expression, reluctance to turn head or move shoulders when increased activity is allowed, restlessness). b. Assess client's perception of the severity of pain using a pain intensity rating scale. c. Assess the client's pain pattern (e.g., location, quality, onset, duration, precipitating factors, aggravating factors, alleviating factors). d. Implement measures *to reduce pain:* 1. perform actions to promote rest (e.g., schedule uninterrupted rest periods, minimize environmental activity and noise, limit number of visitors and their length of stay) *in order to reduce fatigue and subsequently increase the client's threshold and tolerance for pain* 2. perform actions *to prevent or relieve headache:* a. minimize environmental stimuli (e.g., provide a calm environment, dim lights) b. implement measures to reduce psychological stress (see Diagnoses 1, action b; 17; and 18, action b) c. avoid letting any object hit the skull pins, tongs, traction weights, and/or halo frame *(sound transmitted through these objects is intensified by their contact with the skull and loud noise is a noxious stimulus that can cause or intensify headache)* d. apply cool cloth to forehead if client desires 3. perform actions *to prevent or relieve neck, upper arm, and/or shoulder pain:* a. maintain immobilization of the cervical spine as ordered *to reduce nerve root irritation* b. when moving client, provide support to neck and utilize turn sheet rather than pushing or pulling on shoulders and arms c. apply neck support (e.g., soft cervical collar) if ordered following removal of immobilization device d. massage client's upper arms and shoulders, being careful to avoid area around or over cervical spine until the injury has stabilized

Desired Outcome	Nursing Actions *and Selected Purposes/Rationales*

e. consult physician about application of heat and/or cold to upper arms, shoulders, and neck
4. provide or assist with additional nonpharmacologic measures for pain relief (e.g., position change if allowed, progressive relaxation exercises, guided imagery, diversional activities such as watching television or conversing)
5. administer the following medications as ordered:
a. narcotic (opioid) analgesics (used cautiously *because of their respiratory depressant effect)*
b. nonnarcotic analgesics such as acetaminophen and nonsteroidal anti-inflammatory agents
c. muscle relaxants.

e. Consult appropriate health care provider (e.g., pain management specialist, pharmacist, physician) if above measures fail to provide adequate relief of pain.

6. Nursing Diagnosis: INEFFECTIVE THERMOREGULATION

related to:
a. interruption in the feedback system between the area below the level of cord injury and the hypothalamus and loss of vasomotor tone below the level of the injury (these conditions result in the loss of compensatory responses to temperature changes [i.e. vasodilation, sweating, vasoconstriction, shivering, and piloerection]);
b. reduction in heat generation associated with limited body movement (especially during period of spinal shock).

Suggested NOC Outcome: Thermoregulation

Suggested NIC Interventions: Temperature regulation; Environmental management

Desired Outcome	Nursing Actions *and Selected Purposes/Rationales*

6. The client will experience effective thermoregulation as evidenced by:
a. verbalization of comfortable body temperature
b. absence of excessively warm or cool skin below the level of the injury
c. temperature within normal range.

6.a. Assess for signs and symptoms of ineffective thermoregulation (e.g., reports of feeling too warm or too cold, excessively warm or cool skin below the level of the injury, temperature above or below normal range).
b. Implement measures *to maintain effective thermoregulation:*
1. perform actions *to prevent hypothermia:*
a. maintain room temperature at 70° F
b. provide extra clothing and bedding as necessary
c. protect client from drafts
d. apply warming blanket as ordered
e. provide warm liquids for client to drink
f. avoid taking client outdoors when it is very cold
2. perform actions *to prevent hyperthermia:*
a. maintain room temperature at 70° F
b. avoid use of excessive clothing and bedding
c. apply cooling blanket as ordered
d. remove extra clothing during physical and occupational therapy sessions
e. avoid taking client outdoors when it is very hot (especially if the humidity is high).

c. Consult physician if above measures fail to maintain effective thermoregulation.

7. Nursing Diagnosis: RISK FOR IMPAIRED TISSUE INTEGRITY

related to:
a. accumulation of waste products and decreased oxygen and nutrient supply to the skin and subcutaneous tissue associated with reduced blood flow from prolonged pressure on the tissues as a result of decreased mobility

and/or presence of an external device (e.g., halo vest, wrist splint) that is improperly applied or does not fit properly;
b. damage to the skin or subcutaneous tissue associated with friction or shearing;
c. increased fragility of the skin associated with dependent edema and decreased tissue perfusion;
d. frequent contact with irritants if client is incontinent of urine.

Suggested NOC Outcome: Tissue integrity: skin and mucous membranes

Suggested NIC Interventions: Skin surveillance; Pressure management; Positioning: wheelchair; Bed rest care; Pressure ulcer prevention; Skin care: topical treatments; Traction/Immobilization care

Desired Outcome	**Nursing Actions** *and Selected Purposes/Rationales* (see pp. 49–52 for additional rationales)

7. The client will maintain tissue integrity as evidenced by:
   a. absence of redness and irritation
   b. no skin breakdown.

7.a. Inspect the skin (especially bony prominences, dependent and/or edematous areas, perineum, area underneath halo vest, and areas of sensory loss) for pallor, redness, and breakdown.
b. Refer to Care Plan on Immobility, Diagnosis 4, action c (p. 133), for measures to prevent tissue breakdown associated with decreased mobility.
c. Implement additional measures *to prevent tissue breakdown:*
   1. perform actions to maintain adequate tissue perfusion (see Diagnosis 2, action b)
   2. if client is wearing a halo vest:
      a. ensure that vest lining and skin beneath it are kept clean and dry
      b. make sure that clothing worn under the vest is clean, dry, wrinkle-free, and made of cotton (some physicians allow client to wear a T-shirt under the vest; others do not because they feel the shirt promotes slippage of the vest)
      c. cover all rough vest edges with foam tape
      d. consult physician and orthotist about having the vest readjusted if it is placing excessive pressure on any skin area
   3. perform actions to prevent urinary incontinence (see Diagnosis 10, actions e.2–4 and f)
   4. perform actions to decrease spasticity (see Diagnosis 8, action a.8) *because spasms can cause movement and subsequent friction and make it difficult to keep client positioned properly*
   5. ensure that wheelchair is not too small for client and that it is adequately cushioned
   6. ensure that shoes, jewelry, clothing, and straps that secure assistive devices are not too tight
   7. be sure that client wears shoes or sturdy slippers when in wheelchair *to protect feet from trauma*
   8. if fade time (length of time it takes for reddened area to fade after pressure is removed) is greater than 15 minutes, increase frequency of position changes and/or provide more effective methods of cushioning, padding, and positioning.
d. If skin breakdown occurs:
   1. notify appropriate health care provider (e.g., wound care specialist, physician)
   2. perform care of involved area(s) as ordered or per standard hospital procedure.

8. NURSING DIAGNOSIS: ***IMPAIRED PHYSICAL MOBILITY***

related to:
a. activity limitations associated with quadriplegia and immobilization of the spine;
b. spasticity following the period of spinal shock associated with stimulation of the reflex arcs below the level of the injury;

c. decreased motivation associated with fatigue and the psychological response to the extensive motor and sensory losses that have occurred;
d. pain;
e. loss of muscle mass, tone, and strength in areas of existing motor function (biceps, upper shoulders, and neck) associated with prolonged disuse (more likely to occur when client is in skeletal traction and must remain in bed);
f. contractures (if they develop).

Suggested NOC Outcomes: Joint movement: Coordinated movement; Mobility; Transfer performance; Ambulation: wheelchair

Suggested NIC Interventions: Bed rest care; Exercise therapy: joint mobility; Exercise therapy: muscle control

Desired Outcome	Nursing Actions *and Selected Purposes/Rationales*
8. The client will achieve maximum physical mobility within limitations imposed by the injury and the treatment plan.	8.a. Implement measures *to increase mobility:* 1. facilitate client's psychological adjustment to the effects of the spinal cord injury (see Diagnoses 17 and 18, action b) 2. perform actions to reduce pain (see Diagnosis 5, action d) 3. instruct client in and assist with active and active-resistive exercises of neck, shoulders, and biceps when allowed by physician 4. perform actions to prevent contractures (see Diagnosis 15, actions e.2 and 3) *in order to maintain joint mobility* 5. when activity is allowed, instruct client in ways to move body (e.g., hook arm over side rail to assist in turning self, trigger flexor spasm of knees to help swing legs over side of bed during transfer to and from wheelchair) 6. instruct client in and assist with use of mobility aids (e.g., sliding board, electric wheelchair) as activity progresses 7. reinforce instructions, activities, and exercise plan recommended by physical and occupational therapists 8. perform actions *to reduce spasticity (spasms can interfere with attempts to increase mobility):* a. avoid stimulating extremities or muscle groups (e.g., do not jar bed; use slow, steady movements when repositioning client; do not touch easily stimulated areas unnecessarily) b. implement measures to prevent conditions such as urinary tract infection, fecal impaction, pressure ulcers, fatigue, and chills *(these conditions can result in the stimulation of various muscle groups)* c. assist client to change position frequently and perform range of motion exercises *in order to keep muscles stretched (when muscles tighten, spasms are more likely to occur)* d. administer muscle relaxants (e.g., baclofen, dantrolene, tizanidine, diazepam) if ordered e. if undesired muscle spasms occur while moving client, hold the affected area firmly until the spasm subsides 9. provide adequate rest periods before activity sessions. b. Encourage the support of significant others. Allow them to assist with range of motion exercises, positioning, and activity unless contraindicated. c. Consult appropriate health care provider (e.g., physical therapist, physician) if client is unable to achieve expected level of mobility or if range of motion becomes restricted.

9. NURSING DIAGNOSIS: ***SELF-CARE DEFICIT***

related to impaired physical mobility associated with quadriplegia, spasticity, decreased motivation, pain, weakness, and activity restrictions imposed by treatment plan.

Suggested NOC Outcome:
Self-care: activities of daily living

Suggested NIC Intervention: Self-care assistance

Desired Outcome	Nursing Actions *and Selected Purposes/Rationales*

9. The client will demonstrate increased participation in self-care activities within the limitations imposed by the treatment plan and effects of the spinal cord injury.

9.a. With client, develop a realistic plan for meeting daily physical needs. Inform client that with rehabilitation and use of assistive devices, he/she may be able to accomplish activities such as:
   1. feeding self once meal has been set up
   2. washing face and chest
   3. combing front and sides of hair, brushing teeth, and shaving with an electric razor
   4. participating in dressing upper body.

b. When condition stabilizes and physician allows, implement measures *to facilitate client's ability to perform self-care activities:*
   1. perform actions to increase mobility (see Diagnosis 8, action a)
   2. consult occupational therapist regarding assistive devices available; reinforce use of these devices, which may include:
      a. rocker feeder, overhead sling, plate guard, sandwich holder, and broad-handled and/or swivel utensils for feeding self
      b. flexor-hinge splint or universal cuff to aid in brushing teeth, combing hair, and shaving with electric razor
      c. bath mitt for bathing face and chest
      d. Velcro fasteners to facilitate dressing upper body
   3. schedule care at a time when client is most likely to be able to participate (e.g., when analgesics are at peak effect, after rest periods, not immediately after physical therapy sessions or meals)
   4. keep objects client can use independently within easy reach
   5. allow adequate time for accomplishment of self-care activities.

c. Encourage client to perform as much of self-care as possible within physical limitations and activity restrictions imposed by the treatment plan.

d. Perform for client the self-care activities that he/she is unable to accomplish.

e. Inform significant others of client's abilities to participate in own care. Explain the importance of encouraging and allowing client to achieve an optimal level of independence.

10. Nursing Diagnosis:

IMPAIRED URINARY ELIMINATION

a. retention related to:
   1. atony of bladder wall during period of spinal shock
   2. spasticity of the external urinary sphincter and/or loss of ability to coordinate bladder contraction and relaxation of the external urinary sphincter following period of spinal shock
   3. incomplete bladder emptying associated with horizontal positioning (in this position, the gravity needed for complete bladder emptying is lost);

b. incontinence related to:
   1. spasticity of the bladder following period of spinal shock and loss of ability to contract the external urinary sphincter voluntarily (incontinence can occur if the bladder contracts strongly when the external urinary sphincter is relaxed)
   2. inadvertent stimulation of the voiding reflex.

Suggested NOC Outcomes:
Urinary continence; Urinary elimination

Suggested NIC Interventions: Urinary catheterization; Urinary retention care; Urinary incontinence care; Tube care; Urinary

Desired Outcome	**Nursing Actions** *and Selected Purposes/Rationales* (see pp. 59–62 for additional rationales)
10. The client will experience an optimal pattern of urinary elimination as evidenced by: a. absence of bladder distention b. balanced intake and output c. absence of urinary incontinence.	10.a. Assess for and report signs and symptoms of impaired urinary elimination: 1. urinary retention (e.g., bladder distention, intake greater than output) 2. urinary incontinence. b. Catheterize client if ordered *to determine amount of residual urine.* c. Assist with urodynamic studies (e.g., urethral pressure profile, uroflowmetry, cystometrogram) if ordered. d. Monitor client's pattern of fluid intake and urinary elimination (e.g., times and amounts of fluid intake, types of fluids consumed, amount of triggered and involuntary voidings, times of and amount of urine obtained from intermittent catheterizations, activities preceding incontinence). e. Implement measures *to promote optimal urinary elimination:* 1. perform actions *to prevent urinary retention during period of spinal shock:* a. perform intermittent catheterizations or insert indwelling urinary catheter as ordered b. implement measures *to maintain patency of urinary catheter if present* (e.g., keep tubing free of kinks) 2. following the period of spinal shock, perform actions *to promote complete bladder emptying and/or reduce the risk of incontinence:* a. attempt to initiate voiding periodically by stimulating the trigger zones of the reflex sacral arc (e.g., tap suprapubic area, stroke inner thigh, perform anal sphincter stretching, pull pubic hair); if voiding occurs, repeat stimulus as necessary *to empty the bladder* b. if possible, place client on bedside commode or toilet when triggering voiding reflex or performing intermittent catheterization *(gravity facilitates complete bladder emptying)* c. instruct client to space fluid intake evenly throughout the day rather than drinking a large quantity at one time *(if the bladder fills rapidly and frequency of emptying is not increased, bladder distention occurs)* d. instruct client to limit intake of alcohol and beverages containing caffeine such as colas, coffee, and tea *(alcohol and caffeine have a mild diuretic effect and act as irritants to the bladder; the increased urine production can result in bladder distention if the frequency of bladder emptying is not also increased and the bladder irritation can trigger bladder spasms and subsequent incontinence)* e. limit oral fluid intake in the evening *so that the bladder does not become overdistended during the night* (as rehabilitation progresses, most clients do not perform intermittent catheterization or attempt to trigger voiding during the night) 3. instruct client and others to avoid stimulating the voiding reflex trigger zones at times other than during bladder care *in order to reduce the risk of incontinence* 4. administer centrally acting muscle relaxants (e.g., baclofen) or anticholinergics (e.g., tolterodine, oxybutynin) if ordered *to decrease spastic contraction of the bladder and the subsequent risk of incontinence and to decrease tone of the external urinary sphincter (decreased sphincter tone allows for more complete bladder emptying during reflex voiding attempts).* f. If urinary retention or incontinence persists: 1. review and revise bladder training program 2. prepare client for insertion of an indwelling catheter (urethral or suprapubic) if indicated.

11. NURSING DIAGNOSIS: ***RISK FOR CONSTIPATION***

related to:

a. decreased gastrointestinal motility associated with:
   1. loss of autonomic nervous system function below the level of the injury during period of spinal shock
   2. decreased activity;

b. lack of awareness of stool in rectum associated with sensory loss below the level of the injury;
c. loss of central nervous system control over defecation reflex;
d. decreased gravity filling of lower rectum associated with horizontal positioning;
e. decreased intake of fluids and foods high in fiber.

Suggested NOC Outcomes: Bowel elimination; Bowel continence

Suggested NIC Interventions: Constipation/Impaction management; Bowel training; Bowel management

Desired Outcome	**Nursing Actions** *and Selected Purposes/Rationales* (see pp. 24–26 for additional rationales)
11. The client will not experience constipation as evidenced by: a. usual frequency of bowel movements b. passage of soft, formed stool c. absence of abdominal distention.	11.a. Assess for signs and symptoms of constipation (e.g., decrease in frequency of bowel movements; passage of hard, formed stools; abdominal distention). b. Assess bowel sounds. Report a pattern of decreasing bowel sounds. c. Implement measures *to prevent constipation* (the following are usually included in a bowel training program): 1. instruct client to increase intake of foods high in fiber (e.g., bran, whole-grain breads and cereals, fresh fruits and vegetables) unless contraindicated 2. assist client to maintain a minimum fluid intake of 2500 ml/day unless contraindicated 3. encourage client to drink hot liquids before scheduled bowel evacuation *in order to stimulate peristalsis* 4. assist client to eat at scheduled times and adhere to a routine time for defecation; follow client's preinjury pattern if possible 5. increase activity as allowed and tolerated 6. perform digital stimulation and/or insert rectal suppository *to stimulate peristalsis and reflex emptying of rectum* 7. place client on toilet or bedside commode or place in high Fowler's position on bedpan for bowel movements unless contraindicated 8. allow ample time for bowel evacuation (may take up to an hour after rectal stimulation) 9. if an analgesic is needed, encourage use of nonnarcotics rather than narcotics (opioids) *to prevent further decrease in bowel activity* 10. administer laxatives or cathartics and/or enemas if ordered. d. Consult physician about checking for an impaction and digitally removing stool if client has not had a bowel movement in 3 days, if he/she is passing liquid stool, or if other signs and symptoms of constipation are present. e. If constipation occurs, review bowel training program and revise it as needed.

12. NURSING DIAGNOSIS: *RISK FOR INFECTION*

a. pneumonia related to:
   1. stasis of secretions associated with decreased activity and decreased ability to clear tracheobronchial passages (client is unable to cough forcefully as a result of weakness of the diaphragm and paralysis of the abdominal and intercostal muscles)
   2. aspiration of foods/fluids (impaired swallowing can occur as a result of neck hyperextension and/or horizontal body positioning during the time that the cervical spine is immobilized);
b. urinary tract infection related to:
   1. growth and colonization of pathogens associated with urinary stasis
   2. introduction of pathogens associated with presence of an indwelling catheter and/or performance of intermittent catheterizations;
c. skull pin site infection related to introduction of pathogens during or following insertion of skull pins.

Suggested NOC Outcomes: Immune status; Infection severity

Suggested NIC Interventions: Infection protection; Infection control; Cough enhancement; Airway management; Perineal care; Tube care: urinary; Urinary retention care; Traction/Immobilization care

Desired Outcomes	Nursing Actions *and Selected Purposes/Rationales* (see pp. 37–40 for additional rationales)
12.a. The client will not develop pneumonia (see Care Plan on Immobility, Diagnosis 11, outcome a [p. 139], for outcome criteria).	12.a.1. Refer to Care Plan on Immobility, Diagnosis 11, action a (p. 139), for measures related to assessment, prevention, and treatment of pneumonia. 2. Implement additional measures *to prevent pneumonia:* a. perform actions to improve breathing pattern and promote effective airway clearance (see Diagnoses 3 and 4) b. perform actions *to reduce the risk for aspiration* (e.g., place client in high Fowler's or side-lying position during meals unless contraindicated, instruct client to avoid laughing and talking when eating and drinking, instruct client to use a straw for all liquids and to take small sips and sip slowly when drinking).
12.b. The client will remain free of urinary tract infection as evidenced by: 1. clear urine 2. afebrile status 3. no increase in spasticity 4. urinalysis showing fewer than 5 WBCs, negative leukocyte esterase and nitrites, and absence of bacteria 5. negative urine culture.	12.b.1. Assess for and report signs and symptoms of urinary tract infection (e.g., cloudy urine; elevated temperature; increase in spasticity [bladder mucosal irritation triggers muscle spasms]; urinalysis showing a WBC count greater than 5, positive leukocyte esterase or nitrites, or the presence of bacteria; positive urine culture). 2. Refer to Care Plan on Immobility, Diagnosis 11, actions b.2 and 3 (pp. 139–140), for measures related to prevention and treatment of urinary tract infection. 3. Implement measures to prevent urinary retention (see Diagnosis 10, actions e.1, 2, and 4 and f) *in order to further reduce the risk of urinary tract infection.*
12.c. The client will remain free of skull pin site infection as evidenced by: 1. afebrile status 2. absence of redness, heat, swelling, and pain around pin sites 3. absence of unusual drainage from pin sites 4. WBC and differential counts within normal range 5. negative cultures of pin site drainage.	12.c.1. Assess for and report signs and symptoms of skull pin site infection (e.g., fever, redness, heat, swelling, and pain around pin sites; unusual drainage around pin; foul odor from pin site; elevated WBC count and significant change in differential; positive results of cultures of pin site drainage). 2. Implement measures *to prevent skull pin site infection:* a. use good hand washing technique b. keep client's hair clean c. keep hair around pin sites trimmed *so the tissues are not traumatized when hair is combed and hair does not get tangled around the pins* d. instruct persons coming in contact with client to avoid touching pins, tongs, weights, and/or halo ring *in order to reduce movement of the pins and subsequent tissue trauma* e. clean pin sites according to physician's order or standard hospital procedure f. use sterile technique when performing pin site care g. replace equipment and solutions used for pin site care according to hospital policy. 3. If signs and symptoms of skull pin site infection are present, administer antimicrobials and/or apply antimicrobial ointment to pin site(s) if ordered.

13. NURSING DIAGNOSIS: ***RISK FOR INJURY***

a. falls related to loss of motor function, use of kinetic bed, altered sitting balance if wearing a halo device (the structure and weight of the device alter the client's center of gravity), and unexpected body movements resulting from spasticity;

b. burns related to loss of motor and sensory function and unexpected body movements resulting from spasticity.

Suggested NOC Outcome: Fall prevention behavior

Suggested NIC Interventions: Fall prevention; Environmental management; Surveillance: safety; Peripheral sensation management

Desired Outcome	Nursing Actions *and Selected Purposes/Rationales*
13. The client will not experience falls or burns.	13.a. Implement measures *to reduce the risk for injury:* 1. perform actions *to prevent falls:* a. if client is in a standard hospital bed, keep bed in low position with side rails up b. if client is in a kinetic bed, utilize safety measures such as safety straps and padded side pieces c. keep safety belts securely fastened when client is on a stretcher or in a wheelchair d. obtain adequate assistance when moving client; utilize instructions from physical therapist on correct transfer techniques e. implement measures *to increase client's stability when in a wheelchair* (e.g., use wheelchair equipped with an anti-tipping device, fasten safety belt around upper body and chair to stabilize trunk, use H-straps to keep legs positioned properly) f. do not rush client; allow adequate time for the accomplishment of transfers and position changes 2. perform actions *to prevent burns:* a. let hot foods and fluids cool slightly before serving b. supervise client while smoking; do not place ashtray on client's lap *(the cigarette could roll off the ashtray onto client's clothing)* c. assess temperature of bath water before and during use d. when client is in a wheelchair, instruct him/her to avoid placing self next to sources of heat (e.g., heater, stove) 3. encourage client to request assistance whenever needed; have a specially adapted call signal available to client at all times 4. perform actions to decrease spasticity (see Diagnosis 8, action a.8) *in order to reduce the risk of unexpected body movements.* b. Include client and significant others in planning and implementing measures to prevent injury. c. If injury does occur, initiate appropriate first aid and notify physician.

14. NURSING DIAGNOSIS: RISK FOR AUTONOMIC DYSREFLEXIA

related to loss of autonomic nervous system control below the level of the cord injury (can occur once reflex activity returns following period of spinal shock).

Suggested NOC Outcome: Symptom severity

Suggested NIC Intervention: Dysreflexia management

Desired Outcome	Nursing Actions *and Selected Purposes/Rationales*
14. The client will not experience autonomic dysreflexia as evidenced by: a. vital signs within normal range for client b. skin dry and usual color above the level of the injury c. no reports of pounding headache, nasal congestion, and blurred vision.	14.a. Assess for signs and symptoms of autonomic dysreflexia: 1. sudden rise in B/P (systolic pressure may go as high as 300 mm Hg) 2. bradycardia 3. flushing and profuse diaphoresis above level of injury 4. pounding headache 5. nasal congestion 6. blurred vision. b. Implement measures *to prevent stimulation of the sympathetic nervous system below the level of the cord injury in order to prevent autonomic dysreflexia:* 1. perform actions to prevent distention of the bladder and bowel (see Diagnoses 10, actions e.1, 2, and 4 and f and 11, action c)

Desired Outcome	**Nursing Actions** *and Selected Purposes/Rationales*

2. perform actions *to prevent pressure on any area of the client's body below the level of the cord injury:*
   a. instruct and assist client to change position frequently
   b. ensure that overbed tray is not resting on client
   c. ensure that clothing is not constrictive and shoes are not too tight
3. perform good nail care *(ingrown nails can stimulate the sympathetic nervous system)*
4. perform actions to prevent and treat urinary tract infection (see Diagnosis 12, actions b.2 and 3)
5. apply a topical anesthetic agent to any existing pressure ulcer
6. apply a local anesthetic (e.g., Nupercainal ointment) if ordered before performing actions that can result in an exaggerated sympathetic response (e.g., urinary catheterization, removal of a fecal impaction, administration of an enema, care of any wound below the level of the injury).

c. If signs and symptoms of autonomic dysreflexia occur:
   1. immediately implement measures *to promote venous pooling and subsequent decrease in B/P* (e.g., raise head of bed and lower client's legs unless contraindicated; remove abdominal binder, antiembolism stockings, and intermittent pneumatic compression device if present)
   2. monitor B/P and pulse frequently (usually every 3–5 minutes until treatments and/or medication take effect)
   3. assess for and, if possible, alleviate the condition causing sympathetic stimulation; if client needs to be catheterized or have a fecal impaction removed, be sure to use an anesthetic ointment when performing the procedure *in order to decrease the risk of aggravating the autonomic dysreflexia*
   4. administer antihypertensives (e.g., diazoxide, hydralazine, nitroprusside) as ordered
   5. notify physician immediately if signs and symptoms persist or if complications resulting from severe hypertension occur (e.g., seizures, intraocular hemorrhage, cerebrovascular accident, myocardial infarction)
   6. notify all persons participating in client's care of the episode of autonomic dysreflexia *since such episodes can recur.*

15. COLLABORATIVE DIAGNOSES: *POTENTIAL COMPLICATIONS OF SPINAL CORD INJURY*

a. ascending spinal cord injury related to further damage to and/or ischemia of the cord above the C5 level associated with vasospasm of damaged vessels, progressive edema, bleeding, compression of cord by hematoma or bone fragments, and/or ineffective immobilization of an unstable cord injury;
b. paralytic ileus related to absence of neural stimulation of the intestine associated with absence of autonomic nervous system and reflex activity below the level of the spinal cord injury during period of spinal shock;
c. thromboembolism related to:
   1. venous stasis associated with decreased mobility and decreased vasomotor tone below the level of the injury
   2. hypercoagulability associated with increased blood viscosity (if fluid intake is inadequate) and increased levels of calcium in the blood from bone demineralization (can result from prolonged immobility);
d. gastrointestinal (GI) bleeding related to:
   1. erosions of the gastric and duodenal mucosa (can develop as a result of the increased output of hydrochloric acid that occurs with stress)
   2. irritation of the gastric mucosa associated with side effect of certain medications (e.g., corticosteroids);
e. contractures related to:
   1. muscle atrophy and lack of joint movement associated with prolonged immobility and quadriplegia

2. prolonged periods of hip flexion associated with use of wheelchair
3. difficulty putting joints through full range of motion associated with severe spasticity if it occurs and/or heterotopic ossification (excessive bone formation that can begin to develop around joints of paralyzed limbs as early as 1 month after the spinal cord injury).

Desired Outcomes	**Nursing Actions** *and Selected Purposes/Rationales*
15.a. The client will not experience spinal cord injury above the level of C5 as evidenced by: 1. stable respiratory status 2. stable B/P and pulse 3. no further loss of motor and sensory function.	15.a.1. Assess for and report signs and symptoms of ascending spinal cord injury: a. respiratory failure (e.g., rapid, shallow respirations; dusky or cyanotic skin color; drowsiness; confusion) b. significant decrease in B/P and pulse c. further loss of motor and sensory function. 2. Implement measures *to prevent spinal cord injury above the level of C5:* a. perform actions *to maintain immobilization of the spine until stabilization has been accomplished:* 1. do not release or adjust skeletal traction or halo device unless ordered 2. if skeletal traction is present, keep traction rope and weights hanging freely 3. always use turn sheet and adequate assistance when repositioning client; never use the rods of the halo device as handles 4. check pin sites of halo or traction device every shift; notify physician if pins are loose 5. if immobilization device fails (e.g., pins fall out, traction weights drop, rods on halo device disconnect): a. stabilize client's head, neck, and shoulders with hands, sandbags, or cervical collar b. notify physician immediately b. remind staff to utilize the jaw thrust method rather than hyperextending client's neck if respiratory distress occurs c. perform actions *to prevent ascending spinal cord ischemia:* 1. implement measures to maintain adequate tissue perfusion (see Diagnosis 2, action b) 2. administer the following medications if ordered: a. corticosteroids (the administration of high doses of methylprednisolone within the first 8 hours following spinal cord injury appears to be the most effective way of slowing the development of ischemia above the level of the injury) b. calcium-channel blockers (e.g., nimodipine) *to decrease vasospasm* d. prepare client for decompression of the spinal cord (e.g., removal of hematoma or bone fragments) or surgical stabilization (e.g., fusion) if planned. 3. If signs and symptoms of ascending spinal cord injury occur, be prepared to assist with intubation or tracheostomy and mechanical ventilation.
15.b. The client will have resolution of paralytic ileus if it occurs as evidenced by: 1. soft, nondistended abdomen 2. normal bowel sounds 3. passage of flatus.	15.b.1. Assess for and report signs and symptoms of paralytic ileus (e.g., firm, distended abdomen; absent bowel sounds; failure to pass flatus; abdominal x-ray showing distended bowel). 2. If signs and symptoms of paralytic ileus occur: a. withhold all oral intake b. insert nasogastric tube and maintain suction as ordered.

Desired Outcomes	Nursing Actions *and Selected Purposes/Rationales*
15.c.1. The client will not develop a deep vein thrombus as evidenced by: a. absence of swelling and distended superficial vessels in extremities b. usual temperature of extremities.	15.c.1.a. Assess for and report signs and symptoms of a deep vein thrombus (e.g., increase in circumference of extremity, distention of superficial vessels in extremity, unusual warmth of extremity). b. Refer to Care Plan on Immobility, Diagnosis 12, actions a.1.b and c (pp. 140–141), for measures related to prevention and treatment of a deep vein thrombus. c. Implement additional measures *to maintain adequate blood flow in legs and subsequently reduce the risk for thrombus formation:* 1. position firm pillow between client's legs if spasms tend to cause legs to cross 2. instruct client to obtain assistance to reposition legs properly if they cross.
15.c.2. The client will not experience a pulmonary embolism as evidenced by: a. absence of sudden shoulder pain b. unlabored respirations at 12–20/minute c. pulse within normal range for client d. blood gases within normal range.	15.c.2.a. Assess for and report signs and symptoms of pulmonary embolism (e.g., sudden shoulder pain [this is a referred pain], dyspnea, tachypnea, increase in pulse, apprehension, low PaO_2). b. Refer to Care Plan on Immobility, Diagnosis 12, actions a.2.b and c (p. 141), for measures related to prevention and treatment of a pulmonary embolism. c. Implement additional measures *to prevent a pulmonary embolism:* 1. perform actions to prevent and treat a deep vein thrombus (see actions c.1.b and c in this diagnosis) 2. perform actions to prevent autonomic dysreflexia (see Diagnosis 14, action b) *in order to prevent a sudden increase in blood pressure and subsequent dislodgment of a thrombus if present.*
15.d. The client will not experience GI bleeding as evidenced by: 1. no reports of shoulder pain 2. absence of frank and occult blood in stool and gastric contents 3. B/P and pulse within normal range for client 4. RBC, Hct, and Hgb levels within normal range.	15.d.1. Assess for and report signs and symptoms of GI bleeding (e.g., reports of shoulder pain [this is a referred pain]; frank or occult blood in stool or gastric contents; decreased B/P; increased pulse; decreasing RBC, Hct, and Hgb levels). 2. Implement measures *to prevent ulceration of the gastric and duodenal mucosa:* a. perform actions to decrease fear and anxiety (see Diagnosis 1, action b) b. when oral intake is allowed: 1. administer ulcerogenic medications (e.g., corticosteroids) with meals or snacks *to decrease gastric irritation* 2. instruct client to avoid foods/fluids that stimulate hydrochloric acid secretion or irritate the gastric mucosa (e.g., coffee; caffeine-containing tea and colas; spices such as black pepper, chili powder, and nutmeg) c. administer $histamine_2$ receptor antagonists (e.g., ranitidine, famotidine), proton-pump inhibitors (e.g., omeprazole, rabeprazole), antacids, and/or cytoprotective agents (e.g., sucralfate) if ordered. 3. If signs and symptoms of GI bleeding occur: a. insert nasogastric tube and maintain suction as ordered b. administer blood products and/or volume expanders if ordered c. assist with measures to control bleeding (e.g., gastric lavage, endoscopic electrocoagulation) if planned.
15.e. The client will not develop contractures as evidenced by normal or expected range of motion.	15.e.1. Assess for and report: a. statements of shoulder joint stiffness b. limitations in range of motion c. redness, unusual warmth, and swelling of joints in paralyzed limbs (can be indicative of heterotopic ossification, which can cause restricted movement of the involved joint). 2. Refer to Care Plan on Immobility, Diagnosis 12, actions d.2–6 (pp. 142–143), for measures to prevent contractures.

3. Implement additional measures *to reduce the risk of contractures:*
   a. perform actions to reduce spasticity (see Diagnosis 8, action a.8)
   b. position client in prone or supine position routinely unless contraindicated *to counteract prolonged periods of hip flexion resulting from wheelchair use*
   c. administer etidronate (e.g., Didronel) if ordered *to prevent or treat heterotopic ossification*
   d. prepare client for surgical removal of abnormal bone formation around joints if planned *in order to maintain joint mobility.*

16. NURSING DIAGNOSIS: SEXUAL DYSFUNCTION

related to:

a. decreased libido associated with:
   1. loss of sensory and voluntary motor function below the level of spinal cord injury
   2. presence of a urinary catheter and/or fear of urinary and bowel incontinence
   3. depression, disturbed self-concept
   4. fear of rejection by partner
   5. fear of autonomic dysreflexia (genital stimulation can cause dysreflexia);

b. decreased ability to control and maintain an erection associated with loss of ability to have a psychogenic erection (only reflexogenic erection is possible);

c. altered ejaculatory flow associated with impaired nerve function in the bladder neck (can result in retrograde ejaculation).

Suggested NOC Outcomes: Sexual identity; Sexual functioning

Suggested NIC Intervention: Sexual counseling

Desired Outcome	**Nursing Actions** *and Selected Purposes/Rationales*
16. The client will demonstrate beginning acceptance of changes in sexual functioning as evidenced by: a. verbalization of a perception of self as sexually acceptable and adequate b. statements reflecting beginning adjustment to the effects of the spinal cord injury on sexual functioning c. maintenance of relationship with significant other.	16.a. Assess for signs and symptoms of sexual dysfunction (e.g., verbalization of sexual concerns or inability to achieve sexual satisfaction, alteration in relationship with significant other, limitations imposed by quadriplegia). b. Provide accurate information about the effects of the spinal cord injury on sexual functioning. Encourage questions and clarify misconceptions. c. Implement measures *to promote optimal sexual functioning:* 1. facilitate communication between client and partner; focus on the feelings the couple share and assist them to identify changes that affect their sexual relationship 2. discuss ways to be creative in expressing sexuality (e.g., massage, fantasies, cuddling) 3. arrange for uninterrupted privacy if desired by the couple 4. perform actions to improve client's self-concept (see Diagnosis 17) 5. suggest alternative methods of sexual gratification and use of assistive devices if appropriate; encourage partner to explore erogenous areas on the client's lips, neck, and ears 6. inform male client and his partner of techniques for eliciting and maintaining reflexogenic erection (e.g., stimulate genitalia, stroke inner thigh, pull on pubic hairs, stimulate the rectum, manipulate the urinary catheter) 7. if client has difficulty maintaining an erection, encourage him to discuss various treatment options (e.g., vacuum erection aids, penile prosthesis) with physician if desired 8. if client experiences episodes of autonomic dysreflexia, instruct him/her to consult physician about ways to prevent it during sexual activity (e.g., have partner apply a local anesthetic to client's genitalia) 9. inform female client that vaginal lubrication can occur by local stimulation or can be enhanced by using a water-soluble lubricant

Desired Outcome	Nursing Actions *and Selected Purposes/Rationales*

10. if client has an indwelling urethral catheter, instruct him/her on ways to fold and secure the catheter tubing prior to sexual intercourse
11. if incontinence of urine is a concern, instruct client to:
    a. limit fluid intake 2–4 hours before sexual activity
    b. have bladder emptied immediately before sexual activity
12. instruct client to perform bowel care several hours before sexual activity *in order to reduce the risk of bowel incontinence if anal or rectal stimulation occurs during sexual activity*
13. if appropriate, involve partner in care of client *to facilitate partner's adjustment to the changes in client's appearance and body functioning and subsequently decrease the possibility of partner's rejection of client*
14. encourage client to rest before sexual activity
15. instruct client and partner to establish a relaxed, unhurried atmosphere for sexual activity
16. discuss positions that may facilitate sexual activity (e.g., lying on side, client in supine position)
17. provide explicit films and literature if desired by client and/or partner
18. include partner in above discussions and encourage continued support of the client.

d. Consult appropriate health care provider (e.g., sex counselor, physician) when client is ready for sexual counseling and/or sexual counseling appears indicated.

17. Nursing Diagnosis: *DISTURBED SELF-CONCEPT**

related to:
a. dependence on others to meet self-care needs;
b. feelings of powerlessness;
c. change in appearance associated with temporary presence of devices to immobilize the spine, necessity of wheelchair use, and spasticity following period of spinal shock;
d. infertility (in males) associated with:
   1. possibility of retrograde ejaculation (can result from impaired nerve function in the bladder neck)
   2. decreased sperm formation and viability resulting from testicular atrophy and impaired temperature regulation in the testes;
e. changes in body functioning, lifestyle, and roles.

*This diagnostic label includes the nursing diagnoses of disturbed body image, low self-esteem, and ineffective role performance.

Suggested NOC Outcomes: Body image; Self-esteem; Personal autonomy; Psychosocial adjustment: life change

Suggested NIC Interventions: Body image enhancement; Self-esteem enhancement; Emotional support; Support system enhancement; Role enhancement; Counseling

Desired Outcome	Nursing Actions *and Selected Purposes/Rationales* (see pp. 47–49 for additional rationales)
17. The client will demonstrate beginning adaptation to changes in body functioning, appearance, lifestyle, roles, and level of independence (see Care Plan on Immobility, Diagnosis 14 [p. 144], for outcome criteria).	17.a. Refer to Care Plan on Immobility, Diagnosis 14 (pp. 144–145), for measures related to assessment and promotion of a positive self-concept. b. Implement additional measures *to promote a positive self-concept:* 1. reinforce actions to assist client to cope with and adjust to changes resulting from the effects of the spinal cord injury (see Diagnosis 18, action b) 2. perform actions to prevent urinary incontinence (see Diagnosis 10, actions e.2–4 and f) 3. avoid unnecessary exposure of client during care

4. assure client that immobilization device is temporary and will be removed as soon as internal stabilization of the spine occurs; if an upper body brace or cervical collar is needed after removal of the skull pins, assist client to select clothing that makes the spinal support less obvious (e.g., high-collared shirts, loose-fitting shirts)
5. demonstrate acceptance of client using techniques such as touch and frequent visits; encourage significant others to do the same
6. encourage client's participation in activities that can assist him/her to integrate physical changes that have occurred (e.g., exercise, grooming, eating)
7. encourage client contact with others *so that he/she can test and establish a new self-image*
8. reinforce actions to assist client to adjust to alterations in sexual functioning (see Diagnosis 16, action c)
9. discuss alternative methods of becoming a parent (e.g., adoption, sperm harvesting, artificial insemination) if of concern to client
10. perform actions to increase the client's ability to perform self-care (see Diagnosis 9, action b) *in order to increase client's sense of independence*
11. provide privacy during client's attempts at self-care *in order to minimize embarrassment that he/she may feel because of neurological impairments*
12. encourage significant others to allow client to do what he/she is able *so that independence can be re-established and/or self-esteem redeveloped*
13. use the term "disabled" rather than "handicapped," "cripple," or "invalid"; avoid use of slang (e.g., "quad," "gimp").

18. NURSING DIAGNOSIS: INEFFECTIVE COPING OR IMPAIRED ADJUSTMENT*

related to:
a. depression, fear, anxiety, feelings of powerlessness, and ongoing grieving associated with spinal cord injury and its effects on body functioning, lifestyle, and roles;
b. dependence on others to meet basic needs;
c. lack of personal resources to deal with spinal cord injury and its effects;
d. need for extensive rehabilitation.

*The nurse should select the diagnostic label that is most appropriate for the client.

Suggested NOC Outcomes: Acceptance: health status; Psychosocial adjustment: life change; Coping; Compliance behavior; Adaptation to physical disability; Health beliefs: perceived control

Suggested NIC Interventions: Coping enhancement; Crisis intervention; Support system enhancement; Spiritual growth facilitation; Environmental management: home preparation

Desired Outcome	**Nursing Actions** *and Selected Purposes/Rationales* (see pp. 26–28 for additional rationales)
18. The client will demonstrate adjustment to current health status and effective coping skills as evidenced by: a. verbalization of acceptance and ability to cope with the effects of the spinal cord injury b. verbalization of a sense of control over health status	18.a. Assess for and report signs and symptoms of: 1. ineffective coping (e.g., verbalization of inability to cope or ask for help; inability to meet role expectations, problem solve, or meet basic needs; insomnia; withdrawal; reluctance to participate in treatment plan; destructive behavior toward self; inappropriate use of defense mechanisms) 2. impaired adjustment (e.g., denial of health status change, verbalization of lack of control, reluctance to participate in treatment plan and take actions to prevent further health problems). b. Implement measures *to promote effective coping and adjustment to change in health status:*

Desired Outcome	**Nursing Actions** *and Selected Purposes/Rationales*
c. utilization of appropriate problem-solving techniques d. willingness to participate in treatment plan and rehabilitation program e. absence of destructive behavior toward self f. utilization of available support systems.	1. allow time for client to begin to adjust to the diagnosis and planned treatment, residual effects of the spinal cord injury, and anticipated changes in lifestyle and roles 2. perform actions to decrease fear and anxiety (see Diagnosis 1, action b) 3. perform actions *to facilitate the grieving process* (e.g., assist client to acknowledge the changes/losses experienced, assist client to recognize and manage inappropriate denial if present, discuss the grieving process and reinforce that phases may overlap or recur) 4. assist client to identify personal strengths and resources that can be utilized to facilitate adjustment to and coping with the current situation 5. demonstrate acceptance of client but set limits on inappropriate behavior 6. if acceptable to client, arrange for a visit with another individual who has successfully adjusted to a similar injury 7. perform actions *to reduce client's feelings of powerlessness* (e.g., provide information about technical advances that can make independent operation of electronic devices such as lights, radio, television, and specially installed door openers and window shades possible) 8. support realistic hope about the effects of rehabilitation on future independence (with the aid of assistive devices, the client may be able to perform many activities including operating an electric wheelchair, feeding self once meal has been set up, washing face and chest, brushing teeth, and using a computer) 9. stress to persons coming in contact with client that an individual has an enormous potential for adjusting to a disability and that they need to avoid being overly sympathetic *(an overly sympathetic attitude can communicate a feeling of hopelessness)* 10. assist client to select wheelchairs (usually a manual and an electric one) that best meet mobility needs and promote a more active lifestyle 11. encourage client to actively participate in making decisions about his/her living situation; assist him/her to find, hire, and train an attendant before discharge from the extended care or rehabilitation facility 12. if client is experiencing severe spasticity: a. reinforce measures to reduce severity of the spasms (see Diagnosis 8, action a.8) b. reinforce ways that spasms can be beneficial (e.g., help swing legs from bed to wheelchair, initiate arm movements, maintain an erection, evacuate bowels) c. inform client that spasticity usually stabilizes in 1–2 years and may gradually subside after that time 13. inform client that there will be times when spasticity is worse, bowel and bladder programs are less effective, and efforts at self-care are less successful; assure him/her that these are temporary results of physical and/or emotional stress or fatigue rather than an indication of deteriorating neurological status 14. assist client to identify priorities and attainable goals as he/she starts to plan for necessary lifestyle and role changes 15. assist client and significant others to identify ways that personal and family goals can be adjusted rather than abandoned 16. assist client through methods such as role playing to prepare for negative reactions of others to his/her quadriplegia (tetraplegia) 17. administer antianxiety and/or antidepressant agents if ordered 18. if appropriate, assist client to meet spiritual needs (e.g., arrange for a visit from clergy) 19. set up a home evaluation appointment with occupational and physical therapists *so that changes in the home environment (e.g., installation of ramps, widening doorways, altering bathroom facilities) can be completed by discharge*

20. assist client to identify and utilize available support systems; provide information regarding available community resources that can assist client and significant others in adjusting to and coping with effects of the spinal cord injury (e.g., spinal cord injury groups, recreational programs)
21. support behaviors indicative of effective coping and adjustment (e.g., verbalization of ability to cope, utilization of available support systems, participation in rehabilitation program).

c. Consult appropriate health care provider (e.g., psychiatric nurse clinician, physician) if client continues to have difficulty adjusting to and coping with the spinal cord injury and its effects.

19. NURSING DIAGNOSIS: ***INTERRUPTED FAMILY PROCESSES***

related to change in family roles and structure associated with a family member's sudden, catastrophic injury; permanent disability; and need for extensive rehabilitation.

Suggested NOC Outcomes: Family coping; Family functioning; Family resiliency; Family normalization

Suggested NIC Interventions: Family involvement promotion; Family integrity promotion; Family process maintenance; Family support; Family mobilization; Support system enhancement

Desired Outcome

19. The family members* will demonstrate beginning adjustment to changes in functioning of a family member and family roles and structure as evidenced by:
    a. meeting client's needs
    b. verbalization of ways to adapt to required role and lifestyle changes
    c. active participation in decision making and client's rehabilitation
    d. positive interactions with one another.

Nursing Actions *and Selected Purposes/Rationales*

19.a. Assess for signs and symptoms of interrupted family processes (e.g., inability to meet client's needs, statements of not being able to accept client's quadriplegia or make necessary role and lifestyle changes, inability to make decisions, inability or refusal to participate in client's rehabilitation, negative family interactions).

b. Identify components of the family and their patterns of communication and role expectations.

c. Implement measures *to facilitate family members' adjustment to client's diagnosis, changes in client's functioning within the family system, and altered family roles and structure:*
1. encourage verbalization of feelings about client's quadriplegia and the effect of this on family structure; actively listen to each family member and maintain a nonjudgmental attitude about feelings shared
2. reinforce physician's explanations of the effects of the injury and planned treatment and rehabilitation
3. assist family members to gain a realistic perspective of client's situation, conveying as much hope as appropriate
4. provide privacy *so that family members and client can share their feelings with one another;* stress the importance of and facilitate the use of good communication techniques
5. assist family members to progress through their own grieving process; explain that they may encounter times when they need to focus on meeting their own rather than the client's needs
6. emphasize the need for family members to obtain adequate rest and nutrition and to identify and utilize stress management techniques *so that they are better able to emotionally and physically deal with the changes and losses experienced*
7. encourage and assist family members to identify coping strategies for dealing with the client's quadriplegia and its effects on the family
8. assist family members to identify realistic goals and ways of reaching these goals
9. include family members in decision making about client and care; convey appreciation for their input and continued support of client
10. encourage and allow family members to participate in client's care and rehabilitation

---

*The term "family members" is being used here to include client's significant others.

Desired Outcome	**Nursing Actions** *and Selected Purposes/Rationales*
	11. assist family members to identify resources that can assist them in coping with their feelings and meeting their immediate and long-term needs (e.g., counseling and social services; caregiver assistance programs; pastoral care; service, church, and spinal cord injury groups); initiate a referral if indicated. d. Consult appropriate health care provider (e.g., psychiatric nurse clinician, physician) if family members continue to demonstrate difficulty adapting to changes in client's functioning and family structure.

Discharge Teaching/Continued Care

20. Nursing Diagnosis: ***DEFICIENT KNOWLEDGE, INEFFECTIVE THERAPEUTIC REGIMEN MANAGEMENT, OR INEFFECTIVE HEALTH MAINTENANCE* †***

*The nurse should select the diagnostic label that is most appropriate for the client's discharge teaching needs.

†Although the client will not be able to perform many of the following actions independently, he/she must be knowledgeable about them in order to provide proper instruction to significant others and attendant and maintain an active role in the rehabilitation process.

Suggested NOC Outcomes: Knowledge: treatment regimen; Knowledge: health behavior; Knowledge: health resources; Knowledge: treatment procedure(s)

Suggested NIC Interventions: Teaching: individual; Teaching: prescribed activity/exercise; Teaching: psychomotor skills; Health system guidance; Financial resource assistance; Support system enhancement

Desired Outcomes	**Nursing Actions** *and Selected Purposes/Rationales*
20.a. The client will identify ways to prevent complications associated with spinal cord injury and decreased mobility.	20.a.1. Refer to Care Plan on Immobility, Diagnosis 17, action a (pp. 146–147), for instructions related to ways to prevent complications associated with decreased mobility. 2. Instruct client in ways to prevent complications associated with spinal cord injury: a. position firm pillow between legs if spasms tend to cause legs to cross (helps to prevent thrombus formation and adduction contractures) b. wear an abdominal binder when changing from a reclining to a sitting position and take vasoconstrictor drugs if prescribed to prevent dizziness and fainting c. elevate legs periodically during the day to promote venous return d. implement measures to reduce severe spasticity (e.g., avoid fatigue and chills, change position at least every 2 hours, take muscle relaxants as prescribed) in order to increase mobility and prevent contractures e. use full-length and long-handled mirrors to examine all skin surfaces in the morning and the evening; increase pressure relief measures if any areas of redness or pallor develop f. obtain a kinetic bed for home use if possible g. wear shoes when in wheelchair to protect feet from injury h. avoid putting items such as coins, keys, and wallet in skirt or pant pockets (these items can cause pressure on underlying skin areas) i. avoid wearing tight-fitting belts, clothing, shoes, and jewelry; make sure that urine collection leg bag straps are not too tight j. replace wheelchair cushions when they become worn-out

k. implement measures to prevent hyperthermia (e.g., avoid excessive clothing and bedding, limit length of time in direct sunlight in hot weather, wear a wide-brimmed hat when in direct sun, park your car or van in the shade in hot weather and open the doors to let the vehicle cool down before getting inside)
l. implement measures to prevent hypothermia (e.g., wear adequate amounts of clothing, wear a hat when in a cold environment, drink warm liquids)
m. implement measures to prevent falls (e.g., always use safety belt during transfers and when in chair, be certain to have adequate assistance for transfer activity)
n. implement measures to prevent burns:
    1. always check temperature of shower or bath water before use (can use bath water thermometer or have attendant check water temperature)
    2. never smoke when alone; do not place ashtray in lap
    3. let hot foods/fluids cool slightly before attempting to feed self
    4. never position self next to a stove, heater, or other major source of heat; be aware of where feet and legs are in relation to car heater when it is on
    5. never use an electric heating pad or electric blanket
    6. cover plastic or vinyl seat with a blanket before sitting down if seat has been in direct sun
o. implement measures to prevent autonomic dysreflexia:
    1. continue with effective bladder and bowel programs to prevent urinary retention and constipation/impaction
    2. change position frequently
    3. seek medical attention at first sign of infection, persistent pressure area, or ingrown toenail
    4. apply a local anesthetic (e.g., Nupercainal ointment) to area being stimulated prior to procedures/activities that have previously resulted in episodes of autonomic dysreflexia (e.g., urinary catheterization, administration of an enema, sexual activity).

3. Demonstrate the following procedures to client, significant others, and attendant:
    a. assisted coughing technique (quad-cough)
    b. Heimlich maneuver
    c. skin care
    d. proper positioning and padding
    e. transfer techniques
    f. active and passive range of motion exercises
    g. application of elastic stockings, abdominal binder, and heel and elbow protectors
    h. emergency treatment of autonomic dysreflexia (e.g., elevate head of bed and lower client's legs, alleviate causative factor, administer an antihypertensive agent).
4. Allow time for questions, clarification, and return demonstration.

20.b. The client will demonstrate the ability to correctly use and maintain assistive devices.

20.b.1. Reinforce instructions from physical and occupational therapists regarding use of assistive devices. Allow time for questions, clarification, and return demonstration.
2. Instruct client in proper maintenance of assistive devices (e.g., replace parts that are worn-out or broken, clean wheel hubs and crossbars of wheelchairs per manufacturer's instruction, keep wheelchair tires properly inflated).

20.c. The client will identify ways to manage altered bowel and bladder function.

20.c.1. Reinforce bladder and bowel training programs. (Guidelines are included in Diagnoses 10, action e, and 11, action c, but the specific program will vary for each client.)
2. Demonstrate bowel care (e.g., digital stimulation, insertion of suppositories, administration of enemas) and bladder care

Desired Outcomes	Nursing Actions *and Selected Purposes/Rationales*
	(e.g., stimulation techniques, intermittent catheterization, application of leg bag and bedside drainage bag, emptying of urinary collection bag). 3. Allow time for questions, clarification, and return demonstration.
20.d. The client will state signs and symptoms to report to the health care provider.	20.d. Instruct the client to report the following: 1. cloudy or foul-smelling urine 2. nausea and vomiting 3. cough productive of purulent, green, or rust-colored sputum 4. difficulty breathing or increased shortness of breath with activity 5. sudden or persistent shoulder pain (this can be a referred pain) 6. fever 7. chills or profuse sweating (can occur above the level of the injury) 8. increase in spasticity (could indicate an infection below the level of the injury) 9. unsuccessful bowel and/or bladder programs 10. redness in any extremity 11. swelling that appears suddenly, occurs only in one extremity, or does not subside overnight 12. increased restriction of any joint motion 13. persistent swelling over a joint 14. signs and symptoms of autonomic dysreflexia (e.g., pounding headache, sudden rise in blood pressure, blurred vision, slow pulse, flushing and sweating above level of injury, nasal congestion) that do not subside once the stimulus is removed 15. any area of persistent skin irritation or breakdown 16. indications of pregnancy (stress that appropriate prenatal care should be initiated as soon as possible).
20.e. The client will identify resources that can assist with financial needs, home management, and adjustment to changes resulting from spinal cord injury.	20.e.1. Inform client and significant others about resources that can assist with financial needs, home management, and adjustment to changes resulting from spinal cord injury (e.g., spinal cord injury support and social groups; state and federally funded financial programs; home health agencies; community health agencies; local service groups; financial, individual, family, and vocational counselors). 2. Initiate a social service referral if indicated.
20.f. The client will verbalize an understanding of and a plan for adhering to recommended follow-up care including future appointments with health care provider and occupational and physical therapists and medications prescribed.	20.f.1. Reinforce the importance of keeping scheduled follow-up visits with health care provider and occupational and physical therapists. 2. Explain the rationale for, side effects of, and importance of taking prescribed medications. Inform client of pertinent food and drug interactions. 3. Implement measures designed to improve client compliance: a. include significant others and caregivers in teaching sessions b. encourage questions and allow time for reinforcement and clarification of information provided c. provide written instructions on scheduled appointments with health care provider and occupational and physical therapists, medications prescribed, and signs and symptoms to report.

ADDITIONAL NURSING DIAGNOSES

*IMBALANCED NUTRITION: LESS THAN BODY REQUIREMENTS**

related to:

a. decreased oral intake associated with:
   1. dietary restrictions during period of spinal shock if paralytic ileus develops
   2. anorexia resulting from fatigue, depression and social isolation, the effect of negative nitrogen balance, and early satiety that occurs with decreased gastrointestinal motility

---

*See Unit II for outcomes, actions, and rationales.

3. difficulty swallowing resulting from neck hyperextension and/or horizontal body position during the time that the cervical spine is immobilized
4. difficulty feeding self;

b. increased nutritional needs associated with an imbalance in the rate of catabolism and anabolism (catabolic processes occur at a faster rate than anabolic processes in persons who have sustained a spinal cord injury and in those who are immobile).

DISTURBED SENSORY PERCEPTION

a. visual related to decreased ability to move head associated with presence of immobilization device and recumbent position;
b. tactile related to loss of integrity of ascending spinal pathways at the level of the cord injury.

RISK FOR ASPIRATION*

related to:

a. decreased ability to clear tracheobronchial passages associated with inability to cough forcefully resulting from weakness of the diaphragm and paralysis of the abdominal and intercostal muscles;
b. difficulty swallowing associated with neck hyperextension and/or horizontal body positioning during the time that the cervical spine is immobilized.

RISK FOR POWERLESSNESS

related to quadriplegia; dependence on others; and changes in roles, relationships, and future plans.

GRIEVING*

related to extensive loss of motor and sensory function and the effects of this loss on future lifestyle and roles.

RISK FOR LONELINESS

related to inability to participate in usual activities, decreased contact with significant others and friends while in the hospital and extended care or rehabilitation facility, depression, and withdrawal from others.

---

*See Unit II for outcomes, actions, and rationales.

Bibliography

See pages 879 and 881.

UNIT IX

Nursing Care of the Client with Disturbances of Cardiovascular Function

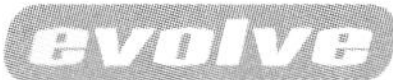

Angina Pectoris

Angina pectoris is transient chest pain or discomfort that is caused by an imbalance between myocardial oxygen supply and demand. The discomfort typically occurs in the retrosternal area; may or may not radiate; and is described as a tight, heavy, squeezing, burning, or choking sensation. The most common cause of angina pectoris is decreased coronary blood supply due to atherosclerosis of a major coronary artery. The atherosclerosis causes narrowing of the vessel lumen and an inability of the vessel to dilate and supply sufficient blood to the myocardium at times when myocardial oxygen needs are increased. Other conditions that can compromise coronary blood flow (e.g., spasm and/or thrombosis of a coronary artery, hypovolemia) and conditions that reduce oxygen availability and/or increase myocardial workload and oxygen demands (e.g., anemia, smoking, exercise, heavy meals, increased altitude, exposure to cold, stress) may precipitate or increase the frequency of angina attacks by widening the gap between oxygen needs and availability.

The two major types of angina pectoris are stable (classic exertional) angina and unstable angina. Stable angina, the most common type, is usually precipitated by physical exertion or emotional stress, lasts 3 to 5 minutes, and is relieved by rest and nitroglycerin. Unstable angina is characterized by an increasing frequency and/or severity of attacks that occur with less provocation or at rest. It is considered to be an acute coronary syndrome, which is associated with thrombus formation in a coronary artery. Persons with unstable angina are usually hospitalized and treated with heparin and antiplatelet agents while decisions regarding medical versus surgical treatment are made. A third type of angina is Prinzmetal's variant angina. It is less common than stable or unstable angina and is caused by severe focal spasm of a coronary artery.

This care plan focuses on the adult client hospitalized during an episode of chest pain/discomfort suspected to be unstable angina.

OUTCOME/DISCHARGE CRITERIA

THE CLIENT WILL:

- perform activities of daily living and ambulate without angina
- have angina controlled by oral medication
- have no signs and symptoms of complications
- verbalize a basic understanding of angina pectoris
- identify factors that may precipitate angina attacks and ways to control these factors
- identify modifiable cardiovascular risk factors and ways to alter these factors
- verbalize an understanding of the rationale for and components of a diet designed to lower serum cholesterol and triglycerides
- demonstrate accuracy in counting pulse
- verbalize an understanding of medications ordered including rationale, food and drug interactions, side effects, schedule for taking, and importance of taking as prescribed
- state signs and symptoms to report to the health care provider
- identify community resources that can assist in making necessary lifestyle changes and adjusting to the effects of angina pectoris
- verbalize an understanding of and a plan for adhering to recommended follow-up care including future appointments with health care provider.

NURSING/COLLABORATIVE DIAGNOSES

DISCHARGE TEACHING

1. Nursing Diagnosis: RISK FOR DECREASED CARDIAC OUTPUT

related to mechanical and/or electrical dysfunction of the heart associated with severe or prolonged myocardial ischemia.

Suggested NOC Outcomes: Circulation status; Cardiac pump effectiveness; Tissue perfusion: cardiac; Tissue perfusion: peripheral

Suggested NIC Interventions: Cardiac care: acute; Hemodynamic regulation; Cardiac precautions; Cardiac care: rehabilitative

Desired Outcome

1. The client will maintain adequate cardiac output as evidenced by:
   a. B/P within normal range for client
   b. apical pulse regular and between 60–100 beats/minute
   c. absence of gallop rhythm
   d. absence of fatigue and weakness
   e. unlabored respirations at 12–20/minute
   f. clear, audible breath sounds
   g. usual mental status
   h. absence of dizziness and syncope
   i. palpable peripheral pulses
   j. skin warm and usual color
   k. capillary refill time less than 2–3 seconds
   l. urine output at least 30 ml/hour
   m. absence of edema and jugular vein distention.

Nursing Actions *and Selected Purposes/Rationales*

(see pp. 20–24 for additional rationales)

1.a. Assess for and report signs and symptoms of decreased cardiac output:
   1. variations in B/P (may be increased because of pain or a compensatory response to low cardiac output; may be decreased when compensatory mechanisms and pump fail)
   2. tachycardia (may also be a response to pain)
   3. presence of gallop rhythm
   4. fatigue and weakness
   5. dyspnea, tachypnea
   6. crackles (rales)
   7. restlessness, change in mental status
   8. dizziness, syncope
   9. diminished or absent peripheral pulses
   10. cool extremities
   11. pallor or cyanosis of skin
   12. capillary refill time greater than 2–3 seconds
   13. oliguria
   14. edema
   15. jugular vein distention (JVD)
   16. chest x-ray results showing pulmonary vascular congestion, pulmonary edema, or pleural effusion
   17. abnormal blood gases
   18. a significant decrease in oximetry results.

b. Monitor for and report the following:
   1. ECG readings showing dysrhythmias or findings indicative of ischemia (e.g., ST segment depression or elevation, inverted T waves)
   2. an elevation in cardiac enzymes (e.g., CK-MB, troponin).

c. Implement measures *to help maintain an adequate cardiac output:*
   1. perform actions *to improve myocardial blood flow and oxygenation and subsequently reduce damage to the myocardium:*
      a. maintain oxygen therapy as ordered
      b. administer the following medications if ordered:
         1. nitrates (e.g., nitroglycerin, isosorbide) *to dilate the coronary and peripheral (primarily venous) blood vessels, thereby improving myocardial blood flow and reducing cardiac workload and myocardial oxygen consumption*
         2. beta-adrenergic blocking agents (e.g., atenolol, nadolol, metoprolol, propranolol) *to reduce myocardial oxygen requirements by decreasing the heart rate and force of myocardial contractility*
         3. calcium-channel blockers (e.g., verapamil, diltiazem, amlodipine, bepridil, nicardipine) *to dilate the coronary arteries and also reduce cardiac workload by dilating peripheral vessels*
         4. anticoagulants (e.g., intravenous heparin, dalteparin, enoxaparin) and antiplatelet agents (e.g., low-dose aspirin, glycoprotein IIb/IIIa receptor inhibitor [e.g., tirofiban, eptifibatide, abciximab], clopidogrel) *to prevent obstruction of the coronary artery(ies) by thrombosis*

c. prepare client for percutaneous coronary intervention (e.g., balloon angioplasty, atherectomy, intracoronary stenting) or coronary artery bypass grafting (CABG) if planned
2. perform additional actions *to reduce cardiac workload:*
   a. implement measures *to promote emotional and physical rest* (e.g., maintain a calm, quiet environment; limit the number of visitors; maintain activity restrictions)
   b. instruct client to avoid activities that create a Valsalva response (e.g., straining to have a bowel movement, holding breath while moving up in bed)
   c. discourage excessive intake of beverages high in caffeine such as coffee, tea, and colas *(caffeine is a myocardial stimulant and can increase myocardial oxygen consumption)*
   d. discourage smoking *(nicotine has a cardiostimulatory effect and causes vasoconstriction; the carbon monoxide in smoke reduces oxygen availability)*
   e. increase activity gradually as allowed and tolerated.

2. NURSING DIAGNOSIS:

ACUTE PAIN: RADIATING OR NONRADIATING CHEST PAIN/DISCOMFORT

related to decreased myocardial oxygenation (an insufficient oxygen supply forces the myocardium to convert to anaerobic metabolism; the end products of anaerobic metabolism act as irritants to myocardial neural receptors).

Suggested NOC Outcomes: Comfort level; Pain control

Suggested NIC Interventions: Pain management; Analgesic administration

Desired Outcome	Nursing Actions *and Selected Purposes/Rationales* (see pp. 45–47 for additional rationales)
2. The client will experience relief of chest pain/discomfort as evidenced by: a. verbalization of same b. relaxed facial expression and body positioning c. increased participation in activities d. stable vital signs.	2.a. Assess for signs and symptoms of pain/discomfort (e.g., verbalization of pain; grimacing; rubbing neck, jaw, or arm; reluctance to move; clutching chest; restlessness; diaphoresis; increased B/P; tachycardia). b. Assess client's perception of the severity of the pain/discomfort using an intensity rating scale. c. Assess the client's pattern of pain/discomfort (e.g., location, quality, onset, duration, precipitating factors, aggravating factors, alleviating factors). d. Implement measures *to relieve pain/discomfort:* 1. administer nitroglycerin as ordered 2. maintain oxygen therapy as ordered *to increase the myocardial oxygen supply* 3. maintain client on bed rest in a semi- to high Fowler's position 4. administer a narcotic (opioid) analgesic (e.g., morphine sulfate) as ordered if pain/discomfort is unrelieved by rest and nitroglycerin within 15–20 minutes (narcotic analgesics are usually administered intravenously *because intramuscular injections are poorly absorbed if tissue perfusion is decreased; intramuscular injections also elevate some serum enzyme levels, which makes assessment of myocardial damage more difficult)* 5. provide or assist with nonpharmacologic measures for relief of discomfort (e.g., position change, relaxation techniques, restful environment). e. Consult physician if pain/discomfort persists or worsens. f. Implement measures to help maintain an adequate cardiac output (see Diagnosis 1, action c) *in order to improve myocardial blood flow and oxygenation and subsequently prevent recurrent episodes of angina.*

3. COLLABORATIVE DIAGNOSES:

POTENTIAL COMPLICATIONS

a. **cardiac dysrhythmias** related to myocardial irritability associated with myocardial hypoxia;
b. **myocardial infarction** related to prolonged myocardial ischemia.

Desired Outcomes	Nursing Actions *and Selected Purposes/Rationales*
3.a. The client will maintain normal sinus rhythm as evidenced by: 1. regular apical pulse at 60–100 beats/minute 2. equal apical and radial pulse rates 3. absence of syncope and palpitations 4. ECG showing normal sinus rhythm.	3.a.1. Assess for and report signs and symptoms of cardiac dysrhythmias (e.g., irregular apical pulse; pulse rate below 60 or above 100 beats/minute; apical-radial pulse deficit; syncope; palpitations; abnormal rate, rhythm, or configurations on ECG). 2. Implement measures to help maintain an adequate cardiac output (see Diagnosis 1, action c) *in order to improve myocardial blood flow and oxygenation and subsequently reduce the risk for dysrhythmias.* 3. If cardiac dysrhythmias occur: a. initiate cardiac monitoring if not already being done b. administer antidysrhythmics (e.g., lidocaine, procainamide, amiodarone, esmolol, adenosine, diltiazem, verapamil) if ordered c. restrict client's activity based on his/her tolerance and severity of the dysrhythmia d. maintain oxygen therapy as ordered e. assess cardiovascular status frequently and report signs and symptoms of inadequate cardiac output (see Diagnosis 1, action a) f. have emergency cart readily available for cardioversion, defibrillation, or cardiopulmonary resuscitation.
3.b. The client will not experience a myocardial infarction as evidenced by: 1. resolution of chest pain within 15–20 minutes 2. stable vital signs 3. cardiac enzymes within normal range 4. absence of ST segment depression or elevation, T wave inversion, and abnormal Q waves on ECG.	3.b.1. Assess for and report signs and symptoms of a myocardial infarction (e.g., chest pain that lasts longer than 20 minutes; increase in pulse rate; significant change in B/P; labored respirations; elevation of cardiac enzymes [e.g., CK-MB, troponin]; ST segment depression or elevation, T wave inversion, and/or abnormal Q waves on ECG [ST segment elevation can also occur in Prinzmetal's angina]). 2. Implement measures to help maintain an adequate cardiac output (see Diagnosis 1, action c) *in order to improve myocardial blood flow and oxygenation and subsequently reduce the risk for a myocardial infarction.* 3. If signs and symptoms of a myocardial infarction occur: a. initiate cardiac monitoring if not already being done b. maintain client on strict bed rest in a semi- to high Fowler's position c. maintain oxygen therapy as ordered d. administer the following medications if ordered: 1. morphine sulfate *to reduce pain and anxiety and decrease cardiac workload* 2. nitrates *to improve coronary blood flow and reduce myocardial oxygen requirements* 3. beta-adrenergic blocking agents *to reduce myocardial oxygen requirements by decreasing the heart rate and force of myocardial contractility* e. prepare client for the following procedures that may be performed *to improve myocardial blood flow:* 1. injection of a thrombolytic agent (e.g., streptokinase, alteplase [tPA], anistreplase [APSAC, Eminase], reteplase, tenecteplase [TNK-tPA]) 2. percutaneous coronary intervention (e.g., balloon angioplasty, atherectomy, intracoronary stenting) or coronary artery bypass grafting [CABG] 3. insertion of an intra-aortic balloon pump (IABP).

4. Nursing Diagnosis: ***FEAR/ANXIETY***

related to discomfort during angina attack and threat of recurrent attacks; lack of understanding of diagnostic tests, diagnosis, and treatment plan; unfamiliar environment; and effect of angina pectoris on future lifestyle and roles.

Suggested NOC Outcomes:
Anxiety self-control; Anxiety level, Fear level; Fear self-control

Suggested NIC Interventions: Anxiety reduction; Calming technique; Emotional support; Presence; Pain management

Desired Outcome	**Nursing Actions** *and Selected Purposes/Rationales* (see pp. 14–16 for additional rationales)

4. The client will experience a reduction in fear and anxiety as evidenced by:
   a. verbalization of feeling less anxious
   b. usual sleep pattern
   c. relaxed facial expression and body movements
   d. stable vital signs
   e. usual perceptual ability and interactions with others.

4.a. Assess client for signs and symptoms of fear and anxiety (e.g., verbalization of feeling anxious, insomnia, tenseness, shakiness, restlessness, diaphoresis, tachycardia, elevated blood pressure, self-focused behaviors).
  b. Implement measures *to reduce fear and anxiety:*
    1. provide care in a calm, supportive, confident manner
    2. if client is having severe pain:
       a. do not leave him/her alone during period of acute distress
       b. perform actions to relieve pain (see Diagnosis 2, action d)
    3. once period of acute distress has subsided:
       a. orient client to environment, equipment, and routines; include an explanation of cardiac monitoring equipment
       b. keep cardiac monitor out of client's view and the sound turned as low as possible
       c. introduce client to staff who will be participating in care; if possible, maintain consistency in staff assigned to his/her care
       d. assure client that staff members are nearby; respond to call signal as soon as possible
       e. encourage verbalization of fear and anxiety; provide feedback
       f. explain all diagnostic tests
       g. reinforce physician's explanations and clarify misconceptions the client has about angina pectoris, the treatment plan, and prognosis; stress to client that he/she has not had a "heart attack"
       h. reinforce physician's explanation of percutaneous coronary intervention procedures (e.g., balloon angioplasty, atherectomy, intracoronary stenting) if planned
       i. initiate preoperative teaching if heart surgery is planned
       j. provide a calm, restful environment
       k. instruct client in relaxation techniques and encourage participation in diversional activities
       l. provide information based on current needs of client at a level he/she can understand; encourage questions and clarification of information provided
       m. assist client to identify specific stressors and ways to cope with them
       n. allow client to discuss concerns about future lifestyle and roles; focus on the need for alteration in rather than elimination of activities
       o. encourage significant others to project a caring, concerned attitude without obvious anxiousness
       p. include significant others in orientation and teaching sessions and encourage their continued support of the client
       q. administer prescribed antianxiety agents if indicated.
  c. Consult appropriate health care provider (e.g., psychiatric nurse clinician, physician) if above actions fail to control fear and anxiety.

Discharge Teaching/Continued Care

5. NURSING DIAGNOSIS: ***DEFICIENT KNOWLEDGE, INEFFECTIVE THERAPEUTIC REGIMEN MANAGEMENT, OR INEFFECTIVE HEALTH MAINTENANCE****

*The nurse should select the diagnostic label that is most appropriate for the client's discharge teaching needs.

Suggested NOC Outcomes: Knowledge: treatment regimen; Knowledge: cardiac disease management

Suggested NIC Interventions: Teaching: individual; Teaching: disease process; Teaching: prescribed activity/exercise; Teaching: prescribed medication; Health system guidance

Desired Outcomes	**Nursing Actions** *and Selected Purposes/Rationales*
5.a. The client will verbalize a basic understanding of angina pectoris.	5.a. Explain angina pectoris in terms that client can understand. Utilize teaching aids (e.g., pamphlets, diagrams) whenever possible.
5.b. The client will identify factors that may precipitate angina attacks and ways to control these factors.	5.b.1. Ask client if there is a pattern to angina attacks and precipitating factors. 2. Inform the client of factors that may precipitate angina pectoris (e.g., strenuous or isometric exercises, change in usual sexual habits and/or partner, consumption of a large meal, exposure to extreme cold, strong emotions, smoking). 3. Provide the following instructions regarding ways to reduce risk of precipitating an angina attack: a. take nitroglycerin before strenuous activity or sexual intercourse and during times of high emotional stress b. gradually increase activity by engaging in a regular aerobic exercise program (e.g., walking, biking, swimming) c. avoid strenuous exercise and activities that involve pushing or lifting heavy objects (e.g., weight lifting) d. avoid exercising for at least an hour after eating and exercise with caution at higher altitude and when the environmental temperature is extremely hot or cold e. avoid tobacco use before exercise f. rest between activities g. stop any activity that causes shortness of breath, palpitations, dizziness, or extreme fatigue or weakness h. begin a cardiovascular fitness program if recommended by physician i. adhere to the following precautions regarding sexual activity: 1. avoid intercourse for at least 1–2 hours after a heavy meal or alcohol consumption and when fatigued or stressed 2. engage in sexual activity in a familiar environment and in a position that minimizes exertion (e.g., side-lying, partner on top); recognize that a new sexual relationship can be started but may result in greater energy expenditure initially 3. avoid hot or cold showers just before and after intercourse.
5.c. The client will identify modifiable cardiovascular risk factors and ways to alter these factors.	5.c.1. Inform client that certain modifiable factors such as elevated serum lipids, a sedentary lifestyle, hypertension, and smoking have been shown to increase the risk for coronary artery disease. 2. Assist client to identify changes in lifestyle that can help him/her to eliminate or reduce the above risk factors and help to manage angina (e.g., dietary modification, physical exercise on a regular basis, moderation of alcohol intake, smoking cessation). 3. Encourage client to limit daily alcohol consumption (daily alcohol intake exceeding 1 oz of ethanol may contribute to the development of hypertension and some forms of heart disease). Current recommendations are no more than 2 drinks/day for men and no more than 1 drink/day for women and lighter weight persons. A "drink" is considered to be ½ oz of ethanol (e.g., 1½ oz of 80-proof whiskey, 12 oz of beer, 5 oz of wine).

Outcome	Intervention
5.d. The client will verbalize an understanding of the rationale for and components of a diet designed to lower serum cholesterol and triglycerides.	5.d.1. Explain the rationale for a diet low in saturated fat and cholesterol. 2. Provide instructions on ways the client can reduce intake of saturated fat and cholesterol: a. reduce intake of meat fat (e.g., trim visible fat off meat; replace fatty meats such as fatty cuts of steak, hamburger, and processed meats with leaner products) b. reduce intake of milk fat (avoid dairy products containing more than 1% fat) c. reduce intake of *trans* fats (e.g., avoid stick margarine and shortening and foods such as commercial baked goods that are prepared with these products) d. use vegetable oil rather than coconut or palm oil in cooking and food preparation e. use cooking methods such as steaming, baking, broiling, poaching, microwaving, and grilling rather than frying f. restrict intake of eggs (recommendations about the number of whole eggs allowed per week vary depending on the client's lipid levels). 3. Encourage client to increase intake of omega-3 fatty acids (e.g., flaxseed, cold water ocean fish such as salmon and halibut) to help lower triglycerides and increase high density lipoproteins (HDLs).
5.e. The client will demonstrate accuracy in counting pulse.	5.e.1. Teach client how to count his/her pulse, being alert to the regularity of the rhythm. 2. Allow time for return demonstration and accuracy check.
5.f. The client will verbalize an understanding of medications ordered including rationale, food and drug interactions, side effects, schedule for taking, and importance of taking as prescribed.	5.f.1. Explain the rationale for, side effects of, and importance of taking the medications prescribed. Inform client of pertinent food and drug interactions. 2. If client is discharged on sublingual or transmucosal nitroglycerin tablets or nitroglycerin translingual spray, instruct to: a. limit intake of alcoholic beverages b. have tablets or spray readily available at all times c. take a tablet or use spray before strenuous activity and in emotionally stressful situations d. take one tablet or spray 1–2 metered doses into mouth when chest pain occurs and repeat every 5 minutes up to a total of 3 times if necessary; notify physician or obtain emergency medical assistance if pain persists e. place sublingual tablet under tongue or transmucosal tablet between the gum and cheek (buccal cavity) or gum and upper lip and allow to dissolve completely; do not chew or swallow tablets f. store tablets in a tightly capped, dark-colored glass container away from heat and moisture g. replace tablets 6 months after the container is opened or sooner if they do not relieve discomfort h. avoid rising to a standing position quickly after taking nitroglycerin in order to reduce dizziness associated with its vasodilatory effect i. recognize that dizziness, flushing, and mild headache may occur after taking nitroglycerin j. report fainting, persistent or severe headache, blurred vision, or dry mouth. 3. If nitroglycerin skin patches are prescribed: a. provide instructions about correct application, skin care, need to rotate sites and remove old patch, and frequency of change; explain that the patch should be removed for an 8–12 hour period of time each day per physician's instructions in order to help prevent the development of nitrate tolerance b. caution client that activities that increase blood flow to the skin (e.g., hot bath or shower, sauna) can cause a sudden reduction in blood pressure c. instruct client to limit intake of alcoholic beverages

Desired Outcomes	Nursing Actions *and Selected Purposes/Rationales*
	d. instruct client to notify health care provider if faintness, dizziness, or flushing occurs following application or if persistent redness or itching occurs at patch site. 4. If client is discharged on a beta-adrenergic blocking agent (e.g., propranolol, metoprolol, atenolol, nadolol), instruct to: a. take the medication at the same time every day b. check pulse before taking medication; consult health care provider if pulse rate is unusually slow (it is expected that pulse will be lower than normal) c. avoid skipping doses, trying to make up for missed doses, altering the prescribed dose, and discontinuing medication without first discussing with health care provider d. change from a lying to a sitting or standing position slowly if dizziness or lightheadedness is a problem e. limit intake of alcoholic beverages f. monitor blood glucose on a regular basis if a diabetic (beta blockers may affect blood sugar and mask symptoms of hypoglycemia) g. wear a medical alert identification bracelet or tag specifying the name of the medication being taken h. report the following: 1. persistent lightheadedness or dizziness 2. significant weight gain, night cough, difficulty breathing, or swelling of feet or ankles (may be indicative of heart failure) 3. cold, painful toes or fingers 4. persistent fatigue, depression, insomnia, or sexual dysfunction 5. worsening of any symptoms of chronic respiratory disease. 5. If client is discharged on a calcium-channel blocker (e.g., amlodipine, bepridil, nicardipine, verapamil, diltiazem), instruct to: a. avoid skipping doses, altering the prescribed dose, and discontinuing medication without first discussing it with health care provider b. change from a lying to a sitting or standing position slowly in order to prevent dizziness c. report any increase in frequency, duration, or severity of angina d. report persistent dizziness, lightheadedness, or headache; swelling of feet or ankles; shortness of breath; or weight gain of more than 2 pounds in a day e. check pulse before taking medication if taking verapamil or diltiazem and report pulse rate that is unusually slow (e.g., less than 50 beats per minute) f. avoid operating dangerous equipment and driving as long as dizziness is present (common in the early treatment period). 6. Instruct client to take lipid-lowering agents (e.g., HMG-CoA reductase inhibitors ["statins"], gemfibrozil, ezetimibe, niacin) and antiplatelet agents (e.g., aspirin, clopidogrel) as prescribed. 7. Instruct client to consult physician before taking other prescription and nonprescription medications. 8. Instruct client to inform all health care providers of medications being taken.
5.g. The client will state signs and symptoms to report to the health care provider.	5.g. Stress the importance of reporting the following signs and symptoms: 1. chest, arm, neck, or jaw discomfort unrelieved by rest and/or nitroglycerin taken every 5 minutes for 15 minutes 2. shortness of breath 3. irregular pulse or a resting pulse less than 56 or greater than 100 beats/minute (the rate the client should report may vary depending on the medication[s] prescribed, the client's baseline pulse, and physician's preference) 4. fainting spells 5. diminished activity tolerance

6. swelling of feet or ankles
7. increase in severity or frequency of angina attacks.

5.h. The client will identify community resources that can assist in making necessary lifestyle changes and adjusting to the effects of angina pectoris.

5.h.1. Provide information about community resources that can assist client in making lifestyle changes and adjusting to effects of angina pectoris (e.g., weight loss, smoking cessation, and stress management programs; American Heart Association; counseling services).
2. Initiate a referral if indicated.

5.i. The client will verbalize an understanding of and a plan for adhering to recommended follow-up care including future appointments with health care provider.

5.i.1. Reinforce the importance of keeping follow-up appointments with health care provider.
2. Implement measures to improve client compliance:
   a. include significant others in teaching sessions if possible
   b. encourage questions and allow time for reinforcement and clarification of information provided
   c. provide written instructions regarding future appointments with health care provider, dietary modifications, activity level, medications prescribed, and signs and symptoms to report.

Bibliography

See pages 879 and 881–882.

evolve

Cardiac Dysrhythmias

Cardiac dysrhythmias are disturbances in the normal heart rate or rhythm that are caused by a disorder in the initiation and/or conduction of intrinsic electrical impulses. Dysrhythmias can be classified according to the site of impulse formation and the site or degree of conduction block. Supraventricular dysrhythmias (e.g., sinus arrhythmia, sinus tachycardia, sinus bradycardia, premature atrial contractions, atrial flutter, atrial fibrillation, junctional rhythm) originate above the ventricle. Ventricular rhythms (e.g., premature ventricular contractions, idioventricular rhythm, ventricular tachycardia, Torsades de pointes, ventricular fibrillation) originate in the ventricle. Impulse conduction defects (e.g., first-degree AV block, second-degree AV block, third-degree AV block, bundle branch block) result from a delay or block in the transmission of impulses. Causes of dysrhythmias include myocardial ischemia, cardiomyopathy, valvular heart disease, hypoxemia, electrolyte and acid-base imbalances, thyroid dysfunction, certain medications, infection, anemia, excessive caffeine or alcohol intake, smoking, pain, and emotional distress.

Dysrhythmias vary in severity and their effect on cardiac function. They can be benign and require no treatment or be life-threatening. The etiological factors and the clinical significance of the dysrhythmia determine the therapeutic management. Drug therapy is often successful at controlling a dysrhythmia. Other treatment options, depending on the type and severity of the dysrhythmia, include electrical cardioversion, a pacemaker, an implantable cardioverter-defibrillator, radiofrequency catheter ablation, surgery (e.g., elimination of offending area of myocardium by surgical excision, cryosurgery, or laser; maze procedure), and cardiopulmonary resuscitation and defibrillation.

This care plan focuses on the adult client needing acute management of a dysrhythmia in a medical setting.

OUTCOME/DISCHARGE CRITERIA

THE CLIENT WILL:

- have fewer or no dysrhythmias
- have adequate cardiac output and tissue perfusion
- tolerate expected level of activity
- have no signs and symptoms of complications
- verbalize a basic understanding of cardiac dysrhythmias
- demonstrate accuracy in counting pulse
- verbalize an understanding of medications ordered including rationale, food and drug interactions, side effects, schedule for taking, and importance of taking as prescribed
- verbalize an understanding of ways to avoid precipitating or exacerbating dysrhythmias
- state signs and symptoms to report to the health care provider
- verbalize an understanding of and a plan for adhering to recommended follow-up care including activity restrictions and future appointments with health care provider.

NURSING/COLLABORATIVE DIAGNOSES

DISCHARGE TEACHING

1. Nursing Diagnosis: *RISK FOR DECREASED CARDIAC OUTPUT*

related to:

a. a slow heart rate (if client has a bradydysrhythmia);
b. decreased ventricular filling and emptying associated with a rapid and/or irregular heart rate.

Suggested NOC Outcomes:
Cardiac pump effectiveness; Circulation status

Suggested NIC Interventions: Cardiac care; Cardiac precautions; Dysrhythmia management

Desired Outcome

1. The client will maintain adequate cardiac output as evidenced by:
   a. B/P within normal range for client
   b. apical pulse between 60–100 beats/minute and more regular
   c. absence of gallop rhythm
   d. no reports of fatigue and weakness
   e. unlabored respirations at 12–20/minute
   f. clear, audible breath sounds
   g. usual mental status
   h. absence of dizziness and syncope
   i. palpable peripheral pulses
   j. skin warm and usual color
   k. capillary refill time less than 2–3 seconds
   l. urine output at least 30 ml/hour
   m. absence of edema and jugular vein distention.

Nursing Actions *and Selected Purposes/Rationales*

(see pp. 20–24 for additional rationales)

1.a. Assess for signs and symptoms of:
   1. dysrhythmias:
      a. ECG showing rate less than 60 or greater than 100 beats/minute, an irregular rhythm, or missed or ectopic beats
      b. palpitations
      c. dizziness or syncope
      d. apical-radial pulse deficit
   2. decreased cardiac output:
      a. variations in B/P (may be increased because of compensatory vasoconstriction; may be decreased when compensatory mechanisms and pump fail)
      b. presence of gallop rhythm
      c. fatigue and weakness
      d. dyspnea, orthopnea, tachypnea
      e. crackles (rales)
      f. restlessness, change in mental status
      g. dizziness, syncope
      h. diminished or absent peripheral pulses
      i. cool extremities
      j. pallor or cyanosis of skin
      k. capillary refill time greater than 2–3 seconds
      l. oliguria
      m. edema
      n. jugular vein distention
      o. chest x-ray results showing pulmonary vascular congestion, pleural effusion, or pulmonary edema
      p. significant decrease in oximetry results.

b. Prepare client for an electrophysiological study (EPS) if planned *to help determine the cause and treatment options for the dysrhythmias.*

c. Implement measures *to maintain an adequate cardiac output:*
   1. perform actions *to treat cardiac dysrhythmias:*
      a. administer antidysrhythmic agents (e.g., lidocaine, procainamide, flecainide, digoxin, amiodarone, sotalol, ibutilide, dofetilide, esmolol, propranolol, diltiazem, verapamil, adenosine, magnesium sulfate)
      b. administer anticholinergic agents (e.g., atropine) or sympathomimetics (e.g., epinephrine) *to increase heart rate if client has a bradydysrhythmia*
      c. assist with vagal maneuvers (e.g., carotid sinus massage) if performed *to slow the heart rate*
      d. assist with cardioversion or defibrillation if performed
      e. prepare client for the following procedures if planned:
         1. insertion of a pacemaker or implantable cardioverter-defibrillator (ICD)
         2. radiofrequency catheter ablation
         3. surgery (e.g., maze procedure, endocardial resection, "corridor" procedure)
   2. perform actions *to reduce cardiac workload:*
      a. place client in a semi- to high Fowler's position
      b. instruct client to avoid activities such as straining to have a bowel movement and holding breath while moving up in bed *(if client has a bradydysrhythmia, the Valsalva maneuver not only increases cardiac workload but can also slow the heart rate)*
      c. implement measures to promote rest and conserve energy (see Diagnosis 2, action b.1)

Desired Outcome	Nursing Actions *and Selected Purposes/Rationales*
	d. maintain oxygen therapy as ordered e. discourage smoking *(nicotine has a cardiostimulatory effect and causes vasoconstriction; the carbon monoxide in smoke reduces oxygen availability, which not only increases cardiac workload but contributes to myocardial irritability)* f. discourage excessive intake of beverages high in caffeine such as coffee, tea, and colas *(caffeine is a myocardial stimulant and can increase myocardial irritability)* g. increase activity gradually as allowed and tolerated. d. Consult physician if signs and symptoms of decreased cardiac output develop and persist or worsen.

2. Nursing Diagnosis: *RISK FOR ACTIVITY INTOLERANCE*

related to:
a. tissue hypoxia if cardiac output is decreased;
b. difficulty resting and sleeping associated with frequent assessments and treatments, fear, and anxiety.

Suggested NOC Outcomes: Activity tolerance; Rest; Energy Conservation; Self-care: activities of daily living

Suggested NIC Interventions: Energy management; Oxygen therapy; Sleep enhancement; Cardiac care

Desired Outcome	Nursing Actions *and Selected Purposes/Rationales* (see pp. 11–12 for additional rationales)
2. The client will not experience activity intolerance as evidenced by: a. no reports of fatigue or weakness b. ability to perform activities of daily living without exertional dyspnea, chest pain, diaphoresis, dizziness, and a significant change in vital signs.	2.a. Assess for signs and symptoms of activity intolerance: 1. statements of fatigue or weakness 2. exertional dyspnea, chest pain, diaphoresis, or dizziness 3. abnormal heart rate response to activity (e.g., increase in rate of 20 beats/minute above resting rate, rate not returning to preactivity level within 3 minutes after stopping activity, change from regular to irregular rate) 4. a significant change (15–20 mm Hg) in blood pressure with activity. b. Implement measures *to prevent activity intolerance:* 1. perform actions *to promote rest and/or conserve energy:* a. maintain activity restrictions as ordered b. minimize environmental activity and noise c. organize nursing care to allow for periods of uninterrupted rest d. limit the number of visitors and their length of stay e. assist client with self-care activities as needed f. keep supplies and personal articles within easy reach g. instruct client in energy-saving techniques (e.g., using shower chair when showering, sitting to brush teeth or comb hair) h. implement measures to reduce fear and anxiety (see Diagnosis 5, action b) i. implement measures *to promote sleep* (e.g., encourage relaxing diversional activities in the evening, allow client to continue usual sleep practices unless contraindicated, reduce environmental distractions, administer prescribed sedative-hypnotics) 2. perform actions to maintain an adequate cardiac output (see Diagnosis 1, action c) 3. maintain oxygen therapy as ordered 4. increase client's activity gradually as allowed and tolerated. c. Instruct client to: 1. report a decreased tolerance for activity

2. stop any activity that causes chest pain, shortness of breath, dizziness, or extreme fatigue or weakness.

d. Consult appropriate health care provider (e.g., cardiac rehabilitation therapist, physician) if signs and symptoms of activity intolerance develop and persist or worsen.

3. NURSING DIAGNOSIS:

RISK FOR FALLS

related to:

a. lightheadedness, dizziness, or syncope associated with inadequate cerebral blood flow resulting from decreased cardiac output and the hypotensive effect of some antidysrhythmic agents;

b. weakness and fatigue that can occur with decreased cardiac output.

Suggested NOC Outcomes: Falls occurrence; Fall prevention behavior

Suggested NIC Intervention: Fall prevention

Desired Outcome	**Nursing Actions** *and Selected Purposes/Rationales*
3. The client will not experience falls.	3.a. Implement measures *to prevent falls:* 1. perform actions *to maintain adequate cerebral blood flow:* a. implement measures to maintain an adequate cardiac output (see Diagnosis 1, action c) b. consult physician before giving diuretics and medications with a negative inotropic or vasodilatory effect if client is hypotensive 2. encourage client to request assistance whenever needed; have call signal within easy reach 3. accompany client during ambulation 4. provide ambulatory aids (e.g., walker) if client is weak or unsteady on feet 5. instruct and assist client to rise and change positions slowly *in order to reduce lightheadedness and dizziness associated with postural hypotension* 6. perform actions to increase strength and help prevent activity intolerance (see Diagnosis 2, action b) 7. make sure that shower has a nonslip bottom surface and that shower chair, secure bath mat, grab bars, and adequate lighting are present. b. Include client and significant others in planning and implementing measures to prevent falls. c. If client falls, initiate first aid measures if appropriate and notify physician.

4. COLLABORATIVE DIAGNOSES:

POTENTIAL COMPLICATIONS OF DYSRHYTHMIAS

a. **systemic arterial embolization** related to:
   1. formation of thrombi in the heart associated with stasis of blood in the heart resulting from ineffective contractions (particularly a risk for clients in atrial fibrillation)
   2. dislodgment of existing thrombi from the heart associated with a sudden restoration of coordinated mechanical contractions (a concern following cardioversion);

b. **heart failure** related to the decreased cardiac output that can occur with a rapid, irregular, or slow heart rate;

c. **sudden cardiac death (SCD)** related to a lack of effective electrical and mechanical activity in the heart.

Desired Outcomes	**Nursing Actions** *and Selected Purposes/Rationales*
4.a. The client will not experience systemic arterial embolization as evidenced by: 1. absence of new or unusual pain in extremities 2. usual temperature and color of extremities 3. palpable and equal peripheral pulses 4. usual mental status 5. usual sensory and motor function 6. absence of sudden chest pain and dyspnea.	4.a.1. Assess for and report signs and symptoms of: a. arterial embolus in an extremity (e.g., diminished or absent peripheral pulses; pallor, coolness, numbness, and/or pain in extremity) b. cerebral embolism (e.g., decreased level of consciousness, alteration in usual sensory and motor function) c. pulmonary embolism (e.g., sudden chest pain, dyspnea, restlessness or apprehension, significant decrease in Sao_2). 2. Implement measures *to reduce the risk of thrombus formation in the heart and the subsequent risk for arterial embolization:* a. perform actions to treat cardiac dysrhythmias (see Diagnosis 1, action c.1) b. administer anticoagulants (e.g., warfarin) and/or antiplatelet agents (e.g., low-dose aspirin) if ordered. 3. If signs and symptoms of an arterial embolus in an extremity occur: a. maintain client on bed rest with affected extremity in a level or slightly dependent position *to improve arterial blood flow* b. prepare client for diagnostic studies (e.g., Doppler or duplex ultrasound, arteriography) if planned c. prepare client for the following if planned: 1. injection of a thrombolytic agent (e.g., streptokinase) 2. embolectomy d. administer anticoagulants (e.g., heparin, warfarin) as ordered. 4. If signs and symptoms of cerebral embolism occur: a. maintain client on bed rest (head of bed should be flat if systolic B/P is less than 90 mm Hg); keep head and neck in neutral, midline position b. maintain oxygen therapy as ordered c. administer anticoagulants (e.g., heparin, warfarin) as ordered. 5. If signs and symptoms of pulmonary embolism occur: a. maintain client on bed rest in a semi- to high Fowler's position b. maintain oxygen therapy as ordered c. prepare client for diagnostic tests (e.g., blood gases, D-dimer level, ventilation-perfusion lung scan, pulmonary angiography) d. administer anticoagulants (e.g., heparin, warfarin) as ordered e. prepare client for the following if planned: 1. injection of a thrombolytic agent (e.g., streptokinase, urokinase, alteplase [tPA]) 2. vena caval interruption (e.g., insertion of an intracaval filtering device) *to prevent further pulmonary emboli* 3. embolectomy.
4.b. The client will not develop heart failure as evidenced by: 1. absence of an S_3 heart sound 2. usual mental status 3. clear, audible breath sounds 4. absence of dyspnea, orthopnea, and a cough 5. no reports of increased fatigue and weakness 6. palpable peripheral pulses 7. urine output at least 30 ml/hour 8. stable weight 9. absence of edema and distended neck veins.	4.b.1. Assess for and report signs and symptoms of heart failure: a. presence of an S_3 heart sound b. restlessness, agitation, confusion, or other change in mental status c. crackles (rales) d. dyspnea, orthopnea e. dry, hacking cough or cough productive of frothy or blood-tinged sputum f. development of or increased weakness and fatigue g. diminished or absent peripheral pulses h. decreased urine output during the day, nocturia i. weight gain j. edema k. distended neck veins l. chest x-ray results showing pulmonary vascular congestion, pleural effusion, or pulmonary edema. 2. Implement measures to maintain adequate cardiac output (see Diagnosis 1, action c) *in order to prevent heart failure.* 3. If signs and symptoms of heart failure occur: a. maintain oxygen therapy as ordered

b. administer the following medications if ordered:
   1. positive inotropic agents (e.g., dopamine, dobutamine, digoxin) *to increase myocardial contractility*
   2. diuretics, vasodilators (e.g., nitroglycerin), and/or ACE inhibitors (e.g., captopril, ramipril) *to decrease cardiac workload*
   3. morphine sulfate *to reduce preload and anxiety* (used primarily in clients with pulmonary edema).

4.c. The client will not experience sudden cardiac death as evidenced by:
1. stable vital signs
2. palpable peripheral pulses
3. usual mental status
4. no evidence of cardiac arrest (flat line) or ventricular defibrillation on ECG.

4.c.1. Assess for and immediately report signs and symptoms of sudden cardiac death:
a. pulselessness (ECG may continue to show electrical activity, which is referred to as pulseless electrical activity)
b. very low or no B/P
c. unresponsiveness
d. ECG showing long pauses, flat line, or ventricular fibrillation.

2. Implement measures to treat cardiac dysrhythmias (see Diagnosis 1, action c.1) *in order to reduce the risk for sudden cardiac death.*
3. If signs and symptoms of sudden cardiac death occur, initiate CPR and call a "code."

5. NURSING DIAGNOSIS: ***FEAR/ANXIETY***

related to:
a. symptoms being experienced as a result of the dysrhythmias (e.g., palpitations, dizziness, shortness of breath);
b. possibility of sudden death;
c. possible changes in lifestyle and roles;
d. unfamiliar environment and separation from significant others;
e. lack of understanding of diagnostic tests, diagnosis, and treatment modalities;
f. financial concerns about the cost of hospitalization, lifelong medication therapy, and/or invasive treatment modalities (e.g., insertion of a pacemaker or implantable cardioverter-defibrillator).

Suggested NOC Outcomes: Anxiety level; Anxiety self-control; Fear level; Fear self-control

Suggested NIC Interventions: Anxiety reduction; Calming technique; Presence; Emotional support

Desired Outcome

Nursing Actions *and Selected Purposes/Rationales* (see pp. 14–16 for additional rationales)

5. The client will experience a reduction in fear and anxiety as evidenced by:
a. verbalization of feeling less anxious
b. usual sleep pattern
c. relaxed facial expression and body movements
d. stable vital signs
e. usual perceptual ability and interactions with others.

5.a. Assess client for signs and symptoms of fear and anxiety (e.g., verbalization of feeling anxious, insomnia, tenseness, shakiness, restlessness, diaphoresis, increased pulse rate, self-focused behaviors).

b. Implement measures *to reduce fear and anxiety:*
   1. orient client to environment, equipment, and routines
   2. introduce client to staff who will be participating in care; if possible, maintain consistency in staff assigned to his/her care
   3. provide care in a calm, supportive, and confident manner
   4. assure client that staff members are nearby; respond to call signal as soon as possible
   5. encourage verbalization of fear and anxiety; provide feedback
   6. keep cardiac monitor out of client's view and the sound turned as low as possible
   7. explain all diagnostic tests
   8. reinforce physician's explanations and clarify misconceptions about cardiac dysrhythmias, the treatment plan, and prognosis
   9. provide a calm, restful environment

Desired Outcome	**Nursing Actions** *and Selected Purposes/Rationales*
	10. instruct client in relaxation techniques and encourage participation in diversional activities 11. assist client to identify specific stressors and ways to cope with them 12. allow client to discuss concerns about possible changes in lifestyle and roles and the possibility of sudden death; focus on the fact that current treatment modalities (e.g., medications, pacemakers, cardioverter-defibrillators, catheter ablation) have greatly improved the prognosis for persons with dysrhythmias 13. provide information based on current needs of client at a level he/she can understand; encourage questions and clarification of information provided 14. encourage significant others to project a caring, concerned attitude without obvious anxiousness 15. include significant others in orientation and teaching sessions and encourage their continued support of the client 16. administer prescribed antianxiety agents if indicated. c. Consult appropriate health care provider (e.g., psychiatric nurse clinician, physician) if the above actions fail to control fear and anxiety.

Discharge Teaching/Continued Care

6. Nursing Diagnosis: ***DEFICIENT KNOWLEDGE, INEFFECTIVE THERAPEUTIC REGIMEN MANAGEMENT, OR INEFFECTIVE HEALTH MAINTENANCE****

*The nurse should select the diagnostic label that is most appropriate for the client's discharge teaching needs.

Suggested NOC Outcome: Knowledge: treatment regimen

Suggested NIC Interventions: Teaching: individual; Teaching: disease process; Teaching: prescribed medications; Health system guidance

Desired Outcomes	**Nursing Actions** *and Selected Purposes/Rationales*
6.a. The client will verbalize a basic understanding of cardiac dysrhythmias.	6.a. Explain cardiac dysrhythmias in terms the client can understand. Use appropriate teaching aids (e.g., pictures, videotapes).
6.b. The client will demonstrate accuracy in counting pulse.	6.b.1. Teach client how to count his/her pulse, being alert to the regularity of the rhythm. 2. Allow time for return demonstration and accuracy check.
6.c. The client will verbalize an understanding of medications ordered including rationale, food and drug interactions, side effects, schedule for taking, and importance of taking as prescribed.	6.c.1. Explain the rationale for and importance of taking the medications prescribed. 2. Provide client with written instructions that include a schedule of times to take medications, the side effects to be alert for, and pertinent food and drug interactions. 3. Caution client to avoid driving and other hazardous activities if experiencing dizziness or lightheadedness. 4. Instruct client to: a. limit intake of alcoholic beverages because of the blood pressure lowering effects of alcohol and many antidysrhythmic agents b. change from a lying to sitting or standing position slowly if dizziness or lightheadedness is a problem c. avoid skipping doses, trying to make up for missed doses, altering the prescribed dose, and discontinuing medication without first discussing it with health care provider

d. check pulse before taking medication if medication prescribed is known to slow pulse (e.g., sotalol, amiodarone, diltiazem, verapamil) and consult health care provider if pulse is unusually slow
e. wear or carry medical identification specifying the name of the medication being taken
f. consult physician before taking other prescription and nonprescription medications
g. inform all health care providers of medications being taken.

6.d. The client will verbalize an understanding of ways to avoid precipitating or exacerbating dysrhythmias.

6.d. Provide client with the following information about ways to reduce the risk for precipitating or exacerbating dysrhythmias:
1. if client has a bradydysrhythmia, instruct to avoid activities that stimulate the vagus nerve (e.g., putting pressure on carotid artery or on eyes, bearing down or straining during a bowel movement, performing activities that involve using arms over head for a prolonged time)
2. if client has a tachydysrhythmia, instruct to:
   a. avoid activities that have a cardiostimulatory effect (e.g., drinking caffeinated beverages, smoking)
   b. avoid stressful situations whenever possible and develop and use stress management techniques (stress has a cardiostimulatory effect)
   c. eat foods high in potassium (e.g., bananas, cantaloupe, potatoes, raisins, avocados) and take prescribed potassium supplement if taking a potassium-depleting diuretic.

6.e. The client will state signs and symptoms to report to the health care provider.

6.e. Instruct the client to report:
1. any significant change in the rate or rhythm of pulse, particularly a rate of less than 50 or greater than 100 and increased irregularity
2. significant weight gain or swelling of feet or ankles
3. shortness of breath or a persistent cough
4. unusual weakness or fatigue
5. persistent lightheadedness or dizziness or any fainting episodes
6. increased awareness of being able to feel the heart beating (palpitations)
7. chest, arm, neck, jaw, or back discomfort.

6.f. The client will verbalize an understanding of and a plan for adhering to recommended follow-up care including activity restrictions and future appointments with health care provider.

6.f.1. Reinforce the importance of keeping follow-up appointments with health care provider.
2. Reinforce instructions from the cardiac rehabilitation therapist and physician about activity level.
3. Implement measures to improve client compliance:
   a. include significant others in teaching sessions if possible
   b. encourage questions and allow time for reinforcement and clarification of information provided
   c. provide written instructions on future appointments with health care provider, activity progression, medications prescribed, and signs and symptoms to report.

Bibliography

See pages 879 and 881–882.

Cardioverter-Defibrillator Implantation

Implantable cardioverter-defibrillators (ICDs) are small battery-powered devices that monitor the heart rate and deliver electrical impulses to the heart to help correct dysrhythmias. An ICD consists of a pulse generator (contains the battery and electronic circuitry) and electrode catheters (leads). It is implanted during a minor surgical procedure under local anesthesia. The leads are inserted into the heart transvenously via the subclavian, jugular, or cephalic vein. The leads are then tunneled under the skin and attached to the pulse generator that is implanted in a subcutaneous pocket created in the subclavicular area or, less commonly, in the abdomen. A combined pacemaker and cardioverter-defibrillator device is also available.

Implantable cardioverter-defibrillators are used to treat life-threatening dysrhythmias. They are indicated for persons who have survived one or more incidents of sudden cardiac death, persons with recurrent ventricular tachycardia or ventricular fibrillation, and for persons with demonstrated risk factors for sudden cardiac death. The sensing lead of an ICD monitors the heart's electrical activity and if the heart rate exceeds the generator's programmed rate, the generator delivers a burst of antitachycardia pacing (ATP) to override the heart's pacemaker. If after a programmed number of ATP therapies, the rate continues to exceed the desired rate, the ICD device then delivers low-energy and high-energy cardioversion shocks. If ventricular fibrillation is present, defibrillation shocks are delivered.

This care plan focuses on the adult client admitted for implantation of a cardioverter-defibrillator.

OUTCOME/DISCHARGE CRITERIA

THE CLIENT WILL:

- have adequate cardiac output
- have no signs and symptoms of postoperative complications
- verbalize a basic understanding of the rationale for and function of an ICD
- demonstrate knowledge of how to monitor ICD function
- verbalize an understanding of appropriate actions to take if the ICD delivers a shock
- verbalize an understanding of recommended activity restrictions
- identify appropriate safety precautions associated with having an ICD
- state signs and symptoms to report to the health care provider
- verbalize an understanding of and a plan for adhering to recommended follow-up care including future appointments with health care provider, medications prescribed, and wound care.

NURSING/COLLABORATIVE DIAGNOSES

Preoperative

1. Risk for decreased cardiac output p. 321
2. Fear/Anxiety p. 321

Postoperative

1. Potential complications p. 322
   a. implantable cardioverter-defibrillator (ICD) malfunction
   b. cardiac tamponade
   c. pneumothorax

DISCHARGE TEACHING

2. Deficient knowledge; Ineffective therapeutic regimen management, or Ineffective health maintenance p. 323

See Standardized Preoperative and Postoperative Care Plans (pp. 97–126) for additional diagnoses.

PREOPERATIVE

Use in conjunction with the Standardized Preoperative Care Plan.

1. NURSING DIAGNOSIS: RISK FOR DECREASED CARDIAC OUTPUT

related to decreased diastolic filling time and ineffective ventricular contractions if client has sustained ventricular tachycardia or ventricular fibrillation.

Suggested NOC Outcomes: Circulation status; Cardiac pump effectiveness

Suggested NIC Interventions: Cardiac care; Cardiac precautions; Dysrhythmia management; Tissue perfusion: cardiac

Desired Outcome

1. The client will maintain an adequate cardiac output as evidenced by:
   a. systolic B/P of at least 90 mm Hg
   b. palpable peripheral pulses
   c. no increase in number or duration of dizziness or syncopal episodes
   d. usual mental status
   e. absence of cyanosis
   f. urine output at least 30 ml/hour.

Nursing Actions *and Selected Purposes/Rationales*

(see pp. 20–24 for additional rationales)

1.a. Assess for and report the following:
   1. ECG showing sustained ventricular tachycardia or ventricular fibrillation
   2. signs and symptoms of a significant decrease in cardiac output:
      a. systolic B/P below 90 mm Hg
      b. absent peripheral pulses
      c. prolonged or increased frequency of dizziness or syncopal episodes
      d. decline in mental status
      e. cool extremities
      f. cyanosis
      g. oliguria
      h. significant decrease in oximetry results.

b. Implement measures *to maintain an adequate cardiac output before surgery:*
   1. perform actions *to reduce cardiac workload:*
      a. place client in a semi- to high Fowler's position unless systolic B/P is less than 90 mm Hg (then head of bed should be flat)
      b. implement measures *to promote rest* (e.g., reduce fear and anxiety, maintain activity restrictions, limit the number of visitors)
      c. maintain oxygen therapy as ordered
      d. discourage smoking *(nicotine has a cardiostimulatory effect and causes vasoconstriction; the carbon monoxide in smoke reduces oxygen availability)*
   2. instruct client to avoid activities that create a Valsalva response (e.g., straining to have a bowel movement, holding breath while moving up in bed) *in order to prevent the sudden increase in cardiac workload that occurs with exhalation*
   3. administer antidysrhythmics (e.g., amiodarone, lidocaine, sotalol, procainamide) if ordered
   4. notify physician if serum potassium level is abnormal *(abnormal potassium levels affect myocardial conductivity)*
   5. consult physician before giving prescribed digitalis preparations *(digitalis preparations can increase ventricular irritability)*
   6. prepare for and assist with cardioversion or defibrillation if performed.

2. NURSING DIAGNOSIS: FEAR/ANXIETY

related to unfamiliar environment, lack of understanding of surgical procedure, anticipated postoperative discomfort, possibility of ICD malfunction, and possible changes in lifestyle as a result of having an ICD.

Suggested NOC Outcomes: Anxiety level; Anxiety self-control; Fear level; Fear self-control

Suggested NIC Interventions: Anxiety reduction; Emotional support; Teaching: preoperative

Desired Outcome	Nursing Actions *and Selected Purposes/Rationales* (see pp. 14–16 for additional rationales)
2. The client will experience a reduction in fear and anxiety (see Standardized Preoperative Care Plan, Diagnosis 1 [pp. 97–98], for outcome criteria).	2.a. Refer to Standardized Preoperative Care Plan, Diagnosis 1 (pp. 97–98), for measures related to assessment and reduction of fear and anxiety. b. Implement additional measures *to reduce fear and anxiety:* 1. explain the rationale for and function of an ICD; utilize diagrams, pamphlets, and show client an actual cardioverter-defibrillator if available 2. explain that the procedure will be performed using local anesthesia 3. if client is to receive an antimicrobial agent before surgery, explain that these medications are often given before and for a short time after surgery to reduce the risk for infection 4. inform client that cardioverter-defibrillators are electrically safe and are not harmed during usual daily activities 5. inform client of the expected life span of the particular cardioverter-defibrillator to be implanted; explain that only the generator will need to be replaced when the battery gets weak 6. discuss the client's concerns regarding whether his/her occupation and hobbies can be continued safely with an ICD in place; if the occupation or interests involve contact sports or contact with high-voltage electrical equipment and large magnets or electromagnetic fields, instruct him/her to consult physician about the safety of continuing these activities.

POSTOPERATIVE

Use in Conjunction with the Standardized Postoperative Care Plan.

1. Collaborative Diagnoses: POTENTIAL COMPLICATIONS OF CARDIOVERTER-DEFIBRILLATOR IMPLANTATION

a. **implantable cardioverter-defibrillator (ICD) malfunction** related to improper placement or dislodgment of the leads, break in or faulty attachment of the leads, or pulse generator malfunction;
b. **cardiac tamponade** related to perforation of the atria or ventricle by the cardioverter-defibrillator leads;
c. **pneumothorax** related to accumulation of air in the pleural space associated with accidental puncture of the pleura during subclavian insertion of the cardioverter-defibrillator leads.

Desired Outcomes	Nursing Actions *and Selected Purposes/Rationales*
1.a. The client will experience normal cardioverter-defibrillator function as evidenced by: 1. absence of sustained ventricular dysrhythmias on ECG 2. client reports of receiving internal shocks when ventricular tachycardia or fibrillation is evident on the ECG.	1.a.1. Ascertain the type of ICD the client has and how it is programmed (including the rate at which pacing should occur if a combination pacemaker/cardioverter-defibrillator was implanted). Have information available about problem-solving techniques and activation and deactivation of the specific device. 2. Assess for and report signs and symptoms of cardioverter-defibrillator malfunction (e.g., ECG showing rapid and/or irregular rate without accompanying antitachycardia pacing, presence of sustained ventricular tachycardia or fibrillation on ECG, client reports of receiving multiple shocks without ECG evidence of tachydysrhythmia). 3. Implement measures *to reduce the risk for breakage and dislodgment of the ICD leads in order to prevent ICD malfunction:* a. maintain activity restrictions as ordered b. instruct client to limit movement of the arm and shoulder on the side that the ICD was inserted for the first 48 hours after surgery. 4. If signs and symptoms of ICD malfunction occur: a. if the device is activated and ventricular fibrillation or pulseless ventricular tachycardia occur: 1. notify the physician

2. proceed with external defibrillation (the defibrillation paddles should be positioned at least 3–4 inches away from the pulse generator)
3. administer antidysrhythmics (e.g., amiodarone, lidocaine) as ordered

b. if the device is activated and delivering inappropriate shocks:
1. notify the physician
2. have the physician or other trained personnel deactivate the device if ordered.

Desired Outcomes	Nursing Actions and Selected Purposes/Rationales
1.b. The client will not experience cardiac tamponade as evidenced by: 1. stable vital signs 2. audible heart sounds 3. absence of jugular vein distention.	1.b.1. Assess for and report signs and symptoms of: a. cardiac perforation (e.g., pericardial pain, pericardial friction rub) b. cardiac tamponade (e.g., significant decrease in B/P, narrowed pulse pressure, pulsus paradoxus, distant or muffled heart sounds, sense of fullness in chest, jugular vein distention). 2. Implement measures to prevent dislodgment of the cardioverter-defibrillator leads (see action a.3 in this diagnosis) *in order to reduce the risk for perforation of the heart wall.* 3. If signs and symptoms of cardiac perforation or tamponade occur: a. prepare client for chest x-ray and echocardiogram b. prepare client for repositioning or replacement of the lead(s), repair of perforation, and/or pericardiocentesis if planned.
1.c. The client will have resolution of pneumothorax if it occurs as evidenced by: 1. audible breath sounds and a resonant percussion note over lungs 2. normal respiratory rate and pattern 3. usual mental status 4. blood gases returning to normal range.	1.c.1. Assess for and immediately report signs and symptoms of pneumothorax (e.g., absent breath sounds with hyperresonant percussion note over involved area; rapid, shallow, and/or labored respirations; tachycardia; sudden onset of chest pain; restlessness; confusion; significant decrease in oximetry results; abnormal blood gases; chest x-ray results showing lung collapse). 2. If signs and symptoms of pneumothorax occur: a. maintain client on bed rest in a semi- to high Fowler's position b. maintain oxygen therapy as ordered c. assess for and immediately report signs and symptoms of tension pneumothorax with mediastinal shift (e.g., severe dyspnea, increased restlessness and agitation, rapid and/or irregular heart rate, hypotension, neck vein distention, shift in trachea from midline) d. prepare client for insertion of chest tube if indicated.

Discharge Teaching/Continued Care

2. NURSING DIAGNOSIS: ***DEFICIENT KNOWLEDGE, INEFFECTIVE THERAPEUTIC REGIMEN MANAGEMENT, OR INEFFECTIVE HEALTH MAINTENANCE****

*The nurse should select the diagnostic label that is most appropriate for the client's discharge teaching needs.

Suggested NOC Outcome: Knowledge: treatment regimen

Suggested NIC Interventions: Teaching: individual; Teaching: prescribed activity/exercise

Desired Outcomes	**Nursing Actions** *and Selected Purposes/Rationales*
2.a. The client will verbalize a basic understanding of the rationale for and function of an ICD.	2.a. Reinforce preoperative teaching regarding the rationale for and basic function of an ICD.

Desired Outcomes	**Nursing Actions** *and Selected Purposes/Rationales*
2.b. The client will demonstrate knowledge of how to monitor ICD function.	2.b.1. If client has a combined pacemaker/cardioverter-defibrillator device, inform him/her of pacemaker's programmed pacing rate and, if appropriate, provide instructions about how to take pulse and monitor both the rate and regularity. (Many physicians prefer that their clients not monitor their own pulse because of the confusion between paced beats and spontaneous beats.) 2. Instruct client with an ICD to monitor for and report the following: a. signs of a heart rhythm disturbance such as dizziness, fainting, shortness of breath, unexplained fatigue, or feeling that heart is fluttering b. shocks received from the ICD (shock is often described as a quick thud or feeling of being kicked in the chest). 3. Instruct client to have ICD function checked regularly per physician's instructions.
2.c. The client will verbalize an understanding of appropriate actions to take if the ICD delivers a shock.	2.c.1. Instruct client to call an ambulance or emergency rescue service and then to lie down if the ICD delivers a shock. 2. Instruct family members to call the client's physician and the ambulance or emergency rescue service if the client's ICD delivers a shock while they are present. Instruct them to get CPR training and to initiate CPR if the client is having symptoms such as an irregular and rapid pulse along with dizziness, shortness of breath, chest pain, sweatiness, or loss of consciousness and the device fails to fire after 30 seconds or if the device fires unsuccessfully 4–7 times.
2.d. The client will verbalize an understanding of recommended activity restrictions.	2.d.1. Provide the following instructions about activity restrictions following ICD insertion: a. limit movement of the arm and shoulder on the side of the ICD insertion for the first 48 hours after surgery b. limit activities that put undue stress on the incision site (e.g., using arms over head, bowling, racquetball, tennis, lifting over 25 pounds) until cleared by physician (usual time is 1–2 months) c. avoid letting anything rub on or hit the ICD d. do not rub or "play with" the ICD under the skin e. avoid immersing the ICD insertion site in water for at least 3 days after surgery f. avoid activities that can cause blunt trauma to the pulse generator (e.g., contact sports, firing a rifle with the butt end of the gun against affected shoulder). 2. Allow adequate time for questions and clarification of information provided.
2.e. The client will identify appropriate safety precautions associated with having an ICD.	2.e. Instruct client to adhere to the following safety precautions: 1. inform all health care providers about the ICD (certain medical equipment such as an MRI machine, radiation therapy machine, and electrocautery equipment may actually damage the pulse generator and/or interfere with normal function of these devices) 2. avoid close proximity with strong magnets (e.g., MRI machine, large industrial magnets), high voltage electrical equipment (e.g., arc welder, running car engine), and large electromagnetic fields (e.g., radio and television transmitters) 3. do not place any electrical device directly over ICD 4. move away from any electrical device if dizziness or lightheadedness occurs 5. if planning to travel, obtain name of a physician and/or pacemaker/ICD clinic at point(s) of destination 6. alert airport personnel to ICD (it may set off the security alarm) 7. always wear a medical alert bracelet or tag and carry an identification card that includes the name of the manufacturer, model number, mode of operation, and insertion date of the ICD

8. adhere to restrictions on driving; typically, clients are not allowed to drive until they have had a 6-month discharge-free period (this is a law in some states for persons with ICDs).

2.f. The client will state signs and symptoms to report to the health care provider.

2.f.1. Refer to Standardized Postoperative Care Plan, Diagnosis 22, action c (p. 125), for signs and symptoms to report to the health care provider.

2. Instruct client to report these additional signs and symptoms:
   a. increased irregularity of pulse (if self-monitoring is being done) or episodes of feeling that heart is fluttering
   b. unexplained fatigue
   c. lightheadedness, dizziness, fainting
   d. shortness of breath
   e. redness, swelling, drainage, or increased soreness at implant site
   f. unexplained fever
   g. swelling of arm on the side of the ICD (may indicate venous thrombosis associated with insertion/presence of leads in vein).

2.g. The client will verbalize an understanding of and a plan for adhering to recommended follow-up care including future appointments with health care provider, medications prescribed, and wound care.

2.g.1. Refer to Standardized Postoperative Care Plan, Diagnosis 22 (pp. 125–126), for routine postoperative instructions and measures to improve client compliance.

2. Remind client of the importance of keeping scheduled appointments with pacemaker/ICD clinic and for chest x-ray verification of lead placement.

Bibliography

See pages 879 and 881–882.

evolve

Heart Failure

Heart failure is a syndrome in which the heart is unable to pump an adequate supply of blood to meet the body's metabolic needs. To compensate for decreased cardiac output, there is an increase in sympathetic nervous system activity and stimulation of renin-angiotensin-aldosterone output and ADH release. These neurohormonal compensatory mechanisms temporarily aid in maintaining an adequate cardiac output but are thought to contribute to cardiac remodeling (changes in the structure of the ventricle [e.g., dilation, hypertrophy]). The increase in fluid volume that results from increased aldosterone and ADH causes elevated pressure in the cardiac chambers, which stimulates the release of natriuretic peptides (atrial natriuretic factor [ANF] and brain natriuretic peptide [BNP]). These hormones counteract the effects of the increased levels of norepinephrine, renin, angiotensin II, and aldosterone and promote sodium and water excretion and vasodilation. Chronic distention of the heart chambers eventually exhausts stores of these natriuretic hormones and the effects of norepinephrine, renin, aldosterone, and ADH prevail, leading to heart failure.

Numerous conditions can lead to heart failure including coronary artery disease, myocardial infarction, cardiomyopathy, cardiac valve malfunction, hypertension, congenital heart defects, and systemic conditions that increase the metabolic rate (e.g., thyrotoxicosis, infection) or cause prolonged or severe hypoxia. Heart failure can be classified in a number of ways. It is often classified as left-sided or right-sided, backward or forward, and/or systolic or diastolic failure. A functional classification system based on the relationship between symptoms and the amount of activity needed to provoke the symptoms was developed by the New York Heart Association and is commonly used by many practitioners. In this system, which has 4 levels or classes, a person is said to have Class I heart failure if no symptoms are experienced with ordinary physical activity and Class IV failure when symptoms occur with any physical activity and possibly at rest.

Signs and symptoms of heart failure are dependent on which side of the heart is failing as well as whether there is forward or backward failure. Symptoms of forward failure are caused by low cardiac output. Symptoms of backward failure are associated with the ventricle failing to empty completely, which results in blood flow backup. In left-sided failure, there is reduced emptying of the left ventricle, which results in decreased systemic tissue perfusion as well as blood flow backup in the left atrium and pulmonary vasculature. Pulmonary vascular congestion leads to pulmonary edema with symptoms such as tachypnea, dyspnea, cough, and abnormal breath sounds. In right-sided failure, the effect of reduced function and emptying of the right ventricle is decreased pulmonary blood flow and backup of blood in the right atrium. This results in systemic venous congestion, which is manifested by peripheral edema and signs of major organ enlargement and dysfunction. Initially only one side of the heart may fail (more commonly the left side), but as failure progresses, both sides are usually affected.

The focus of treatment is to improve performance of the failing heart. Diuretic therapy and an angiotensin converting enzyme (ACE) inhibitor remain the cornerstone of treatment. A positive inotropic agent is often added to ameliorate symptoms. Recent studies have shown that the addition of a beta-adrenergic blocking agent and spironolactone also improve the clinical status of many persons with chronic heart failure. It is thought that ACE inhibitors, beta blockers, and spironolactone interfere with the compensatory neurohormonal activity that occurs with heart failure and alter the course of cardiac remodeling, subsequently slowing disease progression. The pharmacological treatment of heart failure varies somewhat depending on whether the client has systolic failure (an impaired inotropic state characterized by inadequate ventricular emptying) or diastolic failure (impaired filling of the ventricle). Positive inotropic agents are contraindicated for treatment of diastolic failure.

As long as the body's compensatory mechanisms and/ or treatment measures are able to maintain cardiac output that is sufficient to prevent or relieve symptoms, a state of compensated heart failure exists. If the myocardium is severely damaged and intrinsic compensatory mechanisms and treatment measures fail to maintain adequate cardiac output and tissue perfusion, a state of decompensated heart failure exists. When this state persists and is no longer responsive to medical treatment, it is termed intractable or refractory heart failure.

This care plan focuses on the adult client hospitalized for management of heart failure. Much of the information is applicable to clients receiving follow-up care in an extended care facility or home setting.

OUTCOME/DISCHARGE CRITERIA

THE CLIENT WILL:

- have vital signs within a safe range and evidence of adequate peripheral circulation
- tolerate expected level of activity without undue fatigue or dyspnea
- have achieved dry weight and have minimal or no edema
- have clear, audible breath sounds throughout lungs
- have oxygen saturation within normal limits for client's age
- identify modifiable cardiovascular risk factors and ways to alter these factors

- verbalize an understanding of the rationale for and components of a diet low in sodium
- demonstrate accuracy in counting pulse
- verbalize an understanding of medications ordered including rationale, food and drug interactions, side effects, schedule for taking, and importance of taking as prescribed
- state signs and symptoms to report to the health care provider
- identify community resources that can assist with home management and adjustment to changes resulting from heart failure
- share feelings and concerns about changes in body functioning and usual roles and lifestyle
- verbalize an understanding of and a plan for adhering to recommended follow-up care including future appointments with health care provider and activity limitations.

Use in Conjunction with the Care Plan on Immobility.

NURSING/COLLABORATIVE DIAGNOSES

DISCHARGE TEACHING

See pp. 342–343 and Care Plan on Immobility (pp. 129–148) for additional diagnoses.

1. NURSING DIAGNOSIS: ***DECREASED CARDIAC OUTPUT***

related to alterations in preload, afterload, and myocardial contractility associated with:

a. the cardiac condition causing the heart failure (e.g., ischemia of the myocardium, valve malfunction, cardiomyopathy);
b. the effects of sympathetic nervous system and renin-angiotensin-aldosterone stimulation that occur in response to decreased cardiac output;
c. structural changes in the heart (e.g., dilation, hypertrophy) that occur with prolonged activation of neurohormonal adaptive responses.

Suggested NOC Outcomes: Cardiac pump effectiveness; Circulation status; Tissue perfusion: peripheral

Suggested NIC Interventions: Cardiac care: acute; Invasive hemodynamic monitoring; Hemodynamic regulation; Cardiac precautions; Dysrhythmia management; Hypervolemia management; Cardiac care: rehabilitative

Desired Outcome

1. The client will have improved cardiac output as evidenced by:
   a. B/P within normal range for client
   b. apical pulse between 60–100 beats/minute and regular
   c. resolution of gallop rhythm
   d. verbalization of feeling less fatigued and weak
   e. unlabored respirations at 12–20/minute
   f. improved breath sounds
   g. usual mental status
   h. absence of dizziness and syncope
   i. palpable peripheral pulses
   j. skin warm and usual color
   k. capillary refill time less than 2–3 seconds
   l. urine output at least 30 ml/hour
   m. decrease in edema and jugular vein distention
   n. central venous pressure (CVP) within normal range.

Nursing Actions *and Selected Purposes/Rationales*

(see pp. 20–24 for additional rationales)

1.a. Assess for signs and symptoms of heart failure and decreased cardiac output:
   1. variations in B/P (may be increased because of compensatory vasoconstriction; may be decreased when compensatory mechanisms and pump fail)
   2. tachycardia
   3. pulsus alternans (alternating strong and weak pulse)
   4. presence of an S_3 heart sound
   5. fatigue and weakness
   6. dyspnea, orthopnea, tachypnea
   7. dry, hacking cough or cough productive of frothy or blood-tinged sputum
   8. abnormal breath sounds (e.g., crackles [rales], wheezes, diminished sounds)
   9. restlessness, change in mental status
   10. dizziness, syncope
   11. diminished or absent peripheral pulses
   12. cool extremities
   13. pallor or cyanosis of skin
   14. capillary refill time greater than 2–3 seconds
   15. decreased urine output during day, nocturia
   16. edema
   17. jugular vein distention (JVD)
   18. elevated serum levels of atrial natriuretic factor (ANF) and brain natriuretic peptide factor (BNP)
   19. increased CVP (use internal jugular vein pulsation method to estimate CVP if monitoring device not present)
   20. chest x-ray results showing pulmonary vascular congestion, pleural effusion, or pulmonary edema.

b. Implement measures *to improve cardiac output:*
   1. perform actions *to reduce cardiac workload:*
      a. place client in a semi- to high Fowler's position
      b. instruct client to avoid activities that create a Valsalva response (e.g., straining to have a bowel movement, holding breath while moving up in bed)
      c. implement measures *to promote emotional and physical rest* (e.g., maintain a calm, quiet environment; limit the number of visitors; maintain activity restrictions)
      d. implement measures to improve respiratory status (see Diagnosis 2, action b) *in order to improve alveolar gas exchange and promote adequate tissue oxygenation*
      e. discourage smoking *(nicotine has a cardiostimulatory effect and causes vasoconstriction; the carbon monoxide in smoke reduces oxygen availability)*
      f. provide small meals rather than large ones *(large meals can increase cardiac workload because they require a greater increase in blood supply to gastrointestinal tract for digestion)*
      g. discourage excessive intake of beverages high in caffeine such as coffee, tea, and colas *(caffeine is a myocardial stimulant and can increase myocardial oxygen consumption)*
      h. increase activity gradually as allowed and tolerated
      i. implement measures to reduce excess fluid volume (see Diagnosis 3, action a.4.a)
   2. administer the following medications if ordered:
      a. diuretics (e.g., furosemide, torsemide, bumetanide, spironolactone, eplerenone, metolazone) *to reduce sodium and water retention and subsequently reduce cardiac workload*

b. angiotensin-converting enzyme (ACE) inhibitors (e.g., captopril, trandolapril, fosinopril, quinapril, ramipril, enalapril, lisinopril) *to reduce vascular resistance and subsequently decrease cardiac workload; they also alter the course of cardiac remodeling and slow disease progression*
c. positive inotropic agents (e.g., digoxin, dopamine, milrinone, dobutamine) *to improve myocardial contractility*
d. beta-adrenergic blocking agents (e.g., carvedilol, metoprolol) *to blunt the effects of sympathetic nervous system stimulation on the heart and kidney*
e. B-type natriuretic peptide (nesiritide) *to promote diuresis and vasodilation*
f. vasodilators (e.g., nitrates, hydralazine) *to reduce cardiac workload.*

c. Consult physician if signs and symptoms of decreased cardiac output persist or worsen.

2. NURSING DIAGNOSIS: IMPAIRED RESPIRATORY FUNCTION*

a. ineffective breathing pattern related to:
   1. increased rate of respirations associated with fear and anxiety
   2. decreased depth of respirations associated with:
      a. weakness, fatigue, and decreased mobility
      b. decreased lung compliance (distensibility) as a result of pleural effusion or accumulation of fluid in the pulmonary interstitium
      c. pressure on the diaphragm if ascites is present;
b. ineffective airway clearance related to:
   1. increased airway resistance associated with edema of the bronchial mucosa and pressure on the airways resulting from engorgement of the pulmonary vessels
   2. stasis of secretions associated with decreased mobility and poor cough effort;
c. impaired gas exchange related to:
   1. impaired diffusion of gases associated with accumulation of fluid in the pulmonary interstitium and alveoli
   2. decreased pulmonary tissue perfusion associated with decreased cardiac output.

*This diagnostic label includes the following nursing diagnoses: ineffective breathing pattern, ineffective airway clearance, and impaired gas exchange.

Suggested NOC Outcomes: Respiratory status: ventilation; Respiratory status: airway patency; Respiratory status: gas exchange

Suggested NIC Interventions: Respiratory monitoring; Airway management; Chest physiotherapy; Cough enhancement; Ventilation assistance; Oxygen therapy; Anxiety reduction

Desired Outcome	**Nursing Actions** *and Selected Purposes/Rationales* (see pp. 12–14, 18–20, and 33–35 for additional rationales)
2. The client will experience adequate respiratory function as evidenced by: a. normal rate, rhythm, and depth of respirations b. decreased dyspnea c. usual or improved breath sounds d. symmetrical chest excursion e. usual mental status f. oximetry results within normal range g. blood gases within normal range.	2.a. Assess for signs and symptoms of impaired respiratory function: 1. rapid, shallow, slow, or irregular respirations 2. dyspnea, orthopnea 3. use of accessory muscles when breathing 4. adventitious breath sounds (e.g., crackles [rales], wheezes) 5. diminished or absent breath sounds 6. dry, hacking cough or cough productive of frothy or blood-tinged sputum 7. limited chest excursion 8. restlessness, irritability 9. confusion, somnolence 10. central cyanosis (a late sign) 11. significant decrease in oximetry results 12. abnormal blood gases 13. abnormal chest x-ray results.

Desired Outcome	Nursing Actions *and Selected Purposes/Rationales*

b. Implement measures *to improve respiratory status:*
   1. perform actions to improve cardiac output (see Diagnosis 1, action b) *in order to improve pulmonary tissue perfusion and reduce fluid accumulation in the lungs*
   2. perform actions to reduce fear and anxiety (see Diagnosis 10, action b)
   3. instruct client to breathe slowly if hyperventilating
   4. place client in a semi- to high Fowler's position unless contraindicated; position overbed table so client can lean forward on it if desired
   5. instruct client to change position and deep breathe or use incentive spirometer every 1–2 hours
   6. perform actions to increase strength and activity tolerance (see Diagnosis 6, action b) *in order to increase client's willingness and ability to move, cough, deep breathe, and use incentive spirometer*
   7. perform actions *to promote removal of pulmonary secretions:*
      a. instruct and assist client to cough or "huff" every 1–2 hours
      b. humidify inspired air as ordered *to keep secretions thin*
   8. maintain oxygen therapy as ordered
   9. assist with positive airway pressure techniques (e.g., continuous positive airway pressure [CPAP], bilevel positive airway pressure [BiPAP], flutter/positive expiratory pressure [PEP] device) if ordered
   10. instruct client to avoid intake of gas-forming foods (e.g., beans, cauliflower, cabbage, onions), carbonated beverages, and large meals *in order to prevent gastric distention and an increase in pressure on the diaphragm*
   11. discourage smoking *(the irritants in smoke increase mucus production, impair ciliary function, and can cause damage to the bronchial and alveolar walls; the carbon monoxide decreases oxygen availability)*
   12. maintain activity restrictions; increase activity gradually as allowed and tolerated
   13. administer central nervous system depressants judiciously; hold medication and consult physician if respiratory rate is less than 12/minute
   14. administer the following medications if ordered:
      a. diuretics *to decrease fluid accumulation in the lungs*
      b. theophylline *to dilate the bronchioles (it also augments myocardial contractility and increases renal blood flow, which help increase cardiac output and promote diuresis, thereby leading to decreased pulmonary vascular congestion)*
      c. morphine sulfate *to decrease pulmonary vascular congestion in acute pulmonary edema (the vasodilatory action of morphine results in peripheral pooling of blood and a resultant decrease in cardiac workload, which improves left ventricular emptying and allows for increased blood return from the pulmonary veins); morphine also reduces the apprehension associated with dyspnea*
   15. assist with thoracentesis and/or paracentesis if performed *to allow increased lung expansion.*

c. Consult appropriate health care provider (e.g., physician, respiratory therapist) if signs and symptoms of impaired respiratory function persist or worsen.

3. Nursing/Collaborative Diagnosis:

RISK FOR IMBALANCED FLUID AND ELECTROLYTES

a. excess fluid volume related to:
   1. retention of sodium and water associated with a decreased glomerular filtration rate (GFR) and activation of the renin-angiotensin-aldosterone mechanism (both are a result of the reduced renal blood flow that occurs with decreased cardiac output)
   2. decreased excretion of water associated with increased ADH output (a compensatory response to decreased cardiac output);

b. third-spacing of fluid related to:
   1. increased intravascular pressure associated with excess fluid volume

2. low plasma colloid osmotic pressure if serum albumin is decreased as a result of malnutrition or impaired liver function (occurs with hepatic venous congestion);

c. hyponatremia related to:
   1. hemodilution associated with excess fluid volume
   2. sodium loss associated with diuretic therapy and increased release of natriuretic peptide hormones.

Suggested NOC Outcomes: Fluid balance; Fluid overload severity; Electrolyte and acid/base balance

Suggested NIC Interventions: Fluid monitoring; Fluid/electrolyte management; Electrolyte management: hyponatremia; Hypervolemia management

Desired Outcomes

3.a. The client will experience resolution of fluid imbalance as evidenced by:
1. decline in weight toward client's normal
2. B/P and pulse within normal range for client and stable with position change
3. resolution of S_3 heart sound
4. balanced intake and output
5. usual mental status
6. improved breath sounds
7. Hct returning toward normal range
8. decreased dyspnea and orthopnea
9. decrease in edema and ascites
10. resolution of neck vein distention
11. CVP within normal range.

Nursing Actions *and Selected Purposes/Rationales*

(see pp. 31–33 for additional rationales)

3.a.1. Assess for signs and symptoms of the following:
   a. excess fluid volume:
      1. weight gain of 2% or greater in a short period
      2. elevated B/P (B/P may not be elevated if cardiac output is poor or fluid has shifted out of the vascular space)
      3. presence of an S_3 heart sound
      4. intake greater than output
      5. change in mental status
      6. crackles (rales)
      7. low Hct (may be normal or even increased if fluid has shifted out of the vascular space)
      8. dyspnea, orthopnea
      9. edema
      10. distended neck veins
      11. elevated CVP (use internal jugular vein pulsation method to estimate CVP if monitoring device not present)
   b. third-spacing:
      1. ascites
      2. increased dyspnea and diminished or absent breath sounds
      3. evidence of vascular depletion (e.g., postural hypotension; weak, rapid pulse; decreased urine output).

2. Monitor chest x-ray results. Report findings of pulmonary vascular congestion, pleural effusion, or pulmonary edema.
3. Monitor serum albumin levels. Report below-normal levels *(low serum albumin levels result in fluid shifting out of the vascular space because albumin normally maintains plasma colloid osmotic pressure).*
4. Implement measures *to restore fluid balance:*
   a. perform actions *to reduce excess fluid volume:*
      1. restrict sodium intake as ordered
      2. maintain fluid restrictions if ordered
      3. implement measures to improve cardiac output (see Diagnosis 1, action b) *in order to improve renal blood flow and promote the excretion of water*
      4. if client is receiving numerous and/or large volume intravenous medications, consult pharmacist about ways to prevent excessive fluid administration (e.g., stop primary infusion during administration of intravenous medications, dilute medications in the minimum amount of solution)
      5. administer diuretics (e.g., furosemide, bumetanide, torsemide, metolazone, eplerenone, spironolactone) as ordered *to increase excretion of water*
   b. perform actions *to prevent further third-spacing and promote mobilization of fluid back into the vascular space:*
      1. implement measures to reduce excess fluid volume (see action a.4.a in this diagnosis)

Desired Outcomes | **Nursing Actions** *and Selected Purposes/Rationales*

2. administer albumin infusions if ordered *to increase colloid osmotic pressure*
c. assist with thoracentesis or paracentesis if performed *to remove excess fluid from the pleural space or peritoneal cavity.*
5. Consult physician if signs and symptoms of imbalanced fluid persist or worsen.

3.b. The client will maintain a safe serum sodium level as evidenced by:
1. absence of nausea, vomiting, and abdominal cramps
2. usual mental status
3. usual muscle strength
4. absence of seizure activity
5. serum sodium within normal range.

3.b.1. Assess for and report signs and symptoms of hyponatremia (e.g., nausea, vomiting, abdominal cramps, lethargy, confusion, weakness, seizures, low serum sodium level).
2. Implement measures *to treat hyponatremia:*
a. maintain fluid restrictions if ordered
b. consult physician about a decrease in or discontinuation of diuretic and temporary discontinuation of dietary sodium restriction if sodium level is significantly reduced
c. administer intravenous saline solution if ordered (if client's hyponatremia is thought to be due to "salt wasting," treatment includes administration of saline and discontinuation of diuretics).
3. Consult physician if signs and symptoms of hyponatremia persist or worsen.

4. NURSING DIAGNOSIS: *IMBALANCED NUTRITION: LESS THAN BODY REQUIREMENTS*

related to:
a. decreased oral intake associated with:
1. anorexia and nausea (result from venous congestion in the gastrointestinal tract and can occur if digitalis levels exceed a therapeutic level)
2. weakness, fatigue, dyspnea, and dislike of prescribed diet;
b. elevated metabolic rate associated with the increased oxygen needs of the heart and the increased work of breathing;
c. impaired absorption of nutrients associated with poor tissue perfusion.

Suggested NOC Outcome: Nutritional status

Suggested NIC Interventions: Nutritional monitoring; Nutrition management; Nutrition therapy

Desired Outcome | **Nursing Actions** *and Selected Purposes/Rationales* (see pp. 40–43 for additional rationales)

4. The client will maintain an adequate nutritional status as evidenced by:
a. dry weight within normal range for client (dry weight is achieved after excess fluid volume has been resolved)
b. normal BUN and serum albumin, prealbumin, Hct, Hgb, and lymphocyte levels
c. improved strength and activity tolerance
d. healthy oral mucous membrane.

4.a. Assess for and report signs and symptoms of malnutrition:
1. dry weight significantly below client's usual weight or below normal for client's age, height, and body frame
2. abnormal BUN and low serum albumin, prealbumin, Hct, Hgb, and lymphocyte levels
3. weakness and fatigue
4. sore, inflamed oral mucous membrane
5. pale conjunctiva.
b. Monitor percentage of meals and snacks client consumes. Report a pattern of inadequate intake.
c. Implement measures *to maintain an adequate nutritional status:*
1. perform actions *to improve oral intake:*
a. obtain a dietary consult if necessary to assist client in selecting foods/fluids that meet nutritional needs, are appealing, and adhere to personal and cultural preferences as well as the prescribed dietary modifications
b. encourage a rest period before meals *to minimize fatigue*
c. maintain a clean environment and a relaxed, pleasant atmosphere
d. provide oral hygiene before meals *(removes unpleasant tastes, which often improves the taste of foods/fluids)*

e. serve frequent, small meals rather than large ones if client is weak, fatigues easily, and/or has a poor appetite
f. place client in a high Fowler's position for meals and provide supplemental oxygen therapy during meals if indicated *to help relieve dyspnea*
g. instruct client to use herbs, spices, and salt substitutes if approved by physician or dietitian *in order to make low-sodium diet more palatable*
h. allow adequate time for meals; reheat foods/fluids if necessary
i. limit fluid intake with meals (unless the fluid has high nutritional value) *to reduce early satiety and subsequent decreased food intake*
j. increase activity as allowed and tolerated (*activity usually promotes a sense of well-being, which can improve appetite; it also promotes gastric emptying, which reduces feeling of fullness*)

2. perform actions to improve cardiac output (see Diagnosis 1, action b) *in order to increase the absorption of nutrients and reduce venous congestion in the gastrointestinal tract (helps prevent nausea and reduce feeling of fullness)*
3. ensure that meals are well balanced and high in essential nutrients; offer dietary supplements if indicated
4. administer vitamins and minerals if ordered.

d. Perform a calorie count if ordered. Report information to dietitian and physician.
e. Consult physician regarding an alternative method of providing nutrition (e.g., parenteral nutrition, tube feedings) if client does not consume enough food or fluids to meet nutritional needs.

5. NURSING DIAGNOSIS: RISK FOR IMPAIRED TISSUE INTEGRITY

related to:
a. damage to the skin and/or subcutaneous tissue associated with prolonged pressure on the tissues, friction, and/or shearing if mobility is decreased;
b. increased fragility of the skin associated with edema, poor tissue perfusion, and inadequate nutritional status.

Suggested NOC Outcome: Tissue integrity: skin and mucous membrane

Suggested NIC Interventions: Skin surveillance; Skin care: topical treatments; Positioning; Pressure ulcer prevention; Pressure management

Desired Outcome	**Nursing Actions** *and Selected Purposes/Rationales* (see pp. 49–52 for additional rationales)
5. The client will maintain tissue integrity as evidenced by: a. absence of redness and irritation b. no skin breakdown.	5.a. Inspect the skin, especially bony prominences and dependent and edematous areas, for pallor, redness, and breakdown. b. Refer to Care Plan on Immobility, Diagnosis 4, actions c and d (p. 133), for measures to prevent and treat tissue breakdown associated with decreased mobility. c. Implement additional measures *to prevent tissue breakdown:* 1. perform actions *to improve tissue perfusion and reduce edema:* a. implement measures to increase cardiac output (see Diagnosis 1, action b) b. implement measures to restore fluid balance (see Diagnosis 3, action a.4) 2. perform actions to maintain an adequate nutritional status (see Diagnosis 4, action c).

6. NURSING DIAGNOSIS: ACTIVITY INTOLERANCE

related to:
a. tissue hypoxia associated with impaired alveolar gas exchange and decreased cardiac output;
b. inadequate nutritional status;
c. difficulty resting and sleeping associated with dyspnea, frequent assessments and treatments, fear, and anxiety.

Suggested NOC Outcomes:
Activity tolerance; Self-care: activities of daily living; Energy conservation

Suggested NIC Interventions: Energy management; Oxygen therapy; Nutrition management; Sleep enhancement; Cardiac care: rehabilitative

Desired Outcome	Nursing Actions *and Selected Purposes/Rationales* (see pp. 11–12 for additional rationales)
6. The client will demonstrate an increased tolerance for activity as evidenced by: a. verbalization of feeling less fatigued and weak b. ability to perform activities of daily living without exertional dyspnea, chest pain, diaphoresis, dizziness, and a significant change in vital signs.	6.a. Assess for signs and symptoms of activity intolerance: 1. statements of fatigue or weakness 2. exertional dyspnea, chest pain, diaphoresis, or dizziness 3. abnormal heart rate response to activity (e.g., increase in rate of 20 beats/minute above resting rate, rate not returning to preactivity level within 3 minutes after stopping activity, change from regular to irregular rate) 4. a significant change (15–20 mm Hg) in blood pressure with activity. b. Implement measures *to improve activity tolerance:* 1. perform actions *to promote rest and/or conserve energy:* a. maintain activity restrictions as ordered b. minimize environmental activity and noise c. organize nursing care to allow for periods of uninterrupted rest d. limit the number of visitors and their length of stay e. assist client with self-care activities as needed f. keep supplies and personal articles within easy reach g. instruct client in energy-saving techniques (e.g., using shower chair when showering, sitting to brush teeth or comb hair) h. implement measures to reduce fear and anxiety (see Diagnosis 10, action b) i. implement measures to promote sleep (see Diagnosis 7) 2. perform actions to improve respiratory status (see Diagnosis 2, action b) *in order to decrease dyspnea and improve tissue oxygenation* 3. perform actions to increase cardiac output (see Diagnosis 1, action b) 4. perform actions to maintain an adequate nutritional status (see Diagnosis 4, action c) 5. increase client's activity gradually as allowed and tolerated; explain that activity is increased gradually *to prevent a sudden increase in cardiac workload.* c. Instruct client to: 1. report a decreased tolerance for activity 2. stop any activity that causes chest pain, a marked increase in shortness of breath, dizziness, or extreme fatigue or weakness. d. Consult appropriate health care provider (e.g., cardiac rehabilitation therapist, physician) if signs and symptoms of activity intolerance persist or worsen.

7. Nursing Diagnosis: DISTURBED SLEEP PATTERN

related to unfamiliar environment, frequent assessments and treatments, decreased physical activity, fear, anxiety, and inability to assume usual sleep position associated with orthopnea.

Suggested NOC Outcome:
Sleep

Suggested NIC Intervention: Sleep enhancement

Desired Outcome	Nursing Actions *and Selected Purposes/Rationales* (see pp. 52–54 for additional rationales)
7. The client will attain optimal amounts of sleep (see Care Plan on Immobility, Diagnosis 10 [p. 138], for outcome criteria).	7.a. Refer to Care Plan on Immobility, Diagnosis 10 (p. 138), for measures related to assessment and promotion of sleep. b. Implement additional measures *to promote sleep:* 1. perform actions to improve respiratory status (see Diagnosis 2, action b) *in order to relieve dyspnea* 2. if client has orthopnea, assist him/her to assume a position *that facilitates breathing* (e.g., head of bed elevated with arms supported on

pillows, resting forward on overbed table with good pillow support, sitting in chair)
3. maintain oxygen therapy during sleep if indicated
4. perform actions to reduce fear and anxiety (see Diagnosis 10, action b)
5. increase activity as allowed and tolerated during the day and early evening.

8. NURSING DIAGNOSIS:

RISK FOR FALLS

related to:
a. weakness;
b. dizziness and syncope associated with inadequate cerebral blood flow resulting from decreased cardiac output and the hypotensive effect of some medications (e.g., ACE inhibitors, diuretics);
c. getting up without assistance as a result of restlessness, agitation, forgetfulness, and confusion (can result from cerebral hypoxia and imbalanced fluid and electrolytes).

Suggested NOC Outcomes: Falls occurrence; Fall prevention behavior

Suggested NIC Intervention: Fall prevention

Desired Outcome	**Nursing Actions** *and Selected Purposes/Rationales*

8. The client will not experience falls.

8.a. Implement measures *to prevent falls:*
1. keep bed in low position with side rails up when client is in bed
2. keep needed items within easy reach
3. encourage client to request assistance whenever needed; have call signal within easy reach
4. use lap belt when client is in chair if indicated
5. instruct client to wear well-fitting slippers/shoes with nonslip soles and low heels when ambulating
6. keep floor free of clutter and wipe up spills promptly
7. accompany client during ambulation utilizing a transfer safety belt if he/she is weak or dizzy
8. provide ambulatory aids (e.g., walker, cane) if client is weak or unsteady on feet
9. instruct client to ambulate in well-lit areas and to utilize handrails if needed
10. do not rush client; allow adequate time for ambulation to the bathroom and in hallway
11. instruct and assist client to rise and change positions slowly *in order to reduce dizziness associated with postural hypotension*
12. perform actions to improve cardiac output (see Diagnosis 1, action b) *in order to improve cerebral blood flow and subsequently reduce dizziness, syncope, agitation, and confusion*
13. perform actions to restore fluid and electrolyte balance (see Diagnosis 3, actions a.4 and b.2) *in order to reduce the risk for changes in mental status that may result in the client getting up unassisted*
14. perform actions to increase strength and activity tolerance (see Diagnosis 6, action b)
15. make sure that shower has a nonslip bottom surface and that shower chair, secure bath mat, call signal, grab bars, and adequate lighting are present
16. administer central nervous system depressants judiciously
17. if client is confused or irrational:
    a. reorient frequently to surroundings and necessity of adhering to safety precautions
    b. provide appropriate level of supervision
    c. consult physician about the temporary use of a bed alarm or jacket or wrist restraints if necessary

Desired Outcome	Nursing Actions *and Selected Purposes/Rationales*
	d. administer prescribed antianxiety and antipsychotic medications if indicated. b. Include client and significant others in planning and implementing measures to prevent falls. c. If client falls, initiate first aid measures if appropriate and notify physician.

9. Collaborative Diagnoses: POTENTIAL COMPLICATIONS OF HEART FAILURE

a. renal insufficiency related to a prolonged or severe decrease in renal blood flow associated with low cardiac output, volume depletion (may result from third-spacing, increased output of natriuretic hormones, and/or excessive diuretic use), and vasodilator-induced hypotension;
b. cardiac dysrhythmias related to impaired nodal function and/or altered myocardial conductivity associated with hypoxia, sympathetic nervous system stimulation (a compensatory response to low cardiac output), structural changes in the myocardium (e.g., dilation, hypertrophy), and imbalanced electrolytes (particularly the magnesium and potassium depletion that can result from diuretic therapy);
c. acute pulmonary edema related to accumulation of fluid in the lungs associated with increased hydrostatic pressure in the pulmonary vessels as a result of blood flow back up in the left ventricle;
d. thromboembolism related to:
   1. venous stasis in the periphery associated with decreased cardiac output and decreased mobility
   2. stasis of blood in the heart associated with decreased ventricular emptying (risk increases if dysrhythmias are present);
e. cardiogenic shock related to inability of heart, intrinsic compensatory mechanisms, and treatments to maintain adequate tissue perfusion to vital organs.

Desired Outcomes	Nursing Actions *and Selected Purposes/Rationales*
9.a. The client will maintain adequate renal function as evidenced by: 1. urine output at least 30 ml/hour 2. BUN, serum creatinine, and creatinine clearance within normal range.	9.a.1. Assess for and report signs and symptoms of impaired renal function (e.g., urine output less than 30 ml/hour, urine specific gravity fixed at or less than 1.010, elevated BUN and serum creatinine levels, decreased creatinine clearance). 2. Implement measures *to maintain adequate renal blood flow:* a. perform actions to improve cardiac output (see Diagnosis 1, action b) b. perform actions to reduce third-spacing (see Diagnosis 3, action a.4.b) *in order to prevent hypovolemia* c. ensure a minimum fluid intake of 1000 ml/day unless ordered otherwise d. consult physician before giving vasodilators and diuretics if client is hypotensive. 3. If signs and symptoms of impaired renal function occur: a. consult physician about possible need to reduce the digitalis dosage *(digitalis is excreted by the kidney and will quickly reach toxic levels when renal function is impaired)* b. consult physician about lowering the dose of or discontinuing angiotensin-converting enzyme inhibitors and diuretics if BUN and serum creatinine continue to rise significantly (ACE inhibitors and many diuretics should be used cautiously in persons with impaired renal function *because they can have an adverse effect on renal function*) c. assess for and report signs of acute renal failure (e.g., oliguria or anuria; further weight gain; increasing edema; increased B/P; lethargy and confusion; increasing BUN and serum creatinine, phosphorus, and potassium levels) d. prepare client for dialysis if indicated.

9.b. The client will maintain normal sinus rhythm as evidenced by:
1. regular apical pulse at 60–100 beats/minute
2. equal apical and radial pulse rates
3. absence of syncope and palpitations
4. ECG reading showing normal sinus rhythm.

9.b.1. Assess for and report signs and symptoms of cardiac dysrhythmias (e.g., irregular apical pulse; pulse rate below 60 or above 100 beats/minute; apical-radial pulse deficit; syncope; palpitations; abnormal rate, rhythm, or configurations on ECG).
2. Implement measures *to prevent cardiac dysrhythmias:*
   a. perform actions to improve cardiac output (see Diagnosis 1, action b) *in order to promote adequate myocardial tissue perfusion and oxygenation*
   b. perform actions to improve respiratory status (see Diagnosis 2, action b) *in order to improve tissue oxygenation*
   c. consult physician regarding an order for a potassium or magnesium replacement if serum levels of either are below normal.
3. If cardiac dysrhythmias occur:
   a. initiate cardiac monitoring if not already being done
   b. administer antidysrhythmics (e.g., digoxin, amiodarone) if ordered
   c. restrict client's activity based on his/her tolerance and severity of the dysrhythmia
   d. maintain oxygen therapy as ordered
   e. assess cardiovascular status frequently and report signs and symptoms of a further decline in cardiac output and tissue perfusion
   f. prepare client for catheter ablation or insertion of a pacemaker or implantable cardioverter defibrillator (ICD) if planned
   g. have emergency cart readily available for cardioversion, defibrillation, or cardiopulmonary resuscitation.

9.c. The client will not develop acute pulmonary edema as evidenced by:
1. decreased dyspnea
2. usual or improved breath sounds
3. usual mental status
4. blood gases within normal range.

9.c.1. Assess for and report signs and symptoms of acute pulmonary edema:
   a. sudden development of or increased dyspnea or orthopnea
   b. development of or increased crackles (rales) or wheezes
   c. increased restlessness and anxiousness, disorientation
   d. cough productive of frothy or blood-tinged sputum
   e. significant decrease in oximetry results
   f. worsening blood gas results
   g. chest x-ray showing pulmonary edema.
2. Implement measures to improve cardiac output (see Diagnosis 1, action b) *in order to reduce pulmonary vascular congestion.*
3. If signs and symptoms of pulmonary edema occur:
   a. place client in a high Fowler's position unless contraindicated
   b. maintain oxygen therapy as ordered
   c. administer the following medications if ordered:
      1. diuretics (e.g., furosemide, bumetanide) *to reduce fluid accumulation in the lungs*
      2. theophylline *to dilate the bronchioles; it also increases cardiac and urine output, which subsequently reduces pulmonary vascular congestion*
      3. morphine sulfate *to reduce anxiety and decrease pulmonary vascular congestion (increases venous capacitance, which lowers venous return to the heart)*
      4. vasodilators (e.g., sodium nitroprusside, nitroglycerin) *to reduce afterload and improve left ventricular emptying, which reduces pulmonary blood flow backup.*

9.d. The client will not develop a thromboembolism as evidenced by:
1. absence of pain, tenderness, swelling, and numbness in extremities
2. usual temperature and color of extremities
3. palpable and equal peripheral pulses

9.d.1. Assess for and report signs and symptoms of:
   a. deep vein thrombus (e.g., pain, tenderness, swelling, unusual warmth, and/or positive Homans' sign in extremity)
   b. arterial embolus in an extremity (e.g., diminished or absent peripheral pulses; pallor, coolness, numbness, and/or pain in extremity)
   c. cerebral ischemia (e.g., decreased level of consciousness, alteration in usual sensory and motor function)
   d. pulmonary embolism (e.g., sudden onset of chest pain, increased dyspnea, increased restlessness and apprehension, significant decrease in Sao_2).

Desired Outcomes	Nursing Actions *and Selected Purposes/Rationales*
4. usual mental status 5. usual sensory and motor function 6. absence of sudden chest pain and increased dyspnea.	2. Implement measures to prevent and treat a deep vein thrombus and pulmonary embolism (see Care Plan on Immobility, Diagnosis 12, actions a.1.b and c and a.2.b and c [p. 140–141]). 3. Implement additional measures *to prevent the development of thromboemboli:* a. perform actions to improve cardiac output (see Diagnosis 1, action b) b. perform actions to treat cardiac dysrhythmias if present (see action b.3 in this diagnosis) c. administer anticoagulants (e.g., warfarin, low- or adjusted-dose heparin, low-molecular-weight heparin) or antiplatelet agents (e.g., low-dose aspirin) if ordered. 4. If signs and symptoms of an arterial embolus in an extremity occur: a. maintain client on bed rest with affected extremity in a level or slightly dependent position *to improve arterial blood flow* b. prepare client for the following if planned: 1. diagnostic studies (e.g., Doppler or duplex ultrasound, arteriography) 2. injection of a thrombolytic agent (e.g., streptokinase) 3. embolectomy c. administer anticoagulants (e.g., heparin, warfarin) as ordered. 5. If signs and symptoms of cerebral ischemia occur: a. maintain client on bed rest; keep head and neck in neutral, midline position b. administer anticoagulants (e.g., continuous intravenous heparin, warfarin) as ordered.
9.e. The client will not develop cardiogenic shock as evidenced by: 1. stable or improved mental status 2. systolic B/P greater than 80 mm Hg 3. palpable peripheral pulses 4. stable or improved skin temperature and color 5. urine output at least 30 ml/hour.	9.e.1. Assess for and immediately report signs and symptoms of cardiogenic shock: a. increased restlessness, lethargy, or confusion b. systolic B/P below 80 mm Hg c. rapid, weak pulse d. diminished or absent peripheral pulses e. increased coolness and duskiness or cyanosis of skin f. urine output less than 30 ml/hour. 2. Implement measures *to prevent cardiogenic shock:* a. perform actions to improve cardiac output (see Diagnosis 1, action b) b. perform actions to treat cardiac dysrhythmias if present (see action b.3 in this diagnosis). 3. If signs and symptoms of cardiogenic shock occur: a. maintain oxygen therapy as ordered b. administer the following medications if ordered: 1. sympathomimetics (e.g., dopamine, dobutamine, norepinephrine) *to increase cardiac output and maintain arterial pressure* 2. vasodilators (e.g., nitroglycerin) *to decrease cardiac workload* (the use of vasodilators will be determined by the client's blood pressure and pulmonary capillary wedge pressure [PCWP] and are usually not given if the systolic B/P or PCWP is low) c. assist with intubation and insertion of hemodynamic monitoring device (e.g., Swan-Ganz catheter) and intra-aortic balloon pump (IABP) if indicated.

10. Nursing Diagnosis: ***FEAR/ANXIETY***

related to:
a. exacerbation of symptoms and need for hospitalization;
b. lack of understanding of diagnostic tests, the diagnosis, and treatments;
c. cost of hospitalization and lifelong treatment;
d. possibility of early disability and death.

Suggested NOC Outcomes: Anxiety level; Fear level; Anxiety self-control; Fear self-control

Suggested NIC Interventions: Anxiety reduction; Calming technique; Emotional support; Presence; Financial resource assistance

Desired Outcome	**Nursing Actions** *and Selected Purposes/Rationales* (see pp. 14–16 for additional rationales)
10. The client will experience a reduction in fear and anxiety as evidenced by: a. verbalization of feeling less anxious b. usual sleep pattern c. relaxed facial expression and body movements d. stable vital signs e. usual perceptual ability and interactions with others.	10.a. Assess client for signs and symptoms of fear and anxiety (e.g., verbalization of feeling anxious, insomnia, tenseness, shakiness, restlessness, increased dyspnea, diaphoresis, tachycardia, elevated blood pressure, self-focused behaviors). Validate perceptions carefully, remembering that some behavior may result from tissue hypoxia or fluid imbalance. b. Implement measures *to reduce fear and anxiety:* 1. maintain a calm, supportive, confident manner when interacting with client 2. if client is in acute respiratory distress: a. do not leave him/her alone during this period b. perform actions to improve respiratory status (see Diagnosis 2, action b) c. perform actions *to reduce feeling of suffocation:* 1. open curtains and doors 2. limit the number of visitors in room at any one time 3. remove unnecessary equipment from room 4. administer oxygen via nasal cannula rather than mask if possible 3. encourage significant others to project a caring, concerned attitude without obvious anxiousness 4. once the period of acute respiratory distress has subsided: a. orient client to environment, equipment, and routines b. introduce client to staff who will be participating in care; if possible, maintain consistency in staff assigned to his/her care c. assure client that staff members are nearby; respond to call signal as soon as possible d. provide a calm, restful environment e. keep cardiac monitor out of client's view and the sound turned as low as possible f. encourage verbalization of fear and anxiety; provide feedback g. explain all diagnostic tests h. reinforce physician's explanations and clarify misconceptions the client has about heart failure, the treatment plan, and prognosis i. instruct client in relaxation techniques and encourage participation in diversional activities j. initiate a social service referral and/or assist client to identify and contact appropriate community resources if indicated k. provide information based on current needs of client at a level he/she can understand; encourage questions and clarification of information provided l. include significant others in orientation and teaching sessions and encourage their continued support of the client m. administer prescribed antianxiety agents if indicated. c. Consult appropriate health care provider (e.g., psychiatric nurse clinician, physician) if above actions fail to control fear and anxiety.

Discharge Teaching/Continued Care

11. NURSING DIAGNOSIS: ***DEFICIENT KNOWLEDGE, INEFFECTIVE THERAPEUTIC REGIMEN MANAGEMENT, OR INEFFECTIVE HEALTH MAINTENANCE****

*The nurse should select the diagnostic label that is most appropriate for the client's discharge teaching needs.

Suggested NOC Outcomes:
Knowledge: disease process; Knowledge: treatment regimen; Knowledge: cardiac disease management

Suggested NIC Interventions: Teaching: individual; Teaching: disease process; Teaching: prescribed medication; Teaching: prescribed diet; Teaching: prescribed activity/exercise; Health system guidance

Desired Outcomes	Nursing Actions *and Selected Purposes/Rationales*
11.a. The client will identify modifiable cardiovascular risk factors and ways to alter these factors.	11.a.1. Inform client that certain modifiable factors such as elevated serum lipids, excessive alcohol intake, a sedentary lifestyle, hypertension, and smoking have been shown to increase the risk for coronary artery disease and certain forms of heart disease. 2. Assist client to identify changes in lifestyle that can help him/her to manage the above risk factors (e.g., dietary modification, physical exercise on a regular basis, moderation of alcohol intake, smoking cessation). 3. Encourage client to limit daily alcohol consumption (daily alcohol intake exceeding 1 oz of ethanol may contribute to the development of hypertension and some forms of heart disease). Current recommendations are no more than 2 drinks/day for men and no more than 1 drink/day for women and lighter weight persons. A "drink" is considered to be ½ oz of ethanol (e.g., 1½ oz of 80-proof whiskey, 12 oz of beer, 5 oz of wine).
11.b. The client will verbalize an understanding of the rationale for and components of a diet low in sodium.	11.b.1. Explain the rationale for a diet low in sodium. 2. Provide the following information about decreasing sodium intake: a. read labels on foods/fluids and calculate sodium content of items; avoid those products that tend to have a high sodium content (e.g., canned soups and vegetables, tomato juice, commercial baked goods, commercially prepared frozen or canned entrees and sauces) b. do not add salt when cooking foods or to prepared foods; use low-sodium herbs and spices if desired c. avoid cured and smoked foods d. avoid salty snack foods (e.g., crackers, nuts, pretzels, potato chips) e. avoid commercially prepared fast foods f. avoid routine use of over-the-counter medications with a high sodium content (e.g., Alka-Seltzer, some antacids). 3. Obtain a dietary consult to assist client in planning meals that will meet prescribed dietary modifications.
11.c. The client will demonstrate accuracy in counting pulse.	11.c.1. Teach the client how to count his/her pulse, being alert to the regularity of the rhythm. 2. Allow time for return demonstration and accuracy check.
11.d. The client will verbalize an understanding of medications ordered including rationale, food and drug interactions, side effects, schedule for taking, and importance of taking as prescribed.	11.d.1. Explain the rationale for, side effects of, and importance of taking the medications prescribed. Inform client of pertinent food and drug interactions. 2. If client is discharged on a digitalis preparation, instruct to: a. take pulse before taking digitalis (should be a resting pulse rate taken at least 5 minutes after any activity); consult physician before taking medication if pulse rate is more irregular than usual or below 60 or above 100 beats/minute b. avoid taking antacids concurrently with digitalis preparation c. promptly report a loss of usual appetite, nausea, vomiting, confusion, diarrhea, or visual disturbances. 3. If client is discharged on a diuretic, instruct to: a. take once-daily dose in the morning or, if diuretic is to be taken twice each day, take the larger dose in the morning and the second dose no later than 3:00 p.m. (scheduling doses in this manner minimizes nighttime urination)

b. weigh self daily and keep a record of daily weights
c. change from a lying to standing position slowly if experiencing dizziness or lightheadedness with position change
d. increase intake of foods/fluids high in potassium (e.g., orange juice, bananas, potatoes, raisins, avocados, cantaloupe) if taking a potassium-depleting diuretic
e. notify physician if unable to tolerate food or fluids (dehydration can develop rapidly if intake is poor and client continues to take diuretic)
f. avoid salt substitutes with a high potassium content if discharged on a potassium-sparing diuretic (e.g., triamterene, eplerenone, spironolactone)
g. report the following signs and symptoms:
   1. weight loss of more than 5 pounds a week
   2. excessive thirst
   3. severe dizziness or episodes of fainting
   4. muscle weakness or cramping, nausea, vomiting, or increased irregularity of pulse.

4. If client is discharged on an ACE inhibitor, instruct to:
   a. change from a lying to standing position slowly if experiencing dizziness or lightheadedness with position change
   b. avoid hot baths and showers, steam room, and sauna
   c. avoid salt substitutes with a high potassium content
   d. report continued dizziness, lightheadedness, or fainting; a persistent dry cough; or swelling of the tongue, lips, face, or neck.
5. If client is discharged on a beta-adrenergic blocking agent (e.g., carvedilol, metoprolol), instruct to:
   a. take the medication at the same time each day
   b. check pulse before taking medication; consult physician before taking medication if pulse rate is unusually slow (it is expected that pulse will be lower than normal)
   c. change from a lying to sitting or standing position slowly if dizziness or lightheadedness is a problem
   d. limit intake of alcoholic beverages
   e. monitor blood glucose on a regular basis if diabetic (beta blockers may affect blood sugar and mask symptoms of hypoglycemia)
   f. wear or carry medical identification specifying the name of the medication being taken
   g. report the following:
      1. persistent lightheadedness or dizziness
      2. significant weight gain or worsening of symptoms of heart failure (because beta blockers reduce the force of myocardial contractility, they can actually worsen symptoms of heart failure)
      3. cold, painful toes or fingers
      4. persistent fatigue, depression, insomnia, or sexual dysfunction
      5. worsening of any symptoms of chronic respiratory disease.
6. Instruct client to take medications on a regular basis and avoid skipping doses, altering prescribed dose, making up for missed doses, and discontinuing medication without permission of health care provider.
7. Instruct client to consult physician before taking other prescription and nonprescription medications.
8. Instruct client to inform all health care providers of medications being taken.

11.e. The client will state signs and symptoms to report to the health care provider.

11.e. Instruct client to report:
1. weight gain of more than 2 pounds in a day or 4 pounds in a week
2. increased swelling of ankles, feet, or abdomen
3. persistent cough
4. increasing shortness of breath
5. chest discomfort/pain
6. increased weakness and fatigue

Desired Outcomes	**Nursing Actions** *and Selected Purposes/Rationales*
	7. frequent nighttime urination 8. signs and symptoms of digitalis toxicity (see action d.2.c in this diagnosis) 9. side effects of diuretic therapy (see action d.3.g in this diagnosis).
11.f. The client will identify community resources that can assist with home management and adjustment to changes resulting from heart failure.	11.f.1. Provide information regarding community resources that can assist with home management and adjustment to changes resulting from heart failure (e.g., Meals on Wheels, home health agencies, transportation services, American Heart Association, counseling services). 2. Initiate a referral if indicated.
11.g. The client will verbalize an understanding of and a plan for adhering to recommended follow-up care including future appointments with health care provider and activity limitations.	11.g.1. Reinforce the importance of keeping follow-up appointments with health care provider. 2. Provide the following instructions regarding activity: a. progress activity gradually and only as tolerated b. stop any activity that causes chest pain, dizziness, or a significant increase in shortness of breath or fatigue c. plan and adhere to rest periods during the day d. adhere to physician's recommendations about activities that should be avoided e. notify physician if activity tolerance declines f. reduce dyspnea and fatigue during sexual activity by: 1. avoiding sexual activity when unusually fatigued 2. waiting 1–2 hours after a heavy meal or alcohol intake before engaging in sexual activity 3. identifying and using positions that minimize energy expenditure (e.g., side-lying, partner on top) 4. using portable oxygen during sexual activities. 3. Implement measures to improve client compliance: a. include significant others in teaching sessions if possible b. encourage questions and allow time for reinforcement and clarification of information provided c. provide written instructions regarding scheduled appointments with health care provider, medications prescribed, dietary sodium restrictions, and signs and symptoms to report.

ADDITIONAL NURSING DIAGNOSES

NAUSEA

related to stimulation of the vomiting center associated with:

a. stimulation of the visceral afferent pathways resulting from vascular congestion in the heart and gastrointestinal tract;
b. stimulation of the cerebral cortex resulting from stress;
c. stimulation of the chemoreceptor trigger zone by certain medications (e.g., digitalis preparations).

DISTURBED THOUGHT PROCESSES

related to:

a. cerebral hypoxia associated with impaired alveolar gas exchange and inadequate cerebral tissue perfusion (a result of decreased cardiac output);
b. imbalanced fluid and electrolytes.

INEFFECTIVE COPING*

related to fear, anxiety, possible need to alter lifestyle, and knowledge that condition is chronic and will require lifelong medical supervision and medication therapy.

*See Unit II for outcomes, actions, and rationales.

Bibliography

See pages 879 and 881–882.

evolve

Heart Surgery: Coronary Artery Bypass Grafting (CABG) or Valve Replacement

Heart surgery is performed for a variety of reasons including myocardial revascularization, valve repair or replacement, repair of congenital or acquired structural abnormalities, placement of a mechanical assist device, and heart transplantation. Two common heart surgeries are coronary artery bypass grafting (CABG), which is done to treat severe coronary artery disease, and heart valve replacement. CABG involves removing a segment of a vein (e.g., saphenous, cephalic) or an artery (e.g., internal mammary, radial, gastro-epiploic) to create an anastomosis between the aorta or other major artery and a point on the coronary artery distal to the obstruction. Heart valve replacement involves replacing the stenotic or regurgitant valve with a mechanical prosthesis or a biologic (tissue) valve (porcine or bovine valve, human valve).

Heart surgery is usually performed through a median sternotomy. Cardiopulmonary bypass (extracorporeal circulation) is maintained during surgery by a machine that diverts the blood from the heart and lungs, oxygenates the blood and removes carbon dioxide, maintains the desired body temperature, filters the blood, and then recirculates the blood into the arterial system. Systemic hypothermia (provided by the cardiopulmonary bypass machine) can reduce tissue oxygen requirements to 50% of normal, which affords the major organs additional protection from ischemic injury. Cold cardioplegia (infusion of a cold, alkaline solution containing potassium into the coronary circulation) is used to precipitate cardiac arrest and provide additional protection to the myocardium during surgery. An isotonic crystalloid solution is used to prime the bypass machine. This dilutes the client's blood, which improves blood flow and reduces the risk of microemboli formation. Prior to closing the chest, pacing electrodes are usually placed on the epicardial surface of the heart and brought out through the chest wall to be used for temporary pacing if needed. A chest tube is placed in the mediastinum to drain blood and if needed, one is also placed in the pleural space to promote lung re-expansion.

In addition to the traditional sternotomy approach performed on cardiopulmonary bypass (CPB), heart surgery may be performed "off pump" (referred to as off pump coronary bypass [OPCAB]) or using a minimally invasive approach (e.g., small incision in left sternal border, a series of holes or "ports" using video-assisted equipment). Minimally invasive procedures such as a MIDCAB (minimally invasive direct coronary artery bypass) can be performed without cardiopulmonary bypass or with a less invasive, catheter-based system of cardiopulmonary bypass. Several techniques are used to stabilize the operative area during a beating heart procedure (stabilizer device to "still" certain areas of the heart while the rest keeps beating, drugs that decrease the heart rate or cause transient asystole). Because "off pump" and minimally invasive approaches reduce the risk for some of the major complications (e.g., mediastinitis, emboli associated with cross-clamping the aorta) and shorten hospitalization and rehabilitation time, they promise to become more common.

This care plan focuses on the adult client hospitalized for either coronary artery bypass grafting (CABG) or valve replacement surgery. Much of the postoperative information is applicable to clients receiving follow-up care in an extended care facility or home setting.

OUTCOME/DISCHARGE CRITERIA

THE CLIENT WILL:

- have adequate cardiac output and tissue perfusion
- have clear, audible breath sounds throughout lungs
- have evidence of normal healing of surgical wound(s)
- have oxygen saturation within normal limits for client's age
- tolerate expected level of activity
- have surgical pain controlled
- have no signs and symptoms of complications
- identify modifiable cardiovascular risk factors and ways to alter these factors
- verbalize an understanding of the rationale for and components of a diet restricted in sodium, saturated fat, and cholesterol
- verbalize an understanding of activity restrictions and the rate of activity progression
- verbalize an understanding of medications ordered including rationale, food and drug interactions, side effects, schedule for taking, and importance of taking as prescribed
- state signs and symptoms to report to the health care provider

- identify community resources that can assist with cardiac rehabilitation and adjustment to having had heart surgery
- verbalize an understanding of and a plan for adhering to recommended follow-up care including future appointments with health care provider, wound care, and pain management.

NURSING/COLLABORATIVE DIAGNOSES

See Standardized Preoperative and Postoperative Care Plans for additional diagnoses (pp. 97–126).

PREOPERATIVE

Use in conjunction with the Standardized Preoperative Care Plan.

1. NURSING DIAGNOSIS: ***FEAR/ANXIETY***

related to:

a. unfamiliar environment and separation from significant others;
b. lack of understanding of diagnostic tests, preoperative procedures/ preparation, planned surgery, and postoperative course;
c. anticipated loss of control associated with effects of anesthesia;
d. financial concerns associated with surgery and hospitalization;
e. anticipated postoperative discomfort and alterations in lifestyle and roles;
f. risk of disease if blood transfusions are necessary;
g. potential embarrassment or loss of dignity associated with body exposure;
h. possibility of death.

Suggested NOC Outcomes: Anxiety self-control; Anxiety level; Fear self-control; Fear level

Suggested NIC Interventions: Anxiety reduction; Emotional support; Teaching: preoperative

Desired Outcome	Nursing Actions *and Selected Purposes/Rationales* (see pp. 14–16 for additional rationales)
1. The client will experience a reduction in fear and anxiety (see Standardized Preoperative Care Plan, Diagnosis 1 [pp. 97–98], for outcome criteria).	1.a. Refer to Standardized Preoperative Care Plan, Diagnosis 1 (pp. 97–98), for measures related to assessment and reduction of fear and anxiety. b. Implement additional measures *to reduce fear and anxiety:* 1. arrange for a visit from a critical care nurse or a visit to the intensive care unit; assure client and significant others that transfer to the intensive care unit after heart surgery is routine 2. describe and explain the rationale for equipment and tubes that may be present postoperatively (e.g., cardiac monitoring equipment, endotracheal tube and ventilator, chest tube, arterial and venous lines, nasogastric tube, urinary catheter) 3. if bypass grafting is planned, inform client that he/she may have leg or arm incisions as well as a chest incision 4. with client, establish an alternative method of communicating (e.g., Magic Slate, word board, flash cards, signals) to be used while on the ventilator 5. focus on postoperative care *(this promotes a feeling in client that he/she will survive surgery).*

POSTOPERATIVE

Use in Conjunction with the Standardized Postoperative Care Plan.

1. Nursing Diagnosis: *DECREASED CARDIAC OUTPUT*

related to:

a. pre-existing compromise in cardiac function;
b. trauma to the heart during surgery;
c. increased afterload associated with:
   1. vasoconstriction resulting from hypothermia and an increase in catecholamine output and plasma renin levels (these increases occur with cardiopulmonary bypass and the effect of stressors [e.g., pain, anxiety])
   2. fluid overload;
d. decreased preload associated with:
   1. hypovolemia (can result from blood loss, fluid shifting from the intravascular to interstitial space, loss of fluid from nasogastric tube, decreased fluid intake, and excessive diuresis)
   2. hypotension (can occur if body is warmed rapidly following surgery and as a result of the effect of anesthesia and certain medications [e.g., narcotic analgesics, beta-adrenergic blockers, vasodilators]);
e. effects of anesthesia, hypothermia, hypoxemia, and acid-base and/or electrolyte imbalances on contractility and conductivity of the heart.

Suggested NOC Outcomes: Cardiac pump effectiveness; Circulation status; Tissue perfusion: peripheral; Tissue perfusion: cardiac

Suggested NIC Interventions: Cardiac care: acute; Invasive hemodynamic monitoring; Hemodynamic regulation; Cardiac precautions; Dysrhythmia management; Cardiac care: rehabilitative

Desired Outcome

1. The client will maintain adequate cardiac output as evidenced by:
   a. B/P within range of 130–100/80–60
   b. apical pulse regular and between 60–100 beats/minute
   c. absence of or no increase in intensity of gallop rhythm
   d. increased strength and activity tolerance
   e. unlabored respirations at 12–20/minute
   f. absence of adventitious breath sounds
   g. usual mental status
   h. absence of dizziness and syncope
   i. palpable peripheral pulses
   j. skin warm and usual color
   k. capillary refill time less than 2–3 seconds
   l. urine output at least 30 ml/hour
   m. absence of edema and jugular vein distention.

Nursing Actions *and Selected Purposes/Rationales*
(see pp. 20–24 for additional rationales)

1.a. Assess for and report signs and symptoms of:
   1. hypovolemia (e.g., low B/P; resting pulse rate greater than 100 beats/minute; postural hypotension; cool, pale, or cyanotic skin; diminished or absent peripheral pulses; urine output less than 30 ml/hour; low CVP)
   2. hypotension (systolic B/P persistently below 100 mm Hg)
   3. decreased cardiac output:
      a. variations in B/P (may be increased because of compensatory vasoconstriction; may be decreased when compensatory mechanisms and pump fail)
      b. tachycardia
      c. presence of gallop rhythm
      d. fatigue and weakness
      e. dyspnea, tachypnea
      f. crackles (rales)
      g. restlessness, change in mental status
      h. dizziness, syncope
      i. diminished or absent peripheral pulses
      j. cool extremities
      k. pallor or cyanosis of skin
      l. capillary refill time greater than 2–3 seconds
      m. oliguria
      n. edema
      o. jugular vein distention (JVD)
      p. chest x-ray results showing pulmonary vascular congestion, pulmonary edema, or pleural effusion
      q. abnormal blood gases
      r. significant decrease in oximetry results
   4. dysrhythmias (e.g., irregular heart rate; heart rate less than 60 or greater than 100; abnormal rate, rhythm, or configurations on the ECG).

b. Implement measures *to maintain an adequate cardiac output:*
   1. perform actions *to prevent or treat hypovolemia:*
      a. administer blood and/or colloid or crystalloid solutions as ordered
      b. maintain a minimum fluid intake of 1000 ml/day unless ordered otherwise
      c. implement measures to prevent and control bleeding (see Postoperative Diagnosis 6, actions e.4 and 5)
   2. perform actions *to prevent or treat hypotension:*
      a. consult physician before giving negative inotropic agents, diuretics, and vasodilating agents if client is hypotensive
      b. administer narcotic (opioid) analgesics judiciously; in the immediate postoperative period, be alert to the synergistic effect of the narcotic ordered and the anesthetic that was used during surgery
      c. avoid rapid rewarming; gradually bring client's body temperature to normal if he/she is hypothermic
      d. administer sympathomimetics (e.g., dopamine) if ordered
   3. administer positive inotropic agents (e.g., dopamine, dobutamine, digitalis preparations) if ordered *to increase myocardial contractility*
   4. perform actions to prevent or treat cardiac dysrhythmias (see Postoperative Diagnosis 6, actions b.2 and 3)
   5. perform actions *to reduce cardiac workload:*
      a. place client in a semi- to high Fowler's position
      b. perform actions *to prevent or treat hypertension:*
         1. implement measures to gradually rewarm client (e.g., increased room temperature, radiant heat lamp, warm blankets) if he/she is hypothermic *(helps prevent vasoconstriction associated with hypothermia and also prevents shivering, which elevates the metabolic rate and increases cardiac workload)*

Desired Outcome	Nursing Actions *and Selected Purposes/Rationales*

2. implement measures *to reduce stress* (e.g., initiate pain relief measures, reduce fear and anxiety)
3. administer vasodilators (e.g., sodium nitroprusside, nitroglycerin) if ordered

c. instruct client to avoid activities that create a Valsalva response (e.g., straining to have a bowel movement, holding breath while moving up in bed)
d. implement measures *to promote rest* (e.g., maintain activity restrictions, administer prescribed pain medications, limit the number of visitors, reduce anxiety)
e. implement measures to maintain adequate respiratory function (see Postoperative Diagnosis 2, action b) *in order to promote adequate tissue oxygenation*
f. discourage smoking *(nicotine has a cardiostimulatory effect and causes vasoconstriction; the carbon monoxide in smoke reduces oxygen availability)*
g. discourage excessive intake of beverages high in caffeine such as coffee, tea, and colas *(caffeine is a myocardial stimulant and can increase myocardial oxygen consumption)*
h. implement measures to prevent or treat excess fluid volume (see Postoperative Diagnosis 3, action a.4.a)
i. increase activity gradually as allowed and tolerated.

c. Consult physician if signs and symptoms of decreased cardiac output persist or worsen.

2. Nursing Diagnosis: RISK FOR IMPAIRED RESPIRATORY FUNCTION*

a. ineffective breathing pattern related to:
   1. increased rate of respirations associated with fear and anxiety
   2. decreased rate of respirations associated with the depressant effect of anesthesia and some medications (e.g., narcotic [opioid] analgesics)
   3. decreased depth of respirations associated with:
      a. weakness, fatigue, and decreased mobility
      b. depressant effect of anesthesia and some medications (e.g., narcotic [opioid] analgesics)
      c. reluctance to breathe deeply because of chest incision and fear of dislodging chest tube
      d. hemiparesis of the diaphragm if the phrenic nerve was injured
      e. decreased lung compliance (distensibility) if pleural effusion is present;

b. ineffective airway clearance related to:
   1. stasis of secretions associated with decreased activity, depressed ciliary function resulting from the effect of anesthesia, and a weak cough effort
   2. increased secretions associated with irritation of the respiratory tract (can result from inhalation anesthetics and endotracheal intubation);

c. impaired gas exchange related to ventilation/perfusion imbalances associated with:
   1. atelectasis resulting from:
      a. deflation of the alveoli while on the cardiopulmonary bypass machine
      b. decreased surfactant production/function (occurs because of lack of alveolar expansion and decreased pulmonary blood flow during CPB and as a result of a systemic inflammatory response to the bypass machine)
      c. postoperative hypoventilation or ineffective clearance of secretions
   2. accumulation of fluid in the pulmonary interstitium and alveoli (can occur as a result of excess fluid volume)
   3. decreased pulmonary blood flow resulting from decreased cardiac output.

---

*This diagnostic label includes the following nursing diagnoses: ineffective breathing pattern, ineffective airway clearance, and impaired gas exchange.

Suggested NOC Outcomes: Respiratory status: ventilation; Respiratory status: airway patency; Respiratory status: gas exchange

Suggested NIC Interventions: Respiratory monitoring; Airway management; Chest physiotherapy; Cough enhancement; Ventilation assistance; Oxygen therapy; Anxiety reduction

Desired Outcome	**Nursing Actions** *and Selected Purposes/Rationales* (see pp. 12–14, 18–20, and 33–35 for additional rationales)

2. The client will experience adequate respiratory function as evidenced by:
   a. normal rate and depth of respirations
   b. absence of dyspnea
   c. normal breath sounds by 3rd–4th postoperative day
   d. symmetrical chest excursion
   e. usual mental status
   f. oximetry results within normal range
   g. blood gases within normal range.

2.a. Assess for and report signs and symptoms of impaired respiratory function:
   1. rapid, shallow, or slow respirations
   2. dyspnea, orthopnea
   3. use of accessory muscles when breathing
   4. adventitious breath sounds (e.g., crackles [rales], rhonchi)
   5. diminished or absent breath sounds
   6. asymmetrical chest excursion
   7. cough
   8. restlessness, irritability
   9. confusion, somnolence
   10. abnormal blood gases
   11. significant decrease in oximetry results
   12. abnormal chest x-ray results.

b. Implement measures *to maintain adequate respiratory function:*
   1. monitor mechanical ventilation carefully *to ensure that ventilatory rate and pressures are correct*
   2. perform actions to decrease pain (see Standardized Postoperative Care Plan, Diagnosis 6, action d [p. 109]) and increase strength and activity tolerance (see Postoperative Diagnosis 4) *in order to increase client's willingness and ability to move, cough, deep breathe, and use incentive spirometer*
   3. perform actions *to decrease fear and anxiety* (e.g., explain procedures, interact with client in a confident manner, initiate pain relief measures) *in order to prevent the shallow and/or rapid breathing that can occur with fear and anxiety*
   4. perform actions to maintain an adequate cardiac output (see Postoperative Diagnosis 1, action b) *in order to promote adequate pulmonary blood flow*
   5. perform actions to prevent or treat excess fluid volume and third-spacing (see Postoperative Diagnosis 3, action a.4.a) *in order to reduce the risk for pleural effusion and pulmonary edema*
   6. place client in a semi- to high Fowler's position unless contraindicated
   7. if client must remain flat in bed, assist with position change at least every 2 hours
   8. assist with positive airway pressure techniques (e.g., positive end-expiratory pressure [PEEP], continuous positive airway pressure [CPAP], bilevel positive airway pressure [BiPAP], flutter/positive expiratory pressure [PEP] device) if ordered
   9. instruct and assist client to cough and deep breathe or use incentive spirometer every 1–2 hours; assure client that chest tube is sutured in place and that these activities should not dislodge the tube
   10. maintain an adequate fluid intake and humidify inspired air if ordered *to thin tenacious secretions and reduce dryness of the respiratory mucous membrane*
   11. maintain oxygen therapy as ordered
   12. instruct client to avoid intake of gas-forming foods (e.g., beans, cauliflower, cabbage, onions), carbonated beverages, and large meals *in order to prevent gastric distention and subsequent pressure on the diaphragm*
   13. discourage smoking (*the irritants in smoke increase mucus production, impair ciliary function, and can cause damage to the bronchial and alveolar walls; the carbon monoxide decreases oxygen availability*)

Desired Outcome	Nursing Actions *and Selected Purposes/Rationales*
	14. maintain activity restrictions as ordered; increase activity gradually as allowed and tolerated 15. administer central nervous system depressants judiciously; hold medication and consult physician if respiratory rate is less than 12/minute. c. Consult appropriate health care provider (e.g., respiratory therapist, physician) if signs and symptoms of impaired respiratory function persist or worsen.

3. Nursing/Collaborative Diagnosis:

RISK FOR IMBALANCED FLUID AND ELECTROLYTES

a. excess fluid volume related to:
   1. vigorous fluid therapy during and immediately following surgery (the cardiopulmonary bypass machine is primed with a large amount of crystalloid solution to decrease blood viscosity and the risk for embolic complications, decrease hemolysis of cells, and help maintain adequate circulation throughout the body)
   2. increased production of antidiuretic hormone (output of ADH is stimulated by trauma, pain, and anesthetic agents)
   3. reshifting of fluid from the interstitial space back into the intravascular space approximately 3 days after surgery
   4. decreased glomerular filtration rate and activation of the renin-angiotensin-aldosterone mechanism (a result of nonpulsatile renal perfusion while on the bypass machine and the decreased renal blood flow that can occur with decreased cardiac output)
   5. presence of pre-existing heart failure;

b. third-spacing of fluid related to increased capillary permeability (a result of the systemic inflammatory response that occurs with cardiopulmonary bypass) and the subsequent low plasma colloid osmotic pressure associated with decreased plasma proteins;

c. deficient fluid volume related to restricted oral intake before, during, and after surgery; blood loss during surgery and via chest tube after surgery; loss of fluid associated with nasogastric tube drainage and excessive diuresis; and third-spacing of intravascular fluid;

d. hypokalemia, hypochloremia, and/or metabolic alkalosis related to loss of electrolytes and hydrochloric acid associated with nasogastric tube drainage (diuretic therapy and the hemodilution created by priming the bypass machine with large amounts of fluid also contribute to the imbalanced electrolytes).

Suggested NOC Outcomes: Fluid balance; Fluid overload severity; Electrolyte and acid/base balance

Suggested NIC Interventions: Fluid monitoring; Electrolyte monitoring; Acid-base monitoring; Fluid management; Electrolyte management: hypokalemia; Acid-base management: metabolic alkalosis

Desired Outcomes	Nursing Actions *and Selected Purposes/Rationales* (see pp. 30–33 for additional rationales)
3.a. The client will experience resolution of excess fluid volume and third-spacing as evidenced by: 1. decline in weight toward client's normal 2. B/P and pulse within normal range for client and stable with position change	3.a.1. Assess for signs and symptoms of the following: a. excess fluid volume: 1. weight gain of 2% or greater in a short period 2. elevated B/P (B/P may not be elevated if cardiac output is poor or fluid has shifted out of the vascular space) 3. presence of an S_3 heart sound 4. intake greater than output 5. change in mental status 6. crackles (rales) 7. dyspnea, orthopnea

3. resolution of S_3 heart sound
4. balanced intake and output
5. usual mental status
6. improved breath sounds
7. decreased dyspnea and orthopnea
8. decrease in edema and ascites
9. resolution of neck vein distention
10. CVP within normal range.

8. edema, distended neck veins
9. elevated CVP (use internal jugular vein pulsation method to estimate CVP if monitoring device is not present)

b. third-spacing:
1. ascites
2. increased dyspnea and diminished or absent breath sounds
3. evidence of vascular depletion (e.g., postural hypotension; weak, rapid pulse; decreased urine output).

2. Monitor chest x-ray results. Report findings of pulmonary vascular congestion, pleural effusion, or pulmonary edema.
3. Monitor serum albumin levels. Report below-normal levels *(low serum albumin levels result in fluid shifting out of the vascular space because albumin normally maintains plasma colloid osmotic pressure).*
4. Implement measures *to restore fluid balance:*
   a. perform actions *to reduce excess fluid volume:*
      1. refer to Standardized Postoperative Care Plan, Diagnosis 4, action b (p. 107), for measures to prevent and manage excess fluid volume
      2. perform actions to maintain adequate renal blood flow (see Postoperative Diagnosis 6, action h.2)
      3. administer diuretics if ordered
      4. maintain fluid and sodium restrictions as ordered (2500 ml fluid and 3–4 g sodium restrictions are common)
   b. perform actions *to prevent further third-spacing and promote mobilization of fluid back into the vascular space:*
      1. implement measures to reduce excess fluid volume (see action a.4.a in this diagnosis)
      2. administer albumin infusions if ordered *to increase colloid osmotic pressure.*
5. Consult physician if signs and symptoms of excess fluid volume and third-spacing persist or worsen.

3.b. The client will not experience deficient fluid volume, hypokalemia, hypochloremia, or metabolic alkalosis (see Standardized Postoperative Care Plan, Diagnosis 4, outcome a [p. 106], for outcome criteria).

3.b.1. Refer to Standardized Postoperative Care Plan, Diagnosis 4, action a (p. 106), for measures related to assessment, prevention, and treatment of deficient fluid volume, hypokalemia, hypochloremia, and metabolic alkalosis.

2. Administer the following if ordered *to treat deficient fluid volume and hypokalemia:*
   a. blood and/or colloid or crystalloid solutions (colloid solutions may be used rather than crystalloid solutions *because they help maintain colloid osmotic pressure and subsequently reduce shifting of fluid from the intravascular to the interstitial space)*
   b. potassium supplements *(keeping the serum potassium at 4.0–4.5 reduces the risk for dysrhythmias).*

4. NURSING DIAGNOSIS: *ACTIVITY INTOLERANCE*

related to:

a. tissue hypoxia associated with decreased cardiac output, impaired alveolar gas exchange, and anemia (results from hemodilution, blood loss, and red cell hemolysis [red cells are traumatized by the cardiopulmonary bypass machine]);

b. difficulty resting and sleeping associated with frequent assessments and treatments, discomfort, fear, and anxiety.

Suggested NOC Outcomes: Activity tolerance; Energy conservation; Self-care: activities of daily living

Suggested NIC Interventions: Energy management; Oxygen therapy; Nutrition management; Cardiac care: rehabilitative; Blood products administration

Desired Outcome	Nursing Actions and Selected Purposes/Rationales (see pp. 11–12 for additional rationales)
4. The client will demonstrate an increased tolerance for activity (see Standardized Postoperative Care Plan, Diagnosis 11 [p. 113], for outcome criteria).	4.a. Refer to Standardized Postoperative Care Plan, Diagnosis 11 (pp. 113–114), for measures related to assessment and improvement of activity tolerance. b. Implement additional measures *to improve activity tolerance:* 1. perform actions to maintain an adequate cardiac output (see Postoperative Diagnosis 1, action b) 2. perform actions to maintain adequate respiratory function (see Postoperative Diagnosis 2, action b) 3. perform actions *to treat anemia:* a. encourage client to increase intake of foods high in iron (e.g., organ meats, dried fruit, dark green leafy vegetables, whole-grain or iron-enriched breads and cereals) and vitamin C *(enhances the absorption of iron from plant products)* b. autotransfuse blood from the chest drainage device or administer packed red blood cells if ordered c. administer iron supplements if ordered 4. increase client's activity gradually as allowed and tolerated; explain to client that a progressive and gradual increase in activity is necessary *in order to strengthen the myocardium without causing a sudden increase in cardiac workload.*

5. Nursing Diagnosis: RISK FOR INFECTION

a. pneumonia related to stasis of pulmonary secretions associated with decreased activity; depressed ciliary function resulting from the effect of anesthesia; and a poor cough effort resulting from weakness, surgical site pain, and fear of dislodging chest tube;

b. wound infection and mediastinitis related to:
   1. wound contamination associated with introduction of pathogens during or following surgery
   2. decreased resistance to infection associated with factors such as inadequate nutritional status and diminished tissue perfusion to wound area (an increased risk if client is elderly or has diabetes or if on cardiopulmonary bypass a prolonged time or cardiac output is low for a prolonged time).

Suggested NOC Outcomes: Immune status; Infection severity; Wound healing: primary intention

Suggested NIC Interventions: Infection protection; Infection control; Cough enhancement; Airway management; Incision site care

Desired Outcomes	Nursing Actions and Selected Purposes/Rationales (see pp. 37–40 for additional rationales)
5.a. The client will not develop pneumonia (see Standardized Postoperative Care Plan, Diagnosis 17, outcome a [p. 118], for outcome criteria).	5.a.1. Refer to Standardized Postoperative Care Plan, Diagnosis 17, action a (p. 118), for measures related to assessment, prevention, and treatment of pneumonia. 2. Implement additional measures *to reduce the risk for pneumonia:* a. perform actions to maintain adequate respiratory function (see Postoperative Diagnosis 2, action b) b. have client splint chest incision with a pillow when turning, coughing, and deep breathing *in order to increase client's willingness to move, cough, and deep breathe.*

5.b. The client will remain free of wound infection and mediastinitis (see Standardized Postoperative Care Plan, Diagnosis 17, outcome b [pp. 118–119], for outcome criteria).

5.b.1. Refer to Standardized Postoperative Care Plan, Diagnosis 17, action b (pp. 118–119), for measures related to assessment and prevention of wound infection.
2. Assess for and report additional signs and symptoms of sternal wound infection and mediastinitis (e.g., fever persisting beyond the 4th postoperative day, grating sound and/or movement of sternum when client moves or coughs). Be aware that signs and symptoms of sternal infection and mediastinitis are often not manifested until the 2nd week after surgery.
3. If signs and symptoms of a sternal wound infection and mediastinitis occur:
   a. administer antimicrobial agents as ordered
   b. prepare client for surgical debridement, drainage, and antibiotic irrigation of wound if planned.

6. COLLABORATIVE DIAGNOSES: POTENTIAL COMPLICATIONS OF HEART SURGERY

a. **myocardial infarction (MI)** related to an increased myocardial oxygen demand and/or insufficient coronary blood flow (can result from coronary artery spasm, hypotension, or thrombosis or embolism of a native coronary vessel or bypass grafts);
b. **cardiac dysrhythmias** related to impaired nodal function and/or altered myocardial conductivity associated with trauma to the heart during surgery, hypothermia, hypoxia, sympathetic stimulation (can result from anxiety, volume depletion, and pain), or electrolyte and acid-base imbalances;
c. **heart failure** related to pre-existing myocardial dilation or hypertrophy and decreased cardiac output postoperatively associated with damage to and further stress on the heart;
d. **cardiac tamponade** related to accumulation of fluid (usually blood) in the pericardial sac and/or mediastinum associated with excessive bleeding and/or obstructed drainage of the mediastinal tube;
e. **bleeding** related to:
   1. impaired platelet function associated with mechanical damage to the platelets by the bypass machine and possible heparin-induced thrombocytopenia
   2. incomplete neutralization of the heparin used during surgery to prevent thrombus formation in the bypass machine
   3. decreased release and function of clotting factors associated with systemic hypothermia during surgery
   4. anticoagulant therapy (relevant primarily for clients who have had valve replacement and are taking warfarin)
   5. inadequate surgical hemostasis or disruption of suture lines associated with hypertension if it occurs;
f. **thromboembolism** related to:
   1. trauma to the blood vessels associated with bypass grafting, cannulation for cardiopulmonary bypass, and cross-clamping of the aorta
   2. thrombi formation at the prosthetic valve site (with valve replacement surgeries)
   3. formation of microemboli associated with incomplete emptying of cardiac chambers if atrial fibrillation or heart failure occurs
   4. venous stasis associated with diminished cardiac output and decreased activity
   5. hypercoagulability associated with activation of the coagulation cascade during cardiopulmonary bypass (the body does not recognize the nonendothelial surfaces of the bypass machine and initiates the inflammatory and coagulation cascades in response to what it perceives as a foreign substance);
g. **neurological dysfunction** related to:
   1. inadequate cerebral blood flow associated with:
      a. decreased systemic arterial pressure while on cardiopulmonary bypass

b. an embolus (can result from dislodgment of atherosclerotic plaque during cross-clamping of the aorta and cannulation for bypass, dislodgment of debris from calcified valve, incomplete filtration of air by bypass machine, or cardiac thrombus formation on prosthetic valve or as a result of dysrhythmias)
c. hypotension or low cardiac output postoperatively;
2. cerebral edema initiated by a systemic inflammatory response to the cardiopulmonary bypass machine
3. possible poor cerebral protection during cardiopulmonary bypass from inadequate temperature regulation (hypothermia must be adequate in order to help protect the central nervous system);

h. **impaired renal function** related to deposit of hemolyzed red blood cell products in renal tubules or inadequate renal blood flow associated with cardiopulmonary bypass, low cardiac output, hypotension, an embolus, or effect of vasopressor drugs (risk is increased if client is elderly or has pre-existing renal disease);

i. **pneumothorax** related to the accumulation of air in the pleural space if the pleura was opened during surgery.

Desired Outcomes	**Nursing Actions** *and Selected Purposes/Rationales*
6.a. The client will not experience an MI as evidenced by: 1. no episodes of sudden and persistent chest pain 2. stable vital signs 3. cardiac enzyme levels declining toward normal range 4. absence of pathologic Q wave, ST segment depression or elevation, and T-wave inversion on ECG.	6.a.1. Assess for and report signs and symptoms of a myocardial infarction (e.g., sudden and persistent chest pain; significant change in vital signs; further increase in cardiac enzymes; new and persistent ST segment depression or elevation, T wave inversion, and/or abnormal Q waves on ECG). 2. Implement measures to maintain adequate cardiac output (see Postoperative Diagnosis 1, action b) *in order to improve myocardial blood supply and reduce the risk of myocardial infarction.* 3. If signs and symptoms of a myocardial infarction occur: a. initiate cardiac monitoring if not currently being done b. maintain client on bed rest in a semi- to high Fowler's position c. maintain oxygen therapy as ordered d. administer the following medications if ordered: 1. morphine sulfate *to reduce pain and anxiety and decrease cardiac workload* 2. nitrates *to improve coronary blood flow and reduce myocardial oxygen requirements* 3. beta-adrenergic blocking agents *to reduce myocardial oxygen requirements by decreasing heart rate and the force of myocardial contractility.*
6.b. The client will maintain normal sinus rhythm as evidenced by: 1. regular apical pulse at 60–100 beats/minute 2. equal apical and radial pulse rates 3. absence of syncope and palpitations 4. ECG showing normal sinus rhythm.	6.b.1. Assess for and report signs and symptoms of cardiac dysrhythmias (e.g., irregular apical pulse; pulse rate below 60 or above 100 beats/minute; apical-radial pulse deficit; syncope; palpitations; abnormal rate, rhythm, or configurations on ECG). 2. Implement measures *to prevent cardiac dysrhythmias:* a. perform actions to maintain adequate cardiac output and myocardial blood flow (see Postoperative Diagnosis 1, action b) b. maintain oxygen therapy as ordered c. monitor serum electrolyte levels; consult physician about administration of a potassium or magnesium supplement if serum levels of either are low d. perform actions to maintain adequate respiratory function (see Postoperative Diagnosis 2, action b) *in order to improve tissue oxygenation and prevent respiratory acidosis or alkalosis (myocardial conductivity is altered by hypoxia and acid-base imbalance)* e. administer prophylactic antidysrhythmic agents (e.g., beta blockers) if ordered. 3. If cardiac dysrhythmias occur: a. initiate cardiac monitoring if not still being done b. administer antidysrhythmics (e.g., digoxin, diltiazem, verapamil, procainamide, metoprolol, esmolol, lidocaine, adenosine, atropine) if ordered

c. maintain temporary pacemaker function as ordered
d. restrict client's activity based on his/her tolerance and severity of the dysrhythmia
e. maintain oxygen therapy as ordered
f. assess cardiovascular status frequently and report signs and symptoms of inadequate tissue perfusion (e.g., decrease in B/P, cool skin, cyanosis, diminished peripheral pulses, urine output less than 30 ml/hour, restlessness and agitation, shortness of breath)
g. have emergency cart readily available for cardioversion, defibrillation, or cardiopulmonary resuscitation.

6.c. The client will not develop heart failure as evidenced by:
1. pulse 60–100 beats/minute
2. absence of an S_3 heart sound
3. usual mental status
4. absence of adventitious breath sounds
5. absence of dyspnea, orthopnea, and cough
6. palpable peripheral pulses
7. no increase in fatigue and weakness
8. urine output at least 30 ml/hour
9. stable weight
10. absence of edema and distended neck veins
11. CVP within normal limits.

6.c.1. Assess for and report signs and symptoms of heart failure:
a. significant increase in pulse rate
b. presence of an S_3 heart sound
c. restlessness, anxiousness, confusion, or other change in mental status
d. crackles (rales)
e. dyspnea, orthopnea
f. dry, hacking cough or cough productive of blood-tinged or frothy sputum
g. diminished or absent peripheral pulses
h. increased weakness and fatigue
i. decreased urine output during the day, nocturia
j. weight gain
k. edema
l. distended neck veins
m. increased CVP
n. chest x-ray results showing pulmonary vascular congestion, pleural effusion, or pulmonary edema.

2. Implement measures *to prevent heart failure:*
a. perform actions to maintain adequate cardiac output (see Postoperative Diagnosis 1, action b)
b. perform actions to prevent and treat cardiac dysrhythmias (see actions b.2 and 3 in this diagnosis) *because dysrhythmias contribute to the development of heart failure.*

3. If signs and symptoms of heart failure occur:
a. maintain oxygen therapy as ordered
b. administer the following medications if ordered:
   1. positive inotropic agents (e.g., dobutamine, dopamine, digitalis preparations) *to increase myocardial contractility*
   2. diuretics, ACE inhibitors, and/or vasodilators *to decrease cardiac workload*
   3. morphine sulfate *to reduce preload and anxiety* (used primarily in clients with pulmonary edema).

6.d. The client will not experience cardiac tamponade as evidenced by:
1. stable vital signs
2. audible heart sounds
3. absence of jugular vein distention
4. absence of pulsus paradoxus
5. CVP within normal limits.

6.d.1. Assess for and immediately report:
a. a sudden decrease in chest tube drainage
b. chest x-ray reports showing widening of the mediastinum
c. signs and symptoms of cardiac tamponade (e.g., significant decrease in B/P, narrowed pulse pressure, pulsus paradoxus and distant or muffled heart sounds [may be obscured by mechanical ventilation], jugular vein distention, increased CVP).

2. Implement measures *to reduce the risk of cardiac tamponade:*
a. perform actions to maintain patency and integrity of chest drainage system (see action i.3.a in this diagnosis)
b. if chest tube becomes obstructed, assist with clearing of existing tube and/or insertion of a new tube
c. when removing the pacemaker catheter(s), do it carefully *to avoid trauma to the surrounding vessels and subsequent bleeding.*

3. If signs and symptoms of cardiac tamponade occur:
a. prepare client for echocardiography
b. administer intravenous fluids and/or vasopressors if ordered *to maintain mean arterial pressure*
c. prepare client for surgical drainage of pericardial fluid.

Desired Outcomes	Nursing Actions *and Selected Purposes/Rationales*
6.e. The client will not experience unusual bleeding as evidenced by: 1. gradual decrease in amount of bloody drainage from chest tube 2. skin and mucous membranes free of active bleeding, petechiae, purpura, and ecchymoses 3. absence of unusual joint pain 4. no increase in abdominal girth 5. absence of frank and occult blood in stool, urine, and vomitus 6. usual menstrual flow 7. usual mental status 8. vital signs within normal range for client 9. stable or improved Hct and Hgb.	6.e.1. Assess client for and report signs and symptoms of unusual bleeding: a. excessive amount of bloody drainage from chest tube b. continuous oozing of blood from incisions c. prolonged bleeding from puncture sites d. gingival bleeding e. petechiae, purpura, ecchymoses f. epistaxis, hemoptysis g. unusual joint pain h. increase in abdominal girth i. frank or occult blood in stool, urine, or vomitus j. menorrhagia k. restlessness, confusion l. significant drop in B/P accompanied by an increased pulse rate m. decrease in Hct and Hgb levels. 2. Monitor platelet count and coagulation test results (e.g., prothrombin time or International Normalized Ratio [INR], activated partial thromboplastin time, bleeding time). Report abnormal values or values that exceed the therapeutic range if client is on anticoagulant therapy. 3. If platelet count is low, coagulation test results are abnormal, or Hct and Hgb levels decrease, test all stools, urine, and vomitus for occult blood. Report positive results. 4. Implement measures *to prevent bleeding:* a. when giving injections or performing venous and arterial punctures, use the smallest gauge needle possible and apply gentle, prolonged pressure to the site after the needle is removed b. perform actions to prevent and treat hypertension (see Postoperative Diagnosis 1, action b.5.b) *in order to maintain systolic B/P at a level less than 140 mm Hg and subsequently decrease the risk for disruption of suture lines* c. caution client to avoid activities that increase the risk for trauma (e.g., shaving with a straight-edge razor, using stiff bristle toothbrush or dental floss) d. pad side rails if client is confused or restless e. perform actions *to reduce the risk for falls* (e.g., keep bed in low position with side rails up when client is in bed, avoid unnecessary clutter in room, instruct client to wear shoes/slippers with nonslip soles when ambulating) f. instruct client to avoid blowing nose forcefully or straining to have a bowel movement; consult physician regarding order for a decongestant and/or laxative if indicated g. administer the following if ordered: 1. vitamin K (e.g., phytonadione) *to counteract the effect of warfarin therapy* 2. protamine sulfate *to further neutralize the heparin used to prime the bypass machine.* 5. If bleeding occurs and does not subside spontaneously: a. apply firm, prolonged pressure to bleeding area(s) if possible b. maintain oxygen therapy as ordered c. autotransfuse blood from the chest drainage device if ordered d. administer the following if ordered: 1. vitamin K or protamine sulfate 2. whole blood or packed red blood cells 3. blood products (e.g., platelets, FFP, fibrinogen) e. prepare client for return to surgery if planned.

6.f. The client will not develop a thromboembolism as evidenced by:
1. absence of pain, tenderness, swelling, and numbness in extremities
2. usual temperature and color of extremities
3. palpable and equal peripheral pulses
4. usual mental status
5. usual sensory and motor function
6. absence of sudden chest pain and dyspnea.

6.f.1. Assess for and report signs and symptoms of:
- a. deep vein thrombus (e.g., pain, tenderness, swelling, unusual warmth, and/or positive Homans' sign in extremity)
- b. arterial embolus in an extremity (e.g., diminished or absent peripheral pulses; pallor, coolness, numbness, and/or pain in extremity)
- c. neurological dysfunction and cerebral ischemia (see action g.1 in this diagnosis for a list of signs and symptoms)
- d. pulmonary embolism (e.g., sudden onset of chest pain, dyspnea, restlessness and apprehension, significant decrease in $Sa{O_2}$).

2. Implement measures to prevent and treat deep vein thrombus and pulmonary embolism (see Standardized Postoperative Care Plan, Diagnosis 20, actions c.1.b and c and c.2.b and c [pp. 122–123]).
3. Implement measures *to prevent thrombi and microemboli formation in the heart:*
   - a. perform actions *to prevent stasis of blood in the heart:*
     1. implement measures to prevent and treat cardiac dysrhythmias (see actions b.2 and 3 in this diagnosis)
     2. implement measures to maintain an adequate cardiac output (see Postoperative Diagnosis 1, action b)
   - b. administer anticoagulants (e.g., low- or adjusted-dose heparin, low-molecular-weight heparin, warfarin) and antiplatelet agents (e.g., low-dose aspirin) if ordered.
4. If signs and symptoms of an arterial embolus occur:
   - a. maintain client on strict bed rest with affected extremity in a level or slightly dependent position *to improve arterial blood flow*
   - b. prepare client for diagnostic studies (e.g., Doppler or duplex ultrasound, arteriography)
   - c. administer anticoagulants (e.g., heparin, warfarin) if ordered
   - d. prepare client for surgical intervention (e.g., embolectomy, revascularization) if planned
   - e. refer to action g.3 in this diagnosis for additional care measures if signs and symptoms of neurological dysfunction and cerebral ischemia occur.

6.g. The client will maintain usual neurological function as evidenced by:
1. absence of visual disturbances, swallowing difficulties, and speech impairments
2. mentally alert and oriented
3. usual memory and problem-solving abilities
4. normal sensory and motor function.

6.g.1. Assess for and report signs and symptoms of neurological dysfunction:
- a. visual disturbances
- b. swallowing difficulties
- c. slurred speech, expressive or receptive aphasia
- d. decreased level of consciousness, delirium, hallucinations, confusion
- e. impaired memory, lack of ability to concentrate, difficulty problem-solving
- f. paresthesias, weakness of extremity, facial ptosis, paralysis.

2. Implement measures *to promote adequate cerebral blood flow and reduce the risk for neurological dysfunction:*
   - a. keep head of bed flat until B/P is stabilized at a satisfactory level (at least 90 mm Hg systolic)
   - b. keep head and neck in neutral, midline position
   - c. perform actions to maintain adequate cardiac output (see Postoperative Diagnosis 1, action b)
   - d. perform actions to prevent thrombi and microemboli formation in the heart (see action f.3 in this diagnosis)
   - e. perform actions *to reduce the risk for increased intracranial pressure (ICP):*
     1. limit activities that can increase ICP (e.g., excessive suctioning, instruct client to avoid excessive coughing and straining to have a bowel movement)
     2. implement measures to maintain adequate respiratory function and gas exchange (see Postoperative Diagnosis 2, action b) *in order to prevent dilation of the cerebral vessels associated with hypoxia and hypercapnia.*

Desired Outcomes	Nursing Actions *and Selected Purposes/Rationales*
	3. If signs and symptoms of neurological dysfunction occur: a. maintain client on bed rest until physician evaluates symptoms b. maintain oxygen therapy as ordered c. administer anticoagulants (e.g., warfarin, heparin) if ordered.
6.h. The client will maintain adequate renal function as evidenced by: 1. urine output at least 30 ml/hour 2. BUN, serum creatinine, and creatinine clearance within normal range.	6.h.1. Assess for and report signs and symptoms of impaired renal function (e.g., urine output less than 30 ml/hour, urine specific gravity fixed at or less than 1.010, elevated BUN and serum creatinine levels, decreased creatinine clearance). 2. Implement measures *to maintain adequate renal blood flow:* a. maintain a minimum fluid intake of 1000 ml/day unless ordered otherwise b. perform actions to maintain adequate cardiac output (see Postoperative Diagnosis 1, action b) c. perform actions to prevent thrombi and microemboli formation in the heart (see action f.3 in this diagnosis) *in order to reduce the risk for occlusion of the renal artery by an embolus.* 3. If signs and symptoms of impaired renal function occur: a. administer diuretics (e.g., furosemide) if ordered *to increase urine output and subsequently reduce further accumulation of hemolyzed red blood cell products in the renal tubules* b. consult physician about discontinuing any potentially nephrotoxic medications (e.g., NSAIDs, aminoglycosides, loop diuretics) client is receiving c. assess for and report signs of acute renal failure (e.g., oliguria or anuria; weight gain; edema; elevated B/P; lethargy and confusion; increasing BUN and serum creatinine, phosphorus, and potassium levels) d. prepare client for dialysis if indicated.
6.i. The client will experience normal lung re-expansion as evidenced by: 1. audible breath sounds and a resonant percussion note over lungs by 3rd-4th postoperative day 2. unlabored respirations at 12–20/minute 3. blood gases returning toward normal 4. chest x-ray showing lung re-expansion.	6.i.1. Assess for and immediately report signs and symptoms of: a. malfunction of chest drainage system (e.g., respiratory distress, excessive bubbling in water seal chamber, significant increase in subcutaneous emphysema) b. further lung collapse (e.g., extended area of absent breath sounds with hyperresonant percussion note; further increase in pulse rate; rapid, shallow, and/or labored respirations; restlessness; confusion; blood gas values that have worsened). 2. Monitor chest x-ray results. Report findings of delayed lung re-expansion or further lung collapse. 3. Implement measures *to promote lung re-expansion and prevent further lung collapse:* a. perform actions *to maintain patency and integrity of chest drainage system:* 1. maintain fluid level in the water seal and suction chambers as ordered 2. maintain occlusive dressing over chest tube insertion site 3. tape all connections securely 4. tape the tubing to the chest wall close to insertion site *to reduce the risk of inadvertent removal of the tube* 5. position tubing *to promote optimum drainage* (e.g., coil excess tubing on bed rather than allowing it to hang down below the collection device, keep tubing free of kinks) 6. drain any fluid that accumulates in tubing into the collection chamber and milk tube gently if indicated *to dislodge clots* 7. keep drainage collection device below level of client's chest at all times b. perform actions *to facilitate the escape of air from the pleural space* (e.g., maintain suction as ordered, ensure that the air vent is open on the drainage collection device if system is to water seal only)

c. perform actions to maintain adequate respiratory function (see Postoperative Diagnosis 2, action b).

4. If signs and symptoms of further lung collapse occur:
   a. maintain client on bed rest in a semi- to high Fowler's position
   b. maintain oxygen therapy as ordered
   c. assess for and immediately report signs and symptoms of tension pneumothorax (e.g., severe dyspnea, increased restlessness and agitation, rapid and/or irregular pulse rate, hypotension, neck vein distention, shift in trachea from midline)
   d. assist with clearing of existing chest tube and/or insertion of a new tube.

Discharge Teaching/Continued Care

7. NURSING DIAGNOSIS: ***DEFICIENT KNOWLEDGE, INEFFECTIVE THERAPEUTIC REGIMEN MANAGEMENT, OR INEFFECTIVE HEALTH MAINTENANCE****

*The nurse should select the diagnostic label that is most appropriate for the client's discharge teaching needs.

Suggested NOC Outcomes: Knowledge: disease process; Knowledge: treatment regimen; Knowledge: cardiac disease management

Suggested NIC Interventions: Health system guidance; Teaching: individual; Teaching: disease process; Teaching: prescribed activity/exercise; Teaching: prescribed diet; Teaching: prescribed medication

Desired Outcomes	**Nursing Actions** *and Selected Purposes/Rationales*
7.a. The client will identify modifiable cardiovascular risk factors and ways to alter these factors.	7.a.1. Inform client that certain modifiable factors such as elevated serum lipids, a sedentary lifestyle, hypertension, excessive alcohol intake, and smoking have been shown to increase the risk for coronary artery disease and certain forms of heart disease. 2. Assist client to identify changes in lifestyle that can help him/her to eliminate or reduce the above risk factors (e.g., dietary modification, physical exercise on a regular basis, moderation of alcohol intake, smoking cessation). 3. Encourage client to limit daily alcohol consumption (daily alcohol intake exceeding 1 oz of ethanol may contribute to the development of hypertension and some forms of heart disease). Current recommendations are no more than 2 drinks/day for men and no more than 1 drink/day for women and lighter weight persons. A "drink" is considered to be ½ oz of ethanol (e.g., 1½ oz of 80-proof whiskey, 12 oz of beer, 5 oz of wine).
7.b. The client will verbalize an understanding of the rationale for and components of a diet restricted in sodium, saturated fat, and cholesterol.	7.b.1. Explain the rationale for a diet restricting sodium, saturated fat, and cholesterol intake. 2. Provide the following information about decreasing sodium intake: a. read labels on foods/fluids and calculate sodium content of items; avoid those products that tend to have a high sodium content (e.g., canned soups and vegetables, tomato juice, commercial baked goods, commercially prepared frozen or canned entrees and sauces) b. do not add salt when cooking foods or to prepared foods; use low-sodium herbs and spices if desired c. avoid cured and smoked foods d. avoid salty snack foods (e.g., crackers, nuts, pretzels, potato chips) e. avoid commercially prepared fast foods f. avoid routine use of over-the-counter medications with a high sodium content (e.g., Alka-Seltzer, some antacids).

Desired Outcomes	Nursing Actions *and Selected Purposes/Rationales*
	3. Provide instructions on ways the client can reduce intake of saturated fat and cholesterol: a. reduce intake of meat fat (e.g., trim visible fat off meat; replace fatty meats such as fatty cuts of steak, hamburger, and processed meats with leaner products) b. reduce intake of milk fat (avoid dairy products containing more than 1% fat) c. reduce intake of *trans* fats (e.g., avoid stick margarine and shortening and foods such as commercial baked goods that are prepared with these products) d. use vegetable oil rather than coconut or palm oil in cooking and food preparation e. use cooking methods such as steaming, baking, broiling, poaching, microwaving, and grilling rather than frying f. restrict intake of eggs (recommendations about the number of whole eggs allowed per week vary depending on the client's lipid levels). 4. Obtain a dietary consult to assist client in planning meals that will meet the prescribed restrictions of sodium, saturated fat, and cholesterol.
7.c. The client will verbalize an understanding of activity restrictions and the rate of activity progression.	7.c. Reinforce physician's instructions regarding activity. Instruct client to: 1. gradually rebuild activity level by adhering to a planned exercise program (often begins with walking and light household activities) 2. take frequent rest periods for 4–6 weeks following surgery 3. avoid lifting heavy objects in order to allow incision to heal and prevent a sudden increase in cardiac workload 4. avoid driving a car and riding a bicycle, motorcycle, lawn mower, tractor, or a horse for 4–6 weeks; if minimally invasive surgery was performed, these activities will probably be allowed much sooner 5. check with physician or cardiac rehabilitation therapist before resuming sexual activity (usually permitted 3–4 weeks after surgery once able to walk 2 blocks or climb 2 flights of stairs without shortness of breath) 6. stop any activity that causes chest pain, shortness of breath, palpitations, dizziness, or extreme fatigue or weakness 7. participate in a cardiac rehabilitation program if recommended by physician.
7.d. The client will verbalize an understanding of medications ordered including rationale, food and drug interactions, side effects, schedule for taking, and importance of taking as prescribed.	7.d.1. Explain the rationale for, side effects of, and importance of taking medications prescribed. Inform client of pertinent food and drug interactions. 2. If client has had a valve replacement and is discharged on warfarin (e.g., Coumadin), instruct to: a. keep scheduled appointments for periodic blood studies to monitor coagulation times b. take medication at the same time each day, do not stop taking medication abruptly, and do not attempt to make up for missed doses c. avoid regular and/or excessive intake of alcohol (may alter responsiveness to warfarin) d. avoid taking over-the-counter products containing aspirin and other nonsteroidal anti-inflammatory agents (these products enhance the action of warfarin) e. avoid significantly increasing or decreasing consumption of foods high in vitamin K (e.g., green leafy vegetables) f. take the following precautions to minimize the risk of bleeding: 1. use an electric rather than a straight-edge razor 2. floss and brush teeth gently; use waxed floss and soft bristle toothbrush 3. avoid putting sharp objects (e.g., toothpicks) in mouth 4. do not walk barefoot 5. cut nails carefully

6. avoid situations that could result in injury (e.g., contact sports)
7. avoid blowing nose forcefully
8. avoid straining to have a bowel movement

g. report prolonged or excessive bleeding from skin, nose, or mouth; red, rust-colored, or smoky urine; bloody or tarry stools; blood in vomitus or sputum; prolonged or excessive menses; excessive bruising; severe or persistent headache; or sudden abdominal or back pain
h. apply firm, prolonged pressure to any bleeding area if possible
i. wear a medical alert identification bracelet or tag identifying self as being on anticoagulant therapy
j. inform physician immediately if pregnancy is suspected or if you are breastfeeding (warfarin crosses the placental barrier and enters the breastmilk).

3. Instruct client to inform physician before taking other prescription and nonprescription medications.
4. Instruct client to inform all health care providers of medications being taken.

7.e. The client will state signs and symptoms to report to the health care provider.	7.e.1. Refer to Standardized Postoperative Care Plan, Diagnosis 22, action c (p. 125), for signs and symptoms to report to the health care provider. 2. Instruct client to report these additional signs and symptoms: a. chest pain that seems unrelated to incisional discomfort b. development of or increased shortness of breath c. dizziness, fainting d. increased fatigue and weakness e. weight gain of more than 2 pounds in a day or 4 pounds in a week f. swelling of feet or ankles g. persistent cough, especially if productive of yellow, green, rust-colored, or frothy sputum h. significant change in pulse rate or rhythm (check with physician about client's need to monitor pulse at home) i. persistent low-grade temperature or temperature above 101° F (38.3° C) for more than 1 day j. depression or problems with concentration or memory that last more than 6 weeks k. a fever in combination with chest pain and malaise occurring 1 week to 1 month after surgery (may be indicative of postpericardiotomy syndrome and require treatment with anti-inflammatory agents).
7.f. The client will identify community resources that can assist with cardiac rehabilitation and adjustment to having had heart surgery.	7.f.1. Provide information about community resources that can assist client with cardiac rehabilitation and adjustment to having had heart surgery (e.g., American Heart Association, Mended Hearts Club, counseling services). 2. Initiate a referral if indicated.
7.g. The client will verbalize an understanding of and a plan for adhering to recommended follow-up care including future appointments with health care provider, wound care, and pain management.	7.g.1. Refer to Standardized Postoperative Care Plan, Diagnosis 22 (pp. 125–126), for routine postoperative instructions and measures to improve client compliance. 2. If client had a valve replacement, instruct him/her to: a. not have dental work for 6 months b. inform health care providers of valve surgery so prophylactic antimicrobials may be started before any dental work, invasive diagnostic procedures, or surgery c. perform good oral hygiene in order to reduce the risk for infective endocarditis.

Bibliography

See pages 879 and 881–882.

Hypertension

Hypertension is defined by the Joint National Committee on Prevention, Detection, Evaluation, and Treatment of High Blood Pressure as a systolic blood pressure (SBP) of 140 mm Hg or greater, a diastolic blood pressure (DBP) of 90 mm Hg or greater, or taking antihypertensive medication. Isolated systolic hypertension (ISH) is present when the SBP is greater than 140 mm Hg and the DBP is less than 90 mm Hg. The classification of hypertension is based on the level of the blood pressure. The current classification system includes a category designated as prehypertension (SBP of 120–139 or DBP of 80–89) and divides hypertension into two stages. Stage 1 hypertension is an average SBP of 140–159 mm Hg or a DBP of 90–99 mm Hg. Stage 2 hypertension is a SBP of greater than 160 mm Hg or a DBP greater than 100 mm Hg. In addition to classifying the stages of hypertension on the basis of average blood pressure readings, the clinician usually also specifies the presence or absence of target organ disease and the additional risk factors for cardiovascular disease that are present. Hypertensive crisis, urgency, or emergency are terms used to describe a situation in which the pressure elevation poses an immediate threat to the client's life.

The two major types of hypertension are essential (primary or idiopathic) hypertension and secondary hypertension. Essential hypertension, which constitutes approximately 95% of the cases, has an unknown etiology. Secondary hypertension has identifiable causes, which include renal parenchymal or vascular disease, Cushing's syndrome, certain neurological disorders, pheochromocytoma, primary aldosteronism, coarctation of the aorta, and use of certain drugs (e.g., adrenal steroids, oral contraceptives, nonsteroidal anti-inflammatories, cyclooxygenase-2 inhibitors, sympathomimetics such as decongestants and anorexiants, amphetamines, cocaine).

The pathological hallmark of hypertension is an increase in systemic vascular resistance. In order to sustain adequate tissue perfusion when vascular resistance is increased, the heart must pump harder. A prolonged increase in cardiac workload eventually leads to ventricular hypertrophy and heart failure. The prolonged increase in vascular pressure causes widespread pathological changes in the blood vessels. The end result of all the changes in the cardiovascular system is a decreased blood supply to the tissues with target organ damage occurring most often in the eyes, kidneys, brain, and heart. This target organ damage is often what causes the initial symptoms in the person with hypertension.

Initial treatment of hypertension may be nonpharmacologic and consists of lifestyle modifications such as weight reduction, regular aerobic exercise, and moderation of dietary sodium and alcohol intake. If these measures do not achieve the desired control of blood pressure, pharmacologic therapy is initiated. A diuretic alone or in combination with an angiotensin-converting enzyme inhibitor, angiotensin II receptor antagonist, calcium-channel blocking agent, or beta-adrenergic blocking agent are considered appropriate options for initial pharmacologic therapy. If the person's blood pressure is inadequately controlled by the initial drug, a second drug from another class is added or another drug is substituted until the desired control of blood pressure is achieved with a minimum of side effects.

This care plan focuses on the adult client hospitalized with severe hypertension that is either newly diagnosed or uncontrolled.

OUTCOME/DISCHARGE CRITERIA

THE CLIENT WILL:

- have blood pressure within a safe range
- have evidence of adequate tissue perfusion
- have no signs and symptoms of complications
- verbalize a basic understanding of hypertension and its effects on the body
- identify modifiable risk factors for hypertension and ways to alter these factors
- verbalize an understanding of medications ordered including rationale, food and drug interactions, side effects, schedule for taking, and importance of taking as prescribed
- verbalize an understanding of the rationale for and components of the recommended diet
- state signs and symptoms to report to the health care provider
- identify community resources that can assist in making lifestyle changes necessary for effective control of hypertension
- verbalize an understanding of and a plan for adhering to recommended follow-up care including future appointments with health care provider.

NURSING/COLLABORATIVE DIAGNOSES

DISCHARGE TEACHING

1. NURSING DIAGNOSIS: ***INEFFECTIVE TISSUE PERFUSION***

related to:

a. increased peripheral vascular resistance;
b. atherogenic changes in the blood vessels associated with the effects of prolonged or excessive elevation of blood pressure;
c. possible decrease in cardiac output associated with the increased cardiac workload and eventual myocardial hypertrophy that result from elevated blood pressure;
d. excessive lowering of blood pressure by antihypertensive medications.

Suggested NOC Outcomes: Circulation status; Tissue perfusion: cerebral

Suggested NIC Interventions: Vital signs monitoring; Hemodynamic regulation; Cerebral perfusion promotion

Desired Outcome

1. The client will maintain adequate tissue perfusion as evidenced by:
   a. B/P declining toward normal range for client
   b. usual mental status
   c. extremities warm with absence of pallor and cyanosis
   d. palpable peripheral pulses
   e. capillary refill time less than 2–3 seconds
   f. absence of exercise-induced pain
   g. urine output at least 30 ml/hour.

Nursing Actions *and Selected Purposes/Rationales*

(see pp. 57–59 for additional rationales)

1.a. Assess for and report the following:
   1. further increase in B/P, failure of B/P to decline in response to antihypertensive agents, or rapid or excessive decline in B/P
   2. signs and symptoms of diminished tissue perfusion (e.g., restlessness, confusion, cool extremities, pallor or cyanosis of extremities, diminished or absent peripheral pulses, slow capillary refill, angina, increasing BUN and serum creatinine, oliguria).

b. Implement measures *to reduce blood pressure in order to improve tissue perfusion:*
   1. administer the following medications if ordered:
      a. adrenergic inhibiting agents:
         1. centrally acting adrenergic inhibitors (e.g., clonidine, methyldopa, guanabenz, guanfacine)
         2. alpha-adrenergic blockers (e.g., prazosin, terazosin, doxazosin)
         3. peripheral adrenergic inhibitors (e.g., reserpine, guanethidine, guanadrel)
         4. beta-adrenergic blockers (e.g., propranolol, metoprolol, atenolol, nadolol, bisoprolol)
         5. combined alpha- and beta-adrenergic blockers (e.g., labetalol, carvedilol)
      b. vasodilators (e.g., minoxidil, hydralazine, sodium nitroprusside, nitroglycerin, fenoldopam); this group of medications is most often used when immediate reduction of B/P is necessary
      c. angiotensin-converting enzyme inhibitors (e.g., captopril, perindopril, lisinopril, enalapril, fosinopril, quinapril, ramipril, benazepril, moexipril, trandolapril)

Desired Outcome	Nursing Actions *and Selected Purposes/Rationales*

d. calcium-channel blocking agents (e.g., verapamil, isradipine, nicardipine, diltiazem, amlodipine, felodipine; nisoldipine)
e. angiotensin II receptor antagonists (e.g., losartan, valsartan, telmisartan, irbesartan, candesartan)
f. diuretics

2. perform actions *to reduce sympathetic nervous system stimulation:*
    a. implement measures to reduce fear and anxiety (see Diagnosis 4, action b)
    b. implement measures to relieve headache (see Diagnosis 2, action d)
    c. implement measures *to promote rest* (e.g., maintain a calm, quiet environment; limit the number of visitors; maintain activity restrictions)
3. discourage excessive intake of beverages high in caffeine such as coffee, tea, and colas
4. discourage smoking *(nicotine causes vasoconstriction)*
5. maintain dietary sodium restrictions as ordered *to reduce fluid retention.*

c. Consult physician:
1. before administering antihypertensive medications if client has an excessive or rapid drop in B/P *(a rapid drop in B/P of more than 20–25% in a person with severe hypertension can reduce perfusion to vital organs)*
2. if signs and symptoms of diminished tissue perfusion persist or worsen.

2. Nursing Diagnosis: ACUTE PAIN: HEADACHE

related to distention of the cerebral blood vessels associated with increased vascular pressure.

Suggested NOC Outcomes: Comfort level; Pain control

Suggested NIC Interventions: Pain management; Environmental management: comfort; Analgesic administration

Desired Outcome	Nursing Actions *and Selected Purposes/Rationales* (see pp. 45–47 for additional rationales)
2. The client will obtain relief of headache as evidenced by: a. verbalization of same b. relaxed facial expression and body positioning c. increased participation in activities.	2.a. Assess for signs and symptoms of headache (e.g., statements of same, restlessness, irritability, grimacing, rubbing head, avoidance of bright lights and noises, reluctance to move). b. Assess client's perception of the severity of the headache using a pain intensity rating scale. c. Assess the client's pain pattern (e.g., location, quality, onset, duration, precipitating factors, aggravating factors, alleviating factors). d. Implement measures *to relieve headache:* 1. perform actions to reduce blood pressure (see Diagnosis 1, action b) 2. perform actions *to reduce fear and anxiety about the pain experience* (e.g., assure client that his/her need for headache relief is understood, plan methods for relieving headache with client) 3. perform actions to reduce fear and anxiety (see Diagnosis 4, action b) *in order to promote relaxation and subsequently increase the client's threshold and tolerance for pain* 4. administer analgesics as ordered and before headache becomes severe 5. perform actions *to minimize environmental stimuli* (e.g., provide a quiet environment, dim lights) 6. avoid jarring bed or startling client *to minimize risk of sudden movements* 7. provide or assist with nonpharmacologic measures for headache relief (e.g., cool cloth to forehead, back and neck massage, elevation of head, relaxation exercises, diversional activities). e. Consult appropriate health care provider (e.g., pharmacist, physician) if above measures fail to relieve headache.

3. COLLABORATIVE DIAGNOSES: *POTENTIAL COMPLICATIONS OF HYPERTENSION*

a. cerebrovascular accident related to cerebral thrombosis, embolism, or hemorrhage associated with injury to the arterial walls resulting from atherosclerosis and/or a prolonged increase in pressure in the cerebral vessels;
b. hypertensive encephalopathy related to cerebral edema associated with hyperperfusion of the brain (excessive cerebral blood flow results from decompensation of the cerebral blood flow autoregulatory mechanism in response to markedly elevated blood pressure);
c. angina and/or myocardial infarction related to:
   1. insufficient myocardial blood flow associated with coronary artery disease (a sequela of inadequately controlled hypertension)
   2. myocardial oxygen demands exceeding the oxygen supply (a result of the increased cardiac workload that occurs with increased vascular resistance);
d. impaired renal function related to vascular changes in the kidneys associated with effects of prolonged or severe hypertension;
e. heart failure related to the prolonged increase in cardiac workload associated with increased systemic vascular resistance;
f. aortic dissection related to weakening and degeneration of the aortic media associated with a severe or prolonged increase in pressure in the aorta.

Desired Outcomes	**Nursing Actions** *and Selected Purposes/Rationales*
3.a. The client will not experience a cerebrovascular accident or hypertensive encephalopathy as evidenced by: 1. absence of dizziness, syncope, visual disturbances, and speech impairments 2. absence or resolution of headache 3. absence of vomiting 4. mentally alert and oriented 5. pupils equal and normally reactive to light 6. normal sensory and motor function.	3.a.1. Assess for and report signs and symptoms of a cerebrovascular accident and/or hypertensive encephalopathy: a. dizziness, syncope b. visual disturbances (e.g., diplopia, blurred vision, loss of vision) c. slurred speech, aphasia d. persistent or increasing headache e. vomiting f. decreased level of consciousness g. unequal pupils or a sluggish or absent pupillary reaction to light h. paresthesias, facial ptosis, weakness of extremity, paralysis i. seizures. 2. Implement measures *to reduce the risk of a cerebrovascular accident and hypertensive encephalopathy:* a. perform actions to reduce blood pressure (see Diagnosis 1, action b) b. instruct client to avoid activities that create a Valsalva response (e.g., straining to have a bowel movement, holding breath while moving up in bed) *in order to prevent a sudden increase in intracranial pressure and dislodgment of an existing thrombus* c. keep head of bed elevated at least 30° and encourage client to keep head and neck in neutral, midline position *in order to promote adequate venous return from the cerebral vessels.* 3. If signs and symptoms of a cerebrovascular accident or hypertensive encephalopathy occur: a. administer antihypertensive agents that may be ordered to provide rapid blood pressure reduction (e.g., sodium nitroprusside, enalaprilat, labetalol, fenoldopam) b. maintain client on bed rest c. initiate appropriate safety measures (e.g., side rails up, seizure precautions) d. administer osmotic diuretics (e.g., mannitol) and corticosteroids (e.g., dexamethasone) if ordered *to reduce intracranial pressure.*
3.b. The client will not experience episodes of myocardial ischemia as evidenced by: 1. absence of chest pain 2. unlabored respirations at 12–20/minute	3.b.1. Assess for signs and symptoms of myocardial ischemia (e.g., chest pain/discomfort, dyspnea). 2. Implement measures *to prevent myocardial ischemia:* a. perform actions to reduce blood pressure (see Diagnosis 1, action b) b. instruct client to avoid activities that create a Valsalva response (e.g., straining to have a bowel movement, holding breath while moving up in bed)

Desired Outcomes	Nursing Actions *and Selected Purposes/Rationales*
3. cardiac enzymes within normal range 4. absence of ST segment depression or elevation, T wave inversion, and abnormal Q waves on ECG.	c. increase activity gradually as allowed and tolerated. 3. If signs and symptoms of myocardial ischemia occur: a. consult physician about an order for cardiac enzyme levels and ECG; report significant elevation of cardiac enzymes and ST segment depression or elevation, T wave inversion, and/or abnormal Q waves on ECG b. maintain client on strict bed rest in a semi- to high Fowler's position c. maintain oxygen therapy as ordered d. administer the following medications if ordered: 1. nitrates *to improve coronary blood flow and reduce myocardial oxygen requirements* 2. morphine sulfate *to reduce pain and anxiety and decrease cardiac workload* 3. beta-adrenergic blocking agents *to reduce myocardial oxygen requirements by decreasing heart rate and the force of myocardial contractility.*
3.c. The client will maintain adequate renal function as evidenced by: 1. urine output at least 30 ml/hour 2. absence of proteinuria 3. BUN, serum creatinine, and creatinine clearance within normal range.	3.c.1. Assess for and report signs and symptoms of impaired renal function (e.g., nocturia, urine output less than 30 ml/hour, urine specific gravity fixed at or less than 1.010, proteinuria, elevated BUN and serum creatinine levels, decreased creatinine clearance). 2. Implement measures *to maintain adequate renal blood flow:* a. perform actions to reduce blood pressure (see Diagnosis 1, action b) b. maintain an adequate fluid intake *to reduce risk of dehydration.* 3. If signs and symptoms of impaired renal function occur: a. consult physician about lowering the dose of or discontinuing angiotensin-converting enzyme inhibitors if BUN and serum creatinine continue to rise significantly (ACE inhibitors should be used cautiously in persons with impaired renal function *because they can have an adverse effect on renal function)* b. assess for and report signs of acute renal failure (e.g., oliguria or anuria; weight gain; edema; increasing B/P; lethargy and confusion; increasing BUN and serum creatinine, phosphorus, and potassium levels) c. prepare client for dialysis if indicated.
3.d. The client will not develop heart failure as evidenced by: 1. pulse 60–100 beats/minute 2. absence of an S_3 heart sound 3. usual mental status 4. clear, audible breath sounds 5. absence of dyspnea, orthopnea, and cough 6. increased strength and activity tolerance 7. palpable peripheral pulses 8. urine output at least 30 ml/hour 9. stable weight 10. absence of edema and distended neck veins.	3.d.1. Assess for and report signs and symptoms of heart failure: a. tachycardia b. presence of an S_3 heart sound c. restlessness, agitation, confusion, or other change in mental status d. crackles (rales) e. dyspnea, orthopnea f. dry, hacking cough or cough productive of frothy or blood-tinged sputum g. development of or increased weakness and fatigue h. diminished or absent peripheral pulses i. decreased urine output during the day, nocturia j. weight gain k. edema l. distended neck veins m. chest x-ray results showing pulmonary vascular congestion, pleural effusion, or pulmonary edema. 2. Implement measures to reduce blood pressure (see Diagnosis 1, action b) *in order to reduce cardiac workload and prevent heart failure.* 3. If signs and symptoms of heart failure occur: a. maintain oxygen therapy as ordered b. administer the following medications if ordered: 1. positive inotropic agents (e.g., digitalis preparations, dobutamine, inamrinone) *to increase myocardial contractility*

2. diuretics, vasodilators (e.g., nitroglycerin, sodium nitroprusside), and/or ACE inhibitors (e.g., enalaprilat, ramipril, captopril) *to decrease cardiac workload*
3. morphine sulfate *to reduce preload and anxiety* (used primarily in clients with pulmonary edema).

3.e. The client will not experience dissection of the aorta as evidenced by:
1. absence of sudden, severe chest pain
2. palpable peripheral pulses with no change in pulse pattern
3. usual sensory and motor function
4. usual mental status
5. stable vital signs
6. skin warm and usual color.

3.e.1. Assess for and immediately report the following:
a. signs and symptoms of aortic dissection (e.g., sudden, severe chest pain that may radiate to back; abnormal pulse pattern [discrepancies in character, timing, and magnitude]) in extremities; sudden lack of pulse in an extremity; hemianesthesia; hemiplegia; paraplegia)
b. signs and symptoms of hypovolemic shock (e.g., restlessness; agitation; significant decrease in B/P; rapid, weak pulse; cool skin; pallor; diminished or absent pulses).

2. Implement measures *to prevent aortic dissection:*
a. perform actions to reduce blood pressure (see Diagnosis 1, action b)
b. instruct client to avoid activities that create a Valsalva response (e.g., straining to have a bowel movement, holding breath while moving up in bed).

3. If signs and symptoms of aortic dissection occur:
a. maintain client on strict bed rest
b. monitor vital signs frequently
c. administer oxygen as ordered
d. prepare client for diagnostic studies (e.g., transesophageal echocardiogram, computed tomography) if planned
e. administer antihypertensive agents (e.g., beta-adrenergic blocker, nitrate, sodium nitroprusside) if ordered
f. prepare client for surgery if planned.

4. NURSING DIAGNOSIS: *FEAR/ANXIETY*

related to necessity for urgent treatment; possibility of severe disability or sudden death; unfamiliar environment; persistent or severe headache; and lack of understanding of diagnostic tests, diagnosis, and treatment plan.

Suggested NOC Outcomes: Anxiety self-control; Anxiety level; Fear self-control; Fear level

Suggested NIC Interventions: Anxiety reduction; Calming technique; Emotional support; Presence

Desired Outcome

Nursing Actions *and Selected Purposes/Rationales*
(see pp. 14–16 for additional rationales)

4. The client will experience a reduction in fear and anxiety as evidenced by:
a. verbalization of feeling less anxious
b. usual sleep pattern
c. relaxed facial expression and body movements
d. vital signs returning to normal range for client
e. usual perceptual ability and interactions with others.

4.a. Assess client for signs and symptoms of fear and anxiety (e.g., verbalization of feeling anxious, insomnia, tenseness, shakiness, restlessness, diaphoresis, tachycardia, further elevation of blood pressure, self-focused behaviors). Validate perceptions carefully, remembering that some behaviors may result from decreased tissue perfusion and neurological changes.

b. Implement measures *to reduce fear and anxiety:*
1. orient client to environment, equipment, and routines
2. provide a calm, restful environment
3. introduce client to staff who will be participating in care; if possible, maintain consistency in staff assigned to his/her care
4. assure client that staff members are nearby; respond to call signal as soon as possible
5. maintain a calm, supportive, confident manner when interacting with client
6. encourage verbalization of fear and anxiety; provide feedback
7. explain all diagnostic tests

Desired Outcome	Nursing Actions *and Selected Purposes/Rationales*

8. reinforce physician's explanations and clarify misconceptions the client has about hypertension, the treatment plan, and prognosis
9. perform actions to relieve headache (see Diagnosis 2, action d)
10. instruct client in relaxation techniques and encourage participation in diversional activities
11. assist client to identify specific stressors and ways to cope with them
12. provide information based on current needs of client at a level he/she can understand; encourage questions and clarification of information provided
13. encourage significant others to project a caring, concerned attitude without obvious anxiousness
14. include significant others in orientation and teaching sessions and encourage their continued support of client
15. administer prescribed antianxiety agents if indicated.

c. Consult appropriate health care provider (e.g., psychiatric nurse clinician, physician) if above actions fail to control fear and anxiety.

5. Nursing Diagnosis: ***INEFFECTIVE THERAPEUTIC REGIMEN MANAGEMENT***

related to:
a. lack of understanding of the implications of not following the prescribed treatment plan;
b. difficulty modifying personal habits (e.g., alcohol intake, dietary preferences);
c. undesirable side effects of some antihypertensive agents;
d. insufficient financial resources.

Suggested NOC Outcomes: Compliance behavior; Treatment behavior: illness or injury; Knowledge: treatment regimen; Health beliefs: perceived resources; Knowledge: cardiac disease management; Health beliefs: perceived ability to perform

Suggested NIC Interventions: Self-modification assistance; Medication management; Values clarification; Exercise promotion; Smoking cessation assistance; Teaching: prescribed diet; Weight reduction assistance; Financial resource assistance

Desired Outcome	Nursing Actions *and Selected Purposes/Rationales*
5. The client will demonstrate the probability of effective management of the therapeutic regimen as evidenced by: a. willingness to learn about and participate in treatments and care b. statements reflecting ways to modify personal habits c. statements reflecting an understanding of the implications of not following the prescribed treatment plan.	5.a. Assess for indications that the client may be unable to effectively manage the therapeutic regimen: 1. statements reflecting inability to manage care at home 2. failure to adhere to treatment plan (e.g., not adhering to dietary modifications, refusing medications) 3. statements reflecting a lack of understanding of factors that may cause progression of hypertension 4. statements reflecting an unwillingness or inability to modify personal habits 5. statements reflecting view that hypertension will reverse itself or that the situation is hopeless and efforts to comply with the therapeutic regimen are useless 6. statements reflecting that the side effects of medications are too uncomfortable and that he/she feels better when not taking medication 7. statements reflecting that medications are too expensive. b. Implement measures *to promote effective management of the therapeutic regimen:* 1. explain hypertension in terms the client can understand; stress the fact that hypertension is a chronic condition and that adherence to the treatment plan is necessary in order to delay and/or prevent complications

2. encourage questions and clarify misconceptions client has about hypertension and its effects and the side effects of medications
3. provide instructions on and encourage client to participate in the treatment plan (e.g., calculating sodium intake, monitoring blood pressure); determine areas of misunderstanding and reinforce teaching as necessary
4. provide client with written instructions about dietary modifications, signs and symptoms to report, medication therapy, blood pressure monitoring, and exercise regimen
5. assist client to identify ways medication regimen, exercise, and dietary modifications can be incorporated into lifestyle; focus on modifications of lifestyle rather than complete change
6. assist client to identify a reward system for self that will assist him/her to effect necessary change(s)
7. initiate and reinforce discharge teaching outlined in Diagnosis 6 *in order to promote a sense of control*
8. provide information about and encourage utilization of community resources that can assist client to make necessary lifestyle changes (e.g., cardiovascular fitness, weight loss, and smoking cessation programs; stress management classes)
9. encourage client to discuss concerns about the cost of medications and visits with health care provider; obtain a social service consult to assist with financial planning and to obtain financial aid if indicated
10. encourage client to attend follow-up educational classes
11. reinforce behaviors suggesting future compliance with the therapeutic regimen (e.g., statements reflecting plan for adhering to treatment plan, statements reflecting an understanding of hypertension and its long-term effects)
12. include significant others in explanations and teaching sessions and encourage their support; reinforce the need for client to assume responsibility for managing as much of care as possible.

c. Consult appropriate health care provider (e.g., social worker, physician) regarding referrals to community health agencies if continued instruction or support is needed.

Discharge Teaching/Continued Care

6. NURSING DIAGNOSIS: ***DEFICIENT KNOWLEDGE OR INEFFECTIVE HEALTH MAINTENANCE****

*The nurse should select the diagnostic label that is most appropriate for the client's discharge teaching needs.

Suggested NOC Outcomes: Knowledge: treatment regimen; Knowledge: cardiac disease management

Suggested NIC Interventions: Health system guidance; Teaching: individual; Teaching: prescribed medication; Teaching: prescribed diet

Desired Outcomes	Nursing Actions *and Selected Purposes/Rationales*
6.a. The client will verbalize a basic understanding of hypertension and its effects on the body.	6.a.1. Explain hypertension and its effects in terms client can understand. Utilize available teaching aids (e.g., pamphlets, videotapes). 2. Inform client that hypertension is often asymptomatic and that absence of symptoms is not a reliable indication that blood pressure is within a safe range.

Desired Outcomes	Nursing Actions *and Selected Purposes/Rationales*
6.b. The client will identify modifiable risk factors for hypertension and ways to alter these factors.	6.b.1. Inform client that certain modifiable factors such as elevated serum lipids, excessive alcohol intake, a sedentary lifestyle, smoking, and excess body weight have been shown to increase the risk for cardiovascular disease and hypertension. 2. Assist client to identify changes in lifestyle that can help him/her to manage hypertension (e.g., dietary modification, physical exercise on a regular basis, smoking cessation, moderation of alcohol intake, weight loss if overweight). 3. Encourage client to limit daily alcohol consumption (daily alcohol intake exceeding 1 oz of ethanol may contribute to the development of hypertension). Current recommendations are no more than 2 drinks/day for men and no more than 1 drink/day for women and lighter weight persons. A "drink" is considered to be ½ oz of ethanol (e.g., 1½ oz of 80-proof whiskey, 12 oz of beer, 5 oz of wine). 4. Instruct client to participate in a regular aerobic exercise program (e.g., walking, swimming) and avoid isometric exercise (e.g., weight training). Caution client to consult physician before beginning an exercise program.
6.c. The client will verbalize an understanding of medications ordered including rationale, food and drug interactions, side effects, schedule for taking, and importance of taking as prescribed.	6.c.1. Explain the rationale for, side effects of, and importance of taking medications prescribed. Inform client of pertinent food and drug interactions. 2. If client is discharged on a diuretic, instruct to: a. take once-daily dose in the morning or, if diuretic is to be taken twice each day, take the larger dose in the morning and the second dose no later than 3:00 p.m. (scheduling doses in this manner minimizes nighttime urination) b. weigh self as often as instructed (e.g., daily, weekly) and keep a record of weights c. change from a lying to a standing position slowly if experiencing dizziness or lightheadedness with position change d. increase intake of foods/fluids high in potassium (e.g., orange juice, bananas, cantaloupe, potatoes, raisins, avocados) if taking a potassium-depleting diuretic e. notify physician if unable to tolerate food or fluids (dehydration can develop rapidly if intake is poor and client continues to take a diuretic) f. avoid salt substitutes with a high potassium content if discharged on a potassium-sparing diuretic (e.g., triamterene, eplerenone, spironolactone) g. report the following signs and symptoms: 1. weight loss of more than 5 pounds a week 2. excessive thirst 3. severe dizziness or episodes of fainting 4. muscle weakness or cramping, nausea, vomiting, or an irregular pulse. 3. If client is discharged on a beta-adrenergic blocking agent (e.g., propranolol, metoprolol, atenolol, nadolol, bisoprolol), instruct to: a. take the medication at the same time every day b. check pulse before taking medication; consult physician before taking medication if pulse rate is unusually slow (it is expected that pulse will be lower than normal) c. avoid skipping doses, altering the prescribed dose, trying to make up for missed doses, and discontinuing medication without first discussing with health care provider d. change from a lying to a sitting or standing position slowly if dizziness or lightheadedness is a problem e. limit intake of alcoholic beverages f. monitor blood glucose on a regular basis if diabetic (beta blockers may affect blood sugar and mask symptoms of hypoglycemia)

g. wear or carry medical identification specifying the name of the medication being taken
h. report the following:
1. persistent lightheadedness or dizziness
2. significant weight gain or worsening of symptoms of heart failure (because beta blockers reduce the force of myocardial contractility, they can actually worsen symptoms of heart failure)
3. cold, painful toes or fingers
4. persistent fatigue, depression, insomnia, or sexual dysfunction
5. worsening of any symptoms of chronic respiratory disease.

4. If client is discharged on an ACE inhibitor or angiotensin II receptor antagonist, instruct to:
a. change from a lying to a sitting or standing position slowly if experiencing dizziness or lightheadedness with position change
b. avoid hot baths and showers, steam room, and sauna
c. avoid salt substitutes with a high potassium content
d. report continued dizziness, lightheadedness, or fainting; a persistent dry cough; or swelling of the tongue, lips, face, or neck.

5. If client is discharged on a calcium-channel blocker (e.g., amlodipine, verapamil, diltiazem, isradipine, nicardipine, felodipine), instruct to:
a. avoid skipping doses, altering the prescribed dose, and discontinuing medication without first discussing it with health care provider
b. change from a lying to a sitting or standing position slowly in order to prevent dizziness
c. report persistent dizziness, lightheadedness, or headache; swelling of feet or ankles; shortness of breath; or weight gain of more than 2 pounds in a day
d. check pulse before taking medication if taking verapamil or diltiazem and report pulse rate that is unusually slow (e.g., less than 50 beats per minute)
e. avoid operating dangerous equipment and driving as long as dizziness is present (common in the early treatment period).

6. Instruct the client to consult physician before taking other prescription and nonprescription medications.
7. Instruct client to inform all health care providers of medications being taken.

6.d. The client will verbalize an understanding of the rationale for and components of the recommended diet.

6.d.1. Explain the rationale for the recommended dietary modifications.

2. Depending on the physician's recommendations:
a. provide the following information about decreasing sodium intake:
1. read labels on foods/fluids and calculate sodium content of items; avoid those products that tend to have a high sodium content (e.g., canned soups and vegetables, tomato juice, commercial baked goods, commercially prepared frozen or canned entrees and sauces)
2. do not add salt when cooking foods or to prepared foods; use low-sodium herbs and spices if desired
3. avoid cured and smoked foods
4. avoid salty snack foods (e.g., crackers, nuts, pretzels, potato chips)
5. avoid commercially prepared fast foods
6. avoid routine use of over-the-counter medications with a high sodium content (e.g., Alka-Seltzer, some antacids)

b. provide instructions on ways the client can reduce intake of saturated fat and cholesterol:
1. reduce intake of meat fat (e.g., trim visible fat off meat; replace fatty meats such as fatty cuts of steak, hamburger, and processed meats with leaner products)
2. reduce intake of milk fat (avoid dairy products containing more than 1% fat)
3. reduce intake of *trans* fats (e.g., avoid stick margarine and shortening and foods such as commercial baked goods that are prepared with these products)

Desired Outcomes	Nursing Actions *and Selected Purposes/Rationales*
	4. use vegetable oil rather than coconut or palm oil in cooking and food preparation 5. use cooking methods such as steaming, baking, broiling, poaching, microwaving, and grilling rather than frying 6. restrict intake of eggs (recommendations about the number of whole eggs allowed per week vary depending on the client's lipid levels). 3. Instruct client to include the recommended daily allowances of potassium, calcium, and magnesium in diet.
6.e. The client will state signs and symptoms to report to the health care provider.	6.e. Instruct the client to report: 1. persistent headache or headache present upon awakening 2. sudden and continued increase in B/P (if B/P is monitored at home) 3. chest pain 4. shortness of breath 5. significant weight gain or swelling of feet or ankles 6. changes in vision 7. frequent or uncontrollable nosebleeds 8. persistent dizziness, lightheadedness, or fainting 9. persistent side effects experienced from use of antihypertensive medications (e.g., impotence; dry mouth; depression; persistent dry cough; swelling of the tongue, face, or neck) 10. side effects of diuretic therapy (see action c.2.g in this diagnosis).
6.f. The client will identify community resources that can assist in making lifestyle changes necessary for effective control of hypertension.	6.f.1. Provide information regarding community resources and support groups that can assist client in making lifestyle changes that are necessary for effective control of hypertension (e.g., cardiovascular fitness, weight loss, and smoking cessation programs; stress management classes). 2. Initiate a referral if indicated.
6.g. The client will verbalize an understanding of and a plan for adhering to recommended follow-up care including future appointments with health care provider.	6.g.1. Reinforce the importance of keeping follow-up appointments with health care provider and continuing lifelong medical supervision. 2. Refer to Diagnosis 5, action b, for measures to promote client's ability to effectively manage the therapeutic regimen.

Bibliography

See pages 879 and 881–882.

MYOCARDIAL INFARCTION

A myocardial infarction (MI) is an acute coronary syndrome resulting from prolonged ischemia of the heart muscle and occurs when blood flow to an area of the myocardium is insufficient to meet the myocardial oxygen requirements. Sustained ischemia causes tissue necrosis and irreversible cellular damage, which results in disturbances in mechanical, biochemical, and electrical function in the necrotic or infarcted area. The degree of altered function depends on the area of the heart involved and the size of the infarct.

MIs may be classified in a number of ways. A transmural MI involves the full thickness of the myocardium. A significant Q wave develops with a transmural infarction, so this may be referred to as a Q-wave MI. A subendocardial infarction only involves a partial thickness of the myocardium and is often classified as a non–Q-wave MI because a pathologic Q wave does not develop. MIs may also be classified as an ST-elevation MI or a non–ST-elevation MI (NSTEMI). In addition to these classification systems, many practitioners also describe an MI by the area of the heart that has been damaged (e.g., anterior MI, lateral MI, inferior MI).

The majority of MIs are caused by rupture of atherosclerotic plaque in a coronary artery, which leads to the release of substances that activate platelet aggregation and clotting factors and cause local vasoconstriction. Other less common causes include severe, persistent spasm of a coronary artery; severe or prolonged hypotension; a rapid ventricular rate; and cocaine use.

The classic symptom of an MI is intense retrosternal chest pain/discomfort. It is often described as a tight, heavy, squeezing, or crushing sensation or "heartburn"; may radiate to the left arm, neck, jaw, or back; lasts longer than 20 minutes; and is unrelieved by nitroglycerin and rest. However, 15% to 25% of infarctions go unrecognized because clients have only mild or no chest discomfort. Other signs and symptoms may include shortness of breath, diaphoresis, dizziness, weakness, pallor, nausea, and vomiting.

The extent of myocardial damage can be limited by early (within 4–6 hours of the onset of symptoms) restoration of coronary blood flow. This can be accomplished by injection of a thrombolytic agent to dissolve the clot obstructing the coronary artery or by a coronary angioplasty. In addition to early restoration of coronary blood flow, treatment with an antiplatelet agent, a beta blocker, an angiotensin-converting enzyme (ACE) inhibitor, and an HMG-CoA reductase inhibitor has been found to significantly reduce mortality following an MI. The prognosis for a client who has had an MI is largely influenced by size and location of the infarct, concurrent cardiovascular status, and promptness and effectiveness of treatment.

This care plan focuses on the adult client hospitalized during an episode of intense chest pain for definitive diagnosis and management of a myocardial infarction.

OUTCOME/DISCHARGE CRITERIA

THE CLIENT WILL:

- have adequate cardiac output and tissue perfusion
- tolerate prescribed activity without a significant change in vital signs, chest pain, dyspnea, dizziness, or extreme fatigue or weakness
- verbalize a basic understanding of a myocardial infarction
- demonstrate accuracy in counting pulse
- identify modifiable cardiovascular risk factors and ways to alter these factors
- verbalize an understanding of the rationale for and components of a diet designed to lower serum cholesterol and triglycerides
- verbalize an understanding of medications ordered including rationale, food and drug interactions, side effects, schedule for taking, and importance of taking as prescribed
- verbalize an understanding of activity restrictions and the rate at which activity can be progressed
- state signs and symptoms to report to the health care provider
- identify community resources that can assist with cardiac rehabilitation and adjustment to the effects of a myocardial infarction
- share feelings and concerns about changes in body functioning and usual roles and lifestyle
- verbalize an understanding of and a plan for adhering to recommended follow-up care including future appointments with health care provider.

NURSING/COLLABORATIVE DIAGNOSES

See p. 385 for additional diagnoses.

1. Nursing Diagnosis: ***RISK FOR DECREASED CARDIAC OUTPUT***

related to possible decreased contractility and altered conductivity of the heart associated with the myocardial damage that has occurred with infarction.

Suggested NOC Outcomes: Cardiac pump effectiveness; Circulation status; Tissue perfusion: peripheral; Tissue perfusion: cardiac

Suggested NIC Interventions: Cardiac care: acute; Hemodynamic regulation; Cardiac precautions; Dysrhythmia management; Cardiac care: rehabilitative

Desired Outcome

1. The client will have adequate cardiac output as evidenced by:
   a. B/P within normal range for client
   b. apical pulse between 60–100 beats/minute and regular
   c. resolution of gallop rhythm(s)
   d. no reports of fatigue and weakness
   e. unlabored respirations at 12–20/minute
   f. clear, audible breath sounds
   g. usual mental status
   h. absence of dizziness and syncope
   i. palpable peripheral pulses
   j. skin warm and usual color
   k. capillary refill time less than 2–3 seconds
   l. urine output at least 30 ml/hour
   m. absence of edema and jugular vein distention.

Nursing Actions *and Selected Purposes/Rationales*

(see pp. 20–24 for additional rationales)

1.a. Assess for the following:
   1. diagnostic findings indicative of an MI:
      a. elevated CK (CPK)-MB
      b. elevated troponin levels
      c. elevated LDH with an LDH_1 level that is higher than the LDH_2 (a reliable indicator of an acute MI)
      d. ECG showing ST segment elevation or depression, inversion of T waves, and/or presence of abnormal Q waves (there may be no Q waves if client has had a subendocardial infarction)
      e. presence of an S_4 heart sound
   2. signs and symptoms of decreased cardiac output:
      a. variations in B/P (may be increased because of pain or compensatory vasoconstriction; may be decreased when compensatory mechanisms and pump fail)
      b. tachycardia
      c. presence of gallop rhythm(s)
      d. fatigue and weakness
      e. dyspnea, orthopnea, tachypnea
      f. crackles (rales)
      g. restlessness, anxiousness, confusion, or other change in mental status
      h. dizziness, syncope
      i. diminished or absent peripheral pulses
      j. cool extremities
      k. pallor or cyanosis of skin

l. capillary refill time greater than 2–3 seconds
m. oliguria
n. edema
o. jugular vein distention (JVD)
p. chest x-ray results showing pulmonary vascular congestion, pulmonary edema, or pleural effusion
q. abnormal blood gases
r. significant decrease in oximetry results.

b. Implement measures *to maintain an adequate cardiac output:*
   1. prepare client for procedures that may be performed *to improve coronary blood flow:*
      a. injection of a thrombolytic agent (e.g., streptokinase, alteplase [tPA], anistreplase [APSAC, Eminase], reteplase, tenecteplase [TNK-tPA])
      b. percutaneous coronary intervention (e.g., balloon angioplasty, atherectomy, intracoronary stenting)
      c. insertion of an intra-aortic balloon pump (IABP)
   2. perform actions *to reduce cardiac workload:*
      a. place client in a semi- to high Fowler's position
      b. instruct client to avoid activities that create a Valsalva response (e.g., straining to have a bowel movement, holding breath while moving up in bed)
      c. implement measures to promote rest and conserve energy (see Diagnosis 3, action b.1)
      d. maintain oxygen therapy as ordered
      e. discourage smoking *(nicotine has a cardiostimulatory effect and causes vasoconstriction; the carbon monoxide in smoke reduces oxygen availability)*
      f. provide small meals rather than large ones *(large meals require a greater increase in blood supply to gastrointestinal tract for digestion)*
      g. discourage excessive intake of beverages high in caffeine such as coffee, tea, and colas *(caffeine is a myocardial stimulant and can increase myocardial oxygen consumption)*
      h. restrict sodium intake if ordered *to prevent fluid retention*
      i. increase activity gradually as allowed and tolerated
   3. administer the following medications if ordered:
      a. nitrates (e.g., nitroglycerin) *to dilate the coronary and peripheral (primarily venous) blood vessels and subsequently improve coronary blood flow and reduce cardiac workload and myocardial oxygen requirements*
      b. beta-adrenergic blocking agents (e.g., atenolol, propranolol, metoprolol) *to decrease the incidence of dysrhythmias and to reduce myocardial oxygen requirements by decreasing heart rate and the force of myocardial contractility; beta blockers also appear to limit infarct size and reduce short- and long-term cardiac morbidity and mortality*
      c. angiotensin-converting enzyme (ACE) inhibitors such as captopril and ramipril *(have been shown to limit infarct size and reduce ventricular remodeling and the incidence of heart failure following myocardial infarction)*
      d. antidysrhythmics (e.g., lidocaine, procainamide, metoprolol, atenolol, amiodarone, diltiazem, atropine) if dysrhythmias are present
      e. anticoagulants (e.g., intravenous heparin, enoxaparin, dalteparin) and antiplatelet agents (e.g., low-dose aspirin, glycoprotein IIb/IIIa receptor inhibitor [e.g., tirofiban, eptifibatide, abciximab], clopidogrel) *to reduce the incidence of reinfarction and ventricular thrombus formation.*

c. Consult physician if signs and symptoms of decreased cardiac output develop and persist or worsen.

2. Nursing Diagnosis: ACUTE PAIN: CHEST PAIN/DISCOMFORT THAT MAY RADIATE TO ARM, NECK, JAW, OR BACK

related to myocardial ischemia (a decreased oxygen supply forces the myocardium to convert to anaerobic metabolism; the end products of anaerobic metabolism act as irritants to myocardial neural receptors).

Suggested NOC Outcomes: Comfort level; Pain control

Suggested NIC Interventions: Pain management; Analgesic administration; Oxygen therapy

Desired Outcome

2. The client will experience relief of chest pain/discomfort as evidenced by:
   a. verbalization of same
   b. relaxed facial expression and body positioning
   c. increased participation in activities
   d. stable vital signs.

Nursing Actions *and Selected Purposes/Rationales*

(see pp. 45–47 for additional rationales)

2.a. Assess for signs and symptoms of chest pain/discomfort (e.g., verbalization of pain; grimacing; rubbing neck, jaw, or arm; reluctance to move; clutching chest; restlessness; diaphoresis; increased B/P; tachycardia).
  b. Assess client's perception of the severity of the pain/discomfort using an intensity rating scale.
  c. Assess the client's pattern of pain/discomfort (e.g., location, quality, onset, duration, precipitating factors, aggravating factors, alleviating factors).
  d. Implement measures *to relieve pain/discomfort:*
    1. maintain oxygen therapy as ordered *to increase the myocardial oxygen supply*
    2. maintain client on bed rest in a semi- to high Fowler's position
    3. administer the following medications if ordered:
      a. narcotic (opioid) analgesics (e.g., morphine sulfate); an intravenous rather than an intramuscular route should be used *because intramuscular injections are poorly absorbed if tissue perfusion is decreased; intramuscular injections also elevate some serum enzyme levels, which may interfere with assessment of myocardial damage*
      b. nitrates (e.g., nitroglycerin)
    4. implement additional measures to maintain an adequate cardiac output (see Diagnosis 1, action b) *in order to improve myocardial blood flow and oxygenation*
    5. provide or assist with nonpharmacologic measures for pain relief (e.g., relaxation techniques, restful environment).
  e. Consult physician if pain/discomfort persists or worsens.

3. Nursing Diagnosis: RISK FOR ACTIVITY INTOLERANCE

related to:
a. tissue hypoxia if cardiac output is decreased;
b. difficulty resting and sleeping associated with discomfort, frequent assessments and treatments, fear, and anxiety.

Suggested NOC Outcomes: Activity tolerance; Energy conservation; Self-care: activities of daily living

Suggested NIC Interventions: Energy management; Oxygen therapy; Cardiac care: rehabilitative; Sleep enhancement

Desired Outcome

3. The client will not experience activity intolerance as evidenced by:
   a. no reports of fatigue or weakness

Nursing Actions *and Selected Purposes/Rationales*

(see pp. 11–12 for additional rationales)

3.a. Assess for signs and symptoms of activity intolerance:
    1. statements of fatigue or weakness
    2. exertional dyspnea, chest pain, diaphoresis, or dizziness
    3. abnormal heart rate response to activity (e.g., increase in rate of 20 beats/minute above resting rate, rate not returning to preactivity level within 3 minutes after stopping activity, change from regular to irregular rate)

b. ability to perform activities of daily living without exertional dyspnea, chest pain, diaphoresis, dizziness, and a significant change in vital signs.

4. a significant change (15–20 mm Hg) in blood pressure with activity.

b. Implement measures *to prevent activity intolerance:*
   1. perform actions *to promote rest and/or conserve energy:*
      a. maintain activity restrictions as ordered
      b. minimize environmental activity and noise
      c. organize nursing care to allow for periods of uninterrupted rest
      d. limit the number of visitors and their length of stay
      e. assist client with self-care activities as needed
      f. keep supplies and personal articles within easy reach
      g. instruct client in energy-saving techniques (e.g., using shower chair when showering, sitting to brush teeth or comb hair)
      h. implement measures to reduce fear and anxiety (see Diagnosis 5, action b)
      i. implement measures to promote sleep (e.g., encourage relaxing diversional activities in the evening, allow client to continue usual sleep practices unless contraindicated, reduce environmental distractions, administer prescribed sedative-hypnotics)
      j. implement measures to relieve pain/discomfort (see Diagnosis 2, action d)
   2. perform actions to maintain an adequate cardiac output (see Diagnosis 1, action b)
   3. maintain oxygen therapy as ordered
   4. increase client's activity gradually as allowed and tolerated.

c. Instruct client to:
   1. report a decreased tolerance for activity
   2. stop any activity that causes chest pain, shortness of breath, dizziness, or extreme fatigue or weakness.

d. Consult appropriate health care provider (e.g., cardiac rehabilitation therapist, physician) if signs and symptoms of activity intolerance develop and persist or worsen.

4. COLLABORATIVE DIAGNOSES: POTENTIAL COMPLICATIONS OF MYOCARDIAL INFARCTION

a. cardiac dysrhythmias related to impaired nodal function and/or altered myocardial conductivity associated with myocardial ischemia and necrosis, sympathetic nervous system stimulation (a response to low cardiac output, pain, and anxiety), and possible electrolyte and acid-base imbalances;

b. heart failure related to impaired diastolic and systolic function of the heart associated with decreased compliance and contractility of the ischemic/ infarcted area;

c. thromboembolism related to:
   1. stasis of blood in the cardiac chambers associated with incomplete emptying
   2. formation of mural thrombi on the infarcted endocardium
   3. venous stasis associated with peripheral pooling of blood if activity restrictions are prolonged;

d. rupture of a portion of the heart (e.g., ventricular free wall, interventricular septum, papillary muscle) related to thinning and weakening of the necrotic area in the myocardium;

e. pericarditis related to an inflammatory response to epicardial necrosis;

f. infarct extension or recurrence related to insufficient myocardial blood supply to meet the myocardial oxygen requirements associated with decreased cardiac output or reocclusion of coronary artery(ies);

g. cardiogenic shock related to inability of damaged heart, intrinsic compensatory mechanisms, and treatment measures to maintain adequate tissue perfusion to vital organs (can occur as a result of extensive damage to the left ventricle, severe heart failure, severe or prolonged dysrhythmias, or rupture of the ventricle wall).

Desired Outcomes	**Nursing Actions** *and Selected Purposes/Rationales*
4.a. The client will maintain normal sinus rhythm as evidenced by: 1. regular apical pulse at 60–100 beats/minute 2. equal apical and radial pulse rates 3. absence of syncope and palpitations 4. ECG showing normal sinus rhythm.	4.a.1. Assess for and report signs and symptoms of cardiac dysrhythmias (e.g., irregular apical pulse; pulse rate below 60 or above 100 beats/minute; apical-radial pulse deficit; syncope; palpitations; abnormal rate, rhythm, or configurations on ECG). 2. Implement measures to maintain an adequate cardiac output (see Diagnosis 1, action b) *in order to promote adequate myocardial tissue perfusion and oxygenation and reduce the risk of cardiac dysrhythmias.* 3. If cardiac dysrhythmias occur: a. initiate cardiac monitoring if not currently being done b. administer antidysrhythmics (e.g., lidocaine, procainamide, amiodarone, digoxin, metoprolol, atenolol, esmolol, adenosine, diltiazem, verapamil, atropine) if ordered c. restrict client's activity based on his/her tolerance and severity of the dysrhythmia d. maintain oxygen therapy as ordered e. assess cardiovascular status frequently and report signs and symptoms of a further decrease in cardiac output and tissue perfusion f. prepare client for the following if planned: 1. cardioversion 2. insertion of a pacemaker or implantable cardioverter defibrillator (ICD) 3. catheter ablation of irritable site g. have emergency cart readily available for defibrillation or cardiopulmonary resuscitation.
4.b. The client will not develop heart failure as evidenced by: 1. pulse 60–100 beats/minute 2. absence of an S_3 heart sound 3. usual mental status 4. clear, audible breath sounds 5. absence of or no increase in dyspnea and orthopnea 6. absence of cough 7. palpable peripheral pulses 8. no reports of increased fatigue and weakness 9. urine output at least 30 ml/hour 10. stable weight 11. absence of edema and distended neck veins.	4.b.1. Assess for and report signs and symptoms of heart failure: a. tachycardia b. presence of an S_3 heart sound c. increased restlessness or anxiousness, confusion, or other change in mental status d. crackles (rales) e. development of or increased shortness of breath f. dry, hacking cough or cough productive of frothy or blood-tinged sputum g. diminished or absent peripheral pulses h. development of or increased weakness and fatigue i. decreased urine output during the day, nocturia j. weight gain k. edema l. distended neck veins m. chest x-ray results showing pulmonary vascular congestion, pleural effusion, or pulmonary edema. 2. Implement measures *to prevent heart failure:* a. perform actions to maintain an adequate cardiac output (see Diagnosis 1, action b) b. perform actions to treat cardiac dysrhythmias if present (see action a.3 in this diagnosis) *because dysrhythmias contribute to the development of heart failure.* 3. If signs and symptoms of heart failure occur: a. maintain oxygen therapy as ordered b. administer the following medications if ordered: 1. positive inotropic agents (e.g., dobutamine, dopamine, inamrinone) *to increase myocardial contractility* 2. B-type natriuretic peptide (nesiritide) *to promote diuresis and vasodilation* 3. vasodilators (e.g., nitroglycerin) *to decrease cardiac workload* 4. ACE inhibitors (e.g., captopril, ramipril) *to decrease cardiac workload and reduce ventricular remodeling* 5. diuretics (usually not used initially unless pulmonary capillary wedge pressure is above 18 mm Hg *because volume expansion is often not a factor in acute heart failure*)

6. morphine sulfate *to reduce preload and anxiety* (used primarily in clients with pulmonary edema).

4.c. The client will not develop a thromboembolism as evidenced by:
1. absence of pain, tenderness, swelling, and numbness in extremities
2. usual temperature and color of extremities
3. palpable and equal peripheral pulses
4. usual mental status
5. usual sensory and motor function
6. absence of sudden chest pain and dyspnea.

4.c.1. Assess for and report signs and symptoms of:
   a. deep vein thrombus (e.g., pain, tenderness, swelling, unusual warmth, and/or positive Homans' sign in extremity)
   b. arterial embolus in an extremity (e.g., diminished or absent peripheral pulses; pallor, coolness, numbness, and/or pain in extremity)
   c. cerebral ischemia (e.g., decreased level of consciousness, alteration in usual sensory and motor function)
   d. pulmonary embolism (e.g., sudden onset of chest pain, dyspnea, increased restlessness and apprehension, significant decrease in SaO_2).
2. Monitor echocardiogram results and report finding of a cardiac thrombus.
3. Implement measures *to prevent the development of thromboemboli:*
   a. perform actions *to reduce the risk of thrombus formation in the heart:*
      1. implement measures to maintain an adequate cardiac output (see Diagnosis 1, action b)
      2. implement measures to treat dysrhythmias if present (see action a.3 in this diagnosis)
      3. implement measures to treat heart failure if it occurs (see action b.3 in this diagnosis)
   b. if client remains on bed rest or activity is significantly limited for longer than 48 hours, refer to Care Plan on Immobility, Diagnosis 12, actions a.1.b and c and a.2.b and c (pp. 140–141) for measures to prevent and treat a deep vein thrombus and pulmonary embolism
   c. administer anticoagulants (e.g., warfarin, heparin) and antiplatelet agents (e.g., low-dose aspirin, glycoprotein IIb/IIIa receptor inhibitor [e.g., tirofiban, eptifibatide, abciximab], clopidogrel) if ordered.
4. If signs and symptoms of an arterial embolus in an extremity occur:
   a. maintain client on bed rest with affected extremity in a level or slightly dependent position *to improve arterial blood flow*
   b. prepare client for diagnostic studies (e.g., Doppler or duplex ultrasound, arteriography) if planned
   c. prepare client for the following if planned:
      1. injection of a thrombolytic agent (e.g., streptokinase)
      2. embolectomy
   d. administer anticoagulants (e.g., heparin, warfarin) as ordered.
5. If signs and symptoms of cerebral ischemia occur:
   a. maintain client on bed rest; keep head and neck in neutral, midline position
   b. administer anticoagulants (e.g., heparin, warfarin) as ordered.

4.d. The client will not experience rupture of any portion of the heart as evidenced by absence of signs of acute heart failure and/or cardiogenic shock (see outcomes b and g in this diagnosis for outcome criteria).

4.d.1. Assess for and report signs and symptoms of the following:
   a. papillary muscle rupture (e.g., holosystolic murmur, dyspnea, evidence of papillary muscle rupture on echocardiography or cardiac catheterization)
   b. ventricular septal defect (e.g., holosystolic murmur, parasternal thrill, finding of septal defect on echocardiography or cardiac catheterization)
   c. cardiac tamponade resulting from ventricular wall rupture (e.g., significant decrease in B/P, narrowed pulse pressure, pulsus paradoxus, distant or muffled heart sounds, jugular vein distention, increased central venous pressure [CVP]).
2. Assess for and immediately report signs and symptoms of acute heart failure and/or cardiogenic shock (see actions b.1 and g.1 in this diagnosis) that may occur as a result of rupture of a portion of the heart.
3. Implement measures to reduce cardiac workload (see Diagnosis 1, action b.2) *in order to reduce risk of rupture of the papillary muscle and ventricular free wall or septum.*

Desired Outcomes	Nursing Actions *and Selected Purposes/Rationales*
	4. If signs and symptoms of rupture of a portion of the heart occur: a. maintain client on bed rest b. assist with pericardiocentesis if performed c. assist with measures to treat heart failure or cardiogenic shock (see actions b.3 and g.3 in this diagnosis) d. prepare client for surgical intervention (e.g., valve replacement, repair of ventricular septal defect) if planned.
4.e. The client will experience resolution of pericarditis if it develops as evidenced by: 1. fewer reports of precordial pain 2. absence of pericardial friction rub 3. temperature declining toward normal 4. WBC count and sedimentation rate declining toward normal range.	4.e.1. Assess for and report signs and symptoms of pericarditis: a. precordial pain that frequently radiates to shoulder, neck, back, and arm (usually left); is intensified during deep inspiration, movement, and coughing; and usually is relieved by sitting up and leaning forward b. pericardial friction rub (may be transient) c. persistent temperature elevation d. further increase in WBC count and sedimentation rate (both can be elevated as a result of the infarction). 2. If signs and symptoms of pericarditis occur: a. allay client's anxiety (client may believe that symptoms indicate recurrent MI) b. assist client to assume position of comfort (usually sitting up and leaning forward on overbed table) c. administer anti-inflammatory agents (e.g., aspirin) if ordered.
4.f. The client will not experience infarct extension or recurrence as evidenced by: 1. no further episodes of persistent chest pain 2. stable vital signs 3. cardiac enzyme levels declining toward normal range 4. improved ECG readings.	4.f.1. Assess for and report signs and symptoms of infarct extension or recurrence (e.g., recurrent episode of persistent chest pain, significant change in vital signs, further increase in cardiac enzymes, recurrent or further increase in ST segment elevation, and development of abnormal Q waves [if not already present] on ECG). 2. Implement measures to maintain an adequate cardiac output (see Diagnosis 1, action b) *in order to reduce risk of infarct extension or recurrence.* 3. If client experiences signs and symptoms of infarct extension or recurrence: a. administer medications ordered *to reduce infarct expansion* (e.g., a nitrate, ACE inhibitor, beta blocking agent, aspirin, and/or heparin) b. prepare him/her for coronary angiogram, thrombolytic therapy, or revascularization procedure (e.g., PTCA, coronary artery bypass grafting [CABG]) if planned.
4.g. The client will not develop cardiogenic shock as evidenced by: 1. stable or improved mental status 2. systolic B/P greater than 80 mm Hg 3. palpable peripheral pulses 4. stable or improved skin temperature and color 5. urine output at least 30 ml/hour.	4.g.1. Assess for and immediately report signs and symptoms of cardiogenic shock: a. increased restlessness, lethargy, or confusion b. systolic B/P below 80 mm Hg c. rapid, weak pulse d. diminished or absent peripheral pulses e. increased coolness and duskiness or cyanosis of skin f. urine output less than 30 ml/hour. 2. Implement measures *to prevent cardiogenic shock:* a. perform actions to maintain an adequate cardiac output (see Diagnosis 1, action b) b. perform actions to treat cardiac dysrhythmias if present (see action a.3 in this diagnosis) c. perform actions to treat heart failure if it occurs (see action b.3 in this diagnosis) d. perform actions to treat rupture of any portion of the heart if it occurs (see action d.4 in this diagnosis). 3. If signs and symptoms of cardiogenic shock occur: a. maintain oxygen therapy as ordered

b. administer the following if ordered:
   1. sympathomimetics (e.g., dopamine, dobutamine) *to increase cardiac output and maintain arterial pressure*
   2. vasodilators (e.g., nitroglycerin) *to reduce cardiac workload* (vasodilators are usually not given if the systolic B/P or pulmonary capillary wedge pressure [PCWP] are low)
   3. intravenous fluids (may be ordered if signs of hypoperfusion are present and the PCWP is 15 mm Hg or less)
c. assist with intubation and insertion of hemodynamic monitoring device (e.g., Swan-Ganz catheter) and intra-aortic balloon pump (IAPB) if indicated.

5. NURSING DIAGNOSIS: FEAR/ANXIETY

related to:
a. the symptoms being experienced with the MI (e.g., chest discomfort, arm pain, and/or shortness of breath);
b. possible future disability, change in roles and lifestyle, and/or death associated with severe damage to the heart;
c. unfamiliar environment and separation from significant others;
d. lack of understanding of diagnostic tests, diagnosis, and treatment;
e. financial concerns about the cost of hospitalization and future treatment.

Suggested NOC Outcomes: Anxiety self-control; Anxiety level; Fear self-control; Fear level

Suggested NIC Interventions: Anxiety reduction; Calming technique; Emotional support; Presence; Pain management; Financial resource assistance

Desired Outcome	**Nursing Actions** *and Selected Purposes/Rationales* (see pp. 14–16 for additional rationales)
5. The client will experience a reduction in fear and anxiety as evidenced by: a. verbalization of feeling less anxious b. usual sleep pattern c. relaxed facial expression and body movements d. stable vital signs e. usual perceptual ability and interactions with others.	5.a. Assess client for signs and symptoms of fear and anxiety (e.g., verbalization of feeling anxious, insomnia, tenseness, shakiness, restlessness, diaphoresis, tachycardia, self-focused behaviors). Validate perceptions carefully, remembering that some behaviors may result from hypoxia. b. Implement measures *to reduce fear and anxiety:* 1. provide care in a calm, supportive, confident manner 2. if client is experiencing pain/discomfort: a. do not leave alone during period of acute distress b. perform actions to relieve discomfort (see Diagnosis 2, action d) 3. encourage significant others to project a caring, concerned attitude without obvious anxiousness 4. once the period of acute distress has subsided: a. orient client to environment, equipment, and routines; include an explanation of cardiac monitoring devices b. introduce client to staff who will be participating in care; if possible, maintain consistency in staff assigned to his/her care c. assure client that staff members are nearby; respond to call signal as soon as possible d. keep cardiac monitor out of client's view and the sound turned as low as possible e. encourage verbalization of fear and anxiety; provide feedback f. explain all diagnostic tests g. reinforce physician's explanation of invasive measures that are planned to improve coronary blood flow (e.g., infusion of a thrombolytic agent, percutaneous transluminal coronary angioplasty [PTCA], intracoronary stenting, intra-aortic balloon pump [IABP]) h. reinforce physician's explanations and clarify misconceptions client has about an MI, the treatment plan, and prognosis i. provide a calm, restful environment

Desired Outcome	Nursing Actions *and Selected Purposes/Rationales*
	j. instruct client in relaxation techniques and encourage participation in diversional activities k. initiate a social service referral and/or assist client to identify and contact appropriate community resources if indicated l. when appropriate, assist client to meet spiritual needs (e.g., arrange for a visit from clergy) m. assist client to identify specific stressors and ways to cope with them n. provide information based on current needs of client at a level he/she can understand; encourage questions and clarification of information provided o. include significant others in orientation and teaching sessions and encourage their continued support of the client p. administer prescribed antianxiety agents if indicated. c. Consult appropriate health care provider (e.g., psychiatric nurse clinician, physician) if above actions fail to control fear and anxiety.

Discharge Teaching/Continued Care

6. Nursing Diagnosis: DEFICIENT KNOWLEDGE, INEFFECTIVE THERAPEUTIC REGIMEN MANAGEMENT, OR INEFFECTIVE HEALTH MAINTENANCE*

*The nurse should select the diagnostic label that is most appropriate for the client's discharge teaching needs.

Suggested NOC Outcomes: Knowledge: disease process; Knowledge: treatment regimen; Knowledge: cardiac disease management

Suggested NIC Interventions: Health system guidance; Teaching: individual; Teaching: disease process; Teaching: prescribed activity/exercise; Teaching: prescribed medication

Desired Outcomes	Nursing Actions *and Selected Purposes/Rationales*
6.a. The client will verbalize a basic understanding of a myocardial infarction.	6.a. Explain a myocardial infarction in terms the client can understand. Utilize appropriate teaching aids (e.g., pictures, videotapes, heart models). Inform client that it takes approximately 6–8 weeks for the heart to heal after a myocardial infarction.
6.b. The client will demonstrate accuracy in counting pulse.	6.b.1. Teach client how to count his/her pulse, being alert to the regularity of the rhythm. 2. Allow time for return demonstration and accuracy check.
6.c. The client will identify modifiable cardiovascular risk factors and ways to alter these factors.	6.c.1. Inform client that certain modifiable factors such as elevated serum lipids, a sedentary lifestyle, hypertension, and smoking have been shown to increase the risk for coronary artery disease. 2. Assist client to identify changes in lifestyle that can help him/her to eliminate or reduce the above risk factors and to help prevent a recurrent MI (e.g., dietary modification, physical exercise on regular basis, moderation of alcohol intake, smoking cessation). 3. Encourage client to limit daily alcohol consumption (daily alcohol intake exceeding 1 oz of ethanol may contribute to the development of hypertension and some forms of heart disease). Current recommendations are no more than 2 drinks/day for men and no more than 1 drink/day for women and lighter weight persons. A "drink" is considered to be ½ oz of ethanol (e.g., 1½ oz of 80-proof whiskey, 12 oz of beer, 5 oz of wine).

6.d. The client will verbalize an understanding of the rationale for and components of a diet designed to lower serum cholesterol and triglycerides.

6.d.1. Explain the rationale for restricting saturated fat and cholesterol intake.

2. Provide instructions on ways the client can reduce intake of saturated fat and cholesterol:
   a. reduce intake of meat fat (e.g., trim visible fat off meat; replace fatty meats such as fatty cuts of steak, hamburger, and processed meats with leaner products)
   b. reduce intake of milk fat (avoid dairy products containing more than 1% fat)
   c. reduce intake of *trans* fats (e.g., avoid stick margarine and shortening and foods such as commercial baked goods that are prepared with these products)
   d. use vegetable oil rather than coconut or palm oil in cooking and food preparation
   e. use cooking methods such as steaming, baking, broiling, poaching, microwaving, and grilling rather than frying
   f. restrict intake of eggs (recommendations about the number of whole eggs allowed per week vary depending on the client's lipid levels).
3. Encourage client to increase intake of omega-3 fatty acids (e.g., flaxseed, cold water ocean fish such as salmon and halibut) to help lower triglycerides and increase high density lipoproteins (HDLs).

6.e. The client will verbalize an understanding of medications ordered including rationale, food and drug interactions, side effects, schedule for taking, and importance of taking as prescribed.

6.e.1. Explain the rationale for, side effects of, and importance of taking the medications prescribed. Inform client of pertinent food and drug interactions.

2. If client is discharged on sublingual or transmucosal nitroglycerin tablets or nitroglycerin translingual spray, instruct to:
   a. limit intake of alcoholic beverages
   b. have tablets or spray readily available at all times
   c. take a tablet or use spray before strenuous activity and in emotionally stressful situations
   d. take one tablet or spray 1–2 metered doses into mouth when chest pain occurs and repeat every 5 minutes up to a total of 3 times if necessary; notify physician or obtain emergency medical assistance if pain persists
   e. place sublingual tablet under tongue or transmucosal tablet between the gum and cheek (buccal cavity) or gum and upper lip and allow to dissolve completely; do not chew or swallow tablets
   f. store tablets in a tightly capped, dark-colored glass container away from heat and moisture
   g. replace tablets 6 months after the container is opened or sooner if they do not relieve discomfort
   h. avoid rising to a standing position quickly after taking nitroglycerin in order to reduce dizziness associated with its vasodilatory effect
   i. recognize that dizziness, flushing, and mild headache may occur after taking nitroglycerin
   j. report fainting, persistent or severe headache, blurred vision, or dry mouth.
3. If nitroglycerin skin patches are prescribed:
   a. provide instructions about correct application, skin care, need to rotate sites and remove old patches, and frequency of change; explain that the patch should be removed for an 8–12 hour period of time each day per physician's instructions in order to help prevent the development of nitrate tolerance
   b. caution client that activities that increase blood flow to the skin (e.g., hot bath or shower, sauna) can cause a sudden reduction in blood pressure
   c. caution client to limit intake of alcoholic beverages
   d. instruct client to notify health care provider if faintness, dizziness, or flushing occurs following application or if persistent redness or itching occurs at the patch site.

Desired Outcomes	Nursing Actions *and Selected Purposes/Rationales*

4. If client is discharged on a beta-adrenergic blocking agent (e.g., propranolol, metoprolol, atenolol), instruct to:
   a. take the medication at the same time every day
   b. check pulse before taking medication; consult physician before taking medication if pulse rate is unusually slow (it is expected that pulse will be lower than normal)
   c. avoid skipping doses, altering the prescribed dose, trying to make up for missed doses, and discontinuing medication without first discussing it with health care provider
   d. change from a lying to a sitting or standing position slowly if dizziness or lightheadedness is a problem
   e. limit intake of alcoholic beverages
   f. monitor blood glucose on a regular basis if diabetic (beta blockers may affect blood sugar and mask symptoms of hypoglycemia)
   g. wear or carry medical identification specifying the name of the medication being taken
   h. report the following:
      1. persistent lightheadedness or dizziness
      2. significant weight gain, night cough, difficulty breathing, or swelling of feet or ankles (may be indicative of heart failure)
      3. cold, painful toes or fingers
      4. persistent fatigue, depression, insomnia, or sexual dysfunction
      5. worsening of any symptoms of chronic respiratory disease.
5. If client is discharged on an ACE inhibitor:
   a. change from a lying to sitting or standing position slowly if experiencing dizziness or lightheadedness with position change
   b. avoid hot baths and showers, steam room, and sauna
   c. avoid salt substitutes with a high potassium content
   d. report continued dizziness, lightheadedness, or fainting; a persistent dry cough; or swelling of the tongue, lips, face, or neck.
6. Instruct client to take lipid-lowering agents (e.g., HMG-CoA reductase inhibitors ["statins"], gemfibrozil, ezetimibe, niacin) and antiplatelet agents (e.g., aspirin, clopidogrel) as prescribed.
7. Instruct client to consult physician before taking other prescription and nonprescription medications.
8. Instruct client to inform all health care providers of medications being taken.

6.f. The client will verbalize an understanding of activity restrictions and the rate at which activity can be progressed.

6.f.1. Reinforce physician's instructions about activity. Instruct client to:
   a. gradually increase activity by adhering to a regular aerobic exercise program (often begins with walking)
   b. take frequent rest periods for about 4–8 weeks after discharge
   c. avoid physical conditioning programs such as jogging and aerobic dancing until advised by physician
   d. avoid strenuous exercise and activities that involve pushing or lifting heavy objects (e.g., weight lifting)
   e. avoid exercising for at least an hour after eating and when the environmental temperature is extremely hot or cold
   f. avoid tobacco use before exercise
   g. stop any activity that causes chest pain, shortness of breath, palpitations, dizziness, or extreme fatigue or weakness
   h. begin a cardiovascular fitness program if recommended by physician.

2. Reinforce instructions regarding sexual activity:
   a. sexual activity with usual partner can be resumed after the prescribed length of time (many physicians consider a client ready to resume sexual activity when he/she is able to climb 2 flights of stairs briskly without dyspnea or angina)
   b. assume a comfortable and unstrenuous position for intercourse (e.g., side-lying, partner on top)

c. a new sexual relationship can be started but may result in greater energy expenditure until it becomes a more familiar or usual experience
d. take nitroglycerin before sexual activity if angina occurs with sexual activity
e. avoid intercourse for at least 1–2 hours after a heavy meal or alcohol consumption
f. avoid sexual activity when fatigued or stressed
g. avoid hot or cold showers just before and after intercourse.

6.g. The client will state signs and symptoms to report to the health care provider.

6.g. Instruct the client to report:
1. chest, arm, neck, jaw, or back discomfort unrelieved by nitroglycerin
2. shortness of breath
3. significant weight gain or swelling of feet or ankles
4. irregular pulse or a significant unexpected change in the pulse rate
5. persistent impotence or decreased libido (can be a side effect of certain medications or result from anxiety, depression, or fatigue)
6. inability to tolerate prescribed activity
7. increase in severity or frequency of episodes of angina.

6.h. The client will identify community resources that can assist with cardiac rehabilitation and adjustment to the effects of a myocardial infarction.

6.h.1. Provide information on community resources and support groups that can assist client with cardiac rehabilitation and adjustment to the effects of an MI (e.g., American Heart Association, "coronary clubs," counseling services).
2. Initiate a referral if indicated.

6.i. The client will verbalize an understanding of and a plan for adhering to recommended follow-up care including future appointments with health care provider.

6.i.1. Reinforce the importance of keeping follow-up appointments with health care provider and for exercise stress testing and laboratory studies to monitor serum lipid levels.
2. Implement measures to improve client compliance:
a. include significant others in teaching sessions if possible
b. encourage questions and allow time for reinforcement and clarification of information provided
c. provide written instructions on future appointments with health care provider, dietary modifications, activity progression, medications prescribed, and signs and symptoms to report.

Additional Nursing Diagnoses

*DISTURBED SLEEP PATTERN**

related to the symptoms being experienced with the MI (e.g., chest discomfort, shortness of breath), frequent assessments and treatments, fear, and anxiety.

*GRIEVING**

related to loss of normal function of the heart; possible changes in lifestyle, occupation, and roles; and uncertainty of prognosis.

*See Unit II for outcomes, actions, and rationales.

Bibliography

See pages 879 and 881–882.

evolve

Pacemaker Implantation

Pacemakers are small battery-powered devices that monitor the heart rate and deliver electrical impulses to the heart to help correct dysrhythmias. A pacemaker consists of a pulse generator (contains the battery and electronic circuitry) and electrode catheters (leads). It is implanted during a minor surgical procedure under local anesthesia. The leads are inserted into the heart transvenously via the subclavian, jugular, or cephalic vein. The leads are then tunneled under the skin and attached to the pulse generator that is implanted in a subcutaneous pocket created in the subclavicular area or, less commonly, in the abdomen.

A pacemaker is used to stimulate the heart electrically when the heart fails to initiate or conduct intrinsic electrical impulses at a rate that is sufficient to maintain adequate perfusion. Pacemaker insertion is indicated for treatment of symptomatic bradydysrhythmias (e.g., sinus bradycardia, second- and third-degree heart block, sick sinus syndrome) and on some occasions, for treatment of tachydysrhythmias that have been unresponsive to other forms of therapy.

Pacemakers are either temporary or permanent. Temporary pacemakers are used to regulate the heart rate in emergency or short-term situations. In most instances, temporary pacing is done using external transcutaneous pacing electrodes or using temporary pacemaker electrodes that have been placed on the epicardium during thoracic surgery (e.g., heart surgery). Temporary pacemakers are attached to and regulated by an external power source. Permanent pacemakers are utilized for long-term management of certain dysrhythmias. There are a number of permanent pacemakers available. Their functional capabilities are described by a 3- or 5-letter code that specifies the chamber being paced, the chamber being sensed, mode of response, programmability/rate responsiveness, and antitachycardia functions.

The majority of pacemakers used now are dual-chambered pacemakers with leads in both the atrium and ventricle. Dual-chamber pacing allows for the physiological timing between atrial systole and ventricular systole to be maintained, which improves cardiac output. Present day pacemakers can also be programmed externally and the majority operate in a synchronous mode (a chamber of the heart is triggered to fire or is inhibited by the intrinsic activity of the heart) or a rate-responsive mode. The most frequently used rate-responsive systems have an activity sensor in the pulse generator that detects movement and then appropriately increases or decreases the pacing rate. A combined pacemaker and cardioverter-defibrillator device is also available.

This care plan focuses on the adult client with a symptomatic dysrhythmia hospitalized for implantation of a permanent pacemaker.

OUTCOME/DISCHARGE CRITERIA

THE CLIENT WILL:

- have adequate cardiac output
- have no signs and symptoms of postoperative complications
- verbalize a basic understanding of the rationale for and function of a permanent pacemaker
- demonstrate knowledge of how to monitor pacemaker function
- verbalize an understanding of recommended activity restrictions
- identify appropriate safety precautions associated with having a permanent pacemaker
- state signs and symptoms to report to the health care provider
- verbalize an understanding of and a plan for adhering to recommended follow-up care including future appointments with health care provider, medications prescribed, and wound care.

NURSING/COLLABORATIVE DIAGNOSES

Preoperative

1. Decreased cardiac output p. 387
2. Fear/Anxiety p. 388

Postoperative

1. Potential complications p. 388
   a. pacemaker malfunction: failure to fire, capture, or properly sense
   b. cardiac tamponade
   c. pneumothorax
   d. undesirable stimulation of the heart and/or certain nerves and muscles

DISCHARGE TEACHING

2. Deficient knowledge, Ineffective therapeutic regimen management, or Ineffective health maintenance p. 390

See Standardized Preoperative and Postoperative Care Plans (pp. 97–126) for additional diagnoses.

PREOPERATIVE *Use in conjunction with the Standardized Preoperative Care Plan.*

1. NURSING DIAGNOSIS: ***DECREASED CARDIAC OUTPUT***

related to:
a. a slow heart rate (if client has a bradydysrhythmia);
b. decreased diastolic filling time associated with a rapid and/or irregular heart rate (if client has a tachydysrhythmia).

Suggested NOC Outcomes: Circulation status; Cardiac pump effectiveness

Suggested NIC Interventions: Cardiac care; Cardiac precautions; Dysrhythmia management; Temporary pacemaker management

Desired Outcome

1. The client will maintain adequate cardiac output as evidenced by:
   a. systolic B/P of at least 90 mm Hg
   b. palpable peripheral pulses
   c. no increase in number or duration of syncopal episodes
   d. no further decline in mental status
   e. absence of cyanosis
   f. urine output at least 30 ml/hour.

Nursing Actions ***and Selected Purposes/Rationales***
(see pp. 20–24 for additional rationales)

1.a. Assess client upon admission for baseline data regarding status of cardiac output. Expect that many of the following signs and symptoms of dysrhythmias and low cardiac output will be present:
   1. B/P less than 110/70 mm Hg or below normal for client
   2. irregular pulse
   3. pulse rate less than 60 or greater than 100 beats/minute
   4. fatigue and weakness
   5. diminished peripheral pulses
   6. dizziness, lightheadedness, syncope
   7. restlessness, change in mental status
   8. tachypnea, exertional dyspnea
   9. cool, pale skin
   10. capillary refill time greater than 2–3 seconds.

b. Monitor ECG and report worsening of or additional dysrhythmias.

c. Reassess cardiac status frequently and report the following signs and symptoms that may indicate the need for emergency pacemaker/cardioverter-defibrillator insertion:
   1. systolic B/P below 90 mm Hg
   2. absent peripheral pulses
   3. prolonged or increased frequency of syncopal episodes
   4. persistent decline in mental status
   5. cyanosis
   6. urine output less than 30 ml/hour.

d. Implement measures *to maintain an adequate cardiac output before surgery:*
   1. perform actions *to reduce cardiac workload:*
      a. place client in a semi- to high Fowler's position unless systolic B/P is less than 90 mm Hg (then head of bed should be flat)
      b. implement measures *to promote rest* (e.g. reduce fear and anxiety, maintain activity restrictions, limit the number of visitors)
      c. maintain oxygen therapy as ordered
      d. discourage smoking *(nicotine has a cardiostimulatory effect and causes vasoconstriction; the carbon monoxide in smoke reduces oxygen availability)*
   2. instruct client to avoid activities that create a Valsalva response (e.g. straining to have a bowel movement, holding breath while moving up in bed) *in order to reduce vagal stimulation and the subsequent slowing of heart rate and to prevent the sudden increase in cardiac workload that occurs with exhalation*
   3. administer the following if ordered:
      a. medications *to treat tachydysrhythmias if present* (e.g. amiodarone, sotalol, procainamide, ibutilide, esmolol, adenosine, diltiazem)

Desired Outcome	Nursing Actions *and Selected Purposes/Rationales*
	b. anticholinergic agents (e.g. atropine) or sympathomimetics (e.g., epinephrine) *to increase heart rate if client has a bradydysrhythmia* 4. notify physician if serum potassium level is abnormal *(abnormal potassium levels affect myocardial conductivity)* 5. if client has heart block or a ventricular dysrhythmia, consult physician before giving prescribed digitalis preparations *(digitalis preparations delay AV node conductivity and can also increase ventricular irritability)* 6. assist with/maintain temporary pacing if ordered 7. prepare for and assist with cardioversion or defibrillation if performed.

2. Nursing Diagnosis: ***FEAR/ANXIETY***

related to unfamiliar environment, lack of understanding of surgical procedure, anticipated postoperative discomfort, possibility of pacemaker malfunction, and possible changes in lifestyle as a result of having a pacemaker.

Suggested NOC Outcomes: Anxiety self-control; Anxiety level; Fear self-control; Fear level

Suggested NIC Interventions: Anxiety reduction; Emotional support; Teaching: preoperative

Desired Outcome	Nursing Actions *and Selected Purposes/Rationales* (see pp. 14–16 for additional rationales)
2. The client will experience a reduction in fear and anxiety (see Standardized Preoperative Care Plan, Diagnosis 1 [pp. 97–98], for outcome criteria).	2.a. Refer to Standardized Preoperative Care Plan, Diagnosis 1 (pp. 97–98), for measures related to assessment and reduction of fear and anxiety. b. Implement additional measures *to reduce fear and anxiety:* 1. explain the rationale for and function of a pacemaker; utilize diagrams, pamphlets, and show client an actual pacemaker 2. explain that the procedure will be performed using local anesthesia 3. if client is to receive an antimicrobial agent before surgery, explain that these medications are often given before and for a short time after surgery to reduce the risk for infection 4. inform client that pacemakers are electrically safe and are not harmed during usual daily activities 5. inform client of the expected life span of the particular pacemaker to be implanted; explain that only the generator will need to be replaced when the battery gets weak 6. discuss the client's concerns regarding whether his/her occupation and hobbies can be continued safely with a pacemaker in place; if the occupation or interests involve contact sports or contact with high-voltage electrical equipment and large magnets or electromagnetic fields, instruct him/her to consult physician about the safety of continuing these activities.

POSTOPERATIVE

Use in conjunction with the Standardized Postoperative Care Plan.

1. Collaborative Diagnoses: ***POTENTIAL COMPLICATIONS OF PACEMAKER IMPLANTATION***

a. pacemaker malfunction: failure to fire, capture, or properly sense related to break in or faulty attachment of the pacemaker catheter to the generator, pulse generator malfunction, or improper placement or dislodgment of the pacemaker lead(s);

b. cardiac tamponade related to perforation of the atria or ventricle by the pacemaker leads;
c. pneumothorax related to accumulation of air in the pleural space associated with accidental puncture of the pleura during subclavian insertion of the pacemaker leads;
d. undesirable stimulation of the heart and/or certain nerves and muscles related to the presence of a foreign body in the heart and the emission of electrical impulses from the pacemaker lead(s) to nearby muscles and nerves (e.g. diaphragm, intercostal muscles, phrenic nerve).

Desired Outcomes	**Nursing Actions** *and Selected Purposes/Rationales*
1.a. The client will experience normal pacemaker function as evidenced by: 1. regular pulse at a rate equal to or greater than the programmed pacing rate 2. stable B/P 3. absence of dizziness, syncope, and dyspnea 4. ECG showing pacer spikes before the P wave and/or QRS complex when the pulse rate falls below the programmed pacing rate.	1.a.1. Ascertain the method of pacing being used and the rate set by the physician in surgery. Use this information when assessing pacemaker function. 2. Assess for and report signs and symptoms of pacemaker malfunction: a. apical pulse less than programmed pacing rate b. significant decrease in B/P c. dizziness, lightheadedness, syncope d. dyspnea e. ECG showing any of the following: 1. absence of pacer spikes when heart rate falls below the programmed pacing rate 2. pacer spikes present with normal P waves and QRS complexes 3. absence of P wave (if an atrial pacer) or QRS complex (if a ventricular pacer) following a pacer spike 4. presence of ectopic beats (usually premature ventricular beats). 3. Implement measures *to reduce the risk for breakage and dislodgment of the pacemaker lead(s) in order to prevent pacemaker malfunction:* a. maintain activity restrictions as ordered b. instruct client to limit movement of the arm and shoulder on the side of pacemaker insertion for the first 48 hours after surgery. 4. If signs and symptoms of pacemaker malfunction occur: a. turn client to either side (preferably the left) *to help achieve placement of the lead(s) against the endocardium* b. follow manufacturer's suggestions for problem solving (e.g. have a pacemaker magnet readily available to test function and convert pacemaker to asynchronous [fixed rate] mode if necessary; if client has a temporary pacemaker, adjust the sensitivity and/or output [MA] within prescribed limits until capture occurs) c. prepare client for chest x-ray to check placement of the lead(s) d. prepare client for surgical repair or replacement of pulse generator and/or lead(s) if indicated.
1.b. The client will not experience cardiac tamponade as evidenced by: 1. stable vital signs 2. audible heart sounds 3. absence of jugular vein distention.	1.b.1. Assess for and report signs and symptoms of: a. cardiac perforation (e.g. pericardial pain, pericardial friction rub, increasing ventricular pacing threshold, right bundle branch block pattern with pacing) b. cardiac tamponade (e.g. significant decrease in B/P, narrowed pulse pressure, pulsus paradoxus, distant or muffled heart sounds, sense of fullness in chest, jugular vein distention). 2. Implement measures to prevent dislodgment of the pacemaker leads (see action a.3 in this diagnosis) *in order to reduce the risk for perforation of the heart wall.* 3. If signs and symptoms of cardiac perforation or tamponade occur: a. prepare client for chest x-ray and echocardiogram b. prepare client for repositioning or replacement of the lead(s), repair of perforation, and/or pericardiocentesis if planned.

Desired Outcomes	**Nursing Actions** *and Selected Purposes/Rationales*
1.c. The client will have resolution of pneumothorax if it occurs as evidenced by: 1. audible breath sounds and a resonant percussion note over lungs 2. normal respiratory rate and pattern 3. usual mental status 4. blood gases returning to normal range.	1.c.1. Assess for and immediately report signs and symptoms of pneumothorax (e.g. absent breath sounds with hyperresonant percussion note over involved area; rapid, shallow, and/or labored respirations; tachycardia; sudden onset of chest pain; restlessness; confusion; significant decrease in oximetry results; abnormal blood gases; chest x-ray results showing lung collapse). 2. If signs and symptoms of pneumothorax occur: a. maintain client on bed rest in a semi- to high Fowler's position b. maintain oxygen therapy as ordered c. assess for and immediately report signs and symptoms of tension pneumothorax with mediastinal shift (e.g. severe dyspnea, increased restlessness and agitation, rapid and/or irregular heart rate, hypotension, neck vein distention, shift in trachea from midline) d. prepare client for insertion of chest tube if indicated.
1.d. The client will have resolution of ventricular irritability and undesired nerve and muscle stimulation as evidenced by: 1. absence of ventricular ectopic beats 2. absence of hiccups 3. absence of abdominal and intercostal muscle twitching.	1.d.1. Assess for signs and symptoms of ventricular irritability and undesired nerve or muscle stimulation: a. ventricular ectopic beats on ECG b. hiccups c. reports of abdominal or chest wall twitching. 2. If the above signs and symptoms persist: a. consult physician b. turn client to left side c. prepare client for the following procedures if planned: 1. chest x-ray to determine placement of the lead(s) 2. repositioning of the lead(s).

Discharge Teaching/Continued Care

2. Nursing Diagnosis: ***DEFICIENT KNOWLEDGE, INEFFECTIVE THERAPEUTIC REGIMEN MANAGEMENT, OR INEFFECTIVE HEALTH MAINTENANCE****

*The nurse should select the diagnostic label that is most appropriate for the client's discharge teaching needs.

Suggested NOC Outcome: Knowledge: treatment regimen	**Suggested NIC Interventions:** Teaching: individual; Teaching: prescribed activity/exercise

Desired Outcomes	**Nursing Actions** *and Selected Purposes/Rationales*
2.a. The client will verbalize a basic understanding of the rationale for and function of a permanent pacemaker.	2.a. Reinforce preoperative teaching regarding the rationale for and basic function of a permanent pacemaker.
2.b. The client will demonstrate knowledge of how to monitor pacemaker function.	2.b.1. Inform client of pacemaker's programmed pacing rate and, if appropriate, provide instructions about how to take pulse and monitor both the rate and regularity. (Many physicians prefer that their clients not monitor their own pulse because of the confusion between paced beats and spontaneous beats.) 2. Instruct client to have pulse generator function checked regularly per physician's instructions or if experiencing symptoms such as dizziness, fainting, unexplained fatigue, or shortness of breath. Inform client that monitoring may be done at the physician's office or by telephone monitoring device.

2.c. The client will verbalize an understanding of recommended activity restrictions.	2.d.1. Provide the following instructions about activity restrictions following pacemaker insertion: a. limit movement of the arm and shoulder on the side of pacemaker insertion for the first 48 hours after surgery b. limit activities that put undue stress on the incision site (e.g. using arms over head, bowling, racquetball, tennis, lifting over 25 pounds) until cleared by physician (usual time is 1–2 months) c. avoid letting anything rub on or hit the pacemaker d. do not rub or "play with" the pacemaker under the skin e. avoid immersing the pacemaker insertion site in water for at least 3 days after surgery f. avoid activities that can cause blunt trauma to the pulse generator (e.g. contact sports, firing a rifle with the butt end of the gun against affected shoulder). 2. Allow adequate time for questions and clarification of information provided.
2.d. The client will identify appropriate safety precautions associated with having a permanent pacemaker.	2.d. Instruct client to adhere to the following safety precautions: 1. inform all health care providers about the pacemaker (certain medical equipment such as an MRI machine, radiation therapy machine, and electrocautery equipment may actually damage the pulse generator and/or interfere with normal function of the pacemaker) 2. avoid having a digital cellular phone within 6 inches of pacemaker generator while the phone is on 3. avoid close proximity with strong magnets (e.g. MRI machine, large industrial magnets), high voltage electrical equipment (e.g. arc welder, running car engine), and large electromagnetic fields (e.g. radio and television transmitters) 4. do not place any electrical device directly over pacemaker 5. move away from any electrical device if dizziness, lightheadedness, or a significant change in pulse rate occurs or if pulse generator emits a beeping sound (after 30 seconds, the device will deactivate) 6. if planning to travel, obtain name of a physician and/or pacemaker clinic at point(s) of destination 7. alert airport personnel to pacemaker (the pacemaker may set off the security alarm) 8. always wear a medical alert bracelet or tag and carry an identification card that includes the name of the manufacturer, model number, mode of operation, programmed rate, and insertion date of the pacemaker.
2.e. The client will state signs and symptoms to report to the health care provider.	2.e.1. Refer to Standardized Postoperative Care Plan, Diagnosis 22, action c (p. 125), for signs and symptoms to report to the health care provider. 2. Instruct client to report these additional signs and symptoms: a. increased irregularity of pulse or pulse rate lower than the pacemaker's programmed pacing rate (if self-monitoring is being done) b. unexplained fatigue c. lightheadedness, dizziness, fainting d. shortness of breath e. swelling of feet and ankles f. chest pain g. hiccuping lasting more than 2 hours h. redness, swelling, drainage, or increased soreness at implant site i. unexplained fever j. swelling of arm on the side of the pacemaker (may indicate venous thrombosis associated with insertion/presence of leads in vein).

Desired Outcomes	Nursing Actions *and Selected Purposes/Rationales*
2.f. The client will verbalize an understanding of and a plan for adhering to recommended follow-up care including future appointments with health care provider, medications prescribed, and wound care.	2.f.1. Refer to Standardized Postoperative Care Plan, Diagnosis 22 (pp. 125–126), for routine postoperative instructions and measures to improve client compliance. 2. Remind client of the importance of keeping scheduled appointments with pacemaker clinic and for chest x-ray verification of lead placement.

Bibliography

See pages 879 and 881–882.

UNIT X

Nursing Care of the Client with Disturbances of Peripheral Vascular Function

evolve

Abdominal Aortic Aneurysm Repair

An abdominal aortic aneurysm is an abnormal dilation of the wall of the abdominal aorta. The aneurysm usually develops in the segment of the vessel that is between the renal arteries and the iliac branches of the aorta. The most common cause of an abdominal aortic aneurysm is atherosclerosis. The plaque that forms on the wall of the artery causes degenerative changes in the medial layer of the vessel. These changes lead to loss of elasticity, weakening, and eventual dilation of the affected segment. Some other causes of abdominal aortic aneurysm include inflammation (arteritis), trauma, infection, congenital abnormalities of the vessel, and connective tissue disorders that cause vessel wall weakness.

Most abdominal aortic aneurysms are asymptomatic and are discovered during a routine physical examination (signs include palpation of a pulsatile mass in the abdomen and/or auscultation of a bruit over the abdominal aorta) or during a review of x-ray results of the abdomen or lower spine. The presence of symptoms such as mild to severe abdominal, lumbar, or flank pain and/or lower extremity arterial insufficiency is usually indicative of a large aneurysm that is exerting pressure on surrounding tissues or an aneurysm that is leaking.

Surgical repair of an aneurysm is usually performed if the aneurysm is growing rapidly and/or reaches a size of 5–6 cm or larger or if the client experiences symptoms. The procedure often involves the use of a synthetic graft, which is inserted to replace or support the weakened vessel.

This care plan focuses on the adult client hospitalized for surgical repair of an abdominal aortic aneurysm. Much of the postoperative information is applicable to clients receiving follow-up care in an extended care facility or home setting.

OUTCOME/DISCHARGE CRITERIA

THE CLIENT WILL:

- tolerate prescribed diet
- tolerate expected level of activity
- have surgical pain controlled
- have clear, audible breath sounds throughout lungs
- have evidence of normal healing of surgical wounds
- have no signs and symptoms of postoperative complications
- identify ways to prevent or slow the progression of atherosclerosis
- state signs and symptoms to report to the health care provider
- verbalize an understanding of and a plan for adhering to recommended follow-up care including future appointments with health care provider, medications prescribed, activity level, and wound care.

NURSING/COLLABORATIVE DIAGNOSES

Preoperative

1. Fear/Anxiety p. 396
2. Potential complication: hypovolemic shock p. 396

Postoperative

1. Risk for imbalanced fluid and electrolytes p. 397
   a. third-spacing of fluid
   b. excess fluid volume
   c. deficient fluid volume
   d. hypokalemia, hypochloremia, and metabolic alkalosis
2. Potential complications p. 399
   a. hypovolemic shock
   b. lower extremity arterial embolization
   c. cardiac dysrhythmias
   d. ischemic colitis
   e. impaired renal function

DISCHARGE TEACHING

3. Deficient knowledge, Ineffective therapeutic regimen management, or Ineffective health maintenance p. 401

See p. 403 and Standardized Preoperative and Postoperative Care Plans (pp. 97–126) for additional diagnoses.

PREOPERATIVE *Use in conjunction with the Standardized Preoperative Care Plan.*

1. Nursing Diagnosis: FEAR/ANXIETY

related to:
a. unfamiliar environment and separation from significant others;
b. lack of understanding of diagnostic tests, surgical procedure, and postoperative care;
c. anticipated loss of control associated with effects of anesthesia;
d. risk of disease if blood transfusions are necessary;
e. anticipated postoperative discomfort and potential change in sexual functioning;
f. possibility of death.

Suggested NOC Outcomes: Anxiety level; Fear level; Anxiety self-control; Fear self-control

Suggested NIC Interventions: Anxiety reduction; Calming technique; Emotional support; Presence; Teaching: preoperative

Desired Outcome	Nursing Actions *and Selected Purposes/Rationales* (see pp. 14–16 for additional rationales)
1. The client will experience a reduction in fear and anxiety (see Standardized Preoperative Care Plan, Diagnosis 1 [pp. 97–98], for outcome criteria).	1.a. Refer to Standardized Preoperative Care Plan, Diagnosis 1 (pp. 97–98), for measures related to the assessment and reduction of fear and anxiety. b. Implement additional measures *to reduce fear and anxiety:* 1. orient client to critical care unit if appropriate 2. describe and explain the rationale for equipment and tubes that may be present postoperatively (e.g., cardiac monitor, ventilator, intravenous and intra-arterial lines, nasogastric tube, urinary catheter) 3. explain that B/P may be taken in both arms and thighs in order to better evaluate circulatory status 4. reinforce physician's explanations and clarify misconceptions client has about effects of the surgery on sexual functioning (impotence can result from diminished blood flow in the mesenteric or internal iliac arteries during or after surgery and/or from nerve damage during surgery).

2. Collaborative Diagnosis: POTENTIAL COMPLICATION OF ABDOMINAL AORTIC ANEURYSM: HYPOVOLEMIC SHOCK

related to excessive blood loss if the aneurysm ruptures.

Desired Outcome	Nursing Actions *and Selected Purposes/Rationales*
2. The client will not develop hypovolemic shock as evidenced by: a. usual mental status b. stable vital signs c. skin warm and usual color d. palpable peripheral pulses e. urine output at least 30 ml/hour.	2.a. Assess for and immediately report signs and symptoms of conditions that indicate impending aneurysm rupture: 1. leaking aneurysm: a. increasing abdominal girth b. ecchymosis of flank area or perineum c. frank or occult gastrointestinal bleeding *(occurs if the aneurysm ruptures into the duodenum)* d. decreasing RBC, Hct, and Hgb levels e. new or increased reports of lumbar, flank, abdominal, pelvic, or groin pain *(accumulation of blood in the peritoneum and/or retroperitoneal spaces causes irritation of and pressure on the tissues and nerves)* f. diminishing or absent peripheral pulses

g. further decline in thigh B/P as compared with B/P in arm (thigh B/P is usually slightly lower than B/P in arm of a client with an abdominal aortic aneurysm)

2. expanding aneurysm:
   a. new or increased reports of lumbar, flank, or groin pain *(results from pressure on lumbar nerves)*
   b. increased size of pulsating mass in abdomen
   c. increasing sense of abdominal and/or gastric fullness *(results from pressure on duodenum)*
   d. decreasing motor or sensory function of lower extremities *(results from pressure on lumbar and/or sacral nerves).*

b. Assess for and report signs and symptoms of hypovolemic shock:
   1. restlessness, agitation, confusion, or other change in mental status
   2. significant decrease in B/P
   3. postural hypotension
   4. rapid, weak pulse
   5. rapid respirations
   6. cool skin
   7. pallor, cyanosis
   8. diminished or absent peripheral pulses
   9. urine output less than 30 ml/hour.

c. Implement measures *to decrease risk of aneurysm rupture:*
   1. instruct client to avoid elevating legs when in bed, using knee gatch, and crossing legs *in order to prevent restriction of blood flow to the lower extremities and subsequent increase in vascular pressure at the aneurysm site*
   2. perform actions *to prevent an increase in blood pressure:*
      a. limit client's activity as ordered
      b. instruct client to avoid activities that create a Valsalva response (e.g., straining to have a bowel movement, holding breath while moving up in bed, lifting heavy objects)
      c. implement measures to reduce fear and anxiety (see Preoperative Diagnosis 1)
   3. administer antihypertensives if ordered *to reduce pressure in the dilated vessel.*

d. If signs and symptoms of hypovolemic shock occur:
   1. place client flat in bed unless contraindicated
   2. monitor vital signs frequently
   3. administer oxygen as ordered
   4. administer blood and/or volume expanders as ordered (these need to be used with caution *since increased vascular pressure can extend a tear at site of rupture*)
   5. prepare client for insertion of hemodynamic monitoring devices (e.g., central venous catheter, intra-arterial catheter) if indicated
   6. prepare client for emergency surgical repair of aneurysm if indicated.

POSTOPERATIVE

Use in conjunction with the Standardized Postoperative Care Plan.

1. NURSING/COLLABORATIVE DIAGNOSIS:

RISK FOR IMBALANCED FLUID AND ELECTROLYTES

a. third-spacing of fluid related to:
   1. increased capillary permeability in surgical area associated with the inflammation that occurs following extensive dissection of tissue during major abdominal surgery
   2. increased vascular hydrostatic pressure associated with excess fluid volume if present
   3. hypoalbuminemia associated with the escape of proteins from the vascular space into the peritoneum (a result of increased capillary permeability in the surgical area);

b. excess fluid volume related to:
   1. vigorous fluid replacement
   2. fluid retention associated with:
      a. increased secretion of antidiuretic hormone (output of ADH is stimulated by trauma, pain, and anesthetic agents)
      b. renal insufficiency (can occur if there is inadequate blood flow to the kidneys during or after surgery)
   3. reabsorption of third-space fluid (occurs about the 3rd postoperative day);

c. deficient fluid volume related to restricted oral fluid intake before, during, and after surgery; blood loss; and loss of fluid associated with nasogastric tube drainage;

d. hypokalemia, hypochloremia, and metabolic alkalosis related to loss of electrolytes and hydrochloric acid associated with nasogastric tube drainage.

Suggested NOC Outcomes: Fluid balance; Fluid overload severity; Electrolyte and acid/base balance

Suggested NIC Interventions: Fluid monitoring; Fluid management; Electrolyte management: hypokalemia; Fluid/Electrolyte management; Acid-base monitoring; Acid-base management: metabolic alkalosis

Desired Outcomes	**Nursing Actions** *and Selected Purposes/Rationales*
1.a. The client will experience resolution of third-spacing as evidenced by: 1. absence of ascites 2. B/P and pulse within normal range for client and stable with position change.	1.a.1. Assess for and report signs and symptoms of third-spacing: a. ascites (e.g., increase in abdominal girth, dull percussion note over abdomen with finding of shifting dullness) b. evidence of vascular depletion (e.g., postural hypotension; weak, rapid pulse). 2. Monitor serum albumin levels. Report below-normal levels *(low serum albumin levels result in fluid shifting out of vascular space because albumin normally maintains plasma colloid osmotic pressure).* 3. Implement measures *to prevent further third-spacing and/or promote mobilization of fluid back into the vascular space:* a. perform actions to reduce excess fluid volume (see Standardized Postoperative Care Plan, Diagnosis 4, action b.2 [p. 107]) b. administer albumin infusions if ordered *to increase colloid osmotic pressure.* 4. Consult physician if signs and symptoms of third-spacing worsen or fail to resolve within expected length of time (reabsorption usually begins on 3rd postoperative day).
1.b. The client will not experience excess fluid volume (see Standardized Postoperative Care Plan, Diagnosis 4, outcome b [p. 107], for outcome criteria).	1.b. Refer to Standardized Postoperative Care Plan, Diagnosis 4, action b (p. 107), for measures related to assessment, prevention, and treatment of excess fluid volume.
1.c. The client will not experience deficient fluid volume, hypokalemia, hypochloremia, or metabolic alkalosis (see Standardized Postoperative Care Plan, Diagnosis 4, outcome a [p. 106], for outcome criteria).	1.c. Refer to Standardized Postoperative Care Plan, Diagnosis 4, action a (pp. 106–107), for measures related to assessment, prevention, and treatment of deficient fluid volume, hypokalemia, hypochloremia, and metabolic alkalosis.

2. COLLABORATIVE DIAGNOSES: **POTENTIAL COMPLICATIONS OF ABDOMINAL AORTIC ANEURYSM REPAIR**

a. hypovolemic shock related to hypovolemia associated with blood loss during surgery, third-space fluid shift, and hemorrhage (can occur as a result of inadequate wound closure and/or stress on and subsequent leakage or rupture of anastomosis sites);
b. lower extremity arterial embolization related to dislodgment of necrotic debris or clot from surgical site;
c. cardiac dysrhythmias related to altered nodal function and myocardial conductivity associated with:
   1. myocardial hypoxia resulting from:
      a. altered respiratory function
      b. diminished myocardial blood flow that can result from pre-existing coronary artery disease, hypotension (can occur as a result of hypovolemia, vasodilation associated with rapid warming, and effects of some medications), and sympathetic nervous system-mediated vasoconstriction that results from pain, stress, and hypothermia
   2. myocardial damage if a perioperative myocardial infarction has occurred
   3. hypokalemia if present;
d. ischemic colitis related to diminished blood supply to the colon associated with ligation of the inferior mesenteric artery during surgery, hypovolemia, and/or embolization;
e. impaired renal function related to insufficient blood flow to the kidneys associated with hypovolemia and prolonged aortic clamp time.

Desired Outcomes	Nursing Actions *and Selected Purposes/Rationales*
2.a. The client will not develop hypovolemic shock (see Preoperative Diagnosis 2, for outcome criteria).	2.a.1. Assess for and report signs and symptoms of leakage at anastomosis sites: a. new or expanding hematoma at incision site and/or ecchymosis of flank or perineal area b. increased abdominal girth (can also occur with third-spacing) c. new or increased reports of lumbar, flank, abdominal, pelvic, or groin pain d. increasing feeling of abdominal and/or gastric fullness unrelated to oral intake e. diminishing or absent peripheral pulses f. decreased motor or sensory function in lower extremities g. decreasing B/P, increasing pulse h. decreasing RBC, Hct, and Hgb values. 2. Assess for and report signs and symptoms of hypovolemic shock (see Preoperative Diagnosis 2, action b). 3. Implement measures *to prevent hypovolemic shock:* a. perform actions *to prevent or treat hypovolemia:* 1. implement measures to prevent further third-spacing and/or promote mobilization of fluid back into vascular space (see Postoperative Diagnosis 1, action a.3) 2. provide maximum fluid intake allowed (a fluid restriction may be ordered *to prevent fluid overload and subsequent pressure on the anastomosis sites*) 3. administer blood and/or volume expanders as ordered b. perform actions *to reduce stress on and subsequent separation of anastomosis sites:* 1. instruct client to avoid positions that compromise peripheral blood flow (e.g., elevating legs when in bed, use of knee gatch, crossing legs) 2. implement measures to reduce the accumulation of gas and fluid in the gastrointestinal tract and prevent nausea and vomiting (see Standardized Postoperative Care Plan, Diagnoses 7, action b and 8, action b [pp. 110–111])

Desired Outcomes	Nursing Actions *and Selected Purposes/Rationales*
	3. implement measures to prevent or treat excess fluid volume (see Standardized Postoperative Care Plan, Diagnosis 4, action b.2 [p. 107]) 4. instruct client to avoid activities that create a Valsalva response (e.g., straining to have a bowel movement, holding breath while moving up in bed) 5. instruct client to avoid vigorous coughing; consult physician about an order for an antitussive if indicated 6. administer antihypertensives if ordered *to reduce blood pressure.* 4. If signs and symptoms of hypovolemic shock occur: a. place client flat in bed unless contraindicated b. monitor vital signs frequently c. administer oxygen as ordered d. administer blood products and/or volume expanders if ordered (these need to be used with caution if anastomosis site separation is suspected) e. prepare client for surgery if indicated.
2.b. The client will not experience lower extremity arterial embolization as evidenced by: 1. no reports of pain or diminished sensation in lower extremities 2. palpable peripheral pulses 3. usual temperature and color of extremities.	2.b.1. Assess for and report signs and symptoms of lower extremity arterial embolization: a. reports of pain (onset is often sudden and severe) and/or numbness in lower extremity(ies) b. diminishing or absent peripheral pulses (pulses may be absent for a few hours after surgery *as a result of vasospasm)* c. cool, pale, or mottled extremities. 2. Implement measures *to reduce risk of embolization:* a. limit client's activity as ordered b. instruct client to avoid activities that create a Valsalva response (e.g., straining to have a bowel movement, holding breath while moving up in bed) *in order to prevent dislodgment of existing thrombi.* 3. If signs and symptoms of lower extremity arterial embolization occur: a. maintain client on bed rest b. prepare client for the following if planned: 1. diagnostic studies (e.g., Doppler ultrasound, arteriography) 2. embolectomy.
2.c. The client will maintain normal sinus rhythm as evidenced by: 1. regular apical pulse at 60–100 beats/minute 2. equal apical and radial pulse rates 3. absence of syncope and palpitations 4. ECG reading showing normal sinus rhythm.	2.c.1. Assess for and report signs and symptoms of cardiac dysrhythmias (e.g., irregular apical pulse; pulse rate below 60 or above 100 beats/minute; apical-radial pulse deficit; syncope; palpitations; abnormal rate, rhythm, or configurations on ECG). 2. Implement measures *to prevent cardiac dysrhythmias:* a. perform actions to maintain an adequate respiratory status (see Standardized Postoperative Care Plan, Diagnoses 2, action b and 3, action b [pp. 104–105]) *in order to maintain adequate myocardial tissue oxygenation* b. perform actions *to decrease stimulation of the sympathetic nervous system (sympathetic stimulation increases the heart rate and causes vasoconstriction, both of which increase cardiac workload and decrease oxygen availability to the myocardium):* 1. implement measures to reduce pain and anxiety (see Standardized Postoperative Care Plan, Diagnoses 6, action d and 21, action b [pp. 109 and 124]) 2. implement measures *to keep client from getting cold* (e.g., maintain a comfortable room temperature, provide adequate clothing and blankets) c. perform actions to prevent or treat hypokalemia (see Standardized Postoperative Care Plan, Diagnosis 4, action a.2 [p. 106]) d. perform actions *to prevent or treat hypotension:* 1. consult physician before giving negative inotropic agents, diuretics, and vasodilating agents if systolic B/P is below 90–100 mm Hg

2. perform actions to prevent hypovolemic shock (see action a.3 in this diagnosis) *in order to maintain an adequate vascular volume*
3. administer narcotic (opioid) analgesics judiciously, being alert to the synergistic effect of the narcotic ordered and the anesthetic that was used during surgery
4. gradually bring client's body temperature to normal if hypothermic *(rapid warming results in vasodilation)*
5. administer sympathomimetics (e.g., dopamine) if ordered.

3. If cardiac dysrhythmias occur:
   a. administer antidysrhythmics as ordered
   b. restrict client's activity based on his/her tolerance and severity of the dysrhythmia
   c. maintain oxygen therapy as ordered
   d. assess cardiovascular status frequently and report signs and symptoms of inadequate tissue perfusion (e.g., decrease in B/P, cool skin, cyanosis, diminished peripheral pulses, urine output less than 30 ml/hour, restlessness and agitation, shortness of breath)
   e. have emergency cart readily available for cardioversion, defibrillation, or cardiopulmonary resuscitation.

2.d. The client will not develop ischemic colitis as evidenced by:
1. absence of blood in stools
2. absence of diarrhea
3. absence of or decrease in abdominal pain
4. soft, nontender abdomen.

2.d.1. Assess for and report signs and symptoms of ischemic colitis (e.g., blood in stools, diarrhea, reports of new or increasing abdominal pain, distended abdomen).
2. Implement measures to prevent hypovolemic shock and embolization (see actions a.3 and b.2 in this diagnosis) *in order to maintain adequate blood supply to the colon.*
3. If signs and symptoms of ischemic colitis occur:
   a. administer antimicrobials if ordered
   b. prepare client for the following if planned:
      1. colonoscopy
      2. colon resection (usually performed if client has extensive tissue necrosis or gangrenous patches have developed)
      3. embolectomy.

2.e. The client will maintain adequate renal function as evidenced by:
1. urine output at least 30 ml/hour
2. BUN, serum creatinine, and creatinine clearance within normal range.

2.e.1. Assess for and report signs and symptoms of impaired renal function (e.g., urine output less than 30 ml/hour, urine specific gravity fixed at or less than 1.010, elevated BUN and serum creatinine levels, decreased creatinine clearance).
2. Implement measures to prevent hypovolemic shock (see action a.3 in this diagnosis) *in order to maintain adequate renal blood flow.*
3. If signs and symptoms of impaired renal function occur, assess for and report signs of acute renal failure (e.g., oliguria or anuria; weight gain; edema; elevated B/P; lethargy and confusion; increasing BUN and serum creatinine, phosphorus, and potassium levels).

Discharge Teaching/Continued Care

3. Nursing Diagnosis: ***DEFICIENT KNOWLEDGE, INEFFECTIVE THERAPEUTIC REGIMEN MANAGEMENT, OR INEFFECTIVE HEALTH MAINTENANCE****

*The nurse should select the diagnostic label that is most appropriate for the client's discharge teaching needs.

Suggested NOC Outcomes: Knowledge: treatment regimen; Knowledge: cardiac disease management

Suggested NIC Interventions: Health system guidance; Teaching: individual; Teaching: disease process; Teaching: prescribed diet

Desired Outcomes	Nursing Actions *and Selected Purposes/Rationales*
3.a. The client will identify ways to prevent or slow the progression of atherosclerosis.	3.a.1. Inform the client that certain modifiable factors such as elevated serum lipids, a sedentary lifestyle, smoking, and hypertension have been shown to increase the risk of atherosclerosis. 2. Assist client to identify changes in lifestyle that could reduce the risk for atherosclerosis (e.g., dietary modifications, smoking cessation, physical exercise on a regular basis). 3. Provide instructions on ways the client can reduce intake of saturated fat and cholesterol: a. reduce intake of meat fat (e.g., trim visible fat off meat; replace fatty meats such as fatty cuts of steak, hamburger, and processed meats with leaner products) b. reduce intake of milk fat (avoid dairy products containing more than 1% fat) c. reduce intake of *trans* fats (e.g., avoid stick margarine and shortening and foods such as commercial baked goods that are prepared with these products) d. use vegetable oil rather than coconut or palm oil in cooking and food preparation e. use cooking methods such as steaming, baking, broiling, poaching, microwaving, and grilling rather than frying f. restrict intake of eggs (recommendations about the number of whole eggs allowed per week vary depending on the client's lipid levels). 4. Instruct client to take lipid-lowering agents (e.g., HMG-CoA reductase inhibitors ["statins"], ezetimibe, gemfibrozil, niacin) as prescribed.
3.b. The client will state signs and symptoms to report to the health care provider.	3.b.1. Refer to Standardized Postoperative Care Plan, Diagnosis 22, action c (p. 125), for signs and symptoms to report to the health care provider. 2. Instruct client to report these additional signs and symptoms: a. sudden or gradual increase in lower back, flank, groin, or abdominal pain b. chest pain c. coolness, pallor, or blueness of lower extremities d. increased weakness and fatigue e. decreased urine output f. bloody or persistent diarrhea g. increased bruising of incision site, flank area, or perineum h. impotence.
3.c. The client will verbalize an understanding of and a plan for adhering to recommended follow-up care including future appointments with health care provider, medications prescribed, activity level, and wound care.	3.c.1. Refer to Standardized Postoperative Care Plan, Diagnosis 22 (pp. 125–126), for routine postoperative instructions and measures to improve client compliance. 2. Reinforce the physician's instructions regarding: a. importance of scheduling adequate rest periods b. ways to prevent constipation and subsequent straining to have a bowel movement (e.g., drink at least 10 glasses of liquid/day unless contraindicated, increase intake of foods high in fiber, take stool softeners if necessary) c. the need to avoid sexual intercourse, isometric exercise/activity (e.g., lifting objects over 10 pounds, pushing heavy objects), and strenuous exercise for specified length of time (usually 4–12 weeks depending on the activity) d. the need to take prophylactic antimicrobials prior to any dental work or invasive procedure (some physicians recommend this for the first 6–12 months following surgical placement of a synthetic graft).

Additional Nursing Diagnosis

SEXUAL DYSFUNCTION

related to:

a. decreased libido associated with operative site discomfort and fear of surgical site bleeding;
b. impotence associated with prolonged reduction in blood flow in the mesenteric or internal iliac arteries (can occur as a result of prolonged aortic clamp time during surgery, persistent hypovolemia, embolization, or graft occlusion) and/or nerve damage (can occur during surgery).

Bibliography

See pages 879 and 882.

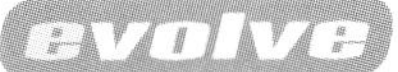

Carotid Endarterectomy

Carotid endarterectomy is the surgical removal of atherosclerotic plaque from the intima of the carotid artery. The most common site of plaque formation in the carotid artery is the bifurcation. Access to this extracranial area is gained through an incision along the anterior sternocleidomastoid muscle. Surgery is performed to improve carotid artery blood flow and to reduce the risk of cerebral embolization and stroke.

This care plan focuses on the adult client hospitalized for a carotid endarterectomy. Much of the postoperative information is applicable to clients receiving follow-up care in an extended care facility or home setting.

OUTCOME/DISCHARGE CRITERIA

THE CLIENT WILL:

- have adequate cerebral blood flow
- have surgical pain controlled
- have evidence of normal wound healing
- identify ways to prevent or slow the progression of atherosclerosis
- identify ways to manage signs and symptoms resulting from cranial nerve damage if it has occurred
- state signs and symptoms to report to the health care provider
- verbalize an understanding of and a plan for adhering to recommended follow-up care including future appointments with health care provider, medications prescribed, activity level, and wound care.

NURSING/COLLABORATIVE DIAGNOSES

Preoperative

1. Ineffective tissue perfusion: cerebral p. 404

Postoperative

1. Potential complications p. 405
   a. cerebral ischemia
   b. respiratory distress
   c. cranial nerve damage (particularly the facial, hypoglossal, glossopharyngeal, vagus, and/or accessory nerves)

DISCHARGE TEACHING

2. Deficient knowledge, Ineffective therapeutic regimen management, or Ineffective health maintenance p. 408

See Standardized Preoperative and Postoperative Care Plans (pp. 97–126) for additional diagnoses.

PREOPERATIVE

Use in conjunction with the Standardized Preoperative Care Plan.

1. Nursing Diagnosis: *INEFFECTIVE TISSUE PERFUSION: CEREBRAL*

related to:

a. partial or complete occlusion of the carotid artery by atherosclerotic plaque and/or a thrombus;
b. a cerebral embolus associated with dislodgment of atherosclerotic plaque or a thrombus from the carotid artery.

Suggested NOC Outcomes:
Tissue perfusion: cerebral; Neurological status; Cognition

Suggested NIC Interventions: Cerebral perfusion promotion; Neurologic monitoring

Desired Outcome	**Nursing Actions** *and Selected Purposes/Rationales*
1. The client will maintain adequate cerebral tissue perfusion as evidenced by: a. mentally alert and oriented b. absence of dizziness, visual disturbances, and speech impairments c. normal motor and sensory function.	1.a. Assess for and report signs and symptoms of carotid artery occlusion and/or cerebral embolization (e.g., agitation, lethargy, confusion, dizziness, diplopia, ipsilateral blindness, homonymous hemianopsia, slurred speech, expressive aphasia, paresthesias, hemiparesis, hemiplegia). b. Implement measures *to maintain adequate cerebral tissue perfusion:* 1. administer anticoagulants (e.g., heparin, warfarin) or antiplatelet agents (e.g., low-dose aspirin, clopidogrel) if ordered *to prevent new or extended thrombus formation and further occlusion of the carotid artery* (these medications might be discontinued before surgery to reduce the risk of intraoperative and postoperative hemorrhage) 2. caution client to avoid activities that create a Valsalva response (e.g., straining to have a bowel movement, holding breath while moving up in bed) *in order to prevent dislodgment of existing thrombi* 3. perform actions *to prevent hypertension in order to reduce the risk of cerebral embolism:* a. implement measures *to reduce stress* (e.g., explain procedures, maintain calm environment) b. administer antihypertensives as ordered (these medications are sometimes discontinued before surgery *to reduce the risk of a critical drop in B/P during and immediately following surgery*). c. If signs and symptoms of decreased cerebral tissue perfusion occur: 1. maintain client on bed rest with head of bed flat unless contraindicated 2. administer anticoagulants (e.g., continuous intravenous heparin, high-dose low-molecular-weight heparin, warfarin) if ordered 3. provide emotional support to client and significant others; be aware that the development of signs and symptoms usually necessitates postponement or cancellation of planned surgery.

POSTOPERATIVE

Use in conjunction with the Standardized Postoperative Care Plan.

1. COLLABORATIVE DIAGNOSES: POTENTIAL COMPLICATIONS OF CAROTID ENDARTERECTOMY

a. cerebral ischemia related to:
   1. prolonged carotid artery clamp time during surgery and/or vasospasm associated with clamping and manipulation of cerebral vessels
   2. compression of carotid vessels associated with inflammation, edema, and/or development of a hematoma in the operative area
   3. hypotension associated with:
      a. hypovolemia resulting from intraoperative and/or postoperative blood loss
      b. stimulation of the carotid sinus baroreceptors resulting from surgical manipulation and/or improved blood flow in the carotid artery following surgery)
   4. increased cerebral vascular dilation and pressure associated with inability of the autoregulatory system to adjust to increased blood flow in cerebral vessels distal to the surgical site (this hyperperfusion syndrome can occur in the initial postoperative period in clients who have had a high-grade, long-term carotid artery blockage that has resulted in chronic cerebral vessel dilation)
   5. embolization during or after surgery and/or formation of a thrombus at surgical site;

b. respiratory distress related to airway obstruction associated with tracheal compression (can occur as a result of inflammation, edema, and/or hematoma formation in the surgical area);

c. cranial nerve damage (particularly the facial, hypoglossal, glossopharyngeal, vagus, and/or accessory nerves) related to surgical trauma and/or compression of the nerves (can occur as a result of inflammation, edema, and/or hematoma formation).

Desired Outcomes	Nursing Actions *and Selected Purposes/Rationales*
1.a. The client will maintain adequate cerebral blood flow as evidenced by: 1. mentally alert and oriented 2. absence of dizziness, visual disturbances, and speech impairments 3. normal sensory and motor function.	1.a.1. Assess for and report signs and symptoms of: a. excessive operative site bleeding (e.g., new or expanding hematoma; continued bright red bleeding from incision or wound drain [a drain is sometimes in place for about 24 hours after surgery]; decreasing RBC, Hct, and Hgb levels) b. hypovolemic shock (see Standardized Postoperative Care Plan, Diagnosis 20, action a.1 [p. 122]) c. cerebral ischemia: 1. agitation, irritability, lethargy, confusion 2. dizziness 3. visual disturbances (e.g., blurred or dimmed vision, diplopia, ipsilateral blindness, homonymous hemianopsia) 4. speech impairments (e.g., slurred speech, expressive aphasia) 5. paresthesias, paresis, paralysis. 2. Implement measures *to prevent cerebral ischemia:* a. perform actions to prevent or treat hypovolemic shock (see Standardized Postoperative Care Plan, Diagnosis 20, actions a.2 and 3 [p. 122]) b. perform actions *to reduce pressure on carotid vessels:* 1. implement measures *to reduce operative site inflammation and/or edema:* a. keep head of bed elevated 30° unless contraindicated b. apply cooling pad or ice pack to incisional area as ordered c. administer corticosteroids if ordered 2. maintain patency of wound drain (e.g., keep tubing free of kinks, empty collection device as often as necessary) if present 3. instruct client to support head and neck with hands during position changes and to avoid turning head abruptly or hyperextending neck *in order to reduce stress on the suture line and prevent subsequent bleeding and hematoma formation* c. caution client to avoid activities that create a Valsalva response (e.g., straining to have a bowel movement, holding breath while moving up in bed) *in order to prevent dislodgment of existing thrombi and reduce stress on and subsequent bleeding from the suture line* d. administer the following medications if ordered *to maintain blood pressure within a safe range:* 1. antihypertensives *to prevent rupture of the operative vessel or reduce the risk of dislodgment of any existing thrombus* (hypertension may occur as a result of factors such as the underlying disease process or damage to the carotid sinus baroreceptors during surgery) 2. sympathomimetics (e.g., dopamine) *to treat hypotension.* 3. If signs and symptoms of cerebral ischemia occur: a. maintain client on bed rest with head of bed flat unless contraindicated b. prepare client for surgical removal of thrombus if planned.
1.b. The client will not experience respiratory distress as evidenced by: 1. usual mental status 2. unlabored respirations at 12–20/minute 3. absence of stridor and sternocleidomastoid muscle retraction 4. oximetry results within normal range 5. blood gases within normal range.	1.b.1. Assess for and report: a. increased edema or expanding hematoma in surgical area b. deviation of trachea from midline c. new or increased difficulty swallowing d. signs and symptoms of respiratory distress (e.g., restlessness, agitation, rapid and/or labored respirations, stridor, sternocleidomastoid muscle retraction) e. abnormal blood gases f. significant decrease in oximetry results. 2. Have tracheostomy and suction equipment readily available. 3. Implement measures *to prevent compression of the trachea and subsequent respiratory distress:* a. perform actions to prevent inflammation, edema, and hematoma formation in the operative area (see action a.2.b in this diagnosis)

b. perform actions *to prevent excessive pressure in the operative vessel and subsequent bleeding and hematoma formation:*
   1. caution client to avoid activities that create a Valsalva response (e.g., straining to have a bowel movement, holding breath while moving up in bed)
   2. administer antihypertensives if ordered.

4. If signs and symptoms of respiratory distress occur:
   a. place client in a high Fowler's position unless contraindicated
   b. loosen neck dressing if it appears tight
   c. administer oxygen as ordered
   d. assist with intubation or tracheostomy if performed
   e. prepare client for evacuation of hematoma or surgical repair of the bleeding vessel if planned.

1.c. The client will experience beginning resolution of cranial nerve damage if it occurs as evidenced by:
1. gradual return of facial symmetry and usual taste sensation
2. increased ability to chew and swallow
3. improved speech
4. return of usual shoulder movements.

1.c.1. Assess for signs and symptoms of the following:
   a. facial nerve damage (e.g., facial ptosis on affected side, impaired sense of taste)
   b. vagus and glossopharyngeal nerve damage (e.g., loss of gag reflex, difficulty swallowing, hoarseness, inability to speak clearly)
   c. hypoglossal nerve damage (e.g., tongue biting when chewing, tongue deviation toward affected side, difficulty swallowing and speaking)
   d. accessory nerve damage (e.g., unilateral shoulder sag, difficulty raising shoulder against resistance).

2. Implement measures to prevent compression of the cranial nerves at the operative site (see actions a.2.b and b.3.b in this diagnosis).

3. If signs and symptoms of cranial nerve damage occur:
   a. if the facial, hypoglossal, vagus, and/or glossopharyngeal nerves are affected:
      1. withhold oral foods/fluids until gag reflex returns and client is better able to chew and swallow *in order to reduce the risk of aspiration;* provide parenteral nutrition or tube feeding if indicated
      2. when oral intake is allowed and tolerated:
         a. implement measures *to improve client's ability to chew and/or swallow:*
            1. place client in high Fowler's position for meals and snacks
            2. assist client to select foods that require little or no chewing and are easily swallowed (e.g., custard, eggs, canned fruits, mashed potatoes)
            3. avoid serving foods that are sticky (e.g., peanut butter, soft bread, honey)
            4. serve thick rather than thin fluids or add a thickening agent (e.g., "Thick-It," gelatin, baby cereal) to thin fluids
            5. moisten dry foods with gravy or sauces (e.g., catsup, sour cream, salad dressing)
         b. instruct client to add extra sweeteners or seasonings to foods/fluids if desired *in order to compensate for impaired sense of taste*
      3. implement measures *to facilitate communication* (e.g., maintain quiet environment; provide pad and pencil, Magic Slate, or word cards; listen carefully when client speaks)
      4. consult speech pathologist about additional ways to facilitate swallowing and communication
   b. if the accessory nerve is affected, instruct client in and assist with exercises *to prevent atrophy of trapezius and sternocleidomastoid muscles* (e.g., range of motion of affected shoulder, wall climbing with fingers, shoulder shrugs)
   c. provide emotional support to client and significant others; assure them that the nerve damage is usually not permanent but caution them that the symptoms may take months to resolve.

Discharge Teaching/Continued Care

2. Nursing Diagnosis: DEFICIENT KNOWLEDGE, INEFFECTIVE THERAPEUTIC REGIMEN MANAGEMENT, OR INEFFECTIVE HEALTH MAINTENANCE*

*The nurse should select the diagnostic label that is most appropriate for the client's discharge teaching needs.

Suggested NOC Outcomes: Knowledge: treatment regimen; Knowledge: cardiac disease management

Suggested NIC Interventions: Health system guidance; Teaching: disease process; Teaching: individual; Teaching: prescribed diet

Desired Outcomes	Nursing Actions *and Selected Purposes/Rationales*
2.a. The client will identify ways to prevent or slow the progression of atherosclerosis.	2.a.1. Inform the client that certain modifiable factors such as elevated serum lipids, a sedentary lifestyle, cigarette smoking, and hypertension have been shown to increase the risk of atherosclerosis. 2. Assist client to identify changes in lifestyle that could reduce the risk for atherosclerosis (e.g., smoking cessation, dietary modifications, physical exercise on a regular basis). 3. Provide instructions on ways the client can reduce intake of saturated fat and cholesterol: a. reduce intake of meat fat (e.g., trim visible fat off meat; replace fatty meats such as fatty cuts of steak, hamburger, and processed meats with leaner products) b. reduce intake of milk fat (avoid dairy products containing more than 1% fat). c. reduce intake of *trans* fats (e.g., avoid stick margarine and shortening and foods such as commercial baked goods that are prepared with these products) d. use vegetable oil rather than coconut or palm oil in cooking and food preparation e. use cooking methods such as steaming, baking, broiling, poaching, microwaving, and grilling rather than frying f. restrict intake of eggs (recommendations about the number of whole eggs allowed per week vary depending on the client's lipid levels). 4. Instruct client to take lipid-lowering agents (e.g., HMG-CoA reductase inhibitors ["statins"], ezetimibe, gemfibrozil, niacin) and antiplatelet agents (e.g., low-dose aspirin) as prescribed.
2.b. The client will identify ways to manage signs and symptoms resulting from cranial nerve damage if it has occurred.	2.b.1. If signs and symptoms of hypoglossal, facial, vagus, and/or glossopharyngeal nerve damage are present: a. reinforce techniques to improve swallowing and speaking b. assist client in identifying foods that are nutritious and easy to chew and swallow; obtain a dietary consult if needed c. instruct client to increase the amount of sweeteners and seasonings usually used and/or to try different seasonings in foods and beverages if sense of taste is altered. 2. If signs and symptoms of accessory nerve damage are present, reinforce exercises that should be performed to maintain shoulder muscle tone and prevent contractures. 3. Allow time for questions, clarification, and return demonstration.
2.c. The client will state signs and symptoms to report to the health care provider.	2.c.1. Refer to Standardized Postoperative Care Plan, Diagnosis 22, action c (p. 125), for signs and symptoms to report to the health care provider. 2. Instruct client to also report: a. increased swelling or purple discoloration at wound site b. new or increased difficulty chewing, swallowing, or speaking

c. any loss of or change in vision
d. dizziness
e. numbness, tingling, or weakness of arm(s) or leg(s)
f. increasing irritability
g. lethargy, confusion
h. failure of signs and symptoms of cranial nerve damage to resolve as expected; remind client that it can take months for reversible signs and symptoms to resolve.

2.d. The client will verbalize an understanding of and a plan for adhering to recommended follow-up care including future appointments with health care provider, medications prescribed, activity level, and wound care.

2.d.1. Refer to Standardized Postoperative Care Plan, Diagnosis 22 (pp. 125–126), for routine postoperative instructions and measures to improve client compliance.
2. Reinforce the physician's instructions regarding:
a. ways to prevent constipation and subsequent straining to have a bowel movement (e.g., drink at least 10 glasses of liquid/day unless contraindicated, increase intake of foods high in fiber, take stool softeners if necessary)
b. the need to avoid isometric exercise/activity (e.g., lifting objects over 10 pounds, pushing heavy objects) and strenuous exercise for specified length of time (usually 4–12 weeks depending on the activity).

Bibliography

See pages 879 and 882.

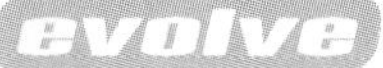

Deep Vein Thrombosis

Venous thrombosis occurs when a thrombus forms in a superficial or deep vein. This condition is often called thrombophlebitis because of the associated inflammation in the involved vessel wall. The predisposing factors for venous thrombus formation are venous stasis, damage to the endothelium of the vein wall, and/or hypercoagulability. Conditions/factors associated with a high risk for venous thrombosis include surgery (especially orthopedic and abdominal surgery), immobility, advanced age, heart failure, certain malignancies, fractures or other injuries of the pelvis or lower extremities, varicose veins, pregnancy, obesity, estrogen and oral contraceptive use, sepsis, venous cannulation, administration of vessel irritants (e.g., hypertonic solutions, chemotherapeutic agents, high-dose antibiotics), history of deep vein thrombosis, and inherited coagulation abnormalities.

Deep vein thrombosis usually develops in a lower extremity; however, the incidence of subclavian venous thrombosis is rising because of the increased use of central venous catheters. Clinical manifestations of deep vein thrombosis are often not distinctive and, in many cases, the client is asymptomatic. Signs and symptoms that may be present include pain, tenderness, swelling, unusual warmth, and/or positive Homans' sign in the involved extremity. The greatest danger associated with deep vein thrombosis is that the clot, or parts of it, will detach and cause embolic occlusion of a pulmonary vessel.

Persons with deep vein thrombosis are usually treated medically rather than surgically unless there is massive occlusion of a vessel and anticoagulation and thrombolytic therapy are contraindicated. With the increasing use of thrombolytic therapy, thrombectomies and embolectomies are rarely performed. Medical treatment varies depending on the location of the thrombus, the person's risk for bleeding and history of previous thrombus, and whether a coagulation abnormality exists. Anticoagulant therapy is not universally used to treat calf vein thrombosis because the incidence of pulmonary embolism is low if there is no proximal vein involvement. However, there is a risk of extension of calf vein thrombi into a proximal venous segment if untreated, and because of this risk, many persons with calf vein thrombosis are treated with anticoagulants. There is also some variation in the anticoagulant regimen in relation to the time that oral anticoagulants are initiated and the route and type of heparin ordered (e.g., continuous intravenous heparin, intermittent intravenous heparin, adjusted-dose subcutaneous heparin, low-molecular-weight heparin).

This care plan focuses on the adult client hospitalized for treatment of deep vein thrombosis in a lower extremity. The information is also applicable to clients receiving follow-up care at home.

OUTCOME/DISCHARGE CRITERIA

THE CLIENT WILL:

- have adequate tissue perfusion in affected extremity
- have no evidence of tissue irritation or breakdown
- have no signs and symptoms of complications
- identify ways to promote venous blood flow and reduce the risk of chronic venous insufficiency and recurrent thrombus formation
- verbalize an understanding of medications ordered including rationale, food and drug interactions, side effects, schedule for taking, and importance of taking as prescribed
- demonstrate the ability to correctly draw up and administer heparin subcutaneously if prescribed
- identify precautions necessary to prevent bleeding associated with anticoagulant therapy
- state signs and symptoms to report to the health care provider
- verbalize an understanding of and a plan for adhering to recommended follow-up care including future appointments with health care provider and activity level.

Use in conjunction with the Care Plan on Immobility.

NURSING/COLLABORATIVE DIAGNOSES

DISCHARGE TEACHING

See Care Plan on Immobility (pp. 129–148) for additional diagnoses.

1. NURSING DIAGNOSIS: *INEFFECTIVE TISSUE PERFUSION: PERIPHERAL*

related to:
a. obstructed venous blood flow in affected extremity associated with the presence of a thrombus and inflammation of the vessel;
b. venous stasis associated with decreased mobility.

Suggested NOC Outcome: Tissue perfusion: peripheral

Suggested NIC Interventions: Embolus care: peripheral; Circulatory care: venous insufficiency; Lower extremity monitoring

Desired Outcome	**Nursing Actions** *and Selected Purposes/Rationales* (see pp. 57–59 for additional rationales)
1. The client will have improved venous blood flow in the affected extremity as evidenced by diminished pain, tenderness, swelling, and distention of superficial blood vessels in extremity.	1.a. Assess for signs and symptoms of impaired venous blood flow in the affected extremity: 1. pain or tenderness in extremity 2. increase in circumference of extremity 3. distention of superficial blood vessels in extremity. b. Implement measures *to improve venous blood flow:* 1. perform actions *to treat the thrombosis:* a. administer anticoagulants (e.g., continuous intravenous heparin, low-molecular-weight heparin, fondaparinux, warfarin) as ordered b. prepare client for intravenous injection of a thrombolytic agent (e.g., streptokinase, tissue plasminogen activator [tPA]) or catheter-directed fibrinolysis (infusion of a fibrinolytic agent into the thrombus) 2. perform actions *to reduce venous stasis:* a. elevate affected extremity 10–20° above the level of the heart b. maintain a minimum fluid intake of 2500 cc (unless contraindicated) *in order to prevent increased blood viscosity* c. apply antiembolism stockings if ordered d. discourage positions that compromise blood flow (e.g., pillows under knees, crossing legs, sitting or standing for long periods). c. Consult physician if signs and symptoms of impaired venous blood flow in affected extremity persist or worsen.

2. NURSING DIAGNOSIS: *ACUTE PAIN: AFFECTED EXTREMITY*

related to:
a. decreased tissue perfusion and swelling associated with obstructed venous blood flow;
b. inflammation of vein.

Suggested NOC Outcomes: Comfort level; Pain control

Suggested NIC Interventions: Pain management; Analgesic administration; Heat/Cold application

Desired Outcome	Nursing Actions *and Selected Purpose/Rationales* (see pp. 45–47 for additional rationales)
2. The client will experience diminished pain in the affected extremity as evidenced by: a. verbalization of a decrease in pain b. relaxed facial expression and body positioning c. increased participation in activities when allowed.	2.a. Assess for signs and symptoms of pain (e.g., verbalization of pain, grimacing, rubbing affected area, restlessness, reluctance to move). b. Assess client's perception of the severity of pain using a pain intensity rating scale. c. Assess client's pain pattern (e.g., location, quality, onset, duration, precipitating factors, aggravating factors, alleviating factors). d. Implement measures *to reduce pain:* 1. perform actions to improve venous blood flow (see Diagnosis 1, action b) 2. apply heat to affected area if ordered 3. perform actions *to protect the affected extremity from trauma, pressure, or excessive movement:* a. avoid jarring the bed b. use a bed cradle or footboard *to relieve pressure from bed linens* c. support extremity during position changes d. maintain activity restrictions as ordered e. instruct client to move affected extremity slowly and cautiously 4. provide or assist with nonpharmacologic methods for pain relief (e.g., position change, relaxation techniques, restful environment, diversional activities); caution client and significant others that the painful extremity should not be rubbed to relieve pain *(rubbing could dislodge the thrombus)* 5. administer analgesics and anti-inflammatory agents if ordered. e. Consult physician if above measures fail to provide adequate pain relief.

3. Nursing Diagnosis: **RISK FOR IMPAIRED TISSUE INTEGRITY**

related to:

a. accumulation of waste products and decreased oxygen and nutrient supply to the skin and subcutaneous tissue associated with prolonged pressure on tissues as a result of decreased mobility;
b. damage to the skin and/or subcutaneous tissue associated with friction or shearing that can occur with movement while on bed rest;
c. increased skin fragility in affected extremity associated with insufficient blood flow and edema.

Suggested NOC Outcome: Tissue integrity: skin and mucous membranes

Suggested NIC Interventions: Skin surveillance; Pressure management; Pressure ulcer prevention

Desired Outcome	Nursing Actions *and Selected Purposes/Rationales* (see pp. 49–52 for additional rationales)
3. The client will maintain tissue integrity as evidenced by: a. absence of redness and irritation b. no skin breakdown.	3.a. Inspect the skin (especially bony prominences, dependent areas, and affected extremity) for pallor, redness, and breakdown. b. Refer to Care Plan on Immobility, Diagnosis 4, action c (p. 133), for measures to prevent tissue breakdown. c. Implement measures *to prevent tissue breakdown in involved extremity:* 1. perform actions to improve venous blood flow (see Diagnosis 1, action b) 2. perform actions *to protect affected extremity from trauma and/or excessive pressure:* a. use a bed cradle or footboard *to relieve pressure from bed linens* b. keep heel off bed by elevating extremity on foam block or pillows or using heel protector c. instruct and assist client to move affected extremity cautiously d. remove antiembolism stockings for 30–60 minutes at least twice daily e. use caution when applying heat to extremity. d. If tissue breakdown occurs: 1. notify appropriate health care provider (e.g., wound care specialist, physician)

2. perform care of involved area(s) as ordered or per standard hospital procedure.

4. COLLABORATIVE DIAGNOSES: **POTENTIAL COMPLICATIONS**

a. pulmonary embolism related to dislodgment of thrombus;
b. bleeding related to prolonged coagulation time associated with anticoagulant therapy and possible heparin-induced thrombocytopenia.

Desired Outcomes	**Nursing Actions** *and Selected Purposes/Rationales*
4.a. The client will not experience a pulmonary embolism as evidenced by: 1. absence of sudden chest pain 2. unlabored respirations at 12–20/minute 3. pulse 60–100 beats/minute 4. blood gases within normal range.	4.a.1. Assess for and report signs and symptoms of a pulmonary embolism (e.g., sudden chest pain, dyspnea, tachypnea, tachycardia, apprehension, low PaO_2). 2. Implement measures *to prevent a pulmonary embolism:* a. perform actions *to prevent dislodgment of thrombus:* 1. maintain client on bed rest as ordered 2. do not exercise or check for Homans' sign in affected extremity during acute phase of deep vein thrombosis 3. never massage affected extremity and caution client not to allow significant others to massage extremity 4. caution client to avoid activities that create a Valsalva response (e.g., straining to have a bowel movement, blowing nose forcefully, holding breath while moving up in bed) b. administer anticoagulants (e.g., continuous intravenous heparin, low-molecular-weight heparin, warfarin) as ordered c. prepare client for a vena caval interruption (e.g., insertion of an intracaval filtering device) if planned. 3. If signs and symptoms of a pulmonary embolism occur: a. maintain client on bed rest in a semi- to high Fowler's position b. maintain oxygen therapy as ordered c. prepare client for diagnostic tests (e.g., blood gases, D-dimer level, ventilation-perfusion lung scan, pulmonary angiography) d. administer anticoagulants (e.g., continuous intravenous heparin, warfarin) as ordered e. prepare client for the following if planned: 1. injection of a thrombolytic agent (e.g., streptokinase, urokinase, tissue plasminogen activator [tPA]) 2. vena caval interruption (e.g., insertion of an intracaval filtering device) *to prevent further pulmonary emboli* 3. embolectomy.
4.b. The client will not experience unusual bleeding as evidenced by: 1. skin and mucous membranes free of petechiae, purpura, ecchymoses, and active bleeding 2. absence of unusual joint pain 3. no increase in abdominal girth 4. absence of frank and occult blood in stool, urine, and vomitus 5. usual menstrual flow 6. vital signs within normal range for client 7. stable Hct and Hgb.	4.b.1. Assess client for and report signs and symptoms of unusual bleeding: a. petechiae, purpura, ecchymoses b. gingival bleeding c. prolonged bleeding from puncture sites d. epistaxis, hemoptysis e. unusual joint pain f. increase in abdominal girth g. frank or occult blood in stool, urine, or vomitus h. menorrhagia i. restlessness, confusion j. decreasing B/P and increased pulse rate k. decrease in Hct and Hgb levels. 2. Monitor platelet count and coagulation test results (e.g., prothrombin time or International Normalized Ratio [INR], activated partial thromboplastin time, partial thromboplastin time). Report a low platelet count and coagulation test results that exceed the therapeutic range. 3. If platelet count is low, coagulation test results are abnormal, or Hct and Hgb levels decrease, test all stool, urine, and vomitus for occult blood. Report positive results.

Desired Outcomes	Nursing Actions *and Selected Purposes/Rationales*
	4. Implement measures *to prevent bleeding:* a. avoid giving injections whenever possible; consult physician about prescribing an alternative route for medications ordered to be given intramuscularly or subcutaneously b. when giving injections or performing venous or arterial punctures, use the smallest gauge needle possible and apply gentle, prolonged pressure to the site after the needle is removed c. caution client to avoid activities that increase the risk for trauma (e.g., shaving with a straight-edge razor, using a stiff bristle toothbrush or dental floss) d. pad side rails if client is confused or restless e. whenever possible, avoid intubations (e.g., nasogastric) and procedures that can cause injury to rectal mucosa (e.g., inserting a rectal suppository or tube, administering an enema) f. perform actions *to reduce the risk for falls* (e.g., keep bed in low position with side rails up when client is in bed, avoid unnecessary clutter in room, instruct client to wear shoes with nonslip soles when ambulating) g. instruct client to avoid blowing nose forcefully or straining to have a bowel movement; consult physician about an order for a decongestant and/or laxative if indicated. 5. If bleeding occurs and does not subside spontaneously: a. apply firm, prolonged pressure to bleeding area(s) if possible b. if epistaxis occurs, place client in a high Fowler's position and apply pressure and ice pack to nasal area c. maintain oxygen therapy as ordered d. administer protamine sulfate (antidote for heparin), vitamin K (e.g., phytonadione), and/or whole blood or blood products (e.g., fresh frozen plasma, platelets) as ordered.

Discharge Teaching/Continued Care

5. Nursing Diagnosis: ***DEFICIENT KNOWLEDGE, INEFFECTIVE THERAPEUTIC REGIMEN MANAGEMENT, OR INEFFECTIVE HEALTH MAINTENANCE****

*The nurse should select the diagnostic label that is most appropriate for the client's discharge teaching needs.

Suggested NOC Outcomes: Knowledge: disease process; Knowledge: treatment regimen

Suggested NIC Interventions: Health system guidance; Teaching: individual; Teaching: prescribed activity/exercise; Teaching: prescribed medication

Desired Outcomes	Nursing Actions *and Selected Purposes/Rationales*
5.a. The client will identify ways to promote venous blood flow and reduce the risk of chronic venous insufficiency and recurrent thrombus formation.	5.a.1. Provide the following instructions on ways to promote venous blood flow and reduce the risk for chronic venous insufficiency (can result from residual vein damage) and recurrent thrombus development: a. avoid wearing constrictive clothing (e.g., garters, girdles, narrow-banded knee-high hose) b. avoid sitting and standing in one position for long periods of time c. wear graduated compression stockings or support hose during the day d. avoid crossing legs and lying or sitting with pillows under knees e. engage in regular aerobic exercise (e.g., swimming, walking, bicycling) f. elevate legs periodically, especially when sitting

g. dorsiflex feet regularly
h. maintain an ideal body weight for age, height, and body frame.
2. Inform client that smoking and the use of estrogen or oral contraceptives can increase the risk for recurrent thrombus formation.

5.b. The client will verbalize an understanding of medications ordered including rationale, food and drug interactions, side effects, schedule for taking, and importance of taking as prescribed.	5.b.1. Explain the rationale for, side effects of, and importance of taking medications prescribed. 2. If client is discharged on warfarin (e.g., Coumadin), instruct to: a. keep scheduled appointments for periodic blood studies to monitor coagulation times b. take medication at the same time each day, do not stop taking medication abruptly, and do not attempt to make up for missed doses c. avoid regular and/or excessive intake of alcohol (may alter responsiveness to warfarin) d. avoid significantly increasing or decreasing consumption of foods high in vitamin K (e.g., green leafy vegetables) e. report prolonged or excessive bleeding from skin, nose, or mouth; red, rust-colored, or smoky urine; bloody or tarry stools; blood in vomitus or sputum; prolonged or excessive menses; excessive bruising; severe or persistent headache; or sudden abdominal or back pain f. inform physician immediately if pregnancy is suspected or if breastfeeding (warfarin crosses the placental barrier and enters the breast milk) g. wear a medical alert bracelet or tag identifying self as being on anticoagulant therapy h. inform physician of any other medications being taken because there are a number of medications that affect the anticoagulant activity of warfarin (e.g., NSAIDs, various antimicrobials, phenytoin) i. notify health care provider immediately of any sudden changes in the skin, such as bruised, darkened, or painful areas (warfarin can cause necrosis of the skin). 3. Instruct client to inform all health care providers of medications being taken.
5.c. The client will demonstrate the ability to correctly draw up and administer heparin subcutaneously if prescribed.	5.c.1. If client is to be discharged on subcutaneous heparin, provide instructions on subcutaneous injection technique. 2. Allow time for questions, practice, and return demonstration.
5.d. The client will identify precautions necessary to prevent bleeding associated with anticoagulant therapy.	5.d.1. Instruct client about ways to minimize risk of bleeding: a. use an electric rather than straight-edge razor b. floss and brush teeth gently; use waxed floss and a soft bristle toothbrush c. avoid putting sharp objects (e.g., toothpicks) in mouth d. do not walk barefoot e. cut nails carefully f. avoid situations that could result in injury (e.g., contact sports) g. avoid blowing nose forcefully h. avoid straining to have a bowel movement. 2. Instruct client to control any bleeding by applying firm, prolonged pressure to the area if possible.
5.e. The client will state signs and symptoms to report to the health care provider.	5.e. Instruct client to report: 1. recurrent tenderness, pain, distention of superficial veins, or swelling in extremity 2. sudden chest pain accompanied by shortness of breath 3. unusual bleeding (see action b.2.e in this diagnosis) 4. discoloration or itching of affected extremity (indicative of stasis dermatitis associated with chronic venous insufficiency) 5. skin breakdown on affected extremity.

Desired Outcomes	**Nursing Actions** *and Selected Purposes/Rationales*
5.f. The client will verbalize an understanding of and a plan for adhering to recommended follow-up care including future appointments with health care provider and activity level.	5.f.1. Reinforce importance of keeping follow-up appointments with health care provider. 2. Reinforce physician's instructions regarding activity limitations. 3. Implement measures to improve client compliance: a. include significant others in teaching sessions if possible b. encourage questions and allow time for reinforcement and clarification of information provided c. provide written instructions regarding future appointments with health care provider, medications prescribed, activity restrictions, signs and symptoms to report, and future laboratory studies.

Bibliography

See pages 879 and 882.

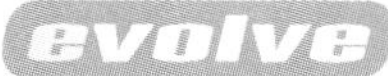

Femoropopliteal Bypass

Lower extremity arterial bypass is performed to treat peripheral artery insufficiency that has not responded well to conservative management. The impaired blood flow can occur as a result of acute conditions (e.g., trauma, embolization) but most often is caused by atherosclerotic changes in the vessels. The femoropopliteal arterial segment is the most common site of occlusion in persons with lower extremity arterial disease. Surgical intervention is usually indicated when the client experiences signs and symptoms of severe occlusion (e.g., intermittent claudication that has become disabling, foot pain that is present at rest, presence of lower extremity ischemic ulcers) and/or when more conservative invasive treatment measures such as balloon angioplasty, laser angioplasty, stent placement, or percutaneous atherectomy have been unsuccessful.

Surgical treatment of the diseased femoropopliteal arterial segment can be accomplished by endarterectomy or removal of the segment and replacement with a synthetic graft, but the most commonly performed procedure is to bypass the segment using a synthetic or an autogenous vein graft. The saphenous vein is the preferred autogenous graft for femoropopliteal bypass because it is thick walled and has an adequate lumen diameter. Prior to grafting the saphenous vein proximal and distal to the occluded arterial segment, reversal of the vein or division of its valve cusps is done to allow unimpeded arterial blood flow.

This care plan focuses on the adult client with atherosclerotic occlusion of the femoropopliteal arterial segment who is hospitalized for a femoropopliteal bypass. Much of the postoperative information is applicable to clients receiving follow-up care in an extended care facility or home setting.

OUTCOME/DISCHARGE CRITERIA

THE CLIENT WILL:

- have adequate circulation in the operative extremity
- have surgical pain controlled
- tolerate expected level of activity
- have evidence of normal wound healing
- have no signs and symptoms of postoperative complications
- identify ways to prevent or slow the progression of atherosclerosis
- identify ways to promote blood flow in the operative extremity
- state signs and symptoms to report to the health care provider
- verbalize an understanding of and a plan for adhering to recommended follow-up care including future appointments with health care provider, medications prescribed, activity level, and wound care.

NURSING/COLLABORATIVE DIAGNOSES

Preoperative

1. Ineffective tissue perfusion: peripheral p. 418
2. Acute/Chronic pain: intermittent claudication and rest pain p. 418

Postoperative

1. Ineffective tissue perfusion: peripheral p. 419
2. Potential complications p. 420
   a. graft occlusion
   b. compartment syndrome
   c. saphenous nerve damage

DISCHARGE TEACHING

3. Deficient knowledge, Ineffective therapeutic regimen management, or Ineffective health maintenance p. 422

See Standardized Preoperative and Postoperative Care Plans (pp. 97–126) for additional diagnoses.

PREOPERATIVE

Use in conjunction with the Standardized Preoperative Care Plan.

1. Nursing Diagnosis: *INEFFECTIVE TISSUE PERFUSION: PERIPHERAL*

related to diminished blood flow in the affected lower extremity associated with:
a. atherosclerotic changes in the femoral and popliteal arteries;
b. thrombus formation in the affected vessel.

Suggested NOC Outcome: Tissue perfusion: peripheral

Suggested NIC Interventions: Circulatory care: arterial insufficiency; Circulatory care: venous insufficiency; Lower extremity monitoring

Desired Outcome	**Nursing Actions** *and Selected Purposes/Rationales* (see pp. 57–59 for additional rationales)
1. The client will not experience further reduction in arterial blood flow in the affected lower extremity as evidenced by: a. no increase in lower extremity pain b. no further decrease in peripheral pulses c. no increase in capillary refill time d. usual temperature and color of extremity.	1.a. Assess for signs and symptoms of a further reduction in arterial blood flow in the affected lower extremity: 1. intermittent claudication occurring with increased intensity and/or with less activity than previously 2. development of or increase in intensity of rest pain (the foot and toe pain that occurs when the client is in a horizontal position results from decreased blood flow to the skin and subcutaneous tissue; because it occurs in the absence of lower extremity muscle activity, it reflects a severe reduction in the femoropopliteal arterial blood flow) 3. diminishing peripheral pulses 4. increase in usual capillary refill time 5. increased coolness and numbness of foot and lower leg 6. increased pallor or blanching of foot and lower leg when extremity is elevated 7. more rapid appearance of rubor or cyanosis in foot and lower leg when extremity is in a dependent position. b. Implement measures *to prevent further reduction in and/or improve blood flow in the affected lower extremity:* 1. discourage positions that compromise blood flow in lower extremities (e.g., crossing legs, pillows under knees, use of knee gatch, elevating legs when in bed, sitting for long periods) 2. perform actions *to prevent vasoconstriction:* a. implement measures *to reduce stress* (e.g., maintain a calm environment, control pain, explain preoperative and postoperative care) b. discourage smoking c. implement measures *to keep client from getting cold* (e.g., maintain a comfortable room temperature; provide adequate clothing, warm socks, and blankets) 3. encourage short walks unless contraindicated 4. administer the following medications if ordered: a. a hemorrheologic agent (e.g., pentoxifylline) *to improve the flow of blood to the ischemic area* b. anticoagulants (e.g., heparin, fondaparinux, warfarin) or antiplatelet agent (e.g., cilostazol, ticlopidine, clopidogrel) *to prevent or treat thrombi.* c. Consult physician if signs and symptoms of further reduction in lower extremity tissue perfusion occur.

2. Nursing Diagnosis: *ACUTE/CHRONIC PAIN: INTERMITTENT CLAUDICATION AND REST PAIN*

related to diminished arterial blood flow in the affected lower extremity (ischemia results in the release of anaerobic metabolites that irritate the nerve endings of the affected lower extremity).

Suggested NOC Outcomes: Comfort level; Pain control

Suggested NIC Intervention: Pain management

Desired Outcome	**Nursing Actions** *and Selected Purposes/Rationales* (see pp. 45–47 for additional rationales)
2. The client will experience diminished lower extremity pain as evidenced by: a. verbalization of same b. relaxed facial expression and body positioning.	2.a. Assess for signs and symptoms of pain in the affected lower extremity: 1. intermittent claudication (e.g., verbalization of pain, aching, and/or cramping [usually in the calf muscle] during ambulation) 2. rest pain (e.g., awakening at night with reports of severe burning or aching in foot or toes) 3. grimacing, restlessness, reluctance to move, and/or rubbing leg or foot. b. Assess client's perception of the severity of pain using a pain intensity rating scale. c. Assess the client's pain pattern (e.g., location, quality, onset, duration, precipitating factors, aggravating factors, alleviating factors). d. Implement measures *to reduce pain in the affected extremity:* 1. perform actions to prevent further reduction in and/or improve blood flow in the affected lower extremity (see Preoperative Diagnosis 1, action b) 2. perform actions *to reduce fear and anxiety about the pain experience* (e.g., assure client that his/her need for pain relief is understood, plan methods for achieving pain control with client) 3. perform actions *to reduce the number of episodes of intermittent claudication:* a. encourage client to stop activity minutes before symptoms are usually experienced (intermittent claudication is predictable and the client is often aware of how far or how long he/she can ambulate before the discomfort begins or intensifies) b. maintain client on bed rest if experiencing severe intermittent claudication *(limiting activity decreases muscle contractions in and subsequent ischemia of the affected lower extremity)* 4. if client is experiencing rest pain in the affected extremity, perform actions *to facilitate gravity flow of arterial blood to the ischemic area:* a. allow client to sleep in a recliner with legs in a dependent position or, if in bed, to hang affected lower leg over the side of bed b. instruct client to avoid horizontal positioning and elevation of affected extremity for prolonged periods 5. provide lightweight blankets or a foot cradle if external pressure aggravates lower extremity pain 6. provide or assist with nonpharmacologic measures for relief of pain (e.g., relaxation techniques; position change; diversional activities such as conversing, watching television, or reading) 7. administer analgesics if ordered. e. Consult physician if above measures fail to provide adequate pain relief.

POSTOPERATIVE

Use in conjunction with the Standardized Postoperative Care Plan

1. NURSING DIAGNOSIS: ***INEFFECTIVE TISSUE PERFUSION: PERIPHERAL***

related to diminished blood flow in the operative extremity associated with:

a. inflammation of the femoral and popliteal arteries at the sites of graft anastomosis;
b. pressure on vessels in the operative extremity resulting from edema that can occur as a result of decreased venous return and dissection of tissue around perivascular lymphatics;
c. venous stasis resulting from decreased mobility and decreased venous return if the saphenous vein was used for the bypass graft (can result in impaired venous return until collateral venous circulation improves);
d. graft occlusion;

e. hypovolemia resulting from blood loss during surgery and decreased fluid intake.

Suggested NOC Outcome: Tissue perfusion: peripheral

Suggested NIC Interventions: Circulatory care: arterial insufficiency; Circulatory care: venous insufficiency; Lower extremity monitoring

Desired Outcome

1. The client will maintain adequate tissue perfusion in the operative extremity as evidenced by:
   a. resolution of leg and foot pain
   b. palpable peripheral pulses
   c. adequate Doppler flow readings in operative extremity
   d. absence of coolness, numbness, and cyanosis in foot and lower leg
   e. resolution of edema in operative extremity
   f. capillary refill time less than 2–3 seconds.

Nursing Actions *and Selected Purposes/Rationales*

(see pp. 57–59 for additional rationales)

1.a. Assess for and report signs and symptoms of ineffective tissue perfusion in operative extremity:
   1. pain unrelieved by prescribed analgesics
   2. diminished or absent pulses (the pulses may be difficult to palpate for 4–12 hours after surgery *because of vasospasm that can occur in the operative extremity*)
   3. diminished or absent Doppler flow readings over operative extremity
   4. coolness, numbness, or cyanosis of foot and lower leg
   5. increase in edema in the operative extremity
   6. capillary refill time greater than 2–3 seconds.

b. Implement measures *to promote adequate tissue perfusion in operative extremity:*
   1. avoid 90° flexion of the hip as much as possible (e.g., place client in high Fowler's position for meals only, limit length of time that client is in straight-back chair, provide recliner for client's use when sitting up)
   2. limit length of time that operative leg is in dependent position (e.g., allow client to sit up for meals only; encourage short, frequent walks rather than long walks)
   3. instruct client to keep knee in a neutral or slightly flexed position
   4. perform actions to prevent graft occlusion (see Postoperative Diagnosis 2, action a.2)
   5. if lower extremity edema is present, elevate foot of bed 15° as ordered *to promote venous return without compromising arterial flow*
   6. place a bed cradle over lower extremities *to minimize pressure from bed linens*
   7. instruct client to perform active foot and leg exercises every 1–2 hours while awake
   8. perform actions *to prevent vasoconstriction:*
      a. implement measures *to reduce stress* (e.g., control pain, maintain a calm environment, explain postoperative care)
      b. discourage smoking
      c. implement measures *to keep client from getting cold* (e.g., maintain a comfortable room temperature; provide adequate clothing, warm socks, and blankets)
   9. maintain a minimum fluid intake of 2500 ml/day unless contraindicated; if oral intake is inadequate or contraindicated, maintain intravenous fluid therapy as ordered
   10. administer blood and blood products as ordered.

c. Consult physician if signs and symptoms of diminished tissue perfusion in the operative extremity persist or worsen.

2. Collaborative Diagnoses: ***POTENTIAL COMPLICATIONS OF FEMOROPOPLITEAL BYPASS***

a. graft occlusion related to thrombus formation, kink in graft, inadequate vessel lumen diameter at sites of anastomosis, or dislodgment of surgical site debris;
b. compartment syndrome related to severe edema of the operative extremity (an infrequent but serious complication that can occur as a result of surgical site inflammation, reperfusion of the ischemic muscles, or dissection of tissue around the perivascular lymphatics);
c. saphenous nerve damage related to:
   1. inadvertent or unavoidable dissection of the nerve during surgery
   2. trauma to the nerve during surgery.

Desired Outcomes	**Nursing Actions** *and Selected Purposes/Rationales*
2.a. The client will maintain a patent graft in the operative extremity as evidenced by: 1. no reports of sudden, severe toe or foot pain 2. palpable peripheral pulses 3. capillary refill time less than 2–3 seconds 4. absence of cyanosis, coolness, and diminishing sensation in the foot.	2.a.1. Assess for and report signs and symptoms of graft occlusion in the operative extremity (e.g., sudden, severe pain in toes or foot; diminishing or absent peripheral pulses; capillary refill time greater than 2–3 seconds; cyanosis, coolness, or diminished sensation in the foot). 2. Implement measures *to prevent graft occlusion:* a. avoid prolonged flexion of the knee on the operative extremity (e.g., limit sitting as ordered, do not place pillows under knees when in bed) *to prevent kinking of graft* b. perform actions *to reduce the risk of thrombus formation:* 1. implement measures to promote adequate tissue perfusion in operative extremity (see Postoperative Diagnosis 1, action b) 2. administer anticoagulants (e.g., warfarin, low- or adjusted-dose heparin, low-molecular-weight heparin) if ordered. 3. If signs and symptoms of graft occlusion occur: a. maintain client on bed rest with operative leg in a level or slightly dependent position *to improve arterial blood flow* b. administer anticoagulants (e.g., heparin, warfarin) as ordered c. prepare client for surgical intervention (e.g., removal of debris or thrombus, straightening of graft, widening of lumen at site[s] of anastomosis) if planned.
2.b. The client will not experience compartment syndrome in the operative extremity as evidenced by: 1. no complaints of increasing leg pain 2. no statements of new or increasing numbness and tingling in foot or leg or tightness and tenseness of thigh or calf muscle 3. ability to move leg and foot 4. no decrease in or absence of peripheral pulses 5. absence of cyanosis and coldness of leg and foot.	2.b.1. Assess for and report signs and symptoms of compartment syndrome in the operative extremity: a. complaints of increasing leg pain b. statements of new or increasing numbness and tingling in foot or leg or tightness and tenseness of thigh or calf muscle c. difficulty moving foot d. diminishing or absent peripheral pulses e. cyanotic, cold foot and leg. 2. Implement measures *to prevent an increase in edema in operative leg in order to reduce the risk of development of compartment syndrome:* a. limit length of time that operative leg is in a dependent position (e.g., limit sitting and walking as ordered) b. elevate operative extremity 15° if ordered c. administer osmotic diuretics (e.g., mannitol) if ordered. 3. If signs and symptoms of compartment syndrome occur: a. maintain client on bed rest b. assess for and report reddish-brown discoloration of urine *(this could indicate myoglobinuria resulting from the release of myoglobin from the damaged muscle cells; if an excessive amount of myoglobin is released, it can get trapped in the renal tubules and cause renal failure)* c. prepare client for a fasciotomy if planned.
2.c. The client will have resolution of or adapt to operative extremity saphenous nerve damage if it has occurred.	2.c.1. Assess for and report signs and symptoms of saphenous nerve damage (e.g., numbness, tingling, or hypersensitivity of the operative extremity). 2. If signs and symptoms of saphenous nerve damage are present: a. adhere to and instruct client in the following safety precautions: 1. wear shoes or slippers whenever out of bed 2. do not apply heat or cold to the affected extremity 3. test temperature of bath water before use 4. protect operative extremity from trauma b. reinforce information from physician regarding permanence of numbness, tingling, or hypersensitivity (these symptoms are permanent if the nerve was severed during surgery; if the nerve was just traumatized, the symptoms are temporary and expected to resolve within 1 year) c. consult physician if signs and symptoms increase in severity.

Discharge Teaching/Continued Care

3. Nursing Diagnosis: ***DEFICIENT KNOWLEDGE, INEFFECTIVE THERAPEUTIC REGIMEN MANAGEMENT, OR INEFFECTIVE HEALTH MAINTENANCE****

*The nurse should select the diagnostic label that is most appropriate for the client's discharge teaching needs.

Suggested NOC Outcomes: Knowledge: treatment regimen; Knowledge: cardiac disease management

Suggested NIC Interventions: Health system guidance; Teaching: individual; Teaching: disease process; Teaching: prescribed diet; Teaching: prescribed activity/exercise

Desired Outcomes	**Nursing Actions** *and Selected Purposes/Rationales*
3.a. The client will identify ways to prevent or slow the progression of atherosclerosis.	3.a.1. Inform the client that certain modifiable factors such as elevated serum lipids, a sedentary lifestyle, smoking, and hypertension have been shown to increase the risk of atherosclerosis. 2. Assist client to identify changes in lifestyle that could reduce the risk for atherosclerosis (e.g., smoking cessation, dietary modifications, physical exercise on a regular basis). 3. Provide instructions on ways the client can reduce intake of saturated fat and cholesterol: a. reduce intake of meat fat (e.g., trim visible fat off meat; replace fatty meats such as fatty cuts of steak, hamburger, and processed meats with leaner products) b. reduce intake of milk fat (avoid dairy products containing more than 1% fat) c. reduce intake of *trans* fats (e.g., avoid stick margarine and shortening and foods such as commercial baked goods that are prepared with these products) d. use vegetable oil rather than coconut or palm oil in cooking and food preparation e. use cooking methods such as steaming, baking, broiling, poaching, microwaving, and grilling rather than frying f. restrict intake of eggs (recommendations about the number of whole eggs allowed per week vary depending on the client's lipid levels). 4. Instruct client to take lipid-lowering agents (e.g., HMG-CoA reductase inhibitor ["statins"], ezetimibe, gemfibrozil, niacin) as prescribed.
3.b. The client will identify ways to promote blood flow in the operative extremity.	3.b. Provide the following instructions about ways to promote blood flow in the operative extremity: 1. avoid wearing constrictive clothing (e.g., garters, girdles, narrow-banded knee-high stockings) 2. avoid positions that compromise blood flow (e.g., pillows under knees, crossing legs, sitting or standing for prolonged periods) 3. do active foot and leg exercises for 5 minutes every hour while awake 4. maintain a regular exercise program (walking and swimming are recommended) 5. stop smoking 6. drink at least 10 glasses of liquid/day unless contraindicated.
3.c. The client will state signs and symptoms to report to the health care provider.	3.c.1. Refer to Standardized Postoperative Care Plan, Diagnosis 22, action c (p. 125), for signs and symptoms to report to the health care provider. 2. Instruct client to report these additional signs and symptoms: a. sudden or gradual increase in operative leg or foot pain b. increased swelling or purple discoloration at incision sites c. pallor, coldness, or bluish color of the operative extremity

d. diminishing or sudden absence of peripheral pulses (client may be instructed to monitor his/her peripheral pulses)
e. significant increase in swelling of operative extremity (edema is expected to resolve gradually within the first 2–8 weeks following surgery)
f. difficulty moving foot on operative side
g. increasing numbness and/or tingling sensation of operative lower leg or foot
h. any area of persistent skin irritation or breakdown of foot on operative side.

3.d. The client will verbalize an understanding of and a plan for adhering to recommended follow-up care including future appointments with health care provider, medications prescribed, activity level, and wound care.

3.d.1. Refer to Standardized Postoperative Care Plan, Diagnosis 22 (pp. 125–126), for routine postoperative instructions and measures to improve client compliance.
2. Reinforce the physician's instructions regarding:
a. importance of scheduling adequate rest periods
b. need to avoid sitting or standing for long periods
c. the need to take prophylactic antimicrobials prior to any dental work or invasive procedure (some physicians recommend this for the first 6–12 months following surgical placement of a synthetic graft).

Bibliography

See pages 879 and 882.

UNIT XI

Nursing Care of the Client with Disturbances of Respiratory Function

Cancer of the Lung

Cancer of the lung, a malignant neoplasm involving lung tissue, is the leading cause of cancer-related deaths in the United States today. The major risk factor in the development of lung cancer is cigarette smoking. Other risk factors include environmental pollution; exposure to carcinogens such as asbestos, radon, arsenic, nickel, iron oxide, chromium, and chloromethyl ether; genetic predisposition; and chronic inflammatory lung conditions (e.g., tuberculosis, bronchiectasis, COPD).

Cancer of the lung can occur as a primary tumor or as a metastasis from a site elsewhere in the body. The majority of primary lung neoplasms fall into one of 4 histological types. The types are small cell (oat cell) lung cancer (SCLC) and three non-small cell types of lung cancer (NSCLC), which include squamous cell (epidermoid) carcinoma, adenocarcinoma, and large cell cancer. These four types vary in relation to where they arise in the lung, responsiveness to the major modes of treatment, pattern of spread, clinical course, and prognosis. Squamous cell carcinoma and adenocarcinoma are the most common types. Squamous cell carcinoma is almost always associated with smoking, usually originates in the central airways, produces early symptoms of local disease because of bronchial obstruction, and generally spreads by direct extension to surrounding tissue. Adenocarcinoma occurs most frequently in the periphery of the lungs, has a slow growth rate, tends to invade the pleura, typically does not produce symptoms until late in the course of the disease, and occurs more frequently in women and nonsmokers. Large cell tumors usually arise in the peripheral area of the lung, grow rapidly, and metastasize early. Small cell lung carcinoma tends to originate in the central portion of the lung and grow rapidly. It has usually metastasized at the time of diagnosis, is the type most frequently associated with paraneoplastic syndromes, and has a very poor prognosis.

The treatment selected depends on the tumor type(s), presence and extent of metastasis, and the client's health status. Surgery is performed to resect the tumor if feasible. Other curative or palliative treatment options that may be performed include chemotherapy, radiation therapy, bronchoscopic laser therapy, phototherapy, and cryotherapy.

The signs and symptoms of cancer of the lung are a result of a variety of factors including the presence of the tumor in the lung, extension of the tumor into the thoracic cavity, metastasis, and paraneoplastic conditions that are associated with the primary tumor. The local manifestations can include dyspnea, cough or change in character of an established cough, change in amount and character of sputum produced (hemoptysis is often present), wheezing, and chest pain. Systemic manifestations of lung cancer include anorexia, weight loss, weakness, and fatigue. If the tumor has extended into the thoracic cavity, signs and symptoms are those resulting from conditions such as pleural effusion, lung abscess, superior vena cava syndrome, and involvement of segments of the cervical and thoracic nerves. The signs and symptoms of metastasis vary depending on the area affected. Common sites of metastasis are the lymph nodes, liver, adrenal glands, brain, bones, and kidneys. Nonmetastatic manifestations (referred to as paraneoplastic syndromes) include metabolic conditions such as Cushing's syndrome, syndrome of inappropriate antidiuretic hormone (SIADH), and hypercalcemia and neuromuscular conditions such as myasthenic (Lambert-Eaton) syndrome. These syndromes may predate x-ray evidence of lung cancer by many months.

This care plan focuses on care of the adult client with cancer of the lung hospitalized either for staging and initiation of treatment or for management of complications that have developed as a result of the disease process or its treatment. Much of the information presented here is also applicable to clients receiving follow-up care in a cancer treatment center, extended care facility, and home setting. If appropriate, this care plan should be used in conjunction with the Care Plans on Chemotherapy, External Radiation Therapy, and/or Thoracic Surgery.

OUTCOME/DISCHARGE CRITERIA

THE CLIENT WILL:

- have an adequate respiratory status
- have no signs and symptoms of complications
- have an adequate or improving nutritional status
- have pain controlled
- tolerate expected level of activity
- identify ways to improve oxygenation status and maximize pulmonary health
- demonstrate proper chest physiotherapy techniques and the ability to use the equipment recommended to maximize pulmonary health
- identify precautions that should be adhered to when using oxygen
- verbalize ways to improve appetite and nutritional status
- verbalize ways to manage chronic syndrome of inappropriate antidiuretic hormone (SIADH) if present
- state signs and symptoms to report to the health care provider
- share thoughts and feelings about the diagnosis of lung cancer, the prognosis, and the effects of the disease process and its treatment on self-concept, lifestyle, and roles

- identify community resources that can assist with home management and adjustment to the diagnosis and the effects of treatment
- verbalize an understanding of and a plan for adhering to recommended follow-up care including future appointments with health care provider, medications prescribed, activity level, and plans for subsequent treatment.

Use in conjunction with the Care Plans on Chemotherapy, External Radiation Therapy, and Thoracic Surgery if appropriate.

NURSING/COLLABORATIVE DIAGNOSES

DISCHARGE TEACHING

See pp. 441–442 and Care Plans on Chemotherapy and External Radiation Therapy (pp. 169–221) for additional diagnoses.

1. NURSING DIAGNOSIS: FEAR/ANXIETY

related to current signs and symptoms; lack of understanding of the diagnosis, diagnostic tests, and treatment plan; unfamiliar environment; financial concerns; anticipated effects of cancer and its treatment on body functioning and usual lifestyle and roles; and probability of premature death.

Suggested NOC Outcomes: Anxiety level; Fear level; Anxiety self-control; Fear self-control

Suggested NIC Interventions: Anxiety reduction; Calming technique; Emotional support; Presence; Financial resource assistance; Teaching: procedure/treatment

Desired Outcome	**Nursing Actions** *and Selected Purposes/Rationales* (see pp. 14–16 for additional rationales)
1. The client will experience a reduction in fear and anxiety as evidenced by: a. verbalization of feeling less anxious b. usual sleep pattern c. relaxed facial expression and body movements d. stable vital signs e. usual perceptual ability and interactions with others.	1.a. Assess client on admission for: 1. fears, misconceptions, and level of understanding about lung cancer, tests to stage the disease, and possible treatment modes 2. perception of anticipated results of diagnostic tests and planned treatment 3. significance of the diagnosis of lung cancer to client 4. availability of an adequate support system 5. past experiences with cancer and its treatment 6. signs and symptoms of fear and anxiety (e.g., verbalization of feeling anxious, insomnia, tenseness, shakiness, restlessness, diaphoresis, tachycardia, elevated blood pressure, self-focused behaviors). b. Refer to Diagnosis 1, action b (p. 171), in Care Plan on Chemotherapy and Diagnosis 2, action b (pp. 198–199) in Care Plan on External Radiation Therapy for measures to reduce fear and anxiety associated with the diagnosis and planned treatment. c. Implement additional measures *to reduce fear and anxiety:* 1. explain all diagnostic tests performed to stage lung cancer 2. perform actions to reduce pain (see Diagnosis 4) 3. perform actions to improve respiratory status (see Diagnosis 2, action b) *in order to reduce dyspnea* 4. if client is experiencing hemoptysis, explain that the amount of blood in sputum does not necessarily correlate with severity of the disease; provide an opaque, covered container for sputum collection *to reduce anxiety resulting from seeing the blood.* d. Consult appropriate health care provider (e.g., oncology nurse specialist, psychiatric nurse clinician, physician) if above actions fail to control fear and anxiety.

2. NURSING DIAGNOSIS: *IMPAIRED RESPIRATORY FUNCTION**

a. ineffective breathing pattern related to:
   1. increased rate of respirations associated with fear and anxiety
   2. decreased rate of respirations associated with the depressant effect of some medications (e.g., narcotic [opioid] analgesics)
   3. decreased depth of respirations associated with:
      a. decreased lung compliance (distensibility) resulting from pleural effusion (if present) and compression of lung tissue by the tumor
      b. weakness, fatigue, fear, anxiety, and reluctance to breathe deeply because of pain
      c. depressant effect of some medications (e.g., narcotic [opioid] analgesics)
      d. paralysis of the diaphragm on involved side (can occur if the tumor has invaded the phrenic nerve);

b. ineffective airway clearance related to:
   1. excessive mucus production associated with inflammation of lung tissue resulting from the disease process
   2. stasis of secretions associated with:
      a. difficulty coughing up secretions resulting from the depressant effect of some medications (e.g., narcotic [opioid] analgesics), pain, weakness, fatigue, and presence of tenacious secretions (can occur if fluid intake is inadequate)
      b. impaired ciliary function resulting from the disease process
      c. decreased mobility
   3. invasion of and/or pressure on airways by tumor;

c. impaired gas exchange related to decrease in effective lung surface associated with replacement of lung tissue by neoplastic cells, accumulation of secretions, and/or atelectasis.

---

*This diagnostic label includes the following nursing diagnoses: ineffective breathing pattern, ineffective airway clearance, and impaired gas exchange.

Suggested NOC Outcomes: Respiratory status: airway patency; Respiratory status: ventilation; Respiratory status: gas exchange

Suggested NIC Interventions: Respiratory monitoring; Airway management; Chest physiotherapy; Cough enhancement; Oxygen therapy; Ventilation assistance; Medication administration

Desired Outcome	Nursing Actions *and Selected Purposes/Rationales* (see pp. 12–14, 18–20, and 33–35 for additional rationales)
2. The client will experience adequate respiratory function as evidenced by: a. normal rate and depth of respirations b. decreased dyspnea c. usual or improved breath sounds d. usual mental status e. oximetry results within normal range for client f. blood gases within normal range.	2.a. Assess for and report: 1. signs and symptoms of impaired respiratory function: a. rapid, shallow, or slow respirations b. dyspnea, orthopnea c. use of accessory muscles when breathing d. abnormal breath sounds (e.g., diminished or absent, rhonchi, crackles [rales], wheezes) e. asymmetrical or limited chest excursion f. cough g. restlessness, irritability h. confusion, somnolence i. significant decrease in oximetry results j. abnormal blood gas values 2. significant abnormalities in chest x-ray reports 3. pulmonary function study results that worsen or fail to improve after treatment begins. b. Implement measures *to improve respiratory status:* 1. place client in a semi- to high Fowler's position unless contraindicated; position overbed table so client can lean on it if desired 2. perform actions to reduce fear and anxiety (see Diagnosis 1, actions b and c) *in order to prevent the shallow and/or rapid breathing that can occur with fear and anxiety* 3. perform actions to reduce pain (see Diagnosis 4) *in order to increase the client's willingness to move, cough, and deep breathe* 4. perform actions to reduce fatigue (see Diagnosis 6) *in order to increase client's willingness and ability to move, cough, deep breathe, and use incentive spirometer* 5. instruct client to breathe slowly if hyperventilating 6. maintain oxygen therapy as ordered 7. if client must remain flat in bed, assist with position change at least every 2 hours 8. instruct client to deep breathe or use incentive spirometer every 1–2 hours 9. assist with positive airway pressure techniques (e.g., continuous positive airway pressure [CPAP], bilevel positive airway pressure [BiPAP], flutter/positive expiratory pressure [PEP] device) if ordered 10. instruct client in and assist with diaphragmatic breathing if appropriate (may be necessary if the tumor has invaded the phrenic nerve) 11. perform actions *to promote removal of pulmonary secretions:* a. instruct and assist client to cough or "huff" every 1–2 hours b. implement measures *to thin tenacious secretions and reduce drying of the respiratory mucous membrane:* 1. maintain a fluid intake of 2500 ml/day unless contraindicated 2. humidify inspired air as ordered c. assist with administration of mucolytics (e.g., acetylcysteine) and diluent or hydrating agents (e.g., water, saline) via nebulizer if ordered d. assist with or perform postural drainage therapy (PDT) if ordered e. perform suctioning if needed f. administer expectorants (e.g., guaifenesin) if ordered 12. instruct client to avoid intake of gas-forming foods (e.g., beans, cauliflower, cabbage, onions), carbonated beverages, and large meals *in order to prevent gastric distention and subsequent pressure on the diaphragm*

13. discourage smoking *(the irritants in smoke increase mucus production, impair ciliary function, and can cause inflammation and damage to the bronchial and alveolar walls; the carbon monoxide decreases oxygen availability)*
14. maintain activity restrictions if ordered; increase activity as allowed and tolerated
15. administer central nervous system depressants judiciously; hold medication and consult physician if respiratory rate is less than 12/minute
16. administer the following medications if ordered:
    a. bronchodilators (e.g., methylxanthines, sympathomimetic [adrenergic] agents)
    b. corticosteroids *(may be given to decrease airway inflammation and thereby improve bronchial airflow)*
17. assist with thoracentesis if performed *to remove excessive pleural fluid and improve lung expansion*
18. prepare client for treatment of the malignancy (e.g., radiation therapy, chemotherapy, surgical resection of tumor) if planned *to reduce the tumor mass.*

c. Consult appropriate health care provider (e.g., respiratory therapist, physician) if signs and symptoms of impaired respiratory function persist or worsen.

3. NURSING DIAGNOSIS: ***IMBALANCED NUTRITION: LESS THAN BODY REQUIREMENTS***

related to:

a. decreased oral intake associated with:
    1. oral, pharyngeal, or esophageal pain (can be a side effect of cytotoxic drugs and/or radiation therapy)
    2. difficulty swallowing resulting from narrowing of the esophagus (can occur if the tumor has invaded or is compressing the esophagus)
    3. anorexia resulting from factors such as depression, fear, anxiety, fatigue, discomfort, dyspnea, early satiety, altered sense of taste and smell (often reported by persons with cancer), and increased levels of certain cytokines that depress appetite (e.g., interleukin-1, tumor necrosis factor)
    4. altered mental status (can result from hypoxia, imbalanced fluid and electrolytes, and metastasis to the brain);

b. loss of nutrients associated with vomiting and diarrhea (can occur as a result of administration of cytotoxic agents);

c. impaired utilization of nutrients associated with:
    1. accelerated and inefficient metabolism of proteins, carbohydrates, and fats resulting from factors such as increased levels of cortisol, glycogen, and certain cytokines (e.g., tumor necrosis factor, interleukin-1)
    2. decreased absorption of nutrients resulting from loss of intestinal absorptive surface if mucositis has developed as a result of the administration of cytotoxic agents;

d. utilization of available nutrients by the malignant cells rather than the host.

Suggested NOC Outcome: Nutritional status

Suggested NIC Interventions: Nutritional monitoring; Nutrition management; Nutrition therapy

Desired Outcome	**Nursing Actions** *and Selected Purposes/Rationales*
3. The client will have or attain an adequate nutritional status (see Care Plan on Chemotherapy, Diagnosis 2 [p. 172], for outcome criteria).	3.a. Refer to Care Plan on Chemotherapy, Diagnosis 2 (pp. 172–173), for measures related to assessment and maintenance or promotion of an adequate nutritional status. b. Implement additional measures *to increase oral intake and subsequently improve nutritional status:* 1. place client in a high Fowler's position for meals and provide supplemental oxygen therapy during meals if indicated *to help relieve dyspnea*

Desired Outcome	Nursing Actions *and Selected Purposes/Rationales*
	2. perform actions to reduce pain (see Diagnosis 4) 3. perform actions to prevent and/or treat conditions such as hypoxia, SIADH, and hypercalcemia (see Diagnoses 2, action b and 8, actions f.2 and g.2) *in order to help maintain adequate mental function.*

4. NURSING DIAGNOSIS: ACUTE/CHRONIC PAIN

a. tissue and skeletal pain related to pressure from the tumor and enlarged lymph nodes, nerve involvement, and metastasis to the bone or other organs if it has occurred;
b. chest pain related to:
   1. inflammation of the parietal pleura associated with extension of the primary tumor
   2. muscle strain associated with excessive coughing (if present)
   3. extension of the primary tumor into the chest wall;
c. pain within the irradiated area related to inflammation and exposure of nerve endings associated with moist desquamation if it occurs;
d. pharyngeal and esophageal pain related to inflammation and/or ulceration of the mucosa associated with the effects of radiation to upper chest and/or administration of cytotoxic drugs;
e. oral pain related to mucositis associated with the effects of cytotoxic drugs on the rapidly dividing cells of the oral mucosa.

Suggested NOC Outcomes: Pain control; Comfort level

Suggested NIC Interventions: Pain management; Environmental management: comfort; Analgesic administration; Patient-controlled analgesia (PCA) assistance

Desired Outcome	Nursing Actions *and Selected Purposes/Rationales*
4. The client will experience diminished pain (see Care Plan on External Radiation Therapy, Diagnosis 5 [pp. 201–202], for outcome criteria).	4.a. Refer to Care Plan on External Radiation Therapy, Diagnosis 5 (pp. 201–202), for measures related to assessment and management of pain. b. Implement additional measures *to reduce pain:* 1. perform actions *to reduce tissue and/or skeletal pain:* a. move client carefully; obtain adequate assistance when needed b. when turning client, logroll and support all extremities c. utilize smooth motions when moving client; avoid pushing or pulling on body parts d. caution client to avoid sudden twisting and turning e. administer the following medications as ordered: 1. narcotic (opioid) analgesics 2. nonnarcotic analgesics such as nonsteroidal anti-inflammatory agents f. encourage client to use patient-controlled analgesia (PCA) device as instructed g. prepare client for radiation therapy to painful skeletal areas if planned *to shrink metastatic tumor and reduce pressure on the bone* 2. perform actions *to reduce chest pain:* a. instruct and assist client to splint chest with hands or pillow when deep breathing, coughing, and changing position b. implement measures to control excessive coughing (see Diagnosis 6, action b.1) c. assist with an intercostal nerve block if performed *for intractable pain.*

5. NURSING DIAGNOSIS: IMPAIRED VERBAL COMMUNICATION

related to pressure on the recurrent laryngeal nerve (can occur if the tumor invades the mediastinum).

Suggested NOC Outcome: Communication

Suggested NIC Interventions: Communication enhancement: speech deficit; Active listening

Desired Outcome	Nursing Actions *and Selected Purposes/Rationales*
5. The client will successfully communicate needs and desires.	5.a. Assess client for impaired verbal communication (e.g., hoarseness, difficulty speaking). b. Implement measures *to facilitate communication:* 1. maintain a patient, calm approach; listen attentively and allow ample time for communication 2. maintain a quiet environment *so that client does not have to speak loudly* 3. ask questions that require short answers or nod of head if client is having difficulty speaking and/or is fatigued 4. provide materials such as Magic Slate, pad and pencil, and/or word cards if appropriate; try to ensure that placement of intravenous line does not interfere with client's use of these communication aids 5. answer call signal in person rather than using intercommunication system. c. Inform significant others and health care personnel of techniques being used to facilitate client's ability to communicate. d. Consult appropriate health care provider (e.g., speech pathologist, physician) if client experiences increasing impairment of verbal communication.

6. NURSING DIAGNOSIS: FATIGUE

related to*:

a. tissue hypoxia associated with impaired alveolar gas exchange and anemia (a result of malnutrition and chemotherapy-induced bone marrow suppression);
b. difficulty resting and sleeping associated with excessive coughing, dyspnea, pain, fear, anxiety, unfamiliar environment, and frequent assessments and treatments;
c. a build up of cellular waste products associated with rapid lysis of cancerous and normal cells exposed to radiation and/or cytotoxic drugs;
d. increased energy expenditure associated with strenuous breathing efforts, persistent coughing, and an increase in the metabolic rate (results from continuous, active tumor growth and increased levels of certain cytokines);
e. overwhelming emotional demands associated with the diagnosis of cancer and its treatment;
f. effects of medications used for control of pain, nausea, and anxiety.

*Some of the etiological factors presented here are under investigation.

Suggested NOC Outcomes: Endurance; Rest; Energy conservation; Psychomotor energy

Suggested NIC Interventions: Energy management; Oxygen therapy; Sleep enhancement; Nutrition management; Pain control; Mood management

Desired Outcome	Nursing Actions *and Selected Purposes/Rationales*
6. The client will experience a reduction in fatigue (see Care Plan on Chemotherapy, Diagnosis 6 [p. 177], for outcome criteria).	6.a. Refer to Care Plan on Chemotherapy, Diagnosis 6 (pp. 177–178), for measures related to assessment and management of fatigue. b. Implement additional measures *to reduce fatigue:* 1. perform actions *to control excessive coughing:* a. instruct client to avoid intake of extremely hot or cold foods/fluids *(these can stimulate cough)* b. protect client from exposure to irritants such as flowers, smoke, and powder

Desired Outcome	Nursing Actions *and Selected Purposes/Rationales*
	c. encourage client not to smoke *(smoke irritates the respiratory tract)* d. administer prescribed antitussives if indicated 2. perform actions to reduce pain (see Diagnosis 4) 3. if oxygen therapy is necessary during activity, keep portable oxygen equipment readily available for client's use 4. perform actions to promote an adequate nutritional status (see Diagnosis 3) 5. instruct client to avoid or limit talking while performing activities that also require energy (e.g., eating, walking, bathing) 6. perform actions to facilitate client's psychological adjustment to the diagnosis of cancer and the treatment regimen and its effects (see Diagnosis 1, actions b and c and Diagnosis 9).

7. NURSING DIAGNOSIS:

RISK FOR INFECTION

related to:

a. stasis of pulmonary secretions associated with airway obstruction, poor cough effort, and decreased activity;
b. lowered natural resistance associated with malnutrition, stress, and immunosuppressive effects of certain drugs (e.g., cytotoxic agents, corticosteroids);
c. break in skin integrity associated with radiation-induced desquamation (if it has occurred) and/or presence of a central venous catheter (may be inserted to administer chemotherapy or total parenteral nutrition);
d. break in mucosal surfaces associated with disrupted cellular renewal resulting from effects of cytotoxic drugs.

Suggested NOC Outcomes: Immune status; Infection severity

Suggested NIC Interventions: Infection protection; Infection control; Cough enhancement; Wound care

Desired Outcome	Nursing Actions *and Selected Purposes/Rationales*
7. The client will remain free of infection (see Care Plan on External Radiation Therapy, Diagnosis 12 [p. 209], for outcome criteria).	7.a. Refer to Care Plan on External Radiation Therapy, Diagnosis 12 (pp. 209–210), for measures related to assessment and prevention of infection. b. Implement additional measures *to reduce the risk for infection:* 1. perform actions to promote removal of pulmonary secretions (see Diagnosis 2, action b.11) *in order to prevent pneumonia* 2. perform actions to reduce stress and pain (see Diagnoses 1, actions b and c; 4; and 9) *in order to prevent an increase in the secretion of cortisol (cortisol interferes with some immune responses).*

8. COLLABORATIVE DIAGNOSES:

POTENTIAL COMPLICATIONS OF LUNG CANCER

a. atelectasis related to stasis of secretions in the alveoli and bronchioles, shallow respirations, and obstructed airflow associated with tumor involvement of major airways;
b. lung abscess related to necrosis of tissue within and around tumor;
c. pleural effusion related to:
   1. increased capillary permeability of pulmonary and pleural vessels associated with inflammation resulting from presence of malignant cells
   2. increased capillary hydrostatic pressure in the visceral pleura associated with obstruction of the pulmonary veins by the tumor
   3. impaired absorption of pleural fluid into the pleural lymphatic channels associated with lymph node obstruction resulting from the presence of a tumor
   4. increased colloid osmotic pressure in the pleural space associated with the presence of necrotic malignant cells;
d. superior vena cava syndrome (SVCS) related to obstruction of the superior vena cava associated with extrinsic pressure by the tumor or

enlarged paratracheal lymph nodes, intraluminal thrombosis, or invasion of the vein wall by tumor cells (occurs most frequently with a superior mediastinal mass);

e. spinal cord compression related to metastasis to the vertebrae and/or epidural space;

f. syndrome of inappropriate antidiuretic hormone (SIADH) related to:
   1. ectopic production and secretion of antidiuretic hormone (ADH) by tumor cells (occurs most frequently with SCLC)
   2. administration of some antineoplastic agents found to stimulate the release of ADH from the pituitary gland or tumor cells (e.g., cyclophosphamide, vincristine)
   3. stimulation of ADH output associated with pain and stress;

g. hypercalcemia related to:
   1. increased bone resorption associated with the release of substances such as parathyroid hormone-related protein (PTHrP) by tumor cells (particularly with squamous cell carcinoma), bone metastasis if present, decreased mobility, and side effect of some cytotoxic agents
   2. increased renal tubular reabsorption of calcium associated with the release of substances such as parathyroid hormone-related protein (PTHrP) by tumor cells (particularly with squamous cell carcinoma);

h. Cushing's syndrome related to ectopic adrenocorticotropic hormone (ACTH) production by tumor cells and/or metastatic lesions of the adrenal glands.

Desired Outcomes	**Nursing Actions** *and Selected Purposes/Rationales*
8.a. The client will not develop atelectasis as evidenced by: 1. audible breath sounds 2. resonant percussion note over lungs 3. no increase in dyspnea or respiratory rate 4. afebrile status.	8.a.1. Assess for and report signs and symptoms of atelectasis (e.g., diminished or absent breath sounds, dull percussion note over affected area, increased dyspnea or respiratory rate, elevated temperature, chest x-ray results showing atelectasis). 2. Implement measures to improve respiratory status (see Diagnosis 2, action b) *in order to prevent atelectasis.* 3. If signs and symptoms of atelectasis occur: a. increase frequency of position change, coughing or "huffing," deep breathing, and use of incentive spirometer b. increase activity as allowed and tolerated c. consult physician if signs and symptoms of atelectasis persist or worsen.
8.b. The client will have resolution of a lung abscess if it occurs as evidenced by: 1. absence of chills and fever 2. improved breath sounds and resonant percussion note over affected area 3. cough productive of clear mucus only 4. decreased chest pain.	8.b.1. Assess for and report signs and symptoms of a lung abscess (e.g., chills; fever; increased respiratory rate; diminished or absent breath sounds and dull percussion note over affected area; cough productive of purulent, foul-smelling sputum; increased chest pain; chest x-ray, computed tomography, or lung scan results showing lung abscess). 2. If signs and symptoms of a lung abscess occur: a. prepare client for surgical drainage of abscess if planned b. administer antimicrobials if ordered.
8.c. The client will experience resolution of pleural effusion if it occurs as evidenced by: 1. decreased dyspnea 2. symmetrical chest excursion 3. improved breath sounds and percussion note throughout lung fields.	8.c.1. Assess for and report signs and symptoms of pleural effusion (e.g., increased dyspnea; decreased chest excursion on affected side; diminished or absent breath sounds and dull percussion note over affected area; chest x-ray, ultrasound, or computed tomography results showing pleural effusion). 2. If signs and symptoms of pleural effusion occur: a. continue with actions to improve respiratory status (see Diagnosis 2, action b) b. prepare client for and assist with procedures to remove excess fluid from the pleural space (e.g., thoracentesis and/or insertion of chest tube)

Desired Outcomes	Nursing Actions *and Selected Purposes/Rationales*
	c. prepare client for the following if planned *to prevent recurrence of the pleural effusion:* 1. radiation therapy and/or chemotherapy *to treat the underlying malignancy* 2. procedures to obliterate the pleural space (e.g., pleurodesis, pleurectomy).
8.d. The client will experience a reduction in signs and symptoms of SVCS if it occurs as evidenced by: 1. decreased dyspnea 2. decreased edema of arms, neck, and face 3. decreased erythema of face, neck, and chest 4. absence of visual changes, headache, and vertigo.	8.d.1. Assess for and report signs and symptoms of SVCS (e.g., increased dyspnea; edema of arms, neck, or face; erythema of face, neck, or chest; distended neck veins; visual changes; headache; vertigo). 2. If signs and symptoms of SVCS occur: a. maintain client on bed rest with head of bed elevated b. prepare client for the following if planned: 1. diagnostic tests (e.g., chest x-ray, computed tomography, venography) 2. radiation therapy and/or chemotherapy *to shrink the obstructing tumor* 3. procedures such as superior vena cava bypass surgery, balloon angioplasty, or placement of intravascular stents if SVCS is caused by thrombosis or if symptoms are severe and have not been controlled by radiation therapy and/or chemotherapy c. administer the following medications if ordered: 1. corticosteroids (e.g., dexamethasone) *to decrease edema at the site of obstruction of superior vena cava* 2. diuretics *to reduce edema,* particularly if client is experiencing respiratory distress (diuretics provide only temporary relief and are used cautiously *because they can further decrease venous return)* 3. thrombolytic agents (e.g., streptokinase) if etiology is intraluminal thrombosis.
8.e. The client will experience a reduction in signs and symptoms of spinal cord compression if it occurs as evidenced by: 1. decreased back and neck pain 2. improved motor and sensory function 3. improved bowel and bladder control.	8.e.1. Assess for and report signs and symptoms of spinal cord compression (e.g., back or neck pain that may or may not radiate, progressive weakness, sensory deficits, loss of bowel and bladder control). Signs and symptoms manifested depend on which segment of the spinal cord is involved and extent of compression. 2. If signs and symptoms of spinal cord compression occur: a. prepare client for the following if planned: 1. diagnostic tests (e.g., computed tomography, magnetic resonance imaging) 2. radiation therapy *to reduce the size of the metastatic tumor* 3. surgical decompression and spine stabilization if neurological deterioration is rapid and relief is not achieved with radiation to affected area b. administer the following medications if ordered: 1. corticosteroids (e.g., dexamethasone) *to reduce edema at the site of metastasis* 2. analgesics *to reduce pain* c. initiate safety measures and assist client with activities of daily living as needed.
8.f. The client will experience resolution of SIADH if it develops as evidenced by: 1. decline in weight toward normal 2. balanced intake and output 3. usual mental status	8.f.1. Assess for and report signs and symptoms of SIADH: a. weight gain of 2% or greater over a short period b. intake greater than output c. lethargy, confusion d. reports of persistent headache e. muscle weakness f. fingerprint edema over sternum (indicative of cellular edema) g. abdominal cramping, nausea, vomiting h. seizures

4. absence of headache, muscle weakness, cellular edema, abdominal cramping, nausea, vomiting, and seizure activity
5. serum and urine sodium and osmolality levels within normal limits.

i. elevated urine sodium and osmolality levels
j. low serum sodium and osmolality levels.

2. If signs and symptoms of SIADH occur:
   a. maintain fluid restrictions if ordered *to prevent further fluid retention* (typically, this is a restriction of free water)
   b. implement measures *to prevent further ADH stimulation:*
      1. perform actions to reduce pain (see Diagnosis 4)
      2. perform actions to reduce fear and anxiety (see Diagnosis 1, actions b and c)
   c. encourage intake of foods/fluids high in sodium (e.g., cured meats, processed cheese, canned soups, catsup, dill pickles, tomato juice, canned vegetables, bouillon)
   d. initiate seizure precautions
   e. administer the following if ordered:
      1. diuretics (usually furosemide) *to promote water excretion*
      2. intravenous infusions of a hypertonic saline solution *to treat severe hyponatremia*
      3. demeclocycline *to promote water excretion (inhibits effect of ADH at the renal tubular level)*
   f. prepare client for treatment of the underlying malignancy if planned.

8.g. The client will maintain a safe serum calcium level as evidenced by:
1. usual mental status
2. usual muscle strength and tone and reflex responses
3. absence of nausea, vomiting, and anorexia
4. regular pulse at 60–100 beats/minute
5. serum calcium within normal range.

8.g.1. Assess for and report signs and symptoms of hypercalcemia (e.g., confusion, muscle weakness, depressed reflexes, nausea, vomiting, anorexia, constipation, polyuria, cardiac dysrhythmias, elevated serum calcium level).

2. Implement measures *to prevent or treat hypercalcemia:*
   a. prepare client for treatment of underlying malignancy
   b. consult physician prior to administering calcium-containing antacids (e.g., Tums, Titralac), vitamin D preparations, or thiazide diuretics *(these can all increase serum calcium levels)*
   c. encourage mobility as tolerated *(weight bearing reduces calcium loss from the bones)*
   d. maintain a minimum fluid intake of 2500 ml/day unless contraindicated *(hydrating the client lowers serum calcium by dilution)*
   e. administer the following if ordered:
      1. medications *to inhibit bone resorption* (e.g., calcitonin, zoledronic acid, pamidronate, gallium nitrate, plicamycin)
      2. loop diuretics (e.g., furosemide) *to increase renal excretion of calcium.*
3. Consult physician if serum calcium levels remain above a safe level.

8.h. The client will experience a reduction in signs and symptoms associated with Cushing's syndrome if it occurs as evidenced by:
1. increased muscle strength
2. resolution of edema
3. usual mental status
4. serum glucose, potassium, ACTH, and cortisol levels within normal range
5. normal urinary cortisol levels.

8.h.1. Assess for and report signs and symptoms of Cushing's syndrome (e.g., weakness, edema, hypertension, change in mental status, hyperglycemia, decreased serum potassium, high serum ACTH and cortisol levels, increased urinary cortisol level. Be aware that the signs and symptoms of Cushing's syndrome associated with lung cancer are usually minimal and do not include the more typical manifestations of glucocorticoid excess (e.g., weight gain, truncal obesity).

2. If signs and symptoms of Cushing's syndrome occur:
   a. ensure that precautions are taken to prevent infection *(the increased cortisol level lowers the client's natural resistance to infection)*
   b. administer the following if ordered:
      1. medications such as mitotane or aminoglutethimide *to inhibit adrenal cortisol synthesis*
      2. potassium supplements *to treat hypokalemia*
   c. prepare client for treatment of the malignancy if planned (e.g., radiation therapy, chemotherapy, bilateral adrenalectomy).

9. Nursing Diagnosis:

GRIEVING*

related to:
a. loss of normal function of the lung;
b. changes in body image and usual lifestyle and roles associated with the disease process and its treatment;
c. diagnosis of cancer with probability of premature death.

*This diagnostic label includes anticipatory grieving and grieving following the actual losses.

Suggested NOC Outcomes: Grief resolution; Psychosocial adjustment: life change

Suggested NIC Interventions: Grief work facilitation; Emotional support; Support system enhancement; Spiritual growth facilitation

Desired Outcome	Nursing Actions and Selected Purposes/Rationales
9. The client will demonstrate beginning progression through the grieving process (see Care Plan on Chemotherapy, Diagnosis 11 [p. 188], for outcome criteria).	9. Refer to Care Plan on Chemotherapy, Diagnosis 11 (p. 188), for measures related to assessment and facilitation of grieving.

Discharge Teaching/Continued Care

10. Nursing Diagnosis:

DEFICIENT KNOWLEDGE, INEFFECTIVE THERAPEUTIC REGIMEN MANAGEMENT, OR INEFFECTIVE HEALTH MAINTENANCE*

*The nurse should select the diagnostic label that is most appropriate for the client's discharge teaching needs.

Suggested NOC Outcomes: Knowledge: disease process; Knowledge: treatment regimen; Knowledge: treatment procedure(s); Knowledge: health resources

Suggested NIC Interventions: Health system guidance; Teaching: individual; Teaching: disease process; Teaching: prescribed diet; Teaching: psychomotor skill

Desired Outcomes	Nursing Actions and Selected Purposes/Rationales
10.a. The client will identify ways to improve oxygenation status and maximize pulmonary health.	10.a. Instruct client in ways to improve oxygenation status and maximize pulmonary health: 1. schedule adequate rest periods 2. avoid exposure to respiratory irritants such as smoke, dust, perfume, aerosol sprays, paint fumes, and solvents whenever possible; wear a mask or scarf over nose and mouth if exposure to high levels of irritants is unavoidable 3. stop smoking 4. avoid high altitudes; if air travel is required, consult physician about the need for supplemental oxygen 5. continue with prescribed chest physiotherapy (e.g., breathing exercises, postural drainage therapy) 6. use supplemental oxygen if prescribed 7. take medications such as bronchodilators and mucolytics as prescribed

8. minimize risk of respiratory tract infections:
   a. avoid contact with persons who have respiratory tract infections
   b. avoid crowds and poorly ventilated areas
   c. maintain good oral hygiene
   d. cleanse all respiratory care equipment properly
   e. drink at least 10 glasses of liquid/day unless contraindicated.

10.b. The client will demonstrate proper chest physiotherapy techniques and the ability to use the equipment recommended to maximize pulmonary health.

10.b.1. Reinforce instructions about proper breathing techniques (e.g., pursed-lip breathing, diaphragmatic breathing) and postural drainage therapy (PDT may be indicated if large amounts of mucus continue to be produced).
2. Reinforce instructions about use of respiratory equipment (e.g., oxygen, incentive spirometer, dry powder inhalers, metered-dose inhalers).
3. Allow time for questions, clarification, and return demonstration.

10.c. The client will identify precautions that should be adhered to when using oxygen.

10.c.1. Instruct client about precautions that should be adhered to when using oxygen:
   a. do not smoke
   b. do not set oxygen flow rate at a level higher than prescribed by physician
   c. do not allow the oxygen system to be within 10 feet of an open flame (e.g., gas stove, kerosene heater or lamp, fireplace, candle) or source of spark (e.g., electric razor, portable radio, wool blanket, hair dryer)
   d. post "No Smoking" signs in and around areas of oxygen use
   e. ensure that all electrical equipment in the area of the oxygen source is grounded
   f. always have a battery-operated oxygen delivery system readily available for use in case a power failure occurs.
2. Instruct client in ways to prevent skin and mucous membrane irritation and breakdown resulting from use of oxygen and/or oxygen delivery devices:
   a. assess areas of skin and mucous membranes that are in contact with oxygen mask or nasal cannula (e.g., nares, bridge of nose, tops of ears) a few times each day for redness and irritation
   b. pad areas of pressure and ensure that straps are not too tight
   c. keep skin areas under straps and mask clean and dry
   d. refill oxygen humidification reservoir as needed, perform frequent oral hygiene, and apply water-based gel to nares and lips to reduce dryness of the mucous membranes.
3. Make sure the client knows how to recognize when the oxygen supply is low and how to get the oxygen source refilled or replaced.
4. Instruct client to have the oxygen delivery system checked regularly by the supplier.

10.d. The client will verbalize ways to improve appetite and nutritional status.

10.d.1. Refer to Care Plan on Chemotherapy, Diagnosis 12, action d (pp. 190–191), for instructions related to improving appetite and maintaining an adequate nutritional status.
2. Encourage client to use supplemental oxygen via nasal cannula during meals if needed.

10.e. The client will verbalize ways to manage chronic SIADH if present.

10.e. If appropriate, provide the following instructions related to management of chronic SIADH:
1. continue to limit water intake if recommended by physician
2. take medications (e.g., furosemide, demeclocycline) as prescribed
3. increase intake of foods/fluids high in sodium (e.g., tomato juice, cured meats, processed cheese, canned vegetables and soups, catsup, dill pickles, bouillon)
4. report new or intensified signs and symptoms of SIADH (e.g., sudden weight gain, decrease in urine output, drowsiness, confusion, weakness, headache, nausea, vomiting, abdominal cramping, seizures).

Desired Outcomes	**Nursing Actions** *and Selected Purposes/Rationales*
10.f. The client will state signs and symptoms to report to the health care provider.	10.f.1. Instruct client to report the following: a. new or increased chest pain b. signs and symptoms of hypercalcemia (e.g., nausea, vomiting, increased urination, muscle weakness, confusion) c. persistent fever d. development of or increased hoarseness or difficulty swallowing e. excessive weight loss f. increasing fatigue, weakness, or shortness of breath g. swollen, painful joints (may indicate the development of hypertrophic pulmonary osteoarthropathy [a paraneoplastic condition]) h. swelling of face, neck, or arms; persistent redness of neck, face, and chest; visual changes; or dizziness (may indicate SVCS) i. persistent headache j. development or worsening of a cough especially if productive of purulent, green, foul-smelling, or blood-tinged sputum k. muscle weakness, numbness or tingling in extremities, or uncoordinated movements (may indicate development of a paraneoplastic neuromuscular syndrome) l. signs and symptoms of Pancoast's syndrome (e.g., pain in shoulder and arm) and Horner's syndrome (e.g., very small pupil, drooping of eyelid, and loss of sweating on one side of face); these two syndromes usually occur together, are a result of extension of the primary tumor into the lower cervical and upper thoracic nerves, and occur most frequently with squamous cell carcinoma m. irritability, drowsiness, or confusion n. signs and symptoms of SIADH (see action e.4 in this diagnosis) o. excessive depression or difficulty coping with the diagnosis and/or treatment. 2. If appropriate, refer to the Care Plan on Chemotherapy, Diagnosis 12, action 1 (pp. 193–194) and/or the Care Plan on External Radiation Therapy, Diagnosis 16, action j (p. 220), for signs and symptoms the client should report if receiving chemotherapy and/or radiation therapy.
10.g. The client will identify community resources that can assist with home management and adjustment to the diagnosis and the effects of treatment.	10.g.1. Provide information about and encourage utilization of community resources that can assist client and significant others with home management and adjustment to the diagnosis of lung cancer and effects of prescribed treatment (e.g., American Cancer Society, counselors, social service agencies, home health agencies, I Can Cope, Meals on Wheels, local support groups, hospice). 2. Initiate a referral if indicated.
10.h. The client will verbalize an understanding of and a plan for adhering to recommended follow-up care including future appointments with health care provider, medications prescribed, activity level, and plans for subsequent treatment.	10.h.1. Reinforce physician's explanation of planned radiation therapy and/or chemotherapy schedule if appropriate. Stress importance of strictly following the prescribed protocol for the treatments and keeping all appointments for follow-up examinations and laboratory work. 2. Explain rationale for, side effects of, and importance of taking medications prescribed. Inform client of pertinent food and drug interactions. 3. Emphasize need for planned rest periods and adjusting activity according to tolerance. 4. Implement measures to improve client compliance: a. include significant others in teaching sessions if possible b. encourage questions and allow time for reinforcement and clarification of information provided c. provide written instructions regarding scheduled appointments with health care provider and for chemotherapy, radiation therapy, and laboratory work; medications prescribed; and signs and symptoms to report.

SELF-CARE DEFICIT

related to:
a. activity limitations imposed by dyspnea, weakness, fatigue, and discomfort associated with the disease process, diagnostic tests, and/or side effects of treatment;
b. disturbed thought processes if present.

DISTURBED SLEEP PATTERN*

related to:
a. fear, anxiety, and grief;
b. decreased activity, unfamiliar environment, and frequent assessments and treatments;
c. excessive coughing and inability to assume usual sleep position associated with orthopnea;
d. discomfort associated with the disease process and/or side effects of treatment.

DISTURBED THOUGHT PROCESSES

related to:
a. cerebral hypoxia associated with impaired alveolar gas exchange and anemia (if present);
b. central nervous system depressant effect of hypercalcemia if present;
c. damage to cerebral tissue (can occur if lung cancer has metastasized to the brain or if client is experiencing certain paraneoplastic neurological conditions).

RISK FOR FALLS

related to:
a. confusion and lethargy associated with hypoxia, hypercalcemia, and brain metastasis (if it has occurred);
b. weakness associated with nutritional and sleep deficits, tissue hypoxia, hypercalcemia, side effects of treatment, and/or presence of paraneoplastic conditions such as myasthenic syndrome.

DISTURBED SELF-CONCEPT*

related to:
a. change in appearance (e.g., excessive weight loss, hair loss associated with chemotherapy, skin changes associated with radiation therapy, gynecomastia associated with ectopic hormone production by tumor cells);
b. temporary or permanent infertility associated with hormonal imbalance resulting from ectopic hormone production by tumor cells and/or cytotoxic drug therapy;
c. changes in sexual functioning associated with weakness, fatigue, dyspnea, pain, and anxiety;
d. increased dependence on others to meet self-care needs;
e. anticipated changes in lifestyle and roles associated with effects of the disease process and its treatment.

INEFFECTIVE COPING*

related to:
a. persistent discomfort associated with the disease process and side effects of treatment;

---

*See Unit II for outcomes, actions, and rationales.

b. guilt associated with the diagnosis of lung cancer if a personal habit such as smoking was the major cause;
c. fear, anxiety, fatigue, feeling of powerlessness, and uncertainty of the effectiveness of treatment.

Bibliography

See pages 879 and 882–883.

CHRONIC OBSTRUCTIVE PULMONARY DISEASE

Chronic obstructive pulmonary disease (COPD) is a term used to describe a disease state characterized by the presence of airflow obstruction in the lungs. The airflow obstruction is chronic, usually progressive, and may be accompanied by airway hyperactivity. Other terms sometimes used to describe this condition are chronic obstructive lung disease (COLD) and chronic airflow limitation (CAL). Signs and symptoms usually include dyspnea, cough, and sputum production that worsen over time and during periodic exacerbations.

The two conditions that comprise COPD are chronic bronchitis and emphysema. Chronic bronchitis is characterized by a cough that persists at least 3 months of the year for 2 consecutive years and an excessive production of mucus in the bronchi due to inflammation of the bronchioles and hypertrophy and hyperplasia of the mucous glands. In contrast, emphysema is characterized by dyspnea and a mild cough. The impaired airflow that occurs with emphysema is related to loss of lung elasticity, narrowing of the terminal nonrespiratory bronchioles, and destructive changes in the walls of the alveolar and/or respiratory bronchioles. Both chronic bronchitis and emphysema are usually present in the person with COPD, although one of the two usually predominates.

Causative factors of COPD include chronic irritation of the lungs by cigarette smoke, exposure to air pollution and chemical irritants, and recurrent respiratory tract infections. In a small percentage of cases of emphysema, the destruction of lung tissue by proteolytic enzymes is a result of a genetic deficiency of alpha$_1$-antitrypsin.

This care plan focuses on care of the adult client with COPD who is hospitalized during an acute exacerbation. Much of the information is applicable to clients receiving follow-up care in an extended care facility or home setting.

OUTCOME/DISCHARGE CRITERIA

THE CLIENT WILL:

- have improved respiratory function
- tolerate expected level of activity
- have no signs and symptoms of complications
- identify ways to prevent or minimize further respiratory problems
- verbalize ways to maintain an optimal nutritional status
- identify ways to conserve energy and/or reduce dyspnea and fatigue
- demonstrate proper chest physiotherapy and use of respiratory equipment
- verbalize an understanding of medications ordered including rationale, food and drug interactions, side effects, methods of administering, and importance of taking as prescribed
- identify precautions that should be adhered to when using oxygen
- state signs and symptoms to report to the health care provider
- share feelings and thoughts about the effects of COPD on lifestyle and roles
- identify resources that can assist with financial needs, home management, and adjustment to changes resulting from COPD
- verbalize an understanding of and a plan for adhering to recommended follow-up care including future appointments with health care provider and graded exercise program.

NURSING/COLLABORATIVE DIAGNOSES

5. Potential complications p. 449
   a. right-sided heart failure (cor pulmonale)
   b. respiratory failure
6. Fear/Anxiety p. 449
7. Ineffective therapeutic regimen management p. 450

DISCHARGE TEACHING

8. Deficient knowledge or Ineffective health maintenance p. 452

See pp. 455–456 for additional diagnoses.

1. Nursing Diagnosis: *IMPAIRED RESPIRATORY FUNCTION**

a. ineffective breathing pattern related to:
   1. increased rate of respirations associated with fear and anxiety
   2. decreased depth of respirations associated with weakness, fatigue, fear, anxiety, and presence of a flattened diaphragm (a result of prolonged hyperinflation of the lungs);
b. ineffective airway clearance related to:
   1. narrowing of the airways associated with:
      a. excessive mucus production and inflammation and hyperplasia of the bronchial walls (especially with chronic bronchitis)
      b. destruction of the elastic fibers in the walls of the small airways (with emphysema)
   2. stasis of secretions associated with:
      a. difficulty coughing up secretions resulting from fatigue, weakness, and presence of tenacious secretions if fluid intake is inadequate
      b. impaired ciliary function resulting from loss of ciliated epithelium (occurs with inflammation, destruction, and fibrosis of bronchial walls)
      c. decreased mobility;
c. impaired gas exchange related to narrowing or obstruction of the small airways and a decrease in effective lung surface (occurs as a result of collapse or destruction of alveolar walls).

*This diagnostic label includes the following nursing diagnoses: ineffective breathing pattern, ineffective airway clearance, and impaired gas exchange.

Suggested NOC Outcomes: Respiratory status: airway patency; Respiratory status: ventilation; Respiratory status: gas exchange

Suggested NIC Interventions: Respiratory monitoring; Airway management; Chest physiotherapy; Cough enhancement; Oxygen therapy; Medication administration; Ventilation assistance

Desired Outcome	**Nursing Actions** *and Selected Purposes/Rationales* (see pp. 12–14, 18–20, and 33–35 for additional rationales)
1. The client will experience adequate respiratory function as evidenced by: a. usual rate and depth of respirations b. decreased dyspnea c. usual or improved breath sounds d. usual mental status e. oximetry results within normal range for client f. blood gases within normal range for client.	1.a. Assess for: 1. signs and symptoms of impaired respiratory function: a. rapid, shallow respirations b. dyspnea, orthopnea c. use of accessory muscles when breathing d. abnormal breath sounds (e.g., diminished or absent, rhonchi, wheezes) e. cough f. restlessness, irritability g. confusion, somnolence h. central cyanosis (a late sign) i. significant decrease in oximetry results j. abnormal blood gas values 2. significant abnormalities in chest x-ray reports

3. pulmonary function study results that worsen or fail to improve after treatment begins.

b. Implement measures *to improve respiratory status:*
   1. perform actions to increase strength and improve activity tolerance (see Diagnosis 3, action b) *in order to increase client's willingness and ability to move, cough, deep breathe, and use incentive spirometer*
   2. perform actions to reduce fear and anxiety (see Diagnosis 6, action b) *in order to prevent the shallow and/or rapid breathing that can occur with fear and anxiety*
   3. place client in a semi- to high Fowler's position; position overbed table so client can lean on it if desired
   4. maintain oxygen therapy as ordered (question any order for high oxygen concentration *since many persons with COPD are dependent on hypoxemia as the stimulus to breathe)*
   5. instruct client in and assist with diaphragmatic and pursed-lip breathing techniques
   6. instruct client to deep breathe or use incentive spirometer every 1–2 hours
   7. perform actions *to promote removal of pulmonary secretions:*
      a. instruct and assist client to cough or "huff" every 1–2 hours
      b. implement measures *to thin tenacious secretions and reduce dryness of the respiratory mucous membrane:*
         1. maintain a fluid intake of at least 2500 ml/day unless contraindicated
         2. humidify inspired air as ordered
      c. assist with administration of mucolytics (e.g., acetylcysteine) and diluent or hydrating agents (e.g., water, saline) via nebulizer if ordered
      d. assist with or perform postural drainage therapy (PDT) if ordered
      e. perform suctioning if needed
      f. administer expectorants (e.g., guaifenesin) if ordered
   8. instruct client to avoid intake of large meals, gas-forming foods (e.g., beans, cauliflower, cabbage, onions), and carbonated beverages *in order to prevent gastric distention and increased pressure on the diaphragm*
   9. discourage smoking *(the irritants in smoke increase mucus production, impair ciliary function, and can cause inflammation and damage to the bronchial and alveolar walls; the carbon monoxide decreases oxygen availability)*
   10. maintain activity restrictions if ordered; increase activity as allowed and tolerated
   11. avoid use of central nervous system depressants *(these further depress respiratory status)*
   12. administer the following medications if ordered:
       a. bronchodilators:
          1. methylxanthines (e.g., theophylline)
          2. beta-adrenergic agonists (e.g., metaproterenol, albuterol, terbutaline)
          3. anticholinergics (e.g., ipratropium)
       b. corticosteroids (e.g., prednisone, methylprednisolone), which may be given *to decrease airway inflammation and thereby improve bronchial air flow*
       c. antimicrobials *(may be given to prevent or treat pneumonia)*
       d. alpha$_1$-proteinase inhibitor (e.g., Prolastin) *if the cause of emphysema is a genetic deficiency of alpha$_1$-antitrypsin.*

c. Consult appropriate health care provider (e.g., respiratory therapist, physician) if signs and symptoms of impaired respiratory function persist or worsen.

2. NURSING DIAGNOSIS: IMBALANCED NUTRITION: LESS THAN BODY REQUIREMENTS

related to:

a. decreased oral intake associated with:
   1. dyspnea, weakness, and fatigue

2. nausea (can occur in response to noxious stimuli such as the sight of expectorated sputum and as a side effect of some medications)
3. early satiety resulting from compression of the stomach by flattened diaphragm;

b. increased metabolic needs associated with increased energy expenditure resulting from strenuous breathing efforts and persistent coughing.

Suggested NOC Outcome:
Nutritional status

Suggested NIC Interventions: Nutritional monitoring; Nutrition management; Nutrition therapy; Nausea management

Desired Outcome

2. The client will maintain an adequate nutritional status as evidenced by:
   a. weight within normal range for client
   b. normal BUN and serum prealbumin and albumin levels
   c. usual strength and activity tolerance
   d. healthy oral mucous membrane.

Nursing Actions *and Selected Purposes/Rationales*

(see pp. 40–43 for additional rationales)

2.a. Assess for and report signs and symptoms of malnutrition:
   1. weight significantly below client's usual weight or less than normal for client's age, height, and body frame
   2. abnormal BUN and low serum prealbumin and albumin levels
   3. increased weakness and fatigue
   4. sore, inflamed oral mucous membrane
   5. pale conjunctiva.

b. Monitor percentage of meals and snacks client consumes. Report a pattern of inadequate intake.

c. Implement measures *to maintain an adequate nutritional status:*
   1. perform actions *to improve oral intake:*
      a. implement measures to improve respiratory status (see Diagnosis 1, action b) *in order to help relieve dyspnea*
      b. schedule treatments that assist in mobilizing mucus (e.g., aerosol treatments, postural drainage therapy) at least 1 hour before or after meals *to prevent nausea*
      c. increase activity as allowed and tolerated *(activity usually promotes a sense of well-being, which can improve appetite)*
      d. obtain a dietary consult if necessary to assist client in selecting foods/fluids that meet nutritional needs, are appealing, and adhere to personal and cultural preferences
      e. encourage a rest period before meals *to minimize fatigue*
      f. eliminate noxious sights and odors from the environment; provide client with an opaque, covered container for expectorated sputum; empty container frequently and remove it from the table during mealtime if it is not needed *(noxious stimuli can cause nausea)*
      g. maintain a clean environment and a relaxed, pleasant atmosphere
      h. provide oral hygiene before meals *(oral hygiene moistens the mouth, which makes it easier to chew and swallow; it also removes unpleasant tastes, which often improves the taste of foods/fluids)*
      i. if client is quite dyspneic, assist him/her to select foods that require little or no chewing
      j. serve frequent, small meals rather than large ones if client is weak, fatigues easily, or has a poor appetite
      k. place client in a high Fowler's position for meals and provide supplemental oxygen therapy during meals if indicated *to help relieve dyspnea*
      l. allow adequate time for meals; reheat foods/fluids if necessary
      m. limit fluid intake with meals (unless the fluid has high nutritional value) *to reduce early satiety and subsequent decreased food intake*
   2. ensure that meals are well balanced and high in essential nutrients; offer dietary supplements if indicated
   3. administer vitamins and minerals if ordered.

d. Perform a calorie count if ordered. Report information to dietitian and physician.

e. Consult physician about an alternative method of providing nutrition (e.g., parenteral nutrition, tube feedings) if client does not consume enough food or fluids to meet nutritional needs.

3. NURSING DIAGNOSIS: ACTIVITY INTOLERANCE

related to:
a. tissue hypoxia associated with impaired gas exchange;
b. inadequate nutritional status;
c. difficulty resting and sleeping associated with dyspnea, excessive coughing, fear, anxiety, frequent assessments and treatments, and side effects of medication therapy (e.g., some bronchodilators, corticosteroids);
d. increased energy expenditure associated with strenuous breathing efforts and persistent coughing.

Suggested NOC Outcomes: Activity tolerance; Endurance; Rest; Energy conservation; Self-care status

Suggested NIC Interventions: Energy management; Oxygen therapy; Sleep enhancement; Nutrition management

Desired Outcome	**Nursing Actions** *and Selected Purposes/Rationales* (see pp. 11–12 for additional rationales)
3. The client will demonstrate an increased tolerance for activity as evidenced by: a. verbalization of feeling less fatigued and weak b. ability to perform activities of daily living without increased dyspnea, chest pain, diaphoresis, dizziness, and a significant change in vital signs.	3.a. Assess for signs and symptoms of activity intolerance: 1. statements of fatigue or weakness 2. exertional dyspnea, chest pain, diaphoresis, or dizziness 3. abnormal heart rate response to activity (e.g., increase in rate of 20 beats/minute above resting rate, rate not returning to preactivity level within 3 minutes after stopping activity, change from regular to irregular rate) 4. a significant change (15–20 mm Hg) in blood pressure with activity. b. Implement measures *to improve activity tolerance:* 1. perform actions *to promote rest and/or conserve energy:* a. maintain activity restrictions as ordered b. minimize environmental activity and noise c. organize nursing care to allow for periods of uninterrupted rest d. limit the number of visitors and their length of stay e. assist client with self-care activities as needed f. keep supplies and personal articles within easy reach g. instruct client in energy-saving techniques (e.g., using shower chair when showering, sitting to brush teeth or comb hair) h. implement measures to reduce fear and anxiety (see Diagnosis 6, action b) i. implement measures *to promote sleep* (e.g., elevate head of bed and support arms on pillows to facilitate breathing; maintain oxygen therapy during sleep; discourage intake of fluids high in caffeine, especially in the evening; encourage use of progressive relaxation techniques or meditation; reduce environmental stimuli) j. implement measures *to control cough:* 1. instruct client to avoid intake of very hot or cold foods/fluids *(these can stimulate cough)* 2. protect client from exposure to irritants such as flowers, smoke, and powder 3. administer prescribed antitussives if indicated *to suppress cough* (when cough is productive, antitussives should be used only when coughing is excessive and interfering significantly with the client's ability to rest and sleep) k. consult occupational therapist about obtaining long-handled assistive devices (e.g., "grabbers," hairbrush, shoehorn) to reduce client's movement of the upper extremities *(activities involving use of the upper extremities can decrease activity tolerance because some of the accessory muscles used for breathing are used instead to control shoulder movement)* l. instruct client to avoid or limit talking while performing activities that also require energy (e.g., eating, walking, bathing)

Desired Outcome	Nursing Actions *and Selected Purposes/Rationales*

2. discourage smoking and excessive intake of beverages high in caffeine such as coffee, tea, and colas *(nicotine and caffeine can increase cardiac workload and myocardial oxygen utilization, thereby decreasing oxygen availability)*
3. perform actions to improve respiratory status (see Diagnosis 1, action b) *in order to improve tissue oxygenation and help relieve dyspnea*
4. perform actions to maintain an adequate nutritional status (see Diagnosis 2, action c)
5. reinforce use of controlled breathing techniques (e.g., inhaling through nose and exhaling slowly through pursed lips) during activity
6. if oxygen therapy is necessary during activity, keep portable oxygen equipment readily available for client's use
7. increase client's activity gradually as allowed and tolerated.

c. Instruct client to:
  1. report a decreased tolerance for activity
  2. stop any activity that causes chest pain, increased shortness of breath, dizziness, or extreme fatigue or weakness.

d. Consult appropriate health care provider (e.g., respiratory therapist, physician) if signs and symptoms of activity intolerance persist or worsen.

4. Nursing Diagnosis: RISK FOR INFECTION: PNEUMONIA

related to:
a. stasis of secretions in the lungs (secretions provide a good medium for bacterial growth);
b. inhalation of pathogens (especially if client is using respiratory equipment or medication delivery devices that are not being cleaned adequately or routinely).

Suggested NOC Outcomes: Infection severity; Immune status

Suggested NIC Interventions: Infection protection; Infection control; Cough enhancement; Airway management

Desired Outcome	Nursing Actions *and Selected Purposes/Rationales*

4. The client will not develop pneumonia as evidenced by:
  a. usual breath sounds and percussion note over lungs
  b. absence of tachypnea
  c. cough productive of clear mucus only
  d. afebrile status
  e. absence of pleuritic pain
  f. WBC count within normal range
  g. blood gases returning to normal range for client
  h. negative sputum culture.

4.a. Assess for and report signs and symptoms of pneumonia:
  1. abnormal breath sounds (e.g., crackles [rales], pleural friction rub, bronchial breath sounds, diminished or absent breath sounds)
  2. dull percussion note over affected lung area
  3. increase in respiratory rate
  4. cough productive of purulent, green, or rust-colored sputum
  5. chills and fever
  6. pleuritic pain
  7. elevated WBC count
  8. significant decrease in oximetry results
  9. worsening of blood gas values
  10. positive sputum culture results
  11. chest x-ray results indicative of pneumonia.

b. Implement measures *to prevent pneumonia:*
  1. perform actions to improve respiratory status (see Diagnosis 1, action b)
  2. protect client from persons with respiratory tract infections
  3. encourage and assist client to perform frequent oral hygiene *in order to remove pathogens and secretions that could be aspirated*
  4. replace or cleanse equipment used for respiratory care as often as needed
  5. instruct and assist client to rinse and clean medication delivery devices (e.g., dry powder inhaler, metered-dose inhaler, spacer) according to manufacturer's instructions.

c. If signs and symptoms of pneumonia occur, administer antimicrobials as ordered.

5. COLLABORATIVE DIAGNOSES: **POTENTIAL COMPLICATIONS OF COPD**

a. right-sided heart failure (cor pulmonale) related to increased cardiac workload associated with:
   1. pulmonary hypertension resulting from pulmonary vasoconstriction that occurs in response to hypoxia
   2. compensatory response to decreased pulmonary blood flow that results from compression of the pulmonary capillaries by hyperinflated alveoli (with emphysema) and loss of large portions of the pulmonary vascular bed (occurs in emphysema as a result of destruction of the alveolar walls);

b. respiratory failure related to severe ventilation/perfusion imbalance associated with end-stage COPD, acute exacerbation of COPD, and/or presence of conditions that further compromise respiratory status (e.g., pneumonia, abdominal or thoracic surgery, pneumothorax).

Desired Outcomes	**Nursing Actions** *and Selected Purposes/Rationales*
5.a. The client will not develop right-sided heart failure as evidenced by: 1. pulse 60–100 beats/minute 2. usual mental status 3. no increase in weakness and fatigue 4. adequate urine output 5. stable weight 6. absence of edema; distended neck veins; and enlarged, tender liver.	5.a.1. Assess for and report signs and symptoms of right-sided heart failure: a. increase in pulse rate b. restlessness, confusion c. increased weakness and/or fatigue d. decreased urine output e. weight gain f. dependent peripheral edema g. distended neck veins h. enlarged, tender liver i. chest x-ray results showing cardiomegaly. 2. Implement measures to improve respiratory status (see Diagnosis 1, action b) *in order to reduce cardiac workload and the subsequent risk for right-sided heart failure.* 3. If signs and symptoms of right-sided heart failure occur: a. maintain oxygen therapy as ordered b. maintain fluid and sodium restrictions if ordered c. maintain client on strict bed rest in a semi- to high Fowler's position d. administer medications that may be ordered *to reduce vascular congestion and/or cardiac workload* (e.g., diuretics, vasodilators).
5.b. The client will not experience respiratory failure as evidenced by: 1. usual skin color 2. usual mental status 3. Pao_2 above 50 mm Hg and $Paco_2$ below 50 mm Hg.	5.b.1. Assess for and report signs and symptoms of severe respiratory distress (e.g., increased sternocleidomastoid and intercostal muscle retraction, cyanotic skin color, drowsiness, confusion, $Paco_2$ of 50 mm Hg or less, $Paco_2$ of 50 mm Hg or greater). 2. Implement measures *to prevent respiratory failure:* a. perform actions to improve respiratory status (see Diagnosis 1, action b) b. perform actions to prevent and treat pneumonia (see Diagnosis 4, actions b and c) *in order to prevent a further compromise in respiratory status.* 3. If signs and symptoms of respiratory failure occur, assist with intubation, mechanical ventilatory support, and transfer to intensive care unit if indicated.

6. NURSING DIAGNOSIS: **FEAR/ANXIETY**

related to:

a. exacerbation of symptoms (e.g., increased dyspnea, feeling of suffocation), need for hospitalization, and concern about prognosis;
b. lack of understanding of the diagnosis, diagnostic tests, treatments, and prognosis;
c. financial concerns about hospitalization and lifelong treatment;
d. feeling of lack of control over the progression of COPD and its effects on lifestyle and roles.

Suggested NOC Outcomes: Anxiety level; Fear level; Anxiety self-control; Fear self-control

Suggested NIC Interventions: Anxiety reduction; Calming technique; Emotional support; Presence; Financial resource assistance

Desired Outcome	Nursing Actions *and Selected Purposes/Rationales* (see pp. 14–16 for additional rationales)
6. The client will experience a reduction in fear and anxiety as evidenced by: a. verbalization of feeling less anxious b. usual sleep pattern c. relaxed facial expression and body movements d. stable vital signs e. usual perceptual ability and interactions with others.	6.a. Assess client for signs and symptoms of fear and anxiety (e.g., verbalization of feeling anxious, insomnia, tenseness, shakiness, restlessness, diaphoresis, elevated blood pressure, tachycardia, self-focused behaviors). Validate perceptions carefully, remembering that some behavior may result from hypoxia and/or hypercapnia. b. Implement measures *to reduce fear and anxiety:* 1. maintain a calm, supportive, confident manner when interacting with client 2. do not leave client alone during period of acute respiratory distress 3. perform actions to improve respiratory status (see Diagnosis 1, action b) *in order to reduce dyspnea* 4. perform actions *to decrease client's feeling of suffocation:* a. open curtains and doors b. approach client from the side rather than face-on *(close face-on contact may make client feel closed in)* c. limit number of visitors in room at any one time d. remove unnecessary equipment from room e. administer oxygen via nasal cannula rather than mask if possible 5. encourage significant others to project a caring, concerned attitude without obvious anxiousness 6. once the period of acute respiratory distress has subsided: a. orient client to environment, equipment, and routines b. introduce client to staff who will be participating in care; if possible, maintain consistency in staff assigned to his/her care c. assure client that staff members are nearby; respond to call signal as soon as possible d. provide a calm, restful environment e. encourage verbalization of fear and anxiety; provide feedback f. reinforce physician's explanations and clarify misconceptions the client has about COPD, the treatment plan, and prognosis g. explain all diagnostic tests h. instruct client in relaxation techniques and encourage participation in diversional activities i. provide information based on current needs of client at a level he/she can understand; encourage questions and clarification of information provided j. perform actions to promote effective therapeutic regimen management (see Diagnosis 7, action b) *in order to increase client's feeling of control over his/her life* k. initiate a social service referral and/or assist client to identify and contact appropriate community resources if indicated l. administer prescribed antianxiety agents if indicated. c. Consult appropriate health care provider (e.g., psychiatric nurse clinician, physician) if above actions fail to control fear and anxiety.

7. Nursing Diagnosis: *INEFFECTIVE THERAPEUTIC REGIMEN MANAGEMENT*

related to:
a. lack of understanding of the implications of not following the prescribed treatment plan;
b. feeling of lack of control over disease progression;
c. difficulty modifying personal habits (e.g., smoking) and integrating necessary treatments into lifestyle;
d. insufficient financial resources.

Suggested NOC Outcomes: Treatment behavior: illness or injury; Compliance behavior; Health beliefs: perceived ability to perform; Knowledge: treatment regimen

Suggested NIC Interventions: Self-modification assistance; Values clarification; Teaching: disease process; Health system guidance; Financial resource assistance; Discharge planning; Medication management; Smoking cessation assistance

Desired Outcome	**Nursing Actions** *and Selected Purposes/Rationales*
7. The client will demonstrate the probability of effective therapeutic regimen management as evidenced by: a. willingness to learn about and participate in treatments and care b. statements reflecting ways to modify personal habits and integrate treatments into lifestyle c. statements reflecting an understanding of the implications of not following the prescribed treatment plan.	7.a. Assess for indications that the client may be unable to effectively manage the therapeutic regimen: 1. statements reflecting inability to manage care at home 2. failure to adhere to treatment plan (e.g., refusing to use proper breathing techniques, refusing medications) 3. statements reflecting a lack of understanding of factors that may cause further progression of COPD 4. statements reflecting an unwillingness or inability to modify personal habits and integrate necessary treatments into lifestyle 5. statements reflecting view that COPD is curable or that the situation is hopeless and efforts to comply with the treatment plan are useless. b. Implement measures *to promote effective therapeutic regimen management:* 1. explain COPD in terms the client can understand; stress the fact that COPD is a chronic condition and adherence to the treatment program is necessary in order to delay and/or prevent complications; caution client that some complications may occur despite strict adherence to treatment plan 2. encourage questions and clarify misconceptions client has about COPD and its effects 3. encourage client to participate in treatment plan (e.g., postural drainage therapy, breathing exercises) 4. consult occupational and/or physical therapist if indicated about a home evaluation to identify assistive devices and environmental modifications that could help the client be more independent in his/her living situation 5. assist client to develop a system for recording frequency of use of medications and respiratory treatments in order to avoid omission of those that should be used routinely and to avoid excessive use of those that should be used on an "as needed" basis (in times of respiratory distress, the client may tend to overuse medications because of fear, anxiety, and impaired cognition) 6. initiate the discharge teaching outlined in Diagnosis 8; determine areas of difficulty and misunderstanding and reinforce teaching as necessary 7. provide client with written instructions about chest physiotherapy, ways to prevent further respiratory problems, prescribed medications, signs and symptoms to report, where to obtain needed equipment and supplies, and future appointments with health care provider 8. assist client to identify ways treatments can be incorporated into lifestyle; focus on modifications of lifestyle rather than complete change 9. encourage client to discuss concerns regarding cost of hospitalization, medications, oxygen equipment, and follow-up care; obtain a social service consult to assist with financial planning and to obtain financial aid if indicated 10. provide information about and encourage utilization of community resources that can assist client to make necessary lifestyle changes (e.g., American Lung Association; pulmonary rehabilitation groups; counseling, vocational, and social services; smoking cessation programs) 11. reinforce behaviors suggesting future compliance with prescribed treatments (e.g., statements reflecting plans for integrating treatments

Desired Outcome	Nursing Actions *and Selected Purposes/Rationales*
	into lifestyle, active participation in treatment plan, changes in personal habits) 12. include significant others in explanations and teaching sessions and encourage their support; reinforce the need for client to assume responsibility for managing as much of care as possible. c. Consult appropriate health care provider about referrals to community health agencies if continued instruction, support, or supervision is needed.

Discharge Teaching/Continued Care

8. Nursing Diagnosis: ***DEFICIENT KNOWLEDGE OR INEFFECTIVE HEALTH MAINTENANCE****

*The nurse should select the diagnostic label that is most appropriate for the client's discharge teaching needs.

Suggested NOC Outcomes: Knowledge: treatment regimen; Knowledge: energy conservation; Knowledge: treatment procedure(s); Knowledge: health resources; Knowledge: illness care

Suggested NIC Interventions: Health system guidance; Teaching: individual; Teaching: disease process; Teaching: prescribed activity/exercise; Teaching: prescribed medication

Desired Outcomes	Nursing Actions *and Selected Purposes/Rationales*
8.a. The client will identify ways to prevent or minimize further respiratory problems.	8.a.1. Instruct client in ways to prevent or minimize further respiratory problems: a. maintain overall general good health (e.g., reduce stress, eat a well-balanced diet, obtain adequate rest, adhere to prescribed graded exercise program) b. stop smoking c. avoid exposure to respiratory irritants such as smoke, dust, some perfumes, aerosol sprays, paint fumes, and solvents d. remain indoors when air pollution levels and/or pollen counts are high and/or outdoor temperatures are extremely hot or cold e. wear a mask or scarf over nose and mouth if exposure to high levels of irritants such as smoke, fumes, and dust is unavoidable f. avoid high altitudes; if air travel is required, consult physician about the need for supplemental oxygen g. adhere to chest physiotherapy (e.g., breathing exercises, postural drainage therapy) as ordered h. take medications such as bronchodilators and mucolytics as prescribed i. decrease the risk of respiratory tract infections: 1. avoid contact with persons who have respiratory tract infections 2. avoid crowds and poorly ventilated areas 3. drink at least 10 glasses of liquid/day unless contraindicated 4. receive immunizations against influenza and pneumococcal pneumonia 5. take antimicrobials as prescribed (some physicians instruct clients to begin antimicrobial therapy if sputum color becomes yellow or green) 6. clean medication administration devices (e.g., metered-dose inhaler, dry powder inhaler, spacer, table-top nebulizer), oxygen delivery devices (e.g., mask, nasal cannula), humidifier, and air filters as instructed by health care provider and manufacturer.

2. Assist client in identifying ways he/she can make appropriate changes in personal habits and lifestyle to reduce modifiable risk factors.

8.b. The client will verbalize ways to maintain an optimal nutritional status.

8.b. Provide instructions regarding ways to maintain an optimal nutritional status:
1. rest prior to meals; do the majority of food preparation in advance rather than just before eating
2. perform good oral hygiene before meals to reduce unpleasant tastes in mouth
3. eat sitting down in a pleasant environment
4. use supplemental oxygen via nasal cannula during meals if needed
5. eat foods that require little or no chewing when energy is low and/or dyspnea is increased
6. eat meals that are well balanced; drink nutritional supplements if needed to maintain an adequate caloric intake
7. take vitamins and minerals as prescribed.

8.c. The client will identify ways to conserve energy and/or reduce dyspnea and fatigue.

8.c. Instruct client in ways to conserve energy and/or reduce dyspnea and fatigue:
1. sit rather than stand during activities such as preparing food, rinsing dishes, ironing, showering, shaving, and talking on the phone
2. have most frequently used food items, dishes, cleaning supplies, and clothing at waist level whenever possible rather than on high or low shelves
3. pace yourself during any activity; stop, relax your muscles, and take a few deep breaths as often as needed
4. simplify your life whenever possible
5. spread large projects over several days or weeks
6. allow others to assist you with or actually do strenuous or lengthy tasks
7. modify activities to avoid bending, reaching, and raising arms whenever possible (e.g., use long-handled assistive devices, simplify hair style so that it does not need to be blown dry or curled, sit with elbows resting on table while shaving)
8. do not try to carry on a conversation during activities that also require energy (e.g., walking, eating, cleaning, gardening)
9. use bronchodilators prior to activity as needed and prescribed
10. use oxygen during activity as needed and prescribed; have portable oxygen system readily available
11. use positions that minimize energy expenditure during sexual activity (e.g., side-lying).

8.d. The client will demonstrate proper chest physiotherapy and use of respiratory equipment.

8.d.1. Reinforce instructions about proper breathing techniques (e.g., pursed-lip breathing, diaphragmatic breathing), postural drainage therapy (PDT may be indicated if large amounts of mucus continue to be produced), and use of respiratory equipment (e.g., oxygen, incentive spirometer).
2. Allow time for questions, clarification, and return demonstration.

8.e. The client will verbalize an understanding of medications ordered including rationale, food and drug interactions, side effects, methods of administering, and importance of taking as prescribed.

8.e.1. Explain the rationale for, side effects of, and importance of taking medications prescribed.
2. Inform client of pertinent food and drug interactions.
3. If client is discharged on theophylline, instruct to:
   a. take it with food to minimize nausea, vomiting, and epigastric pain
   b. take it on a regular basis as ordered to maintain therapeutic blood levels
   c. report signs and symptoms that could indicate a toxic drug level (e.g., persistent nausea, vomiting, dizziness, insomnia, rapid pulse, muscle twitching, seizures)
   d. have blood theophylline levels evaluated periodically.
4. If client is discharged on medications via inhalation:
   a. provide information about the proper use, cleaning, and replacement of the medication delivery devices (e.g., nebulizer, dry powder inhaler, metered-dose inhaler [MDI], spacer)

Desired Outcomes	**Nursing Actions** *and Selected Purposes/Rationales*
	b. instruct to rinse mouth with water after using inhalers (removing remaining drug particles from the mouth helps reduce unpleasant tastes, dryness or irritation of the oral mucosa, and systemic absorption of the drug) c. instruct to observe for and report side effects such as persistent sore throat, increased cough, hoarseness, and/or white patches in mouth (could indicate candidiasis that can occur with corticosteroid use) d. instruct to use the prescribed bronchodilator before inhaling the corticosteroid and to wait 5 minutes between these two medications (this maximizes the effectiveness of the corticosteroid). 5. If client is discharged on a corticosteroid, instruct to: a. take oral preparations with food to reduce gastric irritation b. expect that certain effects such as facial rounding, slight weight gain and swelling, increased appetite, and slight mood changes may occur c. report undesirable effects such as marked swelling in extremities, significant weight gain, extreme emotional and behavioral changes, extreme weakness, tarry stools, bloody or coffee-ground vomitus, frequent or persistent headaches, insomnia, lack of menses, and persistent gastric irritation d. avoid contact with persons who have an infection because corticosteroids lower resistance to infection e. follow recommendations about ways to reduce the risk for developing osteoporosis if long-term corticosteroid use is expected (e.g., take calcium and vitamin D supplements, stop smoking, do 30–60 minutes of weight-bearing exercise each day if able). 6. If client is discharged on a beta-adrenergic agonist (e.g., albuterol, metaproterenol, terbutaline, salmeterol), instruct to: a. take oral preparations with meals to reduce gastric irritation b. expect that certain effects such as nervousness, restlessness, and slight tremor can occur c. report undesirable effects such as persistent or excessive nervousness, restlessness, tremors, headache, and gastric irritation; chest pain; vomiting; irregular heart beat; and wheezing. 7. Instruct client to take regularly scheduled medications as often as prescribed and to avoid skipping doses, altering prescribed dose, making up for missed doses, and discontinuing medication without permission of health care provider. 8. Reinforce instructions about the frequency and dosage of medications prescribed on an "as needed" basis. Emphasize that the client should not increase the frequency or dosage of these medications without permission from health care provider. 9. Instruct client to inform all health care providers of medications being taken. 10. Reinforce the need to consult physician before taking additional prescription and nonprescription medications.
8.f. The client will identify precautions that should be adhered to when using oxygen.	8.f.1. Instruct client about precautions that should be adhered to when using oxygen: a. do not smoke b. do not set oxygen flow rate at a level higher than prescribed by physician c. do not allow the oxygen system to be within 10 feet of an open flame (e.g., gas stove, kerosene heater or lamp, fireplace, candle) or source of spark (e.g., electric razor, portable radio, wool blanket, hair dryer) d. post "No Smoking" signs in and around areas of oxygen use e. ensure that all electrical equipment in the area of the oxygen source is grounded

f. always have a battery-operated oxygen delivery system readily available for use in case a power failure occurs
g. always wear a medical alert identification bracelet or tag to ensure that the appropriate oxygen flow rate is administered in emergency situations.

2. Instruct client in ways to prevent skin and mucous membrane irritation and breakdown resulting from use of oxygen and/or oxygen delivery devices:
   a. assess areas of skin and mucous membranes that are in contact with oxygen mask or nasal cannula (e.g., nares, bridge of nose, tops of ears) a few times each day for redness and irritation
   b. pad areas of pressure and ensure that straps are not too tight
   c. keep skin areas under straps and mask clean and dry
   d. refill oxygen humidification reservoir as needed, perform frequent oral hygiene, and apply water-based gel to nares and lips to reduce dryness of the mucous membranes.
3. Make sure the client knows how to recognize when the oxygen supply is low and how to get the oxygen source refilled or replaced.
4. Instruct client to have the oxygen delivery system checked regularly by the supplier.

8.g. The client will state signs and symptoms to report to the health care provider.

8.g. Instruct client to report:
1. changes in sputum characteristics (e.g., increase in volume or consistency, yellow or green color)
2. sputum that does not return to usual color after 3 days of antimicrobial therapy
3. cough that becomes worse
4. increased fatigue, weakness, and shortness of breath
5. increased need for medications and/or oxygen therapy
6. elevated temperature
7. drowsiness, confusion, new or increased irritability
8. chest pain
9. persistent weight loss or sudden weight gain
10. swelling in ankles and/or feet
11. signs and symptoms of theophylline toxicity and adverse effects of other medications (see actions e.3.c, e.4.c, e.5.c, and e.6.c in this diagnosis).

8.h. The client will identify resources that can assist with financial needs, home management, and adjustment to changes resulting from COPD.

8.h.1. Provide information regarding resources that can assist client and significant others with financial needs, home management, and adjustment to changes resulting from COPD (e.g., American Lung Association; respiratory equipment suppliers; pulmonary rehabilitation programs; counseling, vocational, and social services; Meals on Wheels; transportation services; home health agencies).
2. Initiate a referral if indicated.

8.i. The client will verbalize an understanding of and a plan for adhering to recommended follow-up care including future appointments with health care provider and graded exercise program.

8.i.1. Reinforce importance of lifelong follow-up care.
2. Reinforce physician's instructions about a graded exercise program (e.g., walking for 20 minutes 3 times a week, stationary bicycling).
3. Implement measures to promote effective therapeutic regimen management (see Diagnosis 7, action b).

ADDITIONAL NURSING DIAGNOSES

SELF-CARE DEFICIT

related to weakness, fatigue, and dyspnea.

DISTURBED SLEEP PATTERN*

related to fear, anxiety, unfamiliar environment, excessive coughing, frequent assessments and treatments, side effects of medications (e.g., some bronchodilators, corticosteroids), and inability to assume usual sleep position associated with orthopnea.

DISTURBED SELF-CONCEPT*

related to:

a. change in appearance (e.g., "barrel" chest, clubbing of fingers, retraction of tissues around the neck and shoulders);
b. dependence on others to meet self-care needs;
c. possible alteration in sexual functioning (may result from dyspnea, weakness, fatigue, and persistent cough);
d. stigma associated with chronic illness;
e. possible changes in lifestyle and roles.

RISK FOR POWERLESSNESS

related to physical limitations; disease progression despite efforts to comply with treatment plan; dependence on others to meet self-care needs; and alterations in roles, lifestyle, and future plans.

*See Unit II for outcomes, actions, and rationales.

Bibliography

See pages 879 and 882–883.

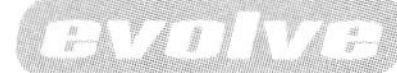

Pneumonia

Pneumonia or pneumonitis is an acute inflammation of lung tissue that can be caused by a variety of infectious agents, chemical irritants, or radiation therapy. Infectious organisms that cause pneumonia reach the lungs by inhalation, aspiration of nasopharyngeal or oropharyngeal contents, or by hematogenous spread of infection from another site in the body.

Pneumonia may be classified according to the causative organism (e.g., pneumococcal pneumonia, staphylococcal pneumonia, viral pneumonia), the area of involvement (e.g., lobar pneumonia), or the etiological factor (e.g., aspiration pneumonia, radiation pneumonitis). Pneumonia may also be classified as community-acquired pneumonia (CAP) or hospital-acquired pneumonia (HAP), the latter often referred to as nosocomial.

The majority of persons hospitalized with pneumonia have bacterial pneumonia. The onset of bacterial pneumonia is often abrupt and manifested by chills, fever, a cough productive of purulent or blood-tinged sputum, and pleuritic chest pain (in some cases). Elderly persons, who often have impaired immune mechanisms, may present with a change in mental status and a recent history of weakness, fatigue, and a decline in appetite rather than the symptoms of typical pneumonia.

This care plan focuses on the adult client hospitalized with bacterial pneumonia. Much of the information is applicable to clients receiving follow-up care in an extended care facility or home setting.

OUTCOME/DISCHARGE CRITERIA

THE CLIENT WILL:

- have improved respiratory function
- tolerate expected level of activity
- have no signs and symptoms of complications
- identify ways to maintain respiratory health
- state signs and symptoms to report to the health care provider
- verbalize an understanding of and a plan for adhering to recommended follow-up care including future appointments with health care provider, medications prescribed, and activity limitations.

NURSING/COLLABORATIVE DIAGNOSES

DISCHARGE TEACHING

See p. 466 for additional diagnoses.

1. Nursing Diagnosis: *IMPAIRED RESPIRATORY FUNCTION**

a. ineffective breathing pattern related to:
   1. decreased depth of respirations associated with:
      a. weakness, fatigue, and reluctance to breathe deeply because of chest pain
      b. decreased lung compliance (distensibility) if pleural effusion is present
   2. increased rate of respirations associated with:
      a. compensation for hypoxia that results from impaired gas exchange
      b. the increase in metabolic rate that occurs with an infectious process;

b. ineffective airway clearance related to:
   1. tracheobronchial inflammation and increased production of mucus associated with the infectious process
   2. stasis of secretions associated with decreased activity, poor cough effort resulting from fatigue and chest pain, and impaired ciliary function (results from the increased viscosity and volume of mucus that occurs with the infectious process);

c. impaired gas exchange related to a decrease in effective lung surface associated with the accumulation of mucus and consolidation of lung tissue.

*This diagnostic label includes the following nursing diagnoses: ineffective breathing pattern, ineffective airway clearance, and impaired gas exchange.

Suggested NOC Outcomes: Respiratory status: airway patency; Respiratory status: ventilation; Respiratory status: gas exchange

Suggested NIC Interventions: Respiratory monitoring; Airway management; Chest physiotherapy; Cough enhancement; Oxygen therapy; Medication administration; Ventilation assistance

Desired Outcome

1. The client will experience adequate respiratory function as evidenced by:
   a. normal rate and depth of respirations
   b. decreased dyspnea
   c. improved breath sounds
   d. symmetrical chest excursion
   e. usual mental status
   f. oximetry results within normal range
   g. blood gases within normal range.

Nursing Actions *and Selected Purposes/Rationales*

(see pp. 12–14, 18–20, and 33–35 for additional rationales)

1.a. Assess for and report signs and symptoms of impaired respiratory function:
   1. rapid, shallow respirations
   2. dyspnea, orthopnea
   3. use of accessory muscles when breathing
   4. abnormal breath sounds (e.g., diminished, bronchial, crackles [rales], wheezes)
   5. asymmetrical or limited chest excursion
   6. cough (usually a productive cough of rust-colored, purulent, or blood-tinged sputum)
   7. restlessness, irritability
   8. confusion, somnolence
   9. significant decrease in oximetry results
   10. abnormal blood gases
   11. abnormal chest x-ray results.

b. Implement measures *to improve respiratory status:*
   1. maintain client on bed rest as ordered during the acute phase *to reduce oxygen needs*
   2. place client in a semi- to high Fowler's position unless contraindicated; position with pillows *to prevent slumping*
   3. instruct client to breathe slowly if hyperventilating
   4. if client must remain flat in bed, assist with position change at least every 2 hours
   5. instruct client to deep breathe or use incentive spirometer every 1–2 hours
   6. assist with positive airway pressure techniques (e.g., continuous positive airway pressure [CPAP], bilevel positive airway pressure [BiPAP], flutter/positive expiratory pressure [PEP] device) if ordered

7. perform actions *to promote removal of pulmonary secretions:*
   a. instruct and assist client to cough or "huff" every 1–2 hours
   b. implement measures *to thin tenacious secretions and reduce dryness of the respiratory mucous membrane:*
      1. maintain a fluid intake of at least 2500 ml/day unless contraindicated
      2. humidify inspired air as ordered
   c. assist with administration of mucolytics (e.g., acetylcysteine) and diluent or hydrating agents (e.g., water, saline) via nebulizer if ordered
   d. assist with or perform postural drainage therapy (PDT) if ordered
   e. perform suctioning if ordered
   f. administer expectorants (e.g., guaifenesin) if ordered
8. perform actions to reduce chest pain (see Diagnosis 4, action d) *in order to increase client's willingness to move, cough, and deep breathe*
9. maintain oxygen therapy as ordered
10. discourage smoking *(the irritants in smoke increase mucus production, impair ciliary function, and can cause inflammation and damage to the bronchial and alveolar walls; the carbon monoxide decreases oxygen availability)*
11. perform actions to increase strength and activity tolerance (see Diagnosis 7, action b) *in order to increase client's willingness and ability to move, cough, and deep breathe*
12. administer central nervous system depressants judiciously; hold medication and consult physician if respiratory rate is less than 12/minute
13. administer the following medications if ordered:
    a. bronchodilators (e.g., methylxanthines, sympathomimetic [adrenergic] agents)
    b. antimicrobials.

c. Consult appropriate health care provider (e.g., respiratory therapist, physician) if signs and symptoms of impaired respiratory function persist or worsen.

2. NURSING DIAGNOSIS: RISK FOR DEFICIENT FLUID VOLUME

related to decreased oral intake and excessive fluid loss (occurs with profuse diaphoresis and hyperventilation if present).

Suggested NOC Outcomes: Fluid balance; Hydration

Suggested NIC Interventions: Fluid monitoring; Fluid management; Intravenous (IV) therapy

Desired Outcome

2. The client will not experience a deficient fluid volume as evidenced by:
   a. normal skin turgor
   b. moist mucous membranes
   c. stable weight
   d. B/P and pulse within normal range for client and stable with position change
   e. capillary refill time less than 2–3 seconds
   f. usual mental status
   g. BUN and Hct within normal range
   h. balanced intake and output
   i. urine specific gravity within normal range.

Nursing Actions *and Selected Purposes/Rationales*

(see pp. 30–31 for additional rationales)

2.a. Assess for and report signs and symptoms of deficient fluid volume:
   1. decreased skin turgor
   2. dry mucous membranes, thirst
   3. weight loss of 2% or greater in a short period
   4. postural hypotension and/or low B/P
   5. weak, rapid pulse
   6. capillary refill time greater than 2–3 seconds
   7. flat neck veins when supine
   8. change in mental status
   9. elevated BUN and Hct
   10. decreased urine output with increased specific gravity (reflects an actual rather than potential fluid volume deficit).

b. Implement measures *to prevent deficient fluid volume:*
   1. perform actions to improve oral intake (see Diagnosis 3, action c.1)
   2. perform actions to reduce fever and resolve the infectious process (see Diagnosis 6, action b) *in order to reduce fluid loss resulting from the diaphoresis and hyperventilation that may accompany an acute infection*

Desired Outcome	Nursing Actions *and Selected Purposes/Rationales*
	3. maintain a fluid intake of at least 2500 ml/day unless contraindicated; if oral intake is inadequate or contraindicated, maintain intravenous and/or enteral fluid therapy as ordered.

3. Nursing Diagnosis: IMBALANCED NUTRITION: LESS THAN BODY REQUIREMENTS

related to:
a. decreased oral intake associated with weakness, fatigue, dyspnea, excessive coughing, and the foul odor and taste of sputum and some aerosol treatments;
b. increased nutritional needs associated with the increase in metabolic rate that occurs with an infectious process.

Suggested NOC Outcome: Nutritional status

Suggested NIC Interventions: Nutritional monitoring; Nutrition management; Nutrition therapy

Desired Outcome	Nursing Actions *and Selected Purposes/Rationales* (see pp. 40–43 for additional rationales)
3. The client will maintain an adequate nutritional status as evidenced by: a. weight within normal range for client b. normal BUN and serum albumin, prealbumin, Hct, and Hgb c. usual strength and activity tolerance d. healthy oral mucous membrane.	3.a. Assess for and report signs and symptoms of malnutrition: 1. weight significantly below client's usual weight or below normal for client's age, height, and body frame 2. abnormal BUN and low serum albumin, prealbumin, Hct, and Hgb 3. increased weakness and fatigue 4. sore, inflamed oral mucous membrane 5. pale conjunctiva. b. Monitor percentage of meals and snacks client consumes. Report a pattern of inadequate intake. c. Implement measures *to maintain an adequate nutritional status:* 1. perform actions *to improve oral intake:* a. consult respiratory therapist about scheduling respiratory treatments at least 1 hour before mealtime *(the foul odor and taste of sputum and some aerosols is likely to decrease appetite)* b. increase activity as allowed and tolerated *(activity usually promotes a sense of well-being, which can improve appetite)* c. obtain a dietary consult if necessary to assist client in selecting foods/fluids that meet nutritional needs, are appealing, and adhere to personal and cultural preferences whenever possible d. encourage a rest period before meals *to minimize fatigue* e. maintain a clean environment and a relaxed, pleasant atmosphere f. assist with oral hygiene before meals *(oral hygiene moistens the mouth, which makes it easier to chew and swallow; it also removes unpleasant tastes, which often improves the taste of foods/fluids)* g. place client in a high Fowler's position for meals and provide supplemental oxygen therapy during meals if indicated *to help relieve dyspnea* h. serve frequent, small meals rather than large ones if client is weak, fatigues easily, or has a poor appetite i. allow adequate time for meals; reheat foods/fluids if necessary 2. ensure that meals are well balanced and high in essential nutrients; offer dietary supplements if indicated 3. administer vitamins and minerals if ordered. d. Perform a calorie count if ordered. Report information to dietitian and physician. e. Consult physician about an alternative method of providing nutrition (e.g., parenteral nutrition, tube feedings) if client does not consume enough food or fluids to meet nutritional needs.

4. NURSING DIAGNOSIS: ACUTE PAIN: CHEST

related to:
a. extension of the inflammatory/infectious process to the pleura;
b. muscle strain associated with excessive coughing.

Suggested NOC Outcomes: Comfort level; Pain control

Suggested NIC Interventions: Pain management; Environmental management: comfort; Analgesic administration

Desired Outcome	**Nursing Actions** *and Selected Purposes/Rationales* (see pp. 45–47 for additional rationales)
4. The client will experience diminished chest pain as evidenced by: a. verbalization of a decrease in or absence of pain b. relaxed facial expression and body positioning c. increased participation in activities.	4.a. Assess for signs and symptoms of pain (e.g., verbalization of pain, grimacing, reluctance to move, restlessness, guarding of affected side of chest). b. Assess client's perception of the severity of pain using a pain intensity rating scale. c. Assess the client's pain pattern (e.g., location, quality, onset, duration, precipitating factors, aggravating factors, alleviating factors). d. Implement measures *to reduce chest pain:* 1. perform actions *to reduce fear and anxiety about the pain experience* (e.g., assure client that chest pain is common with pneumonia and should subside with treatment of the pneumonia, assure client that his/her need for pain relief is understood) 2. administer analgesics prior to any painful procedures (e.g., transtracheal sputum aspiration) 3. instruct and assist client to splint chest with hands or pillow when deep breathing, coughing, or changing position 4. perform actions to promote rest (see Diagnosis 7, action b.1) *in order to reduce fatigue and subsequently increase the client's threshold and tolerance for pain* 5. provide or assist with nonpharmacologic methods for pain relief (e.g., position change, relaxation techniques, restful environment, diversional activities) 6. perform actions to decrease excessive coughing (see Diagnosis 7, action b.1.j) 7. administer analgesics if ordered. e. Consult appropriate health care provider (e.g., pharmacist, physician) if above actions fail to provide adequate relief of chest pain.

5. NURSING DIAGNOSIS: ALTERED COMFORT: CHILLS AND EXCESSIVE DIAPHORESIS

related to persistent fever associated with the infectious process.

Suggested NOC Outcome: Symptom control

Suggested NIC Interventions: Environmental management: comfort; Fever treatment

Desired Outcome	**Nursing Actions** *and Selected Purposes/Rationales*
5. The client will not experience discomfort associated with chills and excessive diaphoresis as evidenced by: a. verbalization of comfort b. ability to rest.	5.a. Assess client for chills and excessive diaphoresis. b. Implement measures to reduce fever (see Diagnosis 6, action b). c. Implement measures *to promote comfort if client is having chills:* 1. maintain a room temperature that is comfortable for client 2. protect client from drafts 3. provide extra blankets and clothing as needed 4. provide warm liquids to drink. d. Implement measures *to promote comfort if excessive diaphoresis is present:* 1. change linen and clothing whenever damp 2. bathe client and sponge his/her face as needed. e. Consult physician if client continues to have chills and excessive diaphoresis.

6. Nursing Diagnosis: *HYPERTHERMIA*

related to stimulation of the thermoregulatory center in the hypothalamus by endogenous pyrogens that are released in an infectious process.

Suggested NOC Outcome: Thermoregulation

Suggested NIC Intervention: Fever treatment

Desired Outcome	**Nursing Actions** *and Selected Purposes/Rationales*
6. The client will experience resolution of hyperthermia as evidenced by: a. skin usual temperature and color b. pulse rate between 60–100 beats/minute c. respirations 12–20/minute d. normal body temperature.	6.a. Assess for signs and symptoms of hyperthermia (e.g., warm, flushed skin; tachycardia; tachypnea; elevated temperature). b. Implement measures *to reduce fever:* 1. perform actions *to resolve the infectious process:* a. implement measures to promote removal of pulmonary secretions (see Diagnosis 1, action b.7) b. implement measures to promote rest and/or conserve energy (see Diagnosis 7, action b.1) c. implement measures to maintain an adequate nutritional status (see Diagnosis 3, action c) d. administer antimicrobials as ordered 2. administer tepid sponge bath and/or apply cool cloths to groin and axillae 3. apply cooling blanket if ordered 4. utilize a room fan *to provide cool circulating air* 5. administer antipyretics if ordered. c. Consult physician if temperature remains elevated.

7. Nursing Diagnosis: *ACTIVITY INTOLERANCE*

related to:

a. tissue hypoxia associated with impaired gas exchange;
b. difficulty resting and sleeping associated with excessive coughing, dyspnea, discomfort, unfamiliar environment, anxiety, and frequent assessments and treatments;
c. inadequate nutritional status;
d. increased energy expenditure associated with persistent coughing and the increased metabolic rate that is present in an infectious process.

Suggested NOC Outcomes: Energy conservation; Rest; Activity tolerance

Suggested NIC Interventions: Energy management; Oxygen therapy; Sleep enhancement; Nutrition management; Infection control

Desired Outcome	**Nursing Actions** *and Selected Purposes/Rationales* (see pp. 11–12 for additional rationales)
7. The client will demonstrate an increased tolerance for activity as evidenced by: a. verbalization of feeling less fatigued and weak b. ability to perform activities of daily living without dizziness; increased dyspnea, chest pain, and diaphoresis; and a significant change in vital signs.	7.a. Assess for signs and symptoms of activity intolerance: 1. statements of fatigue or weakness 2. exertional dyspnea, chest pain, diaphoresis, or dizziness 3. abnormal heart rate response to activity (e.g., increase in rate of 20 beats/minute above resting rate, rate not returning to preactivity level within 3 minutes after stopping activity, change from regular to irregular rate) 4. a significant change (15–20 mm Hg) in blood pressure with activity. b. Implement measures *to improve activity tolerance:* 1. perform actions *to promote rest and/or conserve energy:* a. maintain activity restrictions as ordered b. minimize environmental activity and noise c. organize nursing care to allow for periods of uninterrupted rest d. limit the number of visitors and their length of stay e. assist client with self-care activities as needed f. keep supplies and personal articles within easy reach

g. instruct client in energy-saving techniques (e.g., using shower chair when showering, sitting to brush teeth or comb hair)
h. implement measures *to promote sleep* (e.g., elevate head of bed and support arms on pillows to facilitate breathing, maintain oxygen therapy during sleep, discourage intake of fluids high in caffeine in the evening, reduce environmental stimuli, administer prescribed sedative-hypnotics)
i. implement measures to reduce discomfort (see Diagnoses 4, action d and 5, actions c and d)
j. implement measures *to decrease excessive coughing:*
   1. protect client from exposure to irritants such as smoke, flowers, and powder
   2. instruct client to avoid intake of extremely hot or cold foods/fluids *(these can stimulate cough)*
   3. administer prescribed antitussives if indicated (when cough is productive, antitussives should be used only when coughing is excessive and interfering significantly with the client's ability to rest and sleep)

2. perform actions to reduce fever and resolve the infectious process (see Diagnosis 6, action b) *in order to lower the metabolic rate*
3. discourage smoking and excessive intake of beverages high in caffeine such as coffee, tea, and colas *(nicotine and caffeine can increase cardiac workload and myocardial oxygen utilization, thereby decreasing oxygen availability)*
4. perform actions to improve respiratory status (see Diagnosis 1, action b) *in order to relieve dyspnea and improve tissue oxygenation*
5. if oxygen therapy is necessary during activity, keep portable oxygen equipment readily available for client's use
6. perform actions to maintain an adequate nutritional status (see Diagnosis 3, action c)
7. increase client's activity gradually as allowed and tolerated.

c. Instruct client to:
   1. report a decreased tolerance for activity
   2. stop any activity that causes increased chest pain, increased shortness of breath, dizziness, or extreme fatigue or weakness.

d. Consult appropriate health care provider (e.g., respiratory therapist, physician) if signs and symptoms of activity intolerance persist or worsen.

8. NURSING DIAGNOSIS:

RISK FOR INFECTION: EXTRAPULMONARY (E.G., BACTEREMIA, PERICARDITIS, ENDOCARDITIS, MENINGITIS, SEPTIC ARTHRITIS) AND/OR SUPERINFECTION (E.G., CANDIDIASIS)

related to:
a. spread of infecting organism into the blood and to other sites associated with inadequate host defenses and resistance to antimicrobial agents;
b. interruption in the balance of usual endogenous microbial flora associated with the administration of antimicrobial agents.

Suggested NOC Outcomes: Immune status; Infection severity

Suggested NIC Interventions: Infection protection; Infection control

Desired Outcome	**Nursing Actions** *and Selected Purposes/Rationales* (see pp. 37–40 for additional rationales)
8. The client will not develop an extrapulmonary infection or a superinfection as evidenced by: a. gradual return of vital signs to normal	8.a. Assess for and report signs and symptoms of an extrapulmonary infection or a superinfection: 1. increase in temperature and pulse above previous levels 2. change in mental status 3. pericardial friction rub, precordial pain, or development of a pathologic murmur 4. swollen, red, painful joints

Desired Outcome	Nursing Actions *and Selected Purposes/Rationales*
b. usual mental status c. absence of a pericardial friction rub, precordial pain, and a pathologic murmur d. absence of joint pain and swelling e. absence of unusual drainage from any body cavity f. absence of white patches and ulcerations in mouth g. absence of stiff neck and headache h. WBC and differential counts returning toward normal range for client.	5. unusual color, amount, and odor of vaginal drainage; perineal itching; white patches or ulcerated areas in the mouth *(fungal infections are common superinfections with antimicrobial therapy)* 6. stiff neck, headache 7. increase in WBC count above previous levels and/or significant change in differential. b. Implement measures *to prevent an extrapulmonary infection and/or a superinfection:* 1. perform actions to resolve the infectious process (see Diagnosis 6, action b.1) 2. use good hand hygiene and encourage client to do the same 3. maintain sterile technique during all invasive procedures (e.g., urinary catheterizations, venous and arterial punctures, injections) 4. change peripheral intravenous line sites according to hospital policy 5. protect client from others with infection 6. anchor catheters/tubings (e.g., urinary, intravenous) securely *in order to reduce trauma to the tissues and the risk for introduction of pathogens associated with in-and-out movement of the tubing* 7. change equipment, tubings, and solutions used for treatments such as intravenous infusions and respiratory care according to hospital policy 8. maintain a closed system for drains (e.g., urinary catheter) and intravenous infusions whenever possible 9. instruct and assist client to perform good perineal care routinely and after each bowel movement 10. reinforce importance of frequent oral hygiene. c. If signs and symptoms of an extrapulmonary infection or a superinfection occur: 1. prepare client for and/or assist with diagnostic tests (e.g., lumbar puncture, cultures, joint aspiration) if planned 2. implement appropriate comfort measures for symptoms experienced 3. administer antimicrobials as ordered.

9. Collaborative Diagnoses: *POTENTIAL COMPLICATIONS OF PNEUMONIA*

a. pleural effusion related to an increase in capillary permeability of pulmonary and pleural vessels associated with the inflammatory process;
b. atelectasis related to shallow respirations and stasis of secretions in the alveoli and bronchioles.

Desired Outcomes	Nursing Actions *and Selected Purposes/Rationales*
9.a. The client will not develop pleural effusion as evidenced by: 1. no increase in dyspnea 2. symmetrical chest excursion 3. improved breath sounds and percussion note throughout lung fields.	9.a.1. Assess for and report signs and symptoms of pleural effusion: a. increased dyspnea b. decreased chest excursion on affected side c. dull percussion note and diminished or absent breath sounds over affected area d. chest x-ray, ultrasound, or computed tomography results showing pleural effusion. 2. Implement measures to resolve the infectious process (see Diagnosis 6, action b.1) *in order to reduce the risk for development of pleural effusion.* 3. If signs and symptoms of pleural effusion occur: a. continue with actions to improve respiratory status (see Diagnosis 1, action b) b. prepare client for a thoracentesis if planned.

9.b. The client will not develop atelectasis as evidenced by:
1. improved breath sounds and percussion note over lungs
2. no increase in dyspnea, respiratory rate, or temperature.

9.b.1. Assess for and report signs and symptoms of atelectasis (e.g., diminished or absent breath sounds; dull percussion note over affected area; further increase in respiratory rate, dyspnea, and temperature; chest x-ray results showing atelectasis).
2. Implement measures to improve respiratory status (see Diagnosis 1, action b) *in order to reduce the risk for atelectasis.*
3. If signs and symptoms of atelectasis occur:
   a. increase frequency of position change, coughing or "huffing," deep breathing, and use of incentive spirometer
   b. increase activity as allowed and tolerated
   c. consult physician if signs and symptoms of atelectasis persist or worsen.

Discharge Teaching/Continued Care

10. NURSING DIAGNOSIS: *DEFICIENT KNOWLEDGE, INEFFECTIVE THERAPEUTIC REGIMEN MANAGEMENT, OR INEFFECTIVE HEALTH MAINTENANCE**

*The nurse should select the diagnostic label that is most appropriate for the client's discharge teaching needs.

Suggested NOC Outcomes: Knowledge: disease process; Knowledge: treatment regimen; Knowledge: infection control

Suggested NIC Interventions: Health system guidance; Teaching: individual; Teaching: disease process; Teaching: prescribed medication

Desired Outcomes	Nursing Actions *and Selected Purposes/Rationales*

10.a. The client will identify ways to maintain respiratory health.

10.a. Instruct client in ways to maintain respiratory health:
1. consume a well-balanced diet
2. drink at least 10 glasses of liquid/day unless contraindicated
3. maintain a balanced program of rest and exercise
4. avoid crowds during flu and cold season
5. avoid contact with persons who have respiratory infections
6. consult physician about vaccinations available if at high risk for recurrent pneumonia
7. continue coughing and deep breathing exercises for at least a few weeks after discharge and during any period of decreased physical activity or respiratory infection
8. maintain good oral hygiene in order to reduce the number of organisms in the oropharynx
9. avoid excessive alcohol intake and stop smoking to prevent depression of pulmonary antimicrobial defenses
10. avoid exposure to respiratory irritants (e.g., smoke and other environmental pollutants).

10.b. The client will state signs and symptoms to report to the health care provider.

10.b. Instruct client to report the following signs and symptoms:
1. persistent or recurrent temperature elevation
2. chills
3. difficulty breathing
4. restlessness, irritability, drowsiness, or confusion
5. persistent or increased chest pain
6. persistent weight loss
7. persistent fatigue
8. persistent cough
9. unusual color, amount, and odor of vaginal secretions; white patches or ulcerated areas in the mouth; stiff neck and headache; or swollen,

Desired Outcomes	Nursing Actions *and Selected Purposes/Rationales*
	red, painful joints (indicative of superinfection or extension of infection to another site).
10.c. The client will verbalize an understanding of and a plan for adhering to recommended follow-up care including future appointments with health care provider, medications prescribed, and activity limitations.	10.c.1. Reinforce the importance of keeping follow-up appointments with health care provider. 2. Explain the rationale for, side effects of, and importance of taking medications prescribed (e.g., antimicrobials). Inform client of pertinent food and drug interactions. 3. Implement measures to improve client compliance: a. include significant others in all discharge teaching sessions if possible b. encourage questions and allow time for reinforcement and clarification of information provided c. provide written instructions regarding scheduled appointments with health care provider, medications prescribed, fluid requirements, respiratory care, and signs and symptoms to report.

Additional Nursing Diagnoses

NAUSEA

related to stimulation of the vomiting center associated with noxious stimuli (e.g., foul taste of sputum and some aerosol treatments, sight of sputum).

*DISTURBED SLEEP PATTERN**

related to unfamiliar environment, discomfort, excessive coughing, anxiety, inability to assume usual sleep position because of dyspnea, and frequent assessments and treatments.

*FEAR/ANXIETY**

related to severity of symptoms (e.g., cough, chest pain, shortness of breath) and need for hospitalization, unfamiliar environment, and separation from significant others.

*See Unit II for outcomes, actions, and rationales.

Bibliography

See pages 879 and 882–883.

PNEUMOTHORAX

Pneumothorax occurs when air accumulates in the pleural space and causes complete or partial collapse of a lung. Clinical manifestations vary with the degree of lung collapse but usually include sudden onset of unilateral sharp chest pain, tachypnea, dyspnea, anxiety, agitation, absent or diminished breath sounds, and tachycardia. When the pneumothorax is symptomatic and involves greater than 15% of the lung tissue, it is usually treated with placement of a chest tube into the intrapleural space. The tube is then connected to suction through a closed water-seal drainage system or, less frequently, to a flutter (Heimlich) valve to evacuate the intrapleural air, re-establish negative intrapleural pressure, and re-expand the lung. Following lung re-expansion, obliteration of the pleural space may be necessary in some situations to minimize the risk of a recurrent pneumothorax. Methods for accomplishing this include chemical or mechanical pleurodesis, partial pleurectomy, or pleural stapling.

A pneumothorax can be classified in a variety of ways (e.g., open, closed, iatrogenic, spontaneous [primary, secondary], traumatic [penetrating, blunt]). An open pneumothorax occurs when air enters the pleural space through an opening in the chest wall. This opening can result from a penetrating injury (e.g., gun shot wound, stab wound), surgery involving the chest or diaphragm, or a complication of a diagnostic or therapeutic procedure (e.g., thoracentesis, lung biopsy, insertion of a pacemaker, subclavian venipuncture).

A closed pneumothorax occurs when air enters the pleural space without evidence of an external wound. The most common type of closed pneumothorax occurs in the absence of obvious respiratory disease and is often referred to as a primary spontaneous pneumothorax. Persons at greatest risk for this are men who are tall, 20–40 years of age, smokers, and have a family history of spontaneous pneumothorax. Other causes of a closed pneumothorax include damage to lung tissue as a result of a complication of pulmonary disease (e.g., COPD, cystic fibrosis, lung cancer, tuberculosis), mechanical ventilation, a fractured rib, and migration of a subclavian catheter or pacemaker lead.

This care plan focuses on the adult client hospitalized for diagnosis and treatment of a pneumothorax.

OUTCOME/DISCHARGE CRITERIA

THE CLIENT WILL:

- experience re-expansion of affected lung
- have adequate respiratory function
- identify safety measures related to care of chest tube insertion site and flutter valve (if present)
- identify ways to reduce the risk of another pneumothorax
- state signs and symptoms to report to the health care provider
- verbalize an understanding of and a plan for adhering to recommended follow-up care including future appointments with health care provider and activity restrictions.

NURSING/COLLABORATIVE DIAGNOSES

DISCHARGE TEACHING

1. NURSING DIAGNOSIS: *INEFFECTIVE BREATHING PATTERN*

related to:

a. increased rate of respirations associated with fear and anxiety;
b. decreased rate of respirations associated with the depressant effect of some medications (e.g., narcotic [opioid] analgesics);
c. decreased depth of respirations associated with:
   1. reluctance to breathe deeply resulting from chest pain and fear of dislodging chest tube or experiencing another pneumothorax
   2. complete or partial collapse of the lung
   3. anxiety and the depressant effect of some medications (e.g., narcotic [opioid] analgesics).

Suggested NOC Outcome:
Respiratory status: ventilation

Suggested NIC Interventions: Respiratory monitoring; Ventilation assistance; Anxiety management; Pain management

Desired Outcome	**Nursing Actions** *and Selected Purposes/Rationales* (see pp. 18–20 for additional rationales)
1. The client will experience an effective breathing pattern as evidenced by: a. normal rate and depth of respirations b. decreased dyspnea c. symmetrical chest excursion.	1.a. Assess for signs and symptoms of an ineffective breathing pattern (e.g., shallow respirations, tachypnea, dyspnea, asymmetrical chest excursion, use of accessory muscles when breathing). b. Implement measures *to improve breathing pattern:* 1. perform actions to reduce chest pain (see Diagnosis 3, action d) *in order to increase the client's willingness to move and breathe more deeply* 2. perform actions to reduce fear and anxiety (see Diagnosis 5, action b) *in order to prevent the shallow and/or rapid breathing that can occur with fear and anxiety* 3. place client in semi- to high Fowler's position unless contraindicated; position with pillows *to prevent slumping* 4. instruct client to deep breathe or use incentive spirometer every 1–2 hours 5. assure client that deep breathing and turning should not dislodge the chest tube or increase the risk of another pneumothorax 6. instruct client to breathe slowly if hyperventilating 7. increase activity as allowed and tolerated 8. administer central nervous system depressants judiciously; hold medication and consult physician if respiratory rate is less than 12/minute. c. Consult appropriate health care provider (e.g., respiratory therapist, physician) if ineffective breathing pattern continues.

2. Nursing Diagnosis: *IMPAIRED GAS EXCHANGE*

related to loss of effective lung surface associated with partial or complete lung collapse.

Suggested NOC Outcome:
Respiratory status: gas exchange

Suggested NIC Interventions: Respiratory monitoring; Oxygen therapy; Tube care: chest; Acid-base management

Desired Outcome	**Nursing Actions** *and Selected Purposes/Rationales* (see pp. 33–35 for additional rationales)
2. The client will experience adequate O_2/CO_2 exchange as evidenced by: a. usual mental status b. unlabored respirations at 12–20/minute c. oximetry results within normal range d. blood gases within normal range.	2.a. Assess for and report signs and symptoms of impaired gas exchange: 1. restlessness, irritability 2. confusion, somnolence 3. tachypnea, dyspnea 4. a significant decrease in oximetry results 5. decreased PaO_2 and/or increased $PaCO_2$. b. Implement measures *to improve gas exchange:* 1. perform actions *to promote lung re-expansion:* a. prepare client for and assist with insertion of chest tube (the tube is then connected to a drainage system [with or without suction] or, less commonly, to a flutter valve) b. following chest tube insertion, implement measures *to maintain patency and integrity of chest drainage system:* 1. maintain fluid level in water seal and suction chambers as ordered 2. maintain occlusive dressing over chest tube insertion site 3. tape all connections securely

4. tape the tubing to the chest wall close to insertion site *in order to reduce the risk of inadvertent removal of the tube*
5. position tubing *to promote optimum drainage* (e.g., coil excess tubing on bed rather than allowing it to hang down below the collection device, keep tubing free of kinks)
6. drain fluid that accumulates in tubing into the collection chamber; milk chest tube only if ordered
7. keep drainage collection device below level of client's chest at all times

c. perform actions *to facilitate the escape of air from the pleural space* (e.g., maintain suction as ordered; ensure that the air vent is open on the drainage collection device if system is to water seal only; if a flutter valve is present, ensure that there is no fluid in the valve and that the distal end is open)

2. perform actions to improve breathing pattern (see Diagnosis 1, action b)
3. maintain oxygen therapy as ordered
4. discourage smoking *(the irritants in smoke can damage the bronchial and alveolar walls; the carbon monoxide decreases oxygen availability)*
5. maintain activity restrictions as ordered; increase activity gradually as allowed and tolerated
6. following lung re-expansion, assist with pleurodesis, pleurectomy, or pleural stapling if planned *(may be done to reduce the risk of a recurrent closed pneumothorax)*.

c. Consult appropriate health care provider (e.g., respiratory therapist, physician) if signs and symptoms of impaired gas exchange persist or worsen.

3. NURSING DIAGNOSIS:

ACUTE PAIN: CHEST

related to:

a. irritation of the parietal pleura associated with:
   1. stretching of the pleura resulting from air in the pleural space
   2. inflammatory process if pleurodesis is performed;

b. tissue irritation associated with insertion and presence of chest tube.

Suggested NOC Outcomes: Pain control; Comfort level

Suggested NIC Interventions: Pain management; Analgesic administration

Desired Outcome	**Nursing Actions** *and Selected Purposes/Rationales* (see pp. 45–47 for additional rationales)
3. The client will experience diminished chest pain as evidenced by: a. verbalization of a decrease in or absence of pain b. relaxed facial expression and body positioning c. improved breathing pattern d. increased participation in activities e. stable vital signs.	3.a. Assess for signs and symptoms of chest pain (e.g., verbalization of pain, grimacing, rubbing chest, guarding of affected side of chest, reluctance to move, shallow respirations, restlessness, increased B/P, tachycardia). b. Assess client's perception of the severity of pain using a pain intensity rating scale. c. Assess the client's pain pattern (e.g., location, quality, onset, duration, precipitating factors, aggravating factors, alleviating factors). d. Implement measures *to reduce chest pain:* 1. perform actions to reduce fear and anxiety (see Diagnosis 5, action b) *in order to promote relaxation and subsequently increase the client's threshold and tolerance for pain* 2. perform actions to facilitate the escape of air from the pleural space (see Diagnosis 2, action b.1.c) *in order to reduce stretching of the parietal pleura* 3. administer analgesics before activities and procedures that can cause pain and before pain becomes severe 4. instruct and assist client to splint chest with hands or pillow when deep breathing, coughing, and changing position

Desired Outcome	Nursing Actions *and Selected Purposes/Rationales*
	5. provide or assist with nonpharmacologic methods for pain relief (e.g., position change; progressive relaxation exercises; restful environment; diversional activities such as watching television, reading, or conversing) 6. securely anchor chest tube *to limit its movement and resulting tissue irritation* 7. administer analgesics as ordered. e. Consult appropriate health care provider (e.g., pharmacist, pain management specialist, physician) if the above measures fail to provide adequate pain relief.

4. Collaborative Diagnosis:

POTENTIAL COMPLICATION OF PNEUMOTHORAX: TENSION PNEUMOTHORAX WITH MEDIASTINAL SHIFT

related to a significant increase in intrapleural pressure associated with inability of air to leave pleural space during expiration (can occur as a result of chest tube or flutter valve malfunction).

Desired Outcome	Nursing Actions *and Selected Purposes/Rationales*
4. The client will not develop tension pneumothorax with mediastinal shift as evidenced by: a. no sudden increase in dyspnea b. vital signs within normal range for client c. usual mental status d. absence of neck vein distention e. trachea in midline position f. usual skin color g. blood gases returning toward normal.	4.a. Assess for and immediately report signs and symptoms of: 1. malfunction of chest drainage system (e.g., respiratory distress, lack of fluctuation in the water seal chamber without evidence of lung re-expansion, excessive bubbling in water seal chamber, significant increase in subcutaneous emphysema) 2. malfunction of the flutter valve if present (e.g., respiratory distress, abrupt cessation of air flow from the distal end of the valve during exhalation) 3. extended pneumothorax (e.g., extended area of absent breath sounds with hyperresonant percussion note, increased dyspnea, chest x-ray showing an increase in size of pneumothorax) 4. tension pneumothorax (e.g., severe dyspnea, rapid and/or irregular heart rate, hypotension, restlessness, agitation, confusion, neck vein distention, shift in trachea from midline, blood gas values that have worsened, chest x-ray results showing a mediastinal shift). b. Implement measures to promote lung re-expansion (see Diagnosis 2, action b.1) *in order to reduce the risk of tension pneumothorax with mediastinal shift.* c. If signs and symptoms of tension pneumothorax with mediastinal shift occur: 1. maintain client on bed rest in a semi- to high Fowler's position 2. maintain oxygen therapy as ordered 3. assist with clearing of existing chest tube or flutter valve, insertion of new tube, and/or needle aspiration of air from the pleural space *to reduce intrapleural pressure.*

5. Nursing Diagnosis:

FEAR/ANXIETY

related to difficulty breathing; chest pain; unfamiliar environment; lack of understanding of diagnostic tests, diagnosis, and treatment measures; and possibility of recurrence of pneumothorax.

Suggested NOC Outcomes: Anxiety level; Fear level; Anxiety self-control; Fear self-control

Suggested NIC Interventions: Anxiety reduction; Calming technique; Emotional support; Presence; Pain management

Desired Outcome	Nursing Actions *and Selected Purposes/Rationales* (see pp. 14–16 for additional rationales)
5. The client will experience a reduction in fear and anxiety as evidenced by: a. verbalization of feeling less anxious b. usual sleep pattern c. relaxed facial expression and body movements d. stable vital signs e. usual perceptual ability and interactions with others.	5.a. Assess client for signs and symptoms of fear and anxiety (e.g., verbalization of feeling anxious, insomnia, tenseness, shakiness, restlessness, diaphoresis, tachycardia, elevated blood pressure, self-focused behaviors). Validate perceptions carefully, remembering that some behaviors may be the result of tissue hypoxia and respiratory distress. b. Implement measures *to reduce fear and anxiety:* 1. orient client to hospital environment, equipment, and routines 2. introduce client to staff who will be participating in care; if possible, maintain consistency in staff assigned to his/her care 3. assure client that staff members are nearby; respond to call signal as soon as possible 4. maintain a calm, supportive, confident manner when interacting with client 5. encourage verbalization of fear and anxiety; provide feedback 6. explain all diagnostic tests 7. reinforce physician's explanations and clarify misconceptions the client has about the pneumothorax, treatment plan, and possible recurrence 8. perform actions to reduce chest pain (see Diagnosis 3, action d) 9. perform actions to improve gas exchange (see Diagnosis 2, action b) *in order to relieve respiratory distress* 10. provide a calm, restful environment 11. instruct client in relaxation techniques and encourage participation in diversional activities once the period of acute pain and respiratory distress has subsided 12. provide information based on current needs of client and significant others at a level he/she can understand; encourage questions and clarification of information provided 13. encourage significant others to project a caring, concerned attitude without obvious anxiousness 14. administer prescribed antianxiety agents if indicated. c. Consult appropriate health care provider (e.g., psychiatric nurse clinician, physician) if above actions fail to control fear and anxiety.

Discharge Teaching/Continued Care

6. NURSING DIAGNOSIS: DEFICIENT KNOWLEDGE, INEFFECTIVE THERAPEUTIC REGIMEN MANAGEMENT, OR INEFFECTIVE HEALTH MAINTENANCE*

*The nurse should select the diagnostic label that is most appropriate for the individual client's teaching needs.

Suggested NOC Outcomes: Knowledge: treatment regimen; Knowledge: health promotion

Suggested NIC Interventions: Health system guidance; Teaching: individual; Teaching: procedure/treatment

Desired Outcomes	Nursing Actions *and Selected Purposes/Rationales*
6.a. The client will identify safety measures related to care of chest tube insertion site and flutter valve (if present).	6.a.1. If the chest tube is removed before discharge, explain the importance of keeping a dressing over the insertion site until instructed by physician to remove it. 2. If client is discharged with a flutter valve in place, reinforce the following safety measures: a. maintain an occlusive dressing around the insertion site b. ensure that the connection between the chest tube and flutter valve is taped securely and that it is anchored to the chest wall using tape

Desired Outcomes	**Nursing Actions** *and Selected Purposes/Rationales*
	c. maintain patency of the flutter valve (e.g., avoid occluding the distal end of the flutter valve, contact physician if fluid collects in the valve, avoid activities such as swimming and bathing [the valve should not be submerged in water]). 3. Allow time for questions and clarification of information provided.
6.b. The client will identify ways to reduce the risk of another pneumothorax.	6.b.1. Caution client to avoid activities that involve experiencing marked changes in atmospheric pressure (e.g., scuba diving, flying in unpressurized aircraft, mountain climbing). 2. Encourage client to stop smoking. 3. Instruct client to continue treatment of any underlying lung disease (e.g., COPD, tuberculosis).
6.c. The client will state signs and symptoms to report to the health care provider.	6.c. Instruct client to report the following signs and symptoms: 1. difficulty breathing 2. chest pain 3. elevated temperature 4. chills 5. increased redness and warmth at chest tube insertion site 6. purulent drainage from chest tube insertion site or flutter valve.
6.d. The client will verbalize an understanding of and a plan for adhering to recommended follow-up care including future appointments with health care provider and activity restrictions.	6.d.1. Reinforce importance of keeping follow-up appointments with health care provider. 2. Instruct client to avoid excessive physical exertion and lifting objects over 10 pounds until permitted by physician. 3. Reinforce physician's explanation about the possibility of another pneumothorax. Assist client to develop a plan for obtaining emergency assistance if pneumothorax recurs. 4. Encourage client to continue with deep breathing exercises and use of incentive spirometer for the length of time recommended by physician. 5. Implement measures to improve client compliance: a. include significant others in teaching sessions if possible b. encourage questions and allow time for reinforcement and clarification of information provided c. provide written instructions about precautions related to chest tube insertion site and flutter valve (if present), signs and symptoms to report, future appointments with health care provider, and activity restrictions.

Bibliography

See pages 879 and 882–883.

PULMONARY EMBOLISM

Pulmonary embolism is the partial or complete obstruction of one of the pulmonary arterial vessels by an embolus. The most common source of the embolus is a thrombus that originates in a deep vein of the lower extremities. The embolus can also originate in the right side of the heart; the upper extremities; and vessels that have sustained endothelial injury caused by factors such as trauma, surgery, or presence of an indwelling central venous catheter. Nonthrombotic sources of pulmonary embolism include air, fat, amniotic fluid, tumor cells, and foreign material (e.g., broken intravenous catheter, talc [often used to "cut" drugs injected by intravenous drug abusers]).

The clinical manifestations of pulmonary embolism are varied and nonspecific. The extensiveness of the signs and symptoms depends on the size and number of emboli, size of the vessel that is occluded, extent of vessel occlusion, and presence of pre-existing cardiac or pulmonary disease. The classic signs and symptoms of a moderate-size pulmonary embolism are sudden onset of dyspnea, tachypnea, tachycardia, and a feeling of apprehension or impending doom. The person may also experience chest pain, cough, and low-grade fever.

Medical treatment varies depending on the source of the embolus and its effect on cardiopulmonary function. When the source is a thrombus, treatment usually consists of bed rest and initiation of intravenous anticoagulant therapy. A thrombolytic agent might be administered if the thromboembolus is occluding a large vessel and/or cardiopulmonary status is severely compromised. Anticoagulant therapy (subcutaneous and/or oral) often continues for 3–6 months following discharge. If thrombolytic agents and anticoagulant therapy are contraindicated or unsuccessful or the source of the embolus is nonthrombotic, surgical removal of the embolus may be indicated.

This care plan focuses on the adult client hospitalized for treatment of a pulmonary embolism resulting from a deep vein thrombus. Much of the information is also applicable to clients receiving follow-up care at home.

OUTCOME/DISCHARGE CRITERIA

THE CLIENT WILL:

- have adequate respiratory function
- have no signs and symptoms of complications
- identify ways to reduce the risk of recurrent thrombus formation and pulmonary embolism
- verbalize an understanding of medications ordered including rationale, food and drug interactions, side effects, schedule for taking, and importance of taking as prescribed
- demonstrate the ability to correctly draw up and administer heparin subcutaneously if prescribed
- identify ways to prevent bleeding associated with anticoagulant therapy
- state signs and symptoms to report to the health care provider
- verbalize an understanding of and a plan for adhering to recommended follow-up care including future appointments with health care provider and activity level.

Use in conjunction with the Care Plan on Immobility.

NURSING/COLLABORATIVE DIAGNOSES

DISCHARGE TEACHING

See Care Plan on Immobility (pp. 129–148) for additional diagnoses.

1. Nursing Diagnosis: INEFFECTIVE BREATHING PATTERN

related to:
a. increased rate of respirations associated with fear, anxiety, and stimulant effects of hypoxia;
b. decreased rate of respirations associated with the depressant effect of some medications (e.g., narcotic [opioid] analgesics);
c. decreased depth of respirations associated with:
   1. fear, anxiety, and reluctance to breathe deeply because of chest pain if present
   2. depressant effect of some medications (e.g., narcotic [opioid] analgesics)
   3. decreased mobility.

Suggested NOC Outcome: Respiratory status: ventilation

Suggested NIC Interventions: Respiratory monitoring; Ventilation assistance; Anxiety management; Pain management

Desired Outcome	**Nursing Actions** *and Selected Purposes/Rationales* (see pp. 18–20 for additional rationales)
1. The client will experience an effective breathing pattern as evidenced by: a. normal rate and depth of respirations b. absence of dyspnea.	1.a. Assess for signs and symptoms of an ineffective breathing pattern (e.g., rapid, shallow respirations; dyspnea; use of accessory muscles when breathing; impaired chest excursion). b. Implement measures *to improve breathing pattern:* 1. perform actions to reduce chest pain (see Diagnosis 3, action d) *in order to increase the client's willingness to move and breathe more deeply* 2. perform actions to reduce fear and anxiety (see Diagnosis 5) *in order to prevent the shallow and/or rapid breathing that can occur with fear and anxiety* 3. perform actions to improve gas exchange (see Diagnosis 2, action b) *in order to reduce hypoxia and subsequent stimulation of the respiratory center* 4. place client in a semi- to high Fowler's position unless contraindicated; position with pillows *to prevent slumping* 5. instruct client to breathe slowly if hyperventilating 6. instruct client to deep breathe or use incentive spirometer every 1–2 hours 7. administer central nervous system depressants judiciously; hold medication and consult physician if respiratory rate is less than 12/minute 8. increase activity when allowed. c. Consult appropriate health care provider (e.g., respiratory therapist, physician) if ineffective breathing pattern persists or worsens.

2. Nursing Diagnosis: IMPAIRED GAS EXCHANGE

related to:
a. decreased pulmonary perfusion associated with obstruction of pulmonary arterial blood flow by the embolus and vasoconstriction resulting from the release of vasoactive substances (e.g., serotonin, endothelin, some prostaglandins);
b. decreased bronchial airflow associated with bronchoconstriction resulting from:
   1. the release of substances such as serotonin and some prostaglandins
   2. a compensatory response to an increase in the amount of dead space in the underperfused lung area (the compensatory bronchoconstriction also affects airways in perfused lung areas);
c. loss of effective lung surface associated with atelectasis if it occurs.

Suggested NOC Outcome: Respiratory status: gas exchange

Suggested NIC Interventions: Respiratory monitoring; Oxygen therapy; Airway management; Ventilation assistance; Acid-base management

Desired Outcome	Nursing Actions *and Selected Purposes/Rationales* (see pp. 33–35 for additional rationales)
2. The client will experience adequate O_2/CO_2 exchange as evidenced by: a. usual mental status b. unlabored respirations at 12–20/minute c. oximetry results within normal range d. blood gases within normal range.	2.a. Assess for and report signs and symptoms of impaired gas exchange: 1. restlessness, irritability 2. confusion, somnolence 3. tachypnea, dyspnea 4. significant decrease in oximetry results 5. decreased Pa_{O_2} and/or increased Pa_{CO_2}. b. Implement measures *to improve gas exchange:* 1. maintain client on bed rest *to reduce oxygen demands during acute respiratory distress;* increase activity gradually as allowed and tolerated 2. maintain oxygen therapy as ordered 3. perform actions to improve breathing pattern (see Diagnosis 1, action b) 4. discourage smoking *(the carbon monoxide in smoke decreases oxygen availability and the nicotine can cause vasoconstriction and further reduce pulmonary blood flow)* 5. perform actions *to improve pulmonary blood flow:* a. administer anticoagulants (e.g., continuous intravenous heparin, low-molecular-weight heparin, warfarin) as ordered b. prepare client for the following if planned: 1. injection of a thrombolytic agent (e.g., streptokinase, urokinase, alteplase) 2. embolectomy. c. Consult appropriate health care provider (e.g., respiratory therapist, physician) if signs and symptoms of impaired gas exchange persist or worsen.

3. NURSING DIAGNOSIS:

ACUTE PAIN: CHEST

related to:

a. decreased pulmonary tissue perfusion associated with obstructed pulmonary blood flow;
b. inflammation of the parietal pleura associated with tissue damage if infarction occurs.

Suggested NOC Outcomes: Pain control; Comfort level

Suggested NIC Interventions: Pain management; Analgesic administration; Oxygen administration

Desired Outcome	Nursing Actions *and Selected Purposes/Rationales* (see pp. 45–47 for additional rationales)
3. The client will experience diminished chest pain as evidenced by: a. verbalization of a decrease in pain b. relaxed facial expression and body positioning c. increased participation in activities when allowed d. pulse and B/P within normal range for client.	3.a. Assess for signs and symptoms of pain (e.g., verbalization of pain, grimacing, rubbing chest, reluctance to move, shallow respirations, restlessness, increased B/P, tachycardia). b. Assess client's perception of the severity of pain using a pain intensity rating scale. c. Assess the client's pain pattern (e.g., location, quality, onset, duration, precipitating factors, aggravating factors, alleviating factors). d. Implement measures *to reduce pain:* 1. perform actions to reduce fear and anxiety (see Diagnosis 5) *in order to promote relaxation and subsequently increase the client's threshold and tolerance for pain* 2. perform actions to improve gas exchange (see Diagnosis 2, action b) *in order to reduce tissue hypoxia and the subsequent release of lactic acid (an irritant to nerves) in the involved lung area* 3. instruct and assist client to splint chest with hands or pillow when deep breathing, coughing, and changing position 4. provide or assist with nonpharmacologic methods for pain relief (e.g., position change, relaxation techniques, restful environment, diversional activities)

Desired Outcome	Nursing Actions *and Selected Purposes/Rationales*
	5. administer analgesics if ordered. e. Consult physician if above actions fail to provide adequate pain relief.

4. Collaborative Diagnoses:

POTENTIAL COMPLICATIONS

a. right-sided heart failure related to increased cardiac workload associated with:
   1. pulmonary hypertension (can result from pulmonary vasoconstriction that occurs in response to hypoxia and the release of vasoactive substances)
   2. compensatory response to decreased pulmonary blood flow that results from obstruction of multiple and/or large pulmonary vessels;

b. extended or recurrent pulmonary embolism related to inadequate response to treatment and/or continued presence of predisposing conditions;

c. atelectasis related to:
   1. shallow respirations associated with chest pain, fear, and anxiety
   2. stasis of secretions in the alveoli and bronchioles associated with decreased mobility during time that activity is restricted
   3. decreased surfactant production associated with reduced pulmonary blood flow and inadequate deep breathing;

d. bleeding related to prolonged coagulation time associated with anticoagulant therapy and possible heparin-induced thrombocytopenia.

Desired Outcomes	Nursing Actions *and Selected Purposes/Rationales*
4.a. The client will not develop right-sided heart failure as evidenced by: 1. pulse 60–100 beats/minute 2. usual mental status 3. usual strength and activity tolerance 4. adequate urine output 5. stable weight 6. absence of edema and distended neck veins.	4.a.1. Assess for and report signs and symptoms of right-sided heart failure: a. further increase in pulse b. restlessness, confusion c. weakness and fatigue d. decreased urine output e. weight gain f. dependent peripheral edema g. distended neck veins h. chest x-ray results showing cardiomegaly. 2. Implement measures to improve pulmonary blood flow (see Diagnosis 2, action b.5) *in order to reduce cardiac workload and the subsequent risk for right-sided heart failure.* 3. If signs and symptoms of right-sided heart failure occur: a. maintain oxygen therapy as ordered b. maintain client on strict bed rest in a semi- to high Fowler's position c. maintain fluid and sodium restrictions if ordered d. administer medications that may be ordered *to reduce vascular congestion and/or cardiac workload* (e.g., diuretics, cardiotonics, vasodilators).
4.b. The client will not experience extension or recurrence of a pulmonary embolism as evidenced by: 1. absence of or diminishing chest pain 2. absence of or decrease in dyspnea 3. pulse 60–100 beats/minute 4. blood gases returning toward normal.	4.b.1. Assess for and report signs and symptoms of extended or recurrent pulmonary embolism (e.g., development of, persistent, or increased chest pain, dyspnea, apprehension, tachypnea, or tachycardia; declining PaO_2). 2. Administer anticoagulants (e.g., heparin, warfarin) and/or assist with administration of thrombolytic agents (e.g., alteplase, urokinase, streptokinase) if ordered *to prevent extension of the embolism.* 3. Implement measures *to prevent recurrence of a pulmonary embolism:* a. perform actions to prevent and treat a deep vein thrombus (see Care Plan on Immobility, Diagnosis 12, actions a.1.b and c [pp. 140–141]) b. perform actions *to prevent dislodgment of thrombus:* 1. maintain client on bed rest as ordered 2. do not exercise, check for Homans' sign in, or massage any extremity known to have a thrombus 3. caution client to avoid activities that create a Valsalva response (e.g., straining to have a bowel movement, blowing nose forcefully, holding breath while moving up in bed)

c. prepare client for a vena caval interruption (e.g., insertion of an intracaval filtering device) if planned.

4. If signs and symptoms of extended or recurrent pulmonary embolism occur:
   a. maintain client on strict bed rest in a semi- to high Fowler's position
   b. maintain oxygen therapy as ordered
   c. prepare client for diagnostic tests (e.g., ventilation-perfusion lung scan, blood gases, D-dimer level, pulmonary angiography) if indicated
   d. prepare client for surgical intervention (e.g., embolectomy) if planned
   e. assess for and report signs and symptoms of pulmonary infarction (e.g., hemoptysis, fever, increased WBC count).

4.c. The client will not develop atelectasis (see Care Plan on Immobility, Diagnosis 12, outcome b [p. 141], for outcome criteria).

4.c.1. Refer to Care Plan on Immobility, Diagnosis 12, action b (p. 141), for measures related to assessment, prevention, and treatment of atelectasis.

2. Implement measures to improve breathing pattern and gas exchange (see Diagnoses 1, action b and 2, action b) *in order to further reduce the risk for atelectasis.*

4.d. The client will not experience unusual bleeding as evidenced by:
1. skin and mucous membranes free of petechiae, purpura, ecchymoses, and active bleeding
2. absence of unusual joint pain
3. no increase in abdominal girth
4. absence of frank and occult blood in stool, urine, and vomitus
5. usual menstrual flow
6. vital signs within normal range for client
7. stable Hct and Hgb.

4.d.1. Assess client for and report signs and symptoms of unusual bleeding:
   a. petechiae, purpura, ecchymoses
   b. gingival bleeding
   c. prolonged bleeding from puncture sites
   d. epistaxis, hemoptysis
   e. unusual joint pain
   f. increase in abdominal girth
   g. frank or occult blood in stool, urine, or vomitus
   h. menorrhagia
   i. restlessness, confusion
   j. decreasing B/P and increased pulse rate
   k. decrease in Hct and Hgb levels.

2. Monitor platelet count and coagulation test results (e.g., prothrombin time or International Normalized Ratio [INR], activated partial thromboplastin time). Report a low platelet count and coagulation test results that exceed the therapeutic range.
3. If platelet count is low, coagulation test results are abnormal, or Hct and Hgb levels decrease, test all stools, urine, and vomitus for occult blood. Report positive results.
4. Implement measures *to prevent bleeding:*
   a. avoid giving injections whenever possible; consult physician about prescribing an alternative route for medications ordered to be given intramuscularly or subcutaneously
   b. when giving injections or performing venous or arterial punctures, use the smallest gauge needle possible and apply gentle, prolonged pressure to the site after the needle is removed
   c. caution client to avoid activities that increase the risk for trauma (e.g., shaving with a straight-edge razor, using stiff bristle toothbrush or dental floss)
   d. whenever possible, avoid intubations (e.g., nasogastric) and procedures that can cause injury to the rectal mucosa (e.g., taking temperature rectally, inserting a rectal suppository, administering an enema)
   e. perform actions *to reduce the risk for falls* (e.g., keep bed in low position with side rails up when client is in bed, avoid unnecessary clutter in room, instruct client to wear slippers/shoes with nonslip soles when ambulating)
   f. pad side rails if client is confused or restless

Desired Outcomes	Nursing Actions *and Selected Purposes/Rationales*
	g. instruct client to avoid blowing nose forcefully or straining to have a bowel movement; consult physician about an order for a decongestant and/or laxative if indicated. 5. If bleeding occurs and does not subside spontaneously: a. apply firm, prolonged pressure to bleeding area(s) if possible b. if epistaxis occurs, place client in a high Fowler's position and apply pressure and ice pack to nasal area c. maintain oxygen therapy as ordered d. administer protamine sulfate (antidote for heparin), vitamin K (e.g., phytonadione), and/or whole blood or blood products (e.g., fresh frozen plasma, platelets) as ordered.

5. Nursing Diagnosis: **FEAR/ANXIETY**

related to dyspnea; chest pain; lack of understanding of diagnostic tests, diagnosis, and treatments; unfamiliar environment; possibility of recurrent embolism; and threat of death.

Suggested NOC Outcomes: Anxiety level; Fear level; Anxiety self-control; Fear self-control

Suggested NIC Interventions: Anxiety reduction; Calming technique; Emotional support; Presence

Desired Outcome	Nursing Actions *and Selected Purposes/Rationales*
5. The client will experience a reduction in fear and anxiety (see Care Plan on Immobility, Diagnosis 13 [p. 143], for outcome criteria).	5.a. Refer to Care Plan on Immobility, Diagnosis 13 (pp. 143–144), for measures related to assessment and reduction of fear and anxiety. b. Implement additional measures *to reduce fear and anxiety:* 1. do not leave client alone during period of acute respiratory distress 2. perform actions to improve gas exchange (see Diagnosis 2, action b) *in order to relieve dyspnea* 3. perform actions to reduce chest pain (see Diagnosis 3, action d) 4. explain all diagnostic tests 5. reassure client that extreme apprehension or "sense of doom" is a common symptom of pulmonary embolism and will diminish as condition stabilizes.

Discharge Teaching/Continued Care

6. Nursing Diagnosis: **DEFICIENT KNOWLEDGE, INEFFECTIVE THERAPEUTIC REGIMEN MANAGEMENT, OR INEFFECTIVE HEALTH MAINTENANCE***

*The nurse should select the diagnostic label that is most appropriate for the individual client's teaching needs.

Suggested NOC Outcomes: Knowledge: disease process; Knowledge: treatment regimen

Suggested NIC Interventions: Health system guidance; Teaching: individual; Teaching: prescribed medication; Teaching: prescribed activity/exercise; Teaching: psychomotor skill

Desired Outcomes	Nursing Actions *and Selected Purposes/Rationales*
6.a. The client will identify ways to reduce the risk of recurrent thrombus formation and pulmonary embolism.	6.a.1. Provide the following instructions on ways to promote venous blood flow and reduce the risk of thrombus recurrence: a. avoid wearing constrictive clothing (e.g., garters, girdles, narrow-banded knee-high hose) b. avoid sitting and standing in one position for long periods of time

c. wear graduated compression stockings or support hose during the day
d. avoid crossing legs and lying or sitting with pillows under knees
e. engage in regular aerobic exercise (e.g., swimming, walking, cycling)
f. elevate legs periodically, especially when sitting
g. dorsiflex feet regularly
h. maintain recommended weight for age, height, and body frame.

2. Inform client that smoking and the use of estrogen or oral contraceptives can increase the risk for recurrent thrombus formation.
3. Instruct client to avoid trauma to or massage of any area of suspected thrombus formation in order to decrease risk of pulmonary embolism.
4. Provide information regarding exercise programs and support groups that can assist the client to stop smoking and/or lose weight.

6.b. The client will verbalize an understanding of medications ordered including rationale, food and drug interactions, side effects, schedule for taking, and importance of taking as prescribed.

6.b.1. Explain the rationale for, side effects of, and importance of taking medications prescribed.

2. If client is discharged on warfarin (e.g., Coumadin), instruct to:
   a. keep scheduled appointments for periodic blood studies to monitor coagulation times
   b. take medication at the same time each day, do not stop taking medication abruptly, and do not attempt to make up for missed doses
   c. avoid regular and/or excessive intake of alcohol (may alter responsiveness to warfarin)
   d. avoid significantly increasing or decreasing consumption of foods high in vitamin K (e.g., green leafy vegetables)
   e. report prolonged or excessive bleeding from skin, nose, or mouth; red, rust-colored, or smoky urine; bloody or tarry stools; blood in vomitus or sputum; prolonged or excessive menses; excessive bruising; severe or persistent headache; or sudden abdominal or back pain
   f. inform physician immediately if pregnancy is suspected or if breast-feeding (warfarin crosses the placental barrier and enters the breast milk)
   g. wear a medical alert identification bracelet or tag identifying self as being on anticoagulant therapy
   h. inform physician of any other medications being taken because there are some that affect the anticoagulant activity of warfarin (e.g., NSAIDs, various antimicrobials, phenytoin)
   i. notify health care provider immediately of any sudden changes in the skin, such as bruised, darkened, or painful areas (warfarin can cause necrosis of the skin).
3. Instruct client to inform all health care providers of medications being taken.

6.c. The client will demonstrate the ability to correctly draw up and administer heparin subcutaneously if prescribed.

6.c.1. If client is to be discharged on subcutaneous heparin, provide instructions about subcutaneous injection technique.

2. Allow time for questions, practice, and return demonstration.

6.d. The client will identify ways to prevent bleeding associated with anticoagulant therapy.

6.d.1. Instruct client about ways to minimize the risk of bleeding while on anticoagulant therapy:
   a. use an electric rather than straight-edge razor
   b. floss and brush teeth gently; use waxed floss and a soft bristle toothbrush
   c. avoid putting sharp objects (e.g., toothpicks) in mouth
   d. do not walk barefoot
   e. cut nails carefully
   f. avoid situations that could result in injury (e.g., contact sports)
   g. do not blow nose forcefully
   h. avoid straining to have a bowel movement.

Desired Outcomes	**Nursing Actions** *and Selected Purposes/Rationales*
	2. Instruct client to control any bleeding by applying firm, prolonged pressure to the area if possible.
6.e. The client will state signs and symptoms to report to the health care provider.	6.e. Stress the importance of reporting the following signs and symptoms: 1. tenderness, swelling, or pain in extremity 2. sudden chest pain 3. new or increased shortness of breath 4. extreme anxiousness or restlessness 5. cough productive of blood-tinged sputum 6. unusual bleeding (see action b.2.f in this diagnosis) 7. fever.
6.f. The client will verbalize an understanding of and a plan for adhering to recommended follow-up care including future appointments with health care provider and activity level.	6.f.1. Reinforce the importance of keeping follow-up appointments with health care provider. 2. Reinforce the physician's instructions regarding activity limitations. 3. Implement measures to improve client compliance: a. include significant others in teaching sessions if possible b. encourage questions and allow time for reinforcement and clarification of information provided c. provide written instructions regarding future appointments with health care provider, medications prescribed, activity restrictions, signs and symptoms to report, and future laboratory studies.

Bibliography

See pages 879 and 882–883.

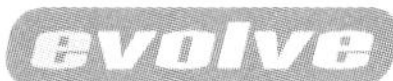

Thoracic Surgery

Thoracic surgery is a term used to refer to surgical procedures that involve entry into the thoracic cavity to gain access to the lungs, heart, aorta, or esophagus. Types of thoracic surgery performed to treat pulmonary disorders include pneumonectomy, lobectomy, segmental resection, and wedge resection. The surgery may be performed to repair lung damage resulting from trauma and to remove benign or malignant tumors; areas of bronchiectasis, fungal infection, or tuberculosis; abscesses; blebs; and bullae. Although some thoracic surgery can be accomplished using an intercostally inserted endoscope, an open thoracic approach is needed to treat conditions requiring surgery deep in the lung and/or extensive removal of lung tissue.

This care plan focuses on the adult client hospitalized for thoracic surgery to remove a portion or all of a lung. Much of the information is applicable to clients receiving follow-up care in an extended care facility or home setting. The care plan will need to be individualized according to the client's diagnosis, extensiveness of the surgery, prognosis, and plans for subsequent treatment. The reader should refer to the Care Plans on Cancer of the Lung, Chronic Obstructive Pulmonary Disease, and Tuberculosis if appropriate.

OUTCOME/DISCHARGE CRITERIA

THE CLIENT WILL:

- have optimal respiratory function
- have evidence of normal healing of surgical wound
- have surgical pain controlled
- have no signs and symptoms of postoperative complications
- identify ways to promote optimal respiratory health
- demonstrate the ability to perform prescribed arm and shoulder exercises
- state signs and symptoms to report to the health care provider
- identify community resources that can assist with home management and adjustment to the diagnosis, effects of surgery, and subsequent treatment if planned
- verbalize an understanding of and a plan for adhering to recommended follow-up care including future appointments with health care provider, medications prescribed, activity level, pain management, wound care, and subsequent treatment of the underlying disorder.

NURSING/COLLABORATIVE DIAGNOSES

Preoperative

1. Fear/Anxiety p. 482

Postoperative

1. Impaired respiratory function p. 482
   a. ineffective breathing pattern
   b. ineffective airway clearance
   c. impaired gas exchange
2. Acute pain: chest p. 484
3. Potential complications p. 484
   a. extended pneumothorax
   b. hemothorax
   c. mediastinal shift
   d. cardiac dysrhythmias
   e. acute pulmonary edema
   f. bronchopleural fistula
   g. restricted arm and shoulder movement

DISCHARGE TEACHING

4. Deficient knowledge, Ineffective therapeutic regimen management, or Ineffective health maintenance p. 487

See Standardized Preoperative and Postoperative Care Plans (pp. 97–126) and, if appropriate, the Care Plans on Cancer of the Lung, Chronic Obstructive Pulmonary Disease, and Tuberculosis for additional diagnoses.

PREOPERATIVE

Use in conjunction with the Standardized Preoperative Care Plan.

1. Nursing Diagnosis: FEAR/ANXIETY

related to:
a. lack of understanding of the diagnosis, surgical procedure, and postoperative management;
b. unfamiliar environment and financial concerns;
c. anticipated loss of control associated with effects of anesthesia;
d. potential embarrassment or loss of dignity associated with body exposure;
e. anticipated pain and/or difficulty breathing;
f. possible changes in usual lifestyle (e.g., activity limitations, cessation of smoking).

Suggested NOC Outcomes: Anxiety level; Fear level; Anxiety self-control; Fear self-control

Suggested NIC Interventions: Anxiety reduction; Calming technique; Emotional support; Presence; Teaching: preoperative

Desired Outcome	Nursing Actions *and Selected Purposes/Rationales*
1. The client will experience a reduction in fear and anxiety (see Standardized Preoperative Care Plan, Diagnosis 1 [pp. 97–98], for outcome criteria).	1.a. Refer to Standardized Preoperative Care Plan, Diagnosis 1 (pp. 97–98), for measures related to assessment and reduction of fear and anxiety. b. Implement additional measures *to reduce fear and anxiety:* 1. reinforce physician's explanations about anticipated effect of loss of lung tissue on activity tolerance; if appropriate, reassure client that the remaining lung tissue should be able to provide adequate respiratory function 2. provide instruction about the purpose of chest drainage system that will be present following removal of a portion of the lung (chest tubes are rarely inserted if a pneumonectomy is performed) 3. assure client that he/she will receive supplemental oxygen following surgery if needed.

POSTOPERATIVE

Use in conjunction with the Standardized Postoperative Care Plan.

1. Nursing Diagnosis: IMPAIRED RESPIRATORY FUNCTION*

a. ineffective breathing pattern related to:
   1. increased rate of respirations associated with fear and anxiety
   2. decreased rate of respirations associated with the depressant effect of anesthesia and some medications (e.g., narcotic [opioid] analgesics, some antiemetics)
   3. decreased depth of respirations associated with:
      a. reluctance to breathe deeply resulting from incisional pain and fear of dislodging chest tube(s) if in place
      b. weakness, fatigue, fear, and anxiety
      c. depressant effect of anesthesia and some medications (e.g., narcotic [opioid] analgesics, some antiemetics)

*This diagnostic label includes the following nursing diagnoses: ineffective breathing pattern, ineffective airway clearance, and impaired gas exchange.

d. limited chest expansion resulting from positioning and elevation of the diaphragm (can occur if abdominal distention is present or if the phrenic nerve was injured during surgery);

b. ineffective airway clearance related to:
   1. occlusion of the pharynx in the immediate postoperative period associated with relaxation of the tongue resulting from the effect of anesthesia and some medications (e.g., narcotic [opioid] analgesics)
   2. stasis of secretions associated with:
      a. decreased activity
      b. depressed ciliary function resulting from effects of anesthesia
      c. difficulty coughing up secretions resulting from the depressant effect of anesthesia and some medications (e.g., narcotic [opioid] analgesics, some antiemetics), pain, weakness, fatigue, and presence of tenacious secretions (can occur as a result of deficient fluid volume)
   3. increased secretions associated with irritation of the respiratory tract (can result from inhalation anesthetics, endotracheal intubation, and surgically induced lung tissue injury and inflammation);

c. impaired gas exchange related to a decrease in alveolar surface area and pulmonary vasculature associated with the extensive removal of lung tissue.

Suggested NOC Outcomes: Respiratory status: airway patency; Respiratory status: ventilation; Respiratory status: gas exchange

Suggested NIC Interventions: Respiratory monitoring; Airway management; Tube care: chest; Cough enhancement; Oxygen therapy; Ventilation assistance

Desired Outcome	**Nursing Actions** *and Selected Purposes/Rationales* (see pp. 12–14, 18–20, and 33–35 for additional rationales)
1. The client will experience adequate respiratory function as evidenced by: a. normal rate and depth of respirations b. absence of dyspnea c. normal breath sounds over remaining lung tissue d. usual mental status e. usual skin color f. oximetry results within normal range g. blood gases within normal range.	1.a. Assess for and report signs and symptoms of impaired respiratory function: 1. rapid, shallow, or slow respirations 2. dyspnea, orthopnea 3. use of accessory muscles when breathing 4. abnormal breath sounds (e.g., diminished or absent breath sounds over remaining lung tissue, rhonchi) 5. development of or increase in cough 6. restlessness, irritability 7. confusion, somnolence 8. significant decrease in oximetry results 9. significant abnormalities of blood gas values 10. significant abnormalities in chest x-ray reports. b. Implement measures *to maintain adequate respiratory function:* 1. perform actions to improve breathing pattern and promote effective airway clearance (see Standardized Postoperative Care Plan, Diagnoses 2, action b and 3, action b [pp. 104 and 105]) 2. perform actions to reduce pain (see Postoperative Diagnosis 2, actions a and b) 3. perform actions to maintain patency and integrity of chest drainage system (see Postoperative Diagnosis 3, action a.2.a) *in order to promote re-expansion of residual lung tissue* 4. if chest tube(s) present, assure client that deep breathing and coughing will not dislodge the tube(s) 5. position client as ordered (e.g., usually on back or operative side after pneumonectomy, on back or either side following removal of a portion of the lung) *to allow full expansion of remaining lung tissue* 6. when positioning client on his/her side, use a 30–45° "tip" position (rather than complete lateral positioning) *to minimize lateral compression of lung tissue* 7. maintain oxygen therapy as ordered

Desired Outcome	Nursing Actions *and Selected Purposes/Rationales*

8. maintain activity restrictions as ordered; increase activity gradually as allowed and tolerated
9. administer bronchodilators (e.g., methylxanthines, sympathomimetics) if ordered.

c. Consult appropriate health care provider (e.g., respiratory therapist, physician) if signs and symptoms of impaired respiratory function persist or worsen.

2. Nursing Diagnosis: ACUTE PAIN: CHEST

related to:

a. tissue trauma, reflex muscle spasm, and disruption of intercostal nerves associated with the surgery;
b. irritation of the parietal pleura associated with surgical trauma and stretching of the pleura (occurs if there is an accumulation of blood or air in the pleural space);
c. tissue irritation associated with presence of chest tube(s);
d. stress on surgical area associated with deep breathing, coughing, and/or movement.

Suggested NOC Outcomes: Pain control; Comfort level

Suggested NIC Interventions: Pain management; Analgesic administration; Environmental management: comfort

Desired Outcome	Nursing Actions *and Selected Purposes/Rationales*
2. The client will experience diminished chest pain (see Standardized Postoperative Care Plan, Diagnosis 6 [p. 109], for outcome criteria).	2.a. Refer to Standardized Postoperative Care Plan, Diagnosis 6 (p. 109), for measures related to assessment and management of pain. b. Implement measures to facilitate the removal of blood and air from the pleural space (see Postoperative Diagnosis 3, actions a.2.a and b) *in order to reduce stretching of the parietal pleura and subsequently reduce chest pain.*

3. Collaborative Diagnoses: POTENTIAL COMPLICATIONS OF THORACIC SURGERY

a. extended pneumothorax related to an increase in intrapleural pressure associated with accumulation of air in pleural space (can occur if the chest drainage system malfunctions and/or air leaks into the pleural space through the incision);
b. hemothorax related to intraoperative or postoperative bleeding and/or malfunction of the chest drainage system;
c. mediastinal shift related to:
    1. a significant increase in intrapleural pressure on the operative side following a lobectomy associated with an accumulation of fluid and air in the pleural space
    2. excessive negative pressure in the operative side following pneumonectomy associated with inadequate serous fluid accumulation in the empty thoracic space (the position of the mediastinum is maintained by accumulation of serous fluid in the empty thoracic space);
d. cardiac dysrhythmias related to altered nodal function and myocardial conductivity associated primarily with myocardial hypoxia (may result from impaired gas exchange and diminished myocardial blood flow that can occur with hypovolemia and sympathetic nervous system-mediated vasoconstriction in the immediate postoperative period);
e. acute pulmonary edema related to:
    1. increased pulmonary capillary permeability associated with hypoxia
    2. increased hydrostatic pressure in the remaining pulmonary vessels associated with reduced size of the pulmonary vasculature bed and decreased effectiveness of lymphatic drainage resulting from extensive removal of pulmonary tissue (especially if pneumonectomy was performed);

f. bronchopleural fistula related to inadequate bronchial closure and healing following a partial or complete resection of the lung (most often associated with preoperative radiation to the lung and/or residual cancer of the bronchial stump);

g. restricted arm and shoulder movement related to decreased activity of the arm and shoulder on the operative side associated with weakness, fatigue, pain, and adhesion formation between incised muscles.

Desired Outcomes	**Nursing Actions** *and Selected Purposes/Rationales*
3.a. The client will experience normal lung re-expansion as evidenced by: 1. audible breath sounds and resonant percussion note over remaining lung tissue by 3rd–4th postoperative day 2. unlabored respirations at 12–20/minute 3. blood gases within normal range 4. chest x-ray showing lung re-expansion.	3.a.1. Assess for and immediately report signs and symptoms of: a. malfunction of chest drainage system (e.g., respiratory distress, lack of fluctuation in water seal chamber without evidence of lung re-expansion, excessive bubbling in water seal chamber, significant increase in subcutaneous emphysema) b. extended pneumothorax (e.g., extended area of absent breath sounds with hyperresonant percussion note; rapid, shallow, and/or labored respirations; restlessness; agitation; confusion; blood gas values that have worsened; chest x-ray results showing delayed lung re-expansion or further lung collapse). 2. Implement measures *to promote lung re-expansion and prevent extended pneumothorax:* a. perform actions *to maintain patency and integrity of chest drainage system if present:* 1. maintain fluid level in the water seal and suction chambers as ordered 2. maintain occlusive dressing over chest tube insertion site(s) 3. tape all connections securely 4. tape the tubing to the chest wall close to insertion site *to reduce the risk of inadvertent removal of the tube* 5. position tubing *to promote optimum drainage* (e.g., coil excess tubing on bed rather than allowing it to hang down below the collection device, keep tubing free of kinks) 6. drain fluid that accumulates in tubing into the collection chamber; milk chest tube(s) only if ordered 7. keep drainage collection device below level of client's chest at all times b. perform actions *to facilitate the escape of air from the pleural space* (e.g., maintain suction as ordered, ensure that the air vent is open on the drainage collection device if system is to water seal only) c. perform actions to maintain adequate respiratory function (see Postoperative Diagnosis 1, action b). 3. If signs and symptoms of extended pneumothorax occur: a. maintain client on bed rest in a semi- to high Fowler's position b. maintain oxygen therapy as ordered c. assist with clearing of existing chest tube(s) and/or insertion of a new tube.
3.b. The client will not develop hemothorax as evidenced by: 1. audible breath sounds and resonant percussion note over remaining lung tissue by 3rd–4th postoperative day 2. unlabored respirations at 12–20/minute 3. blood gases within normal range.	3.b.1. Assess for and immediately report signs and symptoms of: a. thoracic bleeding (e.g., unexpected increase in the amount of bloody drainage from chest tube[s], increase in bloody drainage on dressing, further decrease in Hct and Hgb) b. hemothorax (e.g., diminished or absent breath sounds with dull percussion note over affected area, dyspnea, blood gas values that have worsened). 2. Implement measures to maintain patency and integrity of chest drainage system (see action a.2.a in this diagnosis) *in order to reduce risk of hemothorax.* 3. If signs and symptoms of hemothorax occur: a. maintain client on bed rest in a semi- to high Fowler's position b. maintain oxygen therapy as ordered

Desired Outcomes	Nursing Actions *and Selected Purposes/Rationales*
	c. assist with autotransfusion of blood from chest tube and/or administer blood products and/or volume expanders if ordered d. assist with clearing of existing chest tube(s), thoracentesis, or insertion of chest tube if not already present e. prepare client for surgical intervention to ligate bleeding vessels if indicated.
3.c. The client will not develop a mediastinal shift as evidenced by: 1. absence of or no sudden increase in dyspnea 2. vital signs within normal range for client 3. usual mental status 4. trachea in midline position 5. absence of neck vein distention 6. blood gases within normal range.	3.c.1. Assess for and immediately report signs and symptoms of mediastinal shift (e.g., severe dyspnea, rapid and/or irregular pulse rate, hypotension, restlessness, agitation, confusion, shift in trachea from midline, neck vein distention, blood gas values that have worsened, chest x-ray results showing a deviation of trachea from midline). 2. Implement measures *to reduce risk of mediastinal shift:* a. keep chest tube clamped if one is in place after a pneumonectomy *(serous fluid accumulation is essential to maintain proper pressure gradient on operative side)* b. position client as ordered (e.g., usually on back or on operative side after pneumonectomy) c. perform actions to prevent and treat pneumothorax and hemothorax (see actions a.2 and 3 and b.2 and 3 in this diagnosis). 3. If signs and symptoms of mediastinal shift occur: a. maintain client on bed rest in a semi- to high Fowler's position b. maintain oxygen therapy as ordered c. assist with clearing of existing chest tube(s), thoracentesis, or insertion of new chest tube(s) if indicated.
3.d. The client will maintain normal sinus rhythm as evidenced by: 1. regular apical pulse at 60–100 beats/minute 2. equal apical and radial pulse rates 3. absence of syncope and palpitations 4. ECG showing normal sinus rhythm.	3.d.1. Assess for and report signs and symptoms of cardiac dysrhythmias (e.g., irregular apical pulse; pulse rate below 60 or above 100 beats/minute; apical-radial pulse deficit; syncope; palpitations; abnormal rate, rhythm, or configurations on ECG). 2. Implement measures *to prevent cardiac dysrhythmias:* a. perform actions to maintain adequate respiratory function (see Postoperative Diagnosis 1, action b) *in order to maintain adequate myocardial tissue oxygenation* b. perform actions to reduce pain, fear, and anxiety (see Standardized Postoperative Care Plan, Diagnoses 6, action d and 21, action b [pp. 109 and 124]) *in order to decrease stimulation of the sympathetic nervous system (sympathetic stimulation increases the heart rate and causes vasoconstriction, both of which increase cardiac workload and decrease oxygen availability to the myocardium)* c. perform actions to prevent or treat mediastinal shift (see actions c.2 and 3 in this diagnosis). 3. If cardiac dysrhythmias occur: a. administer antidysrhythmics (e.g., digoxin) as ordered b. restrict client's activity based on his/her tolerance and severity of the dysrhythmia c. maintain oxygen therapy as ordered d. assess cardiovascular status frequently and report signs and symptoms of inadequate tissue perfusion (e.g., decrease in B/P, cool skin, cyanosis, diminished peripheral pulses, urine output less than 30 ml/hour, restlessness and agitation, increased shortness of breath).
3.e. The client will not develop pulmonary edema as evidenced by: 1. unlabored respirations at 12–20/minute	3.e.1. Assess for and report signs and symptoms of pulmonary edema (e.g., severe dyspnea, tachycardia, development of or increase in crackles [rales] or wheezes, dull percussion note over remaining lung tissue, persistent cough productive of frothy and/or blood-tinged sputum, cyanosis, significant decrease in oximetry results, decrease in PaO_2 or increase in $PaCO_2$, chest x-ray results showing pulmonary edema).

2. clear breath sounds and resonant percussion note over unoperative lung tissue
3. absence of productive, persistent cough
4. usual skin color
5. oximetry results within normal range
6. blood gases within normal range.

2. Implement measures *to prevent hypoxia and reduce the risk for pulmonary edema:*
   a. perform actions to maintain adequate respiratory function (see Postoperative Diagnosis 1, action b)
   b. perform actions to maintain patency and integrity of chest drainage system if present (see action a.2.a in this diagnosis) *in order to promote lung re-expansion.*
3. If signs and symptoms of pulmonary edema occur, administer the following medications if ordered:
   a. bronchodilators (e.g., theophylline) *to increase bronchial airflow*
   b. agents *to reduce pulmonary vascular congestion* (e.g., diuretics, morphine sulfate).

3.f. The client will experience resolution of a bronchopleural fistula if it occurs as evidenced by:
1. afebrile status
2. absence of cough
3. absence of continuous bubbling in water seal chamber of chest drainage system
4. unlabored respirations at 12–20/minute
5. WBC and differential counts returning toward normal.

3.f.1. Assess for and report signs and symptoms of a bronchopleural fistula (e.g., fever, cough, purulent sputum, continuous bubbling in water seal chamber of chest drainage system, increasing subcutaneous emphysema around incision and neck, respiratory distress, persistent elevation of WBC count and significant change in differential, chest x-ray results showing presence of bronchopleural fistula).
2. If signs and symptoms of a bronchopleural fistula occur:
   a. turn client to operative side unless contraindicated *(this reduces the risk for aspiration of pleural fluid)*
   b. have tracheostomy tray readily available *(severe subcutaneous emphysema in the neck can compress the trachea and obstruct the airway)*
   c. prepare client for chest tube insertion, thoracentesis, and surgical repair of bronchial stump if planned.

3.g. The client will maintain normal arm and shoulder function as evidenced by ability to move arm and shoulder on operative side through usual range of motion.

3.g.1. Assess for and report signs and symptoms of restricted arm and shoulder movement on operative side (e.g., inability to move arm and shoulder through usual range of motion, inability to use arm in activities of daily living).
2. Implement measures *to prevent restriction of arm and shoulder movement on operative side:*
   a. instruct client in and assist with arm and shoulder exercises as ordered (usually, passive range of motion is started the evening of surgery and active range of motion exercises are started by the second postoperative day)
   b. perform actions to reduce pain (see Diagnosis 2, actions a and b) *in order to increase client's ability and willingness to move arm and shoulder*
   c. encourage client to use arm on operative side to perform self-care activities
   d. place frequently used articles and bed stand on operative side *so that client will be more likely to use that arm*
   e. anchor pull rope at foot of bed; encourage client to use arm on operative side to pull self to sitting position.
3. Consult appropriate health care provider (e.g., physical therapist, physician) if signs and symptoms of restricted arm and shoulder movement occur.

Discharge Teaching/Continued Care

4. NURSING DIAGNOSIS: DEFICIENT KNOWLEDGE, INEFFECTIVE THERAPEUTIC REGIMEN MANAGEMENT, OR INEFFECTIVE HEALTH MAINTENANCE*

*The nurse should select the diagnostic label that is most appropriate for the client's teaching needs.

Suggested NOC Outcomes: Knowledge: health promotion; Knowledge: health resources; Knowledge: treatment regimen

Suggested NIC Interventions: Health system guidance; Teaching: individual; Teaching: prescribed activity/exercise; Teaching: disease process

Desired Outcomes	Nursing Actions *and Selected Purposes/Rationales*
4.a. The client will identify ways to promote optimal respiratory health.	4.a. Instruct client in ways to promote optimal respiratory health: 1. maintain overall general good health (e.g., reduce stress, eat a well-balanced diet, obtain adequate rest, obtain adequate exercise) 2. stop smoking 3. avoid exposure to respiratory irritants such as smoke, dust, aerosol sprays, paint fumes, and solvents 4. remain indoors as much as possible when air pollution levels are high 5. wear a mask or scarf over nose and mouth if exposure to high levels of irritants such as smoke, fumes, and dust is unavoidable 6. take medications as prescribed to treat any underlying respiratory disease such as chronic obstructive pulmonary disease, cancer of the lung, or tuberculosis 7. decrease the risk of respiratory tract infections: a. avoid contact with persons who have respiratory tract infections b. avoid crowds and poorly ventilated areas c. drink at least 10 glasses of liquid/day unless contraindicated d. receive immunizations against influenza and pneumococcal pneumonia.
4.b. The client will demonstrate the ability to perform prescribed arm and shoulder exercises.	4.b.1. Instruct client regarding importance of exercising the arm and shoulder on operative side. Emphasize that the exercises should be performed at least 5 times/day for several weeks. 2. Demonstrate appropriate arm and shoulder exercises (e.g., shoulder shrugs, arm circles). 3. Allow time for questions, clarification, and return demonstration.
4.c. The client will state signs and symptoms to report to the health care provider.	4.c.1. Refer to Standardized Postoperative Care Plan, Diagnosis 22, action c (p. 125), for signs and symptoms to report to the health care provider. 2. Instruct the client to report these additional signs and symptoms: a. increased discomfort in or decreased ability to move arm and shoulder on operative side b. increased shortness of breath c. persistent cough.
4.d. The client will identify community resources that can assist with home management and adjustment to the diagnosis, effects of surgery, and subsequent treatment if planned.	4.d.1. Provide information about community resources that can assist the client and significant others with home management and adjustment to the diagnosis, effects of surgery, and subsequent treatment if planned (e.g., American Lung Association, American Cancer Society, smoking cessation program, Meals on Wheels, counselors, support groups, home health agencies). 2. Initiate a referral if indicated.

4.e. The client will verbalize an understanding of and a plan for adhering to recommended follow-up care including future appointments with health care provider, medications prescribed, activity level, pain management, wound care, and subsequent treatment of the underlying disorder.	4.e.1. Refer to Standardized Postoperative Care Plan, Diagnosis 22 (pp. 125–126), for routine postoperative instructions and measures to improve client compliance. 2. Reinforce physician's instructions about activity level: a. gauge activity according to tolerance and ensure adequate rest periods b. stop any activity that causes excessive fatigue, dyspnea, or chest pain c. avoid lifting heavy objects and doing strenuous upper body exercises until complete healing of chest muscles has occurred (usually 3–6 months). 3. Inform client that numbness and discomfort in the operative area can persist for several weeks but are usually temporary. 4. Clarify plans for subsequent treatment of underlying disorder (e.g., chemotherapy, radiation therapy) if appropriate.

Bibliography

See pages 879 and 882–883.

evolve

Tuberculosis

Tuberculosis (TB) is an infectious disease caused by *Mycobacterium tuberculosis*, a gram-positive, acid-fast bacillus. It is spread by airborne droplets released when a person with active TB disease coughs, sneezes, or speaks. These droplets can cause infection in others if contact with the infected person is close and repeated or prolonged. The inhaled tubercle bacilli implant themselves in the lung, multiply, and can spread to other areas of the body through the lymphatic channels (lymphatic dissemination) and blood (hematogenous dissemination).

Most people who are infected with tubercle bacilli do not develop an active form of TB. Those who do are usually part of high-risk populations that include persons who are immunosuppressed, persons in continued close contact with people with active untreated TB, and those who have been exposed to virulent strains of multi-drug resistant tuberculosis (MDR-TB). In addition, TB that has previously been inactive (latent, dormant) in a person with an effective immune system can become active if that person experiences situations that suppress the immune response (e.g., chemotherapy treatment, long-term corticosteroid use, malnutrition, HIV infection, advanced age).

Signs and symptoms of active TB can include fatigue, anorexia, weight loss, night sweats, fever (usually low-grade), cough (usually progresses from a dry cough to one that is productive of mucopurulent or blood-tinged sputum), dyspnea, and/or pleuritic pain (in some cases).

A person suspected of having active TB is placed on precautions to prevent airborne transmission of the tubercle bacilli and started on a regimen of multiple antitubercular/antimicrobial medications while awaiting results of sputum cultures. If the diagnosis is confirmed, a major health care focus becomes one of promoting compliance with the lengthy (usually 6–18 months), multiple drug treatment regimen.

This care plan focuses on the adult client hospitalized with signs and symptoms of active pulmonary tuberculosis. Much of the information presented here is applicable to clients receiving follow-up care in an extended care facility or home setting.

OUTCOME/DISCHARGE CRITERIA

THE CLIENT WILL:

- have an adequate respiratory status
- tolerate expected level of activity
- have no signs and symptoms of complications
- identify ways to maintain respiratory health
- identify ways to prevent the spread of TB to others
- verbalize an understanding of medications ordered including rationale, food and drug interactions, side effects, and importance of taking as prescribed
- state signs and symptoms to report to the health care provider
- verbalize an understanding of and a plan for adhering to recommended follow-up care including future appointments with health care provider.

NURSING/COLLABORATIVE DIAGNOSES

DISCHARGE TEACHING

See p. 501 for additional diagnoses.

1. NURSING DIAGNOSIS:

IMPAIRED RESPIRATORY FUNCTION*

a. ineffective breathing pattern related to:
   1. decreased depth of respirations associated with weakness, fatigue, and reluctance to breathe deeply if chest pain is present
   2. increased rate of respirations associated with the increase in metabolic rate that occurs with an infectious process;

b. ineffective airway clearance related to:
   1. tracheobronchial inflammation
   2. increase in secretions associated with the infectious process and the necrosis and subsequent liquification of tubercle nodules (the nodules, or caseations, are lesions that consist of tubercle bacilli surrounded by a fibrous capsule)
   3. stasis of secretions associated with decreased activity; poor cough effort resulting from weakness, fatigue, and chest pain (if present); and impaired ciliary function (results from the increased viscosity and volume of mucus that occurs with the infectious process);

c. impaired gas exchange related to a decrease in effective lung surface associated with the accumulation of secretions and destruction of normal lung tissue that occurs with the presence of the tubercle nodules.

*This diagnostic label includes the following nursing diagnoses: ineffective breathing pattern, ineffective airway clearance, and impaired gas exchange.

Suggested NOC Outcomes: Respiratory status: airway patency; Respiratory status: ventilation; Respiratory status: gas exchange

Suggested NIC Interventions: Respiratory monitoring; Ventilation assistance; Airway management; Chest physiotherapy; Cough enhancement; Oxygen therapy; Medication administration

Desired Outcome	**Nursing Actions** *and Selected Purposes/Rationales* (see pp. 12–14, 18–20, and 33–35 for additional rationales)
1. The client will experience adequate respiratory function as evidenced by: a. normal rate and depth of respirations b. decrease in or absence of dyspnea c. normal breath sounds d. usual mental status e. oximetry results within normal range f. blood gases within normal range.	1.a. Assess for and report signs and symptoms of impaired respiratory function: 1. rapid, shallow respirations 2. dyspnea, orthopnea 3. use of accessory muscles when breathing 4. abnormal breath sounds (e.g., diminished, crackles [rales], rhonchi) 5. cough (usually a productive cough of mucopurulent or blood-tinged sputum) 6. limited chest excursion 7. restlessness, irritability 8. confusion, somnolence 9. significant decrease in oximetry results 10. abnormal blood gas values 11. abnormal chest x-ray results. b. Implement measures *to improve respiratory status:* 1. perform actions to increase strength and improve activity tolerance (see Diagnosis 3, action b) *in order to enable the client to breathe more deeply and participate in activities to improve respiratory status* 2. perform actions to reduce chest pain if present (e.g., splint chest with pillow when coughing and deep breathing, administer prescribed analgesics before planned activity) *in order to increase the client's willingness to move, cough, and deep breathe* 3. place client in a semi- to high Fowler's position unless contraindicated; position with pillows *to prevent slumping* 4. if client must remain flat in bed, assist with position change at least every 2 hours 5. instruct client to deep breathe or use inspiratory exerciser every 1–2 hours

Desired Outcome	Nursing Actions *and Selected Purposes/Rationales*

6. assist with positive airway pressure techniques (e.g., continuous positive airway pressure [CPAP], bilevel positive airway pressure [BiPAP], flutter/positive expiratory pressure [PEP] device) if ordered
7. perform actions *to promote removal of pulmonary secretions:*
   a. instruct and assist client to cough or "huff" every 1–2 hours
   b. implement measures *to thin tenacious secretions and reduce dryness of the respiratory mucous membrane:*
      1. maintain a fluid intake of at least 2500 ml/day unless contraindicated
      2. humidify inspired air as ordered
   c. assist with administration of mucolytics (e.g., acetylcysteine) and diluent or hydrating agents (e.g., water, saline) via nebulizer if ordered
   d. assist with or perform postural drainage therapy (PDT) if ordered
   e. perform suctioning if ordered
   f. administer expectorants (e.g., guaifenesin) if ordered
8. maintain oxygen therapy as ordered
9. discourage smoking *(the irritants in smoke increase mucus production, impair ciliary function, and can cause inflammation and damage to the bronchial and alveolar walls; the carbon monoxide decreases oxygen availability)*
10. increase activity as allowed and tolerated
11. administer central nervous system depressants judiciously; hold medication and consult physician if respiratory rate is less than 12/minute
12. administer the following medications as ordered:
    a. bronchodilators (e.g., methylxanthines, sympathomimetic [adrenergic] agents)
    b. antitubercular/antimicrobial agents *to treat the underlying disease process.*

c. Consult appropriate health care provider (e.g., respiratory therapist, physician) if signs and symptoms of impaired respiratory function persist or worsen.

2. Nursing Diagnosis: IMBALANCED NUTRITION: LESS THAN BODY REQUIREMENTS

related to:

a. decreased oral intake associated with weakness, fatigue, frequent cough, the foul odor and taste of sputum and some aerosol treatments, and dyspnea;
b. increased nutritional needs associated with the increase in metabolic rate that occurs with an infectious process.

Suggested NOC Outcome: Nutritional status	**Suggested NIC Interventions:** Nutritional monitoring; Nutrition management; Nutrition therapy

Desired Outcome	Nursing Actions *and Selected Purposes/Rationales* (see pp. 40–43 for additional rationales)
2. The client will maintain an adequate nutritional status as evidenced by: a. weight within normal range for client b. normal BUN and serum albumin, prealbumin, Hct, and Hgb c. usual strength and activity tolerance d. healthy oral mucous membrane.	2.a. Assess for and report signs and symptoms of malnutrition: 1. weight significantly below client's usual weight or less than normal for client's age, height, and body frame 2. abnormal BUN and low serum albumin, prealbumin, Hct, and Hgb 3. increased weakness and fatigue 4. sore, inflamed oral mucous membrane 5. pale conjunctiva. b. Monitor percentage of meals and snacks client consumes. Report a pattern of inadequate intake. c. Implement measures *to maintain an adequate nutritional status:* 1. perform actions *to improve oral intake:* a. consult respiratory therapist about scheduling respiratory treatments at least 1 hour before mealtime *(the foul odor and taste of sputum and some aerosols are likely to decrease appetite)*

b. increase activity as allowed and tolerated *(activity usually promotes a sense of well-being, which can improve appetite)*
c. obtain a dietary consult if necessary to assist client in selecting foods/fluids that meet nutritional needs, are appealing, and adhere to personal and cultural preferences whenever possible
d. encourage a rest period before meals *to minimize fatigue*
e. maintain a clean environment and a relaxed, pleasant atmosphere
f. assist with oral hygiene before meals *(oral hygiene moistens the mouth, which makes it easier to chew and swallow; it also removes unpleasant tastes, which often improves the taste of foods/fluids)*
g. place client in a high Fowler's position for meals and provide supplemental oxygen therapy during meals if indicated *to help relieve dyspnea*
h. serve frequent, small meals rather than large ones if client is weak, fatigues easily, or has a poor appetite
i. allow adequate time for meals; reheat foods/fluids if necessary

2. ensure that meals are well balanced and high in essential nutrients; offer dietary supplements if indicated
3. administer vitamins and minerals if ordered.

d. Perform a calorie count if ordered. Report information to dietitian and physician.
e. Consult physician about an alternative method of providing nutrition (e.g., parenteral nutrition, tube feedings) if client does not consume enough food or fluids to meet nutritional needs.

3. NURSING DIAGNOSIS: ***ACTIVITY INTOLERANCE***

related to:
a. tissue hypoxia associated with impaired gas exchange;
b. difficulty resting and sleeping associated with frequent coughing, dyspnea, and frequent assessments and treatments;
c. inadequate nutritional status;
d. increased energy expenditure associated with persistent coughing and the increased metabolic rate that is present in an infectious process.

Suggested NOC Outcomes: Activity tolerance; Endurance; Rest; Energy conservation

Suggested NIC Interventions: Energy management; Oxygen therapy; Sleep enhancement; Nutrition management; Infection control

Desired Outcome	**Nursing Actions** *and Selected Purposes/Rationales* (see pp. 11–12 for additional rationales)
3. The client will demonstrate an increased tolerance for activity as evidenced by: a. verbalization of feeling less fatigued and weak b. ability to perform activities of daily living without dizziness, increased dyspnea, chest pain, diaphoresis, and a significant change in vital signs.	3.a. Assess for signs and symptoms of activity intolerance: 1. statements of fatigue or weakness 2. exertional dyspnea, chest pain, diaphoresis, or dizziness 3. abnormal heart rate response to activity (e.g., increase in rate of 20 beats/minute above resting rate, rate not returning to preactivity level within 3 minutes after stopping activity, change from regular to irregular rate) 4. a significant change (15–20 mm Hg) in blood pressure with activity. b. Implement measures *to improve activity tolerance:* 1. perform actions *to promote rest and/or conserve energy:* a. maintain activity restrictions as ordered b. minimize environmental activity and noise c. organize nursing care to allow for periods of uninterrupted rest d. limit the number of visitors and their length of stay e. assist client with self-care activities as needed f. keep supplies and personal articles within easy reach g. instruct client in energy-saving techniques (e.g., using shower chair when showering, sitting to brush teeth or comb hair)

Desired Outcome	**Nursing Actions** *and Selected Purposes/Rationales*

h. implement measures *to promote sleep* (e.g., elevate head of bed and support arms on pillows to facilitate breathing; maintain oxygen therapy during sleep; discourage intake of fluids high in caffeine, especially in the evening; encourage use of progressive relaxation techniques or meditation; reduce environmental stimuli)

i. implement measures *to control cough:*

1. instruct client to avoid intake of very hot or cold foods/fluids *(these can stimulate cough)*
2. protect client from exposure to irritants such as flowers, smoke, and powder
3. administer prescribed antitussives if indicated to suppress cough (when cough is productive, antitussives should be used only when coughing is excessive and interfering significantly with the client's ability to rest and sleep)

2. perform actions *to lower the metabolic rate:*
   a. administer antitubercular/antimicrobial medications as ordered *to control the infectious process*
   b. implement measures *to reduce fever if present* (e.g., administer antipyretics as ordered, administer a tepid sponge bath)
3. discourage smoking and excessive intake of beverages high in caffeine such as coffee, tea, and colas *(nicotine and caffeine can increase cardiac workload and myocardial oxygen utilization, thereby decreasing oxygen availability)*
4. perform actions to improve respiratory status (see Diagnosis 1, action b) *in order to relieve dyspnea and improve tissue oxygenation*
5. if oxygen therapy is necessary during activity, keep portable oxygen equipment readily available for client's use
6. perform actions to maintain an adequate nutritional status (see Diagnosis 2, action c)
7. increase client's activity gradually as allowed and tolerated.

c. Instruct client to:
   1. report a decreased tolerance for activity
   2. stop any activity that causes chest pain, increased shortness of breath, dizziness, or extreme fatigue or weakness.

d. Consult appropriate health care provider (e.g., respiratory therapist, physician) if signs and symptoms of activity intolerance persist or worsen.

4. NURSING DIAGNOSIS:

RISK FOR INFECTION: EXTRAPULMONARY (E.G., PERICARDIAL, LARYNGEAL, SKELETAL, JOINT, RENAL, BRAIN, ADRENAL, LYMPHATIC) AND/OR SUPERINFECTION (E.G., CANDIDIASIS)

related to:

a. spread of the tubercle bacilli into the lymph nodes (lymphatic dissemination) and blood (hematogenous dissemination);
b. decreased resistance to infection associated with inadequate nutritional status and/or presence of other diseases (e.g., HIV infection, chronic obstructive pulmonary disease) and side effects of the treatment of those diseases;
c. interruption in the balance of usual endogenous microbial flora associated with the administration of antitubercular/antimicrobial agents.

Suggested NOC Outcomes: Immune status; Infection severity

Suggested NIC Interventions: Infection protection; Infection control

Desired Outcome	Nursing Actions *and Selected Purposes/Rationales* (see pp. 37–40 for additional rationales)
4. The client will not develop extrapulmonary infection or superinfection as evidenced by: a. no increase in temperature b. pulse within client's normal range c. absence of a pericardial friction rub and precordial pain d. absence of heat, pain, redness, swelling, and unusual drainage in any area e. absence of white patches and ulcerations in mouth f. no reports of increased weakness and fatigue g. normal voice quality h. absence of headache i. WBC and differential counts returning toward normal.	4.a. Assess for and report signs and symptoms of extrapulmonary infection or superinfection: 1. further increase in temperature 2. increased pulse 3. pericardial friction rub and/or precordial pain 4. bone pain 5. swollen, red, painful joints 6. swollen lymph node(s) 7. unusual color, amount, and odor of vaginal drainage; perineal itching; white patches or ulcerated areas in the mouth *(fungal infections are common superinfections with antimicrobial therapy)* 8. increased weakness or fatigue 9. hoarseness, sore throat 10. headache 11. increase in WBC count above previous levels and/or significant change in differential. b. Implement measures *to reduce the risk for extrapulmonary infection and/or superinfection:* 1. administer antitubercular/antimicrobial medications as ordered *to resolve the infectious process* 2. use good hand hygiene and encourage client to do the same 3. perform actions to maintain an adequate nutritional status (see Diagnosis 2, action c) 4. maintain sterile technique during all invasive procedures (e.g., venous and arterial punctures, injections, urinary catheterization) 5. change peripheral intravenous line sites according to hospital policy 6. protect client from others with infection 7. anchor catheters/tubings (e.g., urinary, intravenous) securely *in order to reduce trauma to the tissues and the risk for introduction of pathogens associated with the in-and-out movement of the tubing* 8. change equipment, tubing, and solutions used for treatments such as intravenous infusions and respiratory care according to hospital policy 9. maintain a closed system for drains (e.g., urinary catheter) and intravenous infusions whenever possible 10. instruct and assist client to perform good perineal care routinely and after each bowel movement 11. reinforce importance of frequent oral hygiene. c. If signs and symptoms of an extrapulmonary infection or superinfection occur: 1. prepare client for and/or assist with diagnostic tests (e.g., blood, vaginal, pleural fluid, and urine cultures; lumbar puncture; aspiration of joint fluid; bone marrow aspiration) 2. administer additional or alternative antitubercular/antimicrobial medications as ordered 3. implement appropriate comfort measures for symptoms experienced.

5. Collaborative Diagnoses: *POTENTIAL COMPLICATIONS OF PULMONARY TUBERCULOSIS*

a. pleural effusion related to an increase in capillary permeability of the pulmonary and pleural vessels associated with the inflammatory response to the presence of tubercle bacilli in the lung and pleural space;
b. pneumothorax related to accumulation of air in the pleural space associated with formation of a bronchopleural fistula or rupture of a subpleural bleb;
c. atelectasis related to shallow respirations and stasis of secretions in the alveoli and bronchioles.

Desired Outcomes	**Nursing Actions** *and Selected Purposes/Rationales*
5.a. The client will not develop pleural effusion as evidenced by: 1. no increase in dyspnea 2. symmetrical chest excursion 3. improved breath sounds and percussion note throughout lung fields.	5.a.1. Assess for and report signs and symptoms of pleural effusion: a. increased dyspnea b. decreased chest excursion on affected side c. dull percussion note and diminished or absent breath sounds over affected area d. chest x-ray, ultrasound, or computed tomography results showing pleural effusion. 2. Administer antitubercular/antimicrobial medications as ordered *to treat pulmonary TB and subsequently reduce the risk for development of pleural effusion.* 3. If signs and symptoms of pleural effusion occur: a. continue with actions to improve respiratory status (see Diagnosis 1, action b) b. prepare client for a thoracentesis and/or insertion of chest tube if planned.
5.b. The client will have resolution of pneumothorax if it occurs as evidenced by: 1. audible breath sounds and a resonant percussion note over lungs 2. normal rate of respirations 3. usual mental status 4. blood gases returning to normal range.	5.b.1. Assess for and immediately report signs and symptoms of pneumothorax (e.g., absent breath sounds with hyperresonant percussion note over involved area; rapid, shallow, and/or labored respirations; tachycardia; sudden onset of chest pain; restlessness; agitation; confusion; significant decrease in oximetry results; abnormal blood gases; chest x-ray results showing lung collapse). 2. If signs and symptoms of pneumothorax occur: a. maintain client on bed rest in a semi- to high Fowler's position b. maintain oxygen therapy as ordered c. assess for and immediately report signs and symptoms of tension pneumothorax with mediastinal shift (e.g., severe dyspnea, increased restlessness and agitation, rapid and/or irregular heart rate, hypotension, neck vein distention, shift in trachea from midline) d. prepare client for insertion of a chest tube if indicated.
5.c. The client will not develop atelectasis as evidenced by: 1. audible breath sounds and a resonant percussion note over lungs 2. no increase in dyspnea, respiratory rate, or temperature.	5.c.1. Assess for and report signs and symptoms of atelectasis (e.g., diminished or absent breath sounds; dull percussion note over affected area; further increase in respiratory rate, dyspnea, and temperature; chest x-ray results showing atelectasis). 2. Implement measures to improve respiratory status (see Diagnosis 1, action b) *in order to reduce the risk for atelectasis.* 3. If signs and symptoms of atelectasis occur: a. increase frequency of position change, coughing or "huffing," deep breathing, and use of incentive spirometer b. increase activity as allowed and tolerated c. consult physician if signs and symptoms of atelectasis persist or worsen.

6. Nursing Diagnosis: *INEFFECTIVE THERAPEUTIC REGIMEN MANAGEMENT*

related to:

a. lack of understanding of the implications of not following the prescribed treatment plan;
b. difficulty adhering to the prolonged multiple drug regimen;
c. undesirable side effects of some antitubercular/antimicrobial agents;
d. lack of motivation to continue medication regimen once asymptomatic (especially a concern with populations who are homeless, poor, intravenous drug abusers, alcoholics, and/or ill with other conditions such as AIDS);
e. insufficient financial resources.

Suggested NOC Outcomes: Treatment behavior: illness or injury; Compliance behavior; Health beliefs: perceived resources; Health beliefs: perceived ability to perform; Health beliefs: perceived control

Suggested NIC Interventions: Self-modification assistance; Medication management; Values clarification; Teaching: disease process; Support system enhancement

Desired Outcome	Nursing Actions *and Selected Purposes/Rationales*
6. The client will demonstrate the probability of effective therapeutic regimen management as evidenced by: a. willingness to learn about and participate in treatments and care b. statements reflecting ways to incorporate medication regimen into lifestyle c. statements reflecting an understanding of the implications of not following the prescribed treatment plan.	6.a. Assess for indications that the client may be unable to manage the therapeutic regimen effectively: 1. statements reflecting inability to adhere to medication regimen 2. failure to adhere to treatment plan (e.g., not adhering to isolation precautions, refusing respiratory therapy treatments, refusing medications) 3. statements reflecting a lack of understanding of the consequences of not following isolation precautions and prescribed respiratory care and medication regimens 4. statements reflecting an unwillingness or inability to modify personal habits 5. statements reflecting view that TB is cured once the symptoms are gone or that the situation is hopeless and efforts to comply with the therapeutic regimen are useless 6. statements reflecting that the side effects of medications are too uncomfortable and that he/she feels better when not taking the medications 7. statements reflecting that medications are too expensive. b. Implement measures *to promote effective therapeutic regimen management:* 1. explain TB in terms the client can understand; stress that TB is an infectious disease and that adherence to the treatment plan is necessary in order to prevent transmission to others, complications, and reactivation of the disease 2. explain that active TB can be treated successfully but only if the client adheres to the prescribed multiple drug therapy 3. provide instructions about and encourage client to participate in the treatment plan (e.g., protecting others from the infection, adhering to medication regimen, participating in respiratory care treatments) 4. provide client with written instructions about disease transmission, signs and symptoms to report, medication therapy, and follow-up appointments 5. assist client to identify ways the medication regimen can be incorporated into lifestyle 6. assist client to develop a method to promote adherence to the medication schedule (e.g., filling a pill box or empty egg carton with the medications that need to be taken that day/week, setting a timer or alarm as a reminder of when to take medications, using a checklist to document when each medication is due and taken) 7. initiate and reinforce discharge teaching outlined in Diagnosis 7 *in order to promote a sense of control* 8. provide information about and encourage utilization of community resources that can assist client to comply with the medication regimen (e.g., home health agencies, local Department of Health and Human Services, directly observed therapy (DOT) programs, local chapter of the American Lung Association, support groups) 9. encourage client to discuss concerns about the cost of medications and follow-up visits with health care provider; obtain a social service consult to assist with financial planning and to obtain financial aid if indicated

Desired Outcome	Nursing Actions and Selected Purposes/Rationales
	10. reinforce behavior suggesting future compliance with the therapeutic regimen (e.g., statements reflecting plans for adhering to treatment regimen, statements reflecting an understanding of TB and the consequences of inadequate treatment) 11. include significant others in explanations and teaching sessions and encourage their support. c. Consult appropriate health care provider regarding referrals to community health agencies if continued instruction or support is needed.

Discharge Teaching/Continued Care

7. Nursing Diagnosis: ***DEFICIENT KNOWLEDGE OR INEFFECTIVE HEALTH MAINTENANCE****

*The nurse should select the diagnostic label that is most appropriate for the client's discharge teaching needs.

Suggested NOC Outcomes: Knowledge: medication; Knowledge: health promotion; Knowledge: disease process; Knowledge: infection control

Suggested NIC Interventions: Health system guidance; Teaching: individual; Teaching: disease process; Teaching: prescribed medication; Communicable disease management

Desired Outcomes	Nursing Actions and Selected Purposes/Rationales
7.a. The client will identify ways to maintain respiratory health.	7.a. Instruct client in ways to maintain respiratory health: 1. maintain overall general good health (e.g., reduce stress, eat a well-balanced diet, obtain adequate rest) 2. stop smoking 3. avoid exposure to respiratory irritants such as smoke, dust, aerosol sprays, paint fumes, and solvents; wear a mask or scarf over nose and mouth if exposure to high levels of these irritants is unavoidable 4. remain indoors as much as possible when air pollution levels are high 5. avoid prolonged close contact with persons who have active TB or any other respiratory infection 6. avoid crowds and poorly ventilated areas 7. drink at least 10 glasses of liquid/day unless contraindicated 8. receive immunizations against influenza and pneumococcal pneumonia.
7.b. The client will identify ways to prevent the spread of TB to others.	7.b.1. Provide the following instructions on ways to prevent the spread of TB to others: a. cover nose and mouth with a tissue when coughing, sneezing, and laughing b. refrain from spitting or do so into a tissue c. practice good hand hygiene (e.g., wash hands using an antimicrobial soap, use an alcohol-base hand rub), especially after placing hands over mouth or nose and handling soiled tissues d. dispose of soiled tissues properly (e.g., place in paper or plastic bag, flush down toilet) e. avoid close contact with people who are at high risk for infection (e.g., those who are very young or elderly, those with HIV infection); wear a mask if close contact is unavoidable f. adhere strictly to the prescribed medication regimen for the treatment of TB.

2. Inform client that he/she will continue to be infectious until 3 consecutive sputum cultures show absence of the tubercle bacilli (this usually occurs after a couple of weeks of taking the antitubercular/antimicrobial agents) and that in order to not become infectious again, he/she must continue with the medication regimen for the prescribed length of time (usually 6–18 months).

7.c. The client will verbalize an understanding of medications ordered including rationale, food and drug interactions, side effects, and importance of taking as prescribed.

7.c.1. Explain the rationale for, side effects of, and importance of taking medications prescribed.
2. Inform client of pertinent food and drug interactions.
3. Remind client of the consequences of not adhering to the multiple drug regimen (e.g., spread of TB from lungs to other parts of the body, development of a strain of TB that will be very difficult to treat, transmission of TB to others).
4. If client is discharged on isoniazid (INH, Laniazid, Nydrazid) or a drug containing isoniazid (e.g., Rifamate, Rifater), instruct to:
   a. avoid alcohol intake (alcohol interferes with the metabolism of isoniazid and increases the risk of liver damage)
   b. avoid taking an antacid that contains aluminum (e.g., Amphojel, ALternaGEL) within 1 hour of taking isoniazid (aluminum interferes with absorption of isoniazid)
   c. for optimum absorption, take the medication one hour before or two hours after meals; if gastric distress occurs, take it with meals
   d. avoid intake of foods/fluids that contain tyramine (e.g., aged cheese, red wine, beer, bananas, caffeine-containing beverages, chocolate, yogurt, liver) if they cause symptoms such as headache, rapid or pounding heart beat, sweating, flushing, itching, or dizziness
   e. report feeling of heaviness, numbness, tingling, or burning in extremities; ringing in ears; dizziness; rash; fever; and symptoms of possible liver damage (e.g., loss of appetite, dark urine, yellow skin or eyes, fatigue, nausea)
   f. take vitamin B_6 (pyridoxine) as prescribed to prevent or decrease peripheral neuropathy.
5. If client is discharged on rifampin or a drug containing rifampin (e.g., Rifamate, Rifater), instruct to:
   a. expect that body fluids (e.g., urine, sweat, tears, saliva) may turn an orange-red color; stress that this is not permanent or harmful but caution that it could result in permanently stained soft contact lenses
   b. be aware that the drug can decrease the effectiveness of many other drugs (e.g., oral contraceptives, sildenafil [Viagra], warfarin, oral hypoglycemic agents, phenytoin, methadone, corticosteroids, theophylline, digoxin)
   c. monitor for and report side effects such as fever, chills, nausea, vomiting, heartburn, diarrhea, dizziness, excessive drowsiness, generalized itching, facial edema, unusual bruising or bleeding, and symptoms of possible liver damage (e.g., loss of appetite, dark urine, yellow skin or eyes, nausea, fatigue).
6. If client is discharged on ethambutol (Myambutol), instruct to:
   a. take with food to avoid gastric distress
   b. monitor for and immediately report visual changes (e.g., decreased visual field, blurred vision, decreased red-green color discrimination); stress that visual changes will usually resolve within a few months if the drug is discontinued right away
   c. monitor for and report painful joints, rash, nausea, vomiting, headaches, confusion, dizziness, weight gain, and decreased urine output.
7. If client is discharged on pyrazinamide (e.g., PZA) or a drug containing pyrazinamide (e.g., Rifater), instruct to:
   a. take with food to avoid gastric distress
   b. drink at least 8–10 glasses of fluid/day unless contraindicated (helps prevent renal calculi resulting from hyperuricemia)

Desired Outcomes	Nursing Actions *and Selected Purposes/Rationales*
	c. monitor for and report muscle aches, joint pain, nausea, vomiting, and symptoms of possible liver damage (e.g., loss of appetite, dark urine, yellow skin or eyes, nausea, fatigue) d. take allopurinol if prescribed (pyrazinamide raises serum uric acid levels). 8. If client is discharged on streptomycin, instruct to: a. keep scheduled appointments with health care provider to receive the drug (it is administered intramuscularly) b. have hearing checked monthly by health care provider (streptomycin can cause hearing loss) c. monitor for and immediately report dizziness, loss of balance, ringing in ears, hearing loss, swelling in ankles or feet, and decreased urine output (irreversible eighth cranial nerve damage and nephrotoxicity can occur if the drug is not discontinued). 9. Include teaching about any prescribed second-line and uncategorized antitubercular/antimicrobial drugs (e.g., rifapentine, amikacin, cycloserine, capreomycin, ethionamide, levofloxacin, ciprofloxacin, sparfloxacin) and drugs to manage side effects (e.g., antiemetics, vitamin B_6, allopurinol, antipyretics). 10. Instruct client to consult health care provider if considering becoming pregnant, if pregnancy occurs, and if breastfeeding (some of the medications used to treat TB are contraindicated in these situations). 11. Instruct client to take all medications as often as prescribed and avoid skipping doses or altering the prescribed dose; if a dose is missed, instruct client to take it as soon as remembered unless it is almost time for the next dose of the same medication. 12. Reinforce the need to consult physician before discontinuing any medication or taking additional prescription and nonprescription medications. 13. Reinforce the importance of keeping appointments for follow-up tests (e.g., blood work, hearing tests, sputum cultures, chest x-rays) and physical examinations to determine effectiveness of the medication regimen and assess for side effects such as liver and kidney damage.
7.d. The client will state signs and symptoms to report to the health care provider.	7.d. Instruct client to report the following: 1. persistent or recurrent loss of appetite, nausea, weakness, fatigue, or weight loss 2. fever, chills, continued or increased night sweats 3. difficulty breathing, continued or increased cough, or chest pain 4. unusual color, amount, and odor of vaginal secretions; white patches or ulcerated areas in mouth; stiff neck and headache; hoarseness; persistent sore throat; bone pain; swollen, red, painful joints; swollen lymph nodes (can be indicative of superinfection or extension of infection to another site) 5. signs and symptoms of adverse effects of medications (see actions c.4.e, 5.c, 6.c, 7.c, and 8.c in this diagnosis).
7.e. The client will verbalize an understanding of and a plan for adhering to recommended follow-up care including future appointments with health care provider.	7.e.1. Reinforce the importance of continued follow-up with health care provider. 2. Implement measures to promote effective management of the therapeutic regimen (see Diagnosis 6, action b).

Additional Nursing Diagnoses

*FEAR/ANXIETY**

related to unfamiliar environment, separation from significant others, financial concerns, and fear of transmitting disease to others.

*RISK FOR DEFICIENT FLUID VOLUME**

related to decreased oral fluid intake and excessive fluid loss (can occur with night sweats and profuse diaphoresis).

ACUTE PAIN: CHEST*

related to extension of the inflammatory/infectious process to the pleura and muscle strain (can result from excessive coughing).

*DISTURBED SLEEP PATTERN**

related to unfamiliar environment, night sweats, persistent coughing, anxiety, and frequent assessments and treatments.

*See Unit II for outcomes, actions, and rationales.

Bibliography

See pages 879 and 882–883.

UNIT XII

Nursing Care of the Client with Disturbances of the Kidney and Urinary Tract

Bladder Neck Suspension (Vesicourethral Suspension)

A bladder neck suspension is a surgical procedure performed to restore the bladder neck and proximal urethra to a well-supported retropubic position. It is performed to correct anatomic urinary stress incontinence associated with excessive mobility of the urethra and/or lowering of the position of the bladder neck (vesicourethral segment) resulting from pelvic floor weakness. The surgery is indicated when conservative measures for treating stress incontinence (e.g., pelvic floor exercises, biofeedback, estrogen therapy, sympathomimetic agents, periurethral bulking) have failed to produce significant improvement.

A number of techniques can be utilized to suspend the bladder neck and proximal urethra to their proper retropubic position. Most of these techniques involve placement of sutures in the periurethral and/or vaginal fascia and anchoring the sutures to the underside of the pubic symphysis or to an endopelvic ligament or muscle. Another procedure, considered by some authorities to be a bladder neck suspension technique, is called a pubovaginal or suburethral sling and involves the creation of a sling using a ribbon of fascia or synthetic material. This sling is then passed below the urethra and anchored to the urethropelvic ligament and/or vesicopelvic fascia. The approaches that are utilized for bladder suspension surgery include an abdominal approach (e.g., Marshall-Marchetti-Krantz, Burch), a vaginal approach in combination with suprapubic laparoscopy (e.g., Stamey, Raz), or a "no incision" laparoscopic approach (e.g., Gittes). The particular surgery and the approach selected depend on the physiological condition of the client, the type of incontinence present, previous pelvic surgeries the client has had, the presence of associated pelvic floor abnormalities (e.g., uterine prolapse, cystocele, rectocele), and the need for additional abdominal surgery.

This care plan focuses on the adult client having bladder neck suspension surgery. If repair of a cystocele and/or rectocele is planned concurrently, use this care plan in conjunction with the Care Plan on Colporrhaphy.

OUTCOME/DISCHARGE CRITERIA

THE CLIENT WILL:

- have evidence of normal healing of surgical wound(s)
- have clear, audible breath sounds throughout lungs
- have adequate urine output
- have no evidence of wound or urinary tract infection
- have no signs and symptoms of postoperative complications
- demonstrate care of suprapubic catheter if present
- demonstrate the ability to measure residual urine
- state signs and symptoms to report to the health care provider
- verbalize an understanding of and a plan for adhering to recommended follow-up care including future appointments with health care provider, medications prescribed, activity restrictions, and measures to prevent constipation.

NURSING/COLLABORATIVE DIAGNOSES

Postoperative

DISCHARGE TEACHING

See Standardized Preoperative and Postoperative Care Plans (pp. 97–126) for additional diagnoses.

PREOPERATIVE

Refer to the Standardized Preoperative Care Plan.

POSTOPERATIVE *Use in conjunction with the Standardized Postoperative Care Plan.*

1. Nursing Diagnosis: **URINARY RETENTION**

related to:
a. obstruction of the urethral and/or suprapubic catheters if present;
b. impaired urination following removal of the catheter(s) associated with:
   1. edema of the bladder neck and urethra resulting from surgical trauma
   2. increased tone of the urinary sphincters resulting from sympathetic nervous system stimulation (can result from pain, fear, and anxiety)
   3. decreased perception of bladder fullness resulting from the depressant effect of anesthesia and some medications (e.g., narcotic [opioid] analgesics)
   4. relaxation of the bladder muscle resulting from the depressant effect of anesthesia and some medications (e.g., narcotic [opioid] analgesics) and stimulation of the sympathetic nervous system (can result from pain, fear, and anxiety)
   5. urethral obstruction resulting from excessive elevation of the bladder neck.

Suggested NOC Outcome: Urinary elimination

Suggested NIC Interventions: Urinary retention care; Tube care: urinary; Urinary catheterization: intermittent

Desired Outcome

1. The client will not experience urinary retention as evidenced by:
   a. no reports of bladder fullness and suprapubic discomfort
   b. absence of bladder distention
   c. balanced intake and output within 48 hours after surgery
   d. voiding adequate amounts at expected intervals after removal of the catheter(s).

Nursing Actions *and Selected Purposes/Rationales*
(see pp. 61–62 for additional rationales)

1.a. Assess for and report the following:
   1. urinary retention when suprapubic and/or urethral catheters are present (e.g., reports of bladder fullness or suprapubic discomfort, bladder distention, absence of fluid in urinary drainage tubing, output that continues to be less than intake 48 hours after surgery)
   2. urinary retention following catheter removal (e.g., reports of bladder fullness or suprapubic discomfort, bladder distention, output that continues to be less than intake 48 hours after surgery, frequent voiding of small amounts [25–60 ml] of urine).

b. Implement measures *to prevent urinary retention:*
   1. perform actions *to maintain patency of urinary catheter(s):*
      a. keep drainage tubing free of kinks
      b. keep collection container below level of bladder
      c. tape catheter tubing securely (suprapubic catheter tubing to abdomen, urethral catheter tubing to thigh) *in order to prevent inadvertent removal*
      d. irrigate catheter if ordered
   2. after urethral catheter is removed, open suprapubic catheter as scheduled or if client is unable to void voluntarily
   3. when both urethral and suprapubic catheters have been removed, refer to Standardized Postoperative Care Plan, Diagnosis 14, action c (pp. 115–116), for measures related to prevention of urinary retention
   4. perform intermittent catheterization as ordered if post-voiding residual urine exceeds the established parameter (usually 50–100 ml).

2. Nursing Diagnosis: **RISK FOR CONSTIPATION**

related to:
a. decreased gastrointestinal motility associated with manipulation of the bowel (if an abdominal approach was used), decreased activity, and the depressant effect of the anesthetic and narcotic (opioid) analgesics;
b. decreased intake of fluids and foods high in fiber;

c. reluctance to defecate associated with fear of pain and possible disruption of sutures.

Suggested NOC Outcome: Bowel elimination

Suggested NIC Intervention: Constipation/Impaction management

Desired Outcome	**Nursing Actions** *and Selected Purposes/Rationales* (see pp. 24–26 for additional rationales)
2. The client will not experience constipation (see Standardized Postoperative Care Plan, Diagnosis 15 [p. 116], for outcome criteria).	2.a. Refer to Standardized Postoperative Care Plan, Diagnosis 15 (pp. 116–117), for measures related to assessment and prevention of constipation. b. Implement additional measures *to prevent constipation:* 1. consult physician about an order for a stool softener if one has not been ordered 2. instruct client to request an analgesic prior to attempting to defecate *in order to ease the surgical site pain associated with the increased intra-abdominal and perineal pressure that occur with defecation.*

3. Nursing Diagnosis: RISK FOR INFECTION

a. urinary tract infection related to:
   1. increased growth and colonization of microorganisms associated with urinary stasis
   2. introduction of pathogens associated with the presence of urethral and/or suprapubic catheters and performance of intermittent catheterizations if being done;

b. wound infection related to:
   1. wound contamination associated with introduction of pathogens during or following surgery (particularly high risk with a vaginal approach because of the proximity of the incision to the perianal area)
   2. decreased resistance to infection associated with factors such as diminished blood flow to wound area or an inadequate nutritional status.

Suggested NOC Outcomes: Immune status; Infection severity; Wound healing: primary intention

Suggested NIC Interventions: Infection protection; Infection control; Wound care; Urinary retention care; Perineal care

Desired Outcomes	**Nursing Actions** *and Selected Purposes/Rationales* (see pp. 37–40 for additional rationales)
3.a. The client will remain free of urinary tract infection (see Standardized Postoperative Care Plan, Diagnosis 17, outcome c [p. 119], for outcome criteria).	3.a.1. Refer to Standardized Postoperative Care Plan, Diagnosis 17, action c (p. 119), for measures related to assessment, prevention, and treatment of urinary tract infection. 2. Implement measures to prevent urinary retention (see Postoperative Diagnosis 1, action b) *in order to further reduce the risk of urinary stasis and subsequent urinary tract infection.*
3.b. The client will remain free of wound infection (see Standardized Postoperative Care Plan, Diagnosis 17, outcome b [pp. 118–119], for outcome criteria).	3.b.1. Refer to Standardized Postoperative Care Plan, Diagnosis 17, action b (pp. 118–119), for measures related to assessment, prevention, and management of postoperative wound infection. 2. Implement additional measures *to reduce the risk for wound infection if a vaginal incision is present:* a. instruct client to wipe from front to back following urination and defecation b. assist client with perineal care every shift and after each bowel movement.

4. Collaborative Diagnosis: ***POTENTIAL COMPLICATION OF BLADDER NECK SUSPENSION SURGERY: BLADDER, URETHRAL, OR URETERAL INJURY***

related to accidental tear or ligation during the surgical procedure.

Desired Outcome	**Nursing Actions** *and Selected Purposes/Rationales*
4. The client will experience healing of bladder, urethral, or ureteral injury if it occurs as evidenced by: a. gradual resolution of hematuria and backache b. urine output greater than 200 ml within 6–8 hours after surgery.	4.a. Assess for and report signs and symptoms of bladder, urethral, or ureteral injury (e.g., persistent or increasing hematuria or backache, urine output less than 200 ml in first 6–8 hours after surgery). b. If signs and symptoms of bladder, urethral, or ureteral injury are present: 1. continue to monitor output carefully 2. prepare client for surgical repair if indicated.

Discharge Teaching/Continued Care

5. Nursing Diagnosis: ***DEFICIENT KNOWLEDGE, INEFFECTIVE THERAPEUTIC REGIMEN MANAGEMENT, OR INEFFECTIVE HEALTH MAINTENANCE****

*The nurse should select the diagnostic label that is most appropriate for the client's discharge teaching needs.

Suggested NOC Outcome: Knowledge: treatment regimen

Suggested NIC Interventions: Health system guidance; Teaching: individual; Teaching: psychomotor skill; Teaching: disease process

Desired Outcomes	**Nursing Actions** *and Selected Purposes/Rationales*
5.a. The client will demonstrate care of suprapubic catheter if present.	5.a.1. Provide the following instructions about care of suprapubic catheter if client is discharged with one in place: a. tape catheter securely to abdomen b. keep skin around catheter insertion site clean and dry c. keep drainage tubing free of kinks d. keep collection bag below level of bladder. 2. allow time for questions, clarification, and return demonstration.
5.b. The client will demonstrate the ability to measure residual urine.	5.b.1. Provide the following instructions about how to measure residual urine (the client who needs to measure residual urine and does not have a suprapubic catheter will need to be instructed on how to perform self-catheterization): a. unclamp the suprapubic catheter after urinating or at prescribed intervals (usually every 4 hours if unable to urinate) b. leave the suprapubic catheter unclamped for 10 minutes, reclamp the catheter, and then empty the bag and measure the amount of urine c. measure and record the amount of urine voided and the amount of residual urine. 2. Instruct client to contact physician's office once the residual urine amounts are consistently less than 100 ml for 2 consecutive days (most physicians want the suprapubic catheter to be removed at this point). 3. Allow time for questions, clarification, and return demonstration.
5.c. The client will state signs and symptoms to report to the health care provider.	5.c.1. Refer to Standardized Postoperative Care Plan, Diagnosis 22, action c (p. 125), for signs and symptoms to report to the health care provider. 2. Instruct client to report these additional signs and symptoms: a. stress incontinence

b. unusual and continuous abdominal or pelvic pain
c. temperature above 38° C (100.4° F)
d. persistent bright red vaginal bleeding or clots
e. persistent inability to void voluntarily
f. persistent residual urine amounts in excess of 100 ml.

5.d. The client will verbalize an understanding of and a plan for adhering to recommended follow-up care including future appointments with health care provider, medications prescribed, activity restrictions, and measures to prevent constipation.

5.d.1. Refer to Standardized Postoperative Care Plan, Diagnosis 22 (pp. 125–126), for routine postoperative instructions and measures to improve client compliance.
2. Instruct client to avoid vigorous exercise and lifting objects over 15 pounds until healing is complete (about 6 weeks).
3. If client has a vaginal incision, instruct her to:
   a. perform good perineal hygiene, particularly after defecation
   b. avoid inserting anything into vagina (e.g., tampons, douches) or having sexual intercourse until advised by physician (usually for 6 weeks).
4. Reinforce measures to prevent constipation:
   a. drink 8–10 glasses of water a day unless contraindicated
   b. eat foods that are high in fiber (e.g., fresh fruits and vegetables, whole grain cereals)
   c. take 1–2 stool softeners (e.g., Dialose) a day.
5. Instruct client to contact physician's office or follow physician's instructions regarding the appropriate measures to take if there is a two-day span without a bowel movement (at this point, the physician will often recommend that client self-administer a small-volume enema [e.g., Fleet] or laxative suppository [e.g., Dulcolax]).

Bibliography

See pages 879 and 883.

Chronic Renal Failure

Chronic renal failure (CRF) is a progressive, irreversible loss of kidney function that usually develops gradually over many years. The leading causes of CRF are diabetes mellitus, hypertension, and glomerulonephritis. Other causes include pyelonephritis/interstitial nephritis, obstruction of the urinary tract by conditions such as benign prostatic hypertrophy, and hereditary conditions such as polycystic kidney disease. Chronic renal failure can also develop following acute renal failure that has resulted in irreversible renal damage.

Creatinine clearance is the measurement that is used to determine the effectiveness of renal function. As renal failure progresses, creatinine clearance declines, reflecting a decrease in the glomerular filtration rate (GFR) and the percent of functioning nephrons. The severity of CRF can be classified by the proportion of renal function that has been lost and is often divided into stages. In the first stage, diminished renal reserve, the GFR can be as low as 30% of normal but the renal dysfunction usually goes undiagnosed because homeostatic mechanisms are able to maintain fluid balance and keep serum electrolytes, urea nitrogen, and creatinine within normal ranges.

Renal insufficiency, the middle stage, begins when the GFR is about 25% of normal. At this point in the disease process, creatinine clearance continues to decline and azotemia (the retention of nitrogenous substances in the blood) begins. The blood urea nitrogen (BUN) and serum creatinine are elevated but are not high enough to cause symptoms that are problematic for the client. During this stage, the client progresses from a nonoliguric phase, in which the kidneys are unable to concentrate the urine, to a state of oliguria. When this occurs, symptoms become evident and result mainly from a decreased ability of the kidneys to excrete fluid and electrolytes.

The last stage of CRF is end-stage renal disease (ESRD). It occurs when the GFR is less than about 10% of normal and nitrogenous substances (e.g., urea, creatinine) accumulate to levels high enough to cause toxic effects on other body systems. Typical signs and symptoms of ESRD can include lethargy, irritability, extreme fatigue and weakness, pruritus, nausea and vomiting, muscle cramping, and stomatitis. Fluid, electrolyte, and acid-base imbalances also worsen and, in this stage, dialysis or kidney transplantation is necessary for survival.

This care plan focuses on the adult client with renal insufficiency who has progressed from the nonoliguric to the oliguric phase and is hospitalized for treatment and further evaluation of renal function. Much of the information is also applicable to clients in an extended care facility or home setting.

OUTCOME/DISCHARGE CRITERIA

THE CLIENT WILL:

- not have signs and symptoms of uremic syndrome
- have blood pressure within a safe range
- have fluid, electrolyte, and acid-base balance stabilized within a safe range
- tolerate expected level of activity
- have no evidence of infection
- have an adequate nutritional status
- verbalize a basic understanding of chronic renal failure
- identify ways to slow the progression of kidney damage
- verbalize an understanding of fluid restrictions and dietary modifications
- demonstrate the ability to accurately weigh self, measure fluid intake and output, and monitor own blood pressure
- identify ways to reduce the risk of infection
- identify ways to manage signs and symptoms that often occur as a result of chronic renal failure
- share feelings and concerns about the effects of renal failure on lifestyle and roles
- state signs and symptoms to report to the health care provider
- identify community resources that can assist with adjustment to changes resulting from chronic renal failure
- verbalize an understanding of and a plan for adhering to recommended follow-up care including future appointments with health care provider and medications prescribed.

NURSING/COLLABORATIVE DIAGNOSES

See pp. 23–24 for additional diagnoses.

1. NURSING/COLLABORATIVE DIAGNOSIS

RISK FOR IMBALANCED FLUID AND ELECTROLYTES

a. excess fluid volume related to:
   1. retention of sodium and water associated with a decreased glomerular filtration rate (occurs as a result of the decrease in the number of functioning nephrons) and activation of the renin-angiotensin-aldosterone mechanism (can occur if renal blood flow is decreased as a result of the underlying disease process)
   2. fluid intake in excess of prescribed restrictions;
b. hyponatremia related to excessive fluid intake in relation to output (causes a dilutional hyponatremia) and loss of sodium associated with diuretic therapy;
c. hypernatremia related to:
   1. decreased ability of the kidneys to excrete sodium
   2. increased aldosterone output associated with activation of the renin-angiotensin-aldosterone mechanism if decreased renal blood flow has occurred as a result of the underlying disease process
   3. dietary sodium intake in excess of prescribed restrictions;
d. hyperkalemia related to:
   1. decreased ability of the kidneys to excrete potassium
   2. increased cellular release of potassium associated with progressive renal tissue damage and metabolic acidosis
   3. dietary potassium intake in excess of prescribed restrictions
   4. use of potassium-sparing diuretics or medications and salt substitutes containing potassium;
e. hypocalcemia related to:
   1. decreased intestinal absorption of calcium associated with inability of the kidneys to activate vitamin D (the active metabolite of vitamin D is needed to stimulate calcium absorption from the small intestine)
   2. hyperphosphatemia (causes a reciprocal drop in calcium);
f. hyperphosphatemia related to hypocalcemia (an inverse relationship exists between phosphorus and calcium) and decreased ability of the kidneys to excrete phosphorus;
g. hypermagnesemia related to:
   1. decreased ability of the kidneys to excrete magnesium
   2. excessive intake of magnesium-containing antacids, laxatives, or foods;
h. metabolic acidosis related to:
   1. decreased ability of the kidneys to excrete hydrogen ions and reabsorb bicarbonate

2. hyperkalemia (the body attempts to compensate for high serum potassium levels by shifting hydrogen ions into the vascular space in exchange for potassium ions).

Suggested NOC Outcomes: Fluid balance; Electrolyte and acid/base balance; Fluid overload severity; Kidney function

Suggested NIC Interventions: Fluid/Electrolyte monitoring; Fluid management; Hypervolemia management; Electrolyte management: hypocalcemia; Electrolyte management: hypercalcemia; Electrolyte management: hyperphosphatemia; Electrolyte management: hyponatremia; Electrolyte management: hypernatremia; Electrolyte management: hyperkalemia; Electrolyte management: hypermagnesemia; Acid-base monitoring; Acid-base management: metabolic acidosis

Desired Outcomes	**Nursing Actions** *and Selected Purposes/Rationales* (see pp. 31–33 for additional rationales)
1.a. The client will experience resolution of excess fluid volume as evidenced by: 1. decline in weight toward client's normal 2. B/P within normal range for client 3. absence of an S_3 heart sound 4. normal pulse volume 5. balanced intake and output 6. usual mental status 7. normal breath sounds 8. absence of dyspnea, orthopnea, peripheral edema, and distended neck veins.	1.a.1. Assess for and report signs and symptoms of excess fluid volume: a. weight gain of 2% or greater over a short period b. elevated B/P (B/P may not be elevated if fluid has shifted out of vascular space) c. presence of an S_3 heart sound d. bounding pulse e. intake greater than output f. change in mental status g. crackles (rales) and diminished or absent breath sounds h. dyspnea, orthopnea i. peripheral edema j. distended neck veins k. chest x-ray results showing pulmonary vascular congestion, pleural effusion, or pulmonary edema. 2. Implement measures *to reduce excess fluid volume:* a. maintain fluid restrictions as ordered (intake allowed is usually 500–700 ml plus the amount of urine output in the previous 24 hours); instruct client in ways to alleviate thirst and/or keep oral mucous membranes moist (e.g., space fluid intake evenly throughout the hours he/she is awake, rinse mouth frequently with water, breathe through nose rather than mouth) *in order to promote compliance with oral fluid restrictions* b. if client is receiving numerous and/or large volume intravenous medications, consult pharmacist about ways to prevent excessive fluid administration (e.g., stop primary infusion during administration of intravenous medications, dilute medication in the minimum amount of solution) c. restrict sodium intake as ordered d. administer diuretics if ordered *to increase excretion of water.* 3. Consult physician if signs and symptoms of excess fluid volume persist or worsen.
1.b. The client will maintain a safe serum sodium level as evidenced by: 1. absence of nausea, vomiting, abdominal cramps, and thirst 2. moist mucous membranes 3. usual mental status 4. usual muscle strength 5. absence of seizure activity 6. serum sodium within a safe range for client.	1.b.1. Assess for and report signs and symptoms of: a. hyponatremia (e.g., nausea, vomiting, abdominal cramps, lethargy, confusion, weakness, seizures, low serum sodium level) b. hypernatremia (e.g., thirst; dry, sticky mucous membranes; restlessness; lethargy; weakness; elevated temperature; seizures; elevated serum sodium level). 2. Implement measures *to prevent or treat hyponatremia:* a. maintain fluid restrictions as ordered *to prevent dilutional hyponatremia* b. increase dietary allotment of sodium if ordered c. administer loop diuretics (e.g., furosemide) if ordered *to promote excretion of water.* 3. Implement measures *to prevent or treat hypernatremia:* a. maintain maximum fluid intake allowed

b. maintain dietary sodium restrictions if ordered
c. administer thiazide diuretics if ordered.
4. Consult physician if unsafe serum sodium levels persist.

1.c. The client will maintain a safe serum potassium level as evidenced by:
1. regular pulse at 60–100 beats/minute
2. absence of paresthesias
3. usual muscle tone and strength
4. absence of diarrhea and intestinal colic
5. normal ECG
6. serum potassium within a safe range for client.

1.c.1. Assess for and report signs and symptoms of hyperkalemia (e.g., slow or irregular pulse; paresthesias; muscle weakness and flaccidity; diarrhea and intestinal colic; ECG showing peaked T wave, prolonged PR interval, and/or widened QRS; elevated serum potassium level).
2. Implement measures *to prevent or treat hyperkalemia:*
a. maintain dietary restrictions of potassium as ordered by limiting intake of foods/fluids such as bananas, potatoes, raisins, avocados, and orange juice
b. instruct client to consult physician or dietitian about which salt substitute can safely be used *(most salt substitutes contain potassium)*
c. perform actions *to reduce the cellular release of potassium:*
1. implement measures *to spare body proteins and prevent excessive tissue breakdown:*
a. encourage client to consume the amount of dietary protein allotted
b. provide allotted amount of carbohydrates *(spares protein by providing a quick energy source)*
c. perform actions to prevent infection (see Diagnosis 5, action b) *in order to prevent an increase in the metabolic rate and a subsequent increase in protein catabolism*
2. implement measures to prevent or treat metabolic acidosis (see action g.2 in this diagnosis)
d. if signs and symptoms of hyperkalemia are present, consult physician before administering prescribed potassium supplements and other medications that can increase potassium levels (e.g., potassium penicillin G, potassium-sparing diuretics, some beta blockers and angiotensin-converting enzyme [ACE] inhibitors)
e. administer the following medications if ordered:
1. loop diuretics (e.g., ethacrynic acid, furosemide) *to increase renal excretion of potassium*
2. cation-exchange resins (e.g., sodium polystyrene sulfonate [Kayexalate]) *to increase potassium excretion via the intestines (act by exchanging sodium for potassium)*
3. intravenous insulin and hypertonic glucose solutions *to enhance transport of potassium back into cells.*
3. If signs and symptoms of hyperkalemia persist or worsen:
a. consult physician
b. have intravenous calcium preparation (e.g., calcium gluconate) readily available *(may be ordered to counteract the effect of a high potassium level on the heart).*

1.d. The client will maintain a safe serum calcium level as evidenced by:
1. usual mental status
2. negative Chvostek's and Trousseau's signs
3. absence of numbness and tingling in fingers, toes, and circumoral area; hyperreflexia; tetany; and seizure activity
4. serum calcium within a safe range for client.

1.d.1. Assess for and report signs and symptoms of hypocalcemia (e.g., anxiousness; irritability; positive Chvostek's and Trousseau's signs; numbness or tingling of fingers, toes, or circumoral area; hyperactive reflexes; tetany; seizures; serum calcium level that is lower than normal for client).
2. Implement measures *to prevent or treat hypocalcemia:*
a. provide sources of calcium (e.g., milk, milk products) in diet unless contraindicated
b. administer activated vitamin D (e.g., paricalcitol, calcitriol) and calcium supplements if ordered
c. perform actions to prevent or treat hyperphosphatemia (see action e.2 in this diagnosis)
d. avoid rapid or aggressive treatment of acidosis *(rapidly reversing acidosis can result in decreased ionization of calcium).*
3. If signs and symptoms of hypocalcemia occur:
a. institute seizure precautions
b. administer calcium preparations (e.g., calcium gluconate, calcium carbonate) as ordered.

Desired Outcomes	Nursing Actions *and Selected Purposes/Rationales*
1.e. The client will maintain a safe serum phosphorus level as evidenced by: 1. absence of paresthesias, tetany, and seizure activity 2. serum phosphorus within a safe range for client.	1.e.1. Assess for and report signs and symptoms of hyperphosphatemia (e.g., paresthesias, tetany, seizures, higher than normal serum phosphorus level for client). 2. Implement measures *to prevent or treat hyperphosphatemia:* a. restrict dietary intake of phosphorus if ordered by limiting intake of foods/fluids such as poultry, nuts, milk, milk products, eggs, legumes, and some cola beverages b. administer phosphate-binding medications such as sevelamer (e.g., Renagel), aluminum-containing agents (e.g., Amphojel, Basaljel), calcium acetate (e.g., PhosLo), and calcium carbonate (e.g., Tums) if ordered. 3. Consult physician if signs and symptoms of hyperphosphatemia persist or worsen.
1.f. The client will maintain a safe serum magnesium level as evidenced by: 1. absence of flushing, nausea, vomiting, and muscle weakness 2. usual mental status 3. vital signs within normal range for client 4. serum magnesium within a safe range for client.	1.f.1. Assess for and report signs and symptoms of hypermagnesemia (e.g., flushed, warm skin; nausea; vomiting; muscle weakness; drowsiness; lethargy; hypotension; bradypnea; bradycardia; higher than normal serum magnesium level for client). 2. Implement measures *to prevent or treat hypermagnesemia:* a. avoid giving laxatives and antacids that contain magnesium (e.g., Milk of Magnesia, Gelusil, Mylanta, Maalox) b. maintain dietary restrictions of magnesium if ordered by limiting intake of foods/fluids such as seafood; green, leafy vegetables; and legumes. 3. Consult physician if signs and symptoms of hypermagnesemia persist or worsen.
1.g. The client will not experience metabolic acidosis as evidenced by: 1. usual mental status 2. unlabored respirations at 12–20/minute 3. absence of headache, nausea, vomiting, and cardiac dysrhythmias 4. blood gases within a safe range for client 5. anion gap within normal range.	1.g.1. Assess for and report signs and symptoms of metabolic acidosis (e.g., drowsiness; disorientation; stupor; rapid, deep respirations; headache; nausea; vomiting; cardiac dysrhythmias; lower than usual pH and CO_2 content; increased anion gap). 2. Implement measures *to prevent or treat metabolic acidosis:* a. perform actions to prevent or treat hyperkalemia (see action c.2 in this diagnosis) b. administer sodium bicarbonate if ordered. 3. Consult physician if signs and symptoms of acidosis persist or worsen.

2. Nursing Diagnosis: *IMBALANCED NUTRITION: LESS THAN BODY REQUIREMENTS*

related to:

a. decreased oral intake associated with fatigue and dislike of prescribed diet;

b. prescribed dietary modifications (especially protein restrictions that are necessary in order to control the serum levels of nitrogenous substances).

Suggested NOC Outcome: Nutritional status

Suggested NIC Interventions: Nutritional monitoring; Nutrition management; Nutrition therapy

Desired Outcome	Nursing Actions *and Selected Purposes/Rationales* (see pp. 40–43 for additional rationales)

2. The client will maintain an adequate nutritional status as evidenced by:
   a. weight within normal range for client
   b. serum albumin, prealbumin, Hct, Hgb, and lymphocyte levels within normal range
   c. usual or improved strength and activity tolerance
   d. healthy oral mucous membrane.

2.a. Assess for and report signs and symptoms of malnutrition:
1. weight significantly below client's usual weight or below normal for client's age, height, and body frame
2. low serum albumin, prealbumin, Hct, Hgb, and lymphocyte levels (some of these values may be abnormal as a result of decreased renal function)
3. weakness and fatigue (may also be a reflection of decreasing renal function)
4. sore, inflamed oral mucous membrane
5. pale conjunctiva.

b. Monitor percentage of meals and snacks client consumes. Report a pattern of inadequate intake.

c. Implement measures *to maintain an adequate nutritional status:*
1. perform actions *to improve oral intake:*
   a. increase activity as tolerated *(activity usually promotes a sense of well-being, which can improve appetite)*
   b. obtain a dietary consult if necessary to assist client in selecting foods/fluids that meet nutritional needs, are appealing, and adhere to personal and cultural preferences as well as the prescribed dietary modifications
   c. encourage a rest period before meals *to minimize fatigue*
   d. maintain a clean environment and a relaxed, pleasant atmosphere
   e. provide oral hygiene before meals *(removes unpleasant tastes, which often improves the taste of foods/fluids)*
   f. serve frequent, small meals rather than large ones if client is weak, fatigues easily, and/or has a poor appetite
   g. allow adequate time for meals; reheat foods/fluids if necessary
2. encourage client to eat the maximum amount of protein allowed; instruct him/her to satisfy protein requirements with foods/fluids that are complete proteins and contain essential amino acids (e.g., eggs, milk, meat, poultry) if client's serum phosphorus level is not too high
3. offer dietary supplements if indicated
4. administer vitamins and minerals if ordered.

d. Perform a calorie count if ordered. Report information to dietitian and physician.

e. Consult appropriate health care provider (e.g., dietitian, physician) if client does not consume enough food or fluids to meet nutritional needs.

3. Nursing Diagnosis:

ACTIVITY INTOLERANCE

related to:
a. inadequate tissue oxygenation associated with anemia resulting from:
   1. decreased secretion of erythropoietin as a result of impaired renal function (erythropoietin stimulates the bone marrow to produce RBCs)
   2. shortened survival time of RBCs (as renal failure progresses, the nitrogenous substances in the blood increase and cause increased hemolysis of RBCs);
b. inadequate nutritional status.

Suggested NOC Outcomes: Rest; Energy conservation; Self-care status; Self-care: activities of daily living; Activity tolerance

Suggested NIC Interventions: Nutrition management; Energy management

Desired Outcome	Nursing Actions *and Selected Purposes/Rationales* (see pp. 11–12 for additional rationales)
3. The client will demonstrate an increased tolerance for activity as evidenced by: a. verbalization of feeling less fatigued and weak b. ability to perform activities of daily living without exertional dyspnea, chest pain, diaphoresis, dizziness, and a significant change in vital signs.	3.a. Assess for signs and symptoms of activity intolerance: 1. statements of fatigue or weakness 2. exertional dyspnea, chest pain, diaphoresis, or dizziness 3. abnormal heart rate response to activity (e.g., increase in rate of 20 beats/minute above resting rate, rate not returning to preactivity level within 3 minutes after stopping activity, change from regular to irregular rate) 4. a significant change (15–20 mm Hg) in blood pressure with activity. b. Implement measures *to improve activity tolerance:* 1. perform actions *to promote rest and/or conserve energy:* a. maintain activity restrictions if ordered b. minimize environmental activity and noise c. organize nursing care to allow for periods of uninterrupted rest d. limit the number of visitors and their length of stay e. assist client with self-care activities as needed f. keep supplies and personal articles within easy reach g. instruct client in energy-saving techniques (e.g., using shower chair when showering, sitting to brush teeth or comb hair) 2. perform actions to reduce the levels of serum nitrogenous substances (see Diagnosis 6, action a.2) *in order to reduce the rate of RBC hemolysis* 3. perform actions to maintain an adequate nutritional status (see Diagnosis 2, action c) 4. administer the following if ordered *to treat anemia:* a. iron preparations and/or folic acid b. erythropoiesis stimulating growth factor such as epoetin alfa (e.g., Epogen, EPO, Procrit) or darbepoetin alfa (e.g., Aransep) 5. increase client's activity gradually as tolerated. c. Instruct client to: 1. report a decreased tolerance for activity 2. stop any activity that causes chest pain, shortness of breath, dizziness, or extreme fatigue or weakness. d. Consult physician if signs and symptoms of activity intolerance persist or worsen.

4. Nursing Diagnosis: ***RISK FOR CONSTIPATION***

related to:

a. decreased intake of foods high in fiber and fluids associated with prescribed restrictions;
b. decreased gastrointestinal motility associated with decreased activity and the effect of some medications (e.g., those containing aluminum or calcium, iron preparations).

Suggested NOC Outcome: Bowel elimination

Suggested NIC Intervention: Constipation/Impaction management

Desired Outcome	Nursing Actions *and Selected Purposes/Rationales* (see pp. 24–26 for additional rationales)
4. The client will not experience constipation as evidenced by: a. usual frequency of bowel movements b. passage of soft, formed stool c. absence of abdominal distention and pain, rectal fullness or pressure, and straining during defecation.	4.a. Assess for signs and symptoms of constipation (e.g., decrease in frequency of bowel movements; passage of hard, formed stools; anorexia; abdominal distention and pain; feeling of fullness or pressure in rectum; straining during defecation). b. Assess bowel sounds. Report a pattern of diminishing sounds. c. Implement measures *to prevent constipation:* 1. increase activity as tolerated 2. encourage client to consume the allotted amount of fluid 3. encourage client to defecate whenever the urge is felt

4. assist client to bathroom or bedside commode for bowel movements unless contraindicated
5. encourage client to relax, provide privacy, and have call signal within reach during attempts to defecate *(measures to promote relaxation enable client to relax the levator ani muscle and external anal sphincter, which facilitates evacuation of stool)*
6. encourage client to establish a regular time for defecation, preferably an hour after a meal
7. encourage client to drink hot liquids upon arising in the morning *in order to stimulate peristalsis*
8. encourage client to increase intake of bran (bran is recommended *because it is a good source of fiber and is low in phosphorus)*
9. consult physician about alternating antacids that are constipating (e.g., Amphojel, Rolaids, Tums) with those that have a laxative effect (e.g., Milk of Magnesia, Gelusil, Mylanta, Maalox) if client's magnesium level is not too high.

d. Consult appropriate health care provider if signs and symptoms of constipation persist.

5. NURSING DIAGNOSIS: RISK FOR INFECTION

related to:
a. lowered natural resistance associated with:
   1. changes in leukocyte function and a depressed immune response resulting from the effects of increasing levels of serum nitrogenous substances
   2. inadequate nutritional status;
b. stasis of respiratory secretions and urinary stasis if mobility is decreased.

Suggested NOC Outcomes: Immune status; Infection severity

Suggested NIC Interventions: Infection protection; Infection control

Desired Outcome	**Nursing Actions** *and Selected Purposes/Rationales* (see pp. 37–40 for additional rationales)
5. The client will remain free of infection as evidenced by: a. absence of fever and chills b. pulse within normal limits c. normal breath sounds d. usual mental status e. cough productive of clear mucus only f. voiding clear urine without reports of frequency, urgency, and burning g. absence of heat, pain, redness, swelling, and unusual drainage in any area h. no reports of increased weakness and fatigue i. WBC and differential counts within normal range j. negative results of cultured specimens.	5.a. Assess for and report signs and symptoms of infection (be aware that some signs and symptoms vary depending on the site of infection, the causative organism, and the age and immune status of the client): 1. elevated temperature 2. chills 3. increased pulse 4. abnormal breath sounds 5. malaise, lethargy, acute confusion 6. loss of appetite 7. cough productive of purulent, green, or rust-colored sputum 8. cloudy urine 9. reports of frequency, urgency, or burning when urinating 10. urinalysis showing a WBC count greater than 5, positive leukocyte esterase or nitrites, or presence of bacteria 11. heat, pain, redness, swelling, or unusual drainage in any area 12. reports of increased weakness or fatigue 13. increase in WBC count and/or significant change in differential 14. positive results of cultured specimens (e.g., urine, vaginal drainage, sputum, blood). b. Implement measures *to prevent infection:* 1. perform actions to reduce the levels of serum nitrogenous substances (see Diagnosis 6, action a.2) 2. maintain the maximum fluid intake allowed 3. use good hand hygiene and encourage client to do the same

Desired Outcome	Nursing Actions *and Selected Purposes/Rationales*

4. use sterile technique during all invasive procedures (e.g., urinary catheterizations, venous and arterial punctures, injections)
5. anchor catheters/tubings (e.g., urinary, intravenous) securely *in order to reduce trauma to the tissues and the risk for introduction of pathogens associated with the in-and-out movement of the tubing*
6. rotate intravenous sites according to hospital policy
7. change peripheral intravenous line sites according to hospital policy
8. maintain a closed system for drains (e.g., urinary catheter) and intravenous infusions whenever possible
9. protect client from others who have an infection and instruct him/her to continue this after discharge
10. perform actions to maintain an adequate nutritional status (see Diagnosis 2, action c)
11. perform actions to reduce stress (e.g., provide a calm, restful environment; explain procedures; provide for consistency in staff assigned) *in order to prevent an increase in secretion of cortisol (cortisol interferes with some immune responses)*
12. reinforce importance of good oral hygiene
13. perform actions *to prevent stasis of respiratory secretions* (e.g., instruct and assist client to turn, cough, and deep breathe; increase activity as tolerated)
14. perform actions to prevent urinary retention (e.g., instruct client to urinate when the urge is first felt, promote relaxation during voiding attempts) *in order to prevent urinary stasis*
15. instruct and assist client to perform good perineal care routinely and after each bowel movement.

6. COLLABORATIVE DIAGNOSES: POTENTIAL COMPLICATIONS OF CHRONIC RENAL FAILURE

a. **uremic syndrome** related to accumulation of serum nitrogenous substances (e.g., creatinine, urea) associated with extensive loss of renal function (signs and symptoms usually occur when the glomerular filtration rate falls to less than 10% of normal);

b. **hypertension** related to:
   1. excess fluid volume
   2. peripheral vasoconstriction associated with increased stimulation of the renin-angiotensin mechanism (possibly in response to diminished renal blood flow)
   3. cardiovascular changes resulting from the underlying disease process (e.g., diabetes)
   4. effect of some medications (e.g., erythropoietin).

Desired Outcomes	Nursing Actions *and Selected Purposes/Rationales*
6.a. The client will not experience uremic syndrome as evidenced by: 1. pulse regular at 60–100 beats/minute 2. usual mental status 3. usual skin color 4. improved strength and activity tolerance 5. no reports of nausea, insomnia, itching, muscle cramping, joint pain, paresthesias, and taste alterations 6. intact oral mucous membrane	6.a.1. Assess for and report the following: a. increasing BUN and serum creatinine levels b. decreasing creatinine clearance levels c. signs and symptoms of uremic syndrome: 1. cardiac dysrhythmias 2. difficulty concentrating, lethargy, confusion, or hallucinations 3. sallow or grayish-bronze skin color 4. increased weakness or fatigue 5. reports of nausea, insomnia, itching, muscle cramps, joint pain, paresthesias, restless feeling in legs during periods of inactivity, or metallic or bitter taste in mouth 6. stomatitis 7. vomiting 8. unusual bleeding (e.g., ecchymoses; prolonged bleeding from puncture sites; gingival bleeding; frank or occult blood in stool, urine, or vomitus)

7. absence of vomiting, unusual bleeding, pericarditis, asterixis, and seizure activity.

9. pericarditis (e.g., chest pain that frequently radiates to shoulder, neck, back, and arm [usually left]; pericardial friction rub; elevated temperature)
10. asterixis, seizures.

2. Implement measures *to reduce the levels of serum nitrogenous substances in order to prevent uremic syndrome:*
   a. perform actions to maintain an adequate nutritional status (see Diagnosis 2, action c) *in order to reduce catabolism of body proteins*
   b. maintain dietary protein restrictions
   c. perform actions to prevent infection (see Diagnosis 5, action b) *in order to prevent an increase in the metabolic rate and subsequent cellular catabolism*
   d. perform actions *to prevent further renal damage:*
      1. implement measures as ordered to control disease conditions such as diabetes that have caused or contributed to renal failure
      2. consult the physician before administering medications that are known to be nephrotoxic (e.g., NSAIDs, aminoglycosides).
3. If signs and symptoms of uremic syndrome occur:
   a. prepare client for dialysis if planned
   b. maintain a safe environment for client (e.g., side rails up while in bed, assistance with ambulation as needed, constant supervision if indicated, seizure precautions)
   c. perform actions *to treat cardiac dysrhythmias if present* (e.g., administer antidysrhythmics as ordered, restrict activity if indicated)
   d. perform actions *to control nausea and vomiting if present* (e.g., administer antiemetics as ordered; provide small, frequent meals; instruct client to ingest foods/fluids slowly)
   e. perform actions *to reduce pruritus if present* (e.g., use tepid water and mild soap for bathing, apply emollient creams or ointments frequently, administer antihistamines if ordered)
   f. perform actions *to control muscle cramps if they occur* (e.g., instruct client to push feet against a hard surface when leg cramps occur, apply warm packs to affected areas)
   g. perform actions *to reduce the severity of stomatitis if present* (e.g., instruct client to avoid substances such as extremely hot, spicy, or acidic foods/fluids; assist with frequent oral hygiene; apply oral protective pastes as ordered)
   h. perform actions *to prevent bleeding* (e.g., apply gentle, prolonged pressure after injections and venous and arterial punctures; instruct client to use an electric rather than a straight-edge razor and to use a soft bristle toothbrush for oral hygiene)
   i. perform actions *to control bleeding if it occurs* (e.g., apply firm, prolonged pressure to bleeding area if possible; administer clotting factors or vitamin K if ordered)
   j. perform actions *to treat pericarditis if present* (e.g., maintain activity restrictions as ordered, administer an anti-inflammatory agent and analgesics if ordered).

6.b. The client will not experience hypertension as evidenced by:
   1. B/P within a safe range for client
   2. no reports of headache and dizziness.

6.b.1. Assess for and report signs and symptoms of hypertension (e.g., B/P greater than client's usual level [a B/P higher than 140/90 is usually considered to be significant], headache, dizziness).
2. Implement measures *to prevent or control hypertension:*
   a. perform actions to reduce excess fluid volume and prevent or treat hypernatremia (see Diagnosis 1, actions a.2 and b.3)
   b. administer antihypertensives as ordered.
3. Consult physician if hypertension persists or worsens.

7. NURSING DIAGNOSIS: ***INEFFECTIVE THERAPEUTIC REGIMEN MANAGEMENT***

related to lack of understanding of the implications of not following the prescribed treatment plan, difficulty integrating necessary treatments into lifestyle, and lack of financial resources.

Suggested NOC Outcomes: Treatment behavior: illness or injury; Participation in health care decisions; Compliance behavior; Health beliefs: perceived resources; Health beliefs: perceived ability to perform; Health beliefs: perceived control

Suggested NIC Interventions: Self-modification assistance; Medication management; Values clarification; Teaching: prescribed diet

Desired Outcome

7. The client will demonstrate the probability of effective therapeutic regimen management as evidenced by:
   a. willingness to learn about and participate in treatments and care
   b. statements reflecting ways to modify personal habits and integrate prescribed care into lifestyle
   c. statements reflecting an understanding of the implications of not following the prescribed treatment plan.

Nursing Actions *and Selected Purposes/Rationales*

7.a. Assess for indications that the client may be unable to effectively manage the therapeutic regimen:
   1. failure to adhere to treatment plan (e.g., not adhering to dietary modifications and fluid restrictions, refusing medications)
   2. statements reflecting a lack of understanding of factors that will cause further renal damage
   3. statements reflecting an unwillingness or inability to modify personal habits and integrate necessary treatments into lifestyle
   4. statements reflecting view that kidney damage will reverse itself or that the situation is hopeless and efforts to comply with prescribed care are useless.

b. Implement measures *to promote effective therapeutic regimen management:*
   1. explain renal failure in terms client can understand; stress the fact that it is a chronic disease and that adherence to treatment plan is necessary in order to delay and/or prevent complications
   2. initiate and reinforce discharge teaching outlined in Diagnosis 8 *in order to promote a sense of control and self-reliance*
   3. encourage client to participate in prescribed care (e.g., monitoring intake and output, calculating allowed fluid intake, selecting foods and fluids within dietary restrictions)
   4. assist client to identify ways treatments can be incorporated into lifestyle; focus on modifications of lifestyle rather than complete change
   5. obtain a dietary consult to assist client in planning a dietary program based on prescribed modifications and client's likes, dislikes, cultural preferences, and daily routines
   6. provide client with verbal and written instructions about future appointments with health care provider, ways to prevent further kidney damage, dietary modifications, fluid restrictions, medications, and signs and symptoms to report; determine areas of difficulty and misunderstanding and reinforce teaching as necessary
   7. encourage client to discuss concerns about the cost of medications and follow-up medical care; obtain a social service consult to assist with financial planning and to obtain financial aid if indicated
   8. provide information about and encourage use of community resources that can assist client to make necessary lifestyle changes (e.g., local chapter of the American Kidney Association, vocational rehabilitation, counseling services)
   9. reinforce behaviors suggesting future compliance with the therapeutic regimen (e.g., statements reflecting plans for integrating care into lifestyle, active participation in treatment plan, changes in personal habits)
   10. include significant others in explanations and teaching sessions and encourage their support; reinforce the need for client to assume responsibility for managing as much of care as possible.

c. Consult appropriate health care provider (e.g., social worker, physician) regarding referrals to community health agencies if continued instruction, support, or supervision is needed.

Discharge Teaching/Continued Care

8. Nursing Diagnosis: ***DEFICIENT KNOWLEDGE OR INEFFECTIVE HEALTH MAINTENANCE****

*The nurse should select the diagnostic label that is most appropriate for the client's discharge teaching needs.

Suggested NOC Outcomes: Knowledge: treatment regimen; Knowledge: diet; Knowledge: infection control; Knowledge: medication

Suggested NIC Interventions: Health system guidance; Teaching: individual; Teaching: disease process; Teaching: prescribed diet; Teaching: prescribed medication

Desired Outcomes	Nursing Actions *and Selected Purposes/Rationales*
8.a. The client will verbalize a basic understanding of chronic renal failure.	8.a. Explain renal failure in terms that client can understand. Utilize appropriate teaching aids (e.g., pictures, videotapes, kidney models).
8.b. The client will identify ways to slow the progression of kidney damage.	8.b.1. Provide instructions regarding ways to slow the progression of kidney damage: a. control hypertension by adhering to dietary modifications and taking medications as prescribed b. reduce the risk of urinary tract infection by: 1. cleaning perianal area thoroughly after each bowel movement 2. consuming the maximum amount of fluids allowed 3. wiping from front to back after urination and defecation (if female) c. reduce the risk of nephrotoxic reactions by: 1. consulting the appropriate health care provider before: a. taking any additional prescription and nonprescription drugs b. receiving any vaccine c. undergoing diagnostic testing which requires use of a contrast medium d. resuming any occupation or hobby involving exposure to chemicals or fumes 2. avoiding contact with products such as antifreeze, pesticides, carbon tetrachloride, mercuric chloride, lead, arsenic, and creosote. 2. Assist client and significant others to identify ways in which above health care measures can be incorporated into lifestyle.
8.c. The client will verbalize an understanding of fluid restrictions and dietary modifications.	8.c.1. Reinforce the importance of adhering to prescribed fluid restrictions and dietary modifications. 2. Reinforce physician's instructions about specific fluid restrictions and dietary modifications. 3. Reinforce dietitian's instructions on how to calculate and measure dietary allotments. Have client develop sample menus. 4. If client is on a protein- and sodium-restricted diet, inform him/her that numerous salt-free and protein-free products are available. Provide names of local stores that carry these products. 5. If client is on a fluid restriction, instruct to: a. take oral medications with soft foods (e.g., applesauce, pudding) rather than liquids b. reduce thirst by: 1. sucking on hard candy, popsicles, or ice cubes made with favorite juices (caution client that the fluid volume of the popsicles and ice cubes must be considered as oral fluid intake)

Desired Outcomes	**Nursing Actions** *and Selected Purposes/Rationales*
	2. spacing fluids evenly throughout the hours he/she is awake c. set out the 24-hour allotment of liquids in the morning in order to visualize the amount allowed for the day.
8.d. The client will demonstrate the ability to accurately weigh self, measure fluid intake and output, and monitor own blood pressure.	8.d.1. If client needs to monitor weight, instruct him/her to weigh at the same time, on the same scale, and with similar amounts of clothing on. 2. Demonstrate how to measure and record fluid intake and urinary output if indicated. Stress that any substance that is liquid at room temperature is counted as fluid intake. 3. If client needs to monitor blood pressure, provide instructions on how to take, read, and record it. 4. Allow time for questions, clarification, practice, and return demonstration. Instruct client to take record of weights, fluid intake, urinary output, and B/P readings to appointments with health care provider.
8.e. The client will identify ways to reduce the risk of infection.	8.e. Instruct client in ways to reduce the risk of infection: 1. avoid contact with persons who have an infection 2. avoid crowds during the flu or cold season 3. decrease or stop smoking 4. drink allotted amounts of liquids 5. maintain good personal hygiene 6. maintain a good nutritional status 7. maintain an adequate balance between activity and rest 8. take antimicrobials as prescribed before scheduled dental work, invasive diagnostic procedures, or surgery.
8.f. The client will identify ways to manage signs and symptoms that often occur as a result of chronic renal failure.	8.f. Provide instructions regarding ways to manage the following signs and symptoms that often occur as a result of chronic renal failure: 1. weakness and fatigue: a. schedule frequent rest periods throughout the day b. maintain a good nutritional status 2. dry mouth: a. space fluid allotments evenly throughout waking hours b. perform oral hygiene frequently 3. decreased libido (can occur as a result of factors such as weakness, fatigue, depression, and side effects of some medications): a. schedule rest periods before and after sexual activity b. explore creative ways of expressing sexuality (e.g., massage, fantasies, cuddling).
8.g. The client will state signs and symptoms to report to the health care provider.	8.g. Instruct client to report the following: 1. weight gain of more than 0.5 kg (1 pound)/day or a continued weight loss 2. persistent nausea or vomiting 3. increasing fatigue or weakness 4. difficulty concentrating and making decisions 5. confusion 6. persistent or severe headache 7. palpitations or chest pain 8. red, rust-colored, or smoky urine; bloody or tarry stools; blood in sputum or vomitus; persistent bleeding from nose, mouth, or any cut; prolonged or excessive menses; excessive bruising; or sudden abdominal or back pain 9. fever or chills 10. numbness or tingling in extremities, persistent restless feeling in legs during periods of inactivity

11. change in skin color (e.g., bronze, yellow-gray, brownish-gray, increased pallor)
12. impotence, infertility, or amenorrhea (could indicate hormonal imbalances caused by increasing serum levels of nitrogenous substances)
13. increasing blood pressure
14. swelling of feet, ankles, or hands
15. diarrhea or constipation (either can occur as a side effect of some antacid therapy; physicians generally recommend alternating antacids containing magnesium with those containing aluminum or calcium to prevent these bowel problems)
16. persistent itching
17. oral pain or breakdown of oral mucous membrane
18. shortness of breath
19. muscle pain or cramping
20. twitching or seizures
21. joint or bone pain (could indicate renal osteodystrophy resulting from effects of hypocalcemia and hyperphosphatemia).

8.h. The client will identify community resources that can assist with adjustment to changes resulting from chronic renal failure.

8.h.1. Provide information about community resources that can assist the client and significant others to adjust to changes resulting from chronic renal failure (e.g., local chapter of the American Kidney Association, vocational rehabilitation, social services, counseling services).
2. Initiate a referral if indicated.

8.i. The client will verbalize an understanding of and a plan for adhering to recommended follow-up care including future appointments with health care provider and medications prescribed.

8.i.1. Reinforce the importance of keeping follow-up appointments with health care provider.
2. Explain the rationale for, side effects of, and importance of taking prescribed medications (e.g., antihypertensives, antacids, vitamins, electrolyte supplements, diuretics, hematopoietic agents). Inform client of pertinent food and drug interactions.
3. Reinforce the importance of consulting the appropriate health care provider (e.g., pharmacist, nurse practitioner, physician) before taking any prescription and nonprescription drugs. Explain that:
   a. some drugs such as ibuprofen, neomycin, and naproxen are nephrotoxic and can hasten the progression of renal failure
   b. some drugs such as aspirin and digoxin are excreted by the kidneys and can rapidly build to toxic levels in the body (usual dosages may need to be reduced or a different medication may need to be taken)
   c. some drugs contain ingredients that affect electrolyte balance and elevate blood pressure (e.g., many cold remedies).
4. Refer to Diagnosis 7, action b, for measures to promote the client's ability to effectively manage the therapeutic regimen.

ADDITIONAL NURSING DIAGNOSES

IMPAIRED ORAL MUCOUS MEMBRANE: DRYNESS*

related to prescribed fluid restriction.

*FEAR/ANXIETY**

related to:
a. lack of understanding of diagnosis, diagnostic tests, and treatment plan;
b. uncertainty as to extensiveness of loss of renal function;
c. anticipated change in health status, lifestyle, and roles as a result of progressive loss of renal function;
d. awareness of probable future need for dialysis or renal transplantation;
e. financial concerns.

---

*See Unit II for outcomes, actions, and rationales.

*GRIEVING**

related to progressive loss of kidney function and the effects of this on lifestyle and roles.

*See Unit II for outcomes, actions, and rationales.

Bibliography

See pages 879 and 883.

Cystectomy with Urinary Diversion

Cystectomy is the removal of the bladder and is accompanied by a procedure to divert urinary flow. It may be performed to treat a malignancy of the bladder, congenital bladder anomalies, neurogenic bladder, and irreparable bladder trauma. A cystectomy may also be performed to prevent further deterioration of renal function associated with chronic bladder infection. In some cases, the surgery includes removal of just the bladder (simple cystectomy) but when there is an invasive malignancy, a more radical procedure is performed. In men, a radical cystectomy usually includes removal of the bladder, prostate, seminal vesicles, a portion of the vas deferens, and some or all of the pelvic lymph nodes. In women, a radical cystectomy usually includes removal of the bladder, urethra, uterus, fallopian tubes, ovaries, a portion of the anterior vaginal wall, and some or all of the pelvic lymph nodes.

There are several ways to accomplish urinary diversion. The most common surgical method is the conventional conduit (incontinent urinary diversion). In this procedure, the ureters are implanted in a portion of a resected segment of intestine and then the end of the segment is brought through the abdominal wall to create a stoma. Because no valves are incorporated into the construction of the conventional conduit, drops of urine usually flow from the stoma every few seconds, resulting in the client's need to wear a urinary collection appliance at all times.

The second most common surgical method to accomplish urinary diversion is the continent internal reservoir (e.g., Kock pouch, Mainz pouch, Indiana pouch). In this method, the ureters are implanted in a resected portion of intestine that has been remodeled to create a reservoir. Another segment of the reservoir is used to create the stoma that is brought out through the abdominal wall. The reflux of urine from the reservoir back through the ureters and the uncontrolled flow of urine from the reservoir through the stoma are prevented by the surgical positioning of the ureters, reservoir, and stoma or by the construction of one-way valves at these sites. After healing occurs, a catheter is inserted into the stoma at regularly scheduled intervals (usually every 4–6 hours once the reservoir stretches to its full capacity) to drain the reservoir. If the system functions properly, the client does not need to wear a urinary collection appliance over the stoma.

Two less commonly used methods of urinary diversion are cutaneous ureterostomy (direct implantation of the ureters into the abdominal wall) and nephrostomy (insertion of catheters into the kidneys via flank incisions). These methods are usually reserved for clients who cannot tolerate lengthy surgery and/or have a short life expectancy.

The type of urinary diversion selected depends on many factors including the client's preference, age, body build, ability to learn about and participate in care of the urinary diversion, prognosis, and ability to tolerate lengthy surgery; the integrity of the client's ureters, kidneys, and intestinal tract; the advice of the enterostomal therapy (ET) nurse; and the expertise of the surgeon.

This care plan focuses on the adult client hospitalized for a cystectomy with urinary diversion by means of a conventional conduit. Some additional nursing interventions are also included for the client with a continent internal reservoir. Much of the postoperative information is applicable to clients receiving follow-up care in an extended care facility or home setting.

OUTCOME/DISCHARGE CRITERIA

THE CLIENT WILL:

- maintain an adequate urine output via the urinary diversion
- have surgical pain controlled
- have evidence of normal healing of surgical wound
- have a medium pink to red, moist stoma and intact peristomal skin
- have no signs and symptoms of postoperative complications
- verbalize a basic understanding of the anatomical changes that have occurred as a result of the surgery
- demonstrate the ability to change the urostomy appliance and maintain stomal and peristomal skin integrity
- demonstrate the ability to properly clean reusable urostomy equipment
- demonstrate the ability to drain and irrigate a continent internal reservoir if present
- identify ways to control odor of the urostomy drainage and appliance
- identify ways to prevent urinary tract infection
- state signs and symptoms to report to the health care provider
- share thoughts and feelings about altered urinary elimination and its effect on body image and lifestyle

- identify appropriate community resources that can assist with home management and adjustment to changes resulting from the urinary diversion
- verbalize an understanding of and a plan for adhering to recommended follow-up care including future appointments with health care provider, wound care, activity level, and medications prescribed.

NURSING/COLLABORATIVE DIAGNOSES

See pp. 538–539 and Standardized Preoperative and Postoperative Care Plans (pp. 97–126) for additional diagnoses.

PREOPERATIVE

Use in conjunction with the Standardized Preoperative Care Plan.

1. Nursing Diagnosis: FEAR/ANXIETY

related to:
a. unfamiliar environment and separation from significant others;
b. lack of understanding of diagnostic tests, planned surgical procedure, and care that will be required for the urinary diversion;
c. anticipated loss of control associated with effects of anesthesia;
d. anticipated discomfort, surgical findings, changes in appearance and body functioning, and effects of urinary diversion on future lifestyle and roles;
e. financial concerns associated with hospitalization;
f. ability to independently care for urinary diversion following discharge.

Suggested NOC Outcomes: Anxiety level; Fear level; Anxiety self-control; Fear self-control

Suggested NIC Interventions: Anxiety reduction; Calming technique; Emotional support; Presence; Teaching: preoperative

Desired Outcome	Nursing Actions *and Selected Purposes/Rationales* (see pp. 14–16 for additional rationales)
1. The client will experience a reduction in fear and anxiety (see Standardized Preoperative Care Plan, Diagnosis 1 [pp. 97–98], for outcome criteria).	1.a. Refer to Standardized Preoperative Care Plan, Diagnosis 1 (pp. 97–98), for measures related to assessment and reduction of fear and anxiety. b. Implement additional measures *to reduce fear and anxiety:* 1. provide client with information about preoperative routines, the surgical procedure, general postoperative care, the function and

appearance of the stoma, and management of the urinary diversion (see Preoperative Diagnosis 2) *so he/she will know what to expect*
2. explain that every attempt will be made to place the stoma in an area that he/she can easily see and reach and where the appliance will lie flat, adhere well to the skin, and allow freedom of movement (the tentative stoma site is mapped out preoperatively by the physician and/or enterostomal therapy [ET] nurse)
3. inform client that instructions about management of the urinary diversion will be repeated as often as necessary prior to discharge and that there will be resources available to provide assistance/supervision following discharge
4. assure client that stoma has no pain receptors and will not be painful when touched
5. explain that current urostomy collection devices are odorproof and available in sizes to fit various body contours
6. if acceptable to client, arrange for a visit with a person of similar age and same sex who has successfully adapted to a urinary diversion
7. assure client that the urinary diversion need not dramatically alter lifestyle.

Client Teaching

2. NURSING DIAGNOSIS: **DEFICIENT KNOWLEDGE**

regarding hospital routines associated with surgery, physical preparation for the cystectomy with urinary diversion, the surgical procedure, sensations that normally occur following surgery and anesthesia, expected appearance and function of the urostomy, and postoperative care and management of the urinary diversion.

Suggested NOC Outcomes: Knowledge: treatment regimen; Knowledge: treatment procedure(s)

Suggested NIC Interventions: Health system guidance; Teaching: individual; Teaching: procedure/treatment

Desired Outcomes	Nursing Actions *and Selected Purposes/Rationales*
2.a. The client will verbalize an understanding of the surgical procedure, preoperative care, and postoperative sensations and care.	2.a.1. Refer to Standardized Preoperative Care Plan, Diagnosis 4, actions a.1–4 (pp. 100–101), for information to include in preoperative teaching. 2. Provide additional information about specific preoperative care and postoperative sensations and care for clients having a cystectomy with urinary diversion: a. explain the preoperative bowel preparation (e.g., low-residue or clear liquid diet, cleansing enemas, laxatives, antimicrobial therapy); reinforce the fact that bowel preparation is necessary since a portion of the bowel will be used to create the urinary diversion b. if a conventional conduit is the planned method of urinary diversion, explain that ureteral stents (small, firm catheters) may be inserted in surgery to maintain patency of the ureters (the stents will extend from the stoma and are removed once surgical site edema subsides [usually about 5–10 days after surgery]) c. if a continent internal reservoir is the planned method of urinary diversion, inform client that: 1. ureteral stents or a catheter will be inserted in surgery and will extend from the stoma and drain continually into an external collection device; stress that this is a temporary measure (usually for 7–10 days) to maintain urine drainage while surgical site edema subsides and to keep the reservoir from becoming distended while the suture lines are healing 2. the reservoir will need to be irrigated regularly in the early postoperative period to remove mucus that accumulates in the reservoir (the bowel segment used to construct the reservoir initially secretes quite a bit of mucus)

Desired Outcomes	**Nursing Actions** *and Selected Purposes/Rationales*
	3. following removal of the ureteral stents or catheter, a catheter will be inserted into the stoma at regularly scheduled intervals to drain the reservoir and an external collection device will not be needed. 3. Allow time for questions and clarification of information provided.
2.b. The client will demonstrate the ability to perform activities designed to prevent postoperative complications.	2.b. Refer to Standardized Preoperative Care Plan, Diagnosis 4, action b (p. 101), for instructions on ways to prevent postoperative complications.
2.c. The client will verbalize an understanding of the appearance of the stoma and management of the urinary diversion.	2.c.1. Arrange for a visit with an ET nurse if available. 2. Reinforce basic information provided by physician and/or ET nurse regarding: a. expected location of stoma b. expected appearance of stoma postoperatively (moist, red, edematous); assure client that much of the edema will subside within 7 days and that the stoma will continue to gradually decrease in size during the first 6–8 weeks after surgery c. expected drainage (slight bleeding of stoma, some blood in urine for 24–48 hours, mucus in urine [occurs because the urinary diversion is constructed using a section of bowel and the bowel mucosa normally secretes mucus]) d. management of urinary diversion (e.g., peristomal skin care, odor control, use of various types of appliances, irrigation and drainage of an internal reservoir) e. urostomy products that client will be using in the immediate postoperative period. 3. Provide visual aids and allow client to handle appliances that will be used in the immediate postoperative period. 4. Encourage client to try wearing an appliance partially filled with water in order to experience how it feels and to determine if the planned stoma site will be adequate for successful adhesion of appliance. 5. Allow time for questions and clarification of information provided.

POSTOPERATIVE

Use in conjunction with the Standardized Postoperative Care Plan.

1. Nursing Diagnosis: ACTUAL/RISK FOR IMPAIRED TISSUE INTEGRITY

related to:

a. disruption of tissue associated with the surgical procedure;
b. delayed wound healing associated with factors such as decreased nutritional status, inadequate blood supply to wound area, and preoperative radiation therapy (may have been done if the underlying disease process is a malignancy);
c. irritation of skin around suture lines and wound drains associated with contact with wound drainage, pressure from tubes, and use of tape;
d. irritation of peristomal area associated with prolonged contact with urine; soap residue and perspiration under the appliance; allergic reaction to adhesives and other substances used to secure the appliance to the skin; frequent or improper removal of tape, adhesives, and other substances used to secure the appliance to the skin; and/or aggressive cleansing of peristomal area.

Suggested NOC Outcomes:
Ostomy self-care; Wound healing: primary intention; Tissue integrity: skin and mucous membranes

Suggested NIC Interventions: Skin surveillance; Pressure management; Skin care: topical treatments; Incision site care; Ostomy care

Desired Outcomes	**Nursing Actions** *and Selected Purposes/Rationales* (see pp. 49–52 for additional rationales)
1.a. The client will experience normal healing of surgical wounds (see Standardized Postoperative Care Plan, Diagnosis 10, outcome a [p. 112], for outcome criteria).	1.a. Refer to Standardized Postoperative Care Plan, Diagnosis 10, action a (p. 112), for measures related to assessment and promotion of wound healing.
1.b. The client will maintain integrity of the peristomal skin and skin in contact with wound drainage, tape, and tubings as evidenced by: 1. absence of redness and irritation 2. no skin breakdown.	1.b.1. Inspect skin areas that are in contact with wound drainage, tape, and tubings for signs of irritation and breakdown. 2. Assess for signs and symptoms of peristomal irritation or breakdown (e.g., redness, inflammation, and/or excoriation of peristomal skin; reports of itching and burning under the appliance; inability to keep appliance on). 3. Refer to Standardized Postoperative Care Plan, Diagnosis 10, actions b.2 and 3 (pp. 112–113), for measures to prevent and treat tissue irritation and breakdown in areas in contact with wound drainage, tape, and tubings. 4. Implement measures *to prevent peristomal irritation and breakdown:* a. patch test all products that will come in contact with the skin (e.g., adhesives, solvents, sealants, barriers) before initial use; do not use products that cause redness, itching, or burning b. change appliance only when necessary (e.g., if appliance is leaking, if client reports burning or itching of the peristomal skin, when the stoma size changes); appliance is typically changed every 3 days in the early postoperative period and then should be able to remain in place for 5–7 days c. use a 2-piece appliance (faceplate and pouch) in the initial postoperative period *so that the pouch can be removed to assess the stoma without having to remove the adhesive from the skin* d. shave or clip hair from peristomal skin if necessary *to help achieve an adequate appliance seal and to reduce irritation when the appliance is removed* e. perform actions *to reduce peristomal irritation during removal of appliance:* 1. place drops of warm water or solvent where the appliance adheres to the skin *in order to facilitate removal;* allow time for adhesive to loosen before removing appliance 2. remove appliance gently and in direction of hair growth; hold skin adjacent to the skin barrier taut and push down on skin slightly *to facilitate separation* f. perform actions *to prevent urine from coming in contact with the skin when changing appliance:* 1. change appliance when the urostomy is least active (in the morning before drinking liquids or when fluid intake has been reduced for a few hours) 2. place a wick (rolled gauze pad, tampon) on the stoma opening when the appliance is off g. cleanse peristomal skin thoroughly with mild soap and water, rinse completely, and pat dry; use tepid rather than hot water *to prevent burns*

Desired Outcomes	**Nursing Actions** *and Selected Purposes/Rationales*

h. apply skin sealant before application of skin barrier *to protect skin from irritating effect of the adhesive*
i. use a skin barrier composed of synthetic material (e.g., Stomahesive); avoid the use of a hydrophilic barrier (e.g., karaya) *because it will dissolve when in contact with urine*
j. perform actions *to prevent urine from contacting the skin when appliance is on:*
  1. measure diameter of stoma and cut skin barrier and pouch openings no more than 0.3 cm (1/8 inch) larger than stoma (it may be necessary to create a pattern to use for cutting the openings if stoma has an irregular shape)
  2. instruct and assist client to remeasure the stoma size frequently during first 6–8 weeks after surgery and to alter size of skin barrier and pouch openings as stomal edema decreases
  3. implement measures *to achieve an adequate appliance seal:*
     a. avoid use of ointments or lotions on peristomal skin *(these can interfere with adequate adhesive bonding)*
     b. follow manufacturer's instructions when applying products such as skin sealant and barrier and the pouch
     c. apply firm pressure and remove wrinkles and air pockets when applying skin barrier and pouch; place client in a supine position *to increase tautness of skin surface during application*
  4. use a pouch with an antireflux valve
  5. empty pouch when it is about 1/3 full *(the weight of the pouch could cause appliance to separate from the skin)*
  6. position pouch so gravity flow facilitates drainage away from stoma and peristomal skin
  7. tightly close drainage valve or clamp after emptying pouch *to prevent leakage*

k. if a belted appliance is used, fasten the belt so that 2 fingers can easily slip between belt and skin *to prevent excessive pressure on the skin*
l. instruct and assist client to check appliance periodically to ensure that drainage valve or clamp is not placing pressure on the skin.

5. If signs and symptoms of peristomal irritation and breakdown occur:
   a. avoid use of any product that may have caused the peristomal irritation or breakdown
   b. cleanse area gently with warm water
   c. perform skin care as ordered or according to hospital procedure (usual care may include exposing affected area to air for 20–30 minutes when appliance is changed, applying an antifungal agent or corticosteroid preparation to affected skin, and/or covering irritated skin with a solid skin barrier); consult appropriate health care provider (e.g., wound care specialist, ET nurse, physician) if condition of peristomal skin does not improve within 48 hours.

2. NURSING DIAGNOSIS:

RISK FOR INFECTION: URINARY TRACT

related to:

a. increased growth and colonization of microorganisms associated with stasis of urine resulting from:
   1. obstruction of urine flow (can occur as a result of edema of the stoma or ureteral junctions, excessive collection of mucus in the stoma, malfunction of ureteral stents if present, or blockage of stomal catheter [catheter is usually present for 7–10 days postoperatively if client has an internal reservoir and does not have ureteral stents])
   2. incomplete or infrequent emptying of the internal reservoir (if present) following removal of the stomal catheter or ureteral stents;
b. introduction of pathogens into the urinary tract associated with:
   1. reflux of urine from the collection device into the stoma, ureteral stents, or stomal catheter

2. reflux of urine from the conduit or internal reservoir (if present) into the ureters or kidney
3. presence of stomal catheter or ureteral stents
4. incorrect or inadequate cleansing of reusable urostomy appliances or peristomal skin
5. intermittent catheterization and irrigation of the internal reservoir (if present).

Suggested NOC Outcomes: Immune status; Infection severity

Suggested NIC Interventions: Infection protection; Infection control; Tube care: urinary; Urinary catheterization: intermittent

Desired Outcome	Nursing Actions *and Selected Purposes/Rationales*
2. The client will remain free of urinary tract infection as evidenced by: a. no increase in sediment in urine b. no unusual color of urine c. absence of chills and fever d. urinalysis showing fewer than 5 WBCs, negative leukocyte esterase and nitrites, and absence of bacteria e. negative urine culture.	2.a. Assess for and report signs and symptoms of urinary tract infection (e.g., increased sediment in urine; bloody urine; chills; elevated temperature; flank pain; urinalysis showing a WBC count greater than 5, positive leukocyte esterase or nitrites, or the presence of bacteria; positive urine culture). b. Implement measures *to prevent urinary tract infection:* 1. perform actions *to prevent reflux and/or stasis of urine:* a. implement measures to prevent urinary obstruction (see Postoperative Diagnosis 3, action b.2) b. use a pouch with an antireflux valve c. instruct and assist client to empty pouch when it is 1/3 full d. instruct and assist client to connect the pouch to a bedside collection system before lying down for an extended period e. if client has an internal reservoir, instruct and assist him/her to empty it as often as necessary (frequency depends on the reservoir capacity and the client's fluid intake) 2. maintain sterile technique during catheterization and irrigation of the internal reservoir (if present) 3. cleanse peristomal skin thoroughly each time appliance is changed 4. maintain fluid intake of at least 2500 ml/day unless contraindicated *to promote urine formation (if client has a conventional conduit, this increases the amount of urine that passes through the conduit and subsequently flushes pathogens out of the conduit)* 5. ensure that reusable urostomy appliances are cleansed thoroughly, rinsed, and allowed to dry completely between applications 6. if client's urine is too alkaline (pH greater than 6.5): a. encourage client to increase intake of foods/fluids that will make urine more acidic (e.g., cranberry juice, prune juice, plums, poultry, fish, whole grains) b. instruct client to avoid excessive intake of milk, citrus fruits, and carbonated beverages *(these tend to alkalinize urine)* c. administer medications such as ascorbic acid if ordered. c. If signs and symptoms of urinary tract infection occur, administer antimicrobial agents if ordered.

3. COLLABORATIVE DIAGNOSES:

POTENTIAL COMPLICATIONS OF CYSTECTOMY WITH URINARY DIVERSION

a. stomal changes:
   1. prolapse related to pressure around the stoma, poor tissue turgor, and loss of integrity of suture line
   2. excessive bleeding related to irritation associated with aggressive cleansing of stoma and/or improper fit or application of appliance
   3. necrosis related to intraoperative and/or postoperative interruption of blood supply to the stoma;
b. urinary obstruction related to:
   1. loss of patency or dislodgment of stomal catheter or ureteral stents if present

2. edema of stoma and/or ureters associated with surgical trauma
3. collection of mucus in stomal and/or ureteral openings;

c. peritonitis related to:
1. leakage of urine and/or intestinal contents into the peritoneum associated with loss of integrity of the sutures at sites of surgical anastomoses
2. leakage of urine into and/or exposure of the peritoneum associated with retraction of peristomal skin from stoma (mucocutaneous separation) resulting from slippage of the sutures or impaired healing of surgical site
3. accumulation of wound drainage in the peritoneum
4. wound infection.

Desired Outcomes	**Nursing Actions** *and Selected Purposes/Rationales*
3.a. The client will maintain integrity of the stoma as evidenced by: 1. medium pink to red coloring of stoma 2. expected stomal height 3. absence of excessive bleeding and increasing edema of the stoma.	3.a.1. Assess for and report signs and symptoms of impaired stomal integrity (e.g., pale, dark red, dusky blue, or blue-black color of stoma; increased stomal height; increased stomal edema or bleeding). Use clear pouches during immediate postoperative period *to allow easy visibility of stoma.* 2. Implement measures *to maintain integrity of stoma:* a. perform actions *to maintain adequate stomal circulation:* 1. ensure that the openings of the skin barrier, faceplate, and pouch are not too small and that the stoma is centered in the openings *in order to prevent pressure on and around the stoma* 2. instruct client to avoid wearing clothing that puts pressure on the stoma b. apply appliance securely *to prevent it from slipping and irritating or shearing the stoma* c. cleanse stoma gently using a soft cloth, gauze, or tissue. 3. If signs and symptoms of impaired stomal integrity occur: a. perform stomal care as ordered b. prepare client for surgical revision of stoma if indicated.
3.b. The client will not experience urinary obstruction as evidenced by: 1. balanced intake and output beginning 48 hours postoperatively 2. gradual resolution of abdominal tenderness and distention 3. expected volume of drainage from abdominal incision and drain.	3.b.1. Assess for and report signs and symptoms of ureteral or stomal obstruction (e.g., significant decrease in urinary output from stoma, ureteral stents, or stomal catheter; increasing abdominal tenderness and distention; increase in drainage from abdominal incision or drain). 2. Implement measures *to prevent urinary obstruction:* a. encourage a fluid intake of 2500 ml/day unless contraindicated *to maintain adequate urine flow (an adequate urine flow helps flush mucus through the conduit and stoma)* b. flush ureteral stents or irrigate stomal catheter if ordered *(mucus can accumulate in and subsequently obstruct the stents or catheter)* c. if client has an internal reservoir, irrigate the reservoir as ordered *to remove mucus (excessive mucus can obstruct the ureteral openings)* d. change the appliance carefully *in order to avoid dislodgment of the ureteral stents or stomal catheter if present.* 3. If signs and symptoms of urinary obstruction occur, prepare client for dilation of the stoma, surgical revision of stoma or sites of ureteral anastomoses, and/or insertion of ureteral stents.
3.c. The client will not develop peritonitis as evidenced by: 1. gradual resolution of abdominal pain 2. soft, nondistended abdomen 3. temperature declining toward normal 4. stable vital signs 5. absence of nausea and vomiting	3.c.1. Assess for and report signs and symptoms of peritonitis (e.g., increase in severity of abdominal pain; rebound tenderness; distended, rigid abdomen; increase in temperature; tachycardia; tachypnea; hypotension; nausea; vomiting; failure of bowel sounds to return to normal; WBC counts that increase or fail to decline toward normal). 2. Implement measures *to prevent peritonitis:* a. perform actions to prevent wound infection (see Standardized Postoperative Care Plan, Diagnosis 17, action b.2 [pp. 118–119]) b. perform actions *to maintain patency of wound drain if present:* 1. keep tubing free of kinks 2. empty collection device as often as necessary

6. gradual return of normal bowel sounds
7. WBC count declining toward normal.

3. maintain suction as ordered

c. perform actions *to prevent inadvertent removal of wound drain if present:*
   1. use caution when changing dressings surrounding drain
   2. provide extension tubing if necessary *to enable client to move without placing tension on the drain*
   3. instruct client not to pull on drain and drainage tubing
d. perform actions *to prevent distention of the conduit or internal reservoir (distention can cause strain on the suture lines and subsequent leakage of urine into the peritoneal cavity):*
   1. implement measures to prevent urinary obstruction (see action b.2 in this diagnosis)
   2. assist client with intermittent catheterization of the internal reservoir (if present) at scheduled intervals and when he/she feels increased abdominal pressure
e. do not reposition ureteral stents or stomal catheter *(repositioning them could disrupt the suture lines)*
f. if separation of stoma from peristomal skin occurs:
   1. perform wound care as ordered *to facilitate the formation of granulation tissue in retracted area*
   2. prepare client for surgical reconstruction of the stoma if planned.

3. If signs and symptoms of peritonitis occur:
   a. withhold oral intake as ordered
   b. place client on bed rest in a semi-Fowler's position *to assist in pooling or localizing gastrointestinal contents and urine in the pelvis rather than under the diaphragm*
   c. prepare client for diagnostic tests (e.g., abdominal x-ray, peritoneal aspiration, computed tomography, ultrasonography) if planned
   d. insert a nasogastric tube and maintain suction as ordered
   e. administer antimicrobials as ordered
   f. administer intravenous fluids and/or blood volume expanders if ordered *to prevent or treat shock (can result from the increased capillary permeability that occurs with inflammation and the subsequent escape of protein, fluid, and electrolytes from the vascular space into the peritoneal cavity)*
   g. prepare client for surgical intervention (e.g., drainage and irrigation of peritoneum, repair of sites of anastomoses) if indicated.

4. NURSING DIAGNOSIS: ***SEXUAL DYSFUNCTION***

related to:

a. decreased libido associated with feelings of loss of femininity/masculinity and sexual attractiveness, fear of offensive odor or leakage of urine from the stoma (if client has an internal reservoir) or urostomy appliance, fear of rejection by partner, discomfort resulting from surgical incision, and depression;
b. impotence (can occur as a result of nerve damage during a radical cystectomy);
c. decreased potential for orgasm in the female client associated with clitoral injury (can occur with radical cystectomy);
d. dyspareunia associated with narrowing and shortening of the vaginal canal resulting from removal of a portion of the anterior vaginal wall if a radical cystectomy was performed.

Suggested NOC Outcomes: Body image; Personal well-being; Sexual functioning

Suggested NIC Interventions: Body image enhancement; Sexual counseling

Desired Outcome	**Nursing Actions** *and Selected Purposes/Rationales*
4. The client will demonstrate beginning acceptance of changes in sexual functioning as evidenced by: a. verbalization of a perception of self as sexually acceptable and adequate b. statements reflecting beginning adjustment to the effects of the urinary diversion on sexuality c. maintenance of relationship with significant other.	4.a. Assess for signs and symptoms of sexual dysfunction (e.g., verbalization of sexual concerns or inability to achieve sexual satisfaction, alteration in relationship with significant other, limitations imposed by nerve damage and structural changes incurred during surgery). b. Provide accurate information about effects of the surgery and urinary diversion on sexual functioning. Encourage questions and clarify misconceptions. c. Implement measures *to promote optimal sexual functioning:* 1. facilitate communication between client and partner; focus on the feelings the couple share and assist them to identify changes that may affect their sexual relationship 2. perform actions to promote a positive self-concept (see Postoperative Diagnosis 5, actions d–p) 3. instruct client in ways *to reduce risk of leakage of urine during sexual activity:* a. empty the pouch or drain internal reservoir (if present) before sexual activity b. secure appliance seal with tape for added security 4. if client is concerned about odor, instruct him/her to: a. shower or bathe before sexual activity b. use an odorproof pouch or pouch deodorant c. use cologne or perfume if desired d. keep room well ventilated 5. if appropriate, involve partner in urostomy care *to facilitate partner's adjustment to the changes in client's appearance and body functioning and subsequently decrease the possibility of partner's rejection of client* 6. if client is concerned about the presence of the stoma and appliance, discuss the possibility of: a. using opaque or patterned pouches or decorative pouch covers b. wearing underwear with the crotch removed (for females), boxer shorts (for males), or a cummerbund or stretch tube top around abdomen during sexual activity 7. if client is concerned that operative site discomfort will interfere with usual sexual activity: a. assure him/her that discomfort is temporary and will diminish as the incision heals b. encourage alternatives to intercourse or use of positions that decrease pressure on surgical site (e.g., side-lying) 8. if impotence is a problem, encourage client to discuss it and various treatment options (e.g., vacuum erection aids, penile prosthesis) with physician 9. if appropriate, discuss with female client the need for vaginal dilatation after healing has occurred *to prevent further contraction and shortening of the vaginal canal* 10. encourage client to obtain written information regarding sexual activity from the United Ostomy Association and from manufacturers of urostomy appliances 11. include partner in above discussion and encourage continued support of the client. d. Consult appropriate health care provider (e.g., ET nurse, psychiatric nurse clinician, physician) if counseling appears indicated.

5. Nursing Diagnosis: ***DISTURBED SELF-CONCEPT****

related to:

a. loss of ability to urinate normally;
b. dependence (usually temporary) on others for assistance with urostomy management;

*This diagnostic label includes the nursing diagnoses of disturbed body image, low self-esteem, and ineffective role performance.

c. loss of control of urinary elimination if client has a conventional conduit;
d. change in appearance associated with the presence of a stoma and urostomy appliance;
e. changes in usual sexual functioning;
f. embarrassment associated with odor of urostomy drainage and appliance;
g. sterility associated with:
   1. loss of ejaculatory function in the male client resulting from removal of the prostate and seminal vesicles if a radical cystectomy was performed
   2. removal of the ovaries, uterus, and fallopian tubes in the female client if a radical cystectomy was performed.

Suggested NOC Outcomes: Body image; Personal autonomy; Self-esteem; Psychosocial adjustment: life change

Suggested NIC Interventions: Body image enhancement; Self-esteem enhancement; Emotional support; Support system enhancement; Role enhancement; Counseling

Desired Outcome	**Nursing Actions** *and Selected Purposes/Rationales* (see pp. 47–49 for additional rationales)
5. The client will demonstrate beginning adaptation to changes in appearance, body functioning, and lifestyle as evidenced by: a. verbalization of feelings of self-worth b. maintenance of relationships with significant others c. active participation in activities of daily living d. verbalization of a beginning plan for integrating changes in appearance and body functioning into lifestyle.	5.a. Assess for signs and symptoms of a disturbed self-concept (e.g., verbalization of negative feelings about self, withdrawal from significant others, lack of participation in activities of daily living, refusal to look at or touch stoma, lack of plan for adapting to necessary changes in lifestyle). b. Determine the meaning of changes in appearance, body functioning, and lifestyle to the client by encouraging verbalization of feelings and by noting nonverbal responses to the changes experienced. c. Be aware that client may grieve the loss of usual urinary function and change in appearance. Provide support during the grieving process. d. Support realistic hope about the effects of the surgery on the client's life (e.g., increased comfort, improved urinary elimination, treatment of underlying disease process). e. Implement measures to promote optimal sexual functioning (see Postoperative Diagnosis 4, action c). f. Instruct and assist client in ways *to decrease odor of urostomy drainage and appliance:* 1. use odorproof pouches and change appliance regularly 2. use disposable appliances or clean reusable items thoroughly 3. empty appliance regularly 4. perform actions to achieve an adequate appliance seal (see Postoperative Diagnosis 1, action b.4.j.3) 5. drain the internal reservoir (if present) at scheduled intervals and when it feels full to reduce the possibility of urine leakage from stoma 6. maintain an adequate fluid intake (dilute urine has less of an odor than concentrated urine) 7. increase intake of foods/fluids that are known to help reduce odor of urine (e.g., cranberry juice, yogurt, buttermilk) unless contraindicated 8. avoid foods that cause urine to have a strong odor (e.g., asparagus, cabbage) 9. use room or pouch deodorizers 10. change bed linens and clothing as soon as they become soiled. g. Assure client that once the edema and discomfort associated with the surgery have resolved, he/she will be able to dress as before with minor, if any, modifications. h. Show client and significant others some of the attractive urostomy products that are available (e.g., opaque or patterned pouches, pouch covers). i. Encourage client's participation in activities that can assist him/her to integrate physical changes that have occurred (e.g., urostomy care, bathing).

Desired Outcome	Nursing Actions *and Selected Purposes/Rationales*
	j. Demonstrate acceptance of client using techniques such as touch and frequent visits. Encourage significant others to do the same. k. Support behaviors suggesting positive adaptation to changes that have occurred (e.g., willingness to care for urostomy, compliance with the treatment plan, verbalization of feelings of self-worth, maintenance of relationships with significant others). l. Encourage significant others to allow client to do what he/she is able *so that independence can be re-established and/or self-esteem redeveloped.* m. Assist client's and significant others' adjustment by listening, facilitating communication, and providing information. n. Encourage visits and support from significant others. o. If acceptable to client, arrange for a visit with an ostomate of similar age and same sex who has successfully adjusted to a urinary diversion. p. Encourage client to pursue usual roles and interests and to continue involvement in social activities. q. Consult appropriate health care provider (e.g., psychiatric nurse clinician, ET nurse, physician) if client seems unwilling or unable to adapt to changes resulting from the urinary diversion.

Discharge Teaching/Continued Care

6. Nursing Diagnosis: ***DEFICIENT KNOWLEDGE, INEFFECTIVE THERAPEUTIC REGIMEN MANAGEMENT, OR INEFFECTIVE HEALTH MAINTENANCE****

*The nurse should select the diagnostic label that is most appropriate for the client's discharge teaching needs.

Suggested NOC Outcomes: Knowledge: ostomy care; Knowledge: treatment regimen

Suggested NIC Interventions: Health system guidance; Teaching: individual; Teaching: disease process; Teaching: prescribed diet; Teaching: prescribed medication

Desired Outcomes	Nursing Actions *and Selected Purposes/Rationales*
6.a. The client will verbalize a basic understanding of the anatomical changes that have occurred as a result of the surgery.	6.a. Reinforce teaching about the anatomical changes that have occurred as a result of the cystectomy and urinary diversion. Use appropriate teaching aids (e.g., pictures, videotapes, anatomical models).
6.b. The client will demonstrate the ability to change the urostomy appliance and maintain stomal and peristomal skin integrity.	6.b.1. Reinforce teaching regarding application of the appliance, prevention of peristomal skin irritation and breakdown, and maintenance of stomal integrity (see Postoperative Diagnoses 1, action b.4 and 3, action a.2 for appropriate measures). 2. Instruct and assist client to establish a routine for emptying the pouch and changing the appliance. Support client's efforts to maintain integrity of stoma and peristomal skin and keep the pouch from overfilling but discourage excessive emptying of the pouch and changing appliance more often than necessary. 3. Inform client that despite good urostomy care, urine crystals (a result of continued exposure to alkaline urine over time) and encrustations (from mucus accumulation) can form on the stoma and peristomal skin. Explain that if client notices crystals or encrustations, he/she should: a. cleanse the stoma and peristomal skin with prescribed solution (e.g., white vinegar and water) each time appliance is changed

b. replace reusable appliances from which crystals or encrustations cannot be completely removed
c. consult physician or ET nurse about additional care measures.
4. Instruct client to follow special precautions for products used (e.g., skin sealants should be used only on healthy peristomal skin because they can further irritate reddened and excoriated skin).
5. Allow time for questions, clarification, practice, and return demonstration of emptying the pouch, changing the appliance, and performing appropriate stoma and peristomal skin care.

6.c. The client will demonstrate the ability to properly clean reusable urostomy equipment.

6.c.1. Discuss recommended method of cleaning reusable urostomy equipment based on manufacturer's recommendations.
2. Demonstrate appropriate appliance cleansing. Emphasize importance of:
   a. washing and rinsing appliance thoroughly upon removal
   b. soaking pouch according to manufacturer's instructions
   c. allowing appliance to dry thoroughly before reusing
   d. storing appliance according to manufacturer's instructions (e.g., apply powder or cornstarch to inside of pouch; keep items in a clean, dry place).
3. Allow time for questions, clarification, and return demonstration.

6.d. The client will demonstrate the ability to drain and irrigate a continent internal reservoir if present.

6.d.1. Demonstrate the correct method of inserting a catheter through the stoma to drain or irrigate the internal reservoir.
2. Reinforce physician's instructions about the frequency of draining the reservoir (initially the reservoir may need to be emptied every 2–3 hours but, as the incisions heal and the reservoir stretches, the client should be able to extend this to every 4–6 hours during the day and once during the night).
3. Demonstrate correct technique for irrigating an internal reservoir. Caution client to use only the prescribed amount of irrigant in order to avoid overdistending and damaging the reservoir. Inform client that the irrigation is done to remove mucus that is secreted by the bowel segment used to construct the reservoir, that this mucus production decreases over time, and that irrigations will be needed less frequently or not at all as time goes by.
4. Allow time for questions, clarification, practice, and return demonstration of drainage and irrigation of an internal reservoir.

6.e. The client will identify ways to control odor of the urostomy drainage and appliance.

6.e. Provide instructions on ways to control odor of urostomy drainage and appliance (see Postoperative Diagnosis 5, action f).

6.f. The client will identify ways to prevent urinary tract infection.

6.f. Provide instructions on ways to prevent urinary tract infection:
1. drink at least 10 glasses of liquid/day unless contraindicated
2. prevent reflux of urine by:
   a. emptying pouch when it is 1/3 full
   b. attaching a bedside collection system when lying down for an extended period
   c. using a pouch with an antireflux valve
3. maintain urine acidity by:
   a. increasing intake of foods/fluids that acidify the urine (e.g., cranberry juice, prune juice, plums, poultry, fish, whole grains)
   b. avoiding excessive intake of milk, carbonated beverages, and citrus fruit
   c. taking medications such as ascorbic acid as prescribed
4. clean reusable appliances thoroughly (see action c.2 in this diagnosis).

Desired Outcomes	Nursing Actions *and Selected Purposes/Rationales*
6.g. The client will state signs and symptoms to report to the health care provider.	6.g.1. Refer to Standardized Postoperative Care Plan, Diagnosis 22, action c (p. 125), for signs and symptoms to report to the health care provider. 2. Instruct client to also report: a. dark red, dusky blue, blue-black, or pale stoma b. absence of or reduction in urinary output despite an adequate fluid intake c. excessive bleeding of stoma or bloody drainage from stoma d. excessive mucus drainage from urinary meatus (some drainage should be expected for several weeks postoperatively) e. unexpected change in shape, size, or height of stoma (use diagrams and descriptive terms so client does not confuse decreasing stomal size due to resolving edema with actual stomal retraction) f. persistent skin irritation or breakdown of peristomal skin g. persistent presence of urine crystals or encrustations on stoma or peristomal skin h. persistent leakage of urostomy appliance i. persistent leakage of urine from stoma (if client has a continent internal reservoir) j. difficulty draining or irrigating internal reservoir k. signs and symptoms of urinary tract infection (e.g., fever, chills, bloody urine, increased sediment in urine) l. signs and symptoms of renal calculi (e.g., dull, aching or severe, colicky flank pain; blood in urine; nausea; vomiting); stone formation, a late complication of a urinary diversion, may result from persistent urinary stasis, urinary tract infection, or inadequate fluid intake m. difficulty adjusting to change in appearance and body functioning or urostomy care.
6.h. The client will identify appropriate community resources that can assist with home management and adjustment to changes resulting from the urinary diversion.	6.h.1. Provide information about community resources that can assist the client and significant others with home management and adjustment to changes resulting from the urinary diversion (e.g., local ostomy support groups; American Cancer Society; community health agencies; ET nurse; home health agencies; financial, individual, and family counseling services). 2. Initiate a referral if indicated.
6.i. The client will verbalize an understanding of and a plan for adhering to recommended follow-up care including future appointments with health care provider, wound care, activity level, and medications prescribed.	6.i.1. Refer to Standardized Postoperative Care Plan, Diagnosis 22 (pp. 125–126), for routine postoperative instructions and measures to improve client compliance. 2. Reinforce the physician's instructions regarding activity limitations: a. avoid strenuous exercise and lifting heavy objects until permitted by physician b. avoid participating in contact sports. 3. Explain the rationale for, side effects of, and importance of taking medications prescribed (e.g., antimicrobials, ascorbic acid). Inform client of pertinent food and drug interactions. 4. Provide client with a list of urostomy products he/she is using (include product name, size, and number) and where these supplies can be obtained.

Additional Nursing Diagnoses

INEFFECTIVE COPING*

related to:

a. fear, anxiety, and depression associated with the diagnosis, prognosis, loss of control over urinary elimination (especially with a conventional conduit), and possibility of rejection by others;

*See Unit II for outcomes, actions, and rationales.

b. difficulty performing urostomy care and incorporating the care into lifestyle;
c. need for lifelong medical supervision.

*GRIEVING**

related to loss of the ability to urinate normally, change in appearance, and effects of the surgery on sexual functioning.

*See Unit II for outcomes, actions, and rationales.

Bibliography

See pages 879 and 883.

Nephrectomy

Nephrectomy is the surgical removal of the kidney. Conditions that are commonly treated by nephrectomy include renal carcinoma, massive traumatic injury to the kidney, polycystic kidney disease (especially if the kidney is bleeding or severely infected), calculi, renal tuberculosis, pyelonephritis, glomerulonephritis, and renal sclerosis resulting from hypertension. The kidney may also be removed for the purpose of donation.

The surgical approach used to perform a nephrectomy depends on the extensiveness of the planned surgery; the client's age, body build, and physiological status; the underlying pathology; and prior surgical incisions. The approach commonly used for a simple nephrectomy (removal of just the kidney) is the subcostal flank approach. Other approaches (e.g., thoracoabdominal, transabdominal, dorsolumbar) may be necessary when greater visualization, improved access, or a radical nephrectomy (removal of the kidney, renal artery and vein, adrenal gland, proximal ureter, regional lymph nodes, and surrounding fat and fascia) is necessary. Although it is most often necessary to remove the entire kidney, advances in renal imaging, earlier diagnosis of renal disease, and improved surgical techniques have provided surgeons with an option of performing a partial nephrectomy (nephron-sparing nephrectomy) in some instances. In these situations, a laparoscopic, rather than an open, approach is often feasible.

This care plan focuses on the adult client hospitalized for a simple unilateral nephrectomy. Much of the postoperative information is applicable to clients receiving follow-up care in an extended care facility or home setting. The care plan will need to be individualized according to the client's diagnosis, prognosis, and plans for subsequent treatment.

OUTCOME/DISCHARGE CRITERIA

THE CLIENT WILL:

- have evidence of normal healing of surgical wound
- have adequate functioning of the remaining kidney
- have clear, audible breath sounds throughout lungs
- have no signs and symptoms of postoperative complications
- verbalize ways to maintain health of the remaining kidney
- state signs and symptoms to report to the health care provider
- share thoughts and feelings about the loss of the kidney
- verbalize an understanding of and a plan for adhering to recommended follow-up care including future appointments with health care provider, medications prescribed, activity level, wound care, and plans for subsequent treatment of the underlying disorder.

NURSING/COLLABORATIVE DIAGNOSES

Preoperative

1. Fear/Anxiety p. 541

Postoperative

1. Ineffective breathing pattern p. 541
2. Potential complications p. 542
   a. hypovolemic shock
   b. paralytic ileus
   c. pneumothorax

DISCHARGE TEACHING

3. Deficient knowledge, Ineffective therapeutic regimen management, or Ineffective health maintenance p. 543

See Standardized Preoperative and Postoperative Care Plans (pp. 97–126) for additional diagnoses.

PREOPERATIVE

Use in conjunction with the Standardized Preoperative Care Plan.

1. Nursing Diagnosis: **FEAR/ANXIETY**

related to:
a. unfamiliar environment and separation from significant others;
b. anticipated loss of control associated with effects of anesthesia;
c. lack of understanding of diagnostic tests and planned surgical procedure;
d. financial concerns associated with hospitalization;
e. anticipated pain, surgical findings, and change in body functioning as a result of loss of a kidney.

Suggested NOC Outcomes: Anxiety level; Fear level; Anxiety self-control; Fear self-control

Suggested NIC Interventions: Anxiety reduction; Calming technique; Emotional support; Presence

Desired Outcome	Nursing Actions *and Selected Purposes/Rationales* (see pp. 14–16 for additional rationales)
1. The client will experience a reduction in fear and anxiety (see Standardized Preoperative Care Plan, Diagnosis 1 [pp. 97–98], for outcome criteria).	1.a. Refer to Standardized Preoperative Care Plan, Diagnosis 1 (pp. 97–98), for measures related to assessment and reduction of fear and anxiety. b. Implement additional measures *to reduce fear and anxiety:* 1. reinforce physician's explanation that normal kidney function can be maintained by a single healthy kidney 2. begin teaching the client about ways to maintain the health of the kidney that will remain; assure him/her that this information will be reviewed again in detail prior to discharge.

POSTOPERATIVE

Use in conjunction with the Standardized Postoperative Care Plan.

1. Nursing Diagnosis: **INEFFECTIVE BREATHING PATTERN**

related to:
a. increased rate of respirations associated with fear and anxiety;
b. decreased rate of respirations associated with the depressant effect of anesthesia and some medications (e.g., narcotic [opioid] analgesics, some antiemetics);
c. decreased depth of respirations associated with:
   1. depressant effect of anesthesia and some medications (e.g., narcotic [opioid] analgesics, some antiemetics)
   2. reluctance to breathe deeply resulting from incisional pain and fear of dislodging chest tube if present (a chest tube is usually inserted following a thoracoabdominal approach and may be needed following a flank approach)
   3. positioning, weakness, fatigue, and elevation of the diaphragm (can occur if abdominal distention is present).

Suggested NOC Outcome: Respiratory status: ventilation

Suggested NIC Interventions: Respiratory monitoring; Ventilation assistance

Desired Outcome	Nursing Actions *and Selected Purposes/Rationales* (see pp. 18–20 for additional rationales)
1. The client will maintain an effective breathing pattern (see Standardized Postoperative Care Plan, Diagnosis 2 [p. 104], for outcome criteria).	1.a. Refer to Standardized Postoperative Care Plan, Diagnosis 2 (p. 104), for measures related to assessment and management of an ineffective breathing pattern. b. Implement additional measures *to improve breathing pattern:* 1. assure client that deep breathing will not dislodge chest tube if present 2. provide pillow support between lower costal margin and iliac crest when client is lying on operative side *in order to decrease strain on flank incision and subsequently increase ease of deep breathing.*

2. Collaborative Diagnoses:

POTENTIAL COMPLICATIONS OF NEPHRECTOMY

a. **hypovolemic shock** related to excessive blood loss during surgery (the renal area is highly vascular) and hemorrhage following surgery;
b. **paralytic ileus** related to manipulation of the bowel during surgery, the depressant effect of anesthesia and some medications (e.g., narcotic [opioid] analgesics, some antiemetics) on bowel motility, and hypovolemia if it occurs (can cause decreased blood supply to the intestine);
c. **pneumothorax** related to an accumulation of air in the pleural space associated with surgical opening of the pleura (occurs most frequently with thoraco-abdominal and flank approaches) and/or malfunction of chest tube if present.

Desired Outcomes	Nursing Actions *and Selected Purposes/Rationales*
2.a. The client will not develop hypovolemic shock (see Standardized Postoperative Care Plan, Diagnosis 20, outcome a [p. 122], for outcome criteria).	2.a.1. Refer to Standardized Postoperative Care Plan, Diagnosis 20, action a (p. 122), for measures related to assessment, prevention, and treatment of hypovolemic shock. 2. Implement additional measures *to prevent hypovolemic shock:* a. perform actions *to reduce stress on the surgical wound in order to reduce the risk for hemorrhage:* 1. instruct client to splint incisional area with hands or pillow when turning and coughing 2. implement measures to prevent nausea and vomiting (see Standardized Postoperative Care Plan, Diagnosis 8, action b [pp. 110–111]) b. prepare client for surgery (e.g., ligation of bleeding vessels) if indicated.
2.b. The client will have resolution of a paralytic ileus if it occurs (see Standardized Postoperative Care Plan, Diagnosis 20, outcome d [p. 123], for outcome criteria).	2.b. Refer to Standardized Postoperative Care Plan, Diagnosis 20, action d (p. 123), for measures related to assessment and management of a paralytic ileus.
2.c. The client will experience normal lung re-expansion if pneumothorax occurs as evidenced by: 1. audible breath sounds and resonant percussion note by the 3rd–4th postoperative day 2. unlabored respirations at 12–20/minute 3. blood gases returning toward normal 4. chest x-ray showing lung re-expansion.	2.c.1. Assess for and immediately report signs and symptoms of: a. malfunction of the chest drainage system (e.g., respiratory distress, lack of fluctuation in water seal chamber without evidence of lung re-expansion, excessive bubbling in water seal chamber, significant increase in subcutaneous emphysema) b. further lung collapse (e.g., extended area of absent breath sounds with hyperresonant percussion note; rapid, shallow, and/or labored respirations; tachycardia; increased chest pain; restlessness; confusion; blood gas results that have worsened; significant decrease in oximetry results). 2. Monitor chest x-ray results. Report findings of delayed lung re-expansion or further lung collapse.

3. Implement measures *to promote lung re-expansion and prevent further lung collapse:*
   a. perform actions *to maintain patency and integrity of chest drainage system:*
      1. maintain fluid levels in the water seal and suction chambers as ordered
      2. maintain occlusive dressing over chest tube insertion site
      3. tape all connections securely
      4. tape the tubing to the chest wall close to insertion site *to reduce the risk of inadvertent removal of the tube*
      5. position tubing *to promote optimum drainage* (e.g., coil excess tubing on bed rather than allowing it to hang down below the collection device, keep tubing free of kinks)
      6. drain fluid that accumulates in tubing into the collection chamber; milk chest tube gently if indicated *to dislodge clots*
      7. keep drainage collection device below level of client's chest at all times
   b. perform actions *to facilitate the escape of air from the pleural space* (e.g., maintain suction as ordered, ensure that the air vent is open on the drainage collection device if system is to water seal only)
   c. perform actions to improve breathing pattern (see Postoperative Diagnosis 1) and facilitate airway clearance (see Standardized Postoperative Care Plan, Diagnosis 3, action b [p. 105]).
4. If signs and symptoms of further lung collapse occur:
   a. maintain client on bed rest in a semi- to high Fowler's position
   b. maintain oxygen therapy as ordered
   c. assess for and immediately report signs and symptoms of tension pneumothorax (e.g., severe dyspnea, increased restlessness and agitation, rapid and/or irregular pulse rate, hypotension, neck vein distention, shift in trachea from midline)
   d. assist with clearing of existing chest tube and/or insertion of a new tube.

Discharge Teaching/Continued Care

3. NURSING DIAGNOSIS: ***DEFICIENT KNOWLEDGE, INEFFECTIVE THERAPEUTIC REGIMEN MANAGEMENT, OR INEFFECTIVE HEALTH MAINTENANCE****

*The nurse should select the diagnostic label that is most appropriate for the client's discharge teaching needs.

Suggested NOC Outcome: Knowledge: treatment regimen

Suggested NIC Interventions: Health system guidance; Teaching: individual; Teaching: prescribed activity/exercise; Teaching: prescribed medication

Desired Outcomes	**Nursing Actions** *and Selected Purposes/Rationales*
3.a. The client will verbalize ways to maintain health of the remaining kidney.	3.a. Instruct client regarding ways to maintain health of the remaining kidney: 1. adhere to precautions to prevent a urinary tract infection: a. perform actions to prevent urinary stasis: 1. drink at least 10 glasses of liquid/day unless contraindicated 2. urinate whenever the urge is felt 3. avoid long periods of inactivity (if unable to maintain a program of moderate activity, be sure to change positions frequently) b. wipe from front to back after urinating and defecating (if female) c. keep perineal area clean and dry 2. immediately report signs and symptoms of a urinary tract infection (e.g., chills; fever; urgency, frequency, or burning on urination; cloudy or foul-smelling urine)

Desired Outcomes	Nursing Actions *and Selected Purposes/Rationales*
	3. notify physician if a cold or other infection persists for more than 2–3 days or if unable to maintain an adequate fluid intake 4. inform other health care providers about the nephrectomy so that prophylactic antimicrobials may be initiated before dental work and invasive procedures such as cystoscopy and minor surgeries 5. avoid activities that might cause trauma to the remaining kidney (e.g., contact sports, horseback riding) 6. inform physician of all prescription and nonprescription medications being taken and before taking any new medications since they might cause damage to the remaining kidney (e.g., ibuprofen, ciprofloxacin, captopril, quinine, naproxen, lithium, neomycin, gentamicin, pentamidine, vancomycin, cyclosporine) 7. consult health care provider before undergoing any diagnostic test involving the use of contrast media (some of the agents used during these procedures can damage the remaining kidney) 8. if nephrectomy was performed because of renal calculi, reinforce physicians' instructions about diet, drug therapy, and daily fluid requirements to prevent formation of stones in the remaining kidney 9. if surgery was necessary because of renal hypertension, reinforce the physician's instructions about methods of controlling B/P (e.g., dietary modification, medication, physical exercise on regular basis, weight loss if overweight).
3.b. The client will state signs and symptoms to report to the health care provider.	3.b.1. Refer to Standardized Postoperative Care Plan, Diagnosis 22, action c (p. 125), for signs and symptoms to report to the health care provider. 2. Instruct client to report signs and symptoms that could indicate dysfunction of the remaining kidney: a. unexplained weight gain b. decreased urine output c. flank pain on the unoperative side d. blood in the urine.
3.c. The client will verbalize an understanding of and a plan for adhering to recommended follow-up care including future appointments with health care provider, medications prescribed, activity level, wound care, and plans for subsequent treatment of the underlying disorder.	3.c.1. Refer to Standardized Postoperative Care Plan, Diagnosis 22 (pp. 125–126), for routine postoperative instructions and measures to improve client compliance. 2. Reinforce physician's instructions regarding activity: a. gauge activity according to tolerance and allow adequate rest periods b. avoid lifting objects over 7–10 pounds, pushing heavy objects, and exercising strenuously for specified length of time (usually 4–8 weeks). 3. Clarify plans for subsequent treatment of the underlying disorder (e.g., chemotherapy, radiation therapy) if appropriate.

Bibliography

See pages 879 and 883.

UNIT XIII

Nursing Care of the Client with Disturbances of Hematologic and Immune Function

evolve

Human Immunodeficiency Virus (HIV) Infection and Acquired Immune Deficiency Syndrome (AIDS)

Acquired immune deficiency syndrome (AIDS) is an infectious disease of the immune system and is considered to be the last phase of the clinical spectrum of infection by the human immunodeficiency virus (HIV). HIV is a retrovirus that affects the cells in the body that have a CD4 receptor on their surface. The types of cells that have the CD4 receptor and can be infected by the virus include lymphocytes, monocytes, macrophages, glial cells, bone marrow progenitors, and gut-associated lymphoid tissue. The CD4+ T lymphocytes (also called T4 or T-helper cells) have the greatest number of CD4 receptors and are consequently the major target of HIV. These lymphocytes are ultimately destroyed by HIV, which results in severely impaired cell-mediated immunity in the host. Humoral immune function is also impaired because the B lymphocytes are unable to respond appropriately to the presence of a new antigen without the help of normal CD4+ T lymphocytes. The effect of HIV on the monocyte and macrophage further depresses immune system function.

HIV has been isolated from all body fluids but at this point, transmission has been associated only with blood, semen, amniotic fluid, vaginal secretions, and breast milk. The known routes of transmission are by intimate sexual contact, mucous membrane or percutaneous exposure to infected blood or blood products, and perinatal transmission from mother to child. The four high-risk groups for acquiring HIV infection are heterosexuals with multiple sexual partners, men who have sex with men, intravenous drug users, and recipients of blood/blood products. Treating HIV-infected women during pregnancy with an antiretroviral agent (e.g., zidovudine) has significantly reduced the transmission of HIV from mother to child.

Infection with HIV tends to follow a particular course, with the clinical expression being attributed to either the effects of the virus itself or the consequences of CD4+ T lymphocyte depletion. The initial event in the course of the disease is acute retroviral infection, which occurs about 1–6 weeks after exposure to HIV. The person experiences symptoms such as fever, headache, myalgias, lymphadenopathy, rash, fatigue, and sore throat that may persist for a week or longer. Then, the HIV-infected person enters the chronic infection stage. In the early period of chronic infection, the person may be asymptomatic or continue to experience mild symptoms such as fatigue, headache, and lymphadenopathy. This early period often lasts as long as 10–12 years, depending on the rate of viral replication and the rapidity of CD4+ T lymphocyte destruction. The symptomatic stage of HIV infection develops when the CD4+ T lymphocyte count drops below 500 cells/mm^3 and the HIV viral load rises above 10,000 copies/ml. In the early symptomatic stage, the person has various nonspecific symptoms (e.g., unexplained fever and weight loss, fatigue, night sweats, peripheral neuropathy, persistent diarrhea) and persistent localized viral or fungal infections. AIDS is the last stage of HIV infection. In addition to the symptoms experienced in the previous stage, AIDS is heralded by immune suppression (serologically defined as a CD4+ T lymphocyte count less than 200 cells/mm^3) and the presence of a condition that meets the criteria for definition of an AIDS case as specified by the Centers for Disease Control and Prevention (CDC). These AIDS-indicator conditions include HIV-related encephalopathy, HIV wasting syndrome, opportunistic infections (e.g., *Pneumocystis carinii* pneumonia [PCP]; candidiasis of esophagus or bronchi, trachea, or lungs; *Mycobacterium* tuberculosis, *Mycobacterium avium* complex [MAC]; extrapulmonary cryptococcosis; cytomegalovirus infection; *Toxoplasma* encephalitis; coccidioidomycosis), and AIDS-related cancers (e.g., Kaposi's sarcoma, non-Hodgkin's lymphoma, invasive cervical cancer).

At this time, there is no cure for HIV infection. However, there have been significant advances in antiretroviral therapy and prevention of opportunistic infections that have increased the long-term survival of persons with HIV infection. Earlier treatment and the use of highly active antiretroviral therapy (HAART), which consists of a combination of at least 3 antiretroviral agents, have made significant differences in sustaining viral suppression, slowing disease progression, and reducing drug resistance. Because of the side effects of the antiretroviral agents and lack of adherence to the drug regimen, current federal guidelines suggest that treatment be offered early, but that it can be delayed until higher levels of immune suppression are observed. The antiretroviral agents used to control viral replication of HIV include nucleoside reverse transcriptase inhibitors (e.g., zidovudine, lamivudine, zalcitabine, abacavir, didanosine, stavudine), protease inhibitors (e.g., saquinavir, ritonavir, indinavir, amprenavir, nelfinavir), nonnucleoside reverse transcriptase inhibitors (e.g., nevirapine, delavirdine, efavirenz), and fusion inhibitors (e.g., enfuvirtide). Chemoprophylactic therapy to prevent AIDS-defining opportunistic infections has also led to a significant decline in the incidence of certain diseases such as *Pneumocystis carinii* pneumonia, *Mycobacterium avium* complex, tuberculosis, and toxoplasmosis.

This care plan focuses on the adult client with HIV infection hospitalized for treatment of a probable opportunistic infection. Much of the information is applicable to clients receiving follow-up care in an extended care facility or home setting.

OUTCOME/DISCHARGE CRITERIA

THE CLIENT WILL:

- have an adequate respiratory status
- have an adequate or improved nutritional status
- be able to perform activities of daily living without undue fatigue or dyspnea
- demonstrate evidence that opportunistic infection is resolving
- be effectively managing the signs and symptoms of neurological dysfunction
- have discomfort at a manageable level
- show evidence that skin and oral mucous membranes are intact or healing appropriately
- have fewer episodes of diarrhea
- identify ways to prevent the spread of HIV
- identify ways to decrease the risk for developing opportunistic infections
- verbalize ways to maintain an optimal nutritional status
- state signs and symptoms to report to the health care provider
- share feelings about changes in mental and physical functioning and the social isolation and loneliness that may result from having AIDS
- identify resources that can assist with financial needs and adjustment to changes resulting from the diagnosis of AIDS
- verbalize an understanding of and a plan for adhering to recommended follow-up care including regular laboratory studies, future appointments with health care providers, and medications prescribed.

NURSING/COLLABORATIVE DIAGNOSES

1. Impaired respiratory function p. 549
   a. ineffective breathing pattern
   b. ineffective airway clearance
   c. impaired gas exchange
2. Risk for imbalanced fluid and electrolytes p. 550
   a. deficient fluid volume
   b. hypokalemia
   c. hyponatremia
3. Imbalanced nutrition: less than body requirements p. 551
4. Acute/Chronic pain p. 553
   a. oral, pharyngeal, and/or esophageal pain
   b. abdominal pain
   c. neuropathic pain
   d. headache
   e. chest pain
   f. skin and local tissue pain
5. Hyperthermia p. 554
6. Impaired oral mucous membrane p. 555
7. Actual/Risk for impaired tissue integrity p. 556
8. Fatigue p. 557
9. Diarrhea p. 558
10. Disturbed thought processes p. 559
11. Risk for infection: opportunistic infection or sepsis p. 560
12. Risk for injury p. 562
    a. falls
    b. burns
13. Fear/Anxiety p. 563
14. Ineffective coping or Impaired adjustment p. 564
15. Risk for loneliness p. 566
16. Interrupted family processes p. 567

DISCHARGE TEACHING

17. Deficient knowledge, Ineffective therapeutic regimen management, or Ineffective health maintenance p. 568

See p. 572 for additional diagnoses.

1. Nursing Diagnosis: *IMPAIRED RESPIRATORY FUNCTION**

a. ineffective breathing pattern related to:
   1. decreased depth of respirations associated with fear, anxiety, weakness, fatigue, and chest pain if present
   2. increased rate of respirations associated with fear, anxiety, and the increase in metabolic rate that occurs with infection;

b. ineffective airway clearance related to:
   1. increased production of secretions associated with some opportunistic infections of the lungs
   2. stasis of secretions associated with decreased activity and poor cough effort resulting from fatigue and pain;

c. impaired gas exchange related to a decrease in effective lung surface associated with:
   1. the presence of infiltrates and/or cavities in the lung tissue resulting from opportunistic infection of the lungs (e.g., *Pneumocystis carinii* pneumonia, pneumococcal pneumonia, tuberculosis, histoplasmosis)
   2. compression and/or replacement of lung tissue if an AIDS-related cancer such as Kaposi's sarcoma or non-Hodgkin's lymphoma is present.

*This diagnostic label includes the following nursing diagnoses: ineffective breathing pattern, ineffective airway clearance, and impaired gas exchange.

Suggested NOC Outcomes: Respiratory status: airway patency; Respiratory status: ventilation; Respiratory status: gas exchange

Suggested NIC Interventions: Respiratory monitoring; Airway management; Chest physiotherapy; Cough enhancement; Ventilation assistance; Oxygen therapy; Medication administration

Desired Outcome

1. The client will experience adequate respiratory function as evidenced by:
   a. normal rate and depth of respirations
   b. decreased dyspnea
   c. improved breath sounds
   d. symmetrical chest excursion
   e. usual mental status
   f. oximetry results within normal range
   g. blood gases within normal range.

Nursing Actions *and Selected Purposes/Rationales*
(see pp. 12–14, 18–20, and 33–35 for additional rationales)

1.a. Assess for and report signs and symptoms of impaired respiratory function:
   1. rapid, shallow respirations
   2. dyspnea, orthopnea
   3. use of accessory muscles when breathing
   4. abnormal breath sounds (e.g., diminished, bronchial, crackles [rales], wheezes)
   5. asymmetrical chest excursion
   6. cough (can be productive or dry and nonproductive depending on the opportunistic disease present)
   7. restlessness, irritability
   8. confusion, somnolence
   9. significant decrease in oximetry results
   10. abnormal blood gases
   11. abnormal chest x-ray results.

b. Implement measures *to improve respiratory status:*
   1. maintain activity restrictions as ordered *to reduce oxygen needs*
   2. place client in a semi- to high Fowler's position unless contraindicated; position with pillows *to prevent slumping*
   3. instruct client to breathe slowly if hyperventilating
   4. if client must remain flat in bed, assist with position change at least every 2 hours
   5. instruct client to deep breathe or use incentive spirometer every 1–2 hours
   6. assist with positive airway pressure techniques (e.g., continuous positive airway pressure [CPAP], bilevel positive airway pressure [BiPAP], flutter/positive expiratory pressure [PEP] device) if ordered

Desired Outcome	Nursing Actions *and Selected Purposes/Rationales*

7. perform actions *to promote removal of pulmonary secretions:*
   a. instruct and assist client to cough or "huff" every 1–2 hours
   b. implement measures *to thin tenacious secretions and reduce dryness of the respiratory mucous membrane:*
      1. maintain a fluid intake of at least 2500 ml/day unless contraindicated
      2. humidify inspired air as ordered
   c. assist with administration of mucolytics (e.g., acetylcysteine) and diluent or hydrating agents (e.g., water, saline) via nebulizer if ordered
   d. assist with or perform postural drainage therapy (PDT) if ordered
   e. perform suctioning if ordered
   f. administer expectorants (e.g., guaifenesin) if ordered
8. perform actions to reduce pain and fatigue (see Diagnoses 4, action e and 8, action d) *in order to enable the client to breathe more deeply and participate in activities to improve respiratory status*
9. maintain oxygen therapy as ordered
10. discourage smoking *(the irritants in smoke increase mucus production, impair ciliary function, and can cause damage to the bronchial and alveolar walls; the carbon monoxide decreases oxygen availability)*
11. administer central nervous system depressants judiciously; hold medication and consult physician if respiratory rate is less than 12/minute
12. administer the following medications if ordered:
    a. bronchodilators (e.g., theophylline, albuterol, salmeterol, ipratropium)
    b. antimicrobials
    c. corticosteroids *to decrease pulmonary inflammation* (usually reserved for moderate to severe cases of *Pneumocystis carinii* pneumonia *because of the risk for further immunosuppression*).

c. Consult appropriate health care provider (e.g., respiratory therapist, physician) if signs and symptoms of impaired respiratory function persist or worsen.

2. Nursing/Collaborative Diagnosis:

RISK FOR IMBALANCED FLUID AND ELECTROLYTES

a. **deficient fluid volume** related to:
   1. excessive loss of fluid associated with diarrhea, diaphoresis, and vomiting if present
   2. decreased oral intake associated with anorexia, weakness, nausea, and oropharyngeal pain;

b. **hypokalemia** related to:
   1. excessive loss of potassium associated with diarrhea and vomiting if present
   2. decreased oral intake;

c. **hyponatremia** related to:
   1. excessive loss of sodium associated with diarrhea, profuse diaphoresis, and vomiting if present
   2. fluid replacement with hypotonic solutions
   3. water retention associated with increased ADH output resulting from opportunistic disease involvement of the lungs or central nervous system.

Suggested NOC Outcomes: Fluid balance; Hydration; Electrolyte and acid/base balance

Suggested NIC Interventions: Fluid management; Electrolyte management: hypokalemia; Electrolyte management: hyponatremia

Desired Outcome	Nursing Actions *and Selected Purposes/Rationales* (see pp. 30–31 for additional rationales)
2. The client will maintain fluid and electrolyte balance as evidenced by: a. normal skin turgor b. moist mucous membranes c. stable weight d. B/P and pulse within normal range for client and stable with position change e. capillary refill time less than 2–3 seconds f. usual mental status g. balanced intake and output h. usual muscle strength i. soft, nondistended abdomen with normal bowel sounds j. absence of nausea, vomiting, abdominal cramps, and seizure activity k. BUN, Hct, and serum potassium and sodium within normal range.	2.a. Assess for and report signs and symptoms of: 1. deficient fluid volume: a. decreased skin turgor, dry mucous membranes, thirst b. weight loss of 2% or greater over a short period c. postural hypotension and/or low B/P d. weak, rapid pulse e. capillary refill time greater than 2–3 seconds f. change in mental status g. decreased urine output (reflects an actual rather than potential fluid deficit) h. increased BUN and Hct (may not be increased if nutritional status is inadequate) 2. hypokalemia (e.g., cardiac dysrhythmias, postural hypotension, muscle weakness, nausea and vomiting, abdominal distention, hypoactive or absent bowel sounds, low serum potassium level) 3. hyponatremia (e.g., nausea, vomiting, abdominal cramps, lethargy, confusion, weakness, seizures, low serum sodium level). b. Implement measures *to prevent or treat imbalanced fluid and electrolytes:* 1. perform actions to control diarrhea (see Diagnosis 9, action d) 2. perform actions to improve oral intake (see Diagnosis 3, action c.1) 3. perform actions to reduce fever (see Diagnosis 5, action b) 4. administer antiemetics if ordered *to control vomiting* 5. maintain a fluid intake of at least 2500 ml/day unless contraindicated; if oral intake is inadequate or contraindicated, maintain intravenous and/or enteral therapy as ordered 6. administer electrolyte replacements if ordered 7. encourage intake of foods/fluids high in potassium (e.g., bananas, avocado, potatoes, raisins, cantaloupe) and sodium (e.g., processed cheese, canned soups, canned vegetables, bouillon). c. Consult physician if signs and symptoms of imbalanced fluid and electrolytes persist or worsen.

3. NURSING DIAGNOSIS: ***IMBALANCED NUTRITION: LESS THAN BODY REQUIREMENTS***

related to:

a. decreased oral intake associated with:
   1. anorexia resulting from malaise, fatigue, fear, anxiety, pain, depression, increased levels of certain cytokines that depress appetite (e.g., tumor necrosis factor [TNF]), and some antiretroviral agents
   2. nausea, dyspnea, and cognitive impairment if present
   3. oral pain and/or dysphagia resulting from opportunistic lesions in the mouth, pharynx, and esophagus;

b. impaired utilization of nutrients associated with:
   1. accelerated and inefficient metabolism of nutrients resulting from an increased resting energy expenditure that occurs with infection and increased levels of certain cytokines (e.g., TNF, interleukin-1)
   2. decreased absorption of nutrients if HIV and/or opportunistic infection involve the intestine;

c. loss of nutrients associated with persistent diarrhea and vomiting if present.

Suggested NOC Outcomes: Appetite; Nutritional status

Suggested NIC Interventions: Nutritional monitoring; Nutrition management; Nutrition therapy; Exercise promotion: strength training; Nausea management

Desired Outcome	**Nursing Actions** *and Selected Purposes/Rationales* (see pp. 40–43 for additional rationales)

3. The client will maintain an adequate nutritional status as evidenced by:
   a. weight within or returning toward normal range for client
   b. normal BUN and serum prealbumin, albumin, Hct, and Hgb levels
   c. usual strength and activity tolerance
   d. healthy oral mucous membrane.

3.a. Assess for and report signs and symptoms of malnutrition:
  1. weight significantly below client's usual weight or below normal for client's age, height, and body frame
  2. abnormal BUN and low serum prealbumin, albumin, Hct, and Hgb levels
  3. weakness and fatigue
  4. sore, inflamed oral mucous membrane
  5. pale conjunctiva
  6. lower than normal anthropometric measurements such as skinfold thickness, body circumferences (e.g., hip, waist, mid-upper arm), and bioelectrical impedance analysis.

b. Monitor percentage of meals and snacks client consumes. Report a pattern of inadequate intake.

c. Implement measures *to maintain an adequate nutritional status:*
  1. perform actions *to improve oral intake:*
     a. implement measures to prevent breakdown of the oral mucous membrane and promote healing of existing lesions (see Diagnosis 6, action b) *in order to reduce oral/pharyngeal pain and improve swallowing*
     b. implement measures to reduce fear and anxiety and assist client to adjust to and cope with the diagnosis of AIDS (see Diagnoses 13, action b and 14, action b)
     c. implement measures *to reduce nausea* (e.g., administer prescribed antiemetics, encourage client to eat dry foods when nauseated, avoid serving foods with an overpowering aroma)
     d. implement measures to reduce pain (see Diagnosis 4, action e)
     e. increase activity as tolerated *(activity usually promotes a sense of well-being, which can improve appetite)*
     f. obtain a dietary consult if necessary to assist client in selecting foods/fluids that meet nutritional needs, are appealing, and adhere to personal and cultural preferences
     g. if client is having difficulty swallowing, assist him/her to select foods that are easily chewed and swallowed (e.g., eggs, custard, macaroni and cheese, baby foods) and avoid serving foods that are sticky (e.g., peanut butter, soft bread)
     h. encourage a rest period before meals *to minimize fatigue*
     i. maintain a clean environment and a relaxed, pleasant atmosphere
     j. provide oral hygiene before meals *(oral hygiene moistens the mouth, which may make it easier to chew and swallow; it also removes unpleasant tastes, which often improves the taste of foods/fluids)*
     k. serve frequent, small meals rather than large ones if client is weak, fatigues easily, and/or has a poor appetite
     l. if client is dyspneic, place in a high Fowler's position for meals and provide supplemental oxygen therapy during meals
     m. if client's sense of taste is altered, suggest adding extra sweeteners and flavorings/seasonings to foods
     n. encourage significant others to bring in client's favorite foods and eat with him/her *to make eating more of a familiar social experience*
     o. assist client with meals if indicated
     p. allow adequate time for meals; reheat foods/fluids as necessary
  2. perform actions to control diarrhea (see Diagnosis 9, action d)
  3. ensure that meals are well balanced and high in essential nutrients; offer high-protein, high-calorie dietary supplements (e.g., elemental formulas, nutrient-dense candy bars and soups) if indicated
  4. consult physician or physical therapist about a progressive exercise program *(exercise is necessary to promote the maintenance/buildup of lean body mass and help prevent wasting)*
  5. administer the following if ordered:
     a. vitamins and minerals

b. appetite stimulants (e.g., megestrol acetate, dronabinol)
c. anabolic agents (e.g., growth hormone, testosterone, nandrolone, oxandrolone)
d. cytokine inhibitors (e.g., thalidomide) *to improve appetite and promote weight gain by suppressing TNF-α production (use of thalidomide is reserved for persons with severe HIV-related wasting).*

d. Perform a calorie count if ordered. Report information to dietitian and physician.
e. Consult physician about an alternative method of providing nutrition (e.g., parenteral nutrition, tube feedings) if client does not consume enough food or fluids to meet nutritional needs.

4. NURSING DIAGNOSIS:

ACUTE/CHRONIC PAIN

a. oral, pharyngeal, and/or esophageal pain related to the presence of aphthous ulcers in the mouth and/or infections involving the oropharyngeal and esophageal mucosa (e.g., candidiasis, herpes simplex);
b. abdominal pain related to nonspecific gastritis and opportunistic infection or neoplasm involvement of the intestine;
c. neuropathic pain related to the effect of HIV, some opportunistic infections, and some medications (e.g., didanosine, zalcitabine, isoniazid) on the peripheral nerves;
d. headache related to:
   1. cranial inflammation/pressure associated with an opportunistic infection involving the sinuses or brain or the presence of a cerebral neoplasm
   2. vasoactive cytokines that are present with HIV infection;
e. chest pain related to:
   1. inflammation of the parietal pleura associated with an opportunistic infection of the lungs
   2. muscle strain associated with excessive coughing if present;
f. skin and local tissue pain related to:
   1. skin lesions associated with opportunistic infection and/or Kaposi's sarcoma
   2. skin breakdown in perianal area associated with diarrhea.

Suggested NOC Outcomes: Comfort level; Pain control; Pain: disruptive effects

Suggested NIC Interventions: Pain management; Environmental management: comfort; Analgesic administration

Desired Outcome	**Nursing Actions** *and Selected Purposes/Rationales* (see pp. 45–47 for additional rationales)
4. The client will experience diminished pain as evidenced by: a. verbalization of a decrease in or absence of pain b. relaxed facial expression and body positioning c. increased participation in activities d. stable vital signs.	4.a. Assess for signs and symptoms of pain (e.g., verbalization of pain, grimacing, reluctance to move or breathe deeply, rubbing head, reluctance to eat, restlessness, diaphoresis, increased blood pressure, tachycardia). b. Assess client's perception of the severity of pain using a pain intensity rating scale. c. Assess the client's pain pattern (e.g., location, quality, onset, duration, precipitating factors, aggravating factors, alleviating factors). d. Ask the client to describe previous pain experiences and methods used to manage pain effectively. e. Implement measures *to reduce pain:* 1. perform actions *to reduce fear and anxiety about the pain experience* (e.g., assure client that his/her need for pain relief is understood, plan methods for achieving pain control with client) 2. perform actions to reduce fear and anxiety (see Diagnosis 13, action b) *in order to promote relaxation and subsequently increase the client's threshold and tolerance for pain* 3. administer analgesics before activities and procedures that can cause pain and before pain becomes severe

Desired Outcome | **Nursing Actions** *and Selected Purposes/Rationales*

4. perform actions to reduce fatigue (see Diagnosis 8, action d) *in order to increase the client's threshold and tolerance for pain*
5. provide or assist with nonpharmacologic methods for pain relief (e.g., position change; progressive relaxation exercises; guided imagery; restful environment; diversional activities such as watching television, reading, or conversing)
6. plan methods for achieving pain control with client *in order to assist him/her to maintain a sense of control over the pain experience*
7. perform actions to prevent and treat oral mucous membrane and skin lesions (see Diagnoses 6, action b and 7, actions c–e)
8. administer the following if ordered:
   a. nonopioid (nonnarcotic) analgesics such as salicylates and other nonsteroidal anti-inflammatory agents
   b. opioid (narcotic) analgesics
   c. tricyclic antidepressants (e.g., amitriptyline) and/or anticonvulsants (e.g., carbamazepine, gabapentin) *to treat painful neuropathies*
   d. topical anesthetic/analgesic ointments (e.g., capsaicin) *to treat skin and superficial neuropathic pain*
   e. oral anesthetic and/or protective agents (e.g., sucralfate, viscous xylocaine mixed with diphenhydramine elixir and a magnesium or aluminum antacid)
   f. corticosteroids *(may be utilized to relieve pain associated with some CNS lesions, sinusitis, and peripheral neuropathies)*
   g. antimicrobials and/or antineoplastic agents *(may be given to treat HIV infection and/or opportunistic disease[s] causing the pain).*

f. Consult appropriate health care provider (e.g., pharmacist, pain management specialist, physician) if adequate pain relief cannot be achieved with the above measures.

5. Nursing Diagnosis: *HYPERTHERMIA*

related to stimulation of the thermoregulatory center in the hypothalamus by endogenous pyrogens that are released in an infectious process.

Suggested NOC Outcome: Thermoregulation

Suggested NIC Intervention: Fever treatment

Desired Outcome | **Nursing Actions** *and Selected Purposes/Rationales*

5. The client will experience resolution of hyperthermia as evidenced by:
   a. skin usual temperature and color
   b. pulse rate between 60–100 beats/minute
   c. respirations 12–20/minute
   d. normal body temperature.

5.a. Assess for signs and symptoms of hyperthermia (e.g., warm, flushed skin; tachycardia; tachypnea; elevated temperature).

b. Implement measures *to reduce fever:*
   1. perform actions *to resolve the infectious process:*
      a. implement measures to promote rest (see Diagnosis 8, action b.1)
      b. implement measures to maintain an adequate nutritional status (see Diagnosis 3, action c)
      c. implement measures to promote removal of pulmonary secretions (see Diagnosis 1, action b.7) if a respiratory infection is present
      d. maintain a fluid intake of at least 2500 ml/day unless contraindicated
      e. administer antimicrobials as ordered
   2. administer tepid sponge bath and/or apply cool cloths to groin and axillae if indicated
   3. use a room fan *to provide cool circulating air*
   4. apply cooling blanket if ordered
   5. administer antipyretics if ordered.

c. Consult physician if temperature remains higher than 38.5° C.

6. NURSING DIAGNOSIS: IMPAIRED ORAL MUCOUS MEMBRANE

related to:
a. malnutrition and deficient fluid volume;
b. infections such as candidiasis, herpes simplex, oral hairy leukoplakia, and bacterial gingivitis/periodontitis;
c. Kaposi's sarcoma or lymphoma in the oral cavity.

Suggested NOC Outcome: Oral hygiene

Suggested NIC Interventions: Oral health maintenance; Oral health restoration

Desired Outcome

6. The client will have a healthy oral cavity as evidenced by:
   a. absence of inflammation
   b. pink, moist, intact mucosa
   c. absence of lesions
   d. no reports of oral dryness and pain
   e. ability to swallow without discomfort.

Nursing Actions *and Selected Purposes/Rationales*

(see pp. 43–45 for additional rationales)

6.a. Assess client for and report signs and symptoms of impaired oral mucous membrane (e.g., inflamed and/or ulcerated oral mucosa; thickened white patch, particularly on sides of tongue; painful vesicles that ulcerate; white, friable plaques on the buccal mucosa or tongue; cracks and fissures at corner of mouth; reddened and retracted gingivae; reports of oral dryness and pain; dysphagia; positive results of cultured specimens from oral lesions).

b. Implement measures *to prevent breakdown of the oral mucous membrane and promote healing of existing lesions:*
   1. reinforce importance of and assist client with oral hygiene after meals and snacks; avoid use of products that contain lemon and glycerin and mouthwashes containing alcohol *(these products have a drying and irritating effect on the oral mucous membrane)*
   2. have client rinse mouth frequently with salt and warm water; baking soda and warm water; or a solution of salt, baking soda, and warm water
   3. use a soft bristle toothbrush or a sponge-tipped swab for oral hygiene
   4. lubricate client's lips frequently
   5. encourage client to breathe through nose rather than mouth *in order to reduce mouth dryness*
   6. encourage a fluid intake of at least 2500 ml/day unless contraindicated
   7. perform actions to maintain an adequate nutritional status (see Diagnosis 3, action c)
   8. encourage client not to smoke or chew tobacco *(smoking dries the mucosa; tobacco acts as an irritant to the oral mucosa)*
   9. instruct client to avoid substances that might further irritate the oral mucosa (e.g., hot, spicy, or acidic foods/fluids)
   10. administer antimicrobial agents (e.g., clotrimazole troches, nystatin, fluconazole, itraconazole, ketoconazole, acyclovir, foscarnet, cidofovir topical gel) as ordered
   11. if periodontal disease is present, administer the following if ordered:
       a. oral antiseptic rinses (e.g., chlorhexidine gluconate [Peridex, Periogard])
       b. antimicrobial agents (e.g., metronidazole, amoxicillin-clavulanate, clindamycin)
   12. if Kaposi's sarcoma or lymphoma lesions are present in the oral cavity, prepare client for radiation therapy, chemotherapy, and/or excision of lesion(s) if planned
   13. if aphthous ulcers are present, administer the following if ordered:
       a. topical corticosteroid preparations (e.g., fluocinonide [Lidex] ointment mixed with Orabase, Decadron elixir, clobetasol [Temovate] mixed with Orabase)
       b. thalidomide
   14. if stomatitis is not controlled:
       a. increase frequency of oral hygiene
       b. if client has dentures, remove and replace only for meals.

Desired Outcome	**Nursing Actions** *and Selected Purposes/Rationales*
	c. Consult appropriate health care provider (e.g., pharmacist, clinical nurse specialist, physician) if signs and symptoms of impaired oral mucous membrane persist or worsen.

7. NURSING DIAGNOSIS:

ACTUAL/RISK FOR IMPAIRED TISSUE INTEGRITY

related to:
a. presence of cutaneous infections such as folliculitis, herpes zoster or simplex, bullous impetigo, bacillary angiomatosis, molluscum contagiosum, and/or abscesses;
b. presence of certain skin disorders (e.g., seborrheic dermatitis, photodermatitis, psoriasis);
c. skin lesions associated with Kaposi's sarcoma if present;
d. excessive scratching associated with pruritus (can occur with certain skin disorders or as a side effect of some medications such as trimethoprim-sulfamethoxazole);
e. increased skin fragility associated with malnutrition;
f. persistent contact with irritants associated with diarrhea;
g. damage to the skin and/or subcutaneous tissue associated with prolonged pressure on tissues, friction, or shearing if mobility is decreased.

Suggested NOC Outcome: Tissue integrity: skin and mucous membranes

Suggested NIC Interventions: Skin surveillance; Skin care: topical treatments; Pressure ulcer prevention; Medication administration

Desired Outcome	**Nursing Actions** *and Selected Purposes/Rationales* (see pp. 49–52 for additional rationales)
7. The client will maintain and/or regain tissue integrity as evidenced by: a. absence of redness and irritation b. no skin breakdown.	7.a. Assess the client for the presence of cutaneous lesions (e.g., vesicles, pustules, papules, plaques, scaling patches, nodules). b. Assess bony prominences, perineum, and dependent and pruritic areas for pallor, redness, and breakdown. c. Implement measures *to treat existing cutaneous conditions:* 1. administer antimicrobial agents if ordered *to treat cutaneous infections* 2. apply topical corticosteroids if ordered *to treat inflammatory skin conditions* 3. cleanse infected lesions with antibacterial/antifungal solutions if ordered 4. assist with and/or prepare client for procedures such as cryotherapy, electrocautery, curettage, incision and drainage, phototherapy, and radiation that may be performed to remove or reduce the size of cutaneous lesions. d. Implement measures *to prevent additional tissue breakdown:* 1. assist client to turn at least every 2 hours 2. position client properly; use pressure-reducing or pressure-relieving devices (e.g., pillows, gel or foam cushions, alternating pressure mattress, air-fluidized bed) if indicated 3. gently massage around reddened areas at least every 2 hours 4. apply a thin layer of a dry lubricant such as powder or cornstarch to bottom sheet or skin and to opposing skin surfaces (e.g., axillae, beneath breasts) if indicated *to reduce friction* 5. lift and move client carefully using a turn sheet and adequate assistance 6. perform actions to keep client from sliding down in bed (e.g., gatch knees slightly when head of bed is elevated 30° or higher, limit length of time client is in semi-Fowler's position to 30-minute intervals) *in order to reduce the risk of skin surface abrasion and shearing* 7. instruct or assist client to shift weight at least every 30 minutes 8. keep client's skin clean 9. keep bed linens dry and wrinkle-free

10. thoroughly dry skin after bathing and as often as needed, paying special attention to skin folds and opposing skin surfaces (e.g., axillae, perineum); pat skin dry rather than rubbing
11. provide elbow and heel protectors if indicated
12. increase activity as allowed and tolerated
13. perform actions to maintain an adequate nutritional status (see Diagnosis 3, action c)
14. perform actions *to prevent skin irritation resulting from diarrhea:*
    a. implement measures to reduce diarrhea (see Diagnosis 9, action d)
    b. assist client to thoroughly cleanse and dry perineal area with soft tissue or cloth after each bowel movement; apply a protective ointment or cream
    c. apply a fecal incontinence pouch if diarrhea is severe
    d. if use of absorbent products such as pads or undergarments is necessary, select those that effectively absorb moisture and keep it away from the skin
15. perform actions *to prevent skin irritation resulting from scratching:*
    a. implement measures *to relieve pruritus* (e.g., use a mild soap for bathing, add cornstarch or baking soda to bath water, administer prescribed antihistamines)
    b. keep nails trimmed and/or apply mittens if necessary
    c. instruct client to apply firm pressure to pruritic areas rather than scratching
16. apply a protective covering such as a hydrocolloid or transparent membrane dressing to areas of the skin susceptible to breakdown (e.g., coccyx, elbows, heels).

e. If tissue breakdown occurs or existing breakdown progresses:
   1. notify appropriate health care provider (e.g., wound care specialist, physician)
   2. perform care of involved areas as ordered or per standard hospital procedure.

8. NURSING DIAGNOSIS: FATIGUE

related to:
a. difficulty resting and sleeping;
b. increased energy utilization associated with the elevated metabolic rate that is present with infection;
c. malnutrition;
d. tissue hypoxia associated with:
   1. impaired alveolar gas exchange if respiratory infection is present
   2. anemia resulting from:
      a. HIV or opportunistic disease involvement of erythroid precursors in the bone marrow
      b. treatment with medications that can cause bone marrow depression or RBC hemolysis (e.g., zidovudine, antineoplastic agents, trimethoprim-sulfamethoxazole [TMP-SMX])
      c. vitamin B_{12} or folate deficiency (a result of malabsorption if intestinal involvement is present);
e. overwhelming emotional demands associated with the diagnosis of AIDS;
f. side effects of some medications client may be receiving (e.g., narcotic [opioid] analgesics, antiemetics, antianxiety or antipsychotic agents).

Suggested NOC Outcomes: Endurance; Energy conservation; Rest; Psychomotor energy

Suggested NIC Interventions: Energy management; Exercise promotion: strength training; Nutrition management; Sleep enhancement; Mood management

Desired Outcome	Nursing Actions *and Selected Purposes/Rationales*
8. The client will experience a reduction in fatigue as evidenced by: a. verbalization of feelings of increased energy b. ability to perform usual activities of daily living c. increased interest in surroundings and ability to concentrate.	8.a. Assess for signs and symptoms of fatigue (e.g., verbalization of lack of energy and inability to maintain usual routines, lack of interest in surroundings, decreased ability to concentrate, lethargy). b. Inform client that a feeling of persistent fatigue is not unusual and is a result of the disease itself as well as a side effect of certain medications he/she may be taking. c. Assist client to identify personal patterns of fatigue (e.g., time of day, after certain activities) and to plan activities so that times of greatest fatigue are avoided. d. Implement measures *to increase strength and reduce fatigue:* 1. perform actions *to promote rest and/or conserve energy:* a. maintain activity restrictions if ordered b. minimize environmental activity and noise c. organize nursing care to allow for periods of uninterrupted rest d. assist client with self-care activities as needed e. keep supplies and personal articles within easy reach f. instruct client in energy-saving techniques (e.g., using shower chair when showering, sitting to brush teeth or comb hair) g. implement measures to reduce fear and anxiety and assist the client to adjust to and cope with the diagnosis of AIDS (see Diagnoses 13, action b and 14, action b) h. implement measures to reduce pain (see Diagnosis 4, action e) i. implement measures *to promote sleep* (e.g., encourage relaxing diversional activities in the evening, allow client to continue usual sleep practices unless contraindicated, reduce environmental stimuli, administer prescribed sedative-hypnotics) 2. perform actions to resolve the infectious process (see Diagnosis 5, action b.1) 3. perform actions to maintain an adequate nutritional status (see Diagnosis 3, action c) 4. perform actions to improve respiratory status (see Diagnosis 1, action b) 5. discourage smoking and excessive intake of beverages high in caffeine such as coffee, tea, and colas *(nicotine and caffeine can increase cardiac workload and myocardial oxygen utilization, thereby decreasing oxygen availability)* 6. administer the following if ordered *to treat anemia:* a. packed red blood cells b. erythropoiesis stimulating growth factor (e.g., epoetin alfa) *to stimulate RBC production* c. vitamin B_{12}, folic acid, or iron 7. administer stimulants (e.g., dextroamphetamine) if ordered 8. increase client's activity gradually as allowed and tolerated. e. Consult appropriate health care provider (e.g., rehabilitation therapist, psychiatric nurse clinician, physician) if signs and symptoms of fatigue worsen.

9. Nursing Diagnosis: **DIARRHEA**

related to:

a. a direct effect of HIV on the intestine or opportunistic disease involvement of the intestine (e.g., *Mycobacterium avium-intracellulare, Cryptosporidium, Salmonella,* cytomegalovirus, *Escherichia coli, Clostridium difficile, Entamoeba histolytica, Giardia,* Kaposi's sarcoma);
b. side effect of some antiretroviral agents (e.g., protease inhibitors, didanosine).

Suggested NOC Outcome:
Bowel elimination

Suggested NIC Intervention: Diarrhea management

Desired Outcome	Nursing Actions *and Selected Purposes/Rationales* (see pp. 28–30 for additional rationales)
9. The client will have fewer bowel movements and more formed stool.	9.a. Assess for signs and symptoms of diarrhea (e.g., frequent, loose stools; urgency; abdominal cramping; hyperactive bowel sounds). b. Obtain stool specimens for culture and/or examination for ova and parasites. Report positive results. c. Prepare client for endoscopy if planned *to examine intestinal mucosa, obtain specimens for culture, and/or perform biopsies.* d. Implement measures *to control diarrhea:* 1. restrict oral intake if ordered 2. instruct client to avoid the following foods/fluids that may stimulate or irritate the bowel or cause the stool to be more liquid: a. those high in fiber (e.g., whole-grain cereals, raw fruits and vegetables) b. coffee, alcohol, and foods that are spicy or fatty c. extremely hot or cold foods/fluids d. those high in lactose (e.g., milk, milk products) e. those made with synthetic, nonabsorbable sugars (e.g., sorbitol) that are found in many dietetic foods 3. encourage client to drink pectin-containing juices (e.g., apple, pear) 4. administer the following medications if ordered: a. opioids (e.g., paregoric) or synthetic opioids (e.g., loperamide, diphenoxylate) *to decrease gastrointestinal motility* b. adsorbents/protectants (e.g., attapulgite [Kaopectate], bismuth subsalicylate [Pepto-Bismol]) c. antisecretory agents (e.g., octreotide acetate [Sandostatin]) *to suppress the output of gastroenterohepatic peptides and slow intestinal motility* d. antimicrobial agents *to treat the infectious process.* e. Consult physician if diarrhea persists or worsens.

10. NURSING DIAGNOSIS: **DISTURBED THOUGHT PROCESSES***

related to HIV encephalopathy associated with:

a. AIDS dementia complex resulting from a direct effect of HIV on the central nervous system;
b. opportunistic infections and/or neoplasms involving the central nervous system (e.g., toxoplasmic encephalitis, cryptococcal meningitis, progressive multifocal leukoencephalopathy, cytomegalovirus [CMV] encephalitis, primary central nervous system lymphoma);
c. imbalanced fluid and electrolytes and hypoxemia if present.

*The diagnostic label of acute or chronic confusion may be more appropriate depending on the client's symptoms.

Suggested NOC Outcomes: Cognitive orientation; Cognition; Information processing

Suggested NIC Interventions: Dementia management; Behavior modification; Medication administration

Desired Outcome	Nursing Actions *and Selected Purposes/Rationales*
10. The client will experience improvement in thought processes as evidenced by: a. improved verbal response time b. longer attention span	10.a. Assess client for disturbed thought processes (e.g., slowed verbal responses, decreased ability to concentrate, impaired memory, poor reasoning, apathy, agitation, hallucinations, confusion). b. Ascertain from significant others client's usual level of cognitive and emotional functioning. c. Prepare client for diagnostic studies that may be done to determine the cause of disturbed thought processes (e.g., computed tomography [CT]

Desired Outcome	Nursing Actions *and Selected Purposes/Rationales*

c. improved memory
d. improved reasoning ability and judgment
e. decreased apathy
f. decreased agitation
g. absence of hallucinations and confusion.

or magnetic resonance imaging [MRI] of the brain, toxoplasma and cryptococcal serology studies, cerebrospinal fluid analysis, brain biopsy, neuropsychological tests).

d. Implement measures *to improve client's thought processes:*
   1. perform actions to improve tissue oxygenation (see Diagnoses 1, action b and 8, action d.6).
   2. perform actions to prevent or treat imbalanced fluid and electrolytes (see Diagnosis 2, action b)
   3. administer the following medications if ordered:
      a. antimicrobials *to treat HIV and opportunistic infections*
      b. antineoplastic agents *to treat neoplastic conditions affecting the central nervous system*
      c. antipsychotic agents (e.g., haloperidol, perphenazine, risperidone, chlorpromazine) *to reduce restlessness, agitation, or hallucinations*
      d. antimania/mood stabilizing agents (e.g., lithium; anticonvulsants such as carbamazepine, valproic acid, and gabapentin)
      e. central nervous system stimulants (e.g., dextroamphetamine sulfate, methylphenidate [Ritalin]) *to reduce apathy and withdrawn behavior.*
e. If client shows evidence of altered thought processes:
   1. reorient client to person, place, and time as necessary; avoid repeatedly asking questions about orientation that client cannot answer
   2. address client by name
   3. place familiar objects, clock, and calendar within client's view
   4. approach client in a slow, calm manner; allow adequate time for communication
   5. repeat instructions as necessary using clear, simple language and short sentences
   6. keep environmental stimuli to a minimum
   7. avoid touch and proximity if this appears to increase anxiety
   8. maintain a consistent and fairly structured routine and write out schedule of activities for client to refer to if desired
   9. have client perform only one activity at a time and allow adequate time for performance of activities
   10. encourage client to make lists of planned activities, questions, and concerns
   11. use distraction rather than confrontation to manage negative behavior
   12. set limits on negative behavior and avoid arguing about the established limits
   13. if client is confused or experiencing hallucinations, allow significant others to remain with client *in order to provide constant reassurance*
   14. encourage significant others to be supportive of client; instruct them in methods of dealing with client's disturbed thought processes
   15. discuss physiological basis for disturbed thought processes with client and significant others; inform them that cognitive and emotional functioning may improve with drug therapy
   16. consult appropriate health care provider (e.g., psychiatric nurse clinician, physician) if disturbed thought processes persist or worsen.

11. Nursing Diagnosis: RISK FOR INFECTION: OPPORTUNISTIC INFECTION OR SEPSIS

related to:

a. decreased resistance to infection associated with:
   1. cellular and humoral immune deficiencies present in HIV infection
   2. inadequate nutritional status
   3. depletion of immune mechanisms resulting from presenting infection and treatment with antimicrobial agents

4. myelosuppression resulting from certain medications (e.g., zidovudine, antineoplastic agents, trimethoprim-sulfamethoxazole, ganciclovir, pyrimethamine);

b. stasis of respiratory secretions and/or urinary stasis if mobility is decreased;
c. break in integrity of skin associated with frequent venipunctures or placement of a central venous catheter;
d. impaired integrity of skin or mucous membranes if present.

Suggested NOC Outcomes: Immune status; Infection severity

Suggested NIC Interventions: Infection control; Infection protection

Desired Outcome	Nursing Actions *and Selected Purposes/Rationales* (see pp. 37–40 for additional rationales)

11. The client will remain free of additional opportunistic infection and sepsis as evidenced by:
    a. return of temperature toward client's normal range
    b. decrease in episodes of chills and diaphoresis
    c. blood pressure within normal limits and pulse returning toward normal range
    d. normal or improved breath sounds
    e. absence or resolution of dyspnea
    f. stable or improved mental status
    g. voiding clear urine without reports of frequency, urgency, and burning
    h. absence or resolution of painful, pruritic skin lesions
    i. stable or gradual increase in body weight
    j. no reports of increased weakness and fatigue
    k. absence of visual disturbances
    l. absence or resolution of heat, pain, redness, swelling, and unusual drainage in any area
    m. absence or resolution of oral mucous membrane irritation and ulceration
    n. ability to swallow without difficulty
    o. WBC and differential counts returning toward normal range
    p. negative results of cultured specimens.

11.a. Assess for and report signs and symptoms of additional opportunistic infection and sepsis (be alert to subtle changes in client since the signs of infection may be minimal as a result of immunosuppression; also be aware that some signs and symptoms vary depending on the site of infection, the causative organism, and the age of the client):
1. increase in temperature above client's usual level
2. increase in episodes of chills and diaphoresis
3. hypotension (a symptom of sepsis)
4. increased pulse
5. development or worsening of abnormal breath sounds
6. development or worsening of dyspnea
7. development or worsening of cough
8. decline in mental status
9. cloudy urine
10. reports of frequency, urgency, or burning when urinating
11. urinalysis showing a WBC count greater than 5, positive leukocyte esterase or nitrites, or presence of bacteria
12. vesicular lesions particularly on face, lips, and perianal area
13. new or increased reports of pain in and/or itching of skin lesions and surrounding tissue
14. further increase in weight loss, fatigue, or weakness
15. visual disturbances
16. new or increased heat, pain, redness, swelling, or unusual drainage in any area
17. new or increased irritation or ulceration of oral mucous membrane
18. development of or increased dysphagia
19. significant change in WBC count and/or differential
20. positive results of cultured specimens (e.g., urine, vaginal drainage, stool, sputum, blood, drainage from lesions).

b. Implement measures *to prevent further infection:*
1. administer the following if ordered:
    a. antiretroviral agents *to reduce the rate of replication of HIV*
    b. immunomodulating agents (e.g., interleukin-2, colony stimulating factors such as filgrastim and sargramostim) *to stimulate production/enhance activity of the white blood cells*
    c. antimicrobial agents *to treat current infection or prevent additional opportunistic infection* (prophylaxis for *Pneumocystis carinii* pneumonia, *Mycobacterium* tuberculosis, toxoplasmosis, and *Mycobacterium avium* complex is recommended for all patients with a CD4+ cell count below a critical level)
    d. vaccines (e.g., Hepatitis A, Hepatitis B, Pneumococcal pneumonia, influenza)
2. maintain a fluid intake of at least 2500 ml/day unless contraindicated
3. use good hand hygiene and encourage client to do the same
4. protect client from others with infection

Desired Outcome	Nursing Actions *and Selected Purposes/Rationales*

5. perform actions to maintain an adequate nutritional status (see Diagnosis 3, action c)
6. perform actions identified in this care plan to reduce stressors such as discomfort, dyspnea, and fear and anxiety *in order to prevent an increase in secretion of cortisol (cortisol interferes with some immune responses)*
7. perform actions to prevent breakdown of oral mucous membrane and promote healing of existing lesions (see Diagnosis 6, action b); clean or replace oral hygiene items (e.g., denture cup, toothbrush) regularly
8. maintain sterile technique during all invasive procedures (e.g., urinary catheterization, venous and arterial punctures, injections)
9. change peripheral intravenous line sites according to hospital policy
10. anchor catheters/tubings (e.g., urinary, intravenous) securely *in order to reduce trauma to the tissues and the risk for introduction of pathogens associated with the in-and-out movement of the tubing*
11. change equipment, tubings, and solutions used for treatments such as intravenous infusions, respiratory care, irrigations, and enteral feedings according to hospital policy
12. maintain a closed system for drains (e.g., urinary catheter) and intravenous infusions whenever possible
13. provide a low-microbe diet (e.g., thoroughly cooked foods, fruits and vegetables that have been washed thoroughly)
14. perform actions *to prevent stasis of respiratory secretions* (e.g., assist client to turn, cough, and deep breathe; increase activity as allowed and tolerated)
15. perform actions to prevent or treat skin breakdown (see Diagnosis 7, actions c–e)
16. perform actions to prevent urinary retention (e.g., instruct client to urinate when the urge is first felt, promote relaxation during voiding attempts) *in order to prevent urinary stasis*
17. instruct and assist client to perform good perineal care routinely and after each bowel movement
18. if client has open lesions, perform actions *to prevent wound infection* (e.g., maintain sterile technique during wound care, instruct client to avoid touching wounds)
19. if client has a central venous catheter, instruct and assist him/her with proper care of the exit site.

12. Nursing Diagnosis: RISK FOR INJURY

a. falls related to:
   1. weakness and fatigue
   2. decline in cognitive, behavioral, and/or motor function resulting from HIV-associated involvement of the brain and spinal cord (e.g., AIDS dementia complex, vacuolar myelopathy) and/or opportunistic infection or neoplastic involvement of the central nervous system
   3. visual impairment if present (can result from cytomegalovirus retinitis or from an infection and/or neoplasm involving the CNS);

b. burns related to diminished sensation associated with peripheral neuropathy if present (can be a result of the effect of HIV and some opportunistic infections on the peripheral nerves and/or a side effect of some antiretroviral agents).

Suggested NOC Outcome: Fall prevention behavior; Falls occurrence

Suggested NIC Interventions: Fall prevention; Environmental management: safety; Exercise promotion: strength training

Desired Outcome	Nursing Actions *and Selected Purposes/Rationales*
12. The client will not experience falls or burns.	12.a. Implement measures *to reduce the risk for injury:*

1. perform actions *to prevent falls:*
   a. keep bed in low position with side rails up when client is in bed
   b. keep needed items within easy reach
   c. encourage client to request assistance whenever needed; have call signal within easy reach
   d. use lap belt when client is in chair if indicated
   e. instruct client to wear well-fitting slippers/shoes with nonslip soles and low heels when ambulating
   f. keep floor free of clutter and wipe up spills promptly
   g. accompany client during ambulation utilizing a transfer safety belt if he/she is weak or dizzy
   h. provide ambulatory aids (e.g., walker, cane) if client is weak or unsteady on feet
   i. reinforce instructions from physical therapist regarding exercise program and correct transfer and ambulation techniques
   j. instruct client to ambulate in well-lit areas and to use handrails if needed
   k. if vision is impaired, orient client to surroundings and identify obstacles during ambulation
   l. do not rush client; allow adequate time for ambulation to the bathroom and in hallway
   m. make sure that shower has a nonslip bottom surface and that shower chair, secure bath mat, call signal, grab bars, and adequate lighting are present
   n. implement measures to improve strength and reduce fatigue (see Diagnosis 8, action d)
   o. administer central nervous system depressants judiciously
   p. if client is confused or irrational:
      1. reorient frequently to surroundings and necessity of adhering to safety precautions
      2. provide appropriate level of supervision
      3. consult physician about the temporary use of a bed alarm or jacket or wrist restraints if necessary
      4. administer prescribed antianxiety and antipsychotic medications if indicated
2. perform actions *to prevent burns:*
   a. let hot foods and fluids cool slightly before serving
   b. supervise client while smoking if indicated
   c. assess temperature of bath water and direct heat application devices (e.g., heating pad, warm compresses) before and during use
3. administer medications (e.g., antimicrobials, antineoplastic agents) as ordered *to treat the underlying disease condition and subsequently improve mental status and motor and sensory function.*

b. Include client and significant others in planning and implementing measures to prevent injury.
c. If injury does occur, initiate first aid if appropriate and notify physician.

13. NURSING DIAGNOSIS: FEAR/ANXIETY

related to:
a. threat of permanent worsening of health status and possible disability and death;
b. threat to self-concept associated with changes in physical and mental functioning (e.g., wasting syndrome, gait difficulty, poor coordination, dementia);
c. stigma associated with having AIDS;
d. financial concerns;
e. separation from support system;
f. possibility of transmitting disease to others.

Suggested NOC Outcomes: Anxiety self-control; Anxiety level; Fear level; Fear self-control

Suggested NIC Interventions: Anxiety reduction; Calming technique; Emotional support; Presence; Financial resource assistance

Desired Outcome	Nursing Actions *and Selected Purposes/Rationales* (see pp. 14–16 for additional rationales)

13. The client will experience a reduction in fear and anxiety as evidenced by:
    a. verbalization of feeling less anxious
    b. usual sleep pattern
    c. relaxed facial expression and body movements
    d. stable vital signs
    e. usual perceptual ability and interactions with others.

13.a. Assess client for signs and symptoms of fear and anxiety (e.g., verbalization of feeling anxious, insomnia, tenseness, shakiness, restlessness, diaphoresis, tachycardia, elevated blood pressure, self-focused behaviors).

b. Implement measures *to reduce fear and anxiety:*
   1. orient client to environment, equipment, and routines
   2. introduce client to staff who will be participating in care; if possible, maintain consistency in staff assigned to his/her care
   3. assure client that staff members are nearby; respond to call signal as soon as possible
   4. maintain a calm, supportive, confident manner when interacting with client
   5. encourage verbalization of fear and anxiety; provide feedback
   6. explain all tests that may be performed to diagnose the current status of HIV infection and HIV/AIDS-related conditions
   7. reinforce physician's explanation about the current status of HIV infection and prognosis; encourage questions and clarify misconceptions
   8. provide a calm, restful environment
   9. instruct client in relaxation techniques and encourage participation in diversional activities
   10. perform actions to assist client to adjust to and cope with the diagnosis and its implications (see Diagnosis 14, action b)
   11. initiate a social service referral and/or assist client to identify and contact appropriate community resources if indicated
   12. provide information based on current needs of client at a level he/she can understand; encourage questions and clarification of information provided
   13. provide client with a note pad and pencil, printed information, and/or a tape recorder so he/she can review the information presented as often as desired
   14. encourage significant others to project a caring, concerned attitude without obvious anxiousness
   15. include significant others in orientation and teaching sessions and encourage their continued support of the client
   16. administer prescribed antianxiety agents if indicated.

c. Consult appropriate health care provider (e.g., psychiatric nurse clinician, physician) if above actions fail to control fear and anxiety.

14. Nursing Diagnosis: *INEFFECTIVE COPING OR IMPAIRED ADJUSTMENT**

related to:
a. depression, fear, anxiety, and ongoing grieving associated with the diagnosis of AIDS and poor prognosis;
b. need for permanent change in lifestyle associated with impaired immune system functioning and potential for disease transmission to others;
c. uncertainty of disease course and feelings of powerlessness over course of disease;
d. need for disclosure of diagnosis with possibility of subsequent rejection and/or distancing by others and loss of employment and health benefits;
e. guilt associated with past behavior (if it was a factor in contracting HIV) and/or possibility of having transmitted HIV to others;

*The nurse should select the diagnostic label that is most appropriate for the client.

f. lack of personal resources to deal with disability and premature death associated with youth (a significant number of clients are in their twenties or thirties and are not developmentally prepared to acknowledge and cope with disability and their own mortality);
g. multiple losses (e.g., death of close friends with AIDS; loss of normal body functioning, family support, financial security, and/or usual lifestyle and roles);
h. chronic symptoms (e.g., pain, diarrhea, fatigue) if present.

Suggested NOC Outcomes: Acceptance: health status; Psychosocial adjustment: life change; Coping; Compliance behavior; Health beliefs: perceived control

Suggested NIC Interventions: Coping enhancement; Crisis intervention; Support system enhancement; Spiritual growth facilitation

Desired Outcome	**Nursing Actions** *and Selected Purposes/Rationales* (see pp. 26–28 for additional rationales)
14. The client will demonstrate adjustment to current health status and effective coping as evidenced by: a. verbalization of acceptance of having AIDS and ability to cope with the disease b. verbalization of a sense of control over health status c. utilization of appropriate problem-solving techniques d. willingness to participate in treatment plan and meet basic needs e. absence of destructive behavior toward self and others f. utilization of available support systems.	14.a. Assess for and report signs and symptoms of: 1. ineffective coping (e.g., verbalization of inability to cope; inability to ask for help, problem solve, or meet basic needs; insomnia; withdrawal; reluctance to participate in treatment plan; destructive behavior toward self or others; inappropriate use of defense mechanisms) 2. impaired adjustment (e.g., denial of health status change, verbalization of lack of control, reluctance to participate in treatment plan and take actions to prevent further health problems). b. Implement measures *to promote effective coping and adjustment to change in health status:* 1. allow time for client to begin to adjust to the diagnosis and its implications, planned treatment, and anticipated changes in lifestyle and roles 2. perform actions *to facilitate the grieving process* (e.g., assist client to acknowledge the changes/losses experienced, discuss the grieving process and reinforce that phases may overlap or recur, encourage expression of feelings) 3. perform actions to reduce fear and anxiety (see Diagnosis 13, action b) 4. perform actions to reduce pain, control diarrhea, and reduce fatigue (see Diagnoses 4, action e; 9, action d; and 8, action d) 5. assist client to identify personal strengths and resources that can be utilized to facilitate adjustment to and coping with the current situation 6. demonstrate acceptance of client but set limits on inappropriate behavior 7. support realistic hope by providing information about advances in the prevention of disease progression (e.g., HAART) and prevention of opportunistic infections 8. if acceptable to client, arrange for a visit from another individual who is successfully living with AIDS 9. include client in planning care, encourage maximum participation in treatment plan, and allow choices when possible *to enable him/her to maintain a sense of control* 10. assist client to maintain usual daily routines whenever possible 11. assist client to identify priorities and attainable goals as he/she starts to plan for necessary lifestyle and role changes 12. assist client and significant others to identify ways that personal and family goals can be adjusted rather than abandoned

Desired Outcome	Nursing Actions *and Selected Purposes/Rationales*

13. discuss ways to maintain optimal health; focus on methods of altering rather than changing lifestyle
14. assist client through methods such as role playing to prepare for negative reactions from others because of diagnosis of AIDS
15. administer antianxiety and/or antidepressant agents if ordered
16. assist client to identify and utilize available support systems; provide information about resources and support groups that can assist client and significant others in adjusting to and coping with effects of AIDS (e.g., American Foundation for AIDS Research, National AIDS Clearinghouse, National Association of People with AIDS, CDC National AIDS Hotline, Project Inform, hospice programs, drug abuse programs)
17. when appropriate, assist client to meet spiritual needs (e.g., arrange for a visit from clergy)
18. encourage continued emotional support from significant others
19. encourage client to share with significant others the kind of support that would be most beneficial (e.g., listening, inspiring hope, providing reassurance and accurate information)
20. support behaviors indicative of effective coping and adjustment (e.g., participation in treatment plan, verbalization of the ability to cope with diagnosis of AIDS, utilization of effective problem-solving strategies).

c. Consult appropriate health care provider (e.g., psychiatric nurse clinician, physician) if client continues to have difficulty adjusting to and coping with the diagnosis and current situation.

15. Nursing Diagnosis: *RISK FOR LONELINESS*

related to:
a. fear of associating with others because of possibility of contracting an infection;
b. stigma and discrimination associated with the diagnosis of AIDS and others' fear of contracting HIV;
c. decreased participation in usual activities because of weakness, pain, fatigue, and fear of falls;
d. withdrawal from others associated with fear of embarrassment resulting from decline in physical and mental functioning.

Suggested NOC Outcomes: Social involvement; Social support

Suggested NIC Interventions: Socialization enhancement; Visitation facilitation; Family involvement promotion; Family integrity promotion

Desired Outcome	Nursing Actions *and Selected Purposes/Rationales*
15. The client will not experience a sense of isolation and loneliness as evidenced by: a. maintenance of relationships with significant others b. no expression of feelings of isolation and loneliness.	15.a. Assess for indications of isolation and loneliness (e.g., absence of supportive significant others; uncommunicative; withdrawn; expression of feelings of rejection, being different from others, or being lonely; hostility; sad, dull affect). b. Implement measures *to decrease isolation and reduce the risk for loneliness:* 1. assist client to identify reasons for feeling isolated and alone; aid him/her in developing a plan of action to reduce these feelings 2. reinforce physician's explanation about the immune deficiency; assure client that continued social contact with healthy people will not cause disease or infection 3. provide information to client and significant others about how HIV is known to be transmitted; assure them that HIV does not spread through ordinary physical contact 4. demonstrate acceptance of client using techniques such as touch and frequent visits

5. encourage significant others to visit
6. encourage client to maintain telephone contact with significant others
7. schedule time each day to sit and talk with client
8. assist client to identify a few persons he/she feels comfortable with and encourage interactions with them
9. encourage client to allow friends and family to share their feelings and fears *in order to reduce the possibility of their distancing from client*
10. make items such as telephone, TV, radio, greeting cards, and newspapers accessible to client
11. have significant others bring client's favorite objects from home and place in room
12. encourage participation in support groups.

16. NURSING DIAGNOSIS: INTERRUPTED FAMILY PROCESSES

related to:

a. diagnosis of terminal, communicable disease in family member;
b. fear of disclosure of diagnosis with subsequent rejection of family unit;
c. change in family roles and structure associated with progressive disability and eventual death of family member;
d. financial burden associated with extended illness and progressive disability of client;
e. fear of contracting disease from client;
f. decisions made by client and his/her partner about such issues as treatment plan, life support, and disposition of property that may be in conflict with the client's family of origin;
g. anticipatory grief.

Suggested NOC Outcomes: Family coping; Family functioning; Family normalization; Family resiliency

Suggested NIC Interventions: Family involvement promotion; Family integrity promotion; Family process maintenance; Family support; Support system enhancement; Caregiver support

Desired Outcome

16. The family members* will demonstrate beginning adjustment to diagnosis of AIDS in client and changes in functioning of family member and family roles and structure as evidenced by:
    a. meeting client's needs
    b. verbalization of ways to adapt to required role and lifestyle changes
    c. active participation in decision making and client's care
    d. positive interactions with one another.

Nursing Actions *and Selected Purposes/Rationales*

16.a. Assess for signs and symptoms of interrupted family processes (e.g., inability to meet client's needs, statements of not being able to accept client's diagnosis or make necessary role and lifestyle changes, inability to make decisions, inability or refusal to participate in client's care, negative family interactions).

b. Identify components of the family and their patterns of communication and role expectations.

c. Implement measures *to facilitate family members' adjustment to client's diagnosis, changes in his/her functioning within the family system, and the resultant changes in family roles and structure:*
   1. encourage and assist family members to verbalize feelings about client's diagnosis and its effect on their lifestyle and family structure; actively listen to each family member and maintain a nonjudgmental attitude about feelings shared
   2. reinforce physician's explanation about AIDS, how HIV is transmitted, and planned treatment program
   3. assist family members to gain a realistic perspective of client's situation, conveying as much hope as appropriate
   4. provide privacy *so that family members and client can share their feelings with one another;* stress the importance of and facilitate the use of good communication techniques

*The term "family members" is being used here to include client's significant others.

Desired Outcome	Nursing Actions *and Selected Purposes/Rationales*
	5. assist family members to progress through their own grieving process; explain that they may encounter times when they need to focus on meeting their own rather than the client's needs 6. emphasize the need for family members to obtain adequate rest and nutrition and to identify and utilize stress management techniques *so that they are better able to emotionally and physically deal with the changes that are being experienced, physical care of the client, and reactions of others when diagnosis is known* 7. encourage and assist family members to identify coping strategies for dealing with the client's diagnosis and its effect on the family 8. assist family members to identify realistic goals and ways of reaching these goals 9. include family members in decision making about client's care; convey appreciation for their input and continued support of the client 10. encourage and allow family members to participate in client's care as appropriate 11. assist family members to identify resources that can assist them in coping with their feelings and meeting their immediate and long-term needs (e.g., counseling and social services; pastoral care; service, church, and AIDS support groups); initiate a referral if indicated. d. Consult appropriate health care provider (e.g., psychiatric nurse clinician, hospice nurse, physician) if family members continue to demonstrate difficulty adjusting to client's diagnosis and change in client's functioning and family structure.

Discharge Teaching/Continued Care

17. Nursing Diagnosis: ***DEFICIENT KNOWLEDGE, INEFFECTIVE THERAPEUTIC REGIMEN MANAGEMENT, OR INEFFECTIVE HEALTH MAINTENANCE****

*The nurse should select the diagnostic label that is most appropriate for the client's discharge teaching needs.

Suggested NOC Outcomes: Knowledge: disease process; Knowledge: treatment regimen; Knowledge: health behavior; Knowledge: health resources; Knowledge: infection control

Suggested NIC Interventions: Health system guidance; Teaching: disease process; Teaching: prescribed diet; Teaching: prescribed medication; Communicable disease management; Financial resource assistance

Desired Outcomes	Nursing Actions *and Selected Purposes/Rationales*
17.a. The client will identify ways to prevent the spread of HIV.	17.a. Instruct client in ways to prevent spread of HIV to others: 1. if a spill of blood or other body fluids occurs, cleanse area with hot, soapy water or a household detergent and then disinfect with a solution of 1 part bleach to 10 parts water 2. dispose of water used to clean up body fluid spills in the toilet 3. do not share eating utensils, toothbrushes, razors, enema equipment, or sexual devices 4. if sexually active with a partner: a. avoid multiple sexual partners and partners with risky sexual behaviors b. be honest with desired partner about HIV infection c. modify techniques so that both partners are protected from contact with body fluids

d. avoid unsafe sexual practices (e.g., sharing sex toys; allowing ejaculate to come in contact with broken skin or mucous membranes; intercourse without a condom; any activity that could cause tears in lining of vagina, rectum, or penis; mouth contact with penis, vagina, or anal area)
e. avoid vaginal intercourse during menstruation (the contact with blood increases the risk of HIV transmission)
f. use the following guidelines in relation to condom use:
    1. always use a barrier (male and/or female condom) during anal, vaginal, and oral penetration (condom should be applied prior to time a body orifice is entered because HIV is found in preseminal fluid)
    2. use latex or polyurethane condoms (HIV can penetrate other types of materials)
    3. use condoms with a receptacle tip to reduce the risk of spillage of semen; if that type is unavailable, create a receptacle for ejaculate by pinching tip of condom as it is rolled on erect penis
    4. lubricate outside of condom and area to be penetrated to minimize possibility of condom breakage
    5. avoid lubricants made of mineral oil or petroleum distillates such as Vaseline or baby oil (these products weaken latex)
    6. hold condom at base of penis during withdrawal and use caution during removal of condom to prevent spillage of semen (penis should be withdrawn and condom removed before the penis has totally relaxed)
    7. dispose of condom immediately after use (a new one should be used for subsequent sexual activity)
    8. store condoms in a cool place to prevent them from drying out and breaking during use
    9. do not use a condom if the expiration date on the package has passed, the package looks worn or punctured, or if the condom looks brittle or discolored or is sticky
g. consult health care provider if exposed to or experiencing symptoms of a sexually transmitted disease (the presence of genital lesions caused by other STDs increases the shedding of HIV); tell partner to also seek treatment of STD because of the decrease in mucosal resistance to HIV

5. avoid getting pregnant but if pregnancy occurs, consult health care provider about antiretroviral therapy (e.g., zidovudine) to reduce the risk of perinatal transmission of HIV to infant
6. do not breast feed infant
7. do not donate blood, sperm, or body organs
8. if an intravenous drug user:
    a. get involved in a needle and syringe exchange program
    b. do not share drug injecting equipment (e.g., needles, syringes, cookers, cotton, rinse water)
    c. discard disposable needles and syringes after one use or clean them with household bleach and rinse thoroughly with water.

17.b. The client will identify ways to decrease the risk for developing opportunistic infections.

17.b. Instruct client in ways to decrease risk for developing an opportunistic infection:
1. cleanse kitchen and bathroom surfaces regularly with a disinfectant to prevent growth of pathogens
2. use a 1:10 solution of household bleach and water for cleaning and/or disinfecting areas soiled with blood or other body fluids
3. utilize good hand hygiene (e.g., wash hands using an antimicrobial soap, use an alcohol-base hand rub)
4. if respiratory equipment (e.g., inhalers, humidifier) is used at home, cleanse it as instructed and change water in humidifier daily
5. wear gloves when gardening and when in contact with human or pet excreta (e.g., cleaning litter boxes, bird cages, and aquariums)

Desired Outcomes	Nursing Actions *and Selected Purposes/Rationales*
	6. avoid exposure to body fluids during sexual activity and use latex or polyurethane condoms during sexual intercourse 7. avoid oral-anal sex 8. reduce the risk of food-borne illness: a. thoroughly wash hands and food preparation items and surfaces (e.g., knives, cutting board, countertop) before and after cooking, especially when working with raw meat, poultry, and fish b. avoid intake of foods/fluids with a high microorganism content (e.g., raw or undercooked poultry, seafood, meats, or eggs; unwashed fruits and vegetables; unpasteurized dairy products or fruit juices; raw seed sprouts; soft cheeses; anything that has passed its expiration date) c. cook leftover foods or ready-to-eat foods (e.g., hot dogs) until steaming hot before eating d. avoid foods from delicatessen counters (e.g., prepared meats, salads, cheeses) and refrigerated pâtés and other meat spreads or reheat these foods until steaming before eating e. do not drink water directly from lakes or rivers f. boil water for a full minute if a community "boil water" advisory is issued 9. avoid activities such as cleaning, remodeling, or demolishing old buildings; exploring caves; disturbing soil beneath bird-roosting sites or cleaning chicken coops; being around disturbed native soil at building excavation sites or dust storms (considered to be endemic areas for histoplasmosis and coccidioidomycosis) 10. wash hands after handling pets and avoid contact with reptiles (e.g., snakes, lizards, turtles), baby chickens, and ducklings 11. consult health care provider about receiving immunizations (e.g., pneumococcal vaccine, influenza vaccine, hepatitis A and B vaccines) 12. avoid swimming in lakes, rivers, and public pools 13. if traveling to a developing country, consult health care provider about recommended immunizations, prophylactic antimicrobials, and health care practices (e.g., drinking only bottled water; avoiding raw fruits and vegetables, unpasteurized dairy products, and undercooked eggs, fish, and meat) 14. do not share eating utensils, towels, washcloths, toothbrushes, razors, enema equipment, or sexual devices 15. keep living quarters well ventilated and change furnace filters regularly to reduce exposure to airborne disease 16. avoid contact with persons who have an infection and those who have been recently vaccinated 17. maintain an adequate balance between activity and rest 18. inform all health care providers of HIV infection so that drugs that further suppress the immune system (e.g., corticosteroids, immunosuppressants) will not be prescribed unnecessarily 19. maintain an optimal nutritional status 20. drink at least 10 glasses of liquid/day unless contraindicated.
17.c. The client will verbalize ways to maintain an optimal nutritional status.	17.c. Provide instructions regarding ways to maintain an optimal nutritional status: 1. eat foods that are high in protein and calories 2. try to eat a snack or a small meal or drink a nutritional supplement every 2–3 hours 3. take prescribed vitamins, appetite stimulants (e.g., megestrol acetate), and anabolic agents (e.g., oxandrolone) 4. participate in a progressive exercise program if possible.

17.d. The client will state signs and symptoms to report to the health care provider.

17.d. Stress importance of notifying the health care provider if the following signs and symptoms occur or if these existing signs and symptoms worsen:
1. persistent fever or chills
2. night sweats
3. persistent headache or different type of headache
4. swollen glands
5. skin lesions or significant rash
6. reddish-purple patches or nodules on any body area
7. ulcerations or white patches in the mouth
8. difficulty swallowing
9. persistent diarrhea or vomiting
10. perianal or vulvovaginal itching and/or pain
11. frequency, urgency, or burning on urination
12. cloudy or foul-smelling urine
13. dry cough or a cough productive of purulent, green, or rust-colored sputum
14. progressive shortness of breath
15. increasing weakness, fatigue, or weight loss
16. change in vision, spots that appear to drift in front of eye (floaters)
17. decline in mental function or level of consciousness
18. loss of strength and coordination in extremity(ies)
19. numbness, tingling, or pain in extremity(ies)
20. inability to maintain an adequate fluid intake
21. yellow discoloration of skin
22. bleeding from rectum that is not related to hemorrhoids
23. severe depression or anxiousness or feeling of being a danger to self or others
24. seizures.

17.e. The client will identify resources that can assist with financial needs and adjustment to changes resulting from the diagnosis of AIDS.

17.e.1. Provide information to client and significant others about state and federally funded financial program and resources that can assist in adjustment to the diagnosis of AIDS (e.g., American Foundation for AIDS Research, National Association of People with AIDS, hospice programs, community support groups, CDC National AIDS Hotline, Project Inform, counselors).
2. Initiate a referral if indicated.

17.f. The client will verbalize an understanding of and a plan for adhering to recommended follow-up care including regular laboratory studies, future appointments with health care providers, and medications prescribed.

17.f.1. Reinforce the importance of keeping scheduled follow-up appointments for laboratory studies and with health care providers.
2. Explain the rationale for, side effects of, and importance of taking medications prescribed (e.g., antiretroviral agents, antimicrobial agents, hematopoietic agents, anabolic agents, appetite stimulants). Inform client of pertinent food and drug interactions.
3. Reinforce the importance of strictly adhering to the antiretroviral regimen prescribed (usually consists of a combination of at least 3 antiretroviral agents). Explain that not adhering to the prescribed regimen will limit the effectiveness of subsequent regimens.
4. Explain the importance of taking the full dose of any antimicrobial agents prescribed. Reinforce the possibility that life-long treatment with antimicrobials (e.g., TMP-SMX) may be necessary to prevent some opportunistic infections if the CD4+ cell count is critically low.
5. Implement measures to improve client compliance:
   a. include significant others in teaching sessions if possible
   b. encourage questions and allow time for reinforcement and clarification of information provided
   c. provide written instructions regarding scheduled appointments with health care providers and laboratory, medications prescribed, signs and symptoms to report, and ways to prevent infection.

Additional Nursing Diagnoses

ALTERED COMFORT: CHILLS AND EXCESSIVE DIAPHORESIS

related to persistent or recurrent fever associated with HIV and opportunistic infections.

ALTERED COMFORT: PRURITUS

related to:
a. dry skin associated with deficient fluid volume (can occur as a result of decreased oral intake, excessive diaphoresis, and/or persistent diarrhea);
b. pruritic folliculitis (e.g., staphylococcal folliculitis, eosinophilic folliculitis);
c. dermatological disorders such as seborrheic dermatitis, photodermatitis, and psoriasis;
d. a side effect of some antimicrobials (e.g., TMP-SMX);
e. vulvovaginal candidiasis.

SELF-CARE DEFICIT

related to:
a. cognitive and/or motor impairments if present (can result from HIV or opportunistic disease involvement of the central nervous system);
b. fatigue, weakness, and dyspnea;
c. depression;
d. visual impairment if present (can result from cytomegalovirus retinitis or from an infection and/or neoplasm involving the CNS).

DISTURBED SLEEP PATTERN*

related to fear, anxiety, depression, frequent assessments and treatments, pain, diarrhea, pruritus, chills, night sweats, coughing and dyspnea (may occur if respiratory infection is present), unfamiliar environment, and the effect of some medications (e.g., zidovudine).

INEFFECTIVE SEXUALITY PATTERNS

related to:
a. rejection by desired partner associated with his/her fear of contracting AIDS;
b. need to disclose to new partner(s) the diagnosis of AIDS;
c. decreased sexual desire associated with fatigue, pain, weakness, anxiety, depression, and fear of transmitting or contracting disease.

RISK FOR POWERLESSNESS

related to:
a. the disabling and terminal nature of AIDS;
b. increasing dependence on others to meet basic needs;
c. changes in roles, relationships, and future plans.

GRIEVING*

related to:
a. having an incurable illness with an uncertain course and a high probability of premature death;
b. changes in body functioning, appearance, lifestyle, and roles associated with the disease process.

---

*See Unit II for outcomes, actions, and rationales.

Bibliography

See pages 879 and 883–884.

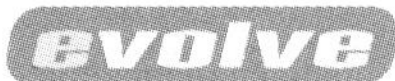

Sepsis

Sepsis is a systemic response to infection. It is defined by the American College of Chest Physicians and Society of Critical Care Medicine as a documented infection with a finding of at least two of the four systemic inflammatory response criteria (i.e., temperature >38° C or below 36° C; heart rate >90 beats/minute; respiratory rate >20/minute or $Paco_2$ <32 mm Hg; WBC count >12,000/mm^3, <4000/mm^3, or >10% immature neutrophils).

Sepsis has become a leading cause of death in the United States. The increase in the number of cases of sepsis is attributed to a number of factors including the increased number of elderly persons and persons who are immunocompromised as a result of HIV infection, more aggressive treatment with chemotherapy and radiation for cancer, and treatment with corticosteroids and immunosuppressive agents. The increased use of invasive diagnostic and therapeutic procedures has also lead to increased exposure to pathogens. In addition, the emergence of resistant organisms is making infections more difficult to treat.

Gram-positive bacteria (e.g., *Staphylococcus aureus, Staphylococcus epidermidis,* enterococci, *Streptococcus pneumoniae*) and gram-negative bacteria (e.g., *E. coli, Haemophilus influenzae, Klebsiella pneumoniae, Pseudomonas aeruginosa, Serratia, Proteus, Enterobacter, Neisseria meningitides*) are the primary organisms that cause sepsis. The most common sites of infection that lead to sepsis are the lungs, blood, abdominal/pelvic cavity, and the urinary tract.

Once the causative organism enters the blood (referred to as septicemia or bacteremia), the toxins produced by the pathogens initiate a widespread inflammatory and immune response commonly referred to as the systemic inflammatory response syndrome (SIRS). This inflammatory response is designed to be a protective process but if uncontrolled, triggers the release of many inflammatory mediators that subsequently cause widespread vasodilation, injury to the endothelium, and increased capillary permeability. This chain of events can lead to maldistribution of circulating blood with hypotension, hypoperfusion, and organ dysfunction. Septic shock, disseminated intravascular coagulation (DIC), and multiple organ dysfunction syndrome (MODS) can develop if this chain of events is not reversed.

This care plan focuses on care of the adult client hospitalized for treatment of sepsis.

OUTCOME/DISCHARGE CRITERIA

THE CLIENT WILL:

- demonstrate evidence that infection is resolving
- have stable vital signs and evidence of adequate organ perfusion
- have no signs and symptoms of complications
- verbalize an understanding of ways to promote continued resolution of existing infection
- identify ways to reduce the risk for recurrent infections
- state signs and symptoms to report to the health care provider
- verbalize an understanding of and a plan for adhering to recommended follow-up care including future appointments with health care provider, medications prescribed, and activity limitations.

NURSING/COLLABORATIVE DIAGNOSES

DISCHARGE TEACHING

1. Nursing Diagnosis: ***INEFFECTIVE TISSUE PERFUSION***

related to:
a. maldistribution of circulating blood associated with the vasodilation, fluid shift that occurs with increased capillary permeability, and selective vasoconstriction that occur in response to inflammatory mediators (e.g., cytokines, complement, histamine, kinins) released in a serious infection;
b. hypovolemia associated with deficient fluid volume resulting from decreased fluid intake, excessive loss of fluid (can occur with diaphoresis, hyperventilation, vomiting, and/or diarrhea if present), and the fluid shift that occurs with increased capillary permeability;
c. decreased cardiac output (occurs late in severe sepsis and shock) associated with the depressant effect of acidosis, myocardial depressant factor, and some inflammatory mediators (e.g., cytokines) on myocardial contractility.

Suggested NOC Outcomes: Circulation status; Tissue perfusion: abdominal organs; Tissue perfusion: cardiac; Tissue perfusion: cerebral; Tissue perfusion: peripheral; Tissue perfusion: pulmonary

Suggested NIC Interventions: Circulatory care: arterial insufficiency; Circulatory care: venous insufficiency; Cerebral perfusion promotion; Hypovolemia management; Cardiac care: acute

Desired Outcome

1. The client will maintain adequate tissue perfusion as evidenced by:
   a. B/P within normal range for client
   b. usual mental status
   c. extremities warm with absence of pallor and cyanosis
   d. palpable peripheral pulses
   e. capillary refill time less than 2–3 seconds
   f. absence of edema
   g. urine output at least 30 ml/hour.

Nursing Actions *and Selected Purposes/Rationales*

1.a. Assess for and report signs and symptoms of diminished tissue perfusion (e.g., decreased blood pressure, restlessness, confusion, cool extremities, pallor or cyanosis of extremities, diminished or absent peripheral pulses, slow capillary refill, edema, oliguria).
b. Implement measures *to maintain adequate tissue perfusion:*
   1. administer intravenous fluids (e.g., crystalloids, colloids) as ordered.
   2. perform actions to prevent or treat deficient fluid volume (see Diagnosis 2, action b)
   3. administer antimicrobial agents as ordered *to treat the infection and subsequently decrease the release of inflammatory mediators*
   4. administer vasopressors (e.g., dopamine, norepinephrine) and positive inotropic agents (e.g., dobutamine) if ordered *to maintain adequate perfusion pressure and cardiac output.*
c. Consult physician if signs and symptoms of diminished tissue perfusion persist or worsen.

2. Nursing Diagnosis: ***RISK FOR DEFICIENT FLUID VOLUME***

related to:
a. decreased oral intake associated with anorexia, fatigue, and nausea if present;
b. increased insensible fluid loss associated with diaphoresis and hyperventilation if present;
c. excessive loss of fluid associated with vomiting and/or diarrhea if present with initial infection or as a side effect of antimicrobial therapy;
d. fluid shifting from the intravascular to extravascular space associated with the increased capillary permeability that occurs with a systemic inflammatory response.

Suggested NOC Outcomes: Fluid balance; Hydration

Suggested NIC Interventions: Fluid monitoring; Fluid management; Hypovolemia management; Intravenous (IV) therapy; Fever treatment; Diarrhea management; Nausea management

Desired Outcome	Nursing Actions *and Selected Purposes/Rationales* (see pp. 30–31 for additional rationales)

2. The client will not experience deficient fluid volume as evidenced by:
   a. normal skin turgor
   b. moist mucous membranes
   c. stable weight
   d. B/P and pulse within normal range for client and stable with position change
   e. usual mental status
   f. BUN and Hct within normal range
   g. balanced intake and output
   h. urine specific gravity within normal range.

2.a. Assess for and report signs and symptoms of deficient fluid volume:
   1. decreased skin turgor
   2. dry mucous membranes, thirst
   3. weight loss of 2% or greater over a short period
   4. postural hypotension and/or low B/P
   5. weak, rapid pulse
   6. neck veins flat when client is supine
   7. change in mental status
   8. elevated BUN and Hct
   9. decrease in urine output with increased specific gravity (reflects an actual rather than a potential deficient fluid volume).

b. Implement measures *to prevent or treat deficient fluid volume:*
   1. perform actions *to reduce nausea and vomiting if present* (e.g., administer antimicrobial agents with food unless contraindicated, administer prescribed antiemetics)
   2. perform actions *to control diarrhea if present* (e.g., consult physician about another antimicrobial agent if onset of diarrhea seems related to initiation of antimicrobial therapy, administer prescribed antidiarrheal agents)
   3. perform actions to reduce fever (see Diagnosis 3, action b) *in order to reduce insensible fluid loss associated with diaphoresis and hyperventilation*
   4. administer antimicrobial agents as ordered to treat the infection and decrease the release of inflammatory mediators *in order to decrease capillary permeability and the resultant fluid shift*
   5. maintain a fluid intake of at least 2500 ml/day unless contraindicated; if oral intake is inadequate or contraindicated, maintain intravenous fluid therapy as ordered.

3. NURSING DIAGNOSIS: HYPERTHERMIA

related to stimulation of the thermoregulatory center in the hypothalamus by endogenous pyrogens that are released in an infectious process.

Suggested NOC Outcome: Thermoregulation

Suggested NIC Intervention: Fever treatment

Desired Outcome	Nursing Actions *and Selected Purposes/Rationales*

3. The client will experience resolution of hyperthermia as evidenced by:
   a. skin usual temperature and color
   b. pulse rate between 60–100 beats/minute
   c. respirations 12–20/minute
   d. normal body temperature.

3.a. Assess for signs and symptoms of hyperthermia (e.g., warm, flushed skin; tachycardia; tachypnea; elevated temperature).

b. Implement measures *to reduce fever:*
   1. perform actions *to resolve the infectious process:*
      a. implement measures *to promote rest* (e.g., assist client with ADLs, provide uninterrupted rest periods, limit visitors)
      b. encourage client to eat a well-balanced diet high in essential nutrients
      c. maintain a fluid intake of at least 2500 ml/day unless contraindicated
      d. administer antimicrobials as ordered
   2. administer tepid sponge bath and/or apply cool cloths to groin and axillae if indicated
   3. use a room fan *to provide cool circulating air*
   4. apply cooling blanket if ordered
   5. administer antipyretics if ordered.

c. Consult physician if temperature remains higher than 38.5° C.

4. Nursing Diagnosis: **IMPAIRED GAS EXCHANGE**

related to:
a. decreased pulmonary blood flow associated with a reduction in systemic tissue perfusion resulting from inflammatory-mediated vasodilation, the fluid shift that occurs with increased capillary permeability, and selective vasoconstriction;
b. loss of effective lung surface associated with:
   1. atelectasis resulting from hypoventilation and the decrease in surfactant production that occurs when blood flow to the lungs is diminished
   2. accumulation of secretions in the lungs resulting from decreased mobility, poor cough effort, and an increased production of secretions if a respiratory tract infection is present
   3. accumulation of fluid in the lungs resulting from the generalized endothelial damage and increase in capillary permeability that occur with a systemic inflammatory response to severe infection.

Suggested NOC Outcome: Respiratory status: gas exchange

Suggested NIC Interventions: Respiratory monitoring; Cough enhancement; Chest physiotherapy; Oxygen therapy

Desired Outcome

4. The client will experience adequate O_2/CO_2 exchange as evidenced by:
   a. usual mental status
   b. unlabored respirations at 12–20/minute
   c. oximetry results within normal range
   d. blood gases within normal range.

Nursing Actions *and Selected Purposes/Rationales*

(see pp. 33–35 for additional rationales)

4.a. Assess for and report signs and symptoms of impaired gas exchange:
   1. restlessness, irritability
   2. confusion, somnolence
   3. tachypnea, dyspnea
   4. significant decrease in oximetry results
   5. decreased Pa_{O_2} and/or increased Pa_{CO_2}.

b. Implement measures *to improve gas exchange:*
   1. perform actions to maintain adequate tissue perfusion (see Diagnosis 1, action b) *in order to maintain adequate pulmonary blood flow*
   2. place client in a semi- to high Fowler's position unless contraindicated
   3. instruct and assist client to change position, deep breathe, and cough at least every 2 hours
   4. assist with positive airway pressure techniques (e.g., continuous positive airway pressure [CPAP], bilevel positive airway pressure [BiPAP], flutter/positive expiratory pressure [PEP] device) if ordered
   5. maintain activity restrictions as ordered; increase activity gradually as allowed and tolerated
   6. discourage smoking *(the irritants in smoke increase mucus production, impair ciliary function, and can damage the bronchial and alveolar walls; the carbon monoxide decreases oxygen availability)*
   7. administer antimicrobial agents as ordered *to resolve the infectious process and control the systemic inflammatory response.*

c. Consult appropriate health care provider (e.g., respiratory therapist, physician) if signs and symptoms of impaired gas exchange persist or worsen.

5. Nursing Diagnosis: **RISK FOR INFECTION: SUPERINFECTION**

related to:
a. decreased resistance to infection associated with depletion of immune mechanisms resulting from the current infection and treatment with antimicrobial agents;
b. stasis of respiratory secretions and/or urinary stasis if mobility is decreased;
c. break in skin integrity associated with frequent venipunctures or presence of invasive lines (e.g., intravenous catheter, hemodynamic monitoring devices).

Suggested NOC Outcomes: Immune status; Infection severity

Suggested NIC Interventions: Infection control; Infection protection

Desired Outcome	Nursing Actions *and Selected Purposes/Rationales* (see pp. 37–40 for additional rationales)
5. The client will have resolution of existing infection and remain free of superinfection as evidenced by: a. return of temperature toward normal range b. decrease in episodes of chills and diaphoresis c. pulse returning toward normal range d. normal or improved breath sounds e. absence or resolution of dyspnea and cough f. stable or improved mental status g. voiding clear urine without reports of frequency, urgency, and burning h. no reports of increased weakness and fatigue i. absence or resolution of heat, pain, redness, swelling, and unusual drainage in any area j. absence of oral mucous membrane lesions and ulceration k. absence or resolution of diarrhea and abdominal pain and cramping l. WBC and differential counts returning toward normal range m. negative results of cultured specimens.	5.a. Assess for and report signs and symptoms of superinfection (be alert to subtle changes in client since the signs of infection may be minimal as a result of immunosuppression; also be aware that some signs and symptoms vary depending on the site of the infection, the causative organism, and the age of the client): 1. increase in temperature 2. increase in episodes of chills and diaphoresis 3. increased pulse 4. development or worsening of abnormal breath sounds 5. development or worsening of dyspnea and/or cough 6. decline in mental status 7. cloudy urine; reports of frequency, urgency, burning when urinating; or urinalysis showing a WBC count greater than 5, positive leukocyte esterase or nitrites, or presence of bacteria 8. further increase in fatigue or weakness 9. new or increased heat, pain, redness, swelling, or unusual drainage in any area 10. development or worsening of lesions or ulceration of oral mucous membrane 11. new or increased episodes of diarrhea and abdominal cramping or pain 12. significant change in WBC count or differential 13. positive results of cultured specimens from suspected new sites of infection. b. Implement measures *to prevent superinfection:* 1. maintain a fluid intake of 2500 ml/day unless contraindicated 2. use good hand hygiene and encourage client to do the same 3. protect client from others with infection 4. encourage client to eat a well-balanced diet high in essential nutrients; provide dietary supplements if indicated 5. maintain sterile technique during all invasive procedures (e.g., urinary catheterization, venous and arterial punctures, injections) 6. consult physician about discontinuing urinary catheter if one is present 7. change intravenous insertion sites according to hospital policy 8. anchor catheter/tubings (e.g., urinary, intravenous) securely *in order to reduce trauma to the tissues and the risk for introduction of pathogens associated with the in-and-out movement of the tubing* 9. change equipment, tubings, and solutions used for treatments such as intravenous infusions, respiratory care, irrigations, and enteral feedings according to hospital policy 10. maintain a closed system for drains (e.g., urinary catheter) and intravenous infusions whenever possible 11. perform actions *to prevent stasis of respiratory secretions* (e.g., assist client to turn, cough, and deep breathe; increase activity as allowed and tolerated) 12. perform actions to prevent urinary retention (e.g., instruct client to urinate when the urge is first felt, promote relaxation during voiding attempts) *in order to prevent urinary stasis* 13. instruct and assist client to perform good perineal care routinely and after each bowel movement 14. if client has open lesions or wound drains, perform actions *to prevent wound infection* (e.g., maintain sterile technique during wound care, instruct client to avoid touching wounds)

Desired Outcome	Nursing Actions *and Selected Purposes/Rationales*
	15. consult physician about: a. enteral feeding rather than TPN if nutritional replacement is necessary *(TPN has a high glucose content, which provides a rich medium for bacterial growth)* b. use of sucralfate rather than antacids and histamine$_2$ receptor antagonists *(these agents increase the pH of the stomach contents, which promotes bacterial overgrowth; aspiration of gastric contents with a high bacteria content increases the risk for pneumonia)* 16. administer antimicrobial agents as ordered.

6. Collaborative Diagnoses: POTENTIAL COMPLICATIONS OF SEPSIS

a. **septic shock** related to systemic hypoperfusion associated with maldistribution of circulating blood, deficient fluid volume, and decreased myocardial contractility resulting from an uncontrolled systemic inflammatory response to severe infection;
b. **disseminated intravascular coagulation** (DIC) related to activation of clotting mechanisms associated with the procoagulant effects of some inflammatory mediators and acidosis;
c. **organ ischemia/dysfunction (multiple organ dysfunction syndrome** [MODS]) related to:
   1. hypoperfusion of major organs associated with septic shock
   2. microvascular thrombosis associated with DIC if it occurs.

Desired Outcomes	Nursing Actions *and Selected Purposes/Rationales*
6.a. The client will not develop septic shock as evidenced by: 1. systolic B/P equal to or higher than 90 mm Hg 2. usual mental status 3. urine output at least 30 ml/hour 4. extremities warm and usual color 5. capillary refill time less than 2–3 seconds 6. palpable peripheral pulses.	6.a.1. Assess for and report signs and symptoms of septic shock: a. hyperdynamic or compensatory phase (e.g., widened pulse pressure with the diastolic pressure dropping and little change in the systolic pressure; restlessness; tachycardia, warm, flushed skin) b. hypodynamic or progressive phase (e.g., systolic B/P less than 90 mm Hg or a reduction of greater than 40 mm Hg from baseline; cool, clammy skin; change in level of consciousness; decreased urine output; rapid, shallow breathing; rapid, thready pulse). 2. Implement measures to maintain adequate tissue perfusion (see Diagnosis 1, action b) *in order to reduce the risk for septic shock.* 3. If signs and symptoms of septic shock occur: a. maintain intravenous fluid therapy as ordered b. maintain oxygen therapy as ordered c. administer antimicrobials as ordered d. administer vasopressors and positive inotropic agents (e.g., dopamine, dobutamine, norepinephrine) as ordered *to maintain adequate perfusion pressure and cardiac output* e. prepare client for transfer to critical care unit.
6.b. The client will not develop DIC as evidenced by: 1. absence of petechiae, ecchymoses, and frank or occult bleeding 2. usual color and temperature of extremities 3. usual mental status 4. fibrin degradation products (FDP) and D-dimer results within normal range 5. fibrinogen, platelets, APTT, PT, and thrombin time within normal range.	6.b.1. Assess for and report signs and symptoms of DIC: a. petechiae, ecchymoses b. frank or occult bleeding (e.g., oozing from venipuncture sites or surgical incisions, epistaxis, hematuria, gingival bleeding, hematemesis, blood in stools) c. cool, mottled extremities d. restlessness, agitation, confusion e. elevated FDP and D-dimer results f. decreased fibrinogen level and platelet count g. prolonged activated partial thromboplastin time (APTT), prothrombin time (PT), and thrombin time (TT). 2. Implement measures *to control infection and reduce the risk for an uncontrolled systemic inflammatory response in order to reduce the risk for DIC:* a. administer antimicrobial agents as ordered

b. perform actions to reduce the risk for superinfection (see Diagnosis 5, action b).
3. If DIC occurs:
a. implement safety precautions *to prevent further bleeding* (e.g., avoid injections, avoid invasive procedures, discontinue any invasive lines with extreme caution, use electric rather than straight-edge razor for shaving)
b. administer fresh frozen plasma, platelets, and/or cryoprecipitate if ordered *to enhance clotting and stop bleeding*
c. administer medications to interrupt clotting (e.g., heparin, antithrombin III) if ordered (heparin is contraindicated if platelet count is less than 50,000).

6.c. The client will not develop organ ischemia/dysfunction as evidenced by:
1. usual mental status
2. urine output at least 30 ml/hour
3. unlabored respirations at 12–20/minute
4. audible breath sounds without an increase in adventitious sounds
5. absence of new or increased abdominal pain, distention, nausea, vomiting, and diarrhea
6. BUN, creatinine, AST, ALT, and LDH within normal range.

6.c.1. Assess for and report signs and symptoms of:
a. cerebral ischemia (e.g., change in mental status)
b. renal insufficiency (e.g., urine output less than 30 ml/hour, elevated BUN and creatinine)
c. acute respiratory distress syndrome (e.g., dyspnea, increase in respiratory rate, low Sao_2, crackles)
d. gastrointestinal ischemia (e.g., hypoactive or absent bowel sounds, abdominal pain and distention, nausea, vomiting, diarrhea, hematemesis, blood in stool)
e. liver dysfunction (e.g., increased AST, ALT, and LDH; jaundice).
2. Implement measures *to reduce the risk for organ ischemia/dysfunction:*
a. perform actions to maintain adequate tissue perfusion (see Diagnosis 1, action b)
b. perform actions to prevent and treat DIC (see actions b.2 and 3 in this diagnosis)
c. administer recombinant activated protein C (drotrecogin alfa) if ordered *(this medication has been found to have antithrombotic, anti-inflammatory, and profibrinolytic activity and may reduce the risk of MODS;* it is only used in persons with severe sepsis who are not having symptoms of DIC).
3. If signs and symptoms of organ ischemia/MODS occur:
a. maintain oxygen therapy
b. prepare client for transfer to critical care unit.

7. NURSING DIAGNOSIS: *FEAR/ANXIETY*

related to unfamiliar environment, separation from significant others, severity of current condition, and threat of death.

Suggested NOC Outcomes: Anxiety self-control; Anxiety level; Fear level; Fear self-control

Suggested NIC Interventions: Anxiety reduction; Calming technique; Presence; Emotional support

Desired Outcome	**Nursing Actions** *and Selected Purposes/Rationales* (see pp. 14–16 for additional rationales)

7. The client will experience a reduction in fear and anxiety as evidenced by:
a. verbalization of feeling less anxious
b. usual sleep pattern
c. relaxed facial expression and body movements
d. usual perceptual ability and interactions with others.

7.a. Assess client for signs and symptoms of fear and anxiety (e.g., verbalization of feeling anxious, insomnia, tenseness, shakiness, restlessness, diaphoresis, tachycardia, elevated blood pressure, self-focused behaviors).
b. Implement measures *to reduce fear and anxiety:*
1. orient client to hospital environment, equipment, and routines
2. introduce client to staff who will be participating in care; if possible, maintain consistency in staff assigned to his/her care
3. assure client that staff members are nearby; respond to call signal as soon as possible
4. maintain a calm, supportive, confident manner when interacting with client

Desired Outcome	Nursing Actions *and Selected Purposes/Rationales*
	5. encourage verbalization of fear and anxiety; provide feedback 6. reinforce physician's explanations and clarify misconceptions the client has about his/her current infection, the treatment plan, and prognosis 7. explain all diagnostic tests and monitoring devices 8. provide information based on current needs of client at a level he/she can understand; encourage questions and clarification of information provided 9. encourage significant others to project a caring, concerned attitude without obvious anxiousness 10. include significant others in orientation and teaching sessions and encourage their continued support of the client 11. administer prescribed antianxiety agents if indicated. c. Consult physician if above actions fail to control fear and anxiety.

Discharge Teaching/Continued Care

8. Nursing Diagnosis: ***DEFICIENT KNOWLEDGE, INEFFECTIVE THERAPEUTIC REGIMEN MANAGEMENT, OR INEFFECTIVE HEALTH MAINTENANCE****

*The nurse should select the diagnostic label that is most appropriate for the client's discharge teaching needs.

Suggested NOC Outcomes: Knowledge: disease process; Knowledge: treatment regimen; Knowledge: health behavior

Suggested NIC Interventions: Health system guidance; Teaching: disease process; Teaching: prescribed medication

Desired Outcomes	Nursing Actions *and Selected Purposes/Rationales*
8.a. The client will verbalize an understanding of ways to promote continued resolution of existing infection.	8.a. Provide the following instructions about ways to promote continued resolution of the existing infection: 1. drink at least 10 glasses of liquid/day unless contraindicated 2. continue with measures to improve respiratory status (e.g., coughing and deep breathing, avoiding smoking) if respiratory infection is present 3. adhere to frequent rest periods 4. eat a well-balanced diet high in calories, protein, vitamins, and minerals 5. take antimicrobials as prescribed; consult health care provider if symptoms of infection get worse or are not resolved at the end of prescribed therapy.
8.b. The client will identify ways to reduce the risk for recurrent infections.	8.b. Instruct client regarding ways to reduce the risk for recurrent infections: 1. avoid contact with persons with infection 2. stop smoking 3. drink at least 10 glasses of liquid/day unless contraindicated 4. wipe from front to back after urinating and defecating (if female) and keep perineal area clean 5. avoid sharing eating and drinking utensils 6. avoid intake of foods with a high microorganism content (e.g., unwashed fruits and vegetables; undercooked meat, poultry, or seafood) 7. eat a well-balanced diet high in essential nutrients 8. maintain an adequate balance between activity and rest 9. practice good hand hygiene (e.g., wash hands using an antimicrobial soap or an alcohol-base hand rub; wash hands before preparing food or eating and after urinating and defecating; wash hands after handling raw meat, poultry, or seafood; wash hands after gardening or cleaning up pet excrement)

10. if tampons are used, change them frequently according to manufacturer's directions; do not use superabsorbent tampons.

8.c. The client will state signs and symptoms to report to the health care provider.

8.c. Instruct client to report the following signs and symptoms:
1. increase in temperature or persistent temperature above 38°C (100.4° F)
2. episodes of chills
3. change in mentation (e.g., agitation, extreme restlessness, confusion)
4. white patches in mouth
5. development of diarrhea with or without abdominal pain and cramping
6. new or persistent cough
7. urine becoming cloudy or foul-smelling and burning with urination
8. increased weakness and fatigue
9. unusual vaginal drainage
10. significant decrease in urine output
11. cool, pale, or bluish-colored extremities
12. difficult breathing.

8.d. The client will verbalize an understanding of and a plan for adhering to recommended follow-up care including future appointments with health care provider, medications prescribed, and activity limitations.

8.d.1. Reinforce the importance of keeping follow-up appointments with health care provider.
2. Explain the rationale for, side effects of, and importance of taking prescribed antimicrobial agents. Inform client of pertinent food and drug interactions.
3. Implement measures to improve client compliance:
   a. include significant others in teaching sessions if possible
   b. encourage questions and allow time for reinforcement and clarification of information provided
   c. provide written instructions regarding scheduled appointments with health care provider, medications prescribed, and signs and symptoms to report.

Bibliography

See pages 879 and 883–884.

Splenectomy

Splenectomy is the surgical removal of the spleen. The most common indication for the surgery is rupture of the spleen. Causes of rupture include penetrating or blunt trauma to the spleen, operative trauma to the spleen during surgery on nearby organs, and damage to the spleen as a result of disease (e.g., mononucleosis, tuberculosis of the spleen). A splenectomy may also be indicated if the spleen is removing excessive quantities of platelets, erythrocytes, or leukocytes from the circulation (hypersplenism). Conditions associated with hypersplenism include leukemia, idiopathic thrombocytopenic purpura, Felty's syndrome, thalassemia major, lymphoma, and hereditary spherocytosis. Additionally, splenectomy may be performed to treat splenic cysts and neoplasm. When feasible, a partial splenectomy is performed so that some of the spleen's immunological function is maintained.

This care plan focuses on the adult client hospitalized for a splenectomy. The care plan will need to be individualized according to the client's underlying disease process or the extensiveness of abdominal trauma necessitating the surgery.

OUTCOME/DISCHARGE CRITERIA

THE CLIENT WILL:

- have surgical pain controlled
- have evidence of normal healing of surgical wound
- have no signs and symptoms of infection
- have no signs and symptoms of postoperative complications
- identify appropriate safety measures to follow because of increased risk for infection
- state signs and symptoms to report to the health care provider
- verbalize an understanding of and a plan for adhering to recommended follow-up care including future appointments with health care provider, medications prescribed, wound care, and activity level.

NURSING/COLLABORATIVE DIAGNOSES

Postoperative

1. Risk for infection p. 583
2. Potential complications p. 584
   a. atelectasis
   b. pancreatitis
   c. subphrenic abscess
   d. thromboembolism
   e. postsplenectomy sepsis

DISCHARGE TEACHING

3. Deficient knowledge, Ineffective therapeutic regimen management, or Ineffective health maintenance p. 586

See Standardized Preoperative and Postoperative Care Plans (pp. 97–126) for additional diagnoses.

PREOPERATIVE

Refer to the Standardized Preoperative Care Plan.

POSTOPERATIVE

Use in conjunction with the Standardized Postoperative Care Plan.

1. NURSING DIAGNOSIS: RISK FOR INFECTION

related to decreased resistance to infection associated with removal of the spleen (the macrophages and lymphocytes in the spleen are responsible for phagocytizing infectious organisms and producing antibodies).

Suggested NOC Outcomes: Immune status; Infection severity; Wound healing: primary intention

Suggested NIC Interventions: Infection protection; Infection control; Cough enhancement; Incision site care

Desired Outcome

1. The client will remain free of infection as evidenced by:
   a. absence of fever and chills
   b. pulse within normal limits
   c. normal breath sounds
   d. usual mental status
   e. cough productive of clear mucus only
   f. voiding clear urine without reports of frequency, urgency, and burning
   g. absence of heat, redness, swelling, and unusual pain and drainage in any area
   h. no further increase in WBC count or significant change in differential
   i. negative results of cultured specimens.

Nursing Actions *and Selected Purposes/Rationales*

(see pp. 37–40 for additional rationales)

1.a. Assess for and report signs and symptoms of infection (be aware that some signs and symptoms vary depending on the site of infection, the causative organism, and the age and immune status of the client):
   1. elevated temperature
   2. chills
   3. increased pulse
   4. abnormal breath sounds
   5. malaise, lethargy, acute confusion
   6. cough productive of purulent, green, or rust-colored sputum
   7. cloudy urine
   8. reports of frequency, urgency, or burning when urinating
   9. urinalysis showing a WBC count greater than 5, positive leukocyte esterase or nitrites, or presence of bacteria
   10. heat, redness, swelling, or unusual pain or drainage in any area
   11. WBC count that continues to increase and/or a significant change in differential
   12. positive results of cultured specimens (e.g., wound drainage, urine, vaginal drainage, sputum, blood).

b. Implement measures *to prevent infection:*
   1. maintain a fluid intake of at least 2500 ml/day unless contraindicated
   2. use good hand hygiene and encourage client to do the same
   3. use sterile technique during all invasive procedures (e.g., urinary catheterizations, venous and arterial punctures, injections, wound care)
   4. anchor catheters/tubings (e.g., urinary, intravenous, wound drainage) securely *in order to reduce trauma to the tissues and the risk for introduction of pathogens associated with the in-and-out movement of the tubing*
   5. change peripheral intravenous line sites according to hospital policy
   6. change equipment, tubings, and solutions used for treatments such as intravenous infusions and respiratory care according to hospital policy
   7. maintain a closed system for drains (e.g., wound, urinary catheter) and intravenous infusions whenever possible
   8. protect client from others with infection and instruct him/her to continue this after discharge
   9. perform actions to maintain an adequate nutritional status (see Standardized Postoperative Care Plan, Diagnosis 5, action d [p. 108])
   10. reinforce importance of good oral hygiene
   11. perform actions *to prevent stasis of respiratory secretions* (e.g., assist client to turn, cough, and deep breathe; increase activity as allowed and tolerated)

Desired Outcome	Nursing Actions *and Selected Purposes/Rationales*
	12. perform actions to prevent urinary retention (e.g., instruct client to urinate when the urge is first felt, promote relaxation during voiding attempts, administer bethanechol as ordered) *in order to prevent urinary stasis* 13. instruct and assist client to perform good perineal care routinely and after each bowel movement 14. perform *actions to prevent wound infection* (e.g., maintain aseptic technique during wound care, instruct client to avoid touching wound, maintain patency of wound drain) 15. administer immunizations (e.g., influenza vaccine, pneumococcal vaccine) if ordered (whenever possible, immunizations are given before the splenectomy *so that immunity has already begun to develop at the time of surgery*) 16. administer antimicrobials if ordered.

2. COLLABORATIVE DIAGNOSES: POTENTIAL COMPLICATIONS OF SPLENECTOMY

a. atelectasis related to:
   1. reluctance to breathe deeply associated with operative site pain and abdominal distention
   2. shallow, slow respirations associated with depressant effect of anesthesia and some medications (e.g., narcotic [opioid] analgesics)
   3. stasis of secretions in alveoli and bronchioles associated with decreased cough effort (can occur as a result of pain, weakness, fatigue, and the depressant effect of anesthesia and some medications such as narcotic [opioid] analgesics)
   4. decreased surfactant production (results from inadequate deep breathing and changes in regional blood flow in the lungs);

b. pancreatitis related to trauma to the pancreas during surgery;

c. subphrenic abscess related to suppuration in the surgical area and decreased resistance to infection;

d. thromboembolism related to:
   1. hypercoagulability associated with:
      a. increase in the number of circulating erythrocytes (contributes to hemoconcentration and increased blood viscosity) and platelets resulting from the spleen no longer being available to destroy the cells that are old or damaged and to store blood (usually stores 150–300 ml of blood including about 30% of the platelet mass)
      b. increased release of tissue thromboplastin into the blood (occurs as a result of trauma from the injury and surgery)
   2. venous stasis associated with decreased activity, increased blood viscosity, and abdominal distention (the distended intestine can put pressure on the abdominal vessels)
   3. trauma to vein walls during surgery;

e. postsplenectomy sepsis related to development of a fulminant infection associated with diminished immune system function following splenectomy.

Desired Outcomes	Nursing Actions *and Selected Purposes/Rationales*
2.a. The client will not develop atelectasis (see Standardized Postoperative Care Plan, Diagnosis 20, outcome b [p. 122], for outcome criteria).	2.a.1. Refer to Standardized Postoperative Care Plan, Diagnosis 20, action b (p. 122), for measures related to assessment, prevention, and treatment of atelectasis. 2. Implement additional measures *to promote effective deep breathing and coughing in order to help prevent atelectasis:* a. instruct client to bend knees while coughing and deep breathing *in order to relieve tension on abdominal muscles and incision* b. instruct and assist client to splint incision with hands or pillow when coughing and deep breathing.

2.b. The client will experience resolution of pancreatitis if it occurs as evidenced by:
1. gradual resolution of abdominal pain
2. temperature declining toward normal
3. stable B/P and pulse
4. serum amylase and lipase levels decreasing toward normal
5. WBC count decreasing toward normal.

2.b.1. Assess for and report signs and symptoms of pancreatitis (e.g., extension of abdominal pain to back, increased midepigastric or left upper quadrant pain, increase in temperature, hypotension, tachycardia, elevated serum amylase and lipase levels, WBC count that increases or fails to decrease toward normal).
2. If signs and symptoms of pancreatitis occur:
   a. assist client to assume position of greatest comfort (e.g., side-lying or sitting with trunk and knees flexed)
   b. maintain food and fluid restrictions as ordered
   c. maintain intravenous fluid therapy as ordered
   d. insert nasogastric tube and maintain suction as ordered *(removal of gastric secretions reduces pancreatic stimulation)*
   e. administer analgesics as ordered.

2.c. The client will experience resolution of a subphrenic abscess if it develops as evidenced by:
1. decrease in abdominal pain
2. temperature declining toward normal
3. WBC count decreasing toward normal.

2.c.1. Assess for and report signs and symptoms of a subphrenic abscess (e.g., increased, persistent abdominal pain; increase in temperature and pulse rate; WBC count that increases or fails to decrease toward normal).
2. If signs and symptoms of subphrenic abscess occur:
   a. administer antimicrobials as ordered
   b. prepare client for surgical intervention (e.g., incision and drainage of abscess) if planned
   c. assess for and report signs and symptoms of peritonitis (e.g., distended, rigid abdomen; increased severity of abdominal pain; rebound tenderness; continued diminished or absent bowel sounds; nausea; vomiting; further increase in temperature; tachycardia; tachypnea; hypotension).

2.d. The client will not experience signs and symptoms of a deep vein thrombus or pulmonary embolism (see Standardized Postoperative Care Plan, Diagnosis 20, outcomes c.1 and 2 [pp. 122–123], for outcome criteria).

2.d.1. Refer to Standardized Postoperative Care Plan, Diagnosis 20, actions c.1 and 2 (pp. 122–123), for measures related to assessment, prevention, and treatment of a deep vein thrombus and pulmonary embolism.
2. Assess for and report increasing abdominal distention and pain *(may indicate portal vein or mesenteric venous thrombus)*.

2.e. The client will not experience postsplenectomy sepsis as evidenced by:
1. absence of nausea, vomiting, and headache
2. usual mental status
3. stable vital signs.

2.e.1. Assess for and report signs and symptoms of postsplenectomy sepsis (e.g., nausea, vomiting, headache, confusion, hypotension, tachycardia, tachypnea). Be aware that client's condition can rapidly progress to shock, coma, and death following the onset of symptoms.
2. Implement measures *to reduce the risk for postsplenectomy sepsis:*
   a. perform actions to prevent infection (see Postoperative Diagnosis 1, action b)
   b. assess for and immediately report signs and symptoms of infection (see Postoperative Diagnosis 1, action a) *so that orders for treatment can be obtained and initiated promptly (a mild infection can develop into sepsis within hours).*
3. If signs and symptoms of postsplenectomy sepsis occur:
   a. monitor vital signs frequently.
   b. obtain specimens (e.g., urine, wound drainage, blood, sputum) for culture as ordered
   c. administer antimicrobials as ordered
   d. prepare client for transfer to critical care unit and insertion of hemodynamic monitoring devices (e.g., central venous catheter, intra-arterial catheter) if planned.

Discharge Teaching/Continued Care

3. NURSING DIAGNOSIS: DEFICIENT KNOWLEDGE, INEFFECTIVE THERAPEUTIC REGIMEN MANAGEMENT, OR INEFFECTIVE HEALTH MAINTENANCE*

*The nurse should select the diagnostic label that is most appropriate for the client's discharge teaching needs.

Suggested NOC Outcomes: Knowledge: treatment regimen; Knowledge: infection control

Suggested NIC Interventions: Health system guidance; Teaching: individual; Teaching: prescribed activity/exercise; Teaching: prescribed medication

Desired Outcomes	Nursing Actions *and Selected Purposes/Rationales*
3.a. The client will identify appropriate safety measures to follow because of increased risk for infection.	3.a.1. Explain to client that he/she is more prone to infection because the rest of the immune system cannot immediately or completely compensate for the loss of the spleen. 2. Instruct client to: a. continue to adhere to measures to prevent infection (see Standardized Postoperative Care Plan, Diagnosis 22, action a [p. 125]) b. consult health care provider about receiving vaccinations periodically to reduce the risk of pneumonia and influenza c. inform all health care providers of being asplenic so that prophylactic antimicrobials can be started before any dental work, invasive diagnostic procedure, or surgery is performed d. carry an identification card and wear a medical alert identification bracelet or tag identifying self as being asplenic and at increased risk for infection.
3.b. The client will state signs and symptoms to report to the health care provider.	3.b.1. Refer to Standardized Postoperative Care Plan, Diagnosis 22, action c (p. 125), for signs and symptoms to report to the health care provider. 2. Instruct client to report these additional signs and symptoms: a. nausea, vomiting, headache, and/or confusion (could indicate postsplenectomy sepsis) b. any febrile illness c. any minor infection.
3.c. The client will verbalize an understanding of and a plan for adhering to recommended follow-up care including future appointments with health care provider, medications prescribed, wound care, and activity level.	3.c. Refer to Standardized Postoperative Care Plan, Diagnosis 22 (pp. 125–126), for routine postoperative instructions and measures to improve client compliance.

Bibliography

See pages 879 and 883–884.

UNIT XIV

Nursing Care of the Client with Disturbances of the Gastrointestinal Tract

APPENDICITIS/APPENDECTOMY

Acute appendicitis is one of the most common indications for emergency abdominal surgery. The appendix is a small fingerlike pouch that extends from the inferior part of the cecum and is usually located in the right iliac region. The most common cause of appendicitis is obstruction of the lumen by a fecalith, a foreign body, an appendiceal calculus, a tumor, or intramural thickening caused by lymphoid hyperplasia. Obstruction of the appendix leads to increased luminal pressure, vascular congestion, bacterial invasion, and ultimately, necrosis and perforation of the appendix.

An appendectomy is the surgical removal of the appendix. It can be done via a laparotomy or laparoscopy. A laparoscopic appendectomy offers the advantage of shorter hospitalization and decreased morbidity and mortality but is contraindicated in persons with extensive intraperitoneal adhesions or other intestinal problems that would impede mobilization and dissection of the appendix.

This care plan focuses on the adult client with suspected appendicitis who is hospitalized for a possible appendectomy.

OUTCOME/DISCHARGE CRITERIA

THE CLIENT WILL:

- have evidence of normal healing of surgical wound
- have clear, audible breath sounds
- tolerate prescribed diet
- have surgical pain controlled
- have no signs and symptoms of postoperative complications
- state signs and symptoms to report to the health care provider
- verbalize an understanding of and a plan for adhering to recommended follow-up care including future appointments with health care provider, medications prescribed, activity level, and wound care.

NURSING/COLLABORATIVE DIAGNOSES

Preoperative

1. Risk for imbalanced fluid and electrolytes: deficient fluid volume, hypokalemia, hypochloremia, and metabolic alkalosis p. 590
2. Acute pain: abdominal (particularly in the periumbilical area or right lower quadrant) p. 590
3. Nausea p. 591
4. Hyperthermia p. 592
5. Potential complications p. 592
   a. abscess formation
   b. peritonitis

Postoperative

1. Potential complications p. 593
   a. abscess formation
   b. peritonitis

DISCHARGE TEACHING

2. Deficient knowledge, Ineffective therapeutic regimen management, or Ineffective health maintenance p. 594

See Standardized Preoperative and Postoperative Care Plans (pp. 97–126) for additional diagnoses.

PREOPERATIVE

Use in conjunction with the Standardized Preoperative Care Plan.

1. Nursing/Collaborative Diagnosis:

RISK FOR IMBALANCED FLUID AND ELECTROLYTES: DEFICIENT FLUID VOLUME, HYPOKALEMIA, HYPOCHLOREMIA, AND METABOLIC ALKALOSIS

related to decreased oral intake (usually NPO) and excessive loss of fluid and electrolytes associated with vomiting and nasogastric tube drainage (if an NG tube is present).

Suggested NOC Outcomes: Fluid balance; Electrolyte and acid/base balance

Suggested NIC Interventions: Fluid management; Electrolyte management: hypokalemia; Acid-base management: metabolic alkalosis

Desired Outcome	Nursing Actions *and Selected Purposes/Rationales* (see pp. 30–31 for additional rationales)
1. The client will maintain fluid and electrolyte balance as evidenced by: a. normal skin turgor b. moist mucous membranes c. stable weight d. B/P and pulse within normal range for client and stable with position change e. capillary refill time less than 2–3 seconds f. usual mental status g. balanced intake and output h. urine specific gravity within normal range i. soft, nondistended abdomen with normal bowel sounds j. absence of cardiac dysrhythmias, muscle weakness, paresthesias, twitching, spasms, and dizziness k. BUN, Hct, serum electrolytes, and blood gases within normal range.	1.a. Assess for signs and symptoms of: 1. deficient fluid volume: a. decreased skin turgor, dry mucous membranes, thirst b. weight loss of 2% or greater in a short period c. postural hypotension and/or low B/P d. weak, rapid pulse e. capillary refill time greater than 2–3 seconds f. neck veins flat when client is supine g. change in mental status h. decreased urine output with increased specific gravity (reflects an actual rather than potential fluid deficit) i. increased BUN and Hct 2. hypokalemia (e.g., cardiac dysrhythmias, postural hypotension, muscle weakness, nausea and vomiting, abdominal distention, hypoactive or absent bowel sounds, low serum potassium) 3. hypochloremia and metabolic alkalosis (e.g., dizziness, irritability, paresthesias, muscle twitching or spasms, hypoventilation, low serum chloride, elevated pH and T_{CO_2}). b. Implement measures *to prevent fluid and electrolyte imbalances:* 1. perform actions to reduce nausea and vomiting (see Preoperative Diagnosis 3, action b) 2. if a nasogastric tube is present and needs to be irrigated frequently and/or with large volumes of solution, irrigate it with normal saline rather than water 3. maintain intravenous therapy as ordered 4. administer electrolyte replacements if ordered. c. Consult physician if signs and symptoms of imbalanced fluid and electrolytes occur.

2. Nursing Diagnosis:

ACUTE PAIN: ABDOMINAL (PARTICULARLY IN THE PERIUMBILICAL AREA OR RIGHT LOWER QUADRANT)

related to:

a. stretching of the appendix associated with obstruction and inflammation of the appendix;
b. irritation of the peritoneum (occurs with transmural involvement of the appendix and subsequent contact of the inflamed serosal surface of the appendix with the peritoneum).

Suggested NOC Outcomes: Comfort level; Pain control

Suggested NIC Interventions: Analgesic administration; Pain management

Desired Outcome	**Nursing Actions** *and Selected Purposes/Rationales* (see pp. 45–47 for additional rationales)

2. The client will experience diminished abdominal pain as evidenced by:
   a. verbalization of a decrease in pain
   b. relaxed facial expression and body positioning
   c. stable vital signs.

2.a. Assess for signs and symptoms of pain (e.g., verbalization of pain, grimacing, reluctance to move, guarding or rubbing of abdomen, restlessness, diaphoresis, increased B/P, tachycardia).
b. Assess client's perception of the severity of pain using a pain intensity rating scale.
c. Assess the client's pain pattern (e.g., location, quality, onset, duration, precipitating factors, aggravating factors, alleviating factors); note that a finding of pain in the right lower quadrant elicited by palpation of the left lower quadrant (Rovsing's sign) and/or localized tenderness over McBurney's point are diagnostic indicators of appendicitis.
d. Implement measures *to reduce pain:*
   1. perform actions *to reduce fear and anxiety about the pain experience* (e.g., assure client that his/her need for pain relief is understood, plan methods for achieving pain control with client)
   2. perform actions to reduce fear and anxiety (see Standardized Preoperative Care Plan, Diagnosis 1, action c [p. 98]) *in order to promote relaxation and subsequently increase the client's threshold and tolerance for pain*
   3. assist client to assume a comfortable position (e.g., side-lying with right knee flexed, head of bed elevated with knees flexed)
   4. apply ice packs or cooling pad to abdomen if ordered
   5. administer analgesics if ordered.
e. Consult physician if above measures fail to provide adequate pain relief.

3. NURSING DIAGNOSIS: *NAUSEA*

related to stimulation of the vomiting center associated with:
a. stimulation of the visceral afferent pathways resulting from inflammation of the appendix;
b. stimulation of the cerebral cortex resulting from pain and stress.

Suggested NOC Outcome: Nausea and vomiting severity

Suggested NIC Interventions: Environmental management: comfort; Nausea management; Vomiting management

Desired Outcome	**Nursing Actions** *and Selected Purposes/Rationales*

3. The client will experience relief of nausea and vomiting as evidenced by:
   a. verbalization of relief of nausea
   b. absence of vomiting.

3.a. Assess client for nausea and vomiting.
b. Implement measures *to reduce nausea and vomiting:*
   1. perform actions to reduce abdominal pain (see Preoperative Diagnosis 2, action d)
   2. perform actions to reduce fear and anxiety (see Standardized Preoperative Care Plan, Diagnosis 1, action c [p. 98])
   3. eliminate noxious sights and odors from the environment *(noxious stimuli can cause stimulation of the vomiting center)*
   4. encourage client to take deep, slow breaths when nauseated
   5. encourage client to change positions slowly *(rapid movement can result in stimulation of the chemoreceptor trigger zone and subsequent excitation of the vomiting center)*
   6. provide oral hygiene after each emesis
   7. restrict oral intake if indicated
   8. administer antiemetics if ordered.
c. If above measures fail to control nausea and vomiting:
   1. consult physician
   2. be prepared to insert a nasogastric tube and maintain suction as ordered.

4. Nursing Diagnosis: HYPERTHERMIA

related to stimulation of the thermoregulatory center in the hypothalamus by endogenous pyrogens that are released in an infectious process.

Suggested NOC Outcome: Thermoregulation

Suggested NIC Intervention: Fever treatment

Desired Outcome	Nursing Actions *and Selected Purposes/Rationales*
4. The client will have hyperthermia adequately controlled as evidenced by: a. skin usual temperature and color b. pulse rate between 60–100 beats/minute c. respirations 12–20/minute d. temperature declining toward normal.	4.a. Assess for signs and symptoms of hyperthermia (e.g., warm, flushed skin; tachycardia; tachypnea; elevated temperature). b. Administer the following medications if ordered *to help reduce fever:* 1. antipyretics 2. antimicrobials *to resolve the infectious process.* c. Consult physician if temperature remains higher than 38° C.

5. Collaborative Diagnoses: POTENTIAL COMPLICATIONS OF APPENDICITIS

a. abscess formation related to perforation of the appendix into a localized, contained area;

b. peritonitis related to release of intestinal contents into the peritoneal cavity associated with perforation of the appendix or leakage of a periappendiceal abscess.

Desired Outcomes	Nursing Actions *and Selected Purposes/Rationales*
5.a. The client will not have formation of an abscess as evidenced by: 1. temperature stable and less than 38° C 2. no increase in abdominal pain or tenderness 3. no further increase in WBC count.	5.a.1. Assess for and report signs and symptoms of abscess formation (e.g., further increase in temperature or temperature above 38° C, increase in abdominal pain and localized tenderness, further increase in WBC count or WBC count greater than 15,000/mm^3). 2. Implement measures *to reduce the risk for perforation of the appendix and subsequent abscess formation:* a. perform actions *to prevent a further increase in intraluminal pressure:* 1. withhold oral intake if ordered 2. insert a nasogastric tube and maintain suction if ordered 3. do not administer an enema b. avoid use of laxatives *(may cause excessive peristalsis)* c. do not apply heat to abdomen *(may speed up the suppurative process and precipitate perforation).* 3. If signs and symptoms of abscess formation occur: a. prepare client for diagnostic studies (e.g., computed tomography, ultrasonography) if planned b. administer antimicrobials as ordered c. prepare client for surgery or percutaneous drainage of abscess.
5.b. The client will not develop peritonitis as evidenced by: 1. temperature stable and less than 38° C 2. soft, nondistended abdomen 3. no increase in abdominal pain and tenderness, nausea, and vomiting	5.b.1. Assess for and report signs and symptoms of peritonitis (e.g., further increase in temperature or temperature above 38° C; distended, rigid abdomen; increase in severity of abdominal pain; rebound tenderness; increased nausea and vomiting; diminished or absent bowel sounds; tachycardia; tachypnea; hypotension; further increase in WBC count or a WBC count greater than 15,000/mm^3). 2. Implement measures to reduce the risk for perforation of the appendix (see action a.2 in this diagnosis) *in order to prevent peritonitis.* 3. If signs and symptoms of peritonitis occur: a. withhold oral intake as ordered

4. normal bowel sounds
5. stable vital signs
6. no further increase in WBC count.

b. place client on bed rest in a semi-Fowler's position *to assist in pooling or localizing gastrointestinal contents in the pelvis rather than under the diaphragm*
c. prepare client for diagnostic tests (e.g., abdominal x-ray, computed tomography, ultrasonography) if planned
d. insert nasogastric tube and maintain suction as ordered
e. administer antimicrobials as ordered
f. administer intravenous fluids and/or blood volume expanders if ordered *to prevent or treat shock (can result from the increased capillary permeability that occurs with inflammation and the subsequent escape of protein, fluid, and electrolytes from the vascular space into the peritoneal cavity)*
g. prepare client for surgery (e.g., appendectomy with drainage and irrigation of peritoneum) if planned.

POSTOPERATIVE

Use in conjunction with the Standardized Postoperative Care Plan.

1. COLLABORATIVE DIAGNOSES: *POTENTIAL COMPLICATIONS OF APPENDECTOMY*

a. **abscess formation** related to suppuration in the inflamed or infected area (more likely to occur following resection of a perforated appendix);
b. **peritonitis** related to entrance of pathogens/irritants into peritoneal cavity associated with wound infection, leakage from an abscess, and/or release of intestinal contents into the peritoneal cavity resulting from preoperative or intraoperative perforation of the appendix and leakage of suture lines postoperatively.

Desired Outcomes	**Nursing Actions** *and Selected Purposes/Rationales*
1.a. The client will not develop or will have resolution of an abscess if it occurs as evidenced by: 1. temperature declining toward normal 2. absence of chills 3. gradual resolution of abdominal pain 4. WBC count declining toward normal.	1.a.1. Assess for and report signs and symptoms of abscess formation (e.g., increase in temperature, chills, increased or more constant abdominal pain, further increase in WBC count). 2. Implement measures to maintain patency and prevent inadvertent removal of wound drain if present (see actions b.2.b and c in this diagnosis) *in order to reduce the risk for abscess formation.* 3. If signs and symptoms of abscess formation occur: a. prepare client for diagnostic tests (e.g., computed tomography, ultrasonography) if planned b. administer antimicrobials as ordered c. prepare client for surgical drainage of the abscess if planned.
1.b. The client will not develop or will have resolution of peritonitis if it occurs as evidenced by: 1. gradual resolution of abdominal pain 2. soft, nondistended abdomen 3. temperature declining toward normal 4. stable vital signs 5. gradual return of normal bowel sounds 6. WBC count declining toward normal.	1.b.1. Assess for and report signs and symptoms of peritonitis (see Preoperative Diagnosis 5, action b.1). 2. Implement measures *to prevent peritonitis:* a. perform actions to treat an abscess if it occurs (see action a.3 in this diagnosis) b. perform actions *to maintain patency of wound drain if present in order to prevent increased pressure on the suture line:* 1. keep tubing free of kinks 2. empty collection device as often as necessary 3. maintain suction as ordered c. perform actions *to prevent inadvertent removal of wound drain if present:* 1. use caution when changing dressings surrounding drain 2. provide extension tubing if necessary *to enable client to move without placing tension on the drain* 3. instruct client not to pull on drain and drainage tubing

Desired Outcomes	Nursing Actions *and Selected Purposes/Rationales*
	d. maintain sterile technique during dressing changes and wound care e. keep abdominal dressing clean and dry f. administer antimicrobials if ordered. 3. If signs and symptoms of peritonitis occur, refer to Preoperative Diagnosis 5, action b.3 for treatment measures.

Discharge Teaching/Continued Care

2. NURSING DIAGNOSIS: ***DEFICIENT KNOWLEDGE, INEFFECTIVE THERAPEUTIC REGIMEN MANAGEMENT, OR INEFFECTIVE HEALTH MAINTENANCE****

*The nurse should select the diagnostic label that is most appropriate for the client's discharge teaching needs.

Suggested NOC Outcome: Knowledge: treatment regimen

Suggested NIC Interventions: Health system guidance; Teaching: individual; Teaching: prescribed activity/exercise; Teaching: prescribed medication

Desired Outcomes	Nursing Actions *and Selected Purposes/Rationales*
2.a. The client will state signs and symptoms to report to the health care provider.	2.a. Refer to Standardized Postoperative Care Plan, Diagnosis 22, action c (p. 125), for signs and symptoms to report to the health care provider.
2.b. The client will verbalize an understanding of and a plan for adhering to recommended follow-up care including future appointments with health care provider, medications prescribed, activity level, and wound care.	2.b. Refer to Standardized Postoperative Care Plan, Diagnosis 22 (pp. 125–126), for routine postoperative instructions and measures to improve client compliance.

Bibliography

See pages 879 and 884.

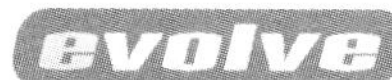

Bowel Diversion: Ileostomy

An ileostomy is the diversion of the ileum from the abdominal cavity through an opening created in the abdominal wall. It may be performed following abdominal trauma or to treat conditions such as familial polyposis, intestinal cancer, and, most commonly, inflammatory bowel disease that is refractory to conservative management. An ileostomy can be temporary or permanent.

A temporary ileostomy is usually created to allow the bowel to heal following traumatic abdominal injury or to permit healing of a newly constructed ileoanal reservoir (pouch). The ileoanal reservoir is a treatment option for some persons with inflammatory bowel disease or familial polyposis. In the initial surgery, the diseased portion of the intestine is removed, a temporary ileostomy is performed, and a reservoir is created in the rectal area using a portion of the ileum. After 2–4 months, the ileostomy is closed and intestinal continuity is established between the remaining intestine and the ileoanal reservoir.

There are two types of permanent ileostomies. The conventional (Brooke) ileostomy is the most common one. It is created by bringing a portion of the terminal ileum through the abdominal wall, usually in the right lower quadrant. The ileostomy drains intermittently but, because it cannot be regulated, a collection device needs to be worn over the stoma at all times. Another type of permanent ileostomy is the continent ileostomy. In this procedure, the terminal ileum is used to construct an intra-abdominal reservoir (Kock pouch). Initially, the reservoir drains via a catheter that is placed through the stoma and a surgically constructed one-way valve. After the surgical area heals, the catheter is removed and the reservoir only needs to be drained periodically. If the system functions properly, the client does not need to wear a collection device over the stoma. The type of permanent ileostomy constructed depends on the client's age, underlying disease process, and preference and expertise of the surgeon. A proctocolectomy (removal of the colon, rectum, and anus) is often done at the same time as a permanent ileostomy to treat the disease process or to prevent future bowel changes that could occur. If a proctocolectomy is not performed, the rectal stump is sutured across the top; the rectum stays intact and secretes mucus that is expelled via the anus.

This care plan focuses on the adult client with inflammatory bowel disease hospitalized for bowel diversion with creation of a permanent ileostomy. Much of the postoperative information is applicable to clients receiving follow-up care in an extended care facility or home setting.

OUTCOME/DISCHARGE CRITERIA

THE CLIENT WILL:

- have surgical pain controlled
- have evidence of normal healing of the surgical wound
- have a medium pink to red, moist stoma and intact peristomal and perianal skin
- have no evidence of fluid and electrolyte imbalances
- maintain an adequate nutritional status
- have no signs and symptoms of postoperative complications
- verbalize a basic understanding of the anatomical changes that have occurred as a result of the bowel diversion
- identify ways to maintain fluid and electrolyte balance
- verbalize ways to maintain an optimal nutritional status
- identify methods of controlling odor and sound associated with ileostomy drainage and gas
- demonstrate the ability to change the pouch system, maintain integrity of the peristomal and perianal skin, and maintain adequate stomal integrity
- demonstrate the ability to properly use, clean, and store ostomy products
- demonstrate the ability to drain and irrigate a continent ileostomy if present
- identify ways to prevent and treat blockage of the stoma
- state signs and symptoms to report to the health care provider
- share thoughts and feelings about the effect of altered bowel function on self-concept and lifestyle
- identify appropriate community resources that can assist with home management and adjustment to changes resulting from the bowel diversion
- verbalize an understanding of and a plan for adhering to recommended follow-up care including future appointments with health care provider, wound care, activity level, and medications prescribed.

NURSING/COLLABORATIVE DIAGNOSES

See p. 611, Care Plan on Inflammatory Bowel Disease (pp. 636–651), and Standardized Preoperative and Postoperative Care Plans (pp. 97–126) for additional diagnoses.

PREOPERATIVE

Use in conjunction with the Care Plan on Inflammatory Bowel Disease and the Standardized Preoperative Care Plan.

1. Nursing Diagnosis: FEAR/ANXIETY

related to:
a. unfamiliar environment and separation from significant others;
b. anticipated loss of control associated with effects of anesthesia;
c. lack of understanding of diagnostic tests, planned surgical procedure, and care that will be required for the ileostomy;
d. financial concerns associated with hospitalization;
e. anticipated discomfort, surgical findings, changes in appearance and body functioning, and effects of ileostomy on future lifestyle;
f. ability to independently perform ileostomy care following discharge.

Suggested NOC Outcomes: Anxiety level; Fear level; Anxiety self-control; Fear self-control

Suggested NIC Interventions: Anxiety reduction; Calming technique; Emotional support; Presence; Teaching: preoperative

Desired Outcome	**Nursing Actions** *and Selected Purposes/Rationales* (see pp. 14–16 for additional rationales)
1. The client will experience a reduction in fear and anxiety (see Standardized Preoperative Care Plan, Diagnosis 1 [pp. 97–98], for outcome criteria).	1.a. Refer to Standardized Preoperative Care Plan, Diagnosis 1 (pp. 97–98), for measures related to assessment and reduction of fear and anxiety. b. Implement additional measures *to reduce fear and anxiety:* 1. provide client with information about preoperative routines, the surgical procedure, general postoperative care, the function and

appearance of the stoma, and management of the ileostomy (see Preoperative Diagnosis 2) *so he/she will know what to expect*

2. explain that every attempt will be made to place the stoma in an area that he/she can easily see and reach and where the appliance will lie flat, adhere well to the skin, and allow freedom of movement (the tentative stoma site is mapped out preoperatively by the physician and/or enterostomal therapy [ET] nurse)
3. inform client that instructions about management of the ileostomy will be repeated as often as necessary prior to discharge and that there will be resources available to provide assistance/supervision following discharge
4. assure client that the stoma has no pain receptors and will not be painful when touched
5. stress that effluent (intestinal drainage from the stoma) usually has a weakly acidic or sweet odor that is not unpleasant
6. assure client that ileostomy pouches are odorproof and available in sizes that fit various body contours
7. if acceptable to client, arrange for a visit with a person of similar age and same sex who has successfully adjusted to an ileostomy.

Client Teaching

2. NURSING DIAGNOSIS: ***DEFICIENT KNOWLEDGE***

regarding the surgical procedure, hospital routines associated with the surgery, physical preparation for the bowel diversion, sensations that normally occur following surgery and anesthesia, expected appearance and function of the ileostomy, and postoperative care and management of the ileostomy.

Suggested NOC Outcomes: Knowledge: treatment regimen; Knowledge: treatment procedure(s)

Suggested NIC Interventions: Health system guidance; Teaching: individual; Teaching: procedure/treatment

Desired Outcomes	Nursing Actions *and Selected Purposes/Rationales*
2.a. The client will verbalize an understanding of the surgical procedure, preoperative care, and postoperative sensations and care.	2.a.1. Refer to Standardized Preoperative Care Plan, Diagnosis 4, actions a.1–4 (pp. 100–101), for information to include in preoperative teaching. 2. Provide additional information regarding specific preoperative care and postoperative sensations and care for clients having a bowel diversion with ileostomy: a. explain the preoperative bowel preparation (e.g., low-residue or clear liquid diet, cleansing enemas, laxatives, antimicrobial therapy) b. if proctocolectomy is planned, inform client that: 1. a perineal wound drain will be present after surgery 2. occasional feelings of pressure in the perineal area are expected after surgery and that these will subside as edema decreases c. if a continent ileostomy is planned, inform client that: 1. a catheter will be inserted into the reservoir during surgery and will extend from the stoma and drain into an external collection device; stress that this is a temporary measure (usually for 2–4 weeks) to keep the reservoir from becoming distended while the suture lines are healing 2. the reservoir will need to be irrigated periodically (especially in the early postoperative period) to remove mucus that accumulates in the reservoir (the bowel used to construct the reservoir initially secretes quite a bit of mucus) 3. following removal of the stomal catheter, a catheter will be inserted into the stoma at regularly scheduled intervals to drain the reservoir and an external collection device will not be needed. 3. Allow time for questions and clarification of information provided.

Desired Outcomes	Nursing Actions *and Selected Purposes/Rationales*
2.b. The client will demonstrate the ability to perform activities designed to prevent postoperative complications.	2.b. Refer to Standardized Preoperative Care Plan, Diagnosis 4, action b (p. 101), for instructions on ways to prevent postoperative complications.
2.c. The client will verbalize an understanding of the appearance, function, and management of the ileostomy.	2.c.1. Arrange for a visit with an ET nurse if available. 2. Reinforce information provided by physician and/or ET nurse about the appearance and function of the ileostomy: a. the stoma will be medium pink to red in color and moist (similar in appearance to healthy oral mucous membrane) b. the stoma will shrink in size as edema resolves during the first 6 weeks after surgery (final stoma height is usually 1.5–2.5 cm [about ½–1 inch] from the skin surface) c. slight bleeding of the stoma is expected when it is wiped with tissue d. for the first day or two after surgery, the stoma will drain a small amount of clear to white, blood-tinged fluid containing some mucus; after a few days, the color of the drainage will change to green and then light to medium brown as the diet progresses e. when the ileostomy begins to function (usually 2–3 days after surgery), the drainage will be watery and high-volume (up to 1–2 liters/day) but within a couple of weeks the amount will begin to decrease (expected amount of output after 2–3 months is 500–800 ml/day) and develop a thicker, paste-like consistency. 3. Provide basic information about peristomal skin care, ways to control intestinal gas and odor of the effluent, products the client will be using after surgery, and irrigation and drainage of the reservoir (if a continent ileostomy is planned). 4. Provide visual aids and allow client to handle ileostomy appliances that will be used in the immediate postoperative period. Provide a pouch clamp so that client can practice putting it on and taking it off of an empty pouch. 5. Encourage client to try wearing a pouch system partially filled with water in order to experience how it feels and to determine if the planned stoma site will be adequate for successful adhesion of the pouch. 6. Allow time for questions and clarification of information provided.

POSTOPERATIVE

Use in conjunction with the Standardized Postoperative Care Plan.

1. Nursing/Collaborative Diagnosis:

RISK FOR IMBALANCED FLUID AND ELECTROLYTES

a. **deficient fluid volume** related to restricted oral fluid intake before, during, and after surgery; blood loss; and loss of fluid associated with vomiting, nasogastric tube drainage, and/or high-volume ileostomy output;

b. **hypokalemia, hypomagnesemia, and hypochloremia** related to loss of electrolytes associated with vomiting, nasogastric tube drainage, decreased oral intake, and/or high-volume ileostomy output;

c. **metabolic alkalosis** related to loss of hydrochloric acid associated with vomiting and nasogastric tube drainage;

d. **metabolic acidosis** related to loss of bicarbonate ions associated with high-volume ileostomy output (effluent contains bicarbonate ions that would normally be absorbed throughout the large intestine).

Suggested NOC Outcomes: Fluid balance; Electrolyte and acid/base balance

Suggested NIC Interventions: Fluid monitoring; Electrolyte management: hypokalemia; Electrolyte management: hypomagnesemia; Fluid/Electrolyte management; Acid-base monitoring; Acid-base management: metabolic alkalosis; Acid-base management: metabolic acidosis

Desired Outcome	**Nursing Actions** *and Selected Purposes/Rationales*
1. The client will not experience deficient fluid volume, hypokalemia, hypochloremia, hypomagnesemia, and acid-base imbalance as evidenced by: a. normal skin turgor b. moist mucous membranes c. stable weight d. B/P and pulse within normal range for client and stable with position change e. capillary refill time less than 2–3 seconds f. balanced intake and output within 48 hours after surgery g. urine specific gravity within normal range h. return of peristalsis within expected time i. usual mental status j. absence of cardiac dysrhythmias, twitching, muscle weakness, paresthesias, dizziness, headache, nausea, and vomiting k. negative Chvostek's and Trousseau's signs l. BUN, serum electrolytes, and blood gases within normal range.	1.a. Assess for and report: 1. excessive ileostomy output (after bowel activity returns, expected output may be as high as 2000 ml/day and then in 10–14 days it should begin to gradually decrease to 500–800 ml/day within 2–3 months) 2. signs and symptoms of deficient fluid volume, hypokalemia, hypochloremia, and metabolic alkalosis (see Standardized Postoperative Care Plan, Diagnosis 4, action a.1 [p. 106]) 3. signs and symptoms of hypomagnesemia (e.g., anxiousness, irritability, cardiac dysrhythmias, tremors, positive Chvostek's and Trousseau's signs, seizures, low serum magnesium) 4. signs and symptoms of metabolic acidosis (e.g., drowsiness; disorientation; stupor; rapid, deep respirations; headache; nausea; vomiting; cardiac dysrhythmias; low pH and T_{CO_2}). b. Refer to Standardized Postoperative Care Plan, Diagnosis 4, action a.2 (p. 106), for measures to prevent or treat deficient fluid volume, hypokalemia, hypochloremia, and metabolic alkalosis. c. Implement additional measures *to prevent or treat deficient fluid volume and electrolyte imbalances:* 1. administer additional electrolyte replacements (e.g., magnesium sulfate, sodium bicarbonate) if ordered 2. as diet advances, perform actions *to prevent or control excessive ileostomy output:* a. instruct client to avoid excessive intake of foods/fluids that may cause diarrhea (e.g., raw fruits and vegetables; prune juice; fatty, spicy, or extremely hot or cold items; coffee) b. encourage intake of foods that may thicken effluent (e.g., applesauce, bananas, boiled rice, tapioca, pretzels, creamy peanut butter, pasta) c. administer antidiarrheal agents (e.g., loperamide, diphenoxylate hydrochloride) if ordered. d. Consult physician if signs and symptoms of deficient fluid volume and electrolyte imbalances persist or worsen.

2. NURSING DIAGNOSIS: IMBALANCED NUTRITION: LESS THAN BODY REQUIREMENTS

related to:

a. decreased oral intake associated with prescribed dietary modifications; pain; weakness; fatigue; nausea; and fear of excessive ileostomy output, gas, and/or odor;
b. inadequate nutritional replacement therapy;
c. loss of nutrients associated with vomiting and excessive ileostomy output;
d. decreased absorption of nutrients associated with loss of absorptive surface of the bowel resulting from surgical removal of a large portion of the intestines;
e. increased nutritional needs associated with the increased metabolic rate that occurs during wound healing.

Suggested NOC Outcome: Nutritional status

Suggested NIC Interventions: Nutritional monitoring; Nutrition management; Nutrition therapy

Desired Outcome	Nursing Actions *and Selected Purposes/Rationales* (see pp. 40–43 for additional rationales)
2. The client will maintain an adequate nutritional status (see Standardized Postoperative Care Plan, Diagnosis 5 [pp. 107–108], for outcome criteria).	2.a. Refer to Standardized Postoperative Care Plan, Diagnosis 5 (pp. 107–108), for measures related to assessment and maintenance of an adequate nutritional status. b. Implement additional measures *to maintain an adequate nutritional status:* 1. perform actions to prevent or control excessive ileostomy output (see Postoperative Diagnosis 1, action c.2) 2. reinforce methods of reducing gas and odor of effluent (see Postoperative Diagnosis 6, actions f and g) *so that this concern does not cause client to limit oral intake* 3. instruct client to chew food thoroughly *in order to enhance digestion and subsequent absorption of nutrients.*

3. NURSING DIAGNOSIS: ***ACTUAL/RISK FOR IMPAIRED TISSUE INTEGRITY***

related to:

a. disruption of tissue associated with the surgical procedure;
b. delayed wound healing associated with factors such as decreased nutritional status and inadequate blood supply to wound area;
c. irritation of skin associated with:
   1. contact with wound drainage, ileostomy output (effluent is rich in proteolytic enzymes), soap residue and perspiration under the pouch, and/or mucous drainage from the anus (occurs if rectum was left intact)
   2. frequent or improper removal of tape, adhesives, or other substances used to secure pouch to the skin
   3. aggressive cleansing of peristomal area
   4. sensitivity to tape, pouch material, ostomy paste, and/or substances used to secure pouch to the skin (e.g., adhesive disk, skin barrier, adhesive spray)
   5. pressure from tubes, appliance belt, and/or pouch drainage valve or clamp.

Suggested NOC Outcomes: Wound healing: primary intention; Ostomy self-care; Tissue integrity: skin and mucous membranes

Suggested NIC Interventions: Skin surveillance; Pressure management; Skin care: topical treatments; Incision site care; Ostomy care

Desired Outcomes	Nursing Actions *and Selected Purposes/Rationales* (see pp. 49–52 for additional rationales)
3.a. The client will experience normal healing of surgical wounds (see Standardized Postoperative Care Plan, Diagnosis 10, outcome a [p. 112], for outcome criteria).	3.a. Refer to Standardized Postoperative Care Plan, Diagnosis 10, action a [p. 112], for measures related to assessment and promotion of wound healing.
3.b. The client will maintain integrity of peristomal and perianal skin and skin in contact with wound drainage, tape, and tubings as evidenced by: 1. absence of redness and irritation 2. no skin breakdown.	3.b.1. Inspect skin areas that are in contact with wound drainage, tape, and tubings for signs of irritation and breakdown. 2. Assess for signs and symptoms of: a. peristomal irritation or breakdown (e.g., redness, inflammation, and/or excoriation of peristomal skin; reports of itching or burning under the pouch seal; inability to keep pouch on) b. perianal irritation or breakdown (e.g., redness, inflammation, and/or excoriation of perianal skin; reports of itching or burning in perianal area).

3. Refer to Standardized Postoperative Care Plan, Diagnosis 10 actions b.2 and 3 (pp. 112–113), for measures to prevent and treat irritation and breakdown in areas in contact with wound drainage, tape, and tubings.
4. Implement measures *to prevent peristomal irritation and breakdown:*
   a. shave or clip hair from peristomal skin if necessary *to help achieve an adequate pouch seal and to reduce irritation when the pouch system is removed*
   b. patch test all products that will come in contact with the skin (e.g., sealant, ostomy paste, barrier, adhesive, solvent) before initial use; do not use products that cause redness, rash, itching, or burning
   c. change entire pouch system only when necessary (e.g., if pouch seal is leaking, if client reports burning or itching of the peristomal skin, when the stoma size changes); pouch system is usually changed every 3 days in the early postoperative period and then should be able to remain in place for 5–7 days
   d. use a 2-piece pouch system (e.g., faceplate and pouch, wafer with flange and pouch) during the initial postoperative period *so that pouch can be removed to assess the stoma without having to remove the adhesive from the skin*
   e. perform actions *to reduce peristomal irritation during removal of the pouch system:*
      1. place drops of warm water or solvent where the pouch system adheres to the skin *in order to facilitate removal;* allow time for adhesive to loosen before removing pouch system
      2. remove pouch system gently and in direction of hair growth; hold skin adjacent to the skin barrier taut and push down on skin slightly *to facilitate separation*
   f. perform actions *to prevent effluent from coming in contact with the skin when changing the pouch system or pouch:*
      1. change the pouch or pouch system when the ileostomy is least active (e.g., upon awakening in the morning, before meals, 2–4 hours after eating, before retiring at night)
      2. place a wick (rolled gauze pad, tampon) on the stoma opening when the pouch system or pouch is off
   g. cleanse peristomal skin thoroughly with mild soap and water, rinse completely, and pat dry; use tepid rather than hot water *to prevent burns*
   h. apply skin sealant to the clean, dry peristomal skin before applying the skin barrier *in order to protect skin from the irritating effect of the adhesive*
   i. always use a skin barrier (e.g., Reliaseal, Stomahesive) *to protect skin from the proteolytic enzymes that are in the effluent*
   j. perform actions *to prevent effluent from contacting the skin when the pouch system is on:*
      1. measure the diameter of the stoma; cut skin barrier the same size as stoma and select a pouch with an opening that is not more than 0.3 cm (⅛ inch) larger than the stoma (it may be necessary to create a pattern to use for cutting barrier and pouch openings if stoma has an irregular shape and cannot be measured using appliance manufacturer's standard measuring guide)
      2. instruct and assist client to remeasure the stoma frequently during the first 6–8 weeks after surgery and to alter size of skin barrier and pouch openings as stomal edema decreases
      3. implement measures *to achieve an adequate pouch seal:*
         a. avoid use of ointments or lotions on peristomal skin *(these can interfere with adequate adhesive bonding)*
         b. follow manufacturer's instructions when applying skin products and pouch system
         c. use products such as ostomy paste (e.g., Stomahesive paste) to fill in irregularities around stoma site (e.g., body folds, scars) before applying pouch system

Desired Outcomes	**Nursing Actions** *and Selected Purposes/Rationales*

d. apply firm pressure and remove air pockets when applying pouch system; place client in a supine position *to increase tautness of skin surface during application*
4. empty pouch when it is ⅓ full of effluent or inflated with gas *(a heavy or inflated pouch can cause the pouch system to separate from the skin)*
5. position pouch so gravity flow facilitates drainage away from stoma and peristomal skin
6. rinse out bottom of drainable pouch after emptying it and then close pouch clamp securely *to prevent leakage*
7. use a drainable pouch, 2-piece pouch system, and/or pouch with release valve if gas is a problem; never puncture or cut the pouch to release gas *because effluent can seep out of the opening*

k. if a belted pouch system is used, fasten the belt so that 2 fingers can slip easily between belt and skin *to prevent excessive pressure on skin*
l. instruct and assist client to check pouch periodically to ensure that pouch clamp is not placing pressure on the skin.

5. Implement measures *to prevent perianal irritation and breakdown:*
   a. keep perianal area clean and dry
   b. instruct client to perform perineal exercises (e.g., relaxing and tightening perineal and gluteal muscles) regularly *to increase anal sphincter tone and reduce the risk of mucus leakage*
   c. place absorbent pads in client's underwear if needed and change pads when they become damp
   d. apply a moisture-barrier ointment to perianal area as ordered *to protect skin.*
6. If signs and symptoms of peristomal or perianal skin irritation or breakdown occur:
   a. cleanse areas gently with warm water
   b. avoid use of any product that may have caused the irritation or breakdown
   c. perform skin care as ordered or according to hospital procedure (usual care may include exposing affected area to air for 20–30 minutes, applying an antifungal agent or corticosteroid preparation to affected skin, and/or covering all irritated skin with a solid skin barrier)
   d. consult appropriate health care provider (e.g., wound care specialist, ET nurse, physician) if areas of irritation or breakdown do not improve within 48 hours.

4. Collaborative Diagnoses:

POTENTIAL COMPLICATIONS OF BOWEL DIVERSION SURGERY

a. **peritonitis** related to:
   1. wound infection (a client with inflammatory bowel disease often has a decreased resistance to infection as a result of long-term preoperative corticosteroid use and decreased nutritional status)
   2. leakage of intestinal contents into the peritoneum during surgery and/or postoperatively associated with loss of integrity of the sutures at sites of anastomoses or separation of the peristomal skin from the stoma (retraction of the stoma can occur as a result of slippage of sutures, impaired healing of surgical site, or shrinkage of the supporting tissues)
   3. accumulation of wound drainage in the peritoneum;

b. **stomal changes:**
   1. **necrosis** related to intraoperative and/or postoperative interruption of blood supply to the stoma
   2. **excessive bleeding** related to irritation associated with aggressive cleansing of stoma and/or improper fit or application of pouch system
   3. **prolapse** related to loss of integrity of the sutures or pressure around the stoma;

c. **stomal obstruction** related to stomal edema and/or blockage of stoma.

Desired Outcomes	Nursing Actions *and Selected Purposes/Rationales*
4.a. The client will not develop peritonitis as evidenced by: 1. gradual resolution of abdominal pain 2. soft, nondistended abdomen 3. temperature declining toward normal 4. stable vital signs 5. absence of nausea and vomiting 6. gradual return of normal bowel sounds 7. WBC count decreasing toward normal.	4.a.1. Assess for and report signs and symptoms of peritonitis (e.g., increase in severity of abdominal pain; generalized abdominal pain; rebound tenderness; distended, rigid abdomen; increase in temperature; tachycardia; tachypnea; hypotension; nausea; vomiting; continued absent or diminished bowel sounds; WBC count that increases or fails to decline toward normal). 2. Implement measures *to prevent peritonitis:* a. perform actions to prevent wound infection (see Standardized Postoperative Care Plan, Diagnosis 17, action b.2 [pp. 118–119]) b. perform actions *to maintain patency of wound drain if present:* 1. keep tubing free of kinks 2. empty collection device as often as necessary 3. maintain suction as ordered c. perform actions *to prevent inadvertent removal of wound drain if present:* 1. use caution when changing dressings surrounding drain 2. provide extension tubing if necessary *to enable client to move without placing tension on drain* 3. instruct client not to pull on drain and drainage tubing d. perform actions *to prevent distention of the internal reservoir (if client has a continent ileostomy) or remaining segment of the ileum (distention can cause strain on the suture lines and subsequent leakage of intestinal contents into the peritoneal cavity):* 1. implement measures to prevent stomal obstruction (see action c.2 in this diagnosis) 2. instruct client to avoid activities such as drinking carbonated beverages, chewing gum, smoking, and eating gas-producing foods (e.g., cabbage, onions, broccoli, beans, cucumbers) *in order to prevent the accumulation of air and gas in the remaining intestine or internal reservoir* 3. use only the prescribed amount of irrigating solution (usually 20–30 ml) when irrigating the stoma or internal reservoir 4. maintain patency of stomal catheter (e.g., keep stomal catheter and drainage bag below level of reservoir *to promote gravity drainage,* keep catheter free of kinks, irrigate catheter as ordered) 5. change pouch system carefully *in order to avoid dislodgment of the stomal catheter* 6. if client has a continent ileostomy and the stomal catheter is removed prior to discharge, assist him/her with drainage of the internal reservoir at scheduled intervals and when he/she feels increased abdominal pressure e. do not reposition the stomal catheter *(repositioning could disrupt the suture line)* f. if the peristomal skin separates from the stoma: 1. perform wound care as ordered *to facilitate the formation of granulation tissue in the affected area* 2. prepare client for surgical reconstruction of the stoma if planned g. administer antimicrobials if ordered. 3. If signs and symptoms of peritonitis occur: a. withhold oral intake as ordered b. place client on bed rest in a semi-Fowler's position *to assist in pooling or localizing gastrointestinal contents in the pelvis rather than under the diaphragm* c. prepare client for diagnostic tests (e.g., abdominal x-ray, computed tomography, ultrasonography) if planned d. insert a nasogastric tube and maintain suction as ordered e. administer antimicrobials as ordered f. administer intravenous fluids and/or blood volume expanders if ordered *to prevent or treat shock (can result from the increased capillary permeability that occurs with inflammation and the subsequent*

Desired Outcomes | **Nursing Actions** *and Selected Purposes/Rationales*

escape of protein, fluid, and electrolytes from the vascular space into the peritoneal cavity)

g. prepare client for surgical intervention (e.g., drainage and irrigation of peritoneum, repair of site of anastomosis) if planned.

4.b. The client will maintain adequate stomal integrity as evidenced by:
1. medium pink to red stomal coloring
2. expected stomal height
3. absence of excessive bleeding and increasing edema of the stoma.

4.b.1. Assess for and report signs and symptoms of impaired stomal integrity (e.g., pale, dark red, dusky blue, blue-black, or purple color of stoma; increased height of stoma; increased stomal edema or bleeding). Use clear pouches during the immediate postoperative period *to allow easy visibility of stoma.*

2. Implement measures *to maintain stomal integrity:*
   a. perform actions *to maintain adequate stomal circulation:*
      1. ensure that openings of the skin barrier and pouch system are not too small and that the stoma is carefully centered in the openings *in order to prevent pressure on and around the stoma*
      2. instruct client to avoid wearing clothing that puts pressure on the stoma
   b. apply pouch system securely *to prevent it from slipping and irritating or shearing stoma*
   c. cleanse stoma gently using a soft cloth, gauze, or tissue.
3. If signs and symptoms of impaired stomal integrity occur:
   a. perform stomal care as ordered
   b. prepare client for surgical revision of stoma if planned.

4.c. The client will not develop stomal obstruction as evidenced by:
1. expected amount and consistency of ileostomy output
2. no reports of abdominal cramping, nausea, or increased feeling of fullness
3. absence of vomiting.

4.c.1. Assess for and report signs and symptoms of stomal obstruction:
   a. less than expected amount of ileostomy output (after return of peristalsis, output may be as high as 2000 ml/day and will gradually decrease to about 500–800 ml/day)
   b. change in effluent consistency from a thicker consistency to a thin, watery liquid (postoperatively, effluent gradually becomes thicker; a return to thin, watery consistency may indicate blockage of stoma)
   c. reports of abdominal cramping, nausea, or increased feeling of fullness
   d. vomiting.
2. Implement measures *to prevent stomal obstruction:*
   a. irrigate stoma if ordered *to remove excessive mucus that could block stoma*
   b. maintain a fluid intake of 2500 ml/day unless contraindicated *to keep effluent from becoming too thick*
   c. administer oral medications crushed and mixed in water or in liquid or chewable form *(undigested pills can block stoma)*
   d. when oral intake is allowed, perform actions *to prevent blockage of stoma by food:*
      1. encourage client to eat small, frequent meals rather than 3 large ones
      2. instruct client to chew food thoroughly
      3. instruct client to avoid or eat only small amounts of foods that are high in fiber *(fibrous foods absorb water in the intestinal tract)* and/or are hard to digest (e.g., popcorn, coconut, raw vegetables, fruits with seeds, celery, bean sprouts, bamboo shoots, whole kernel corn, potato skins, bran, nuts, fruit skins).
3. If stomal edema seems to be obstructing the stoma, consult physician about gently inserting a catheter through the stoma into the ileal segment *to drain effluent until edema decreases.*
4. If food particles or mucus seem to be obstructing the stoma, implement measures *to promote the flow of effluent through the stoma:*
   a. perform actions *to relax the abdominal muscle that surrounds the stoma* (e.g., administer analgesic if ordered, apply warm compress to the abdomen unless contraindicated, encourage participation in relaxing activities such as reading and listening to music)

b. perform actions *to break up or shift food or mucus:*
   1. encourage fluid intake unless contraindicated
   2. instruct and assist client to assume a knee-chest position
   3. gently massage peristomal area unless contraindicated
   4. assist with or gently perform digital dilation of stoma if ordered
   5. irrigate the ileostomy if ordered.

5. If signs and symptoms of stomal obstruction persist:
   a. withhold oral intake as ordered
   b. maintain intravenous fluid therapy as ordered *to prevent fluid volume deficit and increased viscosity of effluent*
   c. insert a nasogastric tube and maintain suction as ordered
   d. prepare client for surgical intervention to remove obstruction if indicated.

5. NURSING DIAGNOSIS: *INEFFECTIVE SEXUALITY PATTERNS*

related to feelings of loss of femininity/masculinity and sexual attractiveness, fear of offensive odor or leakage of effluent and gas, fear of rejection by partner, discomfort associated with surgical incision, and depression.

Suggested NOC Outcomes: Body image; Sexual identity; Personal well-being

Suggested NIC Interventions: Body image enhancement; Sexual counseling

Desired Outcome	Nursing Actions *and Selected Purposes/Rationales*
5. The client will demonstrate beginning adjustment to effects of the ileostomy on sexuality as evidenced by: a. verbalization of a perception of self as sexually acceptable and adequate b. statements reflecting ways to adjust to effects of ileostomy on sexual functioning.	5.a. Assess for signs and symptoms of ineffective sexuality patterns (e.g., verbalization of sexual concerns, reports of anticipated changes in sexual activities or behaviors). b. Implement measures *to promote an optimal sexuality pattern:* 1. facilitate communication between client and partner; focus on feelings the couple share and assist them to identify changes which may affect their sexual relationship 2. perform actions to promote a positive self-concept (see Postoperative Diagnosis 6, actions d–t) 3. instruct client in ways *to reduce risk for leakage of effluent during sexual activity:* a. empty pouch or drain internal reservoir (if present) before sexual activity b. secure pouch seal with tape for added security 4. if client is concerned about odor, instruct to: a. shower or bathe before sexual activity b. use an odorproof pouch or a pouch deodorizer c. use cologne or perfume if desired d. keep room well ventilated 5. if client is concerned about the presence of the stoma and pouch system, discuss the possibility of: a. using opaque or patterned pouches or decorative pouch covers b. wearing underwear with the crotch removed (for females), boxer shorts (for males), or stretch tube top or cummerbund around abdomen during sexual activity 6. if client is concerned that operative site discomfort will interfere with usual sexual activity: a. assure him/her that discomfort is temporary and will diminish as the incision heals b. encourage use of positions that decrease pressure on surgical site (e.g., side-lying) until the incision heals 7. if appropriate, involve partner in ileostomy care *to facilitate partner's adjustment to the changes in client's appearance and body functioning and subsequently decrease the possibility of partner's rejection of client*

Desired Outcome	Nursing Actions *and Selected Purposes/Rationales*

8. encourage client to obtain written information regarding sexual activity and sexuality from the United Ostomy Association and from manufacturers of ostomy products
9. include partner in above discussions and encourage continued support of the client.

c. Consult appropriate health care provider (e.g., ET nurse, psychiatric nurse clinician, physician) if counseling appears indicated.

6. Nursing Diagnosis: *DISTURBED SELF-CONCEPT**

related to:
a. change in appearance associated with presence of stoma and pouch system;
b. embarrassment associated with sound and odor resulting from gas and effluent;
c. dependence (usually temporary) on others for assistance with ileostomy management;
d. loss of control over bowel elimination if client has conventional ileostomy;
e. possibility of impotence if nerve damage occurred during a proctocolectomy (use of nerve-sparing surgical techniques has greatly reduced the occurrence of nerve damage and subsequent impotence).

*This diagnostic label includes the nursing diagnoses of disturbed body image, low self-esteem, and ineffective role performance.

Suggested NOC Outcomes: Body image; Personal autonomy; Self-esteem; Psychosocial adjustment: life change

Suggested NIC Interventions: Body image enhancement; Self-esteem enhancement; Emotional support; Support system enhancement; Role enhancement; Counseling

Desired Outcome	Nursing Actions *and Selected Purposes/Rationales* (see pp. 47–49 for additional rationales)

Desired Outcome

6. The client will demonstrate beginning adaptation to changes in appearance and body functioning as evidenced by:
   a. verbalization of feelings of self-worth
   b. maintenance of relationships with significant others
   c. active participation in activities of daily living
   d. verbalization of a beginning plan for integrating changes in appearance and body functioning into lifestyle.

Nursing Actions

6.a. Assess for signs and symptoms of a disturbed self-concept (e.g., verbalization of negative feelings about self, withdrawal from significant others, lack of participation in activities of daily living, refusal to look at or touch stoma, lack of plan for adapting to necessary changes in lifestyle).
b. Determine the meaning of changes in appearance and body functioning to the client by encouraging verbalization of feelings and by noting nonverbal responses to the changes experienced.
c. Be aware that client may grieve the loss of usual manner of bowel elimination and change in appearance. Provide support during the grieving process.
d. Emphasize the positive effects of the surgery on future lifestyle (e.g., the discomfort and frequent diarrhea associated with inflammatory bowel disease and the side effects of medications such as corticosteroids usually have had a disruptive effect on many aspects of the client's life).
e. Implement measures to promote an optimal sexuality pattern (see Postoperative Diagnosis 5, action b).
f. Instruct client in ways *to reduce gas formation:*
   1. avoid activities that can cause air swallowing (e.g., chewing gum, smoking)
   2. limit intake of carbonated beverages and gas-producing foods (e.g., cabbage, onions, beans, radishes, broccoli, cucumbers).
g. Instruct client in and assist with measures *to reduce odor of ileostomy drainage and/or gas:*
   1. use odorproof pouches, a pouch deodorizer, and/or a pouch with a deodorizing flatus filter

2. empty pouch regularly; rinse inside of pouch and clean off any effluent before closing pouch
3. drain the reservoir of continent ileostomy at scheduled intervals and when it feels full to reduce possibility of leakage from stoma
4. use a disposable pouch and change it regularly or clean reusable pouch thoroughly
5. empty or change pouch in a well-ventilated area; use room deodorizers if desired
6. perform actions to achieve an adequate pouch seal (see Postoperative Diagnosis 3, action b.4.j.3)
7. limit intake of foods that cause effluent to have a strong odor (e.g., onions, fish, eggs, strong cheeses, asparagus)
8. increase intake of foods/fluids that control odor (e.g., spinach, parsley, yogurt, buttermilk)
9. change bed linens and clothing promptly if they become soiled.

h. Inform client that the pouch and clothing muffle sounds of bowel activity.
i. Assure client that once the stomal edema and surgical discomfort have resolved, he/she will be able to dress as before with minor, if any, modifications.
j. Show client and significant others some of the attractive ileostomy products that are available (e.g., opaque or patterned pouches, pouch covers).
k. If nerve damage that could result in impotence is believed to have occurred during a proctocolectomy, encourage client to discuss it and various treatment options (e.g., vacuum erection aids, penile prosthesis) with physician.
l. Encourage client's participation in activities that can assist him/her to integrate physical changes that have occurred (e.g., ileostomy care, bathing).
m. Demonstrate acceptance of client using techniques such as touch and frequent visits. Encourage significant others to do the same.
n. Support behaviors suggesting positive adaptation to changes that have occurred (e.g., willingness to care for ileostomy, compliance with treatment plan, verbalization of feelings of self-worth, maintenance of relationships with significant others).
o. Encourage significant others to allow client to do what he/she is able *so that independence can be re-established and/or self-esteem redeveloped.*
p. Assist client's and significant others' adjustment by listening, facilitating communication, and providing information.
q. Encourage visits and support from significant others.
r. If acceptable to client, arrange for a visit with an ostomate of similar age and same sex who has successfully adjusted to an ileostomy.
s. Encourage client to pursue usual roles and interests and to continue involvement in social activities.
t. Provide information about and encourage utilization of community agencies and support groups (e.g., ostomy groups; sexual, family, individual, and/or financial counseling).
u. Consult appropriate health care provider (e.g., psychiatric nurse clinician, ET nurse, physician) if client seems unwilling or unable to adapt to changes resulting from the bowel diversion.

Discharge Teaching/Continued Care

7. NURSING DIAGNOSIS: ***DEFICIENT KNOWLEDGE, INEFFECTIVE THERAPEUTIC REGIMEN MANAGEMENT, OR INEFFECTIVE HEALTH MAINTENANCE****

*The nurse should select the diagnostic label that is most appropriate for the client's discharge teaching needs.

Suggested NOC Outcomes: Knowledge: ostomy care; Knowledge: treatment regimen; Knowledge: diet

Suggested NIC Interventions: Health system guidance; Teaching: individual; Teaching: disease process; Teaching: prescribed diet; Teaching: prescribed medication

Desired Outcomes	**Nursing Actions** *and Selected Purposes/Rationales*
7.a. The client will verbalize a basic understanding of the anatomical changes that have occurred as a result of the bowel diversion.	7.a. Reinforce teaching regarding the anatomical changes that have occurred as a result of the bowel diversion. Use appropriate teaching aids (e.g., pictures, videotapes, anatomical models).
7.b. The client will identify ways to maintain fluid and electrolyte balance.	7.b. Provide the following instructions on ways to maintain fluid and electrolyte balance: 1. instruct client to drink at least 10 glasses of liquid/day unless contraindicated and to increase fluid intake during hot weather, during and following intense physical activity, when perspiring profusely, if urine is dark yellow, and during episodes of diarrhea; inform client that pale yellow urine is a good indicator of adequate fluid intake 2. instruct client to perform the following actions to prevent excessive ileostomy output: a. avoid excessive intake of foods/liquids that may cause diarrhea (e.g., raw fruits and vegetables, prune juice, fatty foods, spicy foods, coffee) b. do not take laxatives or excessive amounts of magnesium-containing antacids (e.g., Milk of Magnesia, Mylanta, Maalox) c. take antidiarrheal agents (e.g., loperamide, diphenoxylate hydrochloride) as prescribed 3. if ileostomy output increases or becomes more watery, instruct client to: a. increase intake of foods that may thicken effluent (e.g., applesauce, bananas, boiled rice, tapioca, pretzels, creamy peanut butter, pasta) b. increase intake of foods/liquids such as fruit juices, Gatorade, potatoes (without skins), bananas, and bouillon to maintain electrolyte balance c. drink a mixture of baking soda and water (usually ¼–½ teaspoon baking soda in 1 cup of water) if prescribed by physician to maintain acid-base balance.
7.c. The client will verbalize ways to maintain an optimal nutritional status.	7.c. Provide instructions regarding ways to maintain an optimal nutritional status: 1. reinforce ways to prevent excessive ileostomy output (see action b.2 in this diagnosis) 2. stress the need to chew food thoroughly in order to enhance digestion and subsequent absorption of nutrients 3. stress the importance of taking vitamins and minerals as prescribed.
7.d. The client will identify methods of controlling odor and sound associated with ileostomy drainage and gas.	7.d.1. Reinforce instructions regarding ways to reduce gas formation and odor associated with ileostomy drainage and gas (see Postoperative Diagnosis 6, actions f and g). 2. Inform client that the ostomy pouch and clothing will muffle the sounds from the ileostomy.

7.e. The client will demonstrate the ability to change the pouch system, maintain integrity of the peristomal and perianal skin, and maintain adequate stomal integrity.	7.e.1. Reinforce teaching regarding application of the pouch system, prevention of peristomal and perianal skin irritation and breakdown, and maintenance of adequate stomal integrity (see Postoperative Diagnoses 3, actions b.4–5 and 4, action b.2 for appropriate measures). 2. Support client's efforts to decrease odor of effluent and gas but discourage excessive changing and emptying of pouch or pouch system. 3. Instruct and assist client to establish a routine for emptying and changing pouch or emptying continent ileostomy in order to reduce risk of leakage of effluent. 4. Instruct client to follow special precautions for products used (e.g., skin sealants should be used only on healthy peristomal skin because they can further irritate reddened and excoriated skin). 5. Allow time for questions, clarification, practice, and return demonstration of emptying the pouch, changing the pouch system, and performing appropriate stoma and skin care.
7.f. The client will demonstrate the ability to properly use, clean, and store ostomy products.	7.f.1. Instruct client regarding proper use of ostomy products he/she will be using after discharge. 2. Demonstrate appropriate pouch system cleansing. Emphasize importance of: a. rinsing inside of pouch each time it is emptied b. soaking reusable pouch according to manufacturer's instructions and allowing it to dry thoroughly before reusing. 3. Instruct client to avoid reusing disposable products and to discard a reusable pouch if it retains an odor after thorough cleansing or if it becomes brittle. 4. Discuss recommended methods of storing ostomy products based on manufacturer's recommendations. 5. Allow time for questions, clarification, and return demonstration.
7.g. The client will demonstrate the ability to drain and irrigate a continent ileostomy if present.	7.g.1. Explain the gradual and progressive clamping routine if catheter will still be in the stoma of a continent ileostomy at time of discharge. 2. If the stomal catheter has been removed, demonstrate the correct method of and explain the schedule for stomal catheter insertion (initially the reservoir will need to be drained for 5–15 minutes every 3–4 hours but after about 6 months it may need emptying only 2–3 times/day). 3. Demonstrate the correct technique for irrigating a continent ileostomy. Caution client to use only the prescribed amount of irrigant (usually 20–30 ml) in order to avoid overdistending and damaging the internal reservoir. 4. Allow time for questions, clarification, and return demonstration of clamping, draining, and irrigating techniques.
7.h. The client will identify ways to prevent and treat blockage of the stoma.	7.h.1. Instruct client in ways to prevent blockage of the stoma: a. drink at least 10 glasses of liquid/day unless contraindicated b. chew food thoroughly c. avoid or eat only small amounts of foods that are high in fiber and/or hard to digest (e.g., popcorn, coconut, raw vegetables, bean sprouts, bamboo shoots, celery, caraway seeds, whole kernel corn, potato skins, fruit with seeds, nuts, fruit skins) d. ensure that skin barrier and pouch openings are large enough to prevent mechanical constriction of the stoma. 2. Instruct client to do the following if stoma is blocked: a. apply a warm compress to abdomen b. participate in relaxing activities (e.g., warm bath, reading) c. attempt to break up or shift blockage (e.g., assume a knee-chest position, gently massage peristomal area, irrigate the stoma or gently perform digital dilation of the stoma if prescribed).

3. Demonstrate techniques such as massage of abdomen, irrigation of stoma, and digital dilation of stoma if appropriate.
4. Allow time for questions, clarification, and return demonstration.

7.i. The client will state signs and symptoms to report to the health care provider.

7.i.1. Refer to Standardized Postoperative Care Plan, Diagnosis 22, action c (p. 125), for signs and symptoms to report to the health care provider.
2. Instruct client to also report:
   a. dark red, dusky blue, blue-black, purple, or pale stoma
   b. change in color, consistency, or odor of effluent that is not readily identified as a response to food or fluid intake
   c. unexpected change in shape, size, or height of stoma (use diagrams and descriptive terms so client does not confuse decreasing stoma size due to resolving edema with actual stomal retraction)
   d. excessive bleeding of stoma or bloody drainage from stoma
   e. difficulty accomplishing ileostomy care
   f. persistent skin irritation
   g. bright red, bumpy, itchy rash or white-coated area on skin around stoma (may indicate presence of a yeast infection)
   h. skin breakdown
   i. persistent thirst, dry mucous membranes, dizziness, or decreased urine output (may indicate deficient fluid volume)
   j. signs and symptoms of low potassium (e.g., irregular pulse, muscle weakness and cramping, nausea, vomiting)
   k. signs and symptoms of low sodium (e.g., headache, abdominal cramps, fatigue, irritability)
   l. thin, watery ileostomy output; absence of ileostomy output; unusual foul odor of gas; abdominal distention; and/or nausea and vomiting that does not resolve within 2 hours of implementing measures to relieve stomal blockage
   m. persistent leakage of pouch system
   n. persistent leakage of effluent from stoma (if client has a continent ileostomy)
   o. difficulty draining or irrigating internal reservoir
   p. fever; pain or cramping in reservoir area; pain when draining the reservoir; and/or persistent watery, high-volume ileostomy output (these signs and symptoms can indicate inflammation of the internal reservoir [pouchitis], which is a long-term complication that can develop in the client with a continent ileostomy)
   q. difficulty adjusting to changes in appearance and body functioning.

7.j. The client will identify appropriate community resources that can assist with home management and adjustment to changes resulting from the bowel diversion.

7.j.1. Provide information about community resources that can assist the client and significant others with home management and adjustment to changes resulting from the bowel diversion (e.g., local ostomy support groups; community health agencies; ET nurse; home health agencies; financial, individual, and family counseling services).
2. Initiate a referral if appropriate.

7.k. The client will verbalize an understanding of and a plan for adhering to recommended follow-up care including future appointments with health care provider, wound care, activity level, and medications prescribed.

7.k.1. Refer to Standardized Postoperative Care Plan, Diagnosis 22 (pp. 125–126), for routine postoperative instructions and measures to improve client compliance.
2. Reinforce physician's instructions regarding activity limitations:
   a. avoid strenuous exercise and lifting objects over 10 pounds for at least 6 weeks
   b. avoid participating in contact sports.
3. Provide client with a list of ostomy products he/she is using (include product name, size, and number) and where these supplies can be obtained.
4. Explain the rationale for, side effects of, and importance of taking medications prescribed (e.g., electrolyte supplements, vitamins, antimicrobials). Inform client of pertinent food and drug interactions.

5. Stress the fact that oral medications should be crushed or in liquid, chewable, uncoated, or sugar-coated form rather than enteric-coated tablets or timed-release capsules so absorption can take place before the medication is excreted.

ADDITIONAL NURSING DIAGNOSES

*INEFFECTIVE COPING**

related to:

a. fear, anxiety, and depression associated with loss of control over bowel elimination (especially with a conventional ileostomy) and possibility of rejection by others;
b. difficulty performing ileostomy care and incorporating the care into lifestyle;
c. need for lifelong medical supervision.

*GRIEVING**

related to loss of usual manner of bowel elimination and change in appearance associated with the ileostomy.

---

*See Unit II for outcomes, actions, and rationales.

Bibliography

See pages 879 and 884.

Gastrectomy

Gastrectomy is the surgical removal of all or part of the stomach. A total gastrectomy involves removal of the entire stomach and anastomosis of the esophagus to the jejunum (esophagojejunostomy). It may be considered as treatment for advanced stomach cancer or Zollinger-Ellison syndrome that is not controlled by more conservative measures. However, a total gastrectomy is performed infrequently because it is so difficult to maintain an adequate nutritional status postoperatively. The more common type of gastrectomy performed is a partial gastrectomy. This less extensive surgery is most often done to treat peptic ulcer disease that continues to be symptomatic despite conservative management or to treat complications that develop as a result of the disease (e.g., perforation, gastric outlet obstruction, hemorrhage). A partial gastrectomy may also be performed to resect lesions that are believed to be precancerous.

A partial gastrectomy usually involves excision of 40–75% of the distal stomach including the antrum (which contains the gastrin-secreting cells) and a portion of the body of the stomach that contains much of the parietal cell mass. Gastrointestinal continuity is re-established by anastomosis of the remaining stomach to the duodenum (gastroduodenostomy or Billroth I) or jejunum (gastrojejunostomy or Billroth II). In the latter procedure, the duodenal stump is left intact so that bile and pancreatic secretions can enter the jejunum. The decreased output of gastric secretions that results from a partial gastrectomy can be enhanced by a vagotomy (truncal, selective, or highly selective), which is often performed concurrently to further reduce stimulation of gastric secretions. A truncal vagotomy (resection of the vagal nerve trunks at the level of the esophageal hiatus) is the most effective in reducing gastric secretions; however, the extensive denervation also greatly suppresses gastric motility and impairs normal functioning of the pancreas, gallbladder, and small intestine. Because of this, a selective vagotomy (which preserves the hepatic and celiac branches of the vagus nerve) or highly selective vagotomy (which only affects the parietal cell mass) is performed more frequently.

This care plan focuses on the adult client who is hospitalized for a partial gastrectomy. Much of the postoperative information is applicable to clients receiving follow-up care in an extended care facility or home setting.

OUTCOME/DISCHARGE CRITERIA

THE CLIENT WILL:

- have surgical pain controlled
- have evidence of normal healing of the surgical wound
- have clear, audible breath sounds throughout lungs
- have no signs and symptoms of postoperative complications
- tolerate prescribed diet
- verbalize an understanding of ways to maintain an adequate nutritional status
- identify ways to control postvagotomy diarrhea if it occurs
- identify ways to manage dumping syndrome if it occurs
- state signs and symptoms to report to the health care provider
- verbalize an understanding of and a plan for adhering to recommended follow-up care including future appointments with health care provider, medications prescribed, activity level, and wound care.

NURSING/COLLABORATIVE DIAGNOSES

Postoperative

DISCHARGE TEACHING

See Standardized Preoperative and Postoperative Care Plans (pp. 97–126) for additional diagnoses.

PREOPERATIVE *Refer to Standardized Preoperative Care Plan.*

POSTOPERATIVE *Use in conjunction with the Standardized Postoperative Care Plan.*

1. NURSING DIAGNOSIS: ***INEFFECTIVE BREATHING PATTERN***

related to:
a. increased rate of respirations associated with fear and anxiety;
b. decreased rate of respirations associated with the depressant effect of anesthesia and some medications (e.g., narcotic [opioid] analgesics, some antiemetics);
c. decreased depth of respirations associated with:
  1. depressant effects of anesthesia and some medications (e.g., narcotic [opioid] analgesics, some antiemetics)
  2. reluctance to breathe deeply because of pain
  3. fear, anxiety, weakness, and fatigue
  4. restricted chest expansion resulting from positioning and elevation of the diaphragm if abdominal distention is present.

Suggested NOC Outcome: Respiratory status: ventilation

Suggested NIC Interventions: Respiratory monitoring; Ventilation assistance

Desired Outcome	**Nursing Actions** *and Selected Purposes/Rationales* (see pp. 18–20 for additional rationales)
1. The client will maintain an effective breathing pattern (see Standardized Postoperative Care Plan, Diagnosis 2 [p. 104], for outcome criteria).	1.a. Refer to Standardized Postoperative Care Plan, Diagnosis 2 (p. 104), for measures related to assessment and management of an ineffective breathing pattern. b. Implement additional measures *to improve breathing pattern:* 1. instruct client to bend knees while coughing and deep breathing *in order to relieve tension on abdominal muscles and incision* 2. instruct and assist client to splint incision with hands or pillow when coughing and deep breathing.

2. NURSING DIAGNOSIS: ***IMBALANCED NUTRITION: LESS THAN BODY REQUIREMENTS***

related to:
a. decreased oral intake associated with prescribed dietary modifications, pain, weakness, fatigue, nausea, feeling of fullness (can occur as a result of abdominal distention), fear of experiencing dumping syndrome (especially with a gastrojejunostomy) or diarrhea (following a truncal vagotomy), and early satiety resulting from reduced stomach size;
b. decreased absorption of nutrients associated with impaired digestion resulting from:
  1. decreased gastric acid secretion (occurs with vagotomy and removal of gastrin-secreting cells and parietal cells)
  2. rapid entry of food into small intestine (a result of reduced stomach size and removal of pylorus)
  3. decreased stimulation and secretion of pancreatic juice and bile associated with reduction in hydrochloric acid and gastrin secretion and absence of food moving through the duodenum (following gastrojejunostomy);
c. decreased absorption of iron associated with bypassing the duodenum if a gastrojejunostomy was performed;
d. inadequate nutritional replacement therapy;

e. loss of nutrients associated with diarrhea if present;
f. increased nutritional needs associated with the increased metabolic rate that occurs during wound healing.

Suggested NOC Outcome: Nutritional status

Suggested NIC Interventions: Nutritional monitoring; Nutrition management; Nutrition therapy; Diet staging

Desired Outcome	**Nursing Actions** *and Selected Purposes/Rationales* (see pp. 40–43 for additional rationales)
2. The client will maintain an adequate nutritional status (see Standardized Postoperative Care Plan, Diagnosis 5 [pp. 107–108], for outcome criteria).	2.a. Refer to Standardized Postoperative Care Plan, Diagnosis 5 (pp. 107–108), for measures related to assessment and maintenance of an adequate nutritional status. b. Implement additional measures *to maintain an adequate nutritional status when oral intake is allowed:* 1. provide small, frequent meals if client is weak, fatigues easily, has a poor appetite, and/or experiences early satiety 2. instruct client to chew food thoroughly *(small food particles are more easily and completely digested)* 3. perform actions to prevent or control postvagotomy diarrhea and dumping syndrome (see Postoperative Diagnoses 3, action b and 4, actions d.2 and 3) *in order to reduce the client's fear of precipitating these conditions and to promote increased absorption of nutrients* 4. administer the following if ordered: a. vitamins and minerals (may be ordered in liquid or chewable form *to facilitate absorption)* b. pancreatic enzymes (e.g., pancreatin, pancrelipase) and/or bile salts *to facilitate digestion.*

3. Nursing Diagnosis: ***DIARRHEA****

related to dysfunction of the small intestine associated with loss of nervous system regulation of bowel activity if a truncal vagotomy was performed.

*Referred to as "postvagotomy diarrhea."

Suggested NOC Outcome: Bowel elimination

Suggested NIC Interventions: Diarrhea management; Diet staging

Desired Outcome	**Nursing Actions** *and Selected Purposes/Rationales* (see pp. 28–30 for additional rationales)
3. The client will not experience or will have diminished postvagotomy diarrhea as evidenced by: a. passage of formed stool b. no reports of urgency or abdominal cramping.	3.a. Assess for and report signs and symptoms of postvagotomy diarrhea (e.g., watery stools, urgency, and abdominal cramping usually occurring within 1–2 hours after eating). b. When oral intake is allowed, implement measures *to prevent or control postvagotomy diarrhea:* 1. advance diet gradually 2. encourage client to eat small rather than large meals 3. instruct client to drink fluids between rather than with meals 4. administer antidiarrheal agents (e.g., loperamide, diphenoxylate hydrochloride) if ordered. c. Consult physician if postvagotomy diarrhea persists.

4. Collaborative Diagnoses: ***POTENTIAL COMPLICATIONS OF GASTRECTOMY***

a. hypovolemic shock related to excessive blood loss during surgery (many major arteries and veins supply and surround the stomach) and postoperative hemorrhage (can occur if there is excessive stress on the newly ligated operative site vessels);

b. peritonitis related to:
   1. wound infection
   2. leakage of upper gastrointestinal contents into the peritoneal cavity associated with loss of integrity of the suture line at the duodenal stump (with gastrojejunostomy) or the site of anastomosis;

c. afferent loop syndrome related to partial obstruction of the remaining portion of the duodenum associated with factors such as edema or presence of a kink in the efferent jejunal limb after gastrojejunostomy;

d. early dumping syndrome related to rapid emptying of hypertonic food into the jejunum especially after a gastrojejunostomy (the bolus of food is hypertonic and attracts fluid from the vascular space; this distends the bowel lumen and increases intestinal peristalsis and motility);

e. late dumping syndrome (postprandial hypoglycemia) related to rapid emptying of food/fluid high in carbohydrates into the jejunum especially after a gastrojejunostomy (this results in increased absorption of glucose into the blood causing increased release of insulin and subsequent hypoglycemia).

Desired Outcomes	**Nursing Actions** *and Selected Purposes/Rationales*
4.a. The client will not develop hypovolemic shock (see Standardized Postoperative Care Plan, Diagnosis 20, outcome a [p. 122], for outcome criteria).	4.a.1. Refer to Standardized Postoperative Care Plan, Diagnosis 20, action a (p. 122), for measures related to assessment, prevention, and treatment of hypovolemic shock. Be aware that NG drainage may be bright red for a few hours after surgery and then is expected to darken within 24 hours and be a yellow-green color within 2–3 days. 2. Implement additional measures *to prevent hypovolemic shock:* a. perform actions to prevent stress on the newly ligated vessels (see action b.2.d in this diagnosis) b. prepare client for surgery (e.g., ligation of bleeding vessels) if indicated.
4.b. The client will not develop peritonitis as evidenced by: 1. gradual resolution of abdominal pain 2. soft, nondistended abdomen 3. temperature declining toward normal 4. stable vital signs 5. absence of nausea and vomiting 6. gradual return of normal bowel sounds 7. WBC count declining toward normal.	4.b.1. Assess for and report: a. bile in wound drain (indicates leakage from suture lines) b. persistent hiccups (can occur as a result of distention of remaining stomach; distention increases pressure on the suture lines) c. inability to maintain patency of nasogastric tube and/or unexpected decrease in or absence of nasogastric tube drainage (malfunction of nasogastric tube can result in accumulation of gas and fluid and subsequent increased pressure on the suture line) d. signs and symptoms of peritonitis (e.g., increase in severity of abdominal pain; generalized abdominal pain; rebound tenderness; distended, rigid abdomen; increase in temperature; tachycardia; tachypnea; hypotension; nausea; vomiting; continued diminished or absent bowel sounds; WBC count that increases or fails to decline toward normal). 2. Implement measures *to prevent peritonitis:* a. perform actions to prevent wound infection (see Standardized Postoperative Care Plan, Diagnosis 17, action b.2 [pp. 118–119]) b. perform actions *to maintain patency of wound drain if present:* 1. keep tubing free of kinks 2. empty collection device as often as necessary 3. maintain suction as ordered c. perform actions *to prevent inadvertent removal of wound drain if present:* 1. use caution when changing dressings surrounding drain 2. provide extension tubing if necessary *to enable client to move without placing tension on the drain* 3. instruct client not to pull on drain and drainage tubing d. perform actions *to prevent stress on and subsequent leakage from the suture line at site of anastomosis:* 1. do not change position of the nasogastric tube unless ordered *(the tube is positioned during surgery and moving it can traumatize the suture line)* 2. implement measures to prevent nausea and vomiting (see Standardized Postoperative Care Plan, Diagnosis 8, action b [pp. 110–111])

Desired Outcomes	**Nursing Actions** *and Selected Purposes/Rationales*
	3. implement measures *to prevent distention of the remaining portion of the stomach:* a. irrigate nasogastric tube only if ordered and with no more than prescribed amount of solution b. perform actions to reduce the accumulation of gastrointestinal gas and fluid (see Standardized Postoperative Care Plan, Diagnosis 7, action b [p. 110]) c. when oral intake is allowed, progress diet slowly and instruct client to avoid drinking fluids with meals e. perform actions to treat afferent loop syndrome if it occurs (see action c.2 in this diagnosis) *in order to prevent distention of the duodenal stump and subsequently reduce the risk of disruption of the duodenal stump sutures following gastrojejunostomy.* 3. If signs and symptoms of peritonitis occur: a. withhold oral intake as ordered b. place client on bed rest in a semi-Fowler's position *to assist in pooling or localizing gastrointestinal contents in the pelvis rather than under the diaphragm* c. prepare client for diagnostic tests (e.g., abdominal x-ray, computed tomography, ultrasound) if planned d. assist physician with insertion of a nasogastric tube and maintain suction as ordered e. administer antimicrobials as ordered f. administer intravenous fluids and/or blood volume expanders if ordered *to prevent or treat shock (it can result from the increased capillary permeability that occurs with inflammation and the subsequent escape of protein, fluid, and electrolytes from the vascular space into the peritoneal cavity)* g. prepare client for surgical intervention (e.g., repair of anastomosis) if planned.
4.c. The client will have resolution of afferent loop syndrome if it occurs as evidenced by: 1. no reports of intense nausea or epigastric fullness and pain after eating 2. no episodes of vomiting bile after eating.	4.c.1. Assess for and report signs and symptoms of afferent loop syndrome (e.g., reports of intense nausea and/or epigastric fullness and pain after eating, forceful vomiting of large amounts of bile after eating). Signs and symptoms usually occur 20–90 minutes after eating. 2. If signs and symptoms of afferent loop syndrome occur: a. restrict oral intake as ordered b. prepare client for diagnostic tests (e.g., ultrasound, computed tomography) if planned c. assist physician with insertion of a nasogastric tube and maintain suction as ordered d. administer antimicrobials as ordered *(infection can develop as a result of stasis of secretions in the afferent loop)* e. prepare client for surgical intervention if obstruction is caused by kinking of the efferent jejunal limb.
4.d. The client will not experience dumping syndrome after eating as evidenced by: 1. no reports of abdominal cramping 2. normal bowel sounds 3. skin dry and usual color 4. absence of palpitations, weakness, dizziness, and diarrhea 5. usual mental status.	4.d.1. Assess for signs and symptoms of: a. early dumping syndrome (e.g., reports of abdominal cramping, hyperactive bowel sounds, diaphoresis, flushing, palpitations, weakness, dizziness, and/or diarrhea within 30 minutes after meals) b. late dumping syndrome (e.g., anxiety, palpitations, dizziness, weakness, diaphoresis, inability to concentrate, decreased coordination, and/or confusion occurring 1–3 hours after meals). 2. Implement measures *to prevent dumping syndrome:* a. instruct client to avoid intake of simple carbohydrates (e.g., jelly, cake, pie, pudding, candy) *because they are hypertonic and tend to rapidly draw fluid into the intestine and because they are rapidly absorbed into the blood leading to increased insulin release and subsequent hypoglycemia*

b. encourage intake of foods containing moderate to high amounts of fat and protein *(these foods leave the stomach more slowly and are less hypertonic)*
c. instruct client in ways *to delay gastric emptying:*
   1. eat small, dry meals
   2. eat meals slowly
   3. drink fluids between rather than with meals; avoid fluids for at least 1 hour before and after meals
   4. eat in a semi-recumbent position, and then lie down for at least 30 minutes after each meal unless contraindicated.

3. If signs and symptoms of dumping syndrome occur:
   a. provide client with a rapid-acting carbohydrate (e.g., hard candy, sugar-containing soft drink) or glucose tablets *to treat the hypoglycemia that characterizes late dumping syndrome*
   b. consult appropriate health care provider (e.g., dietitian, physician) about revisions in dietary management (e.g., providing smaller meals, further restricting intake of carbohydrates, increasing the amount of fat and protein in diet)
   c. administer the following medications if ordered:
      1. anticholinergics (e.g., propantheline) *to delay gastric emptying*
      2. octreotide *(helps control some of the gastrointestinal symptoms).*

Discharge Teaching/Continued Care

5. NURSING DIAGNOSIS: ***DEFICIENT KNOWLEDGE, INEFFECTIVE THERAPEUTIC REGIMEN MANAGEMENT, OR INEFFECTIVE HEALTH MAINTENANCE****

*The nurse should select the diagnostic label that is most appropriate for the client's discharge teaching needs.

Suggested NOC Outcomes: Knowledge: treatment regimen; Knowledge: diet

Suggested NIC Interventions: Health system guidance; Teaching: individual; Teaching: prescribed diet; Teaching: prescribed activity/exercise; Teaching: prescribed medication

Desired Outcomes	**Nursing Actions** *and Selected Purposes/Rationales*
5.a. The client will verbalize an understanding of ways to maintain an adequate nutritional status.	5.a.1. Instruct client regarding ways to maintain an adequate nutritional status: a. eat regularly scheduled meals and snacks (recommended frequency and amount will vary depending on the size of the remaining stomach); do not skip meals b. eat slowly and chew food thoroughly to enhance digestion and absorption of nutrients c. continue with actions to prevent or control postvagotomy diarrhea and dumping syndrome (see actions b.3 and 4 and c.3–5 in this diagnosis); contact health care provider if these conditions are not controlled since they can result in excessive loss of nutrients d. take vitamin and mineral supplements as prescribed (usually prescribed in liquid or chewable form to ensure maximum absorption) e. take pancreatic enzymes (e.g., pancreatin, pancrelipase) and/or bile salts as prescribed (may be prescribed to facilitate digestion of food). 2. Instruct client to adhere to scheduled follow-up blood studies to determine need for vitamin B_{12} injections (pernicious anemia can develop years after the surgery as a result of decreased secretion of the intrinsic factor resulting from surgical removal of the gastrin-secreting and parietal cells).

Desired Outcomes	**Nursing Actions** *and Selected Purposes/Rationales*
5.b. The client will identify ways to control postvagotomy diarrhea if it occurs.	5.b.1. Inform client that episodes of diarrhea may occur if a truncal vagotomy was performed. 2. Explain that postvagotomy diarrhea usually occurs within 1–2 hours after eating and is often unpredictable (e.g., can be mild or explosive, can occur daily or for a few days every week or two, can occur for 1–2 months then not recur for weeks or months). Emphasize that if this condition occurs, it usually resolves within a year. 3. Instruct client that eating small rather than large meals and drinking liquids between rather than with meals may help prevent postvagotomy diarrhea. 4. Provide teaching regarding antidiarrheal medications recommended or prescribed by physician.
5.c. The client will identify ways to manage dumping syndrome if it occurs.	5.c.1. Reinforce physician's explanation regarding the factors that cause dumping syndrome. Emphasize that if this condition occurs, it usually resolves within 6–12 months. 2. Instruct client to be alert for signs and symptoms of: a. early dumping syndrome (e.g., abdominal cramping, weakness, flushing, palpitations, dizziness, and/or diarrhea within 30 minutes after eating) b. late dumping syndrome (e.g., anxiety, palpitations, dizziness, weakness, sweating, inability to concentrate, and/or decreased coordination 1–3 hours after meals). 3. Reinforce teaching regarding ways to prevent dumping syndrome (see Postoperative Diagnosis 4, action d.2). 4. If the above actions do not prevent dumping syndrome, consult health care provider about taking medications such as propantheline or octreotide. 5. If signs and symptoms of late dumping syndrome (postprandial hypoglycemia) occur, instruct client to drink fluids with high sugar content (e.g., sugar-containing soft drinks), eat candy that contains sugar or graham crackers, or take glucose tablets as instructed by physician.
5.d. The client will state signs and symptoms to report to the health care provider.	5.d.1. Refer to Standardized Postoperative Care Plan, Diagnosis 22, action c (p. 125), for signs and symptoms to report to the health care provider. 2. Instruct client to also report: a. persistent nausea, vomiting, and/or diarrhea b. persistent, increasing, or recurrent abdominal or epigastric discomfort c. abdominal distention or rigidity d. bloody, coffee-ground, or green-yellow vomitus e. foul-smelling, greasy stools that float (indicative of impaired absorption of dietary fat) f. persistent or increasing fatigue and weakness g. persistent weight loss h. signs and symptoms of dumping syndrome (see action c.2 in this diagnosis) that are not controlled using recommended measures i. persistent epigastric burning or aching that gets worse after eating and/or frequent vomiting of bile and food particles (these signs and symptoms are indicative of alkaline reflux gastritis, which can develop when alkaline pancreatic secretions and bile reflux into the remaining portion of the stomach).

5.e. The client will verbalize an understanding of and a plan for adhering to recommended follow-up care including future appointments with health care provider, medications prescribed, activity level, and wound care.	5.e. Refer to Standardized Postoperative Care Plan, Diagnosis 22 (pp. 125–126), for routine postoperative instructions and measures to improve client compliance.

Bibliography

See pages 879 and 884.

Gastric Reduction

Gastric reduction is a surgical procedure performed to control obesity. The methods most frequently used to accomplish gastric reduction are vertical banded gastroplasty and gastric bypass. Both involve reducing the capacity of the stomach to 30–50 ml by partitioning off a small portion of the stomach distal to the gastroesophageal junction to form a gastric pouch. A narrow outlet is then created for the gastric pouch so that it does not empty quickly. As a result of the decreased gastric capacity and delayed pouch emptying, it is expected that the client will experience early satiety and subsequently decrease his/her oral intake and lose weight.

Gastroplasty and gastric bypass differ with regard to the path the ingested food/fluid takes after it enters the gastric pouch. With a vertical banded gastroplasty, the gastric pouch is formed on the lesser curvature side of the stomach by the placement of 2 adjacent rows of vertical staple lines. The narrow channel created between the pouch and remaining stomach is reinforced with a ring of mesh or plastic to reduce the risk of channel widening. Food/fluid then passes from the pouch, through the channel, into the remaining stomach, and through the intestinal tract. Gastric bypass also incorporates gastric partitioning but, in this method of gastric reduction, the gastric pouch is created by the placement of horizontal rows of staples or by actual surgical transection of the stomach. A gastrojejunostomy (Roux-en-Y) is then performed so that foods/fluids pass from the pouch directly into the jejunum.

Clients are carefully screened physically and psychologically and must meet certain criteria before undergoing gastric reduction surgery. The criteria usually include massive obesity for at least 5 years, inability to reduce weight using other forms of treatment, weight that is at least 100 pounds or 100% or more over ideal body weight, and obesity that results from a caloric intake greater than the body's needs rather than an underlying metabolic disorder. The client must also be emotionally stable, have no uncontrolled or severe major illness, verbalize a willingness to adhere to life-long dietary modifications, and have access to adequate follow-up medical care.

This care plan focuses on the adult client hospitalized for gastric reduction surgery. Much of the information is relevant to the client receiving continued care in the home setting.

OUTCOME/DISCHARGE CRITERIA

THE CLIENT WILL:

- have evidence of normal healing of surgical wounds
- have clear, audible breath sounds throughout lungs
- tolerate prescribed diet
- have no signs and symptoms of postoperative complications
- identify ways to prevent excessive stretching of the gastric pouch
- verbalize an understanding of ways to maintain an adequate nutritional status
- identify ways to reduce the risk of consuming excessive amounts of food, fluid, and calories
- demonstrate the ability to accurately calculate and measure the allotted amounts of food and fluid
- state signs and symptoms to report to the health care provider
- identify community resources that can assist in the adjustment to prescribed dietary modifications and future changes in body image
- verbalize an understanding of and a plan for adhering to recommended follow-up care including future appointments with health care provider, activity level, medications prescribed, and wound care.

NURSING/COLLABORATIVE DIAGNOSES

DISCHARGE TEACHING

See Standardized Preoperative and Postoperative Care Plans (pp. 97–126) for additional diagnoses.

PREOPERATIVE

Use in conjunction with the Standardized Preoperative Care Plan.

1. Nursing Diagnosis: **DISTURBED SELF-CONCEPT***

related to obesity and the inability to lose weight by more conventional methods.

*This diagnostic label includes the nursing diagnoses of disturbed body image and low self-esteem.

Suggested NOC Outcomes: Body image; Self-esteem

Suggested NIC Interventions: Body image enhancement; Self-esteem enhancement; Emotional support; Support system enhancement

Desired Outcome	Nursing Actions *and Selected Purposes/Rationales* (see pp. 47–49 for additional rationales)
1. The client will demonstrate a positive self-concept as evidenced by: a. verbalization of feelings of self-worth b. positive statements regarding anticipated effects of surgical procedure c. maintenance of relationships with significant others d. active participation in preoperative care and self-care.	1.a. Assess for signs and symptoms of a disturbed self-concept (e.g., verbalization of negative feelings about self, withdrawal from significant others, lack of participation in preoperative care or self-care). b. Implement measures *to assist client to increase self-esteem* (e.g., limit negative self-assessment, encourage positive comments about self, assist to identify strengths, give positive feedback about accomplishments, provide positive feedback about decision to have the surgery and lose weight). c. Implement measures *to reduce client's embarrassment about obesity:* 1. obtain information from physician regarding client's height and weight so that oversized equipment and supplies (e.g., bed, chair, commode, blood pressure cuff, gowns, bathrobe) can be obtained before client is admitted 2. remove unnecessary furniture and equipment from room so client can move around easily 3. provide privacy when weighing client 4. transfer client to and from operating room in own hospital bed rather than attempting to use a regular-sized stretcher. d. Allow client to wear own clothes rather than hospital gown before and after surgery if desired. e. Assure client that he/she will be assisted with usual grooming and makeup habits after surgery if necessary. f. Arrange for a visit from an individual who has achieved weight loss after gastric reduction surgery if client desires. g. If client is expressing concerns about the amount of excess skin that will be present after the majority of weight loss occurs (usually after 1–1½ years), provide information about various clothing styles that may be most flattering (e.g., long-sleeved shirts or blouses) and reconstructive surgery that is available to remove excess skin from abdomen, breasts, upper arms, and thighs. h. Consult physician if client has unrealistic expectations of postoperative weight loss and dietary management.

POSTOPERATIVE

Use in conjunction with the Standardized Postoperative Care Plan.

1. Nursing Diagnosis: **INEFFECTIVE BREATHING PATTERN**

related to:

a. increased rate of respirations associated with fear and anxiety;
b. decreased rate of respirations associated with the depressant effect of anesthesia (effect lasts longer in the obese client because adipose tissue more readily absorbs and stores anesthetic agents) and some medications (e.g., narcotic [opioid] analgesics, some antiemetics);

c. decreased depth of respirations associated with:
   1. depressant effects of anesthesia and some medications (e.g., narcotic [opioid] analgesics, some antiemetics)
   2. reluctance to breathe deeply because of pain and fear of dislodging tubes
   3. fear, anxiety, weakness, and fatigue
   4. restricted chest expansion resulting from:
      a. limited diaphragmatic excursion (occurs because of the large amount of abdominal adipose tissue and postoperative abdominal distention)
      b. decreased activity (chest expansion is restricted by the bed surface when client is lying in bed)
      c. increased weight of the chest wall of an obese client (especially in women with large, pendulous breasts).

Suggested NOC Outcome: Respiratory status: ventilation

Suggested NIC Interventions: Respiratory monitoring; Ventilation assistance

Desired Outcome	**Nursing Actions** *and Selected Purposes/Rationales* (see pp. 18–20 for additional rationales)
1. The client will maintain an effective breathing pattern (see Standardized Postoperative Care Plan, Diagnosis 2 [p. 104], for outcome criteria).	1.a. Refer to Standardized Postoperative Care Plan, Diagnosis 2 (p. 104), for measures related to assessment and improvement of breathing pattern. b. Implement additional measures *to improve breathing pattern:* 1. position client with head of bed elevated at least 30° at all times 2. instruct and assist client to use overhead trapeze and turn at least every 2 hours 3. add extensions to tubings if necessary *to enable client to turn and move without fear of dislodging tubes* 4. instruct client to bend knees while coughing and deep breathing *in order to relieve tension on abdominal muscles and incision* 5. instruct and assist client to splint incision with hands or pillow when coughing and deep breathing 6. assist with ambulation the evening of surgery and at least 4 times/day as ordered.

2. Nursing Diagnosis: IMBALANCED NUTRITION: LESS THAN BODY REQUIREMENTS

related to:
a. decreased oral intake associated with nausea, pain, weakness, fatigue, prescribed dietary modifications, and early satiety resulting from small gastric pouch and delayed pouch emptying;
b. inadequate nutritional replacement therapy;
c. increased nutritional needs associated with the increased metabolic rate that occurs during wound healing.

Suggested NOC Outcome: Nutritional status

Suggested NIC Interventions: Nutritional monitoring; Nutrition management; Nutrition therapy; Enteral tube feeding; Diet staging

Desired Outcome	**Nursing Actions** *and Selected Purposes/Rationales* (see pp. 40–43 for additional rationales)
2. The client will maintain an adequate nutritional status as evidenced by: a. normal BUN and serum albumin, prealbumin, Hct, and Hgb levels b. usual strength and activity tolerance c. healthy oral mucous membrane.	2.a. Assess for and report signs and symptoms of malnutrition: 1. abnormal BUN and low serum albumin, prealbumin, Hct, and Hgb levels (decreased Hct and Hgb may also result from surgical blood loss) 2. weakness and fatigue 3. sore, inflamed oral mucous membrane 4. pale conjunctiva. b. Assess for return of bowel function every 2–4 hours. Notify physician when client has bowel sounds and is expelling flatus *so that jejunostomy tube feedings and/or oral intake can be started as soon as possible.* c. When oral intake is allowed, monitor the amount and type of fluids consumed.

d. Implement measures *to maintain an adequate nutritional status:*
   1. maintain jejunostomy tube feeding if ordered
   2. when oral intake is allowed:
      a. perform actions to reduce pain (see Standardized Postoperative Care Plan, Diagnosis 6, action d [p. 109])
      b. administer antiemetics and/or gastrointestinal stimulants (e.g., metoclopramide) if ordered *to control nausea*
      c. maintain a clean environment and a relaxed, pleasant atmosphere
      d. provide oral hygiene before offering fluids *(removes unpleasant tastes, which often improves the taste of fluids)*
      e. provide high-protein liquid nourishment as part of fluid allotment as soon as allowed (client is usually allowed to drink dilute liquid protein supplements 4–5 days after surgery)
      f. reinforce the importance of consuming fluids at scheduled frequency and consuming more nutritious fluids and foods as soon as allowed (client is usually allowed to progress from fluids to solids after 6–8 weeks)
   3. administer vitamins and minerals if ordered.

e. Consult physician if client is unable to tolerate or adhere to prescribed diet.

3. NURSING DIAGNOSIS: ACTUAL/RISK FOR IMPAIRED TISSUE INTEGRITY

related to:
a. disruption of tissue associated with the surgical procedure;
b. delayed wound healing associated with factors such as decreased nutritional status and inadequate blood supply to wound area;
c. irritation of skin associated with contact with wound drainage, pressure from tubes, and use of tape;
d. difficulty keeping deep skin fold areas dry;
e. damage to the skin and/or subcutaneous tissue associated with:
   1. friction or shearing when moving in bed
   2. pressure on tissues as a result of excessive body weight and decreased activity.

Suggested NOC Outcomes: Tissue integrity: skin and mucous membranes; Wound healing: primary intention

Suggested NIC Interventions: Skin surveillance; Pressure management; Positioning; Wound care; Incision site care; Pressure ulcer prevention

Desired Outcomes	**Nursing Actions** *and Selected Purposes/Rationales* (see pp. 49–52 for additional rationales)
3.a. The client will experience normal healing of surgical wounds (see Standardized Postoperative Care Plan, Diagnosis 10, outcome a [p. 112], for outcome criteria).	3.a.1. Refer to Standardized Postoperative Care Plan, Diagnosis 10, action a (p. 112), for measures related to assessment and promotion of wound healing. 2. Implement measures to maintain an adequate nutritional status (see Postoperative Diagnosis 2, action d) *in order to further promote wound healing.*
3.b. The client will maintain tissue integrity as evidenced by: 1. absence of redness and irritation 2. no skin breakdown.	3.b.1. Inspect the following sites for pallor, redness, and breakdown: a. skin folds of abdomen and groin and under breasts b. skin areas in contact with wound drainage, tape, and tubings c. back, coccyx, and buttocks d. elbows and heels. 2. Refer to Standardized Postoperative Care Plan, Diagnosis 10, action b.2 (pp. 112–113), for measures to prevent tissue irritation and breakdown in areas in contact with wound drainage, tape, and tubings. 3. Implement additional measures *to reduce the risk for tissue breakdown:* a. assist client to turn at least every 2 hours when in bed; instruct and assist client to use overhead trapeze to lift self off the bed when moving

Desired Outcomes	**Nursing Actions** *and Selected Purposes/Rationales*

b. assist client to position self properly; use pressure-reducing or pressure-relieving devices (e.g., pillows, alternating pressure mattress, air-fluidized bed) if indicated
c. assist client with ambulation as ordered and as frequently as tolerated
d. perform actions to keep client from sliding down in bed (e.g., gatch knees slightly when head of bed is elevated 30° or higher) *in order to reduce the risk of skin surface abrasion and shearing*
e. gently massage heels, elbows, and around reddened areas at least every 2 hours
f. apply a thin layer of a dry lubricant such as powder or cornstarch to bottom sheet or skin and to opposing skin surfaces (e.g., axillae, beneath breasts, abdominal folds) if indicated *to reduce friction*
g. instruct and assist client to thoroughly dry skin after bathing and as often as needed, paying special attention to skin folds and opposing skin surfaces (e.g., axillae, perineum, beneath breasts); pat skin dry rather than rubbing
h. keep bed linens dry and wrinkle-free
i. perform actions *to reduce irritation resulting from friction and pressure on elbows and heels:*
   1. encourage client to use overhead trapeze to move self rather than pushing with heels and elbows
   2. provide elbow and heel protectors if indicated.

4. If tissue breakdown occurs:
   a. notify appropriate health care provider (e.g., physician, wound care specialist)
   b. perform care of involved areas as ordered or per standard hospital procedure.

4. COLLABORATIVE DIAGNOSES:

POTENTIAL COMPLICATIONS OF GASTRIC REDUCTION SURGERY

a. overdistention of the gastric pouch related to:
   1. accumulation of gas and fluid in the pouch associated with:
      a. decreased peristalsis and/or impaired functioning of nasogastric or gastrostomy tube
      b. obstruction of the pouch outlet (the channel between the pouch and distal stomach if gastroplasty performed or the opening between the pouch and jejunal loop if gastric bypass performed) resulting from edema and/or ingestion of medications or fluids that are too thick to pass through pouch outlet
   2. excessive oral intake;

b. peritonitis related to:
   1. wound infection
   2. leakage of gastric contents into the peritoneum associated with disruption of the staple line (if gastroplasty performed) or proximal anastomosis (if gastric bypass performed);

c. thromboembolism related to:
   1. venous stasis associated with decreased activity, increased blood viscosity (can result from deficient fluid volume), and pressure on abdominal vessels from excessive adipose tissue and abdominal distention
   2. hypercoagulability associated with increased release of thromboplastin into the blood (occurs as a result of surgical trauma) and hemoconcentration and increased blood viscosity (can occur as a result of deficient fluid volume)
   3. trauma to vein walls during surgery.

Desired Outcomes	Nursing Actions *and Selected Purposes/Rationales*
4.a. The client will not experience overdistention of the gastric pouch as evidenced by: 1. decreased reports of epigastric fullness 2. absence of nausea and vomiting.	4.a.1. Assess for and report signs and symptoms of overdistention of the gastric pouch (e.g., increasing reports of epigastric fullness, nausea, vomiting). 2. Implement measures *to prevent overdistention of the gastric pouch:* a. maintain patency of nasogastric or gastric tube *to reduce gas and fluid accumulation during period of decreased peristalsis;* irrigate the tube only if ordered and with no more than prescribed amount of solution b. encourage and assist client with frequent position changes and ambulation as soon as allowed and tolerated *(activity stimulates peristalsis)* c. instruct the client to avoid activities such as chewing gum and smoking *in order to reduce air swallowing* d. do not change position of nasogastric or gastric tube unless ordered *(the tube is usually positioned at the pouch outlet to help prevent obstruction of the opening into the distal stomach [if gastroplasty performed] or jejunal loop [if gastric bypass performed])* e. when oral intake is allowed: 1. adhere strictly to prescribed oral intake schedule (clients usually begin with hourly liquid feedings of 30 ml and, over at least 6 weeks, progress to 5 or 6 small [1–2 ounce] liquid meals/day with 1–2 ounces of water allowed periodically between meals) 2. provide client with allotted amounts of fluids at the proper times; discard skipped "meals" *so client does not ingest feedings too close together* 3. instruct client to adhere to the liquid or blenderized diet as ordered *(oral intake that is too thick can block the pouch outlet, which may be narrower in the early postoperative period because of edema)* 4. administer oral medication in liquid or chewable form or crushed thoroughly *to prevent blockage of the pouch outlet* f. encourage client to eructate whenever the urge is felt g. encourage use of nonnarcotic analgesics once severe pain has subsided *(narcotic [opioid] analgesics depress gastrointestinal motility).* 3. If signs and symptoms of overdistention occur: a. withhold all oral intake as ordered b. prepare client for upper abdominal x-rays to check placement of nasogastric or gastric tube if present c. assist physician with adjustment or reinsertion of the nasogastric or gastric tube if indicated.
4.b. The client will not develop peritonitis as evidenced by: 1. gradual resolution of abdominal pain 2. soft, nondistended abdomen 3. temperature declining toward normal 4. stable vital signs 5. absence of nausea and vomiting 6. gradual return of normal bowel sounds 7. WBC count declining toward normal.	4.b.1. Assess for and report signs and symptoms of peritonitis (e.g., increase in severity of abdominal pain; generalized abdominal pain; rebound tenderness; distended, rigid abdomen; increase in temperature; tachycardia; tachypnea; hypotension; nausea; vomiting; continued diminished or absent bowel sounds; WBC count that increases or fails to decline toward normal). 2. Implement measures *to prevent peritonitis:* a. perform actions to prevent wound infection (see Standardized Postoperative Care Plan, Diagnosis 17, action b.2 [pp. 118–119]) b. perform actions *to maintain patency of wound drain if present:* 1. keep tubing free of kinks 2. empty collection device as often as necessary 3. maintain suction as ordered c. perform actions *to prevent inadvertent removal of wound drain if present:* 1. use caution when changing dressing surrounding drain 2. provide extension tubing if necessary *to enable client to move without placing tension on the drain* 3. instruct client not to pull on drain and drainage tubing

Desired Outcomes	Nursing Actions *and Selected Purposes/Rationales*
	d. perform actions *to prevent stress on and subsequent leakage of gastric contents from the staple line or site of proximal anastomosis:* 1. implement measures to prevent overdistention of the gastric pouch (see action a.2 in this diagnosis) 2. implement measures *to prevent nausea and vomiting* (e.g., maintain patency of nasogastric or gastric tube, eliminate noxious sights and odors from the environment, instruct client to change positions slowly, administer antiemetics and/or gastrointestinal stimulants as ordered) 3. do not adjust position of nasogastric or gastric tube unless ordered *(adjustment may cause disruption of staples or perforation at site of proximal anastomosis).* 3. If signs and symptoms of peritonitis occur: a. withhold oral intake and jejunostomy tube feeding as ordered b. place client on bed rest in a semi-Fowler's position *to assist in pooling or localizing gastric contents in the pelvis rather than under the diaphragm* c. prepare client for diagnostic tests (e.g., abdominal x-ray, computed tomography, ultrasound) if planned d. assist physician with insertion of a nasogastric or gastric tube and maintain suction as ordered e. administer antimicrobials as ordered f. administer intravenous fluids and/or blood volume expanders if ordered *to prevent or treat shock (can result from the increased capillary permeability that occurs with inflammation and the subsequent escape of protein, fluid, and electrolytes from the vascular space into the peritoneal cavity)* g. prepare client for surgical intervention (e.g., repair of perforation) if planned.
4.c. The client will not develop a deep vein thrombus and pulmonary embolism (see Standardized Postoperative Care Plan, Diagnosis 20, outcomes c.1 and 2 [pp. 122–123], for outcome criteria).	4.c. Refer to Standardized Postoperative Care Plan, Diagnosis 20, actions c.1 and 2 (pp. 122–123), for measures related to assessment, prevention, and treatment of a deep vein thrombus and pulmonary embolism.

5. Nursing Diagnosis: ***INEFFECTIVE THERAPEUTIC REGIMEN MANAGEMENT***

related to lack of understanding of the implications of not following the prescribed treatment plan and difficulty integrating prescribed dietary modifications into lifestyle.

Suggested NOC Outcomes: Participation: health care decisions; Compliance behavior; Adherence behavior; Health beliefs: perceived ability to perform; Health beliefs: perceived control

Suggested NIC Interventions: Self-modification assistance; Weight reduction assistance; Teaching: prescribed diet; Behavior modification; Support system enhancement

Desired Outcome	**Nursing Actions** *and Selected Purposes/Rationales*
5. The client will demonstrate the probability of effective therapeutic regimen management as evidenced by: a. willingness to learn about and participate in treatments and care b. statements reflecting ways to integrate prescribed dietary plan and exercise program into lifestyle c. statements reflecting an understanding of the implications of not following the prescribed treatment plan.	5.a. Assess for indications that the client may be unable to effectively manage the therapeutic regimen: 1. failure to adhere to treatment plan while in hospital (e.g., not adhering to dietary modifications and fluid restrictions, refusing to increase activity) 2. statements reflecting a lack of understanding of dietary modifications and factors that will cause stretching of the gastric pouch 3. verbalization of an inability to integrate necessary dietary modifications and exercise program into lifestyle 4. statements reflecting the belief that the surgical procedure will result in continued weight loss even without adherence to the prescribed dietary modifications. b. Implement measures *to promote effective therapeutic regimen management:* 1. explain the surgical procedure and importance of dietary modifications and a balanced exercise program in terms the client can understand; emphasize that adherence to the treatment program is necessary if an optimal weight is to be attained 2. inform the client that prescribed food and fluid modifications are not as strict after the surgical area has healed (usually 6–8 weeks) 3. stress the positive effects of compliance with dietary modifications and exercise program (e.g., weight loss resulting in change in appearance; decreased risk of development or worsening of conditions such as diabetes mellitus, cardiovascular disease, respiratory problems, and arthritis) 4. provide a dietary consult to assist client in planning a dietary program based on prescribed modifications and client's personal and cultural preferences and daily routines 5. encourage activities other than eating to cope with stress (e.g., exercise) 6. initiate and reinforce the discharge teaching outlined in Postoperative Diagnosis 6 7. provide written instructions about future appointments with health care provider, dietary modifications, and signs and symptoms to report 8. provide information about and encourage utilization of community resources that can assist client to make necessary lifestyle changes (e.g., weight reduction groups, counseling services, support groups of persons who have had the same or similar surgery, stress management classes) 9. reinforce behaviors suggesting future compliance with the therapeutic regimen (e.g., statements reflecting plans for integrating dietary modifications into lifestyle, active participation in planning dietary program) 10. include significant others in explanations and teaching sessions and encourage their support; reinforce the need for client to assume responsibility for managing as much of care as possible. c. Consult physician regarding referrals to community agencies and/or support groups if continued instruction, support, or supervision is needed.

Discharge Teaching/Continued Care

6. NURSING DIAGNOSIS: **DEFICIENT KNOWLEDGE OR INEFFECTIVE HEALTH MAINTENANCE***

*The nurse should select the diagnostic label that is most appropriate for the client's discharge teaching needs.

Suggested NOC Outcomes:	Suggested NIC Interventions:
Knowledge: diet; Knowledge: treatment regimen	Health system guidance; Teaching: individual; Teaching: prescribed diet; Self-modification assistance; Support system enhancement

Desired Outcomes	**Nursing Actions** *and Selected Purposes/Rationales*
6.a. The client will identify ways to prevent excessive stretching of the gastric pouch.	6.a. Instruct client in ways to prevent excessive stretching of the gastric pouch: 1. decrease risk of blockage of the pouch outlet by: a. limiting oral intake to liquids and blenderized foods for about 6–8 weeks after surgery b. taking all prescription and nonprescription medications in liquid or chewable form or crushing them thoroughly c. chewing food thoroughly 2. do not exceed prescribed volume of food/fluid intake 3. do not make up for skipped meals while on an hourly drinking/eating schedule 4. eat and drink slowly 5. avoid intake of carbonated beverages for 6–8 weeks after surgery and limit intake of these beverages after that time 6. when solid foods are allowed, consume fluids between rather than with meals.
6.b. The client will verbalize an understanding of ways to maintain an adequate nutritional status.	6.b.1. Instruct client regarding ways to maintain an adequate nutritional status: a. do not skip meals b. consume foods/fluids from each food group daily as diet advances c. consume adequate amounts of protein (e.g., blenderized drinks containing peanut butter, pureed meats and fish, cottage cheese) as diet advances d. take vitamin and mineral supplements as prescribed. 2. Obtain dietary consult if indicated to assist client in planning meals.
6.c. The client will identify ways to reduce the risk of consuming excessive amounts of food, fluid, and calories.	6.c. Instruct client in ways to reduce the risk of consuming excessive amounts of food, fluid, and calories: 1. limit food/fluid intake to prescribed volume 2. prepare food ahead of time, freeze in 1-ounce portions using plastic ice cube trays or plastic bags, and then reheat only allowed amounts at mealtime 3. have jars of prepared strained baby food products rather than high-calorie puddings and snacks on hand 4. have only low-calorie drinks available (other than the required high-protein supplements) 5. decrease the risk of hunger by adhering to a schedule of 5 or 6 meals/day as diet advances (each meal will usually consist of 2–4 tablespoons of food) 6. serve food on a small plate (this provides an illusion that meals are larger than they really are) 7. eat and drink very slowly (use techniques such as putting fork down between bites of food and putting glass down between sips of fluid) 8. if going out to dinner, order an appetizer and have it served with everyone else's entrée 9. avoid excessive intake of high-calorie foods/fluids (it is possible to maintain or gain weight if only high-calorie substances are consumed).
6.d. The client will demonstrate the ability to accurately calculate and measure the allotted amounts of food and fluid.	6.d.1. Demonstrate ways to measure foods/fluids accurately using measuring spoons and a cup with 1-ounce markings. 2. Allow time for questions, clarification, and return demonstration.

6.e. The client will state signs and symptoms to report to the health care provider.	6.e.1. Refer to Standardized Postoperative Care Plan, Diagnosis 22, action c (p. 125), for signs and symptoms to report to the health care provider. 2. Instruct client to also report: a. nausea and vomiting after consuming prescribed amount of foods/fluids b. inability to adhere to dietary modifications c. weight gain d. inability to lose weight or excessive weight loss (expected weight loss is usually about 10 pounds/month for the 1st year or 30% of preoperative body weight by the end of the 1st year) e. abdominal cramping, flushing, palpitations, weakness, and/or dizziness within 30 minutes after eating (indicative of dumping syndrome, which sometimes occurs when a client who has had a gastric bypass begins to eat solid food; if dumping syndrome does occur, symptoms are usually mild and self-limiting or easily controlled with minor dietary modifications).
6.f. The client will identify community resources that can assist in the adjustment to prescribed dietary modifications and future changes in body image.	6.f.1. Provide information about community resources that can assist the client with adjustment to prescribed dietary modifications and future changes in body image (e.g., weight reduction groups, counseling services, support groups of persons who have had the same or similar surgery). 2. Initiate a referral if indicated.
6.g. The client will verbalize an understanding of and a plan for adhering to recommended follow-up care including future appointments with health care provider, activity level, medications prescribed, and wound care.	6.g.1. Refer to Standardized Postoperative Care Plan, Diagnosis 22 (pp. 125–126), for routine postoperative instructions. 2. Reinforce the physician's instructions regarding need to adhere to a schedule of moderate exercise (clients are usually instructed to begin a walking program and should be walking 1–2 miles/day by the 4th week after discharge). 3. Refer to Postoperative Diagnosis 5, action b, for measures to promote the client's ability to effectively manage the therapeutic regimen.

Bibliography

See pages 879 and 884.

evolve

Gastrointestinal (GI) Bleed, Acute Upper

Upper GI bleeding accounts for a significant number of hospital admissions each year. Ulcers in the stomach or duodenum are the major cause of GI bleeding. Other causes include esophageal varices, erosive esophagitis or gastritis, gastric cancer, Mallory-Weiss tears, regular use of ulcerogenic medications such as corticosteroids and nonsteroidal anti-inflammatory drugs (NSAIDs), vascular anomalies (e.g., angiodysplasia), and certain blood dyscrasias (e.g., leukemia, aplastic anemia).

The severity of the bleed ranges from slight oozing to frank, profuse hemorrhage and depends on whether the source is arterial, venous, or capillary. Significant bleeding is almost always arterial in nature. A massive GI bleed is generally considered to be a loss of more than 1500 ml of blood. Hematemesis of bright red or "coffee ground" vomitus is often the initial symptom of an upper GI bleed. Melena (dark, tarry stools) can also indicate upper GI bleeding that is occurring at a slower rate.

The majority of people who experience a GI bleed spontaneously stop bleeding. However, treatment is initiated immediately in cases of massive bleeding and consists of endoscopic hemostasis of the bleeding vessel. Vasoactive medications such as epinephrine, octreotide, or vasopressin may also be administered to help stop the bleeding. Gastric lavage may be done prior to endoscopy to remove blood from the stomach and improve endoscopic visualization. If bleeding continues, surgery may be necessary. Subsequent treatment to prevent rebleeding depends on the cause of the bleeding.

This care plan focuses on the adult client hospitalized with a massive upper GI bleed. It should be used in conjunction with the care plans on Peptic Ulcer and Cirrhosis if it is determined that the client's bleed is associated with either of these conditions.

OUTCOME/DISCHARGE CRITERIA

THE CLIENT WILL:

- have adequate tissue perfusion
- tolerate prescribed activity without a significant change in vital signs, chest pain, dizziness, or extreme fatigue or weakness
- have no signs and symptoms of complications
- identify ways to reduce the risk for rebleeding
- state signs and symptoms to report to the health care provider
- verbalize an understanding of and a plan for adhering to recommended follow-up care including future appointments with health care provider, medications prescribed, and dietary restrictions.

NURSING/COLLABORATIVE DIAGNOSES

DISCHARGE TEACHING

See p. 635 and Care Plans on Peptic Ulcer (pp. 658–665) and Cirrhosis (pp. 681–701) for additional diagnoses.

1. Nursing Diagnosis: *INEFFECTIVE TISSUE PERFUSION*

related to hypovolemia associated with gastrointestinal bleeding.

Suggested NOC Outcomes:
Circulation status; Tissue perfusion: abdominal organs; Tissue perfusion: cardiac; Tissue perfusion: cerebral; Tissue perfusion: peripheral; Tissue perfusion: pulmonary

Suggested NIC Interventions: Circulatory Care: arterial insufficiency; Circulatory care: venous insufficiency; Cerebral perfusion promotion; Hypovolemia

Desired Outcome	Nursing Actions *and Selected Purposes/Rationales* (see pp. 57–59 for additional rationales)
1. The client will maintain adequate tissue perfusion as evidenced by: a. B/P within normal range and stable with position change b. usual mental status c. extremities warm with absence of pallor and cyanosis d. palpable peripheral pulses e. capillary refill time less than 2–3 seconds f. BUN and serum creatinine within normal limits g. urine output at least 30 ml/hour.	1.a. Assess for and report signs and symptoms of diminished tissue perfusion: 1. decreased blood pressure 2. decline in systolic B/P of more than 15 mm Hg when client changes from a lying to a sitting or standing position 3. restlessness, confusion, or other change in mental status 4. reports of dizziness or lightheadedness or occurrence of syncopal episodes 5. cool, pale, or cyanotic skin 6. diminished or absent peripheral pulses 7. capillary refill time greater than 2–3 seconds 8. elevated BUN and serum creatinine 9. oliguria. b. Implement measures *to maintain adequate tissue perfusion:* 1. administer intravenous fluids and blood as ordered 2. perform actions to prevent or treat deficient fluid volume (see Diagnosis 2, action b) 3. prepare client for measures which may be performed *to control bleeding:* a. endoscopic thermocoagulation, sclerotherapy, or banding of bleeding varices b. intra-arterial or intravenous administration of vasoactive medications (e.g., epinephrine, octreotide, vasopressin) c. surgery 4. administer the following medications if ordered *to reduce the risk of rebleeding:* a. proton-pump inhibitors (e.g., omeprazole, lansoprazole, pantoprazole, esomeprazole) b. histamine$_2$ receptor antagonists (e.g., famotidine, ranitidine, nizatidine) 5. instruct client to change from a supine to an upright position slowly *(allows time for autoregulatory mechanisms to adjust to the change in distribution of blood associated with an upright position)* 6. maintain a comfortable room temperature and provide client with adequate clothing and blankets *(exposure to cold causes generalized vasoconstriction).* c. Consult appropriate health care provider if signs and symptoms of diminished tissue perfusion persist or worsen.

2. NURSING DIAGNOSIS: *RISK FOR IMBALANCED FLUID AND ELECTROLYTES*

a. deficient fluid volume related to blood loss, decreased oral intake, and loss of fluid associated with vomiting and nasogastric tube drainage;

b. hypokalemia, hypochloremia, and metabolic alkalosis related to loss of electrolytes and hydrochloric acid associated with vomiting and nasogastric tube drainage.

Suggested NOC Outcomes:
Fluid balance; Electrolyte and acid/base balance

Suggested NIC Interventions: Fluid monitoring; Fluid management; Electrolyte management: hypokalemia; Fluid/Electrolyte management; Acid-base monitoring; Acid-base management: metabolic alkalosis

Desired Outcome

Nursing Actions *and Selected Purposes/Rationales*
(see pp. 30–31 for additional rationales)

2. The client will maintain fluid and electrolyte balance as evidenced by:
   a. normal skin turgor
   b. moist mucous membranes
   c. stable weight
   d. B/P and pulse within normal range for client and stable with position change
   e. capillary refill time less than 2–3 seconds
   f. usual mental status
   g. balanced intake and output
   h. urine specific gravity within normal range
   i. soft, nondistended abdomen with normal bowel sounds
   j. absence of cardiac dysrhythmias, muscle weakness, paresthesias, twitching, spasms, and dizziness
   k. BUN, Hct, serum electrolytes, and blood gases within normal range.

2.a. Assess for and report signs and symptoms of:
   1. deficient fluid volume:
      a. decreased skin turgor, dry mucous membranes, thirst
      b. weight loss of 2% or greater over a short period
      c. postural hypotension and/or low B/P
      d. weak, rapid pulse
      e. capillary refill time greater than 2–3 seconds
      f. flat neck veins when supine
      g. change in mental status
      h. decreased urine output with increased specific gravity (reflects an actual rather than a potential fluid deficit)
      i. increased BUN and Hct
   2. hypokalemia (e.g., cardiac dysrhythmias, postural hypotension, muscle weakness, nausea and vomiting, abdominal distention, hypoactive or absent bowel sounds, low serum potassium)
   3. hypochloremia and metabolic alkalosis (e.g., dizziness, paresthesias, muscle twitching or spasms, hypoventilation, low serum chloride, elevated pH and TCO_2).

b. Implement measures *to prevent or treat imbalanced fluid and electrolytes:*
   1. perform actions *to prevent nausea and vomiting:*
      a. insert nasogastric tube and maintain suction and/or perform gastric lavage if ordered *(removal of blood from the stomach reduces the stimulus to vomit)*
      b. administer antiemetics if ordered
   2. if gastric lavage is being done or nasogastric tube is being irrigated frequently with large volumes of solution, consult physician about using saline rather than water *(water is sometimes preferred because it breaks up clots better than saline, but irrigation with large volumes of water may create electrolyte imbalances)*
   3. administer intravenous fluid and electrolytes as ordered
   4. once oral intake is allowed, maintain a fluid intake of at least 2500 ml/day unless contraindicated.

c. Consult physician if signs and symptoms of imbalanced fluid and electrolytes persist or worsen.

RISK FOR ASPIRATION

related to hematemesis and possible decreased level of consciousness.

Suggested NOC Outcomes: Respiratory status: airway patency; Respiratory status: gas exchange

Suggested NIC Interventions: Respiratory monitoring; Aspiration precautions; Airway suctioning

Desired Outcome

Nursing Actions *and Selected Purposes/Rationales*
(see pp. 16–18 for additional rationales)

3. The client will not aspirate as evidenced by:
   a. clear breath sounds
   b. resonant percussion note over lungs
   c. absence of cough, tachypnea, and dyspnea.

3.a. Assess for and report signs and symptoms of aspiration (e.g., rhonchi, dull percussion note over affected lung area, cough, tachypnea, dyspnea, tachycardia, chest x-ray results showing pulmonary infiltrate).

b. Implement measures *to reduce the risk for aspiration:*
   1. keep head of bed elevated at least 45° if vital signs are stable or position client on side (if client is hypotensive, elevating the head of bed is contraindicated)
   2. perform actions to prevent nausea and vomiting (see Diagnosis 2, action b.1)
   3. withhold oral foods/fluids as ordered

4. perform oropharyngeal suctioning and provide oral hygiene as often as needed *to remove blood and vomitus.*

c. If signs and symptoms of aspiration occur:
   1. perform tracheal suctioning
   2. withhold oral intake
   3. prepare client for chest x-ray.

4. NURSING DIAGNOSIS:

RISK FOR ACTIVITY INTOLERANCE

related to:

a. hypoxia associated with anemia resulting from blood loss;
b. difficulty resting and sleeping associated with frequent assessments and treatments, fear, and anxiety.

Suggested NOC Outcomes: Activity tolerance; Energy conservation; Self-care: activities of daily living

Suggested NIC Interventions: Energy management; Oxygen therapy; Sleep enhancement

Desired Outcome

4. The client will not experience activity intolerance as evidenced by:
   a. no reports of fatigue or weakness
   b. ability to perform activities of daily living without exertional dyspnea, chest pain, diaphoresis, dizziness, and a significant change in vital signs.

Nursing Actions *and Selected Purposes/Rationales*
(see pp. 11–12 for additional rationales)

4.a. Assess for signs and symptoms of activity intolerance:
   1. statements of fatigue or weakness
   2. exertional dyspnea, cheat pain, diaphoresis, or dizziness
   3. abnormal heart rate response to activity (e.g., increase in rate of 20 beats/minute above resting rate, rate not returning to preactivity level within 3 minutes after stopping activity, change from regular to irregular rate)
   4. a significant change (15–20 mm Hg) in blood pressure with activity.

b. Implement measures *to prevent activity intolerance:*
   1. perform actions *to promote rest and/or conserve energy:*
      a. maintain activity restrictions as ordered
      b. minimize environmental activity and noise
      c. organize nursing care to allow for periods of uninterrupted rest
      d. limit the number of visitors and their length of stay
      e. assist client with self-care activities as needed
      f. keep supplies and personal articles within easy reach
      g. instruct client in energy-saving techniques (e.g., using shower chair when showering, sitting to brush teeth or comb hair)
      h. implement measures *to reduce fear and anxiety* (e.g., explain diagnostic tests and planned procedures; maintain a calm, confident manner when working with client)
      i. implement measures *to promote sleep* (e.g., allow client to continue usual sleep practices unless contraindicated, reduce environmental distractions, administer prescribed sedative-hypnotics)
   2. administer the following if ordered *to treat anemia:*
      a. iron supplements
      b. packed red blood cells
   3. maintain oxygen therapy as ordered
   4. increase client's activity gradually as allowed and tolerated.

c. Instruct client to:
   1. report a decreased tolerance for activity
   2. stop any activity that causes chest pain, shortness of breath, dizziness, or extreme fatigue or weakness.

d. Consult appropriate health care provider if signs and symptoms of activity intolerance develop and persist or worsen.

5. COLLABORATIVE DIAGNOSIS:

POTENTIAL COMPLICATION OF GI BLEEDING: HYPOVOLEMIC SHOCK

related to excessive loss of blood.

Desired Outcome	Nursing Actions *and Selected Purposes/Rationales*
5. The client will not develop hypovolemic shock as evidenced by: a. usual mental status b. stable vital signs c. skin warm and usual color d. palpable peripheral pulses e. urine output at least 30 ml/hour.	5.a. Assess for and report signs and symptoms of hypovolemic shock: 1. restlessness, agitation, confusion, or other change in mental status 2. significant decrease in B/P 3. postural hypotension 4. rapid, weak pulse 5. rapid respirations 6. cool skin 7. pallor, cyanosis 8. diminished or absent peripheral pulses 9. urine output less than 30 ml/hour. b. Implement measures to control bleeding (see Diagnosis 1, action b.3) *in order to reduce the risk for hypovolemic shock.* c. If signs and symptoms of hypovolemic shock occur: 1. place the client flat in bed with legs elevated unless contraindicated 2. monitor vital signs frequently 3. administer oxygen as ordered 4. administer blood products and/or volume expanders as ordered 5. prepare client for insertion of hemodynamic monitoring devices (e.g., central venous catheter, intra-arterial catheter) if planned.

Discharge Teaching/Continued Care

6. Nursing Diagnosis: DEFICIENT KNOWLEDGE, INEFFECTIVE THERAPEUTIC REGIMEN MANAGEMENT, OR INEFFECTIVE HEALTH MAINTENANCE*

*The nurse should select the diagnostic label that is most appropriate for the client's discharge teaching needs.

Suggested NOC Outcomes: Knowledge: disease process; Knowledge: treatment regimen

Suggested NIC Interventions: Health system guidance; Teaching: individual; Teaching: disease process; Teaching: prescribed diet; Teaching: prescribed medication

Desired Outcomes	Nursing Actions *and Selected Purposes/Rationales*
6.a. The client will identify ways to reduce the risk for rebleeding.	6.a.1. If client's bleed is associated with an ulcer, refer to Care Plan on Peptic Ulcer, Diagnosis 3, actions b and c (pp. 662–664), for teaching regarding ways to promote healing of the ulcer and prevent ulcer recurrence. 2. Provide additional instructions regarding ways to reduce the risk for rebleeding: a. instruct client to avoid activities that increase intra-abdominal pressure (e.g., straining to have a bowel movement, coughing, sneezing, lifting heavy objects) b. inform client that he/she should avoid vigorous exercise or activities that may result in traumatic injury to the abdomen (e.g., contact sports) for at least 4–6 weeks.
6.b. The client will state signs and symptoms to report to the health care provider.	6.b. Instruct client to report: 1. bloody or "coffee-ground" vomitus 2. black or tarry stools 3. persistent epigastric fullness or bloating, nausea, and/or vomiting 4. abdominal distention 5. persistent or increased epigastric or abdominal pain 6. persistent weakness and fatigue.

6.c. The client will verbalize an understanding of and a plan for adhering to recommended follow-up care including future appointments with health care provider, medications prescribed, and dietary restrictions.

6.c.1. Reinforce the importance of keeping follow-up appointments with health care provider.
2. Explain the rationale for, side effects of, and importance of taking medications prescribed (e.g., proton-pump inhibitors, histamine$_2$ receptor antagonists, iron supplement). Inform client of pertinent food and drug interactions.
3. Reinforce physician's instructions regarding dietary restrictions such as caffeinated beverages, alcohol, and spicy foods.
4. Provide written instructions about future appointments with health care provider, medications prescribed, dietary restrictions, and signs and symptoms to report.

ADDITIONAL NURSING DIAGNOSIS

FEAR/ANXIETY*

related to presence of large amount of blood in vomitus and nasogastric tube drainage; concern that bleeding may not be controlled; lack of understanding of the cause of the bleeding, diagnostic tests, treatment plan, and prognosis; unfamiliar environment; and possible need to change lifestyle in order to prevent rebleeding.

*See Unit II for outcomes, actions, and rationales.

Bibliography

See pages 879 and 884.

evolve

Inflammatory Bowel Disease: Ulcerative Colitis and Crohn's Disease

Crohn's disease and ulcerative colitis are idiopathic chronic inflammatory bowel diseases, which are often jointly referred to as inflammatory bowel disease (IBD). These disorders have similarities but can usually be differentiated by clinical, radiological, and pathologic findings. The classic clinical manifestations of inflammatory bowel disease include diarrhea, abdominal pain and cramping, and fever. The severity and pattern of signs and symptoms depend on the portion(s) of the bowel affected and depth of bowel wall involvement. Ulcerative colitis primarily involves the mucosa of the bowel wall, extending to the submucosa only in severe cases. It typically starts in the rectum and sigmoid colon and progresses in a continuous pattern through the colon. It rarely involves the small intestine. Crohn's disease can occur anywhere in the gastrointestinal tract. The most frequent sites of involvement are the terminal ileum and right colon. The entire thickness of the bowel wall is involved and it has a segmental, discontinuous pattern of progression.

Clients with either condition may experience a number of the same complications; however, those with ulcerative colitis have a higher incidence of toxic megacolon and bowel perforation, whereas clients with Crohn's disease have a higher incidence of perianal involvement and fistula formation. Some clients also experience extraintestinal manifestations such as liver and biliary involvement; kidney stones; arthritis; and skin, eye, and oral lesions. Clients with inflammatory bowel disease may require hospitalization during periods of exacerbation or if complications are suspected.

Cornerstones of medical treatment have traditionally included corticosteroids, sulfasalazine, nonsulfa-aminosalicylates, and immunomodulator agents such as azathioprine and mercaptopurine. Research indicates that there may be a defect in immunoregulation of inflammation in Crohn's disease. This has lead to the use of monoclonal antibodies that neutralize a cytokine (specifically tumor necrosis factor-alpha) to treat persons with Crohn's disease who have not been responsive to conventional therapy or who have draining enterocutaneous fistulas.

This care plan focuses on the adult client with severe abdominal pain and diarrhea who is hospitalized for medical management of inflammatory bowel disease. Much of the information is applicable to clients receiving follow-up care in an extended care facility or home setting.

OUTCOME/DISCHARGE CRITERIA

THE CLIENT WILL:

- have decreased abdominal pain
- have fewer episodes of diarrhea
- tolerate prescribed diet and have an improved nutritional status
- be free of signs and symptoms of complications
- identify ways to reduce the incidence of disease exacerbation
- verbalize ways to maintain an optimal nutritional status
- state ways to prevent perianal skin breakdown
- verbalize an understanding of medications ordered including rationale, food and drug interactions, side effects, schedule for taking, and importance of taking as prescribed
- state signs and symptoms to report to the health care provider
- identify resources that can assist in the adjustment to changes resulting from inflammatory bowel disease and its treatment
- share feelings and thoughts about the effects of inflammatory bowel disease on lifestyle and self-concept
- verbalize an understanding of and a plan for adhering to recommended follow-up care including future appointments with health care provider and activity level.

NURSING/COLLABORATIVE DIAGNOSES

1. Risk for imbalanced fluid and electrolytes p. 637
   a. deficient fluid volume, hypokalemia, hypomagnesemia, and hypocalcemia
   b. metabolic acidosis
2. Imbalanced nutrition: less than body requirements p. 638
3. Acute/Chronic pain p. 639
   a. abdominal pain and cramping
   b. joint pain
   c. perianal pain
4. Risk for impaired tissue integrity p. 640
5. Hyperthermia p. 641
6. Activity intolerance p. 642
7. Diarrhea p. 643
8. Risk for infection p. 644
9. Potential complications p. 645
   a. renal calculi
   b. perirectal, rectovaginal, enterovesical, and enteroenteric abscesses and fistulas
   c. toxic megacolon
   d. bowel obstruction
   e. peritonitis
10. Ineffective coping p. 648

DISCHARGE TEACHING

11. Deficient knowledge, Ineffective therapeutic regimen management, or Ineffective health maintenance p. 649

See p. 651 for additional diagnoses.

RISK FOR IMBALANCED FLUID AND ELECTROLYTES

a. deficient fluid volume, hypokalemia, hypomagnesemia, and hypocalcemia related to:
   1. prolonged inadequate oral intake associated with pain, fatigue, prescribed dietary restrictions, and fear of precipitating an attack of abdominal cramping and diarrhea
   2. impaired absorption of fluid and electrolytes associated with inflammation and scarring of the intestine
   3. excessive loss of fluid and electrolytes associated with persistent diarrhea (loss of potassium can also occur as a result of treatment with corticosteroids);

b. metabolic acidosis related to excessive loss of bicarbonate associated with persistent diarrhea.

Suggested NOC Outcomes: Fluid balance; Electrolyte and acid/base balance

Suggested NIC Interventions: Fluid management; Electrolyte management: hypokalemia; Electrolyte management: hypocalcemia; Electrolyte management: hypomagnesemia; Acid-base management: metabolic acidosis; Diarrhea management

Desired Outcome	Nursing Actions and Selected Purposes/Rationales (see pp. 30–31 for additional rationales)
1. The client will maintain fluid and electrolyte balance as evidenced by: a. normal skin turgor b. moist mucous membranes c. stable weight	1.a. Assess for and report signs and symptoms of: 1. deficient fluid volume: a. decreased skin turgor, dry mucous membranes, thirst b. weight loss of 2% or greater over a short period c. postural hypotension and/or low B/P d. weak, rapid pulse e. capillary refill time longer than 2–3 seconds

Desired Outcome	Nursing Actions *and Selected Purposes/Rationales*
d. B/P and pulse within normal range for client and stable with position change e. capillary refill time less than 2–3 seconds f. usual mental status g. balanced intake and output h. urine specific gravity within normal range i. soft, nondistended abdomen with active bowel sounds j. absence of cardiac dysrhythmias, muscle weakness, paresthesias, and seizure activity k. absence of headache, nausea, and vomiting l. negative Chvostek's and Trousseau's signs m. serum electrolytes and blood gases within normal range.	f. neck veins flat when client is supine g. change in mental status h. decreased urine output with increased specific gravity (reflects an actual rather than potential fluid deficit) i. significant increase in BUN and Hct above previous levels 2. hypokalemia (e.g., cardiac dysrhythmias, postural hypotension, muscle weakness, nausea and vomiting, abdominal distention, hypoactive or absent bowel sounds, low serum potassium) 3. hypomagnesemia and/or hypocalcemia (e.g., anxiousness; irritability; cardiac dysrhythmias; positive Chvostek's and Trousseau's signs; numbness or tingling of fingers, toes, or circumoral area; hyperactive reflexes; tetany; seizures; low serum magnesium; low serum calcium) 4. metabolic acidosis (e.g., drowsiness; disorientation; stupor; rapid, deep respirations; headache; nausea and vomiting; cardiac dysrhythmias; low pH and CO_2 content). b. Implement measures *to prevent or treat imbalanced fluid and electrolytes:* 1. perform actions to control diarrhea (see Diagnosis 7, action b) 2. maintain a fluid intake of at least 2500 ml/day unless contraindicated; if oral intake is inadequate or contraindicated, maintain intravenous and/or enteral fluid therapy as ordered 3. when oral intake is allowed: a. perform actions to improve oral intake (see Diagnosis 2, action c.4.c) b. assist client to select foods/fluids within the prescribed dietary regimen that would replenish electrolytes (be aware that many foods/fluids high in potassium and magnesium are contraindicated on a low-residue diet): 1. foods high in potassium (e.g., bananas, avocado, raisins, potatoes, cantaloupe) 2. foods high in magnesium (e.g., seafood) 4. administer the following if ordered: a. electrolyte replacements (e.g., potassium chloride, magnesium sulfate, calcium gluconate, calcium carbonate) b. vitamin D preparations *to increase intestinal absorption of calcium.* c. If signs and symptoms of hypomagnesemia or hypocalcemia occur, institute seizure precautions. d. Consult physician if signs and symptoms of imbalanced fluid and electrolytes persist or worsen.

2. NURSING DIAGNOSIS: *IMBALANCED NUTRITION: LESS THAN BODY REQUIREMENTS*

related to:

a. decreased oral intake associated with pain, fatigue, prescribed dietary restrictions, and the knowledge that eating often precipitates abdominal cramping and diarrhea;
b. decreased absorption of nutrients associated with inflammation and scarring of the bowel;
c. loss of nutrients associated with diarrhea and protein exudation from the inflamed bowel;
d. impaired folate absorption associated with treatment with sulfasalazine;
e. increased metabolism of nutrients associated with the increased metabolic rate that may be present during periods of exacerbation.

Suggested NOC Outcome: Nutritional status

Suggested NIC Interventions: Nutritional monitoring; Nutrition management; Nutrition therapy; Total parenteral nutrition (TPN) administration; Enteral tube feeding

Desired Outcome	Nursing Actions *and Selected Purposes/Rationales* (see pp. 40–43 for additional rationales)
2. The client will have an improved nutritional status as evidenced by: a. weight approaching a normal range for client b. improved BUN and serum prealbumin, albumin, Hct, Hgb, folate, and lymphocyte levels c. increased strength and activity tolerance d. healthy oral mucous membrane.	2.a. Assess for signs and symptoms of malnutrition: 1. weight significantly below client's normal or below normal for client's age, height, and body frame 2. abnormal BUN and low serum prealbumin, albumin, Hct, Hgb, folate, and lymphocyte levels 3. weakness and fatigue 4. sore, inflamed oral mucous membrane 5. pale conjunctiva. b. When oral intake is allowed, monitor the percentage of meals and snacks client consumes. Report a pattern of inadequate intake. c. Implement measures *to improve nutritional status:* 1. administer total parenteral nutrition or enteral tube feeding if ordered 2. perform actions to reduce inflammation and hypermotility of the bowel (see Diagnosis 7, action b) *in order to reduce episodes of diarrhea and increase absorption of nutrients* 3. maintain activity restrictions as ordered (usually bed rest with bedside commode or bathroom privileges) *to reduce caloric requirements* 4. when food or fluid is allowed: a. provide elemental formulas (e.g., Vivonex, Criticare HN) if ordered (these formulas are high in calories and nutrients, free of lactose and fiber, and absorbed in the proximal small bowel) b. progress diet as tolerated (usual progression is from elemental formulas to a low-residue, high-calorie, high-protein diet) c. perform actions *to improve oral intake:* 1. implement measures to reduce pain (see Diagnosis 3, action e) 2. encourage a rest period before meals *to minimize fatigue* 3. maintain a clean environment and a relaxed, pleasant atmosphere 4. provide oral hygiene before meals *(oral hygiene removes unpleasant tastes, which often improves the taste of foods/fluids)* 5. implement measures *to improve the palatability of elemental formulas* (e.g., offer a variety of flavors, serve chilled) 6. obtain a dietary consult if necessary to assist client in selecting foods/fluids that are appealing and adhere to personal and cultural preferences as well as the prescribed dietary modifications 7. serve frequent, small meals rather than large ones if client is weak, fatigues easily, or has a poor appetite 8. allow adequate time for meals; reheat foods/fluids if necessary 5. administer the following if ordered: a. iron preparations (oral iron preparations may not be effective during an acute attack *because they may be poorly absorbed from the inflamed bowel)* b. vitamin preparations (e.g., fat-soluble vitamins, vitamin B_{12}, folic acid). d. Perform a calorie count if ordered. Report information to dietitian and physician. e. Consult physician if nutritional status continues to decline.

3. Nursing Diagnosis: ACUTE/CHRONIC PAIN

a. abdominal pain and cramping related to:
   1. inflammation and ulceration of the bowel
   2. interference with the flow of intestinal contents associated with narrowing of the intestinal lumen as a result of inflammation and hypertrophy and fibrosis of the bowel wall if present;

b. joint pain related to extraintestinal involvement of the joints (peripheral arthritis, ankylosing spondylitis, and sacroiliitis are the most common joint disorders that occur);

c. perianal pain related to irritation and breakdown of skin in the perianal area associated with persistent diarrhea and/or the presence of an anorectal abscess or fistula.

Suggested NOC Outcomes: Comfort level; Pain control

Suggested NIC Interventions: Pain management; Environmental management: comfort; Analgesic administration

Desired Outcome	Nursing Actions and Selected Purposes/Rationales (see pp. 45–47 for additional rationales)
3. The client will experience diminished pain as evidenced by: a. verbalization of same b. relaxed facial expression and body positioning c. increased participation in activities d. stable vital signs.	3.a. Assess for signs and symptoms of pain (e.g., verbalization of pain; grimacing; reluctance to move; rubbing abdomen, back, or joints; restlessness; diaphoresis; increased B/P; tachycardia). b. Assess client's perception of the severity of pain using a pain intensity rating scale. c. Assess the client's pain pattern (e.g., location, quality, onset, duration, precipitating factors, aggravating factors, alleviating factors). d. Ask the client to describe previous pain experiences and methods used to manage pain effectively. e. Implement measures *to reduce pain:* 1. perform actions *to reduce fear and anxiety about the pain experience* (e.g., assure client that his/her need for pain relief is understood, plan methods for achieving pain control with client) 2. administer analgesics before activities and procedures that can cause pain and before pain becomes severe 3. perform actions to promote rest (e.g., minimize environmental activity and noise, limit number of visitors and their length of stay) *in order to reduce fatigue and subsequently increase the client's threshold and tolerance for pain* 4. perform actions to reduce inflammation and hypermotility of the bowel (see Diagnosis 7, action b) *in order to reduce abdominal pain and cramping* 5. consult physician regarding measures *to help relieve joint pain if present* (e.g., application of brace/splint to affected joint, application of heat to affected joint) 6. perform actions *to relieve perianal pain if present:* a. implement measures to control diarrhea (see Diagnosis 7, action b) b. clean perianal area with medicated wipes such as Tucks after each bowel movement c. apply protective ointment or cream to perianal area after each bowel movement d. consult physician about order for sitz baths e. apply anesthetic preparation (e.g., Nupercainal, Tronolane) to perianal area or into rectum if ordered f. administer corticosteroid foam or enema or mesalamine suppository or enema if ordered 7. provide or assist with nonpharmacologic measures for pain relief (e.g., position change; relaxation exercises; restful environment; diversional activities such as watching television, reading, or conversing) 8. administer analgesics if ordered (narcotic [opioid] analgesics must be administered judiciously *because they slow gastrointestinal motility and can cause toxic megacolon*). f. Consult appropriate health care provider (e.g., pharmacist, physician) if above measures fail to provide adequate pain relief.

RISK FOR IMPAIRED TISSUE INTEGRITY

related to:

a. damage to the skin and/or subcutaneous tissue associated with prolonged pressure on the tissues, friction, and shearing that can occur when mobility is decreased;

b. frequent contact with irritants associated with persistent diarrhea;
c. increased fragility of skin associated with malnutrition.

Suggested NOC Outcome: Tissue integrity: skin and mucous membrane

Suggested NIC Interventions: Skin surveillance; Skin care: topical treatments; Pressure management

Desired Outcome	**Nursing Actions** *and Selected Purposes/Rationales* (see pp. 49–52 for additional rationales)
4. The client will maintain tissue integrity as evidenced by: a. absence of redness and irritation b. no skin breakdown.	4.a. Inspect the skin (especially bony prominences, dependent areas, and perianal area) for pallor, redness, and breakdown. b. Implement measures *to prevent tissue breakdown:* 1. instruct and/or assist client to turn at least every 2 hours 2. position client properly; use pressure-reducing or pressure-relieving devices (e.g., pillows, gel or foam cushions, alternating pressure mattress, air-fluidized bed) if indicated 3. gently massage around reddened areas at least every 2 hours 4. apply a thin layer of a dry lubricant such as powder or cornstarch to bottom sheet or skin and to opposing skin surfaces if indicated *to reduce friction* 5. perform actions to keep client from sliding down in bed (e.g., gatch knees slightly when head of bed is elevated 30° or higher, limit length of time client is in semi-Fowler's position to 30 minute intervals) *in order to reduce the risk for skin surface abrasion and shearing* 6. instruct or assist client to shift weight at least every 30 minutes 7. keep client's skin clean 8. keep bed linens dry and wrinkle-free 9. increase activity as allowed and tolerated 10. perform actions to improve nutritional status (see Diagnosis 2, action c) 11. perform actions *to prevent skin irritation resulting from diarrhea:* a. implement measures to control diarrhea (see Diagnosis 7, action b) b. assist client to gently cleanse and dry perianal area with a soft tissue or cloth after each bowel movement; apply a protective ointment or cream c. if use of absorbent products such as pads or undergarments is necessary, select those that effectively absorb moisture and keep it away from the skin 12. apply a protective covering such as a hydrocolloid or transparent membrane dressing to areas of the skin susceptible to breakdown (e.g., coccyx). c. If tissue breakdown occurs: 1. notify appropriate health care provider (e.g., physician, wound care specialist) 2. perform care of involved areas as ordered or per standard hospital procedure.

5. NURSING DIAGNOSIS: HYPERTHERMIA

related to stimulation of the thermoregulatory center in the hypothalamus by endogenous pyrogens that are released in an inflammatory process.

Suggested NOC Outcome: Thermoregulation

Suggested NIC Intervention: Fever treatment

Desired Outcome	Nursing Actions and Selected Purposes/Rationales
5. The client will experience resolution of hyperthermia as evidenced by: a. skin usual temperature and color b. pulse rate between 60–100 beats/minute c. respirations 12–20/minute d. normal body temperature.	5.a. Assess for signs and symptoms of hyperthermia (e.g., warm, flushed skin; tachycardia; tachypnea; elevated temperature). b. Implement measures *to reduce fever:* 1. perform actions *to reduce inflammation of the bowel* (e.g., administer corticosteroids, aminosalicylates, and/or immunomodulating agents as ordered) 2. administer antipyretics if ordered. c. Consult physician if temperature remains higher than 38° C.

6. Nursing Diagnosis: ACTIVITY INTOLERANCE

related to:
a. inadequate nutritional status;
b. difficulty resting and sleeping associated with pain, frequent need to defecate, fear, and anxiety;
c. tissue hypoxia associated with anemia resulting from:
  1. blood loss from the ulcerated bowel
  2. decreased oral intake and impaired absorption of iron, vitamin B_{12}, and folate;
d. increased energy expenditure associated with the increased metabolic rate that may be present during period of exacerbation.

Suggested NOC Outcomes: Activity tolerance; Rest; Energy conservation; Self-care: activities of daily living

Suggested NIC Interventions: Energy management; Nutrition management; Sleep enhancement

Desired Outcome	Nursing Actions and Selected Purposes/Rationales (see pp. 11–12 for additional rationales)
6. The client will demonstrate an increased tolerance for activity as evidenced by: a. verbalization of feeling less fatigued and weak b. ability to perform activities of daily living without exertional dyspnea, chest pain, diaphoresis, dizziness, and a significant change in vital signs.	6.a. Assess for signs and symptoms of activity intolerance: 1. statements of fatigue or weakness 2. exertional dyspnea, chest pain, diaphoresis, or dizziness 3. abnormal heart rate response to activity (e.g., increase in rate of 20 beats/minute above resting rate, rate not returning to preactivity level within 3 minutes after stopping activity, change from regular to irregular rate) 4. a significant change (15–20 mm Hg) in blood pressure with activity. b. Implement measures *to improve activity tolerance:* 1. perform actions *to promote rest and/or conserve energy:* a. maintain activity restrictions as ordered b. minimize environmental activity and noise c. organize nursing care to allow for periods of uninterrupted rest d. limit the number of visitors and their length of stay e. assist client with self-care activities as needed f. keep supplies and personal articles within easy reach g. instruct client in energy-saving techniques (e.g., using shower chair when showering, sitting to brush teeth or comb hair) h. implement measures *to reduce fear and anxiety* (e.g., maintain a calm, confident manner when working with client; explain procedures/treatments) i. implement measures *to promote sleep* (e.g., encourage relaxing diversional activities in the evening, allow client to continue usual sleep practices unless contraindicated, reduce environmental stimuli, administer prescribed sedative-hypnotics) j. implement measures to reduce pain (see Diagnosis 3, action e)

2. perform actions to reduce inflammation and hypermotility of the bowel (see Diagnosis 7, action b) *in order to reduce excess energy demands associated with inflammation, improve absorption of nutrients, reduce pain, and increase client's ability to rest and sleep*
3. perform actions to improve nutritional status (see Diagnosis 2, action c)
4. perform actions *to treat anemia if present:*
   a. administer iron, folic acid, and/or vitamin B_{12} as ordered
   b. administer epoetin alfa if ordered *to stimulate erythropoiesis*
   c. administer packed red blood cells if ordered
5. perform actions to reduce fever (see Diagnosis 5, action b) *in order to prevent the increased metabolic rate that occurs with hyperthermia*
6. increase client's activity gradually as allowed and tolerated.

c. Instruct client to:
   1. report a decreased tolerance for activity
   2. stop any activity that causes chest pain, shortness of breath, dizziness, or extreme fatigue or weakness.

d. Consult appropriate health care provider (e.g., physician) if signs and symptoms of activity intolerance persist or worsen.

7. NURSING DIAGNOSIS: DIARRHEA

related to increased peristalsis and a disturbance in intestinal secretion and absorption associated with inflammation of the bowel.

Suggested NOC Outcome: Bowel elimination

Suggested NIC Intervention: Diarrhea management

Desired Outcome	Nursing Actions *and Selected Purposes/Rationales* (see pp. 28–30 for additional rationales)
7. The client will have fewer bowel movements and more formed stool.	7.a. Assess for signs and symptoms of diarrhea (e.g., frequent, loose stools; urgency; abdominal cramping; hyperactive bowel sounds).

b. Implement measures *to reduce inflammation and hypermotility of the bowel in order to control diarrhea:*
   1. perform actions *to rest the bowel:*
      a. restrict oral intake if ordered (usually NPO during acute stage)
      b. maintain activity restrictions as ordered (may initially be limited to bed rest with bedside commode or bathroom privileges)
      c. implement measures *to reduce stress* (e.g., explain procedures, provide for consistency in staff assigned, perform actions to reduce pain)
      d. when oral intake is allowed:
         1. progress diet as ordered (diet usually progresses from elemental formulas *[these formulas are absorbed in the proximal small bowel and thereby minimize stimulation of the bowel]* to a low-residue diet)
         2. instruct client to avoid the following foods/fluids that may be poorly digested or can act as irritants to the inflamed bowel:
            a. milk and milk products *(clients with Crohn's disease may have an intolerance to lactose-rich foods because of a deficiency of lactase)*
            b. those high in fat (e.g., fried foods, gravies)
            c. those high in fiber or residue (e.g., whole-grain cereals, nuts, raw fruits and vegetables)
            d. those high in caffeine (e.g., coffee, tea, colas)
            e. spicy foods
            f. extremely hot or cold foods/fluids
         3. instruct client to add new foods one at a time
         4. provide small, frequent meals rather than 3 large ones
   2. administer the following medications if ordered:
      a. corticosteroids (e.g., prednisone, budesonide) *to reduce inflammation of the bowel*

Desired Outcome	Nursing Actions *and Selected Purposes/Rationales*
	b. sulfasalazine or a nonsulfa-aminosalicylate (e.g., olsalazine, controlled-release mesalamine) *to reduce inflammation of the bowel* c. antidiarrheal agents (e.g., diphenoxylate, loperamide) *to slow intestinal motility* (these medications must be used cautiously in severe disease *because of the risk for toxic megacolon*) d. immunomodulators: 1. azathioprine or mercaptopurine *to suppress the immune system and down-regulate inflammation* 2. monoclonal antibodies (e.g., infliximab) *to neutralize tumor necrosis factor-alpha and help decrease bowel inflammation.* c. Consult physician if diarrhea persists.

8. NURSING DIAGNOSIS:

RISK FOR INFECTION

related to:
a. ulcerations in the bowel wall;
b. lowered resistance to infection associated with malnutrition and treatment with corticosteroids and/or immunosuppressive agents;
c. stasis of respiratory secretions and urine associated with decreased mobility if activity restrictions are prescribed.

Suggested NOC Outcomes: Immune status; Infection severity

Suggested NIC Interventions: Infection protection; Infection control

Desired Outcome	Nursing Actions *and Selected Purposes/Rationales* (see pp. 37–40 for additional rationales)
8. The client will remain free of infection as evidenced by: a. temperature declining toward normal b. absence of chills c. pulse within normal limits d. normal breath sounds e. usual mental status f. cough productive of clear mucus only g. voiding clear urine without reports of frequency, urgency, and burning h. no increase in episodes of diarrhea and abdominal cramping and pain i. absence of heat, pain, redness, swelling, and unusual drainage in any area j. no reports of increased weakness and fatigue k. WBC and differential counts returning toward normal l. negative results of cultured specimens.	8.a. Assess for and report signs and symptoms of infection (be aware that some signs and symptoms vary depending on the site of infection, the causative organism, and the age and immune status of the client): 1. significant increase in temperature (an elevated temperature may be present due to the bowel inflammation) 2. chills 3. increased pulse 4. abnormal breath sounds 5. lethargy, acute confusion 6. cough productive of purulent, green, or rust-colored sputum 7. cloudy urine 8. reports of frequency, urgency, or burning when urinating 9. reports of increased weakness or fatigue 10. urinalysis showing a WBC count greater than 5, positive leukocyte esterase or nitrites, or presence of bacteria 11. increase in episodes of diarrhea and abdominal cramping and pain 12. heat, pain, redness, swelling, or unusual drainage in any area 13. increase in WBC count above previous levels (WBC count will usually be elevated as a result of bowel inflammation) and/or significant change in differential 14. positive results of cultured specimens (e.g., urine, vaginal drainage, stool, sputum, blood). b. Implement measures *to prevent infection:* 1. maintain a fluid intake of at least 2500 ml/day unless contraindicated 2. use good hand hygiene and encourage client to do the same 3. adhere to the appropriate precautions established to prevent transmission of infection to the client (standard precautions, transmission-based precautions on other clients)

4. use sterile technique during all invasive procedures (e.g., urinary catheterizations, venous and arterial punctures, injections)
5. protect client from others with infection
6. change peripheral intravenous line sites according to hospital policy
7. anchor catheter/tubings (e.g., urinary, intravenous) securely *in order to reduce trauma to the tissues and the risk for introduction of pathogens associated with the in-and-out movement of the tubing*
8. change equipment, tubings, and solutions used for treatments such as intravenous infusions and enteral feedings according to hospital policy
9. maintain a closed system for drains (e.g., urinary catheter) and intravenous infusions whenever possible
10. perform actions to improve nutritional status (see Diagnosis 2, action c)
11. reinforce importance of good oral hygiene
12. perform actions *to reduce stress* (e.g., explain procedures, provide for consistency in staff assigned, perform actions to reduce pain) *in order to prevent an increase in secretion of cortisol (cortisol interferes with some immune responses)*
13. perform actions *to prevent stasis of respiratory secretions* (e.g., instruct client to turn, cough, and deep breathe; increase activity as allowed and tolerated)
14. perform actions to prevent tissue breakdown (see Diagnosis 4, action b)
15. perform actions to prevent urinary retention (e.g., instruct client to urinate when the urge is first felt, promote relaxation during voiding attempts) *in order to prevent urinary stasis*
16. instruct and assist client to perform good perineal care routinely and after each bowel movement
17. perform actions to reduce inflammation of the bowel (e.g., administer corticosteroids, aminosalicylates, and/or immunomodulating agents as ordered) *to prevent further ulceration of the bowel and subsequently reduce the risk for intestinal infection*
18. administer antimicrobials if ordered (antimicrobials are generally given only if surgery is planned or if the client has severe colitis and is at high risk for infection; however, metronidazole or ciprofloxacin may be prescribed by some practitioners for the relief of symptoms).

a. related to crystalline deposits in the urine associated with:
   1. increased serum oxalate (dietary oxalate normally binds with calcium in the intestine and is excreted in the stool; in clients with inflammatory bowel disease, calcium is bound with the poorly absorbed fat and oxalate becomes available for absorption)
   2. decreased flushing of solutes from the urinary tract if urine formation is reduced as a result of deficient fluid volume
   3. treatment with sulfasalazine;

b. related to extension of a mucosal fissure or ulcer through the intestinal wall;

c. related to loss of colonic muscle tone associated with the effects of widespread inflammation in the bowel, use of some medications (e.g., opiates, anticholinergics), and hypokalemia;

d. related to narrowing of the intestinal lumen associated with inflammation and scar tissue formation in the bowel;

e. related to perforation of the bowel or leakage from an abscess or fistula.

Desired Outcomes	**Nursing Actions** *and Selected Purposes/Rationales*
9.a. The client will not develop renal calculi as evidenced by: 1. absence of flank pain, hematuria, nausea, and vomiting 2. clear urine without calculi.	9.a.1. Assess for and report signs and symptoms of renal calculi (e.g., dull, aching or severe, colicky flank pain; hematuria; nausea; vomiting). 2. Implement measures *to prevent renal calculi:* a. maintain a minimum fluid intake of 2500 ml/day unless contraindicated b. encourage client to decrease intake of foods/fluids high in oxalate (e.g., tea, instant coffee, peanuts, chocolate, spinach) *in order to decrease absorption of oxalate from the intestine* c. encourage client to adhere to a low-fat diet *(this reduces the amount of fat available to bind calcium, thereby freeing calcium to bind with oxalate).* 3. If signs and symptoms of renal calculi occur: a. strain all urine and save any calculi for analysis; report finding to physician b. maintain a minimum fluid intake of 2500 ml/day unless contraindicated c. administer analgesics and antispasmodic agents (e.g., oxybutynin) as ordered d. prepare client for removal of calculi (e.g., extracorporeal shock wave lithotripsy [ESWL], percutaneous nephrolithotomy, ureteroscopy with lithotripsy and stone extraction) if planned.
9.b. The client will have resolution of any abscesses and fistulas that develop as evidenced by: 1. temperature declining toward normal 2. resolution of abdominal pain 3. absence of perianal redness, swelling, and pain 4. no unusual vaginal drainage 5. clear, yellow urine 6. WBC count declining toward normal.	9.b.1. Assess for and report signs and symptoms of abscess and/or fistula formation (e.g., further increase in temperature; increased or more constant abdominal pain; perianal redness, swelling, and pain; foul vaginal discharge or passage of stool from vagina; dysuria; fecaluria; further increase in WBC count). 2. Implement measures to reduce inflammation of the bowel (e.g., administer corticosteroids, aminosalicylates, and/or immunomodulating agents as ordered) *to promote healing of the intestinal mucosa and subsequently decrease the risk for development of abscesses and fistulas and promote healing of any that exist.* 3. If signs and symptoms of abscesses or fistulas occur: a. prepare client for diagnostic studies (e.g., computed tomography, ultrasonography, barium enema) b. administer the following medications if ordered: 1. antimicrobial agents (e.g., metronidazole, ciprofloxacin) 2. immunomodulator agents such as azathioprine, mercaptopurine, or a monoclonal antibody (e.g., infliximab) c. if a cutaneous fistula is present, perform wound care as ordered d. prepare client for surgical intervention (e.g., incision and drainage of abscess, resection of involved area) if planned.
9.c. The client will not develop toxic megacolon as evidenced by: 1. absence of abdominal distention 2. gradual resolution of abdominal pain 3. active bowel sounds 4. gradual resolution of diarrhea 5. temperature and WBC count declining toward normal.	9.c.1. Assess for and report signs and symptoms of toxic megacolon: a. abdominal distention and increased abdominal pain and tenderness b. hypoactive or absent bowel sounds with tympanic percussion note over abdomen c. sudden decrease in episodes of diarrhea d. fever (usually greater than 38.6° C) and tachycardia e. increase in WBC count f. abdominal x-ray results showing colonic dilation. 2. Implement measures *to prevent development of toxic megacolon:* a. perform actions *to reduce inflammation of the bowel* (e.g., administer corticosteroids, aminosalicylates, and/or immunomodulating agents as ordered) b. administer medications that slow gastrointestinal motility (e.g., narcotic analgesics, antidiarrheal agents, anticholinergics) judiciously c. perform actions to prevent or treat hypokalemia (see Diagnosis 1, action b).

3. If signs and symptoms of toxic megacolon occur:
   a. withhold oral intake as ordered
   b. consult physician about discontinuing any medications that slow gastrointestinal motility (e.g., narcotic analgesics, antidiarrheal agents, anticholinergics)
   c. insert nasogastric tube and maintain suction as ordered
   d. administer the following if ordered:
      1. intravenous fluids *to maintain adequate vascular volume (third-space fluid shifting occurs as a result of increased capillary permeability associated with the inflammation and increased intraluminal pressure that are present with toxic megacolon)*
      2. corticosteroids *to reduce intestinal inflammation*
      3. antimicrobials (e.g., metronidazole) *to prevent infection (the risk of perforation is increased when toxic megacolon develops)*
   e. prepare client for surgical intervention (e.g., colectomy) if planned.

9.d. The client will not develop a bowel obstruction as evidenced by:
1. gradual resolution of abdominal pain
2. absence of vomiting and abdominal distention
3. gradual return of normal bowel sounds.

9.d.1. Assess for and report signs and symptoms of a bowel obstruction:
   a. increased abdominal cramping and pain
   b. vomiting
   c. abdominal distention
   d. change in bowel sounds (bowel sounds can be high-pitched and more hyperactive if the bowel is partially obstructed or they can be absent once there is complete obstruction)
   e. abdominal x-ray results showing partial or complete bowel obstruction.
2. Implement measures to reduce inflammation of the bowel (e.g., administer corticosteroids, aminosalicylates, and/or immunomodulating agents as ordered) *to reduce intestinal narrowing and scar tissue formation.*
3. If signs and symptoms of a bowel obstruction occur:
   a. withhold oral intake as ordered
   b. insert nasogastric tube and maintain suction as ordered
   c. administer intravenous fluids if ordered *to maintain an adequate vascular volume (dehydration occurs with prolonged vomiting and third-spacing occurs due to the increased capillary permeability that results from increased intraluminal pressure in a bowel obstruction)*
   d. prepare client for endoscopic balloon dilatation of strictures or surgical intervention (e.g., stricturoplasty, bowel resection) if planned.

9.e. The client will not develop peritonitis as evidenced by:
1. temperature declining toward normal
2. soft, nondistended abdomen
3. gradual resolution of abdominal pain
4. gradual return of normal bowel sounds
5. absence of nausea and vomiting
6. stable vital signs
7. WBC count declining toward normal.

9.e.1. Assess for and report signs and symptoms of peritonitis (e.g., further increase in temperature; distended, rigid abdomen; increased abdominal pain; rebound tenderness; diminished or absent bowel sounds; nausea; vomiting; tachycardia; tachypnea; hypotension; WBC count that increases or fails to decline toward normal).
2. Implement measures to prevent and treat abscesses, fistulas, toxic megacolon, and/or bowel obstruction (see actions b.2 and 3, c.2 and 3, and d.2 and 3 in this diagnosis) *in order to reduce the risk for peritonitis.*
3. If signs and symptoms of peritonitis occur:
   a. withhold oral intake as ordered
   b. place client on bed rest in a semi-Fowler's position *to assist in pooling or localizing intestinal contents in the pelvis rather than under the diaphragm*
   c. prepare client for diagnostic tests (e.g., abdominal x-ray, computed tomography, ultrasonography) if planned
   d. insert nasogastric tube and maintain suction as ordered
   e. administer antimicrobials (e.g., metronidazole) as ordered
   f. administer intravenous fluids and/or blood volume expanders if ordered *to prevent or treat shock (it can result from the increased capillary permeability that occurs with inflammation and the subsequent escape of protein, fluid, and electrolytes from the vascular space into the peritoneal cavity)*
   g. prepare client for surgical intervention (e.g., repair of perforation, bowel resection) if planned.

10. Nursing Diagnosis: INEFFECTIVE COPING

related to:
a. chronicity of condition and effect of inflammatory bowel disease on lifestyle;
b. pain;
c. concern about eventual need for an ileal diversion;
d. feeling of lack of control over disease progression.

Suggested NOC Outcomes: Coping; Acceptance: health status

Suggested NIC Interventions: Coping enhancement; Support system enhancement

Desired Outcome	Nursing Actions *and Selected Purposes/Rationales* (see pp. 26–28 for additional rationales)

10. The client will demonstrate effective coping as evidenced by:
    a. verbalization of ability to cope with inflammatory bowel disease and its effects
    b. utilization of appropriate problem-solving techniques
    c. willingness to participate in treatment plan and meet basic needs
    d. absence of destructive behavior toward self and others
    e. appropriate use of defense mechanisms
    f. utilization of available support systems.

10.a. Assess for and report signs and symptoms of ineffective coping (e.g., verbalization of inability to cope or ask for help; inability to meet role expectations, problem solve, or meet basic needs; insomnia; withdrawal; reluctance to participate in treatment plan; destructive behavior toward self or others; inappropriate use of defense mechanisms).
b. Assess client's perception of current situation.
c. Implement measures *to promote effective coping:*
   1. assist client to recognize and manage inappropriate denial if it is present
   2. perform actions to reduce pain (see Diagnosis 3, action e)
   3. encourage verbalization about current situation and ways comparable situations have been handled in the past
   4. assist client to identify personal strengths and resources that can be used to facilitate coping with the current situation
   5. if acceptable to client, arrange for a visit with another individual who has successfully adjusted to inflammatory bowel disease
   6. provide consistency in caregivers when possible; inform client if there will be a change in caregivers *so he/she will not interpret the change as rejection*
   7. include client in planning of care, encourage maximum participation in treatment plan, and allow choices when possible *to enable him/her to maintain a sense of control*
   8. instruct client in effective problem-solving techniques (e.g., accurate identification of stressors, determination of various options to solve problem)
   9. assist client to maintain usual daily routines whenever possible
   10. assist client to identify priorities and attainable goals as he/she starts to plan for necessary lifestyle and role changes
   11. assist client to prepare for negative reactions from others because of diarrhea and odor of flatus
   12. assist client to identify and utilize available support systems; provide information regarding available community resources that can assist client and significant others in coping with inflammatory bowel disease (e.g., support groups, counseling services, Crohn's and Colitis Foundation of America)
   13. administer antianxiety and/or antidepressant agents if ordered
   14. encourage continued emotional support from significant others; reinforce the importance of maintaining a calm, nonstressful atmosphere during visits
   15. encourage client to share with significant others the kind of support that would be the most beneficial (e.g., listening, inspiring hope, providing reassurance and accurate information)
   16. support behaviors indicative of effective coping (e.g., increased participation in self-care activities and treatment plan, verbalization of ways to adapt to necessary changes in lifestyle).

d. Consult appropriate health care provider (e.g., psychiatric nurse clinician, physician) if client continues to have difficulty coping with his/her situation.

Discharge Teaching/Continued Care

11. NURSING DIAGNOSIS: ***DEFICIENT KNOWLEDGE, INEFFECTIVE THERAPEUTIC REGIMEN MANAGEMENT, OR INEFFECTIVE HEALTH MAINTENANCE****

*The nurse should select the diagnostic label that is most appropriate for the client's discharge teaching needs.

Suggested NOC Outcome: Knowledge: diet; Knowledge: medication; Knowledge: treatment regimen

Suggested NIC Interventions: Health system guidance; Teaching: individual; Teaching: disease process; Teaching: prescribed diet; Teaching: prescribed medication

Desired Outcomes	**Nursing Actions** *and Selected Purposes/Rationales*
11.a. The client will identify ways to reduce the incidence of disease exacerbation.	11.a.1. Reinforce the importance of adhering to the prescribed treatment regimen in order to reduce the incidence of disease exacerbation. 2. Instruct the client regarding ways to reduce bowel irritation: a. reduce intake of or avoid foods/fluids likely to be poorly digested or that may irritate the bowel (e.g., raw fruits and vegetables, whole-grain cereals, gravy, fried foods, spicy foods, milk and milk products, caffeine-containing beverages, extremely hot drinks, iced drinks, alcohol) b. avoid use of laxatives. 3. Explain that stress can precipitate periods of exacerbation. Provide information about stress management classes and counseling services that may assist client to manage stress.
11.b. The client will verbalize ways to maintain an optimal nutritional status.	11.b. Provide instructions regarding ways to maintain an optimal nutritional status: 1. reinforce instructions regarding prescribed diet (a low-residue, high-calorie, high-protein diet is often recommended) 2. inform client that eating small, frequent meals rather than 3 large meals may help achieve the recommended high-calorie intake 3. reinforce the benefits of eating when rested and in a relaxed atmosphere 4. stress the importance of taking vitamins and minerals as prescribed.
11.c. The client will state ways to prevent perianal skin breakdown.	11.c. Provide the following instructions about ways to prevent perianal skin breakdown: 1. use soft toilet tissue for wiping after each bowel movement 2. cleanse perianal area with a mild soap and warm water after each bowel movement; dry thoroughly 3. apply a protective ointment or cream to perianal area after skin has been cleansed.
11.d. The client will verbalize an understanding of medications ordered including rationale, food and drug interactions, side effects, schedule for taking, and importance of taking as prescribed.	11.d.1. Explain rationale for, side effects of, and importance of taking medications prescribed. Inform client of pertinent food and drug interactions. 2. If client is discharged on sulfasalazine, instruct to: a. drink at least 10 glasses of liquid/day to reduce risk of kidney stone formation b. expect that urine might be an orange-yellow color c. take medication with food or after meals if gastric upset occurs; do not chew, crush, or break tablets

Desired Outcomes	**Nursing Actions** *and Selected Purposes/Rationales*
	d. report a sore throat or mouth, fever, unusual fatigue, continuous headache or aching joint(s), unusual bruising or bleeding, nausea, vomiting, rash, or confusion e. avoid direct exposure of skin to sun and sun lamps f. inform physician if pregnancy is suspected or if breast-feeding (sulfasalazine crosses the placenta and also enters the breast milk) g. notify health care provider if unable to impregnate partner (sulfasalazine can cause a reduction in sperm count or a change in sperm morphology) h. keep scheduled appointments for blood and urine studies. 3. If client is discharged on a corticosteroid preparation, instruct to: a. take medication exactly as prescribed b. adjust dosage only if prescribed by physician c. gradually taper off medication as directed; do not discontinue medication suddenly or of own accord d. take with food or antacids to reduce gastric irritation e. expect that certain effects such as facial rounding, slight weight gain and swelling, increased appetite, and slight mood changes may occur f. report undesirable effects of corticosteroid therapy such as marked swelling in extremities, significant weight gain, extreme emotional and behavioral changes, extreme weakness, tarry stools, bloody or coffee-ground vomitus, frequent or persistent headaches, insomnia, lack of menses, and persistent gastric irritation g. avoid contact with persons who have an infection because corticosteroids lower resistance to infection h. follow recommendations about ways to reduce the risk for developing osteoporosis (e.g., take calcium and vitamin D supplements, stop smoking, do 30–60 minutes of a weight-bearing exercise daily) if long-term corticosteroid use is expected. 4. If client is to administer corticosteroid enemas or rectal foam or mesalamine enemas or rectal suppositories at home, instruct in technique, schedule (it is usually recommended that these products be administered at bedtime), and length of time the solution or suppository should be retained. Allow time for questions, clarification, and return demonstration. 5. Instruct client to inform physician before taking other prescription and nonprescription medications. 6. Instruct client to inform all health care providers of medications being taken.
11.e. The client will state signs and symptoms to report to the health care provider.	11.e. Instruct client to report the following signs and symptoms: 1. recurrent episodes of diarrhea and abdominal pain and cramping 2. increasing abdominal distention 3. persistent vomiting 4. unusual rectal or vaginal drainage 5. burning on urination or brownish, foul-smelling urine 6. pain, swelling, or open sores in perianal area 7. continued weight loss 8. constipation 9. yellowing of skin, flank pain, change in vision, eye pain, or joint pain or swelling (can indicate extraintestinal involvement).
11.f. The client will identify resources that can assist in the adjustment to changes resulting from inflammatory bowel disease and its treatment.	11.f.1. Provide information about resources that can assist the client and significant others in adjusting to inflammatory bowel disease and its effects (e.g., local support groups, Crohn's and Colitis Foundation of America, counseling services, stress management classes). 2. Initiate a referral if indicated.

11.g. The client will verbalize an understanding of and a plan for adhering to recommended follow-up care including future appointments with health care provider and activity level.

11.g.1. Reinforce importance of keeping follow-up appointments with health care provider.
2. Reinforce importance of frequent rest periods throughout the day.
3. Implement measures to improve client compliance:
   a. include significant others in teaching sessions if possible
   b. encourage questions and allow time for reinforcement and clarification of information provided
   c. provide written instructions on future appointments with health care provider, medications prescribed, signs and symptoms to report, and future laboratory studies.

ADDITIONAL NURSING DIAGNOSES

DISTURBED SLEEP PATTERN*

related to frequent need to defecate, pain, fear, and anxiety.

FEAR/ANXIETY*

related to:
a. symptoms being experienced (e.g., abdominal pain, persistent diarrhea, fever);
b. lack of understanding of diagnosis, diagnostic tests, and treatments;
c. concern about need for surgery if disease condition cannot be medically controlled;
d. anticipated changes in future lifestyle because of inability to control symptoms;
e. concern about expense of hospitalization and treatment for a chronic disease.

DISTURBED SELF-CONCEPT*

related to:
a. dependence on others to meet self-care needs;
b. embarrassment associated with diarrhea;
c. changes in sexual functioning associated with pain, fatigue, and weakness;
d. changes in lifestyle associated with pain and chronic diarrhea.

*See Unit II for outcomes, actions, and rationales.

Bibliography

See pages 879 and 884.

Intestinal Obstruction

Intestinal (bowel) obstruction is a condition in which the intestinal contents fail to move through the bowel. The obstruction can be partial or complete and can develop slowly or rapidly. It can occur as a result of any factor that narrows the lumen of the intestine or interferes with peristalsis. Narrowing of the lumen results in a mechanical obstruction and can be caused by factors such as adhesions, tumors, inflammatory bowel disease, hernias, fecal impaction, intussusception, a volvulus, and strictures. In a nonmechanical obstruction, the bowel lumen remains open but the intestinal contents are not propelled forward. Factors that can cause this paralytic (adynamic) ileus include abdominal surgery, effects of anesthesia and some medications (e.g., narcotic [opioid] analgesics, some antiemetics, anticholinergics, antidiarrheals), electrolyte imbalances such as hypokalemia, decreased blood flow to the intestine (can occur with conditions such as hypovolemia or blockage of mesenteric vessels as a result of an embolus, thrombus, or arteriosclerosis), spinal cord injury, and peritonitis.

Signs and symptoms of intestinal obstruction vary depending on the location, cause, and degree of the obstruction. Common clinical manifestations include abdominal pain and distention, nausea, and vomiting. Hyperactive, high-pitched bowel sounds are present early in the development of a mechanical obstruction. Bowel sounds are absent or hypoactive in nonmechanical obstruction and as mechanical obstruction worsens.

Treatment of intestinal obstruction is directed toward relieving symptoms, managing fluid and electrolyte imbalances, preventing complications, and determining and treating the cause of the obstruction. Most cases of nonmechanical obstruction do not necessitate surgery. Some mechanical obstructions can be treated nonsurgically (e.g., enemas and laxatives to remove fecal impaction, dilatation of obstructed portion of bowel via endoscopy, radiation or chemotherapy to reduce tumor size, gentle instillation of barium to resolve an intussusception or reverse a sigmoid volvulus). Surgical intervention (intestinal resection with reanastomosis or creation of an ileostomy or colostomy) is indicated when it is necessary to remove an obstruction that persists despite conservative management or to remove a segment of bowel that is strangulated or necrotic.

This care plan focuses on the adult client hospitalized with an intestinal obstruction. Some of the information is applicable to clients receiving follow-up care in an extended care facility or home setting.

Outcome/Discharge Criteria

THE CLIENT WILL:

- have absence of or minimal abdominal pain
- have gradual return of normal bowel function
- tolerate prescribed diet
- have no signs and symptoms of complications
- verbalize an understanding of ways to reduce the risk for recurrent intestinal obstruction
- state signs and symptoms to report to the health care provider
- verbalize an understanding of and a plan for adhering to recommended diet, prescribed medications, ways to prevent recurrent intestinal obstruction, and future appointments with health care provider.

Nursing/Collaborative Diagnoses

See p. 657 for additional diagnoses.

1. NURSING/COLLABORATIVE DIAGNOSIS

IMBALANCED FLUID AND ELECTROLYTES

a. deficient fluid volume, hypokalemia, hypochloremia, and metabolic alkalosis related to:
   1. decreased absorption of intestinal fluid into the vascular space associated with inflammation and distention of the bowel (the sequestering of fluid in the intestine is a major factor with obstructions of the small intestine and proximal portion of the large intestine)
   2. restricted oral intake
   3. excessive loss of fluid and electrolytes associated with vomiting and nasogastric tube drainage;

b. third spacing related to the increased capillary permeability that results from increased intraluminal pressure in the distended bowel.

Suggested NOC Outcomes: Fluid balance; Electrolyte and acid-base balance

Suggested NIC Interventions: Fluid monitoring; Fluid management; Electrolyte management: hypokalemia; Fluid/Electrolyte management; Acid-base monitoring; Acid-base management: metabolic alkalosis

Desired Outcome

1. The client will maintain fluid and electrolyte balance as evidenced by:
   a. normal skin turgor
   b. moist mucous membranes
   c. stable weight
   d. B/P and pulse within normal range for client and stable with position change
   e. capillary refill time less than 2–3 seconds
   f. usual mental status
   g. balanced intake and output
   h. urine specific gravity within normal range
   i. abdomen less distended and bowel sounds returning toward normal
   j. absence of cardiac dysrhythmias, muscle weakness, paresthesias, twitching, spasms, and dizziness
   k. BUN, Hct, serum electrolytes, and blood gases within normal range.

Nursing Actions *and Selected Purposes/Rationales*

(see pp. 30–31 for additional rationales)

1.a. Assess for and report signs and symptoms of:
   1. deficient fluid volume:
      a. decreased skin turgor, dry mucous membranes, thirst
      b. weight loss of 2% or greater over a short period
      c. postural hypotension and/or low B/P
      d. weak, rapid pulse
      e. capillary refill time greater than 2–3 seconds
      f. flat neck veins when supine
      g. change in mental status
      h. decreased urine output with increased specific gravity (reflects an actual rather than a potential fluid deficit)
      i. increased BUN and Hct
   2. hypokalemia (e.g., cardiac dysrhythmias, postural hypotension, muscle weakness, nausea and vomiting, abdominal distention, hypoactive or absent bowel sounds, low serum potassium)
   3. hypochloremia and metabolic alkalosis (e.g., dizziness, paresthesias, muscle twitching or spasms, hypoventilation, low serum chloride, elevated pH and T_{CO_2})
   4. third-spacing:
      a. ascites
      b. evidence of vascular depletion (e.g., postural hypotension; weak, rapid pulse; decreased urine output).

b. Implement measures *to prevent or treat imbalanced fluid and electrolytes:*
   1. perform actions to reduce nausea and vomiting (see Diagnosis 3, action b)
   2. if nasogastric tube is present and needs to be irrigated frequently and/or with large volumes of solution, irrigate it with normal saline rather than water
   3. maintain intravenous fluid therapy as ordered
   4. administer electrolyte replacements as ordered
   5. administer albumin infusions if ordered *to increase colloid osmotic pressure and promote mobilization of third-space fluid back into the vascular space*
   6. when oral intake is allowed, assist client to select foods/fluids high in potassium (e.g., bananas, potatoes, raisins, orange juice, cantaloupe).

c. Consult physician if signs and symptoms of imbalanced fluid and electrolytes persist or worsen.

2. Nursing Diagnosis: ACUTE PAIN: ABDOMINAL

related to:
a. distention of the intestinal lumen associated with the accumulation of gas and fluid;
b. inflammation of the intestine (can occur as a result of the underlying cause of the obstruction [e.g., inflammatory bowel disease]).

Suggested NOC Outcomes: Pain control; Comfort level

Suggested NIC Interventions: Analgesic administration; Pain management

Desired Outcome	Nursing Actions *and Selected Purposes/Rationales* (see pp. 45–47 for additional rationales)
2. The client will experience diminished pain as evidenced by: a. verbalization of same b. relaxed facial expression and body positioning c. increased participation in activities d. stable vital signs.	2.a. Assess for signs and symptoms of pain (e.g., verbalization of pain, grimacing, reluctance to move, guarding of abdomen, restlessness, diaphoresis, increased B/P, tachycardia). b. Assess client's perception of the severity of pain using a pain intensity scale. c. Assess the client's pain pattern (e.g., location, quality, onset, duration, precipitating factors, aggravating factors, alleviating factors). d. Implement measures *to reduce pain:* 1. perform actions *to reduce fear and anxiety about the pain experience* (e.g., assure client that his/her need for pain relief is understood, plan methods for achieving pain control with client) 2. perform actions *to decrease the accumulation of intestinal gas and fluid:* a. maintain food and oral fluid restrictions as ordered b. insert nasogastric tube and maintain suction as ordered c. administer gastrointestinal stimulants (e.g., metoclopramide) if ordered *to promote intestinal motility* (may be ordered if obstruction is not complete or is the result of a paralytic ileus) d. instruct client to avoid chewing gum, sucking on ice or hard candy, and smoking *in order to reduce air swallowing* e. when oral intake is allowed, advance diet slowly and instruct client to avoid intake of carbonated beverages and gas-producing foods (e.g., cabbage, onions, beans) 3. perform actions to reduce fear and anxiety (e.g., explain treatments and diagnostic procedures; provide care in a calm, confident manner) *in order to promote relaxation and subsequently increase the client's threshold and tolerance for pain* 4. provide or assist with nonpharmacologic measures for pain relief (e.g., position change; restful environment; diversional activities such as watching television, reading, or conversing) 5. administer analgesics as ordered (the use of narcotic [opioid] analgesics is often avoided until the cause of the obstruction is determined). e. Consult appropriate health care provider (e.g., pharmacist, physician) if above measures fail to provide adequate pain relief.

3. Nursing Diagnosis: NAUSEA

related to stimulation of the vomiting center associated with:
a. stimulation of the visceral afferent pathways resulting from inflammation and distention of the intestine;
b. stimulation of the cerebral cortex resulting from pain and stress.

Suggested NOC Outcome: Nausea and vomiting severity

Suggested NIC Interventions: Nausea management; Vomiting management; Environmental management: comfort

Desired Outcome	**Nursing Actions** *and Selected Purposes/Rationales*

3. The client will experience relief of nausea and vomiting as evidenced by:
   a. verbalization of relief of nausea
   b. absence of vomiting.

3.a. Assess client for nausea and vomiting.
  b. Implement measures *to reduce nausea and vomiting:*
    1. maintain food and oral fluid restrictions as ordered
    2. insert nasogastric tube and maintain suction as ordered
    3. eliminate noxious sights and odors from the environment *(noxious stimuli can cause stimulation of the vomiting center)*
    4. instruct client to change positions slowly *(rapid movement can result in chemoreceptor trigger zone stimulation and subsequent excitation of the vomiting center)*
    5. provide oral hygiene after each emesis
    6. perform actions to reduce pain (see Diagnosis 2, action d)
    7. perform actions *to reduce fear and anxiety* (e.g., assure client that staff are nearby; provide a calm, restful environment; explain all tests and procedures)
    8. encourage client to take deep, slow breaths when nauseated
    9. administer antiemetics as ordered
    10. when oral intake is allowed, advance diet slowly.
  c. Consult physician if above measures fail to control nausea and vomiting.

4. COLLABORATIVE DIAGNOSES: POTENTIAL COMPLICATIONS OF INTESTINAL OBSTRUCTION

a. peritonitis related to release of intestinal contents into the peritoneal cavity associated with perforation of the bowel if it occurs;
b. intestinal necrosis related to obstruction of blood flow in the affected area associated with:
   1. inflammation and distention of the bowel lumen
   2. hypovolemia
   3. mesenteric vessel thrombosis or embolus (can be a cause of nonmechanical obstruction)
   4. strangulation of a portion of the intestine (especially if obstruction is a result of a hernia, strictures, adhesions, or a volvulus).

Desired Outcomes	**Nursing Actions** *and Selected Purposes/Rationales*

4.a. The client will not develop peritonitis as evidenced by:
   1. temperature stable and less than 38° C
   2. abdomen less distended and firm
   3. no increase in abdominal pain and tenderness, nausea, and vomiting
   4. gradual return of normal bowel sounds
   5. stable vital signs
   6. no increase in WBC count.

4.a. Assess for and report signs and symptoms of peritonitis (e.g., further increase in temperature or temperature above 38° C, abdomen more distended and firm, increase in severity of abdominal pain, rebound tenderness, increased nausea and vomiting, tachycardia, hypotension, increase in WBC count).
  b. Implement measures *to prevent peritonitis:*
    1. perform actions *to reduce the risk for perforatiom of the bowel:*
       a. implement measures to decrease the accumulation of intestinal gas and fluid (see Diagnosis 2, action d.2)
       b. continue with actions to treat the underlying cause of the obstruction (e.g., anti-inflammatory agents to treat inflammatory bowel disease, chemotherapeutic agents to reduce tumor size)
    2. administer antimicrobials if ordered *(may be ordered prophylactically).*
  c. If signs and symptoms of peritonitis occur:
    1. withhold oral food and fluids as ordered
    2. place client on bed rest in a semi-Fowler's position *to assist in pooling or localizing gastrointestinal contents in the pelvis rather than the diaphragm*
    3. prepare client for diagnostic tests (e.g., abdominal x-ray, computed tomography) if planned
    4. administer antimicrobials as ordered
    5. administer fluids and/or blood volume expanders if ordered *to prevent or treat shock (it can result from the increased capillary permeability that occurs with inflammation and the subsequent escape of protein, fluid, and electrolytes from the vascular space into the peritoneal cavity)*
    6. prepare client for surgery (e.g., drainage and irrigation of the peritoneum, bowel resection) if planned.

Desired Outcomes	Nursing Actions and Selected Purposes/Rationales
4.b. The client will not experience intestinal necrosis as evidenced by: 1. decreased abdominal pain 2. absence of bloody diarrhea 3. no increase in WBC count.	4.b.1. Assess for and report signs and symptoms of intestinal necrosis (e.g., severe continuous abdominal pain; bloody diarrhea; WBC count that increases or fails to decline toward normal). 2. Implement measures *to improve blood flow to the intestine in order to prevent intestinal necrosis:* a. perform actions to prevent and treat deficient fluid volume (see Diagnosis 1, action b) b. perform actions to reduce the accumulation of intestinal gas and fluid (see Diagnosis 2, action d.2) c. prepare client for treatment of the underlying cause of vascular obstruction (e.g., mesenteric thrombectomy or embolectomy; surgery to repair hernia, release adhesions, or correct volvulus) if planned. 3. If signs and symptoms of intestinal necrosis occur: a. administer antimicrobials if ordered b. prepare client for surgical resection of the affected bowel (usually performed if the client has extensive tissue necrosis or gangrenous patches have developed).

*The nurse should select the diagnostic label that is most appropriate for the client's discharge teaching needs.

Suggested NOC Outcomes: Knowledge: disease process; Knowledge: treatment regimen

Suggested NIC Interventions: Health system guidance; Teaching: individual; Teaching: disease process; Teaching: prescribed diet; Teaching: prescribed medication

Desired Outcomes	Nursing Actions and Selected Purposes/Rationales
5.a. The client will state signs and symptoms to report to the health care provider.	5.a. Instruct client to report the following signs and symptoms: 1. recurrent episodes of abdominal pain 2. increasing abdominal distention 3. nausea or vomiting 4. constipation 5. elevated temperature.
5.b. The client will verbalize an understanding of ways to minimize the risk of recurrence of intestinal obstruction.	5.b. Reinforce physician's instructions regarding ways to prevent the risk for recurrent intestinal obstruction. For example: 1. follow-up radiation and/or chemotherapy if obstruction was caused by a tumor 2. dietary and medication management if obstruction was caused by inflammatory bowel disease 3. bowel care regimen if obstruction was caused by a fecal impaction.
5.c. The client will verbalize an understanding of and a plan for adhering to recommended follow-up care including recommended diet, prescribed medications, ways to prevent recurrent intestinal obstruction, and future appointments with health care provider.	5.c.1. Reinforce the importance of keeping follow-up appointments with health care provider. 2. Reinforce physician's instructions regarding dietary restrictions and advancement of diet. 3. Reinforce physician's instructions regarding prescribed medications. 4. Implement measures to improve client compliance: a. include significant others in teaching sessions if possible b. encourage questions and allow time for reinforcement and clarification of information provided c. provide written instructions on future appointments with health care provider, dietary restrictions, medications prescribed, and signs and symptoms to report.

Additional Nursing Diagnoses

IMBALANCED NUTRITION: LESS THAN BODY REQUIREMENTS*

related to:
a. decreased oral intake associated with nausea, pain, and prescribed dietary restrictions;
b. loss of nutrients associated with vomiting.

IMPAIRED ORAL MUCOUS MEMBRANE:* DRYNESS

related to:
a. deficient fluid volume associated with restricted oral intake and fluid loss resulting from vomiting and nasogastric tube drainage;
b. decreased salivation associated with deficient fluid volume, restricted oral intake, and the effect of some medications (e.g., narcotic [opioid] analgesics, some antiemetics);
c. mouth breathing when nasogastric tube is in place.

INEFFECTIVE BREATHING PATTERN*

related to:
a. increased rate of respirations associated with pain, fear, and anxiety;
b. decreased rate of respirations associated with the depressant effect of some medications (e.g., narcotic [opioid] analgesics, some antiemetics);
c. decreased depth of respirations associated with:
   1. depressant effect of some medications (e.g., narcotic [opioid] analgesics, some antiemetics)
   2. fear, anxiety, and reluctance to breathe deeply because of pain
   3. restricted chest expansion resulting from elevation of the diaphragm (occurs with abdominal distention).

FEAR AND ANXIETY*

related to discomfort; lack of understanding of the diagnosis, diagnostic tests, treatments, and prognosis; and possibility of surgery.

---

*See Unit II for outcomes, actions, and rationales.

Bibliography

See pages 879 and 884.

evolve

Peptic Ulcer

A peptic ulcer is a break in the continuity of the gastrointestinal mucosa that is exposed to acidic digestive secretions. The areas most often involved are the stomach and duodenum. Erosion of these areas can result from direct damage to the mucosa or from an increase in mucosal permeability, which allows gastric acids to diffuse through the mucosal barrier into the underlying tissue. The two most common causes of peptic ulcers are infection with *Helicobacter pylori (H. pylori)* and use of aspirin or other nonsteroidal anti-inflammatory agents (NSAIDs). Other factors believed to have a role in ulcer development, exacerbation, and/or recurrence include ingestion of alcohol, coffee, certain foods and spices, and caffeine; medications such as corticosteroids and some chemotherapeutic agents; smoking; stress; hypovolemia (can result in ischemia of the gastrointestinal mucosa and subsequent alteration in mucosal permeability); certain disease conditions (e.g., Zollinger-Ellison syndrome, chronic obstructive pulmonary disease, pancreatitis, chronic renal failure); and genetic predisposition.

Peptic ulcers are usually classified by location (e.g., gastric, duodenal) and by the extensiveness of erosion (e.g., acute [superficial erosion with minimal inflammation], chronic [erosion of mucosa and submucosa with scar tissue formation]). Causative factors and the relationship between eating and occurrence of pain vary depending on the location and extensiveness of the ulcer. The characteristic symptom of a peptic ulcer is chronic, intermittent epigastric pain that is described as burning, aching, gnawing, or cramping.

Medical treatment of a peptic ulcer focuses on eradicating *H. pylori* infection if present, decreasing the degree of gastric acidity, and promoting mucosal integrity and regeneration. Surgical intervention (e.g., vagotomy, pyloroplasty, partial gastrectomy) may be indicated if symptoms cannot be medically controlled; if ulcers recur frequently; or if complications such as hemorrhage, perforation, or obstruction occur in the ulcerated area(s).

This care plan focuses on the adult client hospitalized for evaluation and medical treatment of a peptic ulcer that has become increasingly symptomatic. Much of the information presented here is applicable to client's receiving care in an extended care facility or home setting.

OUTCOME/DISCHARGE CRITERIA

THE CLIENT WILL:

- have pain controlled
- have no signs and symptoms of complications
- verbalize a basic understanding of peptic ulcer disease and the importance of adhering to the prescribed treatment plan
- identify ways to promote healing of the existing ulcer and prevent recurrence of peptic ulcer
- verbalize an understanding of medications ordered including rationale, food and drug interactions, side effects, schedule for taking, and importance of taking as prescribed
- state signs and symptoms to report to the health care provider
- verbalize an understanding of and a plan for adhering to recommended follow-up care including future appointments with health care provider.

NURSING/COLLABORATIVE DIAGNOSES

DISCHARGE TEACHING

See pp. 664–665 for additional diagnoses.

1. NURSING DIAGNOSIS:

ACUTE PAIN: EPIGASTRIC

related to:

a. inflammation and edema in the ulcerated area;
b. stimulation of exposed nerve endings and reflex muscle spasm (occurs when gastric secretions or other irritants come in contact with the ulcer).

Suggested NOC Outcomes: Pain control; Comfort level

Suggested NIC Interventions: Pain management; Analgesic administration; Medication management

Desired Outcome	Nursing Actions *and Selected Purposes/Rationales* (see pp. 45–47 for additional rationales)

1. The client will experience diminished pain as evidenced by:
   a. verbalization of a decrease in or absence of pain
   b. relaxed facial expression and body positioning
   c. increased participation in activities.

1.a. Assess for signs and symptoms of pain (e.g., verbalization of pain [may be described as a sharp, burning, aching, cramp-like, or gnawing epigastric pain that sometimes radiates to the back and/or chest], guarding of abdomen, rubbing epigastric area, grimacing, reluctance to move, restlessness).

b. Assess client's perception of the severity of pain using a pain intensity rating scale.

c. Assess the client's pain pattern (e.g., location, quality, onset, duration, precipitating factors, aggravating factors, alleviating factors).

d. Implement measures *to reduce epigastric pain:*
   1. perform actions *to prevent further tissue irritation and/or promote healing of the ulcer:*
      a. withhold oral intake as ordered *to reduce stimulation of gastric acid secretion*
      b. insert a nasogastric tube and maintain suction as ordered *to remove gastric secretions*
      c. administer the following medications if ordered:
         1. histamine$_2$ receptor antagonists (e.g., famotidine, ranitidine, nizatidine) and/or proton-pump inhibitors (e.g., omeprazole, esomeprazole, lansoprazole, pantoprazole) *to inhibit gastric acid secretion*
         2. antimicrobials (e.g., amoxicillin, clarithromycin, tetracycline, metronidazole) *to treat H. pylori infection if present;* the usual treatment regimen includes antimicrobials plus a proton-pump inhibitor or bismuth subsalicylate (e.g., Pepto-Bismol); *the bismuth subsalicylate is believed to have an antibacterial effect, promote ulcer healing, and protect the ulcerated area*
         3. cytoprotective agents (e.g., sucralfate) *to protect the ulcerated area*
         4. synthetic prostaglandins (e.g., misoprostol) *to inhibit gastric acid secretion and protect the ulcerated area*
         5. antacids *to neutralize gastric secretions* (because antacids can provide rapid relief of symptoms, they are often given initially to supplement treatment with histamine$_2$ receptor antagonists and proton-pump inhibitors)
      d. implement measures to reduce fear and anxiety (e.g., provide a calm, restful environment; explain all diagnostic tests and treatment plan) *in order to reduce stimulation of the vagus nerve and subsequent increase in gastric acid output*
      e. when foods/fluids are allowed:
         1. instruct client to:
            a. avoid intake of coffee, caffeine-containing tea and colas, spices such as black pepper and chili powder, and extremely hot foods/fluids *(these substances typically cause irritation of the gastric mucosa)*
            b. chew food thoroughly and eat slowly *(a large bolus of food causes an increased output of hydrochloric acid and pepsin)*
            c. avoid intake of foods/fluids that cause epigastric pain

Desired Outcome	Nursing Actions *and Selected Purposes/Rationales*
	2. provide regularly scheduled meals and snacks as ordered *to neutralize gastric acid* (moderate-sized meals are usually recommended rather than large ones *to help prevent the stimulation of excessive amounts of gastric acid*) f. encourage client to stop smoking g. if client must take medications that are known to be ulcerogenic (e.g., aspirin or other NSAIDs, corticosteroids), administer them with meals or snacks *to decrease gastric irritation* 2. provide or assist with nonpharmacologic measures for pain relief (e.g., position change; progressive relaxation exercises; restful environment; diversional activities such as watching television, reading, or conversing) 3. administer analgesics if ordered. e. Consult physician if above measures fail to provide adequate pain relief.

2. Collaborative Diagnoses: POTENTIAL COMPLICATIONS OF PEPTIC ULCER

a. hypovolemic shock related to upper gastrointestinal (GI) bleeding associated with:
   1. erosion of numerous small blood vessels (the gastric and duodenal mucosa have a rich blood supply)
   2. erosion of a major blood vessel (can occur if the ulcer is deep);

b. peritonitis related to leakage of gastrointestinal contents into the peritoneal cavity associated with perforation of the wall of the stomach or duodenum (can occur if the ulcer is deep);

c. gastric outlet obstruction related to narrowing of the pylorus associated with inflammation, spasm, and/or scar tissue formation (can occur if the ulcer is at or near the gastric outlet).

Desired Outcomes	Nursing Actions *and Selected Purposes/Rationales*
2.a. The client will not develop hypovolemic shock as evidenced by: 1. usual mental status 2. stable vital signs 3. skin warm and usual color 4. palpable peripheral pulses 5. urine output at least 30 ml/hour.	2.a.1. Assess for and report signs and symptoms of: a. upper GI bleeding (e.g., hematemesis; bright red or coffee-ground drainage from nasogastric tube; melena; decreased B/P; increased pulse rate; decreasing RBC, Hct, and Hgb levels) b. hypovolemic shock: 1. restlessness, agitation, confusion, or other change in mental status 2. significant decrease in B/P 3. postural hypotension 4. rapid, weak pulse 5. rapid respirations 6. cool skin 7. pallor, cyanosis 8. diminished or absent peripheral pulses 9. urine output less than 30 ml/hour. 2. Implement measures to prevent further tissue irritation and/or promote healing of the ulcer (see Diagnosis 1, action d.1) *in order to prevent upper GI bleeding.* 3. If signs and symptoms of upper GI bleeding occur: a. insert nasogastric tube if not already present and maintain suction as ordered b. prepare client for diagnostic tests (e.g., endoscopy) if planned c. assist with measures to control bleeding (e.g., gastric lavage, endoscopic electrocoagulation, selective arterial embolization) if ordered d. prepare client for surgical intervention (e.g., ligation of bleeding vessels, partial gastrectomy) if planned. 4. If signs and symptoms of hypovolemic shock occur: a. place client flat in bed with legs elevated unless contraindicated

b. monitor vital signs frequently
c. administer oxygen as ordered
d. administer blood products and/or volume expanders if ordered
e. prepare client for insertion of hemodynamic monitoring devices (e.g., central venous catheter, intra-arterial catheter) if planned.

2.b. The client will not develop peritonitis as evidenced by:
1. no reports of new or increased abdominal pain and tenderness
2. soft, nondistended abdomen
3. afebrile status
4. stable vital signs
5. absence of nausea and vomiting
6. normal bowel sounds
7. WBC count within normal range.

2.b.1. Assess for and report signs and symptoms of:
a. perforation of the gastric or duodenal wall (e.g., sudden, sharp, severe upper abdominal pain; extreme abdominal tenderness; shoulder pain [can occur as a result of phrenic nerve irritation]; abdominal x-ray showing free air in peritoneal cavity)
b. peritonitis (e.g., reports of new or increased abdominal pain; rebound tenderness; distended, rigid abdomen; elevated temperature; tachycardia; tachypnea; hypotension; nausea; vomiting; diminished or absent bowel sounds; increase in WBC count).

2. Implement measures to prevent further tissue irritation and/or promote healing of the ulcer (see Diagnosis 1, action d.1) *in order to reduce the risk for perforation.*
3. If signs and symptoms of peritonitis occur:
a. withhold oral intake as ordered
b. place client on bed rest in a semi-Fowler's position *to assist in pooling or localizing gastrointestinal contents in the pelvis rather than under the diaphragm*
c. prepare client for diagnostic tests (e.g., abdominal x-ray, computed tomography, ultrasonography) if planned
d. insert a nasogastric tube and maintain suction as ordered
e. administer antimicrobials as ordered
f. administer intravenous fluids and/or blood volume expanders if ordered *to prevent or treat shock (can result from the increased capillary permeability that occurs with inflammation and the subsequent escape of protein, fluid, and electrolytes from the vascular space into the peritoneal cavity)*
g. prepare client for surgical repair of the perforation if indicated.

2.c. The client will not experience gastric outlet obstruction as evidenced by:
1. soft, nondistended epigastric area
2. no reports of epigastric fullness or bloating
3. absence of anorexia, nausea, and vomiting.

2.c.1. Assess for and report signs and symptoms of gastric outlet obstruction (e.g., epigastric distention, reports of epigastric fullness or bloating, anorexia, nausea, vomiting, foul-smelling vomitus containing particles of food ingested many hours earlier).

2. Implement measures to prevent further tissue irritation and/or promote healing of the ulcer (see Diagnosis 1, action d.1) *in order to reduce the risk of narrowing of the pylorus if the ulcer is at or near the gastric outlet.*
3. If signs and symptoms of gastric outlet obstruction occur:
a. withhold oral intake as ordered
b. prepare client for diagnostic tests (e.g., endoscopy, barium swallow) if planned
c. insert a nasogastric tube and maintain suction as ordered
d. administer intravenous fluid and electrolyte replacements as ordered
e. prepare client for endoscopic balloon dilatation or surgical intervention (e.g., partial gastrectomy, pyloroplasty) if planned.

Discharge Teaching/Continued Care

3. NURSING DIAGNOSIS: DEFICIENT KNOWLEDGE OR INEFFECTIVE HEALTH MAINTENANCE*

*The nurse should select the diagnostic label that is most appropriate for the client's discharge teaching needs.

Suggested NOC Outcomes: Knowledge: disease process; Knowledge: medication; Knowledge: treatment regimen

Suggested NIC Interventions: Health system guidance; Teaching: individual; Teaching: disease process; Teaching: prescribed diet; Teaching: prescribed medication

Desired Outcomes	Nursing Actions *and Selected Purposes/Rationales*
3.a. The client will verbalize a basic understanding of peptic ulcer disease and the importance of adhering to the prescribed treatment plan.	3.a. Explain peptic ulcer disease in terms the client can understand; stress that complications such as hemorrhage, perforation, and obstruction can occur and/or the ulcer will recur if the treatment plan is not followed.
3.b. The client will identify ways to promote healing of the existing ulcer and prevent recurrence of peptic ulcer.	3.b. Instruct client in ways to promote healing of the existing ulcer and prevent recurrence of peptic ulcer: 1. drink decaffeinated or caffeine-free tea and colas rather than those containing caffeine 2. avoid drinking coffee and alcohol or drink these beverages only in small amounts during or immediately following a meal 3. avoid ingestion of foods that are known to irritate gastric mucosa directly or increase gastric acid production (e.g., whole grains, chocolate, rich pastries, spicy foods, meat extracts, extremely hot foods) 4. avoid intake of any foods and fluids that cause gastric distress 5. eat three regularly scheduled meals (moderate-sized, rather than large) and snacks each day; do not skip meals 6. eat slowly and chew food thoroughly 7. maintain a calm, pleasant atmosphere at mealtime and whenever possible 8. stop smoking 9. maintain a balance of physical activity and rest 10. avoid stressful situations whenever possible 11. avoid ingestion of over-the-counter medications such as aspirin and ibuprofen; if it is necessary to take these or other ulcerogenic medications (e.g., corticosteroids), take them with antacids or food unless contraindicated and/or take enteric-coated or buffered preparations of the drugs if available 12. if it is necessary to take an NSAID, consult health care provider about taking it with a medication that helps protect the gastric mucosa (e.g., misoprostol, sucralfate) and/or switching to an NSAID that is known to be less irritating to the mucosa (e.g., a COX-2 inhibitor selective agent such as celecoxib, valdecoxib, and rofecoxib) 13. take medications for ulcer treatment as prescribed.
3.c. The client will verbalize an understanding of medications ordered including rationale, food and drug interactions, side effects, schedule for taking, and importance of taking as prescribed.	3.c.1. Explain the rationale for, side effects of, schedule for taking, and importance of taking medications prescribed. Inform client of pertinent food and drug interactions. 2. If client is discharged on antacid therapy, instruct to: a. take as prescribed (usually 7 times/day [1 hour and 3 hours after each meal and at bedtime] or 4 times/day [1 hour after each meal and at bedtime] for 4–6 weeks) b. take antacid suspensions rather than tablets whenever possible (suspensions neutralize gastric acid more effectively) c. thoroughly chew tablets that are labeled as "chewable" d. shake antacid suspensions vigorously before taking dose e. check the sodium content of antacids and avoid intake of those high in sodium (e.g., Amphojel, Basaljel, Delcid) if hypertensive or on a sodium-restricted diet

f. alternate aluminum-containing antacids (e.g., Amphojel, ALternaGEL) and magnesium-containing antacids (e.g., Milk of Magnesia, Mag-Ox) periodically or take aluminum and magnesium hydroxide combination antacids (e.g., Maalox, Gaviscon, Mylanta) if constipation or diarrhea develops
g. avoid excessive intake of antacids high in calcium (e.g., Titralac, Tums) and sodium bicarbonate (e.g., baking soda, Alka-Seltzer)
h. expect that stool may be speckled or whitish
i. observe for and report:
   1. thirst, dry mouth, weakness, lethargy (may indicate hypernatremia resulting from excessive amounts of antacids containing sodium) and/or swelling of extremities and weight gain (can occur with the subsequent water retention)
   2. constipation not resolved by increased fluid intake, laxatives, and switching to an antacid containing magnesium
   3. diarrhea not controlled by antidiarrheal medication and switching to an antacid containing aluminum.

3. If client is discharged on sucralfate (Carafate), instruct to:
   a. take it an hour before meals and at bedtime
   b. avoid taking antacids for at least 30 minutes before and after taking the medication
   c. monitor for and report persistent constipation, nausea, or indigestion.
4. If client is discharged on a histamine$_2$ receptor antagonist (e.g., nizatidine, famotidine, ranitidine) or proton-pump inhibitor (e.g., pantoprazole, esomeprazole, omeprazole, lansoprazole) instruct to:
   a. consult physician or pharmacist about appropriate scheduling in relation to other medications and meals
   b. do not crush or chew the granules that are in capsules
   c. monitor for and report persistent sleepiness, headache, dizziness, rash, diarrhea, or nausea.
5. If client is discharged on misoprostol (e.g., Cytotec), instruct to:
   a. avoid taking it with food or antacids
   b. monitor for and report persistent diarrhea, abdominal pain, or menstrual irregularities (e.g., spotting, cramps, excessive bleeding)
   c. notify physician it pregnancy is suspected (misoprostol may induce miscarriage).
6. If client is discharged on a bismuth-containing agent (e.g., Pepto-Bismol), instruct to:
   a. be aware that the medication can cause a temporary grey-black discoloration of the tongue and stool
   b. shake suspension vigorously before taking dose
   c. thoroughly chew tablets that are labeled as "chewable"
   d. monitor for and report taste disturbances that interfere with adequate nutritional intake or constipation that is not resolved by increasing intake of fluids and high fiber foods or taking a laxative.
7. If client is discharged on antimicrobial medications for treatment of *H. pylori* infection (e.g., amoxicillin, clarithromycin, tetracycline, metronidazole), instruct to:
   a. take them for the prescribed length of time (usually 2 weeks) and frequency (antimicrobials should be spaced as evenly as possible over a 24 hour period to maintain optimal serum levels); avoid skipping doses or adjusting doses
   b. monitor for and report nausea, vomiting, diarrhea, rash, itching, white patches in mouth, vaginal itching or discharge, fever, chills, joint pain or swelling
   c. complete follow-up testing (e.g., blood test, urea breath test, endoscopy) as prescribed (testing is usually done about 4 weeks after completion of the antimicrobial regimen to determine if it has effectively cured the infection).
8. Instruct client to consult physician before taking any additional antacids or other nonprescription medications that are advertised for the treatment of peptic ulcers.

Desired Outcomes	Nursing Actions *and Selected Purposes/Rationales*
	9. Caution client to consult physician before stopping any medication prescribed for peptic ulcer treatment. 10. Instruct client to inform health care providers of medications being taken for the treatment of peptic ulcer (many of these drugs can alter the absorption of other medications).
3.d. The client will state signs and symptoms to report to the health care provider.	3.d. Instruct client to report: 1. black or tarry stools 2. bloody or coffee-ground vomitus 3. abdominal distention 4. persistent epigastric fullness or bloating, nausea, and/or vomiting 5. persistent weight loss 6. persistent or increased epigastric or abdominal pain 7. weakness and fatigue 8. undesirable side effects of medications prescribed (see actions c.2.i, 3.c, 4.c, 5.b, 6.d, and 7.b in this diagnosis) 9. persistent high stress levels 10. difficulty taking medications as prescribed.
3.e. The client will verbalize an understanding of and a plan for adhering to recommended follow-up care including future appointments with health care provider.	3.e.1. Reinforce the importance of keeping follow-up appointments with health care provider. 2. Implement measures to improve client compliance: a. include significant others in teaching sessions if possible b. encourage questions and allow time for reinforcement and clarification of information provided c. if client has concerns regarding the cost of medications, obtain a social service consult to assist with financial planning and to obtain financial aid if indicated d. obtain a dietary consult if client needs assistance planning meals that meet nutritional needs and incorporating the recommended dietary modifications into his/her daily routines and personal and cultural preferences e. if appropriate, provide information about and encourage use of community resources that can assist the client to make necessary lifestyle changes (e.g., smoking cessation programs, stress management classes, counseling services) f. if client is being treated for *H. pylori* infection, inform him/her that the treatment regimen, which involves taking multiple medications on various schedules is not a long-term situation (it is usually effective after just 2 weeks) g. provide written instructions about future appointments with health care provider, medications prescribed, dietary modifications, signs and symptoms to report, and follow-up tests.

Additional Nursing Diagnoses

IMBALANCED NUTRITION: LESS THAN BODY REQUIREMENTS*

related to:

a. decreased oral intake associated with pain (especially with a gastric ulcer because pain often increases after eating);

b. failure to eat a well-balanced diet associated with dietary modifications.

FEAR/ANXIETY*

related to pain; lack of understanding of the diagnosis, diagnostic tests, treatment plan, and prognosis; unfamiliar environment; financial concerns; and possible need to change lifestyle in order to control symptoms and prevent ulcer recurrence.

---

*See Unit II for outcomes, actions, and rationales.

INEFFECTIVE THERAPEUTIC REGIMEN MANAGEMENT

related to lack of understanding of the implications of not following the prescribed treatment plan and difficulty modifying personal habits.

Bibliography

See pages 879 and 884.

UNIT XV

Nursing Care of the Client with Disturbances of the Liver, Biliary Tract, and Pancreas

Cholecystectomy

A cholecystectomy is the surgical removal of the gallbladder. It is commonly performed to treat symptomatic cholecystitis and/or cholelithiasis. A cholecystectomy can be done via laparoscopy or through a right subcostal incision (open cholecystectomy). A laparoscopic cholecystectomy is usually the procedure of choice because of the short hospitalization (less than 2 days), reduced pain, and a more rapid return to usual activities. An open cholecystectomy is warranted when the client is in the last trimester of pregnancy or has a gangrenous or perforated gallbladder, a suspected gallbladder malignancy, severe inflammation that obscures the structures of the hepatobiliary triangle, or large stones in the biliary ducts. An open cholecystectomy may also be performed when problems are encountered during a laparoscopic cholecystectomy. If stones are present in the common bile duct, they can often be extracted endoscopically but a choledocholithotomy may be necessary if the stones are large. Following a choledocholithotomy, a T tube is placed in the common bile duct to maintain adequate flow or drainage of bile until ductal edema subsides.

This care plan focuses on the adult client hospitalized for an open cholecystectomy with common bile duct exploration.

OUTCOME/DISCHARGE CRITERIA

- have pain controlled
- tolerate prescribed diet
- have evidence of normal healing of surgical wound(s) and normal skin integrity around T tube site
- have clear, audible breath sounds throughout lungs
- have no signs and symptoms of postoperative complications
- demonstrate the ability to appropriately care for T tube and surrounding skin if T tube is present
- verbalize an understanding of the rationale for and components of a low- to moderate-fat diet if prescribed
- state signs and symptoms to report to the health care provider
- verbalize an understanding of and a plan for adhering to recommended follow-up care including future appointments with health care provider, wound care, medications prescribed, and activity level.

NURSING/COLLABORATIVE DIAGNOSES

Postoperative

1. Ineffective breathing pattern p. 670
2. Potential complications p. 670
   a. abscess formation
   b. peritonitis
   c. continued obstruction of bile flow

DISCHARGE TEACHING

3. Deficient knowledge, Ineffective therapeutic regimen management, or Ineffective health maintenance p. 672

See Care Plan on Cholelithiasis/Cholecystitis (pp. 674–680) and the Standardized Preoperative and Postoperative Care Plans (pp. 97–126) for additional diagnoses.

PREOPERATIVE

Refer to the Care Plan on Cholelithiasis/Cholecystitis and the Standardized Preoperative Care Plan.

POSTOPERATIVE

Use in conjunction with the Standardized Postoperative Care Plan.

1. Nursing Diagnosis: INEFFECTIVE BREATHING PATTERN

related to:
a. increased rate of respirations associated with fear and anxiety;
b. decreased rate of respirations associated with the depressant effect of anesthesia and some medications (e.g., narcotic [opioid] analgesics, some antiemetics);
c. decreased depth of respirations associated with:
   1. depressant effect of anesthesia and some medications (e.g., narcotic [opioid] analgesics, some antiemetics)
   2. reluctance to breathe deeply because of pain
   3. fear, anxiety, weakness, and fatigue
   4. restricted chest expansion resulting from positioning and elevation of the diaphragm if abdominal distention is present.

Suggested NOC Outcome: Respiratory status: ventilation

Suggested NIC Interventions: Respiratory monitoring; Ventilation assistance; Pain management

Desired Outcome	Nursing Actions *and Selected Purposes/Rationales*
1. The client will maintain an effective breathing pattern (see Standardized Postoperative Care Plan, Diagnosis 2 [p. 104], for outcome criteria).	1.a. Refer to Standardized Postoperative Care Plan, Diagnosis 2 (p. 104), for measures related to assessment and management of an ineffective breathing pattern. b. Implement additional measures *to improve breathing pattern:* 1. instruct client to bend knees while coughing and deep breathing *in order to relieve tension on abdominal muscles and incision* 2. instruct and assist client to splint incision with hands or pillow when coughing and deep breathing.

2. Collaborative Diagnoses: POTENTIAL COMPLICATIONS OF CHOLECYSTECTOMY

a. **abscess formation** related to accumulation of drainage in the surgical area and subsequent invasion of the area by microorganisms and neutrophils;
b. **peritonitis** related to escape of bile into the peritoneal cavity associated with surgical trauma to the gallbladder and biliary duct;
c. **continued obstruction of bile flow** related to residual stones in the biliary duct system or persistent inflammation and/or strictures of the common bile duct associated with surgical trauma.

Desired Outcomes	Nursing Actions *and Selected Purposes/Rationales*
2.a. The client will not develop an abscess as evidenced by: 1. gradual resolution of abdominal pain 2. temperature declining toward normal 3. WBC count declining toward normal.	2.a.1. Assess for and report signs and symptoms of an abscess (e.g., increased or more constant abdominal pain, increase in temperature and pulse rate, further increase in WBC count). 2. Implement measures *to prevent accumulation of drainage in the surgical area in order to reduce the risk for abscess formation:* a. perform actions *to maintain patency of wound drain and/or T tube if present:* 1. implement measures *to prevent stasis and reflux of drainage:* a. keep drainage tubing free of dependent loops and kinks (prevent kinking by placing a gauze roll under the drain tube and anchoring it to the skin or dressing with tape) b. keep collection device(s) below drain insertion site(s) unless ordered otherwise (physician may order T tube collection

device to be positioned just slightly below, level with, or above drain insertion site *in order to reduce loss of bile*)
c. empty collection device(s) as often as necessary and at least every shift
2. implement measures *to prevent inadvertent removal of wound drain and/or T tube:*
a. instruct client not to pull on drain(s) and drainage tubing
b. use caution when changing dressings surrounding drain(s)
c. attach collection device(s) securely to abdominal dressing
b. maintain client in a semi- to high-Fowler's position as much as possible when in bed.
3. If signs and symptoms of an abscess occur:
a. prepare client for diagnostic tests (e.g., ultrasonography, computed tomography)
b. administer antimicrobials if ordered
c. prepare client for surgical intervention (e.g., incision and drainage of abscess) if planned.

2.b. The client will not develop peritonitis as evidenced by:
1. gradual resolution of abdominal pain
2. soft, nondistended abdomen
3. temperature declining toward normal
4. stable vital signs
5. absence of nausea and vomiting
6. gradual return of normal bowel sounds
7. WBC count declining toward normal.

2.b.1. Assess for and report signs and symptoms of peritonitis (e.g., increase in severity of abdominal pain; generalized abdominal pain; rebound tenderness; distended, rigid abdomen; increase in temperature; tachycardia; tachypnea; hypotension; nausea; vomiting; continued diminished or absent bowel sounds; WBC count that increases or fails to decline toward normal).
2. Implement measures *to prevent peritonitis:*
a. perform actions to maintain patency and prevent inadvertent removal of wound drain and/or T tube if present (see action a.2.a in this diagnosis) *in order to reduce the risk for wound drainage and bile accumulating and leaking into the peritoneum*
b. administer antimicrobials if ordered.
3. If signs and symptoms of peritonitis occur:
a. withhold oral intake as ordered
b. place client on bed rest in a semi-Fowler's position *to assist in pooling or localizing gastrointestinal contents in the pelvis rather than under the diaphragm*
c. prepare client for diagnostic tests (e.g., abdominal x-ray, computed tomography, ultrasonography)
d. insert a nasogastric tube and maintain suction as ordered
e. administer antimicrobials as ordered
f. administer intravenous fluids and/or blood volume expanders if ordered *to prevent or treat shock (can result from the increased capillary permeability that occurs with inflammation and the subsequent escape of protein, fluid, and electrolytes from the vascular space into the peritoneal cavity)*
g. prepare client for surgical intervention (e.g., drainage and irrigation of peritoneum, repair of leakage site) if planned.

2.c. The client will have resolution of bile flow obstruction within 7–10 days after surgery as evidenced by:
1. decline in output of bile in T tube to less than 400 ml/day
2. absence of pain, nausea, and feeling of fullness when T tube is clamped
3. absence of jaundice, clay-colored stools, and dark amber urine.

2.c.1. Assess for and report signs and symptoms of continued bile flow obstruction (e.g., T tube draining more than 1000 ml in 24 hours; a marked increase in T tube drainage after it has started to decline; persistent pain, nausea, or feeling of fullness when T tube is clamped; jaundice; clay-colored stools; dark amber urine).
2. Implement measures to maintain patency of T tube (see action a.2.a. in this diagnosis) *in order to promote drainage of bile.*
3. If signs and symptoms of bile flow obstruction occur:
a. leave T tube unclamped
b. implement measures to maintain patency of T tube (see action a.2.a in this diagnosis)
c. prepare client for diagnostic tests (e.g., ultrasound, cholangiogram) if planned
d. prepare client for removal of residual stones (e.g., extraction via T tube, endoscopic sphincterotomy with basket removal of stones)

Desired Outcomes	Nursing Actions and Selected Purposes/Rationales
	or treatment of bile duct stricture (e.g., endoscopic or percutaneous balloon dilatation with or without stent placement, surgical resection of stricture site) if planned.

Discharge Teaching/Continued Care

3. Nursing Diagnosis: ***DEFICIENT KNOWLEDGE, INEFFECTIVE THERAPEUTIC REGIMEN MANAGEMENT, OR INEFFECTIVE HEALTH MAINTENANCE****

*The nurse should select the diagnostic label that is most appropriate for the client's discharge teaching needs.

Suggested NOC Outcomes: Knowledge: treatment regimen; Knowledge: diet

Suggested NIC Interventions: Health system guidance; Teaching: prescribed diet; Teaching: procedure/treatment; Teaching: prescribed medication

Desired Outcomes	Nursing Actions and Selected Purposes/Rationales
3.a. The client will demonstrate the ability to appropriately care for T tube and surrounding skin if T tube is present.	3.a.1. If the client is to be discharged with a T tube in place, instruct regarding care of the T tube and surrounding skin: a. cleanse the skin around the T tube insertion site daily and cover the site with a dry sterile dressing; apply zinc oxide cream to skin around insertion site if skin is irritated b. keep the T tube drainage collection device in the position prescribed (usually slightly below the insertion site) c. keep the tubing pinned to the dressing and avoid any kinks or tension on the tubing d. empty the drainage collection device at least twice daily or more often if needed; keep a record of the amount of drainage e. when emptying the drainage collection device, check to see that the tube has not become dislodged (this can be easily monitored if the tube is marked at the skin line before discharge) f. clamp T tube only as instructed. 2. Allow time for questions, clarification, and return demonstration of care of T tube and surrounding skin.
3.b. The client will verbalize an understanding of the rationale for and components of a low- to moderate-fat diet if prescribed.	3.b.1. Explain the rationale for avoiding excessive fat intake for the first 4–6 weeks after surgery (many physicians instruct client to just avoid foods that cause epigastric discomfort). 2. Instruct client to increase fat intake gradually and introduce foods/fluids high in fat (e.g., butter, cream, whole milk, ice cream, fried foods, gravies, nuts) one at a time.
3.c. The client will state signs and symptoms to report to the health care provider.	3.c.1. Refer to Standardized Postoperative Care Plan, Diagnosis 22, action c (p. 125), for signs and symptoms to report to health care provider. 2. Instruct client to report these additional signs and symptoms: a. development of increased itchiness or yellowing of skin b. clay-colored stools or dark amber urine when the T tube drainage subsides or after the T tube has been removed c. purulent drainage from the T tube or green-brown drainage around T tube or from wound site d. a significant increase in or more than 500 ml/day of drainage from T tube e. a sudden marked decrease in T tube drainage or increase in length of the T tube (may indicate that the T tube has become dislodged)

f. recurrent or persistent abdominal pain
g. abdominal distention or rigidity
h. recurrent or persistent temperature elevation
i. persistent heartburn, feeling of bloating, or nausea
j. loose stools that continue for longer than 2–3 months.

3.d. The client will verbalize an understanding of and a plan for adhering to recommended follow-up care including future appointments with health care provider, wound care, medications prescribed, and activity level.

3.d.1. Refer to Standardized Postoperative Care Plan, Diagnosis 22 (pp. 125–126), for routine postoperative instructions and measures to improve client compliance.
2. Instruct client to avoid heavy lifting for 4–6 weeks after surgery.
3. Inform client who has had a laparoscopic cholecystectomy that mild shoulder pain may persist for a week after surgery until the carbon dioxide used during surgery is completely absorbed. Tell client that lying on his/her left side with right knee flexed may help relieve this pain.

Bibliography

See pages 879 and 884.

evolve

Cholelithiasis/Cholecystitis

Cholelithiasis refers to the presence of gallstones in the gallbladder. Factors that contribute to gallstone formation are abnormal bile composition; biliary stasis or slow emptying of the gallbladder resulting from factors such as fasting, pregnancy, prolonged parenteral nutrition, or an obstructive lesion in the biliary system; and inflammation of the gallbladder. Cholesterol stones are the most prevalent type of gallstone. They are most often associated with a high-cholesterol diet or cholesterol-lowering drugs and form when bile becomes supersaturated with cholesterol, which then precipitates and starts to form stones. Other components of bile that precipitate into stones are bile salts, bilirubin, calcium, and protein. Stones either remain in the gallbladder or migrate into the duct system where they may cause partial or complete obstruction. The severity of the client's symptoms depends on the degree of bile flow obstruction.

Cholecystitis is inflammation of the gallbladder wall. The majority of cases of cholecystitis result from bile stasis, which is most commonly due to obstruction of the cystic duct by a gallstone. The bile trapped in the gallbladder acts as a chemical irritant causing inflammation and edema of the gallbladder wall. Cholecystitis in the absence of stones (acalculous cholecystitis) is thought to result from a buildup of mucus or sludge in the gallbladder associated with biliary stasis. This stasis can result from factors such as prolonged fasting or total parenteral nutrition, ischemia of the gallbladder associated with vasculitis, or bacterial invasion of the gallbladder via the blood or lymph system. Following the period of acute inflammation, scarring often develops, resulting in loss of normal gallbladder function.

In most cases, the treatment of choice for symptomatic cholelithiasis and cholecystitis is cholecystectomy and choledocholithotomy if stones have migrated into the biliary duct system. A percutaneous cholecystostomy may be done to relieve symptoms if the client has severe symptoms and is a poor surgical risk. Nonsurgical treatment of gallstones includes endoscopic sphincterotomy with basket removal of stones, dissolution of stones using oral bile acids, percutaneous or endoscopic instillation of a dissolution agent into the gallbladder, and extracorporeal shock-wave lithotripsy. These nonoperative modalities are only performed on a small percentage of patients (e.g., high-risk surgical candidates, persons who refuse surgery) because of the high incidence of recurrence of gallstones with nonsurgical treatments and the increasing popularity of laparoscopic surgery.

This care plan focuses on the adult client hospitalized with probable cholelithiasis and/or cholecystitis.

OUTCOME/DISCHARGE CRITERIA

THE CLIENT WILL:

- have relief of severe pain
- tolerate prescribed diet
- have no signs and symptoms of complications
- verbalize an understanding of ways to reduce the risk for recurrent gallbladder attacks
- state signs and symptoms to report to the health care provider
- verbalize an understanding of and a plan for adhering to recommended follow-up care including future appointments with health care provider and medications prescribed.

NURSING/COLLABORATIVE DIAGNOSES

1. Imbalanced fluid and electrolytes: deficient fluid volume, hypokalemia, hypochloremia, and metabolic alkalosis p. 675
2. Acute pain: epigastric area or right upper quadrant of abdomen with radiation to interscapular area or right scapula or shoulder p. 675
3. Nausea p. 676
4. Altered comfort: dyspepsia p. 677
5. Potential complications p. 677
   a. abscess or fistula formation
   b. peritonitis
   c. pancreatitis
   d. cholangitis

DISCHARGE TEACHING

6. Deficient knowledge, Ineffective therapeutic regimen management, or Ineffective health maintenance p. 679

See p. 680 for additional diagnoses.

1. NURSING/COLLABORATIVE DIAGNOSIS:

IMBALANCED FLUID AND ELECTROLYTES: DEFICIENT FLUID VOLUME, HYPOKALEMIA, HYPOCHLOREMIA, AND METABOLIC ALKALOSIS

related to decreased oral intake and excessive loss of fluid and electrolytes associated with vomiting and nasogastric tube drainage.

Suggested NOC Outcomes: Fluid balance; Electrolyte and acid/base balance

Suggested NIC Interventions: Fluid monitoring; Fluid management; Electrolyte management: hypokalemia; Fluid/Electrolyte management; Acid-base monitoring; Acid-base management: metabolic alkalosis

Desired Outcome

1. The client will maintain fluid and electrolyte balance as evidenced by:
   a. normal skin turgor
   b. moist mucous membranes
   c. stable weight
   d. B/P and pulse within normal range for client and stable with position change
   e. capillary refill time less than 2–3 seconds
   f. usual mental status
   g. balanced intake and output
   h. urine specific gravity within normal range
   i. soft, nondistended abdomen with normal bowel sounds
   j. absence of cardiac dysrhythmias, muscle weakness, paresthesias, twitching, spasms, and dizziness
   k. BUN, Hct, serum electrolytes, and blood gases within normal range.

Nursing Actions *and Selected Purposes/Rationales*
(see pp. 30–31 for additional rationales)

1.a. Assess for and report signs and symptoms of:
   1. deficient fluid volume:
      a. decreased skin turgor, dry mucous membranes, thirst
      b. weight loss of 2% or greater over a short period
      c. postural hypotension and/or low B/P
      d. weak, rapid pulse
      e. capillary refill time greater than 2–3 seconds
      f. flat neck veins when supine
      g. change in mental status
      h. decreased urine output with increased specific gravity (reflects an actual rather than potential fluid deficit)
      i. increased BUN and Hct
   2. hypokalemia (e.g., cardiac dysrhythmias, postural hypotension, muscle weakness, nausea and vomiting, abdominal distention, hypoactive or absent bowel sounds, low serum potassium)
   3. hypochloremia and metabolic alkalosis (e.g., dizziness, paresthesias, muscle twitching or spasms, hypoventilation, low serum chloride, elevated pH and TCO_2).

b. Implement measures *to prevent or treat imbalanced fluid and electrolytes:*
   1. perform actions to reduce nausea and vomiting (see Diagnosis 3, action b)
   2. if a nasogastric tube is present and needs to be irrigated frequently and/or with large volumes of solution, irrigate it with normal saline rather than water
   3. maintain a fluid intake of at least 2500 ml/day unless contraindicated; if oral intake is inadequate or contraindicated, maintain intravenous therapy as ordered
   4. administer electrolyte replacements if ordered
   5. when oral intake is allowed, assist client to select foods/fluids high in potassium (e.g., bananas, potatoes, raisins, orange juice, cantaloupe).

c. Consult physician if signs and symptoms of imbalanced fluid and electrolytes persist or worsen.

2. NURSING DIAGNOSIS:

ACUTE PAIN: EPIGASTRIC AREA OR RIGHT UPPER QUADRANT OF ABDOMEN WITH RADIATION TO INTERSCAPULAR AREA OR RIGHT SCAPULA OR SHOULDER

related to:
a. inflammation and distention of the gallbladder;
b. ductal spasms associated with blockage of bile flow if gallstones are present in the duct system.

Suggested NOC Outcomes: Pain control; Comfort level

Suggested NIC Interventions: Analgesic administration; Pain management; Patient-controlled analgesia (PCA) assistance

Desired Outcome	Nursing Actions *and Selected Purposes/Rationales* (see pp. 45–47 for additional rationales)

2. The client will experience diminished pain as evidenced by:
   a. verbalization of same
   b. relaxed facial expression and body positioning
   c. increased participation in activities
   d. stable vital signs.

2.a. Assess for signs and symptoms of pain (e.g., verbalization of pain, grimacing, reluctance to move, guarding of abdomen, rubbing right shoulder, restlessness, diaphoresis, increased B/P, tachycardia).
  b. Assess client's perception of the severity of pain using a pain intensity rating scale.
  c. Assess the client's pain pattern (e.g., location, quality, onset, duration, precipitating factors, aggravating factors, alleviating factors); note that a finding of increased pain with transient inspiratory arrest upon deep palpation of the right upper quadrant (Murphy's sign) is indicative of cholecystitis.
  d. Implement measures *to reduce pain:*
    1. perform actions *to reduce fear and anxiety about the pain experience* (e.g., assure client that his/her need for pain relief is understood, plan methods for achieving pain control with client)
    2. perform actions *to reduce stimulation of gallbladder contractions:*
       a. maintain NPO status as ordered
       b. insert nasogastric tube and maintain suction if ordered
       c. when oral intake is allowed, maintain dietary restrictions of fat as ordered (avoid foods/fluids high in fat such as butter, cream, whole milk, ice cream, fried foods, gravies, and nuts)
    3. provide or assist with nonpharmacologic measures for pain relief (e.g., position change; restful environment; diversional activities such as watching television, reading, or conversing)
    4. administer the following if ordered:
       a. analgesics
       b. antimicrobials *to prevent or treat infection and subsequently reduce inflammation of the gallbladder wall*
    5. if client has a patient-controlled analgesia device, encourage him/her to use it as instructed.
  e. Consult appropriate health care provider (e.g., pharmacist, physician) if above measures fail to provide adequate pain relief.

3. Nursing Diagnosis: *NAUSEA*

related to stimulation of the vomiting center associated with:
a. stimulation of the visceral afferent pathways as a result of the visceral irritation that occurs with gallbladder and bile duct inflammation;
b. stimulation of the cerebral cortex resulting from pain and stress.

Suggested NOC Outcome: Nausea and vomiting severity

Suggested NIC Interventions: Nausea management; Vomiting management; Environmental management: comfort

Desired Outcome	Nursing Actions *and Selected Purposes/Rationales*

3. The client will experience relief of nausea and vomiting as evidenced by:
   a. verbalization of relief of nausea
   b. absence of vomiting.

3.a. Assess client for nausea and vomiting.
  b. Implement measures *to reduce nausea and vomiting:*
    1. maintain NPO status if ordered
    2. insert nasogastric tube and maintain suction if ordered
    3. eliminate noxious sights and odors from the environment *(noxious stimuli can cause stimulation of the vomiting center)*
    4. instruct client to change positions slowly *(rapid movement can result in stimulation of the chemoreceptor trigger zone and subsequent excitation of the vomiting center)*
    5. provide oral hygiene after each emesis
    6. perform actions to reduce pain (see Diagnosis 2, action d)
    7. encourage client to take deep, slow breaths when nauseated

8. when oral intake is allowed:
   a. advance diet as tolerated
   b. avoid serving foods with an overpowering aroma; remove lids from hot foods before entering room
   c. provide small, frequent meals; instruct client to ingest foods and fluids slowly
   d. instruct client to eat dry foods (e.g., toast, crackers) and avoid drinking liquids with meals if nauseated
   e. instruct client to avoid the following:
      1. foods/fluids high in fat (e.g., butter, cream, whole milk, ice cream, fried foods, gravies, nuts)
      2. foods/fluids that irritate the gastric mucosa (e.g., spicy foods; caffeine-containing beverages such as tea, coffee, and colas)
9. administer antiemetics if ordered (phenothiazines should be used cautiously *because of their potential cholestatic effect*).

c. Consult physician if above measures fail to control nausea and vomiting.

4. NURSING DIAGNOSIS: ALTERED COMFORT: DYSPEPSIA

related to impaired fat digestion associated with bile flow obstruction.

Suggested NOC Outcome: Comfort level	**Suggested NIC Interventions:** Flatulence reduction; Nausea management

Desired Outcome	Nursing Actions and Selected Purposes/Rationales
4. The client will verbalize relief of dyspepsia.	4.a. Assess client for signs and symptoms of dyspepsia (e.g., reports of epigastric discomfort, heartburn, nausea, or feeling of fullness or bloating; frequent eructation). b. Determine if particular foods/fluids contribute to dyspepsia (client usually reports an intolerance of fatty foods). c. Implement measures *to reduce dyspepsia:* 1. perform actions to reduce nausea (see Diagnosis 3, action b) 2. perform actions *to reduce the accumulation of gas in the gastrointestinal tract:* a. encourage and assist client with frequent position changes and ambulation as allowed and tolerated *(activity stimulates peristalsis and expulsion of flatus)* b. instruct client to avoid activities such as chewing gum, drinking through a straw, and smoking *in order to reduce air swallowing* c. encourage client to avoid the following foods/fluids: 1. those high in fat (e.g., fried foods, gravies, butter, cream, whole milk, ice cream, nuts) 2. carbonated beverages 3. gas-producing foods (e.g., cabbage, onions, beans) d. encourage client to eructate and expel flatus whenever the urge is felt e. administer antiflatulents (e.g., simethicone) if ordered 3. administer antacids if ordered. d. Consult physician if above measures fail to control dyspepsia.

5. COLLABORATIVE DIAGNOSIS: POTENTIAL COMPLICATIONS OF CHOLELITHIASIS/CHOLECYSTITIS

a. abscess or fistula formation related to presence of increased cholecystic and ductal pressure (can cause perforation of the gallbladder into localized, contained area [abscess] or wall of an adjacent organ [fistula]);

b. [illegible] related to escape of bile into the peritoneal cavity associated with perforation of the gallbladder;

c. [illegible] related to obstruction of the flow of pancreatic secretions as a result of a stone or inflammation in the common bile duct;

d. cholangitis related to proliferation of bacteria in the biliary ducts associated with obstructed bile flow and stasis of bile.

Desired Outcomes	**Nursing Actions** *and Selected Purposes/Rationales*
5.a. The client will experience resolution of any abscess or fistula that develops as evidenced by: 1. decrease in abdominal pain 2. temperature and pulse declining toward normal 3. WBC count declining toward normal.	5.a.1. Assess for and report signs and symptoms of abscess and/or fistula formation (e.g., increased abdominal pain, further increase in temperature and pulse rate, further increase in WBC count). 2. If signs and symptoms of an abscess or fistula occur: a. prepare client for diagnostic studies (e.g., ultrasonography, computed tomography) b. administer antimicrobials as ordered c. prepare client for surgical intervention (e.g., cholecystectomy or cholecystostomy with incision and drainage of abscess or closure of fistula) if planned.
5.b. The client will have resolution of peritonitis if it occurs as evidenced by: 1. gradual resolution of abdominal pain 2. soft, nondistended abdomen 3. temperature declining toward normal 4. stable vital signs 5. decreased nausea and vomiting 6. gradual return of normal bowel sounds 7. WBC count declining toward normal.	5.b.1. Assess for and report signs and symptoms of peritonitis (e.g., diffuse abdominal pain; rebound tenderness; distended, rigid abdomen; further increase in temperature; tachycardia; tachypnea; hypotension; increased nausea and vomiting; diminished or absent bowel sounds; WBC count that increases or fails to decline toward normal). 2. If signs and symptoms of peritonitis occur: a. withhold oral intake as ordered b. place client on bed rest in a semi-Fowler's position *to assist in pooling or localizing gastrointestinal contents in the pelvis rather than under the diaphragm* c. prepare client for diagnostic tests (e.g., abdominal x-ray, computed tomography, ultrasonography) if planned d. insert a nasogastric tube and maintain suction as ordered e. administer antimicrobials as ordered f. administer intravenous fluids and/or blood volume expanders if ordered *to prevent or treat shock (can result from the increased capillary permeability that occurs with inflammation and the subsequent escape of protein, fluid, and electrolytes from the vascular space into the peritoneal cavity)* g. prepare client for surgery (e.g., cholecystectomy or cholecystostomy with peritoneal lavage) if planned.
5.c. The client will experience resolution of pancreatitis if it occurs as evidenced by: 1. gradual resolution of abdominal pain 2. temperature declining toward normal 3. stable B/P and pulse 4. serum amylase and lipase levels declining toward normal 5. WBC count declining toward normal.	5.c.1. Assess for and report signs and symptoms of pancreatitis (e.g., extension of pain to left upper quadrant or back, further increase in temperature, tachycardia, hypotension, elevated serum amylase and lipase levels, WBC count that increases or fails to decline toward normal). 2. If signs and symptoms of pancreatitis occur: a. assist client to assume position of greatest comfort (e.g., side-lying or sitting with trunk and knees flexed) b. maintain food and fluid restrictions as ordered c. maintain intravenous fluid therapy as ordered d. insert nasogastric tube if not already present and maintain suction as ordered *(removal of gastric secretions reduces pancreatic stimulation)* e. administer analgesics as ordered f. prepare client for endoscopic sphincterotomy and stone extraction or surgery to relieve ductal obstruction if planned.
5.d. The client will experience resolution of cholangitis if it occurs as evidenced by: 1. gradual resolution of abdominal pain 2. absence of jaundice and chills	5.d.1. Assess for signs and symptoms of cholangitis (e.g., increased abdominal pain, jaundice, chills, increase in temperature, increased WBCs and serum bilirubin and alkaline phosphatase). 2. If signs and symptoms of cholangitis occur: a. prepare client for diagnostic studies (e.g., computed tomography, ultrasonography, endoscopic retrograde cholangiopancreatography [ERCP])

3. temperature declining toward normal
4. WBC count declining toward normal.

b. assess for and report signs and symptoms such as lethargy, confusion, hypotension, and positive blood cultures (could indicate sepsis, which can develop with suppurative cholangitis)
c. administer antimicrobials as ordered
d. prepare client for endoscopic sphincterotomy and stone extraction, insertion of a percutaneous transhepatic catheter (to decompress duct) or surgical removal of ductal stone if planned.

Discharge Teaching/Continued Care

6. NURSING DIAGNOSIS: DEFICIENT KNOWLEDGE, INEFFECTIVE THERAPEUTIC REGIMEN MANAGEMENT, OR INEFFECTIVE HEALTH MAINTENANCE*

*The nurse should select the diagnostic label that is most appropriate for the client's discharge teaching needs.

Suggested NOC Outcomes: Knowledge: disease process; Knowledge: treatment regimen

Suggested NIC Interventions: Health system guidance; Teaching: disease process; Teaching: prescribed medication; Teaching: prescribed diet

Desired Outcomes	Nursing Actions *and Selected Purposes/Rationales*
6.a. The client will verbalize an understanding of ways to reduce the risk for recurrent gallbladder attacks.	6.a. Instruct client regarding ways to reduce the risk for recurrent gallbladder attacks: 1. adhere to a low- to moderate-fat diet (avoid foods/fluids high in fat such as butter, cream, whole milk, ice cream, fried foods, gravies, and nuts) 2. lose weight if obese but avoid rapid weight loss (rapid weight loss has been shown to increase biliary cholesterol saturation) 3. exercise regularly 4. consult physician before starting or resuming use of lipid-lowering agents or estrogen preparations/oral contraceptives (some estrogen preparations and lipid-lowering agents [e.g., clofibrate] increase the risk for gallstones).
6.b. The client will state signs and symptoms to report to the health care provider.	6.b. Instruct client to report the following signs and symptoms: 1. persistent indigestion, flatulence, and loose stools 2. nausea and vomiting 3. recurrent episodes of abdominal pain 4. development of or persistent itching, yellow coloring of skin or eyes, dark color of urine, or clay-colored stools (indicative of bile flow obstruction) 5. persistent or recurrent temperature elevation.
6.c. The client will verbalize an understanding of and a plan for adhering to recommended follow-up care including future appointments with health care provider and medications prescribed.	6.c.1. Reinforce importance of keeping follow-up appointments with health care provider. 2. Explain the rationale for, side effects of, and importance of taking prescribed medications (e.g., fat-soluble vitamins, bile salts, gallstone dissolution agents such as ursodiol [Actigall], antimicrobials). Inform client of pertinent food and drug interactions. 3. Implement measures to improve client compliance: a. include significant others in teaching sessions if possible b. encourage questions and allow time for reinforcement and clarification of information provided c. provide written instructions on future appointments with health care provider, medications prescribed, and signs and symptoms to report.

Additional Nursing Diagnoses:

IMBALANCED NUTRITION: LESS THAN BODY REQUIREMENTS*

related to:
a. decreased oral intake associated with nausea, dyspepsia, pain, and self-imposed or prescribed dietary restrictions;
b. loss of nutrients associated with vomiting;
c. decreased absorption of fats and fat-soluble vitamins associated with bile flow obstruction.

ALTERED COMFORT: PRURITUS

related to stimulation of itch fibers in the skin by bile acid metabolites that accumulate in the blood as a result of bile flow obstruction.

IMPAIRED ORAL MUCOUS MEMBRANE*: DRYNESS

related to:
a. deficient fluid volume associated with restricted oral intake and fluid loss resulting from vomiting and nasogastric tube drainage;
b. decreased salivation associated with deficient fluid volume, restricted oral intake, and the effect of some medications (e.g., narcotic [opioid] analgesics);
c. mouth breathing when nasogastric tube is in place.

FEAR/ANXIETY*

related to discomfort, unknown diagnosis, unfamiliar environment, lack of understanding of diagnostic tests and treatments, and possibility of surgery.

*See Unit II for outcomes, actions, and rationales.

Bibliography

See pages 879 and 884.

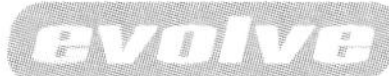

Cirrhosis

Cirrhosis is a chronic disease of the liver that occurs as a result of extensive destruction of the parenchymal cells in the liver. These cells are eventually replaced by fibrous scar tissue with subsequent change in the structure and functioning of the liver. The structural changes impair portal blood flow which results in venous congestion in other organs and systems such as the spleen and gastrointestinal tract.

There are numerous causes of cirrhosis. Over half of the cases of cirrhosis are associated with alcohol and chronic viral hepatitis. Other causes of cirrhosis include exposure to toxic chemicals or drugs, hereditary metabolic disorders (e.g., $alpha_1$-antitrypsin deficiency, Wilson's disease, hemochromatosis), heart failure, and conditions that cause persistent bile flow obstruction (e.g., primary biliary cirrhosis, primary sclerosing cholangitis). In approximately 15–20% of cases, no cause is identified.

All types of cirrhosis have similar signs and symptoms, which are manifestations of impaired liver function and the venous congestion that occurs with portal hypertension. Alcohol-related cirrhosis may have additional manifestations such as cerebral degeneration and demyelinating neuropathies that are thought to be a direct result of the toxic effects of alcohol or certain associated vitamin deficiencies. Treatment of cirrhosis is supportive and directed at slowing the progression of liver failure and reducing the incidence and/or severity of complications. The primary goals of treatment are to eliminate or manage the factors/conditions that contributed to the development of cirrhosis, provide a diet that is high in nutrients and will reduce the risk for further liver damage, and encourage rest to reduce the metabolic demands on the liver. A liver transplant may be indicated to treat end-stage liver disease.

This care plan focuses on the adult client with alcoholic (Laennec's) cirrhosis hospitalized for management of increasing ascites and peripheral edema. Much of the information is applicable to clients receiving follow-up care in an extended care facility or home setting.

OUTCOME/DISCHARGE CRITERIA

THE CLIENT WILL:

- have an adequate nutritional intake
- perform activities of daily living without extreme fatigue or dyspnea
- have a reduction in or resolution of ascites and edema
- have no evidence of life-threatening complications
- identify ways to prevent further liver damage
- verbalize an understanding of the rationale for and components of the recommended diet
- identify ways to reduce stress on or trauma to the esophageal blood vessels
- identify ways to prevent bleeding
- identify ways to reduce the risk of infection
- identify ways to relieve pruritus
- state signs and symptoms to report to the health care provider
- identify community resources that can assist with home management and adjustment to lifestyle changes necessary for effective management of cirrhosis
- share concerns and feelings about the diagnosis of cirrhosis; prognosis; and effects of the disease process and its treatment on self-concept, lifestyle, and roles
- verbalize an understanding of and a plan for adhering to recommended follow-up care including future appointments with health care provider, medications prescribed, and activity level.

Use in Conjunction with the Care Plan on Immobility.

NURSING/COLLABORATIVE DIAGNOSES

See p. 701 and Care Plan on Immobility (pp. 129–148) for additional diagnoses.

1. Nursing Diagnosis: *INEFFECTIVE BREATHING PATTERN*

related to:
a. increased rate of respirations associated with fear and anxiety;
b. decrease depth of respirations associated with:
   1. weakness and fatigue
   2. decreased lung compliance (distensibility) resulting from pleural effusion (hepatic hydrothorax) that occurs because of excess fluid volume and passage of ascitic fluid into the pleural space through a probable pressure-related defect in the diaphragm
   3. restricted chest expansion resulting from positioning and pressure on the diaphragm as a result of ascites.

Suggested NOC Outcome: Respiratory status: ventilation

Suggested NIC Interventions: Respiratory monitoring; Ventilation assistance

Desired Outcome	**Nursing Actions** *and Selected Purposes/Rationales* (see pp. 18–20 for additional rationales)
1. The client will have an improved breathing pattern as evidenced by: a. normal rate and depth of respirations b. decreased dyspnea c. symmetrical chest excursion.	1.a. Assess for signs and symptoms of an ineffective breathing pattern (e.g., shallow respirations, dyspnea, tachypnea, use of accessory muscles when breathing, limited chest excursion). b. Implement measures *to improve breathing pattern:* 1. perform actions to increase strength and activity tolerance (see Diagnosis 7, action b) *in order to increase client's willingness and ability to move, deep breathe, and use incentive spirometer* 2. perform actions to restore fluid balance (see Diagnosis 2, action a.2) *in order to reduce fluid accumulation in the peritoneal cavity and pleural space*

3. place client in a semi-Fowler's position (a high Fowler's position is uncomfortable if ascites is severe)
4. instruct client to deep breathe or use incentive spirometer every 1–2 hours
5. instruct client to avoid intake of gas-forming foods (e.g., beans, cauliflower, cabbage, onions), carbonated beverages, and large meals *in order to prevent gastric distention and additional pressure on the diaphragm*
6. assist with positive airway pressure techniques (e.g., continuous positive airway pressure [CPAP], bilevel positive airway pressure [BiPAP], flutter/positive expiratory pressure [PEP] device) if ordered
7. increase activity as allowed and tolerated
8. administer central nervous system depressants judiciously; hold medication and consult physician if respiratory rate is less than 12/minute
9. assist with thoracentesis and/or paracentesis if performed *to remove pleural and/or peritoneal fluid in order to allow increased chest and lung expansion.*

c. Consult appropriate health care provider (e.g., respiratory therapist, physician) if:
1. ineffective breathing pattern continues
2. signs and symptoms of impaired gas exchange (e.g., restlessness, irritability, confusion, significant decrease in oximetry results, decreased PaO_2 and increased $PaCO_2$ levels) are present.

2. NURSING/COLLABORATIVE DIAGNOSIS:

RISK FOR IMBALANCED FLUID AND ELECTROLYTES

a. excess fluid volume related to sodium and water retention associated with an increased aldosterone level resulting from:
1. inability of the liver to metabolize aldosterone
2. activation of the renin-angiotensin-aldosterone mechanism as a result of decreased renal blood flow (occurs because of a decrease in intravascular volume that results from vasodilation and from third-spacing and sequestration of fluid in the splanchnic system);

b. third-spacing related to:
1. low plasma colloid osmotic pressure associated with hypoalbuminemia (a result of decreased hepatic synthesis of albumin and prolonged inadequate nutrition)
2. increased pressure in the portal system and hepatic lymph system associated with blood flow backup resulting from structural changes in the liver
3. a generalized increase in hydrostatic pressure associated with excess fluid volume;

c. hypokalemia related to excessive potassium loss associated with an increased aldosterone level (aldosterone causes potassium excretion) and diuretic therapy;

d. hyponatremia related to hemodilution associated with excess fluid volume, sodium loss associated with diuretic therapy, and dietary sodium restriction.

Suggested NOC Outcomes: Fluid balance; Fluid overload severity; Electrolyte and acid/base balance

Suggested NIC Interventions: Fluid monitoring; Fluid/electrolyte management; Electrolyte management: hyponatremia; Electrolyte management: hypokalemia; Hypervolemia management

Desired Outcomes	Nursing Actions *and Selected Purposes/Rationales*
2.a. The client will experience resolution of imbalanced fluid as evidenced by: 1. decline in weight toward client's normal	2.a.1. Assess for and report: a. signs and symptoms of excess fluid volume: 1. weight gain of 2% or greater in a short period 2. elevated B/P (B/P may not be elevated if fluid has shifted out of the vascular space) 3. development or worsening of S_3 heart sound

Desired Outcomes	Nursing Actions *and Selected Purposes/Rationales*
2. B/P and pulse within normal range for client and stable with position change 3. absence or resolution of S_3 heart sound 4. balanced intake and output 5. usual mental status 6. serum sodium returning toward normal range 7. decreased dyspnea, peripheral edema, and neck vein distention 8. improved breath sounds 9. resolution of ascites.	4. intake greater than output 5. change in mental status (may also reflect impending hepatic encephalopathy) 6. low serum sodium (may also result from diuretic therapy and a low sodium diet) 7. dyspnea, orthopnea 8. peripheral edema 9. distended neck veins 10. crackles (rales), diminished or absent breath sounds b. signs and symptoms of third-spacing: 1. ascites 2. dyspnea and diminished or absent breath sounds 3. evidence of vascular depletion (e.g., postural hypotension; weak, rapid pulse; decreased urine output) c. chest x-ray results showing pulmonary vascular congestion, pleural effusion, or pulmonary edema d. low serum albumin levels *(results in fluid shifting out of the vascular space because albumin normally maintains plasma colloid osmotic pressure).* 2. Implement measures *to restore fluid balance:* a. perform actions *to reduce excess fluid volume:* 1. restrict sodium intake as ordered 2. maintain fluid restrictions if ordered 3. encourage client to rest periodically in a recumbent position *(lying down reduces peripheral pooling of blood, which increases effective circulating volume and renal blood flow and subsequently promotes diuresis)* 4. implement measures to promote mobilization of fluid back into the vascular space (see action a.2.b in this diagnosis) *in order to improve renal blood flow, which increases water excretion and reduces activation of the renin-angiotensin-aldosterone mechanism* 5. administer diuretics if ordered (potassium-sparing diuretics such as spironolactone and amiloride are often used initially) b. perform actions *to prevent further third-spacing and promote mobilization of fluid back into the vascular space:* 1. implement measures to reduce excess fluid volume (see action a.2.a in this diagnosis) 2. administer albumin infusions if ordered *to increase colloid osmotic pressure.* 3. Consult physician if signs and symptoms of imbalanced fluid persist or worsen.
2.b. The client will maintain a safe serum potassium level as evidenced by: 1. regular pulse at 60–100 beats/minute 2. B/P within normal range for client and stable with position change 3. usual muscle tone and strength 4. absence of nausea and vomiting 5. soft, nondistended abdomen with normal bowel sounds 6. normal ECG reading 7. serum potassium within normal range.	2.b.1. Assess for and report signs and symptoms of hypokalemia (e.g., cardiac dysrhythmias; postural hypotension; muscle weakness; nausea and vomiting; abdominal distention; hypoactive or absent bowel sounds; ECG reading showing ST segment depression, T wave inversion or flattening, and presence of U waves; low serum potassium level). 2. Implement measures *to prevent or treat hypokalemia:* a. administer intravenous and oral potassium replacements as ordered (monitor serum potassium and urine output closely when giving supplemental potassium; consult physician if potassium level increases above normal and/or urine output is less than 30 ml/hour) b. if client is taking a potassium-depleting diuretic or if signs and symptoms of hypokalemia are present, encourage intake of foods/fluids high in potassium (e.g., bananas, potatoes, raisins, cantaloupe). 3. Consult physician if signs and symptoms of hypokalemia persist or worsen.

2.c. The client will maintain a safe serum sodium level as evidenced by:
1. absence of nausea, vomiting, and abdominal cramps
2. usual mental status
3. usual muscle strength
4. absence of seizure activity
5. serum sodium within normal range.

2.c.1. Assess for and report signs and symptoms of hyponatremia (e.g., nausea, vomiting, abdominal cramps, lethargy, confusion, weakness, seizures, low serum sodium level).
2. Implement measures *to treat hyponatremia:*
   a. maintain fluid restrictions if ordered
   b. administer hypertonic saline solutions if ordered (is not commonly given until hyponatremia is severe *because of the risk of hypernatremia and intravascular volume overload);* furosemide may be given concurrently *to promote water excretion and reduce the risk for intravascular volume overload.*
3. Consult physician if signs and symptoms of hyponatremia persist or worsen.

3. NURSING DIAGNOSIS

IMBALANCED NUTRITION: LESS THAN BODY REQUIREMENTS

related to:
a. poor eating habits prior to admission;
b. decreased oral intake associated with dyspepsia, fatigue, dyspnea, dislike of the prescribed diet, and feeling of fullness (a result of increased intra-abdominal pressure that occurs with ascites);
c. reduced metabolism and storage of nutrients by the liver associated with a reduction of functional liver tissue;
d. malabsorption of fats and fat-soluble vitamins associated with impaired bile production and flow.

Suggested NOC Outcome: Nutritional status

Suggested NIC Interventions: Nutritional monitoring; Nutrition management; Nutrition therapy; Nutritional counseling

Desired Outcome

Nursing Actions *and Selected Purposes/Rationales*

(see pp. 40–43 for additional rationales)

3. The client will have an improved nutritional status as evidenced by:
   a. dry weight approaching normal range for client (dry weight is achieved after excess fluid volume has been resolved)
   b. improved serum prealbumin, albumin, Hct, Hgb, and lymphocyte levels
   c. improved strength and activity tolerance
   d. healthy oral mucous membrane.

3.a. Assess for and report signs and symptoms of malnutrition:
   1. dry weight significantly below client's usual weight or below normal for client's age, height, and body frame
   2. decreased serum prealbumin, albumin, Hct, Hgb, and lymphocyte levels
   3. weakness and fatigue
   4. sore, inflamed oral mucous membrane
   5. pale conjunctiva.

b. Monitor percentage of meals and snacks client consumes. Report a pattern of inadequate intake.

c. Implement measures *to improve nutritional status:*
   1. perform actions *to improve oral intake:*
      a. implement measures to reduce dyspepsia (see Diagnosis 5, action c)
      b. implement measures to restore fluid balance (see Diagnosis 2, action a.2) *in order to reduce fluid accumulation in the peritoneal cavity and subsequently reduce the feeling of fullness*
      c. obtain a dietary consult if necessary to assist the client in selecting foods/fluids that are appealing and adhere to personal and cultural preferences as well as the prescribed dietary modifications
      d. encourage a rest period before meals *to minimize fatigue*
      e. maintain a clean environment and a relaxed, pleasant atmosphere
      f. serve frequent, small meals rather than large ones if client is weak, fatigues easily, and/or has a poor appetite
      g. elevate head of bed as tolerated for meals *to help relieve dyspnea and feeling of fullness* (a high Fowler's position may be too uncomfortable if ascites is severe)
      h. instruct client to use herbs, spices, and salt substitutes (if approved by physician) *in order to make low-sodium diet more palatable*

Desired Outcome	Nursing Actions *and Selected Purposes/Rationales*

i. allow adequate time for meals; reheat foods/fluids if necessary
j. increase activity as allowed and tolerated *(activity usually promotes a sense of well-being, which can improve appetite)*
k. limit fluid intake with meals (unless the fluid has high nutritional value) *to reduce early satiety and subsequent decreased food intake*

2. assist and instruct client to adhere to the following dietary recommendations:
   a. avoid skipping meals
   b. consume a diet high in calories (2000–3000 calories/day) and carbohydrates
   c. maintain a moderate to high protein intake (generally at least 1 g of protein/kg of body weight is recommended unless the serum ammonia level is high or clinical evidence of encephalopathy is present)
   d. consume meals that are well balanced and high in essential nutrients; offer dietary supplements if client's caloric intake is inadequate
3. administer vitamins and minerals (e.g., fat-soluble vitamins, thiamine, folic acid, iron) if ordered.

d. Perform a calorie count if ordered. Report information to dietitian and physician.
e. Consult physician about an alternative method of providing nutrition (e.g., parenteral nutrition, tube feedings) if client does not consume enough food or fluids to meet nutritional needs.

4. Nursing Diagnosis: ALTERED COMFORT: PRURITUS

related to stimulation of itch receptors in the skin by bile acid metabolites that accumulate in the blood as a result of bile flow obstruction.

Suggested NOC Outcomes: Comfort level; Symptom control

Suggested NIC Intervention: Pruritus management

Desired Outcome	Nursing Actions *and Selected Purposes/Rationales*
4. The client will experience relief of pruritus as evidenced by: a. verbalization of same b. no scratching or rubbing of skin.	4.a. Assess for the following: 1. reports of itchiness 2. persistent scratching or rubbing of skin. b. Instruct client in and/or implement measures *to relieve pruritus:* 1. apply cool, moist compresses to pruritic areas 2. apply emollient creams or ointments frequently *to prevent dryness* 3. add emollients, cornstarch, or baking soda to bath water 4. use tepid water and mild soaps for bathing 5. pat skin dry after bathing, making sure to dry thoroughly 6. maintain a cool environment 7. encourage participation in diversional activity 8. utilize relaxation techniques 9. utilize cutaneous stimulation techniques (e.g., massage, pressure, vibration, stroking with soft brush) at sites of itching or acupressure points 10. encourage client to wear loose cotton garments and avoid clothes or blankets made from wool 11. administer the following medications if ordered: a. antihistamines (e.g., diphenhydramine, hydroxyzine [Atarax]) b. bile acid sequestering agents (e.g., cholestyramine). c. Consult appropriate health care provider (e.g., clinical nurse specialist, physician) if above measures fail to alleviate pruritus or if the skin becomes excoriated.

5. NURSING DIAGNOSIS:

ALTERED COMFORT: DYSPEPSIA

related to:
a. impaired fat digestion associated with bile flow obstruction;
b. reflux of gastric contents associated with increased intra-abdominal pressure resulting from ascites;
c. impaired gastrointestinal functioning associated with venous congestion in the gastrointestinal tract (portal hypertensive gastropathy) resulting from portal hypertension;
d. esophagitis/gastritis associated with the irritant effect of chronic alcohol ingestion on the esophageal and gastric mucosa.

Suggested NOC Outcomes: Comfort level; Symptom control

Suggested NIC Interventions: Flatulence reduction; Nausea management

Desired Outcome	**Nursing Actions** *and Selected Purposes/Rationales*
5. The client will verbalize relief of dyspepsia.	5.a. Assess client for signs and symptoms of dyspepsia (e.g., reports of epigastric discomfort, heartburn, nausea, or feeling of fullness or bloating; frequent eructation). b. Determine if particular foods/fluids contribute to dyspepsia. c. Implement measures *to reduce dyspepsia:* 1. perform actions *to reduce gastroesophageal reflux:* a. keep head of bed elevated for 2–3 hours after meals b. provide small, frequent meals rather than large ones 2. perform actions to restore fluid balance (see Diagnosis 2, action a.2) *in order to promote the resolution of ascites and subsequently reduce abdominal pressure and the associated gastroesophageal reflux and feeling of fullness and bloating* 3. instruct client to ingest foods and fluids slowly 4. encourage client not to smoke 5. encourage client to avoid the following foods/fluids: a. those high in fat (e.g., fried foods, gravies, butter, cream, ice cream) b. carbonated beverages c. gas-producing foods (e.g., beans, onions, cabbage) d. those that may cause gastric irritation (e.g., spicy foods; caffeine-containing beverages such as coffee, tea, and colas; alcohol) 6. administer the following medications if ordered: a. antacids, histamine$_2$ receptor antagonists (e.g., famotidine, nizatidine, ranitidine), or proton-pump inhibitors (e.g., omeprazole, lansoprazole, pantoprazole, esomeprazole) *to reduce acidity of gastric contents and subsequently also reduce esophageal irritation if reflux occurs* b. cytoprotective agents (e.g., sucralfate, misoprostol) *to protect the gastric mucosa* c. antiflatulents (e.g., simethicone) d. antiemetics (phenothiazines should be used cautiously). d. Consult appropriate health care provider (e.g., clinical nurse specialist, physician) if above measures fail to control dyspepsia.

6. NURSING DIAGNOSIS:

RISK FOR IMPAIRED TISSUE INTEGRITY

related to:
a. damage to the skin and/or subcutaneous tissue associated with prolonged pressure on the tissues, friction, and/or shearing if mobility is decreased;
b. increased fragility of the skin associated with edema and malnutrition;
c. excessive scratching associated with pruritus.

Suggested NOC Outcome: Tissue integrity: skin and mucous membrane

Suggested NIC Interventions: Skin surveillance; Pressure ulcer prevention; Positioning; Pruritus management

Desired Outcome	Nursing Actions and Selected Purposes/Rationales
6. The client will maintain tissue integrity as evidenced by: a. absence of redness and irritation b. no skin breakdown.	6.a. Inspect the skin (especially bony prominences and dependent, edematous, and pruritic areas) for pallor, redness, and breakdown. b. Refer to Care Plan on Immobility, Diagnosis 4, action c (p. 133), for measures to prevent tissue breakdown. c. Implement additional measures *to prevent tissue breakdown:* 1. perform actions *to prevent skin irritation resulting from scratching:* a. implement measures to relieve pruritus (see Diagnosis 4, action b) b. keep nails trimmed and/or apply mittens if necessary c. instruct client to apply firm pressure to pruritic areas rather than scratching 2. perform actions to improve nutritional status (see Diagnosis 3, action c) 3. perform actions to reduce excess fluid volume (see Diagnosis 2, action a.2.a) *in order to reduce edema.*

7. NURSING DIAGNOSIS: ACTIVITY INTOLERANCE

related to:

a. tissue hypoxia associated with anemia resulting from:
   1. decreased production of RBCs resulting from a decreased intake and absorption of vitamins and minerals and an inability of the liver to store vitamins and minerals
   2. excessive RBC destruction resulting from hypersplenism (if venous congestion has resulted in splenomegaly, the spleen will destroy RBCs faster than usual)
   3. blood loss if bleeding has occurred;

b. loss of muscle mass, tone, and strength associated with malnutrition and disuse if mobility has been limited for an extended period;

c. decrease in available energy associated with inability of the liver to metabolize glucose, fats, and proteins properly;

d. difficulty resting and sleeping associated with dyspnea, discomfort, frequent assessments and treatments, fear, anxiety, and unfamiliar environment.

Suggested NOC Outcomes: Rest; Energy conservation; Activity tolerance

Suggested NIC Interventions: Energy management; Oxygen therapy; Nutrition management; Sleep enhancement

Desired Outcome	Nursing Actions and Selected Purposes/Rationales (see pp. 11–12 for additional rationales)
7. The client will demonstrate an increased tolerance for activity as evidenced by: a. verbalization of feeling less fatigued and weak b. ability to perform activities of daily living without exertional dyspnea, chest pain, diaphoresis, dizziness, and a significant change in vital signs.	7.a. Assess for signs and symptoms of activity intolerance: 1. statements of fatigue or weakness 2. exertional dyspnea, chest pain, diaphoresis, or dizziness 3. abnormal heart rate response to activity (e.g., increase in rate of 20 beats/minute above resting rate, rate not returning to preactivity level within 3 minutes after stopping activity, change from regular to irregular rate) 4. a significant change (15–20 mm Hg) in blood pressure with activity. b. Implement measures *to improve activity tolerance:* 1. perform actions *to promote rest and/or conserve energy:* a. maintain activity restrictions as ordered b. minimize environmental activity and noise c. organize nursing care to allow for periods of uninterrupted rest d. limit the number of visitors and their length of stay

e. assist client with self-care activities as needed
f. keep supplies and personal articles within easy reach
g. instruct client in energy-saving techniques (e.g., using shower chair when showering, sitting to brush teeth or comb hair)
h. implement *measures to reduce fear and anxiety* (e.g., assure client that staff are nearby, explain all tests and procedures, encourage verbalization of fear and anxiety)
i. implement measures *to promote sleep* (e.g., elevate head of bed and support arms on pillows to facilitate breathing; maintain oxygen therapy during sleep; discourage intake of fluids high in caffeine, especially in the evening; encourage relaxing diversional activities in the evening)
j. implement measures to reduce discomfort (see Diagnoses 4, action b and 5, action c)

2. discourage smoking and excessive intake of beverages high in caffeine such as coffee, tea, and colas *(nicotine and caffeine can increase cardiac workload and myocardial oxygen utilization, thereby decreasing oxygen availability)*
3. perform actions to improve breathing pattern (see Diagnosis 1, action b) *in order to decrease dyspnea and improve tissue oxygenation*
4. maintain oxygen therapy as ordered
5. perform actions to improve nutritional status (see Diagnosis 3, action c)
6. perform actions *to treat anemia* (e.g., administer prescribed iron, folic acid, and/or vitamin B_{12}; administer packed red blood cells if ordered)
7. increase client's activity gradually as allowed and tolerated.

c. Instruct client to:
1. report a decreased tolerance for activity
2. stop any activity that causes chest pain, a marked increase in shortness of breath, dizziness, or extreme fatigue or weakness.

d. Consult physician if signs and symptoms of activity intolerance persist or worsen.

8. NURSING DIAGNOSIS: DISTURBED THOUGHT PROCESSES*

related to disturbances in central nervous system functioning associated with accumulation of toxic substances (e.g., ammonia) in the brain, toxic effects of long-term alcohol use, deficiencies of certain vitamins (e.g., thiamine), and hypoxia if anemia is moderate to severe.

*The diagnostic label of acute or chronic confusion might be more appropriate depending on the client's symptoms.

Suggested NOC Outcomes: Cognitive ability; Cognitive orientation; Concentration; Information processing

Suggested NIC Interventions: Cognitive stimulation; Reality orientation

Desired Outcome

8. The client will demonstrate improvement in thought processes as evidenced by:
a. improved ability to grasp ideas
b. improved memory
c. longer attention span
d. absence or resolution of inappropriate behavior
e. oriented to person, place, and time.

Nursing Actions *and Selected Purposes/Rationales*

8.a. Assess client for disturbed thought processes (e.g., impaired ability to grasp ideas, impaired memory, shortened attention span, inappropriate affect or behavior, disorientation).

b. Ascertain from significant others client's usual level of cognitive and emotional functioning and whether personality changes have occurred.

c. Implement measures *to maintain optimal thought processes:*
1. perform actions to improve nutritional status (see Diagnosis 3, action c) *in order to provide vitamins and minerals that are essential for normal neurological functioning and treatment of anemia*
2. perform actions to prevent or manage hepatic coma (see Diagnosis 11, actions e.3 and 4) *and subsequently reduce levels of cerebral toxins*

Desired Outcome	Nursing Actions *and Selected Purposes/Rationales*

3. administer central nervous system depressants such as opioids (narcotics), sedative-hypnotics, and antianxiety agents with extreme caution *(many of these agents are metabolized in the liver)*; question any order for a normal adult dose of these medications
4. administer thiamine if ordered *to prevent progression of neurological manifestations*
5. maintain oxygen therapy as ordered.

d. If client shows evidence of disturbed thought processes:
1. reorient client to person, place, and time as necessary
2. address client by name
3. place familiar objects, clock, and calendar within client's view
4. approach client in a slow, calm manner; allow adequate time for communication
5. repeat instructions as necessary using clear, simple language and short sentences
6. maintain a consistent and fairly structured routine and write out a schedule of activities for client to refer to if desired
7. have client perform only one activity at a time and allow adequate time for performance of activities
8. encourage client to make lists of planned activities, questions, and concerns
9. assist client to problem solve if necessary
10. maintain realistic expectations of client's ability to learn, comprehend, and remember information provided; provide client with a written copy of instructions
11. encourage significant others to be supportive of client. Instruct them in methods of dealing with client's disturbed thought processes
12. inform client and significant others that cognitive and emotional functioning are likely to improve with treatment
13. consult physician if disturbed thought processes worsen.

9. Nursing Diagnosis: *RISK FOR INFECTION*

related to:

a. lowered resistance to infection associated with:
1. diminished function of the Kupffer cells in the liver (these cells normally phagocytize bacteria)
2. malnutrition
3. leukopenia resulting from hypersplenism (if venous congestion has resulted in splenomegaly, the spleen will destroy leukocytes faster than usual)
4. serum complement deficiency resulting from decreased production of complement proteins by the liver;

b. colonization of bacteria in the ascitic fluid (spontaneous bacterial peritonitis);

c. stasis of secretions in the lungs and urinary stasis if mobility is decreased.

Suggested NOC Outcomes: Immune status; Infection severity

Suggested NIC Interventions: Infection protection; Infection control

Desired Outcome	Nursing Actions *and Selected Purposes/Rationales* (see pp. 37–40 for additional rationales)
9. The client will remain free of infection as evidenced by: a. absence of fever and chills b. pulse within normal limits	9.a. Assess for signs and symptoms of infection (be aware that some signs and symptoms vary depending on the site of infection, the causative organism, and the age and immune status of the client): 1. elevated temperature 2. chills

c. normal breath sounds
d. usual mental status
e. cough productive of clear mucus only
f. voiding clear urine without reports of frequency, urgency, and burning
g. absence of heat, pain, redness, swelling, and unusual drainage in any area
h. no reports of increased weakness and fatigue
i. WBC and differential counts within normal range
j. negative results of cultured specimens
k. ascitic fluid polymorphonuclear (PMN) leukocyte count within normal limits.

3. increased pulse
4. abnormal breath sounds
5. change in mental status
6. loss of appetite
7. cough productive of purulent, green, or rust-colored sputum
8. cloudy urine
9. reports of frequency, urgency, or burning when urinating
10. urinalysis showing greater than 5 WBCs, positive leukocyte esterase or nitrites, or presence of bacteria
11. heat, pain, redness, swelling, or unusual drainage in any area
12. reports of increased weakness or fatigue
13. abdominal pain and tenderness
14. elevated WBC count and/or significant change in differential
15. positive results of cultured specimens (e.g., urine, vaginal drainage, sputum, blood, ascitic fluid)
16. ascitic fluid showing greater than 250 PMNs/μl.

b. Implement measures *to prevent infection:*
   1. perform actions to prevent tissue breakdown (see Diagnosis 6, actions b and c)
   2. maintain the maximum fluid intake allowed
   3. use good hand hygiene and encourage client to do the same
   4. use sterile technique during all invasive procedures (e.g., urinary catheterization, venous and arterial punctures, injections)
   5. change peripheral intravenous line sites according to hospital policy
   6. change equipment, tubings, and solutions used for treatments such as intravenous infusions and respiratory care according to hospital policy
   7. anchor catheters/tubings (e.g., urinary, intravenous) securely *in order to reduce trauma to the tissues and the risk for introduction of pathogens associated with the in-and-out movement of the tubing*
   8. maintain a closed system for drains (e.g., urinary catheter) and intravenous infusions whenever possible
   9. protect client from others with infection
   10. perform actions to improve nutritional status (see Diagnosis 3, action c)
   11. provide or assist with good oral hygiene
   12. perform actions to reduce stress (e.g., relieve discomfort; explain procedures and treatments; provide a quiet, restful environment) *in order to prevent an increase in secretion of cortisol (cortisol interferes with some immune responses)*
   13. perform actions *to prevent stasis of respiratory secretions* (e.g., assist client to turn, cough, and deep breathe; increase activity as allowed and tolerated)
   14. perform actions to prevent urinary retention (e.g., instruct client to urinate when the urge is first felt, promote relaxation during voiding attempts) *in order to prevent urinary stasis*
   15. instruct and assist client to perform good perineal care routinely and after each bowel movement
   16. administer prophylactic antimicrobials if ordered (norfloxacin or trimethoprim-sulfamethoxazole may be ordered for clients with ascites *to help prevent spontaneous bacterial peritonitis*).

c. If signs and symptoms of infection occur:
   1. notify physician
   2. administer antimicrobials as ordered; question any order for aminoglycosides *because they can precipitate the hepatorenal syndrome.*

10. NURSING DIAGNOSIS: RISK FOR INJURY

a. falls related to:
   1. weakness
   2. dizziness (can result from anemia and the postural hypotension that occurs with third-spacing)

3. balance and gait disturbances that can occur with deficiencies of thiamine and/or vitamin B_{12}
4. disturbed thought processes (e.g., agitation, confusion);

b. **burns and lacerations** related to:
1. paresthesias that can occur with deficiencies of thiamine and vitamin B_{12}
2. tremors and jerky, restless movements associated with delirium tremens ("DTs") if present.

Suggested NOC Outcome: Fall prevention behavior: Fall occurrence

Suggested NIC Interventions: Fall prevention; Environmental management: safety

Desired Outcome	**Nursing Actions** *and Selected Purposes/Rationales*

10. The client will not experience falls, burns, or lacerations.

10.a. Implement measures *to reduce the risk for injury:*
1. perform actions *to prevent falls:*
   a. keep bed in low position with side rails up when client is in bed
   b. keep needed items within easy reach
   c. encourage client to request assistance whenever needed; have call signal within easy reach
   d. instruct and assist client to rise and change positions slowly *in order to reduce dizziness associated with postural hypotension*
   e. use lap belt when client is in chair if indicated
   f. instruct client to wear well-fitting slippers/shoes with nonslip soles and low heels when ambulating
   g. keep floor free of clutter and wipe up spills promptly
   h. accompany client during ambulation using a transfer safety belt if he/she is weak or dizzy
   i. provide ambulatory aids (e.g., walker, cane) if the client is weak or unsteady on feet
   j. instruct client to ambulate in well-lit areas and to use handrails if needed
   k. do not rush client; allow adequate time for ambulation to the bathroom and in hallway
   l. perform actions to increase strength and activity tolerance (see Diagnosis 7, action b)
   m. reinforce instructions from physical therapist on correct transfer and ambulation techniques if client has gait disturbances
   n. make sure that shower has a nonslip bottom surface and that shower chair, secure bath mat, call signal, grab bars, and adequate lighting are present
2. perform actions *to prevent burns:*
   a. let hot foods and fluids cool slightly before serving
   b. supervise client while smoking if indicated
   c. assess temperature of bath water and direct heat application device (e.g., heating pad, warm compress) before and during use
3. assist client with tasks that require fine motor skills (e.g., shaving) *in order to prevent lacerations*
4. if client is confused or irrational:
   a. reorient frequently to surroundings and necessity of adhering to safety precautions
   b. provide appropriate level of supervision
   c. consult physician about the temporary use of a bed alarm or jacket or wrist restraints if necessary
   d. administer prescribed antianxiety and antipsychotic medications if indicated
5. administer central nervous system depressants with extreme caution *(many of these agents are metabolized in the liver);* question any order for a normal adult dose of these medications.

b. Include client and significant others in planning and implementing measures to prevent injury.
c. If injury does occur, initiate appropriate first aid and notify physician.

11. COLLABORATIVE DIAGNOSES: POTENTIAL COMPLICATIONS OF CIRRHOSIS

a. bleeding related to:
   1. decreased production of clotting factors associated with impaired liver function and decreased available vitamin K (can occur from malnutrition, antimicrobials that suppress activity of intestinal flora, and impaired absorption of vitamin K as a result of bile flow obstruction)
   2. thrombocytopenia associated with hypersplenism (if venous congestion has resulted in splenomegaly, the spleen will destroy platelets faster than usual);
b. ascites related to:
   1. low plasma colloid osmotic pressure associated with hypoalbuminemia (a result of decreased hepatic synthesis of albumin and prolonged inadequate nutrition)
   2. increased pressure in the portal system and hepatic lymph system associated with blood flow backup resulting from structural changes in the liver
   3. a generalized increase in hydrostatic pressure associated with excess fluid volume;
c. hepatorenal syndrome related to decreased renal blood flow possibly associated with:
   1. a decrease in intravascular volume resulting from:
      a. third-spacing and sequestration of fluid in the splanchnic system
      b. treatment-induced fluid loss (e.g., paracentesis, diuretic therapy)
   2. intrarenal vasoconstriction that may result from increased levels of certain renal arteriolar vasoconstrictors (e.g., angiotensin, endothelin), increased sympathetic nervous system activity, and impaired synthesis of renal vasodilators such as prostaglandin E_2;
d. bleeding esophageal varices related to:
   1. tortuosity and increased fragility of small vessels in the esophagus associated with portal hypertension
   2. increased bleeding tendency;
e. hepatic (portal-systemic) encephalopathy (hepatic coma) related to altered brain function associated with:
   1. the effect of toxic end products of intestinal protein digestion (e.g., ammonia) on the brain
   2. replacement of true neurotransmitters by false neurotransmitters
   3. increased brain sensitivity to certain substances (e.g., benzodiazepines, gamma-aminobutyric acid [GABA])
   4. decreased activity of urea-cycle enzymes if zinc deficiency is present.

Desired Outcomes	**Nursing Actions** *and Selected Purposes/Rationales*
11.a. The client will not experience unusual bleeding as evidenced by: 1. skin and mucous membranes free of petechiae, purpura, ecchymoses, and active bleeding 2. absence of unusual joint pain 3. no further increase in abdominal girth 4. absence of frank and occult blood in stool, urine, and vomitus	11.a.1. Assess client for and report signs and symptoms of unusual bleeding: a. petechiae, purpura, ecchymoses b. gingival bleeding c. prolonged bleeding from puncture sites d. epistaxis, hemoptysis e. unusual joint pain f. further increase in abdominal girth g. frank or occult blood in the stool, urine, or vomitus h. menorrhagia i. restlessness, confusion j. decreasing B/P and increased pulse rate k. decrease in Hct and Hgb levels. 2. Monitor platelet count and coagulation test results (e.g., prothrombin time or International Normalized Ratio [INR], activated partial thromboplastin time, bleeding time). Report abnormal values.

Desired Outcomes	**Nursing Actions** *and Selected Purposes/Rationales*
5. usual menstrual flow 6. vital signs within normal range for client 7. stable or improved Hct and Hgb.	3. Implement measures *to prevent bleeding:* a. perform actions to reduce risk of bleeding from esophageal varices (see action d.2 in this diagnosis) b. avoid giving injections whenever possible; consult physician about prescribing an alternative route for medications ordered to be given intramuscularly or subcutaneously c. when giving injections or performing venous or arterial punctures, use the smallest gauge needle possible and apply gentle, prolonged pressure to the site after the needle is removed d. caution client to avoid activities that increase the risk for trauma (e.g., shaving with a straight-edge razor, using stiff bristle toothbrush or dental floss) e. whenever possible, avoid intubations (e.g., nasogastric) and procedures that can cause injury to the rectal mucosa (e.g., taking temperature rectally, inserting a rectal suppository, administering an enema) f. pad side rails if client is confused or restless g. perform actions to prevent injury (see Diagnosis 10) h. instruct client to avoid blowing nose forcefully or straining to have a bowel movement; consult physician about an order for a decongestant and/or laxative if indicated i. administer the following if ordered *to improve clotting ability:* 1. vitamin K (e.g., phytonadione) injections 2. platelets 3. fresh frozen plasma (FFP) 4. cryoprecipitate. 4. If bleeding occurs and does not subside spontaneously: a. apply firm, prolonged pressure to bleeding area(s) if possible b. if epistaxis occurs, place client in a high Fowler's position and apply pressure and ice pack to nasal area c. maintain oxygen therapy as ordered d. implement measures identified in action d.3 in this diagnosis if esophageal bleeding occurs e. administer vitamin K (e.g., phytonadione) injections, whole blood, or blood products (e.g., fresh frozen plasma, platelets) as ordered f. assess for and report signs and symptoms of hypovolemic shock (e.g., restlessness; confusion; significant decrease in B/P; rapid, weak pulse; rapid respirations; cool skin; urine output less than 30 ml/hour).
11.b. The client will have decreased ascites if present as evidenced by: 1. decrease in abdominal girth 2. abdominal percussion note more tympanic.	11.b.1. Assess for signs and symptoms of ascites: a. increase in abdominal girth (abdominal girth should be measured daily at the same time and in the same location on the abdomen with client in the same position) b. dull percussion note over abdomen with finding of shifting dullness c. presence of abdominal fluid wave d. protruding umbilicus and bulging flanks. 2. Implement measures to reduce excess fluid volume, promote mobilization of fluid back into the vascular space, and prevent further third-spacing (see Diagnosis 2, action a.2) *in order to promote the resolution of ascites.* 3. If signs and symptoms of ascites are present and persist or worsen: a. consult physician b. assist with paracentesis and administer albumin infusions if ordered c. prepare client for a portal systemic shunt procedure (e.g., transjugular intrahepatic portosystemic shunt [TIPS]) if planned *to treat portal hypertension and subsequently reduce ascites.*

11.c. The client will maintain adequate renal function as evidenced by:
1. serum creatinine level within normal range
2. creatinine clearance and urine sodium within normal range
3. urine output at least 30 ml/hour.

11.c.1. Assess for and report signs and symptoms of hepatorenal syndrome (e.g., increased serum creatinine, decreased creatinine clearance, low urine sodium, urine output less than 30 ml/hour).
2. Implement measures *to reduce the risk for hepatorenal syndrome:*
   a. perform actions *to maintain adequate renal blood flow:*
      1. maintain an adequate fluid intake; if client is on a fluid restriction, maintain the maximum fluid intake allowed
      2. administer albumin infusions if ordered *to increase the intravascular volume*
      3. consult physician about reducing the dose of diuretic ordered if client loses more than 1 kg of weight/day *(vigorous diuresis can reduce the intravascular volume enough to decrease renal blood flow and precipitate the hepatorenal syndrome)*
   b. consult physician regarding discontinuation of prescribed medications that can be nephrotoxic (e.g., nonsteroidal anti-inflammatory agents, aminoglycosides).
3. If signs and symptoms of the hepatorenal syndrome occur:
   a. administer intravenous infusions of dopamine, ornipressin, and/or albumin if ordered
   b. prepare client for dialysis if indicated.

11.d. The client will not experience bleeding of esophageal varices as evidenced by:
1. absence of hematemesis and melena
2. B/P and pulse within normal range for client
3. stable or improved RBC, Hct, and Hgb levels.

11.d.1. Assess for and report signs and symptoms of bleeding esophageal varices (e.g., hematemesis; melena; decreased B/P; increased pulse; decreasing RBC, Hct, and Hgb levels).
2. Implement measures *to reduce risk of bleeding from esophageal varices:*
   a. perform actions to reduce excess fluid volume (see Diagnosis 2, action a.2.a) *in order to reduce pressure in esophageal vessels*
   b. instruct client to avoid activities such as straining to have a bowel movement, coughing, sneezing, and lifting heavy objects *in order to prevent a sudden increase in intra-abdominal pressure;* consult physician about an order for a laxative, antitussive, and/or decongestant if indicated
   c. instruct client to avoid eating foods that might cause mechanical trauma to the esophageal varices (e.g., chips)
   d. administer a nonselective beta-adrenergic blocker (e.g., propranolol, nadolol) *to reduce portal pressure* (a nitrate such as isosorbide may be given with the beta blocker *to further reduce portal pressure*)
   e. administer vitamin K and blood products if ordered *to improve clotting ability.*
3. If signs and symptoms of bleeding esophageal varices occur:
   a. turn client on side and suction as necessary *to reduce risk of aspiration*
   b. maintain oxygen therapy as ordered
   c. assist with administration of octreotide (Sandostatin) or vasopressin if ordered *to constrict splanchnic vessels and reduce blood flow to the portal vein* (nitroglycerin is often given with vasopressin *to lower portal pressure and also reduce the vasoconstrictor side effects of vasopressin*)
   d. prepare client for endoscopic sclerotherapy or ligation of varices if planned
   e. assist with insertion of a gastroesophageal balloon tube (e.g., Sengstaken-Blakemore tube, Minnesota tube); maintain balloon pressure and suction and perform lavage as ordered
   f. administer vitamin K (e.g., phytonadione) injections, whole blood, or blood products (e.g., fresh frozen plasma, platelets) as ordered
   g. prepare client for a transjugular intrahepatic portosystemic shunt (TIPS) or surgery (e.g., esophageal transection with reanastomosis, distal splenorenal shunt) if planned.

Desired Outcomes	Nursing Actions *and Selected Purposes/Rationales*
11.e. The client will not develop hepatic encephalopathy as evidenced by: 1. usual speech and handwriting 2. usual mental status 3. absence of asterixis and fetor hepaticus 4. serum ammonia level within normal range.	11.e.1. Assess for and report signs and symptoms of hepatic encephalopathy (e.g., change in handwriting, inability to draw simple figures or numbers, asterixis, slow or slurred speech, inability to concentrate, emotional lability, disordered sleep, agitation, belligerence, disorientation, lethargy, fetor hepaticus [musty or fruity odor on breath], unresponsiveness). 2. Monitor serum ammonia results. Report elevated values. 3. Implement measures *to reduce the risk for hepatic coma:* a. perform actions *to eliminate or control the following factors that increase levels of ammonia and other nitrogenous substances:* 1. constipation *(results in increased formation and absorption of ammonia and mercaptans from the gut)* 2. gastrointestinal hemorrhage *(intestinal bacteria convert the protein in blood to ammonia and other nitrogenous substances)* 3. hypokalemia and/or metabolic alkalosis *(both conditions contribute to increased cerebral levels of ammonia)* 4. renal failure *(results in decreased excretion of ammonia)* 5. excessive protein intake *(intestinal bacteria convert protein to ammonia and other nitrogenous substances)* 6. infection *(bacteria that produce urease break urea into ammonia)* 7. dehydration/hypovolemia *(reduced blood flow to the liver results in decreased detoxification of ammonia and other toxins)* 8. if client is to receive blood transfusions, request fresh rather than stored blood *(stored blood contains more ammonia and citrate)* b. consult physician about discontinuation of prescribed medications that are potential hepatotoxins (e.g., isoniazid, amiodarone, 6-mercaptopurine, erythromycin, phenytoin) *in order to prevent further liver damage* c. administer central nervous system depressants such as narcotics, sedative-hypnotics, and antianxiety agents with extreme caution *(many of these agents are metabolized in the liver and may precipitate nonnitrogenous coma).* 4. If signs and symptoms of hepatic encephalopathy occur: a. maintain client on strict bed rest *to reduce metabolic demands on the liver* b. maintain dietary protein restrictions as ordered; increase protein intake slowly as encephalopathy resolves and encourage intake of vegetable proteins rather than animal proteins *(vegetable proteins are less ammoniagenic)* c. ensure a high carbohydrate intake or administer intravenous glucose or tube feedings as ordered *to provide a rapid energy source and decrease metabolism of endogenous proteins* d. administer enemas and/or cathartics as ordered *to hasten expulsion of intestinal contents so that bacteria have less time to convert proteins to ammonia and other nitrogenous substances* e. administer the following medications if ordered: 1. antimicrobials that suppress activity of the intestinal flora (e.g., neomycin, metronidazole) *to decrease protein breakdown in the intestine and subsequently reduce the formation of nitrogenous substances* 2. lactulose *to stimulate catharsis and create an acidic medium in the intestine (the acidity reduces bacterial growth and the resultant formation of nitrogenous substances and also traps ammonia in the colon by promoting the conversion of* NH_3 *to the poorly absorbed* NH_4*)* 3. benzodiazepine receptor antagonists (e.g., flumazenil) *to block benzodiazepine uptake in the brain*

4. zinc supplements *to stimulate ureagenesis (several enzymes in the urea cycle are zinc dependent)*

f. institute general safety precautions.

12. NURSING DIAGNOSIS:

*DISTURBED SELF-CONCEPT**

related to:
a. changes in appearance (e.g., edema, ascites, jaundice, spider angiomas, gynecomastia);
b. alterations in sexual functioning (e.g., impotence, decreased libido);
c. dependence on others to meet self-care needs;
d. disturbed thought processes;
e. stigma of having a chronic illness;
f. possible changes in lifestyle and roles.

*This diagnostic label includes the nursing diagnoses of disturbed body image, low self-esteem, and ineffective role performance.

Suggested NOC Outcomes: Body image; Personal autonomy; Self-esteem; Psychosocial adjustment: life change

Suggested NIC Interventions: Body image enhancement; Self-esteem enhancement; Emotional support; Support system enhancement; Role enhancement; Counseling

Desired Outcome	**Nursing Actions** *and Selected Purposes/Rationales* (see pp. 47–49 for additional rationales)
12. The client will demonstrate beginning adaptation to changes in appearance, level of independence, body functioning, lifestyle, and roles (see Care Plan on Immobility, Diagnosis 14 [p. 144], for outcome criteria).	12.a. Refer to Care Plan on Immobility, Diagnosis 14 (pp. 144–145), for measures related to assessment and promotion of a positive self-concept. b. Implement additional measures *to assist client to adapt to changes in appearance, level of independence, body functioning, lifestyle, and roles:* 1. inform client that many of changes in appearance may be lessened by adherence to treatment regimen 2. discuss techniques the client can use *to adapt to disturbed thought processes:* a. make lists and jot down messages and refer to these notes rather than relying on memory b. place self in a calm environment when making decisions c. validate decisions, clarify information, and seek assistance to problem solve 3. assist client *to attain and maintain optimal independence:* a. perform actions to increase strength and activity tolerance (see Diagnosis 7, action b) b. consult social services and occupational therapist about a home evaluation to identify ways that home environment can be modified so that client can function more independently c. reinforce benefits of using portable oxygen if it has been prescribed 4. encourage maximum participation in self-care within the prescribed activity restrictions and encourage significant others to allow client to do what he/she is able *so that independence can be re-established and self-esteem redeveloped.*

13. NURSING DIAGNOSIS:

INEFFECTIVE THERAPEUTIC REGIMEN MANAGEMENT

related to:
a. lack of understanding of the implications of not following the prescribed treatment plan;
b. difficulty modifying personal habits (e.g., dietary habits, alcohol intake);
c. insufficient financial resources.

Suggested NOC Outcomes: Compliance behavior; Treatment behavior: illness or injury; Knowledge: treatment regimen; Health beliefs: perceived resources; Health beliefs: perceived ability to perform

Suggested NIC Interventions: Self-modification assistance; Values clarification; Substance use treatment; Teaching: prescribed diet; Financial resource assistance; Support system enhancement

Desired Outcome

13. The client will demonstrate the probability of effective therapeutic regimen management as evidenced by:
    a. willingness to learn about and participate in treatment plan and care
    b. statements reflecting ways to modify personal habits and integrate treatments into lifestyle
    c. statements reflecting an understanding of the implications of not following the prescribed treatment plan.

Nursing Actions *and Selected Purposes/Rationales*

13.a. Assess for indications that the client may be unable to manage the therapeutic regimen effectively:
1. statements reflecting inability to manage care at home
2. failure to adhere to treatment plan (e.g., not adhering to dietary modifications and fluid restrictions, refusing medications)
3. statements reflecting a lack of understanding of the factors that will cause further progression of liver failure
4. statements reflecting an unwillingness or inability to modify personal habits and integrate necessary treatments into lifestyle
5. statements reflecting the view that cirrhosis has resolved once he/she is feeling better or that there is no way to control the disease and efforts to comply with treatments are useless.

b. Implement measures *to promote effective therapeutic regimen management:*
1. explain cirrhosis in terms the client can understand; stress that cirrhosis is a chronic disease and adherence to the treatment plan is necessary in order to delay and/or prevent complications
2. encourage questions and clarify misconceptions client has about cirrhosis and its effects
3. encourage client to participate in the treatment plan
4. initiate and reinforce the discharge teaching outlined in Diagnosis 14 *in order to promote a sense of control and self-reliance*
5. provide instructions on weighing self and calculating dietary sodium and protein content; allow time for return demonstration; determine areas of difficulty and misunderstanding and reinforce teaching as necessary
6. provide client with written instructions about scheduled appointments with health care provider, medications, signs and symptoms to report, weighing self, and dietary modifications
7. assist client to identify ways treatments can be incorporated into lifestyle; focus on modifications of lifestyle rather than complete change
8. encourage client to discuss concerns about the cost of hospitalization, medications, and lifelong follow-up care; obtain a social service consult to assist with financial planning and to obtain financial aid if indicated
9. provide information about and encourage utilization of community resources that can assist client to make necessary lifestyle changes (e.g., drug and alcohol rehabilitation programs)
10. reinforce behaviors suggesting future compliance with the therapeutic regimen (e.g., statements reflecting plans for integrating treatments into lifestyle, participation in diet planning, statements reflecting an understanding of the importance of eliminating alcohol intake)
11. include significant others in explanations and teaching sessions and encourage their support; reinforce the need for client to assume responsibility for managing as much of care as possible.

c. Consult appropriate health care provider (e.g., social worker, physician) about referrals to community agencies if continued instruction, support, or supervision is needed.

Discharge Teaching/Continued Care

14. NURSING DIAGNOSIS: ***DEFICIENT KNOWLEDGE OR INEFFECTIVE HEALTH MAINTENANCE****

*The nurse should select the diagnostic label that is most appropriate for the client's discharge teaching needs.

Suggested NOC Outcomes: Knowledge: diet; Knowledge: disease process; Knowledge: treatment regimen

Suggested NIC Interventions: Health system guidance; Teaching: individual; Teaching: disease process; Teaching: prescribed diet; Teaching: prescribed activity/exercise; Substance use treatment

Desired Outcomes	Nursing Actions *and Selected Purposes/Rationales*
14.a. The client will identify ways to prevent further liver damage.	14.a. Provide the following instructions regarding ways to prevent further liver damage: 1. avoid the following hepatotoxic agents: a. alcohol b. cleaning agents containing carbon tetrachloride and solvents (these are toxic even when inhaled) c. industrial chemicals such as nitrobenzene, disulfide, and tetrachloroethane 2. take acetaminophen (e.g., Tylenol) only when necessary and do not exceed the recommended dose because of its potential toxic effect on the liver 3. adhere to the following precautions to prevent hepatitis: a. eat only in restaurants that have been inspected and approved by health authorities b. if blood transfusions are anticipated, arrange to donate and receive autologous blood rather than commercially obtained blood if possible c. avoid sharing food or eating utensils and handling toiletry items of others d. practice safe sex (e.g., condom use for intercourse) e. avoid anal sex f. do not share drug paraphernalia (e.g., needles, syringes, cookers, rinse water, straws for intranasal inhalation) g. get vaccinations for hepatitis A and B if recommended by health care provider h. if traveling to a developing country: 1. receive immune globulin and vaccines for hepatitis (e.g., hepatitis B vaccine, hepatitis A vaccine) as recommended by health care provider 2. drink only bottled water and avoid eating raw fruits and vegetables washed or prepared with local water when in the country 4. inform all health care providers of history of hepatitis because a number of medications (e.g., chlorpromazine, acetaminophen, allopurinol, amiodarone, erythromycin, 6-mercaptopurine, phenytoin) can be hepatotoxic and should not be prescribed if alternatives are available.
14.b. The client will verbalize an understanding of the rationale for and components of the recommended diet.	14.b.1. Reinforce the dietary instructions outlined in Diagnosis 3, action c.2. 2. Explain the rationale for a diet low in sodium and provide information about decreasing sodium intake: a. read food labels and calculate sodium content of items; avoid those products that tend to have a high sodium content (e.g., canned soups and vegetables, tomato juice, commercial baked goods, commercially prepared frozen or canned entrees and sauces)

Desired Outcomes	**Nursing Actions** *and Selected Purposes/Rationales*
	b. do not add salt when cooking foods or to prepared foods; use low-sodium herbs and spices if desired c. avoid cured and smoked foods d. avoid salty snack foods e. avoid commercially prepared fast foods f. avoid routine use of over-the-counter medications with a high sodium content (e.g., some antacids, Alka-Seltzer). 3. Obtain a dietary consult to assist client in planning meals that will meet prescribed dietary modifications.
14.c. The client will identify ways to reduce stress on or trauma to the esophageal blood vessels.	14.c. Provide the following instructions about ways to reduce stress on or trauma to the esophageal blood vessels: 1. adhere to prescribed measures to reduce fluid retention (e.g., fluid restriction, low-sodium diet, diuretics) 2. avoid activities that increase intra-abdominal pressure (e.g., straining to have a bowel movement, coughing, sneezing, lifting heavy objects) 3. avoid eating foods that might cause mechanical trauma to the esophageal varices (e.g., chips).
14.d. The client will identify ways to prevent bleeding.	14.d.1. Instruct client about ways to minimize risk of bleeding: a. avoid taking aspirin and other nonsteroidal anti-inflammatory agents (e.g., ibuprofen) on a regular basis b. use an electric rather than a straight-edge razor c. floss and brush teeth gently d. cut nails carefully e. avoid situations that could result in injury (e.g., contact sports) f. avoid blowing nose forcefully g. avoid straining to have a bowel movement h. avoid putting sharp objects (e.g., toothpicks) in mouth i. do not walk barefoot. 2. Instruct client to control any bleeding by applying firm, prolonged pressure to the area if possible.
14.e. The client will identify ways to reduce the risk of infection.	14.e. Instruct client in ways to reduce risk of infection: 1. continue with coughing and deep breathing or use of incentive spirometer every 2 hours while awake as long as activity is limited 2. increase activity as tolerated 3. avoid contact with persons who have an infection 4. avoid crowds, especially during flu and cold seasons 5. decrease or stop smoking 6. drink at least 10 glasses of liquid/day unless on a fluid restriction 7. adhere to recommended diet 8. take supplemental vitamins and minerals as prescribed 9. maintain good personal hygiene 10. receive immunizations (e.g., influenza vaccine, pneumococcal vaccine, hepatitis vaccines) if approved by health care provider.
14.f. The client will identify ways to relieve pruritus.	14.f.1. Reinforce instructions in Diagnosis 4, action b, regarding ways to relieve itching. 2. Instruct client to take bile acid sequestering agents (e.g., cholestyramine) or an antihistamine as prescribed.
14.g. The client will state signs and symptoms to report to the health care provider.	14.g. Stress the importance of reporting the following signs and symptoms: 1. rapid weight gain or loss 2. increasing size of abdomen 3. increased swelling of lower extremities 4. increasing shortness of breath 5. increased itchiness or yellowing of skin

6. temperature elevation that lasts more than 2 days
7. red, rust-colored, or smoky urine; bloody or tarry stools; blood in sputum or vomitus; persistent bleeding from nose, mouth, or skin; prolonged or excessive menses; excessive bruising; severe or persistent headache; or sudden abdominal or back pain
8. persistent impotence or decrease in libido
9. tremors or changes in behavior, speech, or handwriting.

14.h. The client will identify community resources that can assist with home management and adjustment to lifestyle changes necessary for effective management of cirrhosis.

14.h.1. Provide information regarding community resources that can assist client and significant others with home management and adjustment to changes necessary for effective management of cirrhosis (e.g., Meals on Wheels, home health agencies, transportation services, drug and alcohol rehabilitation programs, counseling services).
2. Initiate a referral if indicated.

14.i. The client will verbalize an understanding of and a plan for adhering to recommended follow-up care including future appointments with health care provider, medications prescribed, and activity level.

14.i.1. Reinforce the importance of keeping follow-up appointments with health care provider.
2. Explain the rationale for, side effects of, and importance of taking medications prescribed. Inform client of pertinent food and drug interactions.
3. Reinforce physician's instructions regarding activity level. Stress the importance of rest.
4. Implement measures outlined in Diagnosis 13, action b, to promote the client's ability to effectively manage the therapeutic regimen.

ADDITIONAL NURSING DIAGNOSES:

SELF-CARE DEFICIT

related to weakness, fatigue, dyspnea, and disturbed thought processes.

DISTURBED SLEEP PATTERN*

related to unfamiliar environment, frequent assessments and treatments, decreased physical activity, discomfort, fear, anxiety, and inability to assume usual sleep position because of orthopnea.

FEAR/ANXIETY*

related to difficulty breathing; unfamiliar environment and separation from significant others; lack of understanding of the diagnosis, diagnostic tests, and treatments; uncertainty of prognosis; financial concerns; and possibility of changes in lifestyle and roles.

*See Unit II for outcomes, actions, and rationales.

Bibliography

See pages 879 and 884.

Hepatitis

Hepatitis is widespread inflammation of the liver. It is most commonly caused by a virus but can also be caused by bacteria; an autoimmune reaction; or toxic injury to the liver by drugs, alcohol, industrial chemicals, or plant poisons. The five major viruses that cause hepatitis are the hepatitis A virus (HAV), hepatitis B virus (HBV), hepatitis C virus (HCV), hepatitis E virus (HEV), and the delta virus or hepatitis D virus (HDV). Several other viruses (e.g., hepatitis G virus) have been identified but occur rarely and do not appear to cause significant liver disease.

Hepatitis A and E are both spread by the fecal-oral route. Hepatitis A is the most common cause of acute hepatitis in the United States. Hepatitis E is similar in many respects to hepatitis A but is seen predominantly in persons who live in or have traveled to developing countries. Hepatitis B is transmitted sexually, perinatally, and parenterally (primarily in intravenous drug users who share needles). In the United States and many developed countries, sexual transmission is now the prevalent mode of transmission of hepatitis B. Hepatitis C is the most common blood-borne disease in the United States and the cause of chronic hepatitis in the majority of cases. End-stage liver disease associated with chronic hepatitis C is now the leading indication for liver transplants in the United States. Hepatitis C is transmitted predominantly by the parenteral route with intravenous drug use and sharing of drug paraphernalia being the most common risk factors. The risk for perinatal and sexual transmission is relatively low. Hepatitis D appears to require the presence of the hepatitis B virus for its replication and is therefore only seen in HBV-infected persons.

The various forms of hepatitis have similar clinical manifestations. Signs and symptoms vary in severity and many cases (particularly of hepatitis C) go undetected because the person either has very mild symptoms or is asymptomatic. Elevated serum aminotransferases (ALT and AST) are hallmarks of acute hepatitis. Other signs and symptoms include flu-like symptoms, mild-to-moderate right upper quadrant pain, and symptoms of bile flow obstruction (e.g., jaundice, pruritus, dark amber urine, light-colored stools). The only definitive way to distinguish the various forms of viral hepatitis is by the presence of antigens and antigenic subtypes and the subsequent development of antibodies to these antigens.

Hospitalization of persons with hepatitis is usually not indicated except for certain high-risk persons (e.g., the elderly, immunocompromised persons, persons with other disease conditions that may be difficult to manage with hepatitis) and persons with severe disease. Signs and symptoms of severe disease include a marked prolongation of prothrombin time, serum bilirubin more than 10 times normal, symptoms of encephalopathy, the presence of edema and/or ascites, or an inability to maintain adequate hydration.

Acute viral hepatitis is a major public health problem because it is highly communicable and because there is currently no effective treatment. The majority of cases are self-limited and resolve completely without complications but a small percentage of cases of hepatitis B and as many as 70-85% of cases of hepatitis C do progress to a chronic state which can then progress to cirrhosis or hepatocellular carcinoma. The treatment of acute hepatitis is primarily supportive and directed toward reducing the metabolic demands on the liver and promoting cell regeneration. If the client has hepatitis B, C, or D, close follow-up should be encouraged to determine if medication therapy (e.g., interferon, ribavirin, adefovir) is indicated to prevent and treat chronic hepatitis.

This care plan focuses on the adult client with acute viral hepatitis hospitalized because of persistent nausea, worsening of liver function test results, and a prolonged prothrombin time. Much of the information is applicable to clients receiving follow-up care in an extended care facility or home setting.

OUTCOME/DISCHARGE CRITERIA

THE CLIENT WILL:

- have resolution of nausea
- have no evidence of bleeding or progressive liver degeneration
- have an adequate nutritional intake
- perform activities of daily living without fatigue
- identify ways to prevent the spread of hepatitis to others
- identify ways to prevent further liver damage
- verbalize an understanding of the rationale for and components of the recommended diet
- state signs and symptoms to report to the health care provider
- verbalize an understanding of and a plan for adhering to recommended follow-up care including activity level, medications prescribed, and future appointments with health care provider and for laboratory studies.

NURSING/COLLABORATIVE DIAGNOSES

1. NURSING DIAGNOSIS: *RISK FOR DEFICIENT FLUID VOLUME*

related to:
a. decreased oral intake associated with anorexia and nausea;
b. excessive loss of fluid if diaphoresis and/or persistent vomiting is present.

Suggested NOC Outcomes: Fluid balance; Hydration

Suggested NIC Interventions: Fluid monitoring; Fluid management; Intravenous (IV) therapy; Nausea management

Desired Outcome

1. The client will not experience deficient fluid volume as evidenced by:
   a. normal skin turgor
   b. moist mucous membranes
   c. stable weight
   d. B/P and pulse within normal range for client and stable with position change
   e. capillary refill time less than 2–3 seconds
   f. balanced intake and output
   g. urine specific gravity within normal range
   h. usual mental status
   i. BUN and Hct within normal range.

Nursing Actions *and Selected Purposes/Rationales*
(see pp. 30–31 for additional rationales)

1.a. Assess for and report signs and symptoms of deficient fluid volume:
   1. decreased skin turgor, dry mucous membranes, thirst
   2. weight loss of 2% or greater over a short period
   3. postural hypotension and/or low B/P
   4. weak, rapid pulse
   5. capillary refill time greater than 2–3 seconds
   6. flat neck veins when supine
   7. decreased urine output with increased specific gravity (reflects an actual rather than potential fluid deficit)
   8. change in mental status
   9. increased BUN and Hct.

b. Implement measures *to prevent deficient fluid volume:*
   1. perform actions to reduce nausea and prevent vomiting (see Diagnosis 5, action b)
   2. perform actions to improve oral intake (see Diagnosis 2, action c.1)
   3. perform actions to reduce fever if present (e.g., administer tepid sponge bath, administer antipyretics if ordered) *in order to reduce fluid loss from diaphoresis*
   4. maintain a fluid intake of at least 2500 ml/day unless contraindicated; if oral intake is inadequate or contraindicated, maintain intravenous and/or enteral fluid therapy as ordered.

2. NURSING DIAGNOSIS: *IMBALANCED NUTRITION: LESS THAN BODY REQUIREMENTS*

related to:
a. decreased oral intake associated with anorexia and nausea;
b. loss of nutrients associated with persistent vomiting if present;
c. reduced metabolism and storage of nutrients by the liver associated with an alteration in normal liver function as a result of inflammation;

d. malabsorption of fats and fat-soluble vitamins associated with impaired bile flow resulting from inflammation of the liver;
e. increased utilization of nutrients associated with the increased metabolic rate that is present with infection.

Suggested NOC Outcome: Nutritional status

Suggested NIC Interventions: Nutritional monitoring; Nutrition management; Nutrition therapy; Nutritional counseling; Nausea management

Desired Outcome

2. The client will maintain an adequate nutritional status as evidenced by:
   a. weight within normal range for client
   b. normal BUN and serum prealbumin, albumin, Hct, and Hgb levels
   c. improved strength and activity tolerance
   d. healthy oral mucous membrane.

Nursing Actions *and Selected Purposes/Rationales*

(see pp. 40–43 for additional rationales)

2.a. Assess for and report signs and symptoms of malnutrition:
   1. weight significantly below client's usual weight or below normal for client's age, height, and body frame
   2. abnormal BUN and low serum prealbumin, albumin, Hct, and Hgb levels (some of these values also reflect impaired liver function)
   3. weakness and fatigue
   4. sore, inflamed oral mucous membrane
   5. pale conjunctiva.

b. Monitor percentage of meals and snacks client consumes. Report a pattern of inadequate intake.

c. Implement measures *to maintain an adequate nutritional status:*
   1. perform actions *to improve oral intake:*
      a. implement measures to reduce nausea and prevent vomiting (see Diagnosis 5, action b)
      b. obtain a dietary consult if necessary to assist client in selecting foods/fluids that are appealing and adhere to personal and cultural preferences as well as prescribed dietary modifications
      c. encourage a rest period before meals *to minimize fatigue*
      d. maintain a clean environment and a relaxed, pleasant atmosphere
      e. provide oral hygiene before meals *(oral hygiene removes unpleasant tastes, which often improves the taste of foods/fluids)*
      f. serve frequent, small meals rather than large ones if client is weak, fatigues easily, or has a poor appetite
      g. allow adequate time for meals; reheat foods/fluids if necessary
      h. limit fluid intake with meals (unless the fluid has high nutritional value) *to reduce early satiety and subsequent decreased food intake*
      i. increase activity as allowed and tolerated *(activity usually promotes a sense of well-being, which can improve appetite)*
   2. encourage client to consume meals that are well balanced and high in essential nutrients; offer dietary supplements if client's caloric intake is inadequate
   3. assist and instruct client to adhere to the following dietary recommendations:
      a. avoid skipping meals
      b. consume a diet high in calories (2000–3000 calories/day) and carbohydrates; if unable to tolerate food, suck on hard candy and drink fruit juices and regular soft drinks
      c. maintain a moderate to high protein intake (unless the serum ammonia level is high or clinical evidence of encephalopathy is present) *in order to promote healing of the liver*
   4. administer vitamin preparations (e.g., fat-soluble vitamins, thiamine, folic acid, iron) if ordered.

d. Perform a calorie count if ordered. Report information to dietitian and physician.

e. Consult physician about an alternative method of providing nutrition (e.g., parenteral nutrition, tube feeding) if client does not consume enough food or fluids to meet nutritional needs.

3. NURSING DIAGNOSIS:

ACUTE PAIN

a. right upper quadrant related to inflammation of the liver;
b. myalgias/arthralgias related to the presence of circulating immune complexes and activation of the complement system associated with viral infection.

Suggested NOC Outcomes: Comfort level; Pain control

Suggested NIC Interventions: Pain management; Environmental management: comfort; Analgesic administration

Desired Outcome	**Nursing Actions** *and Selected Purposes/Rationales* (see pp. 45–47 for additional rationales)
3. The client will experience diminished pain as evidenced by: a. verbalization of a decrease in or absence of pain b. relaxed facial expression and body positioning c. increased participation in activities.	3.a. Assess for signs and symptoms of pain (e.g., verbalization of pain, reluctance to move, grimacing, rubbing joints or muscles, guarding of abdomen). b. Assess client's perception of the severity of pain using a pain intensity rating scale. c. Assess the client's pain pattern (e.g., location, quality, onset, duration, precipitating factors, aggravating factors, alleviating factors). d. Implement measures *to reduce pain:* 1. perform actions to promote rest (see Diagnosis 6, action b.1) *in order to reduce fatigue and subsequently increase the client's threshold and tolerance for pain* 2. perform actions to reduce fear and anxiety (see Diagnosis 8, action b) *in order to promote relaxation and subsequently increase the client's threshold and tolerance for pain* 3. provide or assist with nonpharmacologic measures for pain relief (e.g., position change; relaxation exercises; restful environment; diversional activities such as watching television, reading, or conversing) 4. administer analgesics if ordered; be aware of the following: a. narcotics are usually not ordered or ordered only in low doses *because the liver cannot detoxify narcotics at a normal rate* b. acetaminophen may be ordered (despite its potential hepatotoxic effect) rather than acetylsalicylic acid *because of the increased risk of bleeding with acetylsalicylic acid.* e. Consult appropriate health care provider (e.g., pharmacist, physician) if above measures fail to provide adequate pain relief.

4. NURSING DIAGNOSIS:

ALTERED COMFORT: PRURITUS

related to stimulation of itch fibers in the skin by bile acid metabolites that accumulate in the blood as a result of bile flow obstruction.

Suggested NOC Outcomes: Comfort level; Symptom control

Suggested NIC Intervention: Pruritus management

Desired Outcome	**Nursing Actions** *and Selected Purposes/Rationales*
4. The client will experience relief of pruritus as evidenced by: a. verbalization of same b. no scratching or rubbing of skin.	4.a. Assess for the following: 1. reports of itchiness 2. persistent scratching or rubbing of skin. b. Instruct client in and/or implement measures *to relieve pruritus:* 1. apply cool, moist compresses to pruritic areas 2. apply emollient cream or ointment frequently *to prevent dryness* 3. add emollients, cornstarch, or baking soda to bath water 4. use tepid water and mild soaps for bathing 5. pat skin dry after bathing, making sure to dry thoroughly 6. maintain a cool environment

Desired Outcome	Nursing Actions *and Selected Purposes/Rationales*

7. encourage participation in diversional activity
8. utilize relaxation techniques
9. utilize cutaneous stimulation techniques (e.g., massage, pressure, vibration, stroking with a soft brush) at the sites of itching or acupressure points
10. encourage client to wear loose cotton garments and avoid clothes or blankets made from wool
11. administer the following medications if ordered:
    a. antihistamines (e.g., diphenhydramine, hydroxyzine [Atarax])
    b. bile acid sequestering agents (e.g., cholestyramine).

c. Consult appropriate health care provider (e.g., clinical nurse specialist, physician) if above measures fail to alleviate pruritus or if the skin becomes excoriated.

5. Nursing Diagnosis: NAUSEA

related to stimulation of the vomiting center associated with stimulation of the visceral afferent pathways as a result of:
a. inflammation of the gastrointestinal tract resulting from immune complex-mediated tissue responses to the viral infection;
b. gaseous distention resulting from impaired fat digestion if bile flow is obstructed;
c. venous congestion in the gastrointestinal tract if portal hypertension has developed.

Suggested NOC Outcome: Nausea and vomiting severity

Suggested NIC Interventions: Nausea management; Environmental management: comfort

Desired Outcome	Nursing Actions *and Selected Purposes/Rationales*
5. The client will experience relief of nausea as evidenced by verbalization of same.	5.a. Assess client for nausea. b. Implement measures *to reduce nausea and prevent vomiting:* 1. eliminate noxious sights and odors from the environment *(noxious stimuli can cause stimulation of the vomiting center)* 2. instruct client to change positions slowly *(rapid movement can result in stimulation of the chemoreceptor trigger zone and subsequent excitation of the vomiting center)* 3. encourage client to take deep, slow breaths when nauseated 4. encourage client to avoid intake of foods/fluids high in fat (e.g., butter, cream, whole milk, ice cream, fried foods, gravies, nuts) *to prevent a delay in gastric emptying and reduce nausea associated with impaired fat digestion* 5. avoid serving foods with an overpowering aroma; remove lids from hot foods before entering room 6. instruct client to eat dry foods (e.g., toast, crackers) and avoid drinking liquids with meals if nauseated 7. provide small, frequent meals; instruct client to ingest foods and fluids slowly 8. instruct client to avoid foods/fluids that irritate the gastric mucosa (e.g., spicy foods; caffeine-containing beverages such as tea, coffee, and colas) 9. administer antiemetics if ordered (phenothiazines are contraindicated *because of their potential cholestatic effects*). c. Consult physician if above measures fail to control nausea.

6. Nursing Diagnosis: ACTIVITY INTOLERANCE

related to:
a. inadequate nutritional status;

b. increased energy utilization associated with the increased metabolic rate present in an infectious process;
c. difficulty resting and sleeping associated with frequent assessments and treatments, discomfort, anxiety, and unfamiliar environment.

Suggested NOC Outcomes: Rest; Energy conservation; Activity tolerance

Suggested NIC Interventions: Energy management; Nutrition management; Sleep enhancement

Desired Outcome	**Nursing Actions** *and Selected Purposes/Rationales* (see pp. 11–12 for additional rationales)
6. The client will demonstrate an increased tolerance for activity as evidenced by: a. verbalization of feeling less fatigued and weak b. ability to perform activities of daily living without exertional dyspnea, chest pain, diaphoresis, dizziness, and a significant change in vital signs.	6.a. Assess for signs and symptoms of activity intolerance: 1. statements of fatigue or weakness 2. exertional dyspnea, chest pain, diaphoresis, or dizziness 3. abnormal heart rate response to activity (e.g., increase in rate of 20 beats/minute above resting rate, rate not returning to preactivity level within 3 minutes after stopping activity, change from regular to irregular rate) 4. a significant change (15–20 mm Hg) in blood pressure with activity. b. Implement measures *to improve activity tolerance:* 1. perform actions *to promote rest and/or conserve energy:* a. maintain activity restrictions as ordered b. minimize environmental activity and noise c. organize nursing care to allow for periods of uninterrupted rest d. limit the number of visitors and their length of stay e. assist client with self-care activities as needed f. keep supplies and personal articles within easy reach g. instruct client in energy-saving techniques (e.g., using shower chair when showering, sitting to brush teeth or comb hair) h. implement measures to reduce discomfort (see Diagnoses 3, action d; 4, action b; and 5, action b) i. implement measures *to promote sleep* (e.g., encourage relaxing diversional activities in the evening; allow client to continue usual sleep practices unless contraindicated; reduce environmental stimuli; discourage intake of fluids high in caffeine, especially in the evening) 2. perform actions to maintain an adequate nutritional status (see Diagnosis 2, action c) 3. increase client's activity gradually as allowed and tolerated. c. Instruct client to: 1. report a decreased tolerance for activity 2. stop any activity that causes chest pain, shortness of breath, dizziness, or extreme fatigue or weakness. d. Consult physician if signs and symptoms of activity intolerance persist or worsen.

7. COLLABORATIVE DIAGNOSES: POTENTIAL COMPLICATIONS OF HEPATITIS

a. **bleeding** related to:
   1. decreased production of clotting factors associated with impaired liver function and impaired vitamin K absorption if bile flow is obstructed (normal bile flow is necessary for absorption of vitamin K)
   2. thrombocytopenia associated with hypersplenism (if venous congestion has resulted in splenomegaly, the spleen will destroy platelets faster than usual);

b. **progressive liver degeneration (e.g., fulminant hepatitis, chronic active hepatitis)** related to continued degeneration/necrosis of liver cells.

Desired Outcomes	**Nursing Actions** *and Selected Purposes/Rationales*

Desired Outcomes

7.a. The client will not experience unusual bleeding as evidenced by:
1. skin and mucous membranes free of petechiae, purpura, ecchymoses, and active bleeding
2. absence of unusual joint pain
3. no increase in abdominal girth
4. absence of frank and occult blood in stool, urine, and vomitus
5. usual menstrual flow
6. vital signs within normal range for client
7. stable or improved Hct and Hgb.

Nursing Actions *and Selected Purposes/Rationales*

7.a.1. Assess client for and report signs and symptoms of unusual bleeding:
- a. petechiae, purpura, ecchymoses
- b. gingival bleeding
- c. prolonged bleeding from puncture sites
- d. epistaxis, hemoptysis
- e. unusual joint pain
- f. increase in abdominal girth
- g. frank or occult blood in stool, urine, or vomitus
- h. menorrhagia
- i. restlessness, confusion
- j. decreasing B/P and an increased pulse rate
- k. decrease in Hct and Hgb levels.

2. Monitor platelet count and coagulation test results (e.g., prothrombin time or International Normalized Ratio [INR], activated partial thromboplastin time, bleeding time). Report abnormal values.
3. Implement measures *to prevent bleeding:*
   - a. avoid giving injections whenever possible; consult physician about prescribing an alternative route for medications ordered to be given intramuscularly or subcutaneously
   - b. when giving injections or performing venous or arterial punctures, use the smallest gauge needle possible and apply gentle prolonged pressure to the site after the needle is removed
   - c. caution client to avoid activities that increase the risk for trauma (e.g., shaving with a straight-edge razor, using stiff bristle toothbrush or dental floss)
   - d. pad side rails if client is confused or restless
   - e. whenever possible, avoid intubations (e.g., nasogastric) and procedures that can cause injury to the rectal mucosa (e.g., inserting a rectal suppository or tube, administering an enema)
   - f. perform actions *to reduce the risk for falls* (e.g., avoid unnecessary clutter in room, instruct client to wear shoes/slippers with nonslip soles when ambulating)
   - g. instruct client to avoid blowing nose forcefully or straining to have a bowel movement; consult physician about an order for a decongestant and/or laxative if indicated
   - h. administer the following if ordered *to improve clotting ability:*
     1. vitamin K (e.g., phytonadione) injections
     2. platelets
     3. fresh frozen plasma (FFP).
4. If bleeding occurs and does not subside spontaneously:
   - a. apply firm, prolonged pressure to bleeding area(s) if possible
   - b. if epistaxis occurs, place client in a high Fowler's position and apply pressure and ice pack to nasal area
   - c. maintain oxygen therapy as ordered
   - d. if esophageal bleeding occurs:
     1. turn client on side and suction as necessary *to reduce the risk for aspiration*
     2. assist with administration of octreotide (Sandostatin) or vasopressin if ordered *to constrict splanchnic vessels and reduce blood flow to the portal vein*
     3. prepare client for endoscopic sclerotherapy or ligation of varices if planned
     4. assist with insertion of a gastroesophageal balloon tube (e.g., Sengstaken-Blakemore tube, Minnesota tube); maintain balloon pressure, suction client, and perform lavage if ordered
   - e. administer vitamin K (e.g., phytonadione) injections, whole blood, or blood products (e.g., fresh frozen plasma [FFP], platelets) as ordered
   - f. assess for and report signs and symptoms of hypovolemic shock (e.g., restlessness; confusion; significant decrease in B/P; rapid, weak pulse; rapid respirations; cool skin; urine output less than 30 ml/hour).

7.b. The client will not experience progressive liver degeneration as evidenced by:
1. resolution of signs and symptoms of hepatitis
2. absence of edema, ascites, and bleeding
3. usual mental status
4. coagulation test results and serum AST, ALT, alkaline phosphatase, bilirubin, and albumin levels within or returning toward normal limits.

7.b.1. Assess for signs and symptoms of progressive liver degeneration:
a. worsening of signs and symptoms (e.g., increased jaundice, weakness, and pruritus)
b. edema, ascites
c. bleeding (see action a.1 in this diagnosis)
d. encephalopathy (e.g., change in handwriting, slow or slurred speech, emotional lability, agitation, asterixis, disorientation, lethargy)
e. further increase in prothrombin time
f. further elevation of serum AST, ALT, alkaline phosphatase, and bilirubin
g. low serum albumin.
2. Implement measures identified in this care plan to promote healing of the liver.
3. If signs and symptoms of progressive liver degeneration occur:
a. implement measures to prevent bleeding (see action a.3 in this diagnosis)
b. implement measures to prevent an increase in levels of ammonia and other nitrogenous substances (e.g., administer neomycin if ordered, administer lactulose if ordered, maintain prescribed dietary protein restrictions) *in order to prevent or treat hepatic encephalopathy (hepatic coma)*
c. implement measures *to reduce the risk for injury* (e.g., keep side rails up, maintain seizure precautions)
d. prepare client for liver transplant if planned.

8. NURSING DIAGNOSIS: FEAR/ANXIETY

related to:
a. unfamiliar environment and lack of understanding of diagnosis and diagnostic tests;
b. lack of definitive treatment for hepatitis and the possibility of serious complications;
c. discomfort associated with nausea, pain, and pruritus;
d. possible transmission of disease to others and rejection by others because of their fear of contracting hepatitis;
e. temporary restrictions of some of usual activities (e.g., vigorous exercise, contact sports, sexual activity, alcohol consumption).

Suggested NOC Outcomes: Anxiety self-control; Anxiety level; Fear level; Fear self-control

Suggested NIC Interventions: Anxiety reduction; Calming technique; Emotional support; Presence

Desired Outcome	**Nursing Actions** *and Selected Purposes/Rationales* (see pp. 14–16 for additional rationales)

8. The client will experience a reduction in fear and anxiety as evidenced by:
a. verbalization of feeling less anxious
b. usual sleep pattern
c. relaxed facial expression and body movements
d. stable vital signs
e. usual perceptual ability and interactions with others.

8.a. Assess client for signs and symptoms of fear and anxiety (e.g., verbalization of feeling anxious, insomnia, tenseness, shakiness, restlessness, diaphoresis, tachycardia, elevated blood pressure, self-focused behaviors).
b. Implement measures *to reduce fear and anxiety:*
1. orient client to environment, equipment, and routines
2. introduce client to staff who will be participating in care; if possible, maintain consistency in staff assigned to his/her care
3. assure client that staff members are nearby; respond to call signal as soon as possible
4. maintain a calm, supportive, confident manner when interacting with client
5. encourage verbalization of fear and anxiety; provide feedback
6. reinforce physician's explanations and clarify misconceptions the client has about hepatitis, the treatment plan, and prognosis

Desired Outcome	Nursing Actions *and Selected Purposes/Rationales*

7. explain all diagnostic tests
8. perform actions to reduce discomfort (see Diagnoses 3, action d; 4, action b; and 5, action b)
9. provide a calm, restful environment
10. instruct client in relaxation techniques and encourage participation in diversional activities
11. convey acceptance of client
12. provide information based on current needs of client at a level he/she can understand; encourage questions and clarification of information provided
13. encourage significant others to visit and to convey a caring, concerned attitude without obvious anxiousness
14. include significant others in orientation and teaching sessions and encourage their continued support of the client
15. administer prescribed antianxiety agents if indicated (use caution when administering these agents *because many are metabolized by the liver*).

c. Consult appropriate health care provider (e.g., psychiatric nurse clinician, physician) if above actions fail to control fear and anxiety.

Discharge Teaching/Continued Care

9. Nursing Diagnosis: ***DEFICIENT KNOWLEDGE, INEFFECTIVE THERAPEUTIC REGIMEN MANAGEMENT, OR INEFFECTIVE HEALTH MAINTENANCE****

*The nurse should select the diagnostic label that is most appropriate for the client's discharge teaching needs.

Suggested NOC Outcomes: Knowledge: disease process; Knowledge: treatment regimen; Knowledge: health behavior; Knowledge: infection control

Suggested NIC Interventions: Health system guidance; Teaching: disease process; Teaching: prescribed diet; Teaching: prescribed medication; Communicable disease management; Teaching: individual

Desired Outcomes	Nursing Actions *and Selected Purposes/Rationales*

9.a. The client will identify ways to prevent the spread of hepatitis to others.

9.a.1. Provide the following instructions on ways to prevent the spread of hepatitis to others:

a. if client has hepatitis A, instruct him/her to adhere to the following precautions for 1–2 weeks after the onset of jaundice:
   1. wash hands thoroughly after having a bowel movement
   2. use separate toilet facilities if possible; if separate toilet facilities are not available, clean toilet seat with a chlorine solution after use
   3. wash bedding, towels, and underwear in hot, soapy water; wash them separately from other articles
   4. do not donate blood or work in food services until approved by physician

b. if client has hepatitis B, C, or D, instruct him/her to adhere to the following precautions until health care provider states that transmitting hepatitis to others is no longer a risk:
   1. wash hands thoroughly after urinating and having a bowel movement
   2. do not share personal articles (e.g., toothbrush, straight-edge razor, thermometer, washcloth)
   3. use disposable eating utensils or wash utensils separately in hot, soapy water

4. do not share food, cigarettes, or eating utensils
5. if any injections (e.g., insulin, vitamin B_{12}) are given at home, use disposable equipment and dispose of it properly to reduce the risk of others coming in contact with contaminated needles
6. do not share drug paraphernalia (e.g., needles, straws for intranasal inhalation)
7. avoid intimate sexual contact; once sexual activity is resumed, avoid intercourse during menstruation and intermenstrual bleeding and make sure that a condom is used during intercourse
8. do not donate blood.

2. Instruct client to inform household and sexual contacts to see health care provider for appropriate immunization and testing for early detection of hepatitis.

9.b. The client will identify ways to prevent further liver damage.

9.b. Provide the following instructions regarding ways to prevent further liver damage:
1. avoid alcohol intake for a minimum of 6 months (many sources recommend a year)
2. avoid contact with substances known to be injurious to the liver (e.g., cleaning agents containing carbon tetrachloride, solvents, industrial chemicals such as nitrobenzene, disulfide, and tetrachloroethane)
3. take acetaminophen (e.g., Tylenol) only when necessary and do not exceed the recommended dose or take it after drinking alcohol because of its potential toxic effect on the liver
4. take precautions to prevent recurrent hepatitis (client is immune only to the viral type he/she has had):
   a. avoid unnecessary transfusions; if transfusions are necessary, arrange to donate and receive autologous blood rather than commercially obtained blood if possible
   b. practice safe sex (e.g., condom use during intercourse); if sexual partner is a carrier, consult health care provider about receiving a hepatitis B vaccination
   c. avoid sharing food, eating utensils, and toiletry items
   d. avoid sharing drug paraphernalia (e.g., needles, syringes, cookers, rinse water, straws for intranasal inhalation)
   e. eat only in restaurants that have been inspected and approved by health authorities
   f. get vaccinations for hepatitis A and B if recommended by health care provider
   g. avoid anal sex
   h. if traveling to a developing country:
      1. receive immune globulin and vaccines for hepatitis (e.g., hepatitis B vaccine, hepatitis A vaccine) as recommended by health care provider
      2. drink only bottled water and avoid eating raw fruits and vegetables washed or prepared with local water when in the country
5. inform all health care providers of history of hepatitis because a number of medications (e.g., chlorpromazine, acetaminophen, allopurinol, amiodarone, erythromycin, 6-mercaptopurine, phenytoin) can be hepatotoxic and should not be prescribed if alternatives are available.

9.c. The client will verbalize an understanding of the rationale for and components of the recommended diet.

9.c.1. Explain to client that adherence to the recommended diet will promote healing of the liver and reduce the risk of further liver damage.
2. Reinforce the dietary instructions outlined in Diagnosis 2, action c.3.
3. Instruct client to avoid intake of foods high in fat (e.g., butter, cream, ice cream, pork, fried foods, gravy) until gastrointestinal symptoms such as nausea and indigestion subside.

Desired Outcomes	**Nursing Actions** *and Selected Purposes/Rationales*
9.d. The client will state signs and symptoms to report to the health care provider.	9.d. Stress the importance of reporting the following signs and symptoms: 1. persistent or recurrent loss of appetite, nausea, fatigue, or weight loss 2. vomiting 3. increased itchiness or yellowing of skin 4. swelling of lower extremities, rapid weight gain, or increased size of abdomen 5. red, rust-colored, or smoky urine; bloody or tarry stools; blood in sputum or vomitus; prolonged or excessive bleeding from nose, mouth, or skin; prolonged or excessive menses; excessive bruising; severe or persistent headache; or sudden abdominal or back pain 6. changes in behavior, speech, or handwriting.
9.e. The client will verbalize an understanding of and a plan for adhering to recommended follow-up care including activity level, medications prescribed, and future appointments with health care provider and for laboratory studies.	9.e.1. Reinforce physician's instructions regarding activity level. Stress the importance of rest during convalescent phase (from 6 weeks to 6 months). 2. Reinforce the importance of keeping follow-up appointments with health care provider and for laboratory studies (liver enzyme levels and serological markers provide information about immunity, presence of a carrier state, and chronicity, which helps determine the need for additional treatment [e.g., interferon, ribavirin, adefovir] and teaching). 3. If medication is prescribed to prevent/treat chronic hepatitis, explain the rationale for, side effects of, and importance of taking the medications prescribed (e.g., interferon, ribavirin, adefovir). If client is to administer own interferon, provide instructions on subcutaneous injection technique. 4. Provide client with information about and encourage participation in drug and alcohol rehabilitation programs if indicated. 5. Implement measures to improve client compliance: a. include significant others in teaching sessions if possible b. encourage questions and allow time for reinforcement and clarification of information provided c. provide written instructions regarding scheduled appointments with health care provider and for laboratory studies, medications prescribed, activity restrictions, and signs and symptoms to report.

Bibliography

See pages 879 and 884.

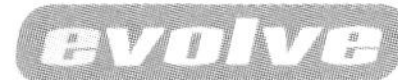

PANCREATITIS, ACUTE

Acute pancreatitis is an inflammation of the pancreas that occurs when the enzymes it produces become activated in the pancreas rather than in the duodenum. The subsequent autodigestion causes pathologic changes that range from a mild local inflammatory response to extensive tissue and vascular damage that can result in life-threatening complications such as shock and multiple organ failure. Following an episode of mild to moderate acute pancreatitis, the structure and function of the pancreas often return to normal. However, with more severe and/or recurrent episodes of acute pancreatitis, irreversible changes can occur and chronic pancreatitis can develop.

It is theorized that pancreatic duct obstruction, pancreatic ischemia, direct injury to the acinar cells, and reflux of bile into the pancreatic duct are among the mechanisms that trigger the activation of enzymes in the pancreas. The most common causes of acute pancreatitis are biliary tract disease and heavy alcohol intake. Some less frequent causes include external trauma to the abdomen, trauma to the pancreas during pancreatic endoscopy or abdominal surgery, infections, drugs (e.g., azathioprine, mercaptopurine, didanosine, pentamidine, estrogen, thiazides, valproic acid), and metabolic disorders such as chronic hypercalcemia and genetic hyperlipidemia.

Signs and symptoms of acute pancreatitis usually include severe, continuous epigastric pain that radiates to the back; nausea; vomiting; fever (usually low-grade); and abdominal tenderness and distention. The focus of medical treatment is to prevent further autodigestion of the pancreas and prevent systemic complications by decreasing stimulation of the pancreatic enzymes until normal outflow resumes. If the cause of the pancreatitis is biliary tract disease, surgery (e.g., removal of gallstones that may be blocking the pancreatic duct) is usually performed after pancreatic inflammation has subsided and the client is in stable condition.

This care plan focuses on the adult client hospitalized with acute pancreatitis. Some of the information is applicable to clients receiving follow-up care in an extended care facility or home setting.

OUTCOME/DISCHARGE CRITERIA

THE CLIENT WILL:

- have no signs and symptoms of complications
- have relief of severe pain
- have an adequate nutritional intake
- identify ways to prevent overstimulation of and further trauma to the pancreas
- verbalize an understanding of recommended dietary modifications
- state signs and symptoms to report to the health care provider
- verbalize an understanding of and a plan for adhering to recommended follow-up care including future appointments with health care provider and medications prescribed.

NURSING/COLLABORATIVE DIAGNOSES

DISCHARGE TEACHING

See p. 725 for additional diagnoses.

1. Nursing Diagnosis: INEFFECTIVE BREATHING PATTERN

related to:
a. increased rate of respirations associated with fear and anxiety;
b. decreased rate of respirations associated with the depressant effect of some medications (e.g., narcotic [opioid] analgesics, some antiemetics);
c. decreased depth of respirations associated with:
   1. depressant effects of some medications (e.g., narcotic [opioid] analgesics, some antiemetics)
   2. fear, anxiety, decreased activity, and reluctance to breathe deeply because of pain
   3. restricted chest expansion resulting from positioning (client often positions self on side with knees and trunk flexed to reduce pain) and pressure on the diaphragm (can occur as a result of accumulation of gastrointestinal gas and fluid and ascites if present)
   4. decreased lung compliance (distensibility) if pleural effusion is present.

Suggested NOC Outcome:
Respiratory status: ventilation

Suggested NIC Interventions: Respiratory monitoring; Ventilation assistance; Pain management

Desired Outcome

1. The client will maintain an effective breathing pattern as evidenced by:
   a. normal rate and depth of respirations
   b. absence of dyspnea
   c. symmetrical chest excursion.

Nursing Actions *and Selected Purposes/Rationales*

(see pp. 18–20 for additional rationales)

1.a. Assess for signs and symptoms of an ineffective breathing pattern (e.g., shallow respirations, dyspnea, tachypnea, use of accessory muscles when breathing, limited chest excursion).
  b. Implement measures *to improve breathing pattern:*
     1. perform actions to reduce fear and anxiety (e.g., assure client that staff are nearby; provide a calm, restful environment; explain all tests and procedures) *in order to prevent the shallow and/or rapid breathing that can occur with fear and anxiety*
     2. perform actions to reduce pain (see Diagnosis 4, action d) *in order to increase the client's willingness to move and breathe more deeply*
     3. perform actions *to reduce pressure on the diaphragm:*
        a. implement measures to reduce the accumulation of gas and fluid in the gastrointestinal tract (see Diagnosis 6, action b)
        b. implement measures to prevent further third-spacing and/or promote mobilization of fluid back into vascular space (see Diagnosis 2, action b.3) *in order to reduce ascites*
     4. perform actions to prevent and treat pleural effusion (see Diagnosis 8, actions d.2 and 3)
     5. when severe pain has subsided, place client in a semi- to high Fowler's position unless contraindicated; position with pillows *to prevent slumping*
     6. if client must remain flat in bed, assist with position change at least every 2 hours
     7. instruct client to deep breathe or use incentive spirometer every 1–2 hours
     8. assist with positive airway pressure techniques (e.g., continuous positive airway pressure [CPAP], bilevel positive airway pressure [BiPAP], flutter/positive expiratory pressure [PEP] device) if ordered
     9. increase activity as allowed and tolerated
     10. administer central nervous system depressants judiciously; hold medication and consult physician if respiratory rate is less than 12/minute.
  c. Consult appropriate health care provider (e.g., respiratory therapist, physician) if:
     1. ineffective breathing pattern continues
     2. signs and symptoms of atelectasis (e.g., diminished or absent breath sounds, dull percussion note over affected area, increased respiratory rate, dyspnea, tachycardia, elevated temperature) develop

3. signs and symptoms of impaired gas exchange (e.g., restlessness, irritability, confusion, significant decrease in oximetry results, decreased Pa_{O_2} and increased Pa_{CO_2} levels) are present.

2. NURSING/COLLABORATIVE DIAGNOSIS:

IMBALANCED FLUID AND ELECTROLYTES

a. **deficient fluid volume** related to:
   1. decreased oral intake
   2. excessive loss of fluid associated with vomiting and nasogastric tube drainage
   3. third-spacing of intravascular fluid;
b. **hypokalemia, hypochloremia, and metabolic alkalosis** related to loss of electrolytes and hydrochloric acid associated with vomiting and nasogastric tube drainage;
c. **hypocalcemia** related to:
   1. binding of calcium to the undigested fats in the intestine (enzymes such as lipase and phospholipase A are not released into the intestinal tract to digest fats so calcium binds with the free fats and is excreted in the stool)
   2. hypoalbuminemia associated with increased vascular permeability that occurs with inflammation (albumin is needed to transport nonionized calcium in the blood)
   3. binding of calcium to free fatty acids in areas of tissue necrosis;
d. **third-spacing** related to increased vascular permeability associated with the inflammatory response and activation of kinin peptides such as bradykinin and kallidin (occurs when the pancreatic enzyme trypsin enters systemic circulation).

Suggested NOC Outcomes: Fluid balance; Electrolyte and acid-base balance

Suggested NIC Interventions: Fluid monitoring; Fluid/Electrolyte management; Electrolyte management: hypokalemia; Electrolyte management: hypocalcemia; Acid-base monitoring; Acid-base management: metabolic alkalosis

Desired Outcomes	**Nursing Actions** *and Selected Purposes/Rationales* (see pp. 30–31 for additional rationales)
2.a. The client will not experience deficient fluid volume, hypokalemia, hypochloremia, hypocalcemia, or metabolic alkalosis as evidenced by: 1. normal skin turgor 2. moist mucous membranes 3. stable weight 4. B/P and pulse within normal range for client and stable with position change 5. capillary refill time less than 2–3 seconds 6. usual mental status 7. balanced intake and output 8. urine specific gravity within normal range 9. soft, nondistended abdomen with normal bowel sounds	2.a.1. Assess for and report signs and symptoms of: a. deficient fluid volume: 1. decreased skin turgor, dry mucous membranes, thirst 2. weight loss of 2% or greater over a short period 3. postural hypotension and/or low B/P 4. weak, rapid pulse 5. capillary refill time greater than 2–3 seconds 6. flat neck veins when supine 7. change in mental status 8. decreased urine output with increased specific gravity (reflects an actual rather than potential fluid volume deficit) 9. increased BUN and Hct b. hypokalemia (e.g., cardiac dysrhythmias, postural hypotension, muscle weakness, nausea and vomiting, abdominal distention, hypoactive or absent bowel sounds, low serum potassium) c. hypochloremia and metabolic alkalosis (e.g., dizziness, paresthesias, muscle twitching or spasms, hypoventilation, low serum chloride, elevated pH and T_{CO_2}) d. hypocalcemia (e.g., anxiousness; irritability; numbness or tingling of fingers, toes, or circumoral area; positive Chvostek's and Trousseau's signs; hyperactive reflexes; tetany; seizures; low serum calcium). 2. Implement measures *to prevent or treat deficient fluid volume, hypokalemia, hypochloremia, hypocalcemia, and metabolic alkalosis:* a. perform actions to reduce nausea and vomiting (see Diagnosis 5, action b)

Desired Outcomes	Nursing Actions *and Selected Purposes/Rationales*
10. absence of cardiac dysrhythmias, muscle weakness, paresthesias, muscle twitching or spasms, dizziness, tetany, and seizure activity 11. negative Chvostek's and Trousseau's signs 12. BUN, Hct, serum electrolytes, and blood gases within normal range.	b. if a nasogastric tube is present and needs to be irrigated frequently and/or with large volumes of solution, irrigate it with normal saline rather than water c. administer fluid and electrolyte replacements if ordered d. maintain a fluid intake of at least 2500 ml/day unless contraindicated e. when oral intake is allowed: 1. assist client to select the following foods/fluids: a. those high in potassium (e.g., bananas, potatoes, cantaloupe, avocados, raisins) b. those high in calcium such as milk and milk products (if client is on a low-fat diet, items such as ice cream, whole milk, butter, and cream should be omitted) 2. administer pancreatic enzymes (e.g., pancreatin, pancrelipase) if ordered *to promote fat digestion so that there is less fat available for calcium to bind to.* 3. Consult physician if signs and symptoms of deficient fluid volume and electrolyte imbalances persist or worsen.
2.b. The client will experience resolution of third-spacing as evidenced by: 1. resolution of ascites 2. absence of dyspnea 3. audible breath sounds 4. B/P and pulse within normal range for client and stable with position change 5. balanced intake and output.	2.b.1. Assess for and report signs and symptoms of third-spacing: a. ascites b. dyspnea and diminished or absent breath sounds c. evidence of vascular depletion (e.g., postural hypotension; weak, rapid pulse; decreased urine output) d. chest x-ray results showing pleural effusion. 2. Monitor serum albumin levels. Report below-normal levels *(low serum albumin levels result in fluid shifting out of vascular space because albumin normally maintains plasma colloid osmotic pressure).* 3. Implement measures *to prevent further third-spacing and/or promote mobilization of fluid back into vascular space:* a. administer albumin infusions if ordered *to increase colloid osmotic pressure* b. perform actions to decrease pancreatic stimulation (see Diagnosis 4, action d.5) *in order to decrease inflammation and activation of vasoactive plasma peptides and subsequently decrease vascular permeability.* 4. Consult physician if signs and symptoms of third-spacing persist or worsen.

3. Nursing Diagnosis:

IMBALANCED NUTRITION: LESS THAN BODY REQUIREMENTS

related to:

a. decreased oral intake associated with nausea, pain, prescribed dietary restrictions, and feeling of fullness resulting from abdominal distention;
b. loss of nutrients associated with vomiting;
c. decreased utilization of nutrients associated with impaired digestion of fats, proteins, and carbohydrates resulting from loss of normal outflow of pancreatic enzymes;
d. increased nutritional needs associated with the increased metabolic rate that occurs with pancreatitis.

Suggested NOC Outcome: Nutritional status

Suggested NIC Interventions: Nutritional monitoring; Nutrition management; Nutrition therapy; Nausea management; Pain management; Total parenteral nutrition (TPN) administration

Desired Outcome	**Nursing Actions** *and Selected Purposes/Rationales* (see pp. 40–43 for additional rationales)
3. The client will maintain an adequate nutritional status as evidenced by: a. weight within normal range for client b. normal BUN and serum prealbumin, albumin, Hct, Hgb, and lymphocyte levels c. usual strength and activity tolerance d. healthy oral mucous membrane.	3.a. Assess for and report signs and symptoms of malnutrition: 1. weight significantly below client's usual weight or less than normal for client's age, height, and body frame 2. abnormal BUN and low serum prealbumin, albumin, Hct, Hgb, and lymphocyte levels (albumin levels can also be low because of increased vascular permeability) 3. weakness and fatigue 4. sore, inflamed oral mucous membrane 5. pale conjunctiva. b. When oral intake is allowed, monitor percentage of meals and snacks client consumes. Report a pattern of inadequate intake. c. Implement measures *to maintain an adequate nutritional status:* 1. administer total parenteral nutrition if ordered 2. limit activity as ordered *to decrease energy utilization and metabolic rate* 3. when food or oral fluids are allowed: a. perform actions *to improve oral intake:* 1. implement measures to reduce pain (see Diagnosis 4, action d) 2. implement measures to reduce ascites and the accumulation of gas and fluid in the gastrointestinal tract (see Diagnoses 2, action b.3 and 6, action b) *in order to reduce abdominal distention and the subsequent feeling of fullness and early satiety* 3. implement measures to reduce nausea and vomiting (see Diagnosis 5, action b) 4. increase activity as allowed and tolerated *(activity usually promotes a sense of well-being, which can improve appetite)* 5. obtain a dietary consult if necessary to assist client in selecting foods/fluids that meet nutritional needs, are appealing, and adhere to personal and cultural preferences as well as the prescribed dietary modifications 6. maintain a clean environment and a relaxed, pleasant atmosphere 7. allow adequate time for meals; reheat foods/fluids if necessary 8. limit fluid intake with meals (unless the fluids have high nutritional value) *to reduce early satiety and subsequent decreased food intake* b. ensure that meals are well balanced and high in essential nutrients; offer dietary supplements if indicated c. administer the following if ordered: 1. vitamins and minerals 2. pancreatic enzymes (e.g., pancreatin, pancrelipase) *to facilitate the digestion of proteins, fats, and carbohydrates.* d. Perform a calorie count if ordered. Report information to dietitian and physician. e. Reassess nutritional status on a regular basis and report decline.

4. NURSING DIAGNOSIS: ***ACUTE PAIN: EPIGASTRIC WITH RADIATION TO THE BACK***

related to:
a. distention of the pancreas associated with inflammation and obstruction of pancreatic ducts;
b. peritoneal irritation associated with escape of activated pancreatic enzymes into the peritoneum.

Suggested NOC Outcomes: Pain control; Comfort level

Suggested NIC Interventions: Pain management; Analgesic administration; Patient-controlled analgesia (PCA) assistance

Desired Outcome	**Nursing Actions** *and Selected Purposes/Rationales* (see pp. 45–47 for additional rationales)
4. The client will experience diminished pain as evidenced by: a. verbalization of a decrease in or absence of pain b. relaxed facial expression and body positioning c. increased participation in activities d. stable vital signs.	4.a. Assess for signs and symptoms of pain (e.g., verbalization of pain, guarding of abdomen, rubbing epigastric or flank area, grimacing, reluctance to move, restlessness, diaphoresis, increased B/P, tachycardia). b. Assess client's perception of the severity of pain using a pain intensity rating scale. c. Assess the client's pain pattern (e.g., location, quality, onset, duration, precipitating factors, aggravating factors, alleviating factors). d. Implement measures *to reduce pain:* 1. perform actions *to reduce fear and anxiety about the pain experience* (e.g., assure client that his/her need for pain relief is understood, plan methods for achieving pain control with client) 2. perform actions to reduce fear and anxiety (e.g., assure client that staff are nearby; provide a calm, restful environment; explain all tests and procedures) *in order to promote relaxation and subsequently increase the client's threshold and tolerance for pain* 3. administer analgesics before activities and procedures that can cause pain and before pain becomes severe 4. perform actions to promote rest (e.g., minimize environmental activity and noise) *in order to reduce fatigue and subsequently increase the client's threshold and tolerance for pain* 5. perform actions *to reduce pancreatic stimulation:* a. withhold all food and oral fluid as ordered *(food and fluid [especially those that are acidic or have a high protein or fat content] entering the duodenum cause the release of secretin and/or cholecystokinin, which stimulate the output of pancreatic secretions)* b. implement measures *to reduce the amount of hydrochloric acid in the stomach (as the hydrochloric acid enters the duodenum, it stimulates the release of secretin; some physicians believe that the secretin released stimulates a significant output of pancreatic secretions):* 1. insert a nasogastric tube and maintain suction if ordered 2. administer histamine$_2$ receptor antagonists (e.g., famotidine, ranitidine, nizatidine) if ordered c. minimize client's exposure to odor and sight of food until oral intake is allowed *in order to prevent stimulation of gastric secretions and the subsequent output of pancreatic secretions* d. when oral intake is allowed: 1. advance diet slowly 2. provide small, frequent meals rather than 3 large ones 3. avoid foods/fluids high in fat (e.g., butter, cream, whole milk, ice cream, fried foods, gravies, nuts), spicy foods, and caffeine-containing beverages (e.g., coffee, tea, colas) if ordered 6. allow client to sit or lie with knees and trunk flexed *(this position relieves pressure on the inflamed pancreas)* 7. provide or assist with additional nonpharmacologic measures for pain relief (e.g., massage; position change; progressive relaxation exercises; restful environment; diversional activities such as watching television, reading, or conversing) 8. administer analgesics as ordered and encourage client to use patient-controlled analgesia (PCA) device as instructed 9. if client is receiving epidural analgesia, perform actions *to maintain patency of the system* (e.g., keep tubing free of kinks, tape catheter securely, use caution when moving client to avoid dislodging catheter) 10. assist with peritoneal lavage if performed *(may be done to remove some of the activated pancreatic enzymes and debris that cause peritoneal irritation and subsequent pain).* e. Consult appropriate health care provider (e.g., pharmacist, pain management specialist, physician) if above measures fail to provide adequate pain relief.

5. NURSING DIAGNOSIS:

NAUSEA

related to stimulation of the vomiting center associated with:
a. stimulation of the visceral afferent pathways resulting from abdominal distention and inflammation of the pancreas;
b. stimulation of the cerebral cortex resulting from pain and stress.

Suggested NOC Outcome: Nausea and vomiting severity

Suggested NIC Interventions: Nausea management; Vomiting management; Environmental management: comfort

Desired Outcome	**Nursing Actions** *and Selected Purposes/Rationales*
5. The client will experience relief of nausea and vomiting as evidenced by: a. verbalization of relief of nausea b. absence of vomiting.	5.a. Assess client for nausea and vomiting. b. Implement measures *to reduce nausea and vomiting:* 1. maintain food and oral fluid restrictions as ordered 2. insert nasogastric tube and maintain suction if ordered 3. perform actions *to reduce fear and anxiety* (e.g., assure client that staff are nearby; provide a calm, restful environment; explain all tests and procedures) 4. perform actions to reduce pain (see Diagnosis 4, action d) 5. perform actions to reduce the accumulation of gas and fluid in the gastrointestinal tract (see Diagnosis 6, action b) *in order to prevent abdominal distention and subsequent visceral irritation* 6. eliminate noxious sights and odors from the environment *(noxious stimuli can cause stimulation of the vomiting center)* 7. encourage client to take deep, slow breaths when nauseated 8. instruct client to change positions slowly *(rapid movement can result in chemoreceptor trigger zone stimulation and subsequent excitation of the vomiting center)* 9. provide oral hygiene after each emesis 10. when oral intake is allowed: a. avoid serving foods with an overpowering aroma; remove lids from hot foods before entering room b. provide small, frequent meals rather than 3 large ones; instruct client to ingest foods and fluids slowly c. instruct client to eat dry foods (e.g., toast, crackers) and avoid drinking liquids with meals if nauseated d. instruct client to avoid foods/fluids that irritate the gastric mucosa (e.g., spicy foods; caffeine-containing beverages such as tea, coffee, and colas) e. instruct client to avoid foods/fluids high in fat (e.g., butter, cream, whole milk, ice cream, fried foods, gravies, nuts) *in order to prevent a delay in gastric emptying and reduce nausea associated with impaired fat digestion* 11. administer antiemetics if ordered. c. Consult physician if above measures fail to control nausea and vomiting.

6. NURSING DIAGNOSIS:

ALTERED COMFORT: ABDOMINAL DISTENTION AND GAS PAIN

related to accumulation of gas and/or fluid in the gastrointestinal tract associated with:
a. an inability to digest fats properly resulting from obstruction of the flow of lipase;
b. decreased gastrointestinal motility resulting from the depressant effect of some medications (e.g., narcotic [opioid] analgesics, some antiemetics) and decreased activity.

Suggested NOC Outcomes: Comfort level; Symptom control

Suggested NIC Intervention: Flatulence reduction

Desired Outcome	Nursing Actions *and Selected Purposes/Rationales*
6. The client will experience diminished abdominal distention and gas pain as evidenced by: a. verbalization of same b. relaxed facial expression and body positioning c. decrease in abdominal girth.	6.a. Assess for signs and symptoms of abdominal distention or gas pain (e.g., verbal reports of abdominal fullness or gas pain, grimacing, clutching or guarding of abdomen, restlessness, reluctance to move, increasing abdominal girth). b. Implement measures *to reduce the accumulation of gas and fluid in the gastrointestinal tract in order to decrease abdominal distention and gas pain:* 1. encourage and assist client with frequent position changes and ambulation as allowed and tolerated *(activity stimulates peristalsis and expulsion of flatus)* 2. instruct client to avoid activities such as chewing gum, drinking through a straw, and smoking *in order to reduce air swallowing* 3. maintain food and oral fluid restrictions as ordered 4. maintain patency of nasogastric tube if present 5. when oral intake is allowed, instruct client to avoid the following: a. carbonated beverages and gas-producing foods (e.g., cabbage, onions, baked beans) b. foods/fluids high in fat (e.g., butter, cream, whole milk, ice cream, fried foods, gravies, nuts) 6. encourage client to eructate and expel flatus whenever the urge is felt 7. administer the following medications if ordered: a. antiflatulents (e.g., simethicone) *to reduce gas accumulation* b. pancreatic enzymes (e.g., pancreatin, pancrelipase) *to improve fat digestion* 8. encourage use of nonnarcotic analgesics once the period of severe pain has subsided *(narcotic [opioid] analgesics depress gastrointestinal motility).* c. Consult physician if signs and symptoms of abdominal distention and gas pain persist or worsen.

7. Nursing Diagnosis: ***RISK FOR INFECTION: SEPSIS***

related to:

a. release of bacteria into the blood associated with:
   1. presence of infected necrotic areas or leakage of infected pseudocysts or abscesses (necrotic areas, pseudocysts, and abscesses can develop as a result of destruction of pancreatic and surrounding tissue by the activated proteolytic enzymes)
   2. peritonitis (if it occurs);

b. decreased resistance to infection associated with decreased nutritional status;

c. break in skin integrity associated with frequent venipunctures or presence of invasive lines (e.g., intravenous catheter, hemodynamic monitoring devices).

Suggested NOC Outcomes: Immune status; Infection severity

Suggested NIC Interventions: Infection protection; Infection control

Desired Outcome	Nursing Actions *and Selected Purposes/Rationales* (see pp. 37–40 for additional rationales)
7. The client will not experience sepsis as evidenced by: a. no further increase in temperature b. absence of chills and diaphoresis c. pulse and respiratory rate within normal range for client	7.a. Assess for and report signs and symptoms of sepsis (e.g., increase in temperature, chills, diaphoresis, tachypnea, tachycardia, increase in WBC count above previous levels and/or significant change in differential, positive blood cultures). b. Implement measures *to prevent sepsis:* 1. perform actions to decrease pancreatic stimulation (see Diagnosis 4, action d.5) *in order to reduce destruction of pancreatic and peripancreatic tissue and subsequent development of necrotic areas, pseudocysts, and abscesses* 2. perform actions to prevent and treat peritonitis (see Diagnosis 8, actions b.2 and 3)

d. WBC and differential counts returning to normal
e. negative blood culture results.

3. prepare client for drainage of an abscess or pseudocyst or surgical resection of necrotic tissue if planned
4. maintain sterile technique during all invasive procedures (e.g., venous and arterial punctures)
5. perform actions to maintain an adequate nutritional status (see Diagnosis 3, action c)
6. perform actions to reduce stress (e.g., reduce pain and nausea; provide a calm, restful environment; explain diagnostic tests and treatment plan) *in order to prevent an increase in secretion of cortisol (cortisol interferes with some immune responses)*
7. change intravenous line sites, tubing, and solutions according to hospital policy and maintain a closed system for intravenous infusions whenever possible
8. anchor catheters/tubings (e.g., intravenous) securely *in order to reduce trauma to the tissues and the risk for introduction of pathogens associated with in-and-out movement of the tubing*
9. administer antimicrobials as ordered.

c. If signs and symptoms of sepsis occur, assess for and immediately report signs and symptoms of septic shock (e.g., systolic blood pressure less than 90 mm Hg; rapid, weak pulse; restlessness; agitation; confusion; urine output less than 30 ml/hour; cool, pale, mottled, and/or cyanotic extremities; capillary refill time greater than 3 seconds; diminished or absent peripheral pulses).

8. COLLABORATIVE DIAGNOSES: POTENTIAL COMPLICATIONS OF ACUTE PANCREATITIS

a. **hypovolemic shock** related to:
   1. deficient fluid volume associated with restricted oral intake and fluid loss resulting from vomiting and nasogastric tube drainage
   2. peripheral vasodilation and increased vascular permeability with subsequent third-spacing associated with activation of kinin peptides such as bradykinin and kallidin (occurs when the pancreatic enzyme trypsin enters systemic circulation)
   3. hemorrhage associated with destruction of elastic fibers of the blood vessels by the proteolytic enzyme elastase (elastase is activated in the pancreas by trypsin and causes localized vessel damage in addition to the vessel wall destruction that occurs when it enters the systemic circulation);

b. **peritonitis** related to:
   1. escape of activated pancreatic enzymes from the pancreas into the peritoneum
   2. leakage of necrotic substances into the peritoneum associated with rupture of an infected pancreatic or peripancreatic abscess or pseudocyst
   3. suppuration in areas of pancreatic and peripancreatic necrosis;

c. **hyperglycemia** related to:
   1. increased glucagon and decreased insulin output associated with damage to the pancreatic islet cells resulting from activation of pancreatic enzymes in the pancreas
   2. the increased glucagon, cortisol, and catecholamine output that occurs with stress;

d. **pleural effusion** related to:
   1. increased capillary permeability of and damage to the pleural vessels associated with the escape of activated pancreatic enzymes into systemic circulation
   2. passage of exudate from the peritoneal cavity to the pleural cavity through the transdiaphragmatic lymph channels;

e. **organ ischemia/dysfunction (multiple organ dysfunction syndrome [MODS])** related to:
   1. hypoperfusion of major organs associated with hypovolemic and/or septic shock if present and decreased myocardial contractility (can occur as a result of the release of myocardial depressant factor in response to the inflammatory process that occurs in pancreatitis)

2. microvascular thrombosis associated with disseminated intravascular coagulation (DIC) if it occurs (activation of clotting mechanisms can occur in response to the presence of activated proteolytic enzymes in the blood vessels and/or the procoagulant effects of some inflammatory mediators).

Desired Outcomes	**Nursing Actions** *and Selected Purposes/Rationales*
8.a. The client will not develop hypovolemic shock as evidenced by: 1. usual mental status 2. stable vital signs 3. skin warm and usual color 4. palpable peripheral pulses 5. urine output at least 30 ml/hour.	8.a.1. Assess for and report signs and symptoms of: a. deficient fluid volume and third-spacing (see Diagnosis 2, actions a.1.a and b.1 for signs and symptoms) b. bleeding (e.g., gray-blue discoloration around umbilicus [Cullen's sign], green-blue or purple-blue discoloration of flanks [Grey Turner's sign], increased abdominal or back pain, increased abdominal girth, decreasing B/P and increased pulse rate, decreased Hct and Hgb levels) c. hypovolemic shock: 1. restlessness, agitation, confusion, or other change in mental status 2. significant decrease in B/P 3. postural hypotension 4. rapid, weak pulse 5. rapid respirations 6. cool skin 7. pallor, cyanosis 8. diminished or absent peripheral pulses 9. urine output less than 30 ml/hour. 2. Implement measures *to prevent hypovolemic shock:* a. perform actions to prevent or treat imbalanced fluid and electrolytes (see Diagnosis 2, actions a.2 and b.3) b. perform actions to reduce pancreatic stimulation (see Diagnosis 4, action d.5) *in order to decrease the amount of elastase that is activated and released into the tissue and systemic circulation and thereby reduce the risk for bleeding.* 3. If signs and symptoms of hypovolemic shock occur: a. place client flat in bed with legs elevated unless contraindicated b. monitor vital signs frequently c. administer oxygen as ordered d. administer whole blood, blood products, and/or volume expanders if ordered e. prepare client for transfer to the critical care unit and insertion of hemodynamic monitoring devices (e.g., central venous catheter, intra-arterial catheter) if indicated.
8.b. The client will not develop peritonitis as evidenced by: 1. gradual resolution of abdominal pain 2. soft, nondistended abdomen 3. temperature declining toward normal 4. stable vital signs 5. decreased nausea and vomiting 6. gradual return of normal bowel sounds 7. WBC count declining toward normal.	8.b.1. Assess for and report signs and symptoms of peritonitis (e.g., increase in severity of abdominal pain; generalized abdominal pain; rebound tenderness; distended, rigid abdomen; further increase in temperature; tachycardia; tachypnea; hypotension; increased nausea and vomiting; diminished or absent bowel sounds; WBC count that increases or fails to decline toward normal). 2. Implement measures *to prevent peritonitis:* a. perform actions to reduce pancreatic stimulation (see Diagnosis 4, action d.5) *in order to decrease activation of pancreatic enzymes within the pancreas and reduce the risk for their escape into the peritoneum* b. administer antimicrobials if ordered *(may be ordered prophylactically or if culture of drainage from a necrotic area, pseudocyst, or abscess is positive)* c. prepare client for drainage or removal of infected pseudocysts and abscesses and resection of necrotic tissue if planned. 3. If signs and symptoms of peritonitis occur: a. withhold oral intake as ordered b. place client on bed rest in a semi-Fowler's position *to assist in pooling or localizing gastrointestinal contents in the pelvis rather than under the diaphragm* c. prepare client for diagnostic tests (e.g., abdominal x-ray, computed tomography, ultrasonography) if planned

d. insert a nasogastric tube and maintain suction as ordered
e. administer antimicrobials as ordered
f. administer intravenous fluids and/or blood volume expanders if ordered *to prevent or treat shock (can result from the increased capillary permeability that occurs with inflammation and the subsequent escape of protein, fluid, and electrolytes from the vascular space into the peritoneal cavity)*
g. prepare client for and assist with peritoneal lavage if performed *to remove toxins from the peritoneal cavity.*

8.c. The client will maintain a safe blood glucose level as evidenced by:
1. absence of polydipsia, polyuria, and polyphagia
2. usual mental status
3. serum glucose between 60–200 mg/dl.

8.c.1. Assess for and report signs and symptoms of hyperglycemia (e.g., polydipsia, polyuria, polyphagia, change in mental status, blood glucose levels above 200 mg/dl or greater than the parameter specified by physician).
2. Implement measures *to prevent hyperglycemia:*
a. perform actions to reduce pancreatic stimulation (see Diagnosis 4, action d.5) *in order to prevent further damage to the pancreatic islet cells*
b. perform actions such as relieving discomfort, explaining all tests and procedures, and providing a restful environment *in order to reduce stress (stress causes an increased output of epinephrine, norepinephrine, glucagon, and cortisol, which results in a further increase in blood glucose).*
3. If signs and symptoms of hyperglycemia occur:
a. administer insulin or oral hypoglycemic agents if ordered
b. assess for and report signs and symptoms of ketoacidosis (e.g., warm, flushed skin; thirst; weakness; lethargy; hypotension; increased abdominal pain; fruity odor on breath; Kussmaul respirations; blood glucose above 250 mg/dl; ketones in blood and urine; low serum pH and CO_2 content)
c. if client does not have a history of diabetes or chronic pancreatitis, assure him/her that the hyperglycemia is expected to resolve as the pancreatitis does.

8.d. The client will not experience pleural effusion as evidenced by:
1. unlabored respirations at 12–20/minute
2. symmetrical chest excursion
3. resonant percussion note throughout lung fields
4. normal breath sounds.

8.d.1. Assess for and report signs and symptoms of pleural effusion (e.g., dyspnea, chest pain, decreased chest excursion on affected side, dull percussion note and diminished or absent breath sounds over the affected area, chest x-ray results showing pleural effusion).
2. Implement measures to reduce pancreatic stimulation (see Diagnosis 4, action d.5) *in order to reduce the release of activated pancreatic enzymes into the systemic circulation and transdiaphragmatic lymph channels.*
3. If signs and symptoms of pleural effusion occur, prepare client for thoracentesis if planned.

8.e. The client will not develop organ ischemia/dysfunction as evidenced by:
1. usual mental status
2. urine output at least 30 ml/hour
3. unlabored respirations at 12–20/minute
4. audible breath sounds without an increase in adventitious sounds
5. absence of new or increased abdominal pain, distention, nausea, vomiting, and diarrhea
6. BUN, creatinine, AST, ALT, and LDH within normal range.

8.e.1. Assess for and report signs and symptoms of organ ischemia/dysfunction:
a. cerebral ischemia (e.g., change in mental status)
b. renal insufficiency (e.g., urine output less than 30 ml/hour, elevated BUN and creatinine)
c. acute respiratory distress syndrome (e.g., dyspnea, increase in respiratory rate, low SaO_2, crackles)
d. gastrointestinal ischemia (e.g., increased abdominal pain, nausea, and abdominal distention; continued hypoactive or absent bowel sounds; development of or increased episodes of vomiting; diarrhea; hematemesis; blood in stool)
e. liver dysfunction (e.g., increased AST, ALT, and LDH).
2. Implement measures *to reduce the risk for organ ischemia/dysfunction:*
a. perform actions to prevent hypovolemic shock (see action a.2 in this diagnosis)
b. perform actions to prevent sepsis (see Diagnosis 7, action b) *in order to prevent septic shock and the subsequent systemic hypoperfusion*
c. perform actions *to treat DIC if it occurs* (e.g., implement safety precautions to prevent further bleeding; administer fresh frozen plasma, platelets, and/or cryoprecipitate if ordered; administer

Desired Outcomes	Nursing Actions *and Selected Purposes/Rationales*
	medications such as heparin and antithrombin III if ordered to interrupt clotting) d. maintain intravenous therapy as ordered e. maintain oxygen therapy as ordered f. administer vasopressors (e.g., dopamine, norepinephrine) and/or positive inotropic agents (e.g., dobutamine) as ordered *to maintain adequate tissue perfusion and cardiac output.* 3. If signs and symptoms of organ ischemia/MODS occur, prepare client for transfer to critical care unit.

Discharge Teaching/Continued Care

9. Nursing Diagnosis: DEFICIENT KNOWLEDGE, INEFFECTIVE THERAPEUTIC REGIMEN MANAGEMENT, OR INEFFECTIVE HEALTH MAINTENANCE*

*The nurse should select the diagnostic label that is most appropriate for the client's discharge teaching needs.

Suggested NOC Outcomes: Knowledge: treatment regimen; Knowledge: diet; Knowledge: disease process

Suggested NIC Interventions: Health system guidance; Teaching: individual; Teaching: disease process; Teaching: prescribed diet; Teaching: prescribed medication

Desired Outcomes	Nursing Actions *and Selected Purposes/Rationales*
9.a. The client will identify ways to prevent overstimulation of and further trauma to the pancreas.	9.a.1. Instruct client in importance of avoiding overstimulation of the pancreas for the length of time specified by the physician (may be for a few months or for life depending on the cause of the pancreatitis and if permanent pancreatic damage has occurred). 2. Instruct client in ways to prevent overstimulation of and further trauma to the pancreas: a. maintain a balanced program of rest and exercise b. avoid drinking alcohol c. adhere to recommended dietary modifications (see action b.1 in this diagnosis). 3. If indicated, provide information about and encourage use of community resources that can assist client to make necessary lifestyle changes (e.g., alcohol rehabilitation program).
9.b. The client will verbalize an understanding of recommended dietary modifications.	9.b.1. Instruct client regarding dietary modifications necessary to prevent overstimulation of the pancreas during the recovery period: a. eat small, frequent meals rather than 3 large ones b. avoid foods/fluids high in fat (e.g., butter, cream, whole milk, ice cream, fried foods, gravies, nuts) c. avoid spicy foods and caffeine-containing beverages (e.g., coffee, tea, colas). 2. Obtain a dietary consult if client needs assistance in planning meals that incorporate dietary modifications.
9.c. The client will state signs and symptoms to report to the health care provider.	9.c. Instruct client to report: 1. stools that float and are grayish, greasy, and foul-smelling (indicates a very high fat content resulting from impaired flow of the pancreatic enzyme lipase into the intestinal tract) 2. persistent or recurrent abdominal or back pain 3. nausea or vomiting 4. abdominal distention or increasing feeling of fullness

5. excessive thirst or excessive urination
6. irritability or confusion
7. continued or unexplained weight loss
8. bluish areas on the back or abdomen
9. persistent or recurrent temperature elevation
10. fever, chills
11. difficulty breathing
12. reddened, tender nodules on skin (could be indicative of destruction of superficial fatty tissue by activated pancreatic enzymes such as lipase and phospholipase A that have entered the systemic circulation and tissue; if this relatively rare condition occurs, it is usually weeks to months after the episode of acute pancreatitis).

9.d. The client will verbalize an understanding of and a plan for adhering to recommended follow-up care including future appointments with health care provider and medications prescribed.

9.d.1. Reinforce the importance of keeping follow-up appointments with health care provider.
2. Explain the rationale for, side effects of, and importance of taking medications prescribed (e.g., vitamins, antimicrobials, pancreatic enzymes). Inform client of pertinent food and drug interactions.
3. Implement measures to improve client compliance:
   a. include significant others in teaching sessions if possible
   b. encourage questions and allow time for reinforcement and clarification of information provided
   c. provide written instructions on scheduled appointments with health care provider, medications prescribed, and signs and symptoms to report.

ADDITIONAL NURSING DIAGNOSES:

IMPAIRED ORAL MUCOUS MEMBRANE: DRYNESS*

related to:

a. deficient fluid volume associated with restricted oral intake and fluid loss resulting from vomiting and nasogastric tube drainage;
b. decreased salivation associated with deficient fluid volume, restricted oral intake, and the side effect of some medications (e.g., narcotic [opioid] analgesics, some antiemetics);
c. mouth breathing if nasogastric tube is in place.

*FEAR/ANXIETY**

related to severe pain; unfamiliar environment; and lack of understanding of diagnostic tests, treatment plan, and prognosis.

---

*See Unit II for outcomes, actions, and rationales.

Bibliography

See pages 879 and 884.

UNIT XVI

Nursing Care of the Client with Disturbances of Metabolic Function

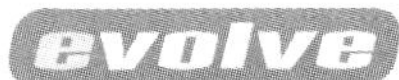

Diabetes Mellitus

Diabetes mellitus is a chronic multisystem disease characterized by alterations in carbohydrate, fat, and protein metabolism resulting from abnormal insulin production, impaired insulin utilization, or both. The hallmark of this metabolic disorder is hyperglycemia.

Diabetes* is often complicated by structural and functional abnormalities in the blood vessels and nerves. The atherosclerotic changes that frequently occur in the large vessels (macroangiopathy) affect the cardiac, cerebral, and peripheral circulation. Thickening of the basement membrane of the capillaries (microangiopathy) can also occur and is especially significant when it involves the vessels in the eyes and kidneys. The neurological involvement can be manifested in a wide variety of ways and is referred to as diabetic neuropathy. There are several different mechanisms that are thought to contribute to the development of diabetic neuropathy. These include reduced blood flow to the nerves as a result of angiopathies and a metabolic defect in the polyol pathway resulting in accumulation of sorbitol in the nerves, which subsequently alters nerve function. The most common neuropathy is peripheral sensorimotor polyneuropathy, which has a gradual onset of sensory manifestations such as numbness and tingling, burning or shooting pain sensations, and/or hyperesthesia. Neuropathy of the autonomic nervous system is also common. Parasympathetic involvement often occurs earlier and is more profound than sympathetic nervous system involvement and manifestations vary depending on the system involved.

The two major types of diabetes are type 1 and type 2. Type 1 diabetics have an absolute insulin deficiency and are dependent on insulin replacement. The insulin deficiency is usually due to an immune-mediated destruction of the pancreatic B-cells in a person with a genetic predisposition and a triggering environmental insult (e.g., viral infection). Type 2 diabetics have a relative deficiency of insulin caused by decreased tissue responsiveness to insulin (insulin resistance), a defect in insulin secretion, and inappropriate hepatic glucose production. Heredity plays a role in development of type 2 diabetes. Additional risk factors for type 2 diabetes include a history of gestational diabetes mellitus or impaired glucose tolerance, increasing age, obesity, and a sedentary lifestyle.

A sequence of pathophysiological events occurs in diabetes. When an insulin deficiency exists, glucose cannot be transported into the cells for energy metabolism. As a result, glucose accumulates in the blood and starts to spill into the urine once the level exceeds the renal threshold (180 mg/dl or greater). The high blood glucose acts as an osmotic diuretic, which leads to excessive diuresis and subsequent deficient fluid volume. Because the glucose cannot be utilized as an energy source by many cells, fat and protein are broken down to provide a source of energy for the starving cells. The free fatty acids that are mobilized from adipose tissue are converted by the liver to ketones to be used as an energy source. The ketones are strong acids and eventually deplete the body's buffer system and respiratory compensatory ability, leading to a state of metabolic acidosis. The simultaneous increase in glucagon and epinephrine release that occurs with an insulin deficiency exacerbates the hyperglycemia and ketogenesis. Continuation of these metabolic derangements leads to life-threatening imbalances.

This care plan focuses on the adult client who has had diabetes for many years and is being hospitalized because of difficulty stabilizing blood glucose levels. Many of the long-term vascular and neurological complications have been included in this care plan and should be individualized based on the client's current status. Much of the information in this care plan is applicable to clients receiving follow-up care in an extended care facility or home setting. This care plan should be used in conjunction with the care plans on Heart Failure, Myocardial Infarction, Cerebrovascular Accident, Hypertension, and/or Chronic Renal Failure if the client is also being treated for one of these vascular complications of diabetes.

*Diabetes mellitus will be referred to as diabetes throughout this care plan.

OUTCOME/DISCHARGE CRITERIA

THE CLIENT WILL:

- have blood glucose stabilized within a desired range
- have signs and symptoms of vascular and neurological complications at a manageable level
- verbalize a basic understanding of diabetes mellitus
- verbalize an understanding of medications ordered and demonstrate the ability to correctly draw up and administer insulin if prescribed
- verbalize an understanding of the principles of dietary management and be able to calculate and plan meals within the prescribed caloric distribution
- demonstrate the ability to perform blood glucose and urine tests correctly and interpret results accurately

- verbalize an understanding of the role of exercise in the management of diabetes
- identify health care and hygiene practices that should be integrated into lifestyle
- identify appropriate safety measures to follow because of the diagnosis of diabetes
- state signs and symptoms of hypoglycemia and ketoacidosis and appropriate actions for prevention and treatment
- state signs and symptoms to report to the health care provider
- share feelings and concerns about diabetes and its effect on lifestyle
- identify resources that can assist in the adjustment to and management of diabetes
- verbalize an understanding of and a plan for adhering to recommended follow-up care including future appointments with health care provider and for laboratory studies.

NURSING/COLLABORATIVE DIAGNOSES

DISCHARGE TEACHING

See pp. 749–750 for additional diagnoses.

1. Nursing Diagnosis: *INEFFECTIVE TISSUE PERFUSION*

related to:

a. vascular abnormalities (atherosclerosis, microangiopathies) that commonly develop with diabetes;
b. postural hypotension if autonomic neuropathy involving the cardiovascular system has developed.

Suggested NOC Outcomes: Circulation status; Tissue perfusion: peripheral

Suggested NIC Interventions: Circulatory care: arterial insufficiency; Circulatory care: venous insufficiency; Lower extremity monitoring

Desired Outcome	**Nursing Actions** *and Selected Purposes/Rationales* (see pp. 57–59 for additional rationales)
1. The client will maintain adequate tissue perfusion as evidenced by: a. B/P within normal range for client b. usual mental status c. extremities warm with absence of pallor and cyanosis	1.a. Assess for and report signs and symptoms of: 1. autonomic neuropathy involving the cardiovascular system: a. lightheadedness, dizziness, or syncope upon standing b. decline in systolic B/P of 30 mm Hg or more when client changes from a lying to a sitting or standing position 2. diminished tissue perfusion (e.g., significant decrease in B/P, restlessness, confusion, cool extremities, pallor or cyanosis of extremities, diminished or absent peripheral pulses, slow capillary refill, edema, claudication, angina, oliguria).

d. palpable peripheral pulses
e. capillary refill time less than 2–3 seconds
f. absence of edema
g. absence of exercise-induced pain
h. urine output at least 30 ml/hour.

b. Implement measures *to maintain adequate tissue perfusion:*
   1. perform actions *to promote adequate circulation in lower extremities:*
      a. increase activity as allowed; instruct client with intermittent claudication to walk slowly and alternate activity with periods of rest
      b. discourage positions that compromise blood flow in lower extremities (e.g., crossing legs, pillows under knees, use of knee gatch, prolonged sitting or standing)
      c. instruct client in and assist with active foot and leg exercises every 1–2 hours
   2. perform actions *to reduce postural hypotension:*
      a. instruct client to change from a supine to an upright position slowly *in order to allow time for autoregulatory mechanisms to adjust to the change in the distribution of blood associated with an upright position*
      b. keep head of bed elevated at least 30°
      c. administer fludrocortisone acetate (Florinef) if ordered *to increase intravascular volume*
      d. consult physician about an order for antiembolism stockings or an intermittent pneumatic compression device
   3. instruct client to avoid foods high in saturated fat and cholesterol (e.g., butter, cheese, ice cream, eggs, red meat) and *trans* fats (e.g., stick margarine and shortening and foods such as commercial baked goods that are prepared with these products) *in order to reduce progression of atherogenesis*
   4. perform actions to maintain blood glucose at a near-normal level (see Diagnosis 3, action d); *maintaining blood glucose at a near-normal level may prevent or delay development of some of the vascular complications*
   5. perform actions to prevent deficient fluid volume (see Diagnosis 2, action b) *in order to maintain adequate intravascular volume*
   6. perform actions *to prevent vasoconstriction:*
      a. implement measures *to reduce stress* (e.g., explain procedures, maintain a calm environment, reduce discomfort)
      b. discourage smoking
      c. implement measures *to keep client from getting cold* (e.g., maintain a comfortable room temperature, provide adequate clothing and blankets)
   7. administer the following medications if ordered:
      a. lipid-lowering agents (e.g., HMG-CoA reductase inhibitors ["statins"], ezetimibe, gemfibrozil) *to prevent further atherogenesis*
      b. hemorrheologic agents (e.g., pentoxifylline) *to increase erythrocyte flexibility and reduce blood viscosity, which improves peripheral blood flow*
      c. antihypertensives (e.g., ACE inhibitors, angiotensin II receptor antagonists) *to control hypertension if present and subsequently reduce atherogenesis (hypertension accelerates atherosclerosis);* ACE inhibitors and angiotensin II receptor antagonists are also being used *to reduce the incidence of or slow progression of nephropathy and cardiovascular disease*
      d. thiazolidinediones *(have been found to have an antiatherogenic effect).*

c. Consult physician if signs and symptoms of diminished tissue perfusion persist or worsen.

2. Nursing Diagnosis: ***RISK FOR DEFICIENT FLUID VOLUME***

related to excessive loss of fluid associated with the osmotic diuresis that can result from hyperglycemia.

Suggested NOC Outcomes: Fluid balance; Hydration

Suggested NIC Interventions: Fluid monitoring; Fluid management; Intravenous (IV) therapy; Hyperglycemia management

Desired Outcome	Nursing Actions *and Selected Purposes/Rationales*
2. The client will not experience a deficient fluid volume as evidenced by: a. normal skin temperature and turgor b. moist mucous membranes c. stable weight d. B/P within normal range for client and stable with position change e. capillary refill time less than 2–3 seconds f. usual mental status g. balanced intake and output h. urine specific gravity within normal range i. Hct within normal range.	2.a. Assess for and report signs and symptoms of deficient fluid volume: 1. warm, flushed skin 2. decreased skin turgor 3. dry mucous membranes, thirst 4. weight loss of 2% or greater in a short period (many clients with diabetes are on weight reduction diets, so some weight loss is expected) 5. postural hypotension and/or low B/P 6. capillary refill time greater than 2–3 seconds 7. flat neck veins when supine 8. change in mental status 9. decreased urine output with increased specific gravity (reflects an actual rather than potential fluid deficit; if client has diabetic nephropathy, specific gravity may not be a useful indicator of hydration status) 10. elevated Hct. b. Implement measures *to prevent deficient fluid volume:* 1. perform actions to prevent or treat hyperglycemia (see Diagnosis 10, action a.2) *in order to prevent osmotic diuresis* 2. maintain a fluid intake of at least 2500 ml/day unless contraindicated; if oral intake is inadequate or contraindicated, maintain intravenous therapy as ordered.

3. Nursing Diagnosis: ***IMBALANCED NUTRITION: LESS THAN BODY REQUIREMENTS***

related to:

a. decreased cellular uptake and utilization of glucose and a compensatory increase in metabolism of fat and protein stores associated with insulin deficiency;

b. decreased oral intake associated with nausea and feeling of fullness resulting from delayed gastric emptying if diabetic gastroparesis is present.

Suggested NOC Outcomes: Nutritional status; Blood glucose control

Suggested NIC Interventions: Nutritional monitoring; Nutrition management; Nutritional counseling; Hyperglycemia management; Weight management

Desired Outcome	Nursing Actions *and Selected Purposes/Rationales*
3. The client will maintain an adequate nutritional status as evidenced by: a. maintenance of or return toward normal weight b. serum albumin, prealbumin, Hct, Hgb, and lymphocyte levels within normal range c. usual strength and activity tolerance.	3.a. Assess for signs and symptoms of an altered nutritional status: 1. abnormal weight for client's age, height, and body frame (many clients with type 2 diabetes are overweight) 2. low serum albumin, prealbumin, Hct, Hgb, and lymphocyte levels 3. weakness and fatigue. b. Monitor blood glucose levels regularly. Report values below 60 mg/dl, above 200 mg/dl, or outside of the parameters specified by physician. c. Monitor percentage of meals and snacks client consumes. Report a pattern of inadequate or excessive intake. d. Implement measures *to maintain blood glucose at a near-normal level, achieve ideal weight, and provide necessary nutrients in order to maintain an adequate nutritional status:* 1. obtain a dietary consult to reinforce teaching about the diet prescribed and ways to adapt it to personal and cultural preferences and specific needs (dietary restrictions will vary but are most often prescribed as specific percentages of carbohydrate, fat, and protein within an optimal calorie level; it is recommended that 45–60% of calories be derived from carbohydrate [the majority of which should be complex carbohydrates], 20–30% from fat [saturated fats should be restricted to 10% and cholesterol intake should be less than 300 mg], and 12–20% from protein; increasing soluble fiber intake [e.g., fruits, legumes, whole-grain cereals, green leafy vegetables] is also often recommended *because of its lipid-lowering effect*)

2. encourage client to adhere to the diabetic diet prescribed and assist him/her with the selection of appropriate foods
3. provide meals and snacks on time and at evenly spaced intervals *to maintain desired balance between insulin and glucose*
4. administer the following glucose-lowering agents if ordered *to enhance the cellular utilization of glucose and prevent abnormal metabolism of fats and proteins:*
   a. insulin
   b. oral agents
      1. sulfonylureas (e.g., glipizide, glyburide, glimepiride)
      2. meglitinides (e.g., repaglinide [Prandin], nateglinide [Starlix])
      3. biguanides (e.g., metformin [Glucophage]); be aware that practitioners may withhold metformin in hospitalized persons since many acute illnesses compromise cardiorenal function *(metformin is excreted by the kidneys and increased levels of metformin increase the risk of lactic acidosis)*
      4. thiazolidinediones or "glitazones" (e.g., rosiglitazone [Avandia], pioglitazone [Actos])
      5. alpha-glucosidase inhibitors (e.g., acarbose [Precose], miglitol [Glyset])
      6. combination agents (e.g., metformin and glyburide [Glucovance], metformin and glipizide [Metaglip], metformin and rosiglitazone [Avandamet])
5. perform actions to treat gastroparesis and the resultant gastric discomfort if present (see Diagnosis 4.B, action 2) *in order to promote even absorption of nutrients and an adequate oral intake*
6. reinforce importance of weight loss if client is obese *(studies have shown that obesity is a cause of insulin resistance).*

e. Perform a calorie count if ordered. Report information to dietitian and physician.

4.A. NURSING DIAGNOSIS:

ALTERED COMFORT: BURNING, ACHING, CRAMPING, HYPERESTHESIA, NUMBNESS, AND/OR TINGLING (PARTICULARLY IN LOWER EXTREMITIES)

related to peripheral polyneuropathy and/or peripheral vascular insufficiency.

Suggested NOC Outcomes: Comfort level; Pain control

Suggested NIC Interventions: Pain management; Environmental management: comfort; Analgesic administration; Hyperglycemia management

Desired Outcome	**Nursing Actions** *and Selected Purposes/Rationales*
4.A. The client will experience diminished discomfort in extremities as evidenced by: 1. verbalization of same 2. relaxed facial expression and body positioning 3. increased participation in activities 4. stable vital signs.	4.A.1. Assess for: a. signs and symptoms of peripheral neuropathy (e.g., reports of persistent burning; sharp, shooting pain; numbness; tingling; or increased sensitivity to sensory stimuli [hyperesthesia]) b. signs and symptoms of peripheral vascular insufficiency (e.g., reports of cramping in calves precipitated by ambulation [intermittent claudication], delayed capillary refill, cold feet, dependent rubor, diminished or absent pulses) c. nonverbal signs of discomfort (e.g., grimacing, guarding of affected area, reluctance to move, restlessness, diaphoresis, increased B/P, tachycardia). 2. Assess client's perception of the severity of the discomfort using an intensity rating scale. 3. Assess the client's pattern of discomfort (e.g., location, quality, onset, duration, precipitating factors, aggravating factors, alleviating factors). 4. Ask the client to describe methods he/she has used to manage the discomfort effectively.

Desired Outcome	Nursing Actions *and Selected Purposes/Rationales*

5. Implement measures *to reduce discomfort:*
   a. perform actions *to reduce fear and anxiety about discomfort* (e.g., assure client that his/her need for relief of discomfort is understood; plan methods for control of discomfort with client)
   b. perform actions to reduce stress (e.g., explain procedures, maintain a calm environment) *in order to promote relaxation and subsequently increase the client's threshold and tolerance for discomfort*
   c. administer analgesics before pain becomes severe and before bedtime if discomfort is typically worse at night
   d. if client has hyperesthesia, provide a bed cradle *to keep bedding off affected extremities*
   e. assist client with ambulation if walking relieves discomfort (walking often relieves lower extremity discomfort associated with neuropathies of the lower extremities); if client is experiencing intermittent claudication, encourage short, more frequent walks *since longer walks exacerbate pain associated with vascular insufficiency*
   f. provide or assist with additional nonpharmacologic measures for relief of discomfort (e.g., position change, relaxation exercises, guided imagery, quiet conversation, restful environment)
   g. perform actions to maintain blood glucose at a near-normal level (see Diagnosis 3, action d); *maintaining optimal glycemic control can actually alleviate or reduce neuropathic discomfort and the progression of neuropathy*
   h. administer the following medications if ordered *to control discomfort:*
      1. analgesics (narcotic [opioid] analgesics are avoided as long as possible *because the pain may be chronic*)
      2. tricyclic antidepressants (e.g., amitriptyline, imipramine, desipramine, nortriptyline)
      3. anticonvulsants such as gabapentin or carbamazepine (have been useful in treatment of some sharp or stabbing neuralgia pain)
      4. capsaicin cream (useful in treatment of superficial burning pain)
      5. hemorrheologic agents (e.g., pentoxifylline) *to improve peripheral blood flow and reduce discomfort associated with intermittent claudication*
      6. skeletal muscle relaxants or quinine sulfate (sometimes useful for treating painful leg cramps).
6. Consult appropriate health care provider (e.g., pharmacist, pain management specialist, physician) if above measures fail to provide adequate relief of discomfort.

4.B. Nursing Diagnosis: ***ALTERED COMFORT: GASTRIC DISCOMFORT***

related to delayed emptying of the stomach associated with autonomic neuropathy involving the gastrointestinal tract.

Suggested NOC Outcomes: Comfort level; Symptom control

Suggested NIC Interventions: Environmental management: comfort; Nausea management; Hyperglycemia management

Desired Outcome	Nursing Actions *and Selected Purposes/Rationales*
4.B. The client will experience a reduction in gastric discomfort as evidenced by: 1. verbalization of same 2. relaxed facial expression and body positioning.	4.B.1. Assess client for: a. verbal reports of gastric discomfort (e.g., gastric fullness, postprandial bloating, nausea) b. nonverbal signs of discomfort (e.g., grimacing, rubbing upper abdomen, restlessness, reluctance to move). 2. Implement measures *to reduce gastric discomfort:* a. perform actions *to reduce the accumulation of gas and fluid in the stomach:* 1. encourage and assist client with frequent position changes and ambulation as tolerated *(activity stimulates gastrointestinal motility)*

2. have client sit up during meals and for 1–2 hours after meals *(gravity promotes passage of food and fluid through the gastrointestinal tract)*
3. provide small, frequent meals rather than 3 large ones; instruct client to ingest foods and fluids slowly
4. instruct client to avoid foods high in fat *(fat further delays gastric emptying)*
5. instruct client to avoid activities such as chewing gum, drinking through a straw, and smoking *in order to reduce air swallowing*
6. instruct client to avoid intake of carbonated beverages and gas-producing foods (e.g., cabbage, onions, beans)
7. encourage client to eructate whenever the urge is felt
8. administer medications that enhance gastric motility (e.g., metoclopramide) if ordered

b. perform actions *to reduce nausea if present:*
1. encourage client to take deep, slow breaths when nauseated
2. instruct client to avoid foods/fluids that irritate the gastric mucosa (e.g., spicy foods; caffeine-containing beverages such as coffee, tea, and colas)
3. eliminate noxious sights and odors from the environment *(noxious stimuli can cause stimulation of the vomiting center)*
4. instruct client to change positions slowly *(rapid movement can result in stimulation of the chemoreceptor trigger zone and subsequent excitation of the vomiting center)*
5. avoid serving foods with an overpowering aroma; remove lids from hot foods before entering room
6. instruct client to eat dry foods (e.g., toast, crackers) and avoid drinking liquids with meals when feeling nauseated
7. administer antiemetics if ordered

c. perform actions to maintain blood glucose at a near-normal level (see Diagnosis 3, action d); *maintaining optimal glycemic control seems to improve gastric emptying and reduce the progression of neuropathy.*

3. Consult physician if gastric discomfort persists or worsens.

5. NURSING DIAGNOSIS: DISTURBED SENSORY PERCEPTION: VISUAL

related to:
a. osmotic swelling of the lens associated with hyperglycemia;
b. changes in the retinal vessels (retinopathy);
c. presence of cataracts (there is an increased incidence of cataract formation in persons with diabetes).

Suggested NOC Outcomes: Vision compensation behavior; Risk control: visual impairment

Suggested NIC Interventions: Communication enhancement: visual deficit; Environmental management

Desired Outcome	**Nursing Actions** *and Selected Purposes/Rationales*
5. The client will not experience further progression of visual disturbances and will demonstrate adaptation to existing ones.	5.a. Assess for visual disturbances (e.g., reports of blurred vision; partial or total loss of vision; the presence of "floaters," spots, or flashing lights). b. Implement measures identified in Diagnosis 3, action d, to maintain blood glucose at a near-normal level *in order to reduce further progression of visual disturbances (studies show that the incidence and progression of changes in the eye can be reduced by optimal glycemic control).* c. If vision is impaired: 1. implement measures *to reduce the risk for injury* (e.g., orient client to surroundings and identify obstacles during ambulation, instruct client to ambulate in well-lit areas and use handrails if available) 2. avoid startling client (e.g., speak client's name and identify yourself when entering room and before any physical contact, describe activities and reasons for various noises in the room)

Desired Outcome	Nursing Actions *and Selected Purposes/Rationales*
	3. assist client with personal hygiene he/she is unable to perform independently 4. if client has glasses, make sure they are clean and within reach 5. identify where items are placed on plate and tray, cut food, open packages, and feed client if necessary 6. assist with activities such as filling out menus and reading mail and legal documents as needed 7. instruct client in use of appropriate self-help devices (e.g., magnifier for insulin syringe, syringe with a plunger lock, insulin pen that delivers fixed amount of insulin, needle guide for insulin vial, glucometer that displays blood glucose values in bold numbers); monitor client's accuracy in testing blood glucose and administering insulin 8. provide auditory rather than visual diversionary activities 9. inform client of resources available if he/she desires additional information about visual aids (e.g., American Federation for the Blind) 10. encourage client to discuss options available for treatment of retinopathy (e.g., laser photocoagulation) and cataracts with physician. d. Reassess visual status regularly and consult physician if visual status worsens.

6. Nursing Diagnosis: *RISK FOR IMPAIRED TISSUE INTEGRITY*

related to:

a. increased fragility of the skin associated with inadequate tissue perfusion (a result of the vascular changes that frequently develop in persons with diabetes);
b. damage to the skin and/or subcutaneous tissue associated with prolonged pressure on the tissues, friction, or shearing if mobility is decreased;
c. abnormal pressure distribution on plantar aspect of feet associated with muscle weakness and the subsequent joint deformity in the feet that may occur as a result of peripheral neuropathy;
d. undetected foot injuries associated with the diminished sensation that may be present with peripheral polyneuropathy.

Suggested NOC Outcomes: Tissue integrity: skin and mucous membranes; Wound healing: secondary intention

Suggested NIC Interventions: Skin surveillance; Skin care: topical treatments; Pressure management; Pressure ulcer prevention; Wound care

Desired Outcome	Nursing Actions *and Selected Purposes/Rationales* (see pp. 49–52 for additional rationales)
6. The client will maintain tissue integrity as evidenced by: a. absence of redness and irritation b. no skin breakdown.	6.a. Determine client's risk for skin breakdown using a risk assessment tool (e.g., Norton Scale, Braden Scale, Gosnell Scale). b. Inspect skin for areas of pallor, redness, and breakdown with particular attention to: 1. spaces between toes 2. feet and lower legs 3. dependent areas 4. bony prominences 5. areas where sensation is diminished *(client may be unaware of development of blisters and ulcerations).* c. Implement measures *to prevent tissue breakdown:* 1. assist client to turn every 2 hours if activity is limited 2. gently massage around reddened areas at least every 2 hours 3. apply a thin layer of a dry lubricant such as powder or cornstarch to bottom sheet or skin and to opposing skin surfaces (e.g., axillae, beneath breasts) if indicated *to reduce friction*

4. perform actions to keep client from sliding down in bed (e.g., gatch knees slightly when head of bed is elevated 30° or higher, limit length of time client is in semi-Fowler's position to 30 minute intervals) *in order to reduce the risk of skin surface abrasion and shearing*
5. instruct or assist client to shift weight at least every 30 minutes
6. position client properly; use pressure-reducing or pressure-relieving devices (e.g., pillows, gel or foam cushions, alternating pressure mattress) if indicated
7. keep client's skin clean
8. keep bed linens dry and wrinkle-free
9. increase activity as allowed and tolerated
10. perform actions to maintain adequate tissue perfusion (see Diagnosis 1, action b)
11. perform meticulous foot care:
    a. wash feet daily with warm water and a mild soap
    b. dry feet thoroughly using a soft towel or cloth, paying particular attention to interdigital spaces
    c. apply lanolin or other lubricating lotion to feet (except between toes) daily
12. perform actions *to prevent injury to feet:*
    a. caution client to always wear socks and shoes or sturdy slippers when ambulating
    b. do not place heating pad on feet
    c. check the temperature of bath water before client immerses feet.

d. If tissue breakdown is present:
1. notify appropriate health care provider (e.g., wound care specialist, physician)
2. perform care of involved area(s) as ordered or per hospital procedure
3. implement measures *to promote wound healing:*
    a. perform actions *to maintain adequate circulation to the wound area:*
        1. implement measures to maintain adequate tissue perfusion (see Diagnosis 1, action b)
        2. do not apply dressings tightly *(excessive pressure impairs circulation to the area)*
    b. perform actions to prevent infection in wound (see Diagnosis 9, action b.12)
    c. perform actions to maintain an adequate nutritional status (see Diagnosis 3, action d)
    d. assist with tissue debridement if performed
    e. encourage client to wear immobilization device (e.g., cast, boot) if ordered.

7. NURSING DIAGNOSIS: URINARY RETENTION

related to loss of bladder sensation and diminished contractility of the detrusor muscle associated with autonomic neuropathy involving the genitourinary system.

Suggested NOC Outcome: Urinary elimination

Suggested NIC Interventions: Urinary elimination management; Urinary retention care

Desired Outcome	**Nursing Actions** *and Selected Purposes/Rationales* (see pp. 61–62 for additional rationales)
7. The client will not experience urinary retention as evidenced by: a. voiding at normal intervals b. no reports of bladder fullness and suprapubic discomfort	7.a. Assess for signs and symptoms of urinary retention: 1. frequent voiding of small amounts (25–60 ml) of urine 2. reports of bladder fullness or suprapubic discomfort 3. bladder distention 4. dribbling of urine 5. output less than intake. b. Assist with urodynamic studies (e.g., urethral pressure profile, uroflowmetry, cystometrogram) if ordered.

Desired Outcome	**Nursing Actions** *and Selected Purposes/Rationales*
c. absence of bladder distention and dribbling of urine d. balanced intake and output.	c. Implement measures *to prevent urinary retention:* 1. offer bedpan or urinal or assist client to bedside commode or bathroom every 2–4 hours if indicated 2. instruct client to urinate when the urge is first felt 3. perform actions *that may help trigger the micturition reflex* (e.g., run water, place client's hands in warm water, pour warm water over perineum) 4. allow client to assume a normal position for voiding unless contraindicated 5. instruct client to lean upper body forward and/or gently press downward on lower abdomen during voiding attempts unless contraindicated *in order to put pressure on the bladder area (pressure helps create a sensation of bladder fullness, which stimulates the micturition reflex)* 6. administer cholinergic (parasympathomimetic) drugs (e.g., bethanechol) if ordered *to stimulate bladder contraction.* d. Consult physician about intermittent catheterization or insertion of an indwelling catheter if above actions fail to alleviate urinary retention.

8. Nursing Diagnosis: *CONSTIPATION*

related to colonic atony or dilatation associated with autonomic neuropathy involving the large bowel.

Suggested NOC Outcome: Bowel elimination

Suggested NIC Interventions: Constipation/Impaction management; Bowel management

Desired Outcome	**Nursing Actions** *and Selected Purposes/Rationales* (see pp. 24–26 for additional rationales)
8. The client will not experience or will have resolution of constipation as evidenced by: a. passage of soft, formed stool every 1–3 days b. absence of abdominal distention and pain, rectal fullness or pressure, and straining during defecation.	8.a. Assess for signs and symptoms of constipation (e.g., decrease in frequency of bowel movements; passage of hard, formed stools; anorexia; abdominal distention and pain; feeling of fullness or pressure in rectum; straining during defecation). b. Assess bowel sounds. Report a pattern of decreasing bowel sounds. c. Implement measures *to prevent or treat constipation:* 1. encourage client to defecate whenever the urge is felt 2. assist client to toilet or bedside commode or place in a high Fowler's position on bedpan for bowel movements unless contraindicated 3. encourage client to relax, provide privacy, and have call signal within reach during attempts to defecate *(measures to promote relaxation enable client to relax the levator ani muscle and external anal sphincter, which facilitates evacuation of stool)* 4. encourage client to establish a regular time for defecation, preferably within an hour after a meal 5. instruct client to increase intake of foods high in fiber (e.g., bran, whole-grain breads and cereals, fresh fruits and vegetables) unless contraindicated; obtain a dietary consult if indicated to assist client with ways to incorporate high-fiber foods into prescribed diabetic diet 6. instruct client to maintain a minimum fluid intake of 2500 ml/day unless contraindicated 7. increase activity as allowed and tolerated 8. administer laxatives and/or enemas if ordered. d. Consult appropriate health care provider if signs and symptoms of constipation persist.

9. Nursing Diagnosis: *RISK FOR INFECTION*

related to:

a. decreased efficiency of leukocyte function in a hyperglycemic environment;

b. delayed healing of any break in skin integrity associated with decreased tissue perfusion and altered nutritional status (there is diminished protein synthesis and tissue repair when insulin is deficient);
c. increased growth and colonization of microorganisms in the urinary tract associated with glycosuria (creates a good medium for growth of pathogens) and urinary stasis (can result from retention and decreased mobility if present).

Suggested NOC Outcomes: Immune status; Infection severity

Suggested NIC Interventions: Infection control; Infection protection; Wound care

Desired Outcome	**Nursing Actions** *and Selected Purposes/Rationales* (see pp. 37–40 for additional rationales)

9. The client will remain free of infection as evidenced by:
   a. absence of fever and chills
   b. pulse within normal limits
   c. normal breath sounds
   d. usual mental status
   e. cough productive of clear mucus only
   f. absence of any unusual vaginal discharge
   g. voiding clear urine without reports of frequency, urgency, and burning
   h. absence of heat, pain, redness, swelling, and unusual drainage in any area
   i. WBC and differential counts within normal range
   j. negative results of cultured specimens.

9.a. Assess for and report signs and symptoms of infection (be aware that some signs and symptoms vary depending on the site of infection, the causative organism, and the age and immune status of the client):
   1. elevated temperature
   2. chills
   3. increased pulse
   4. abnormal breath sounds
   5. malaise, lethargy, acute confusion
   6. loss of appetite
   7. cough productive of purulent, green, or rust-colored sputum
   8. unusual vaginal discharge and pruritus in vulvovaginal area
   9. cloudy urine
   10. reports of frequency, urgency, or burning when urinating
   11. urinalysis showing a WBC count greater than 5, positive leukocyte esterase or nitrites, or presence of bacteria
   12. heat, pain, redness, swelling, or unusual drainage in any area
   13. elevated WBC count and/or significant change in differential
   14. positive results of cultured specimens (e.g., urine, vaginal drainage, sputum, blood).

b. Implement measures *to prevent infection:*
   1. maintain a fluid intake of at least 2500 ml/day unless contraindicated
   2. perform actions to maintain an adequate nutritional status and a near-normal blood glucose level (see Diagnosis 3, action d)
   3. instruct and assist client with good oral hygiene
   4. use good hand hygiene and encourage client to do the same
   5. use sterile technique during all invasive procedures (e.g., urinary catheterizations, venous and arterial punctures, injections)
   6. change equipment, tubings, and solutions used for treatments such as intravenous infusions, irrigations, and wound care according to hospital policy
   7. change peripheral intravenous line sites according to hospital policy
   8. anchor catheters/tubings (e.g., urinary, intravenous) securely *in order to reduce trauma to the tissues and the risk for introduction of pathogens associated with the in-and-out movement of the tubing*
   9. maintain a closed system for drains (e.g., urinary catheter) and intravenous infusions whenever possible
   10. protect client from others with infection
   11. perform actions to prevent and treat tissue breakdown (see Diagnosis 6, actions c and d)
   12. perform actions *to prevent infection in any existing wound:*
       a. instruct client to avoid touching dressings or open wounds
       b. maintain sterile technique during all dressing changes and wound care
       c. administer antimicrobials if ordered
   13. perform actions *to prevent stasis of respiratory secretions* (e.g., assist client to turn, cough, and deep breathe; increase activity as allowed and tolerated)

Desired Outcome	Nursing Actions *and Selected Purposes/Rationales*
	14. perform actions to prevent urinary retention (see Diagnosis 7, action c) *in order to prevent urinary stasis* 15. instruct and assist client to perform good perineal care routinely and after each bowel movement.

10. Collaborative Diagnoses: ***POTENTIAL ACUTE METABOLIC COMPLICATIONS OF DIABETES MELLITUS***

a. diabetic ketoacidosis (DKA) related to hyperglycemia and accelerated ketogenesis associated with the combined effect of severe insulin deficiency and excess secretion of counterregulatory hormones such as glucagon and epinephrine (DKA may be precipitated by administration of inadequate amounts of insulin and/or the presence of stressors such as illness, trauma, or infection);
b. hypoglycemia related to administration of too much insulin or oral hypoglycemic agent, inadequate food intake, and/or decreased excretion of insulin and some oral hypoglycemic agents if renal function is impaired;
c. hyperglycemic hyperosmolar nonketotic coma related to severe dehydration associated with sustained osmotic diuresis resulting from uncontrolled hyperglycemia.

Desired Outcomes	Nursing Actions *and Selected Purposes/Rationales*
10.a. The client will not experience ketoacidosis as evidenced by: 1. stable vital signs 2. usual skin temperature and color 3. absence of unusual weakness, lethargy, nausea, vomiting, abdominal pain, and fruity odor on breath 4. unlabored respirations at 12–20/minute 5. blood glucose less than 250 mg/dl 6. absence of ketones in blood and urine 7. blood pH and bicarbonate level within normal range.	10.a.1. Assess for and report signs and symptoms of ketoacidosis (clients at greatest risk are type 1 [insulin-dependent] diabetics): a. evidence of deficient fluid volume (e.g., hypotension; weak, rapid pulse; warm, flushed skin; thirst) b. weakness, lethargy c. nausea, vomiting, abdominal pain d. acetone (fruity) odor on breath e. Kussmaul respirations f. blood glucose above 250 mg/dl g. ketones in blood and urine h. low blood pH and bicarbonate (CO_2 content) level. 2. Implement measures to prevent or treat hyperglycemia *in order to prevent ketoacidosis:* a. encourage client to adhere to the diabetic diet prescribed (e.g., consistent carbohydrate diet, exchange list, Food Guide Pyramid) b. administer insulin as ordered and in an area where maximum absorption will occur *(the absorption of insulin can be erratic if it is administered in an area where tissue is hypertrophied)*; if client has an insulin pump, maintain prescribed infusion rate and ensure that client receives preprandial boluses as ordered c. if client is hypotensive, consult health care provider about administering insulin intravenously rather than subcutaneously *(subcutaneous insulin absorption will be delayed if client's B/P is low enough to cause inadequate tissue perfusion)* d. if client is receiving continuous intravenous insulin, do not discontinue the infusion until subcutaneous insulin has been administered and had time to reach its onset of action e. administer oral glucose-lowering agent(s) as ordered f. minimize client's exposure to emotional and physiological stress *(stress causes an increased output of epinephrine, glucagon, and cortisol, all of which increase blood sugar).* 3. If signs and symptoms of ketoacidosis occur: a. maintain client on bed rest b. administer the following if ordered: 1. insulin (regular insulin is administered intravenously in the initial phase of treatment)

2. intravenous fluid and electrolyte replacements:
   a. isotonic or half-strength normal saline (usually rapidly infused until B/P is stabilized and urine output is adequate)
   b. combination saline and glucose solutions once blood sugar falls to 250–300 mg/dl *(prevents hypoglycemia that can result with a rapid drop in blood sugar)*
   c. potassium chloride or potassium phosphate *(hypokalemia and hypophosphatemia result from osmotic diuresis and a shift of potassium and phosphorus into the cells during insulin therapy)*
   d. sodium bicarbonate if the serum pH drops to 7.0 or below; if bicarbonate is administered, it should be discontinued when the pH reaches 7.1–7.2 *because reversing acidosis too quickly has harmful physiological effects.*

10.b. The client will not experience hypoglycemia as evidenced by:
1. pulse rate between 60–100 beats/minute
2. absence of palpitations
3. warm, dry skin
4. usual mental status
5. absence of slurred speech, gait abnormalities, mood swings, and seizures
6. blood glucose above 60 mg/dl.

10.b.1. Assess for and report signs and symptoms of hypoglycemia (at greatest risk are clients taking insulin or long-acting sulfonylureas, those having adjustments in insulin dosages or having difficulty maintaining an adequate oral intake, and clients with liver disease or end-stage renal failure):
   a. adrenergic-mediated signs and symptoms: tachycardia; palpitations; cool, pale skin; diaphoresis; weakness; nervousness; shakiness *(these signs and symptoms reflect the sympathetic nervous system response to hypoglycemia)*; be aware that early sympathetic warning symptoms may not be present in some type 1 diabetics *because of a decrease in epinephrine output* and that early warning symptoms may also be diminished if client is taking a beta-adrenergic blocking agent
   b. neuroglycopenic symptoms (signs and symptoms reflecting central nervous system fuel deprivation): headache, inability to concentrate, somnolence, slurred speech, staggering gait, mood swings, irrational behavior, double or blurred vision, confusion, seizures, coma
   c. blood glucose below 60 mg/dl.

2. Determine from client whether he/she has night sweats, nightmares, or an early-morning headache *(these symptoms are indicative of hypoglycemia occurring during sleep).*
3. Implement measures *to prevent hypoglycemia:*
   a. administer insulin as ordered being careful to inject it into an area that has adequate subcutaneous tissue
   b. perform actions *to ensure that client has an adequate caloric intake:*
      1. provide a meal within 1 hour after administering insulin (especially routine morning dose) or oral hypoglycemic agent; if client has gastroparesis and the subsequent delayed gastric emptying and intestinal absorption of nutrients, administer insulin just before client eats or right after the meal
      2. provide snacks in midafternoon and at bedtime if client is receiving an intermediate or long-acting insulin
      3. consult dietitian about appropriate supplements if client does not eat all the meals and snacks provided
   c. consult physician about altering prescribed insulin dose and/or providing alternative forms of intake (e.g., intravenous therapy) if client is to receive nothing by mouth in preparation for a diagnostic test or surgery or is unable to maintain an adequate oral intake.
4. If signs and symptoms of hypoglycemia occur, administer the following depending on the severity of hypoglycemia and hospital protocol:
   a. for a blood glucose less than 70 mg/dl but greater than 45 mg/dl, give 3 glucose tablets **OR** 4 oz of a regular soft drink **OR** instant glucose; double these amounts if the blood glucose is less than 45 mg/dl; repeat in 10–15 minutes if symptoms persist; once blood glucose is above 70 mg/dl, give client a complex carbohydrate and protein snack (e.g., glass of milk and 2–3 graham cracker squares, peanut butter and crackers, or cheese and crackers) if it will be longer than 30 minutes until the next scheduled meal

Desired Outcomes	Nursing Actions *and Selected Purposes/Rationales*
	b. for a severe reaction (client unresponsive or having difficulty swallowing), give glucagon **OR** 25 ml of 50% glucose intravenously and repeat in 2–5 minutes if no response; contact physician immediately; when blood glucose is above 70 mg/dl and client can swallow without difficulty, give client a snack (e.g., glass of milk and 2–3 graham cracker squares, peanut butter and crackers, or cheese and crackers) or a meal.
10.c. The client will not experience hyperglycemic hyperosmolar nonketotic coma as evidenced by: 1. stable vital signs 2. usual skin temperature and color 3. absence of motor and sensory deficits and seizure activity 4. blood glucose less than 600 mg/dl.	10.c.1 Assess for and report signs and symptoms of hyperglycemic hyperosmolar nonketotic coma (clients at greatest risk are persons over 60 years of age; type 2 [non–insulin-dependent] diabetics; clients with inadequate fluid intake or excessive fluid loss; those who are experiencing unusual emotional or physical stress [e.g., acute illness, infection, surgery]; and clients receiving corticosteroids, diuretics, hyperalimentation, or dialysis treatments): a. evidence of deficient fluid volume (e.g., hypotension; weak, rapid pulse; warm, flushed skin; decreased skin turgor; thirst) b. high serum osmolality (above 320 mOsm/liter) c. neurological signs such as hemiparesis, aphasia, lethargy, disorientation, and seizures d. blood glucose above 600 mg/dl with absent or only slight elevation of ketones in urine and serum. 2. Implement measures *to prevent hyperglycemic hyperosmolar nonketotic coma:* a. perform actions to prevent or treat hyperglycemia (see action a.2 in this diagnosis) *in order to prevent hyperosmolarity and the subsequent osmotic diuresis* b. notify physician if client is unable to take in an adequate amount of oral fluids, develops signs and symptoms of infection, has persistent diarrhea or vomiting, or is experiencing unusual emotional stress. 3. If signs and symptoms of hyperglycemic hyperosmolar nonketotic coma occur, administer the following if ordered: a. fluid replacement (isotonic or half-strength saline is infused rapidly until B/P is stabilized and urine output is adequate; once blood sugar falls to 250–300 mg/dl, 5% glucose is added *to prevent hypoglycemia that can result from the rapid drop in blood sugar*) b. insulin (regular insulin is administered intravenously in the initial phase of treatment) c. intravenous potassium chloride or potassium phosphate (*hypokalemia and hypophosphatemia result from osmotic diuresis and a shift of potassium and phosphorus into the cells during insulin therapy*).

11. NURSING DIAGNOSIS: *INEFFECTIVE THERAPEUTIC REGIMEN MANAGEMENT*

related to:
a. lack of understanding of the implications of not following the prescribed treatment plan;
b. feeling of lack of control over disease progression despite efforts to follow prescribed treatment plan;
c. difficulty modifying personal habits and integrating necessary treatments and dietary regimen into lifestyle;
d. insufficient financial resources.

Suggested NOC Outcomes: Compliance behavior; Diabetes self-management; Treatment behavior: illness or injury; Knowledge: treatment regimen; Health beliefs: perceived resources; Health beliefs: perceived ability to perform

Suggested NIC Interventions: Self modification assistance; Medication management; Values clarification; Teaching: disease process; Teaching: prescribed diet; Weight reduction assistance; Financial resource assistance; Support system enhancement

Desired Outcome	Nursing Actions *and Selected Purposes/Rationales*
11. The client will demonstrate the probability of effective therapeutic regimen management as evidenced by: a. willingness to learn about and participate in treatments and care b. statements reflecting ways to modify personal habits and integrate treatments into lifestyle c. statements reflecting an understanding of the implications of not following the prescribed treatment plan.	11.a. Assess for indications that client may be unable to effectively manage the therapeutic regimen: 1. statements reflecting inability to manage care at home 2. failure to adhere to treatment plan (e.g., refusing medications, not adhering to dietary restrictions) 3. statements reflecting a lack of understanding of factors that contribute to acute and chronic complications 4. statements reflecting an unwillingness or inability to modify personal habits and integrate necessary treatments into lifestyle 5. statements reflecting the view that diabetes is curable or that the situation is hopeless and that efforts to comply with treatments are useless. b. Implement measures *to promote effective therapeutic regimen management:* 1. determine client's understanding of diabetes; clarify misconceptions and stress the fact that diabetes is a chronic condition and adherence to the treatment plan may delay and/or prevent complications; caution client that some complications may occur despite strict adherence to treatment plan 2. encourage client to participate in assessments and treatments (e.g., blood glucose monitoring, selection of diet, insulin administration) 3. review prescribed diet with client and his/her technique for drawing up and administering insulin and testing blood glucose; determine areas of difficulty and misunderstanding and reinforce teaching as necessary 4. provide client with written instructions about future appointments with health care provider, diet, medications, exercise, signs and symptoms to report, foot care, and sick day management 5. discuss with client difficulties he/she has had incorporating treatments into lifestyle; assist client to identify ways to modify lifestyle rather than completely change it 6. encourage client to discuss concerns about the cost of medications, food, and supplies; obtain a social service consult to assist with financial planning and obtain financial aid if indicated 7. initiate and reinforce the discharge teaching outlined in Diagnosis 12 *in order to promote a sense of control and self-reliance* 8. encourage client to attend follow-up diabetic education classes 9. provide information about and encourage utilization of resources that can assist client to make necessary lifestyle changes (e.g., diabetes support groups, counseling services, American Diabetes Association, diabetic cookbooks, publications such as *Diabetes Forecast*) 10. reinforce behaviors suggesting future compliance with the therapeutic regimen (e.g., participation in the treatment plan, statements reflecting plans for integrating treatments into lifestyle) 11. include significant others in explanations and teaching sessions and encourage their support; reinforce the need for client to assume responsibility for managing as much of care as possible. c. Consult appropriate health care provider (e.g., social worker, physician) about referrals to community health agencies if continued instruction or supervision is needed.

12. NURSING DIAGNOSIS: ***DEFICIENT KNOWLEDGE OR INEFFECTIVE HEALTH MAINTENANCE****

*The nurse should select the diagnostic label that is most appropriate for the client's discharge teaching needs.

Suggested NOC Outcomes: Knowledge: disease process; Knowledge: diabetes management

Suggested NIC Interventions: Teaching: individual; Teaching: disease process; Teaching: prescribed medication; Teaching: prescribed diet; Teaching: foot care; Teaching: prescribed activity/exercise; Teaching: procedure/treatment; Teaching: psychomotor skill; Health system guidance

Desired Outcomes	**Nursing Actions** *and Selected Purposes/Rationales*
12.a. The client will verbalize a basic understanding of diabetes mellitus.	12.a.1. Determine client's understanding of diabetes mellitus. 2. Clarify misconceptions and reinforce teaching as necessary. Utilize available teaching aids (e.g., pamphlets, videotapes).
12.b. The client will verbalize an understanding of medications ordered and demonstrate the ability to correctly draw up and administer insulin if prescribed.	12.b.1. Explain the rationale for, side effects of, and importance of taking medications prescribed. 2. Provide the following instructions if client is to administer own insulin injections after discharge: a. store insulin and prefilled syringes in refrigerator b. let refrigerated insulin return to room temperature before use if possible c. if traveling, store insulin at room temperature unless the room temperature is above 86° F (insulin is stable for up to 1 month at room temperature) d. periodically check expiration date and discard bottle(s) and cartridges of insulin that are outdated e. do not use insulin that has changed color or contains granules or clumped particles f. do not change the type of insulin unless directed by physician g. mix insulin before use by gently rotating or rolling bottle between palms or palm and thigh; do not vigorously shake the bottle h. read the label on the insulin bottle(s) carefully, making sure the correct type of insulin (e.g., regular, NPH) is being used i. clean the top of the bottle(s) with alcohol before withdrawing insulin j. withdraw the correct amount of insulin making sure to remove air bubbles k. if mixing two insulins, withdraw in the same order every time (usually recommended that the rapid-acting insulin be drawn up first in order to reduce the risk of contaminating the vial of rapid-acting insulin with a longer-acting insulin) l. if mixing lente and regular insulin in one syringe, give injection immediately after drawing up the insulins m. select injection sites using the following guidelines: 1. injections should be given in the same region at the same time each day (e.g., abdomen in the morning, leg or buttock at night) and sites should be rotated within a region with no site being used more than once every 2–3 weeks 2. there should be at least 2.5 cm (1 inch) between sites 3. avoid giving injections right at the waistline or within 2.5 cm (1 inch) of the umbilicus 4. avoid using an area that will be heavily exercised or to which heat will be applied that day (insulin will be more rapidly absorbed from that area) 5. do not give injections into areas where the skin appears raised, thickened, or "wasted" n. to administer insulin, insert needle into subcutaneous tissue and inject insulin o. following insulin injection, apply gentle pressure to site rather than rubbing p. dispose of syringes in approved biohazard device

q. plan meals and snacks keeping the onset, peak action, and length of action of the insulin(s) prescribed in mind
r. adjust insulin dosage based on blood sugar results and parameters established by physician
s. if local reaction such as itching, redness, tenderness, or burning continues to occur after injections, consult health care provider
t. always have a rapid-acting carbohydrate readily available and know actions to take if signs and symptoms of hypoglycemia occur (see action h.1.c in this diagnosis)
u. consult health care provider if repeated episodes of sweating, nervousness, weakness, hunger, shakiness, slurred speech, blurred or double vision, nightmares, and difficulty concentrating occur (may indicate need to reduce insulin dose)
v. consult health care provider if experiencing unusual emotional or physical stress (e.g., acute illness, physical trauma, pregnancy) so that insulin dose can be increased to provide adequate coverage.

3. If client is discharged with an insulin pump device, provide instructions regarding its management (e.g., changing the insertion site, filling syringes, changing batteries in pump). Allow time for practice and return demonstration.
4. If client is discharged on an oral glucose-lowering agent, instruct to:
   a. take medication exactly as prescribed
   b. notify health care provider if unable to tolerate food and fluid
   c. adhere strictly to the prescribed diet (oral agents are not a substitute for good dietary management)
   d. consult health care provider if experiencing unusual emotional or physical stress so that dosage may be adjusted to provide adequate coverage
   e. consult health care provider if pregnant or lactating and be aware that some oral agents may interfere with the effectiveness of oral contraceptives
   f. store medication at room temperature and out of exposure to direct sunlight.
5. Instruct client to consult pharmacist or health care provider before taking other prescription and nonprescription medications (e.g., over-the-counter cold preparations).
6. Instruct client to inform all health care providers of medications being taken.

12.c. The client will verbalize an understanding of the principles of dietary management and be able to calculate and plan meals within the prescribed caloric distribution.

12.c.1. Reinforce dietary instructions regarding the prescribed diabetic diet and methods of calculating the foods/fluids allowed (e.g., exchange list, consistent carbohydrate diet, Food Guide Pyramid).
2. Have client plan sample menus before discharge to ensure that he/she is able to calculate the diet correctly.
3. Explain the purpose of weight reduction if client has been placed on a caloric restriction to reduce weight. Reinforce need to avoid fasting and fad diets.
4. Instruct client on appropriate dietary adjustments that should be made if meal schedule or activity level has been significantly altered.
5. Reinforce the following principles of good dietary management:
   a. eat 3 meals each day about 4–5 hours apart and close to the same time each day; do not skip meals
   b. limit intake of concentrated sweets (e.g., sugar, candy, syrups, jams, jellies, cakes, pies, pastries, fruits packed in heavy syrup)
   c. avoid foods high in saturated fat and cholesterol (e.g., butter, cheese, eggs, ice cream, red meat) and *trans* fats (e.g., stick margarine and shortening and foods such as commercial baked goods that are prepared with these products)
   d. increase intake of foods high in soluble fiber (e.g., fruits, whole-grain cereals, green leafy vegetables)
   e. read food/fluid labels and limit intake of those that contain significant amounts of sugar, honey, and nutritive sweeteners

Desired Outcomes	Nursing Actions *and Selected Purposes/Rationales*
	such as xylitol, sorbitol, and fructose (nutritive sweeteners are usually labeled as "sugar free" but are only "sucrose free," not carbohydrate free; however, they are not digested and absorbed as well as other carbohydrates and therefore contribute only 2 kcal/g as compared to 4 kcal/g of other carbohydrates) f. use artificial (nonnutritive or noncaloric) sweeteners such as saccharin (e.g., Sweet and Low), acesulfame (e.g., Sunnette), and aspartame (e.g., Equal, NutraSweet) when possible g. eat an afternoon carbohydrate snack (e.g., fresh fruit, ½ bagel, 1 cup skim milk) if taking an intermediate-acting insulin in the morning and a snack at bedtime that includes protein and carbohydrate (e.g., milk and graham crackers, ½ meat sandwich, cheese and crackers) if taking an oral glucose-lowering agent or insulin in the evening h. if alcoholic beverages are consumed: 1. drink alcohol with food (alcohol can cause low blood sugar) 2. avoid liqueurs, sweet wines, wine coolers, and sweet mixes that contain large amounts of carbohydrates 3. do not substitute alcohol for anything in prescribed diet 4. limit alcohol intake to 2 drinks/day for men and 1 drink/day for women (a "drink" is considered to be 1½ oz of liquor, 12 oz of beer, or 5 oz of wine).
12.d. The client will demonstrate the ability to perform blood glucose and urine tests correctly and interpret results accurately.	12.d.1. Review with client how and when to perform a blood glucose measurement, test urine for ketones, and calibrate and maintain a glucose monitoring device. 2. Have client demonstrate blood and urine tests. Reinforce teaching as necessary. 3. Instruct client to keep a record of test results and take the record of results to appointments with the health care provider. 4. Provide instructions on actions client should take when test results are abnormal (some clients are instructed to adjust insulin dose and dietary intake; others are instructed to notify appropriate health care provider).
12.e. The client will verbalize an understanding of the role of exercise in the management of diabetes.	12.e.1. Explain how exercise affects blood sugar levels. 2. Provide the following instructions about exercise and diabetes management: a. maintain a regular exercise program making sure to start exercise slowly and build up gradually b. avoid exercising during insulin peak action time c. try to exercise about 1 hour after a meal and about the same time of the day d. avoid giving insulin in a site that will be heavily exercised e. adjust insulin dosage before exercise according to physician's instructions f. consume extra carbohydrates before vigorous exercise and supplement carbohydrate intake (15–30 g) at 30–60 minute intervals during vigorous prolonged exercise g. maintain adequate hydration during periods of intense exercise h. consume an extra bedtime snack on days that exercise has been prolonged or unusually vigorous i. do not exercise in extreme heat or cold j. do not exercise at times when blood sugar is greater than 250 and ketones are present in urine or if blood sugar is greater than 300 (strenuous exercise is perceived as a stressor leading to an increased output of counterregulatory hormones and a further increase in blood sugar) k. perform blood glucose tests more frequently during periods of significant variation in activity level

l. carry a rapid-acting carbohydrate source (e.g., hard candy, glucose tablets) during exercise (especially if using insulin and if exercise is expected to be prolonged or vigorous)
m. stop any activity that causes extreme weakness, trembling, incoordination, or nausea.

12.f. The client will identify health care and hygiene practices that should be integrated into lifestyle.	12.f.1. Reinforce the importance of adhering to the following health care practices: a. perform oral hygiene including brushing and flossing at least twice a day b. have regular dental appointments at least every 6 months c. have annual eye examinations (beginning 5 years post-onset for type 1 and at onset for type 2) d. avoid smoking (smoking contributes to the risk for cardiovascular disease) e. have feet examined by health care provider annually f. have annual urine testing (for microalbuminuria) and fasting blood work for lipid panel g. if female, reduce the risk for a vaginal infection by maintaining good personal hygiene, wiping from front to back after voiding, wearing cotton underwear, avoiding douching, and avoiding tight jeans and nylon pantyhose h. limit alcohol intake j. perform meticulous care of cuts, burns, and scratches. 2. Provide instructions about foot care: a. inspect feet daily for cuts, redness, cracks, blisters, corns, and calluses; use a mirror to check bottoms of feet if necessary b. wash feet daily with a mild soap and warm water and dry gently but thoroughly c. apply lanolin or other lubricating lotion to feet (except between toes) daily d. keep feet dry by wearing cotton socks and avoiding shoes with rubber or plastic soles (cause feet to sweat) e. cut nails after a bath or shower; cut them straight across and smooth them with an emery board after cutting f. see a podiatrist rather than using home remedies to treat corns, calluses, and ingrown nails or if help is needed with routine nail care g. avoid wearing socks, stockings, or garters that are tight (may further compromise peripheral blood flow) h. buy shoes that fit well and break them in gradually; it is best to buy shoes in the late afternoon when feet are at their largest i. do not wear open-toed shoes, sandals, high heels, or thongs because they increase the risk for trauma j. do not walk barefoot; wear shoes or slippers when walking to protect feet from injury k. do not use a heating pad or hot water bottle on feet (if paresthesias are present, burns may occur); test bath water with bath thermometer, wrist, or elbow before immersing feet (temperature should be between 30–32° C [84–90° F]) l. protect feet from extreme cold to prevent vasoconstriction and possible frostbite.
12.g. The client will identify appropriate safety measures to follow because of the diagnosis of diabetes.	12.g. Teach client the following safety precautions: 1. always carry an identification card or wear a medical alert bracelet or tag identifying self as a diabetic; identification card should have the name of health care provider, the type and dose of insulin and/or oral agent(s), and measures to take if found behaving abnormally or unconscious 2. always carry a rapid-acting carbohydrate such as glucose tablets or instant glucose gel

Desired Outcomes	**Nursing Actions** *and Selected Purposes/Rationales*
	3. if insulin-dependent, always have insulin readily available (carry in purse or briefcase) 4. if traveling by plane, bus, or train: a. carry a letter from health care provider indicating the necessity of having syringes, blood glucose monitoring equipment, and medication b. keep snack items; a quick-acting source of carbohydrate; a full day's supply of food; blood glucose monitoring equipment; and an extra supply of insulin, injection equipment, and oral agents in carry-on luggage 5. consult physician about plans for pregnancy and maintain close prenatal supervision 6. keep a glucagon kit readily available and know how and when to use it; make sure significant other is also trained in how to use it 7. if ill but able to tolerate some foods/fluids: a. take usual dose of insulin or oral glucose-lowering agent unless blood glucose is low b. check blood glucose every 4 hours or a minimum of 4 times a day c. if blood glucose is greater than 240, test urine for ketones d. drink 8–12 oz of caffeine-free and alcohol-free fluid every hour (e.g., broth, fruit juice, regular or diet soda, water, Gatorade) e. if not able to tolerate solid foods, substitute liquids and easily digested soft foods f. do not exercise 8. notify physician if: a. unable to eat for more than 24 hours b. vomiting or severe diarrhea persists for more than 4 hours c. blood sugar is greater than 300 or ketones are present in urine d. having difficulty breathing or a change in mental status occurs e. symptoms of dehydration such as unusual thirst, dry mouth, or fever occur 9. inform all health care providers of diabetic condition.
12.h. The client will state signs and symptoms of hypoglycemia and ketoacidosis and appropriate actions for prevention and treatment.	12.h.1. Reinforce the following information about hypoglycemia: a. factors that precipitate hypoglycemia (e.g., too much insulin or oral hypoglycemic agent, insufficient oral intake, excessive exercise, excessive alcohol intake) b. signs and symptoms of hypoglycemia (e.g., shakiness, nervousness, weakness, hunger, sweating, nightmares, early-morning headache, incoordination, blood sugar less than 70) c. actions to take if signs and symptoms of hypoglycemia occur: 1. test blood glucose if possible and if less than 70 (or if symptoms are present but glucose testing is not possible), take 15 grams of rapid-acting carbohydrate (e.g., half a glass of regular [sugar-containing] soft drink, 3 glucose tablets, half a tube of instant glucose); if taking acarbose (Precose) or miglitol (Glyset), only the glucose tablets or instant glucose will correct hypoglycemia quickly 2. retest glucose level in 15 minutes and if still less than 70, take another 15 grams of rapid-acting carbohydrate; if blood glucose level remains below 70 and/or symptoms persist for more than 30 minutes, consult health care provider 3. after the hypoglycemic episode, consume a snack (e.g., graham crackers and a glass of milk, half a sandwich and half a glass of milk) if it will be longer than 30 minutes until the next meal. 2. Teach significant others how to treat hypoglycemia: a. if client is awake but groggy, put corn syrup, honey, cake icing, or instant glucose in his/her mouth between cheek and gum b. if client loses consciousness, administer glucagon injection.

3. Reinforce the following information about ketoacidosis:
   a. factors that precipitate ketoacidosis (e.g., emotional stress, infection, failure to take insulin or oral glucose-lowering agent)
   b. signs and symptoms of impending or actual ketoacidosis (e.g., unusual thirst; excessive urination; weakness; warm, flushed skin; blood sugar higher than 250; ketones in urine; abdominal pain; nausea and vomiting)
   c. immediate actions to take if signs and symptoms of ketoacidosis occur:
      1. drink a cup or more of broth or sugar-free liquid if able to tolerate it
      2. administer insulin (if previously instructed in insulin coverage based on blood glucose results)
      3. consult health care provider.

12.i. The client will state signs and symptoms to report to the health care provider.

12.i. Instruct client to report the following:
1. unexplained episodes of hypoglycemia and ketoacidosis (see actions h.1.b and h.3.b in this diagnosis for signs and symptoms)
2. unusual variations in blood glucose results
3. a cut, scratch, or burn that becomes red, swollen, tender, or does not start to heal within 24 hours
4. nausea and vomiting or severe diarrhea that lasts more than 4 hours
5. temperature elevation that lasts more than 2 days
6. change in vision
7. development or worsening of symptoms that are indicative of long-term complications (e.g., burning or aching pain in extremity, decreased sensation in extremity, persistent gastric discomfort, frequent urination of small amounts, impotence, gait disturbances, chest pain, extreme fatigue, persistent dizziness or lightheadedness).

12.j. The client will identify resources that can assist in the adjustment to and management of diabetes.

12.j.1. Provide information about resources that can assist client and significant others in adjustment to and management of diabetes (e.g., American Diabetes Association, diabetic education classes, weight loss programs, diabetes support groups, counseling services, publications such as *Diabetes Forecast*, internet sites [www.diabetes.org]).
2. Initiate a referral if indicated.

12.k. The client will verbalize an understanding of and a plan for adhering to recommended follow-up care including future appointments with health care provider and for laboratory studies.

12.k.1. Reinforce the importance of keeping follow-up appointments with health care provider and for laboratory studies.
2. Refer to Diagnosis 11, action b, for measures to promote the client's ability to effectively manage the therapeutic regimen.

ADDITIONAL NURSING DIAGNOSES

DIARRHEA*

related to the effects of autonomic neuropathy on intestinal motility.

RISK FOR INJURY

a. falls related to:
   1. gait abnormalities (may result from impaired proprioception and muscle weakness and loss of normal structure of the foot) and muscle weakness and diminished reflexes in lower extremity(ies) associated with motor and sensory neuropathies that may be present
   2. dizziness and syncope associated with postural hypotension that may be present as a result of autonomic neuropathy
   3. diminished visual acuity;

b. burns related to decreased sensation in extremities (may be present as a result of peripheral polyneuropathy).

SEXUAL DYSFUNCTION

related to autonomic neuropathy and angiopathies that may occur (men may experience impotence and ejaculatory changes; women may experience changes in arousal pattern, vaginal lubrication, and orgasm.

INEFFECTIVE COPING* OR IMPAIRED ADJUSTMENT

related to fear of complications and inability to manage them; discomfort; need to alter lifestyle; feeling of powerlessness; and knowledge that condition is chronic and will require lifelong medical supervision, dietary regulation, and medication therapy.

---

*See Unit II for outcomes, actions, and rationales.

Bibliography

See pages 879 and 884–885.

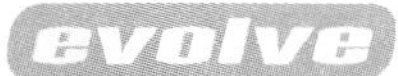

Thyroidectomy

Thyroidectomy is the surgical removal of the thyroid gland. It may be performed to treat a benign or malignant tumor, an unusually large goiter, or hyperthyroidism that has been refractory to medical treatment. A subtotal thyroidectomy (removal of up to 90% of the thyroid gland) is the preferred procedure unless the surgery is being done to treat a malignancy, in which case a total thyroidectomy will usually be performed. Following a subtotal thyroidectomy, the remaining gland tissue usually hypertrophies enough to eventually supply adequate amounts of thyroid hormone.

The client is often given antithyroid agents for 6–8 weeks prior to hospitalization for a thyroidectomy in order to achieve a euthyroid state and minimize the risk of thyroid crisis. Iodine preparations may also be administered for 7–10 days prior to surgery to reduce vascularity of the thyroid gland and the risk for hemorrhage in the intraoperative and postoperative period. During this presurgical period, it is also important that an optimal nutritional state and cardiovascular status be attained.

This care plan focuses on the adult client with hyperthyroidism whose condition has been medically stabilized and who is being hospitalized for a thyroidectomy.

OUTCOME/DISCHARGE CRITERIA

THE CLIENT WILL:

- have surgical pain controlled
- have evidence of normal healing of surgical wound
- have no signs and symptoms of complications
- verbalize an understanding of range of motion exercises of the neck
- state signs and symptoms to report to the health care provider
- verbalize an understanding of and a plan for adhering to recommended follow-up care including future appointments with health care provider, medications prescribed, dietary recommendations, activity level, and wound care.

NURSING/COLLABORATIVE DIAGNOSES

Preoperative

1. Deficient knowledge p. 751

Postoperative

1. Ineffective airway clearance p. 752
2. Potential complications p. 753
   a. hemorrhage
   b. respiratory distress
   c. hypocalcemia
   d. thyroid storm (thyrotoxic crisis)
   e. laryngeal nerve damage

DISCHARGE TEACHING

3. Deficient knowledge, Ineffective therapeutic regimen management, or Ineffective health maintenance p. 755

See Standardized Preoperative and Postoperative Care Plans (pp. 97–126) for additional diagnoses.

PREOPERATIVE

Use in conjunction with the Standardized Preoperative Care Plan.

Client Teaching

1. Nursing Diagnosis: **DEFICIENT KNOWLEDGE**

regarding the surgical procedure, routines associated with surgery, physical preparation for a thyroidectomy, sensations that normally occur following surgery and anesthesia, and postoperative care.

Suggested NOC Outcomes: Knowledge: treatment regimen; Knowledge: prescribed activity

Suggested NIC Interventions: Teaching: individual; Teaching: preoperative; Teaching: prescribed activity/exercise

Desired Outcomes	Nursing Actions *and Selected Purposes/Rationales*
1.a. The client will verbalize an understanding of the surgical procedure, preoperative care, and postoperative sensations and care.	1.a.1. Refer to Standardized Preoperative Care Plan, Diagnosis 4, actions a.1–4 (pp. 100–101), for information to include in preoperative teaching. 2. Inform client that he/she will be assessed for voice changes routinely after surgery. Explain that hoarseness is expected for a few days and unnecessary talking should be avoided during that time. 3. Allow time for questions and clarification of information provided.
1.b. The client will demonstrate the ability to perform activities designed to prevent postoperative complications.	1.b.1. Refer to Standardized Preoperative Care Plan, Diagnosis 4, action b.1 (p. 101), for instructions on ways to prevent postoperative complications. 2. Provide additional instructions on ways to prevent complications after a thyroidectomy: a. instruct client on ways to minimize stress on the suture line: 1. support head and neck with hands when turning head and coughing for first few days after surgery 2. avoid turning head abruptly and hyperextending neck b. inform client that he/she will need to do neck range of motion exercises beginning 2–4 days after surgery; demonstrate flexion, extension, rotation, and lateral movement of head and neck. 3. Allow time for questions, clarification, and return demonstration.

POSTOPERATIVE

Use in conjunction with the Standardized Postoperative Care Plan.

1. Nursing Diagnosis: ***INEFFECTIVE AIRWAY CLEARANCE***

related to:

a. occlusion of the pharynx in the immediate postoperative period associated with relaxation of the tongue resulting from the effect of anesthesia and some medications (e.g., narcotic [opioid] analgesics);

b. stasis of secretions associated with:
   1. decreased activity
   2. poor cough effort resulting from the depressant effect of anesthesia and some medications (e.g., narcotic [opioid] analgesics), pain, weakness, and fear of disrupting incision;

c. increased secretions associated with irritation of the respiratory tract (can result from inhalation anesthetics and endotracheal intubation);

d. tracheal compression associated with swelling and/or bleeding in the surgical area.

Suggested NOC Outcomes: Respiratory status: airway patency; Respiratory status: ventilation

Suggested NIC Interventions: Respiratory monitoring; Airway management

Desired Outcome	**Nursing Actions** *and Selected Purposes/Rationales*
1. The client will maintain clear, open airways (see Standardized Postoperative Care Plan, Diagnosis 3 [p. 105], for outcome criteria).	1.a. Refer to Standardized Postoperative Care Plan, Diagnosis 3 (p. 105), for measures related to assessment and promotion of effective airway clearance. b. Implement additional measures *to promote effective airway clearance:* 1. perform actions *to minimize swelling in the surgical area and subsequently reduce pressure on the trachea:* a. keep head of bed elevated at least 30° b. apply cooling pad or ice packs to neck if ordered *to reduce inflammation* 2. perform actions to reduce stress on the incision (see Postoperative Diagnosis 2, action a.2.b) *in order to reduce the risk of bleeding and a subsequent increase in pressure on the trachea.*

2. COLLABORATIVE DIAGNOSES: POTENTIAL COMPLICATIONS OF THYROIDECTOMY

a. **hemorrhage** related to surgery in a highly vascular area;
b. **respiratory distress** related to airway obstruction associated with:
   1. tracheal compression resulting from swelling and/or bleeding in the surgical area
   2. closure of the glottis resulting from paralysis of the vocal cords (can occur with injury to the bilateral recurrent laryngeal nerves) or laryngeal spasm that can occur with calcium deficiency;
c. **hypocalcemia** related to disruption of blood supply to parathyroid gland(s) or damage to or inadvertent removal of the parathyroid gland(s) during surgery;
d. **thyroid storm (thyrotoxic crisis)** related to excessive amounts of thyroid hormone in the blood associated with surgical manipulation of a hyperactive thyroid gland (can occur if a euthyroid state was not achieved preoperatively);
e. **laryngeal nerve damage** related to trauma to the nerve(s) during surgery and/or pressure on the nerve(s) associated with swelling and/or bleeding in the surgical area.

Desired Outcomes	**Nursing Actions** *and Selected Purposes/Rationales*
2.a. The client will not have excessive bleeding in the surgical area as evidenced by: 1. absence of feeling of tightness of neck dressing and sensation of pressure or fullness at incision site 2. expected amount of drainage on dressing 3. increasing ease of swallowing 4. absence of choking sensation and respiratory distress 5. stable vital signs.	2.a.1. Assess for and report signs and symptoms of hemorrhage (e.g., increased tightness of neck dressing; complaints of fullness or pressure in neck; excessive bloody drainage on dressing, pillow, or back of neck; statements of persistent or increased difficulty swallowing or a choking sensation; difficulty breathing; tachycardia; decrease in B/P). 2. Implement measures *to reduce the risk of hemorrhage:* a. maintain pressure dressing over incision site as ordered b. perform actions *to reduce stress on the incision:* 1. place client in a semi-Fowler's position with small pillow under head 2. maintain client's head and neck in proper alignment using pillows or sandbags if necessary 3. support client's head and neck during position change until client is able to do so independently 4. reinforce preoperative instructions about supporting head and neck and remind client to avoid turning head abruptly and hyperextending neck 5. perform actions to prevent nausea and vomiting (see Standardized Postoperative Care Plan, Diagnosis 8, action b [pp. 110–111]) 6. place personal articles and call signal within easy reach *so client does not have to turn head and neck or strain to reach them* 7. focus on deep breathing, use of incentive spirometer, and "huff" coughing rather than vigorous coughing to promote an effective breathing pattern and airway clearance *(vigorous coughing increases stress on suture line)* 8. stress importance of doing neck range of motion exercises gently (exercises are usually started 2–4 days postoperatively)

Desired Outcomes	**Nursing Actions** *and Selected Purposes/Rationales*
	c. perform actions *to decrease venous pressure in the surgical area:* 1. keep head of bed elevated at least 30° 2. discourage vigorous coughing d. apply cooling pad or ice packs to neck if ordered. 3. If signs and symptoms of bleeding occur: a. loosen dressing *to promote drainage of blood and reduce the risk of respiratory distress* b. assist with suture/staple removal and drainage of hematoma if indicated c. assist with emergency tracheostomy if respiratory distress develops d. prepare client for surgical intervention (e.g., ligation of bleeding vessels) if planned.
2.b. The client will not experience respiratory distress as evidenced by: 1. unlabored respirations at 12–20/minute 2. absence of stridor and sternocleidomastoid muscle retraction 3. usual mental status 4. usual skin color 5. oximetry results within normal range 6. blood gases within normal range.	2.b.1. Assess for and immediately report: a. increased swelling of the neck or bulging of the wound b. persistent or increased difficulty swallowing or choking sensation c. signs and symptoms of respiratory distress (e.g., rapid and/or labored respirations, stridor, sternocleidomastoid muscle retraction, restlessness, agitation, cyanosis) d. significant decrease in oximetry results e. abnormal blood gases. 2. Have oxygen and staple or suture removal, tracheostomy, and suction equipment readily available. 3. Implement measures *to prevent respiratory distress:* a. perform actions *to minimize swelling in the surgical area:* 1. keep head of bed elevated at least 30° 2. apply cooling pad or ice packs to neck if ordered b. perform actions to reduce the risk of hemorrhage or treat bleeding if it occurs (see actions a.2 and 3 in this diagnosis) c. assess for and immediately report signs and symptoms of hypocalcemia (see action c.1 in this diagnosis) *so that treatment can be initiated and the risk of laryngeal spasm can be reduced.* 4. If signs and symptoms of respiratory distress occur: a. place client in a high Fowler's position unless he/she is hypotensive b. loosen dressing on neck *to prevent further compression of trachea* c. maintain oxygen therapy as ordered d. suction client if indicated e. assist with emergency tracheostomy if performed.
2.c. The client will experience resolution of hypocalcemia if it occurs as evidenced by: 1. absence of numbness and tingling in fingers, toes, and circumoral area 2. negative Chvostek's and Trousseau's signs 3. absence of muscle twitching and spasms and seizure activity 4. serum calcium level within normal range.	2.c.1. Assess for and report signs and symptoms of hypocalcemia (e.g., numbness or tingling of fingers, toes, or circumoral area; positive Chvostek's and Trousseau's signs; muscle twitching or spasms; seizures; low serum calcium). 2. If signs and symptoms of hypocalcemia occur: a. institute seizure precautions b. administer calcium preparations (e.g., intravenous calcium gluconate, calcium carbonate) as ordered.
2.d. The client will not develop thyroid storm as evidenced by: 1. stable vital signs 2. usual mental status 3. absence of tremors, nausea, and vomiting.	2.d.1. Assess for and report signs and symptoms of thyroid storm: a. fever greater than 38° C (100.4° F) b. marked increase in client's usual pulse rate c. increasing restlessness d. agitation, irritability, tremors e. nausea, vomiting f. delirium, coma.

2. If signs and symptoms of thyroid storm occur:
   a. utilize hypothermia techniques (e.g., cooling blanket, tepid sponge bath) *to reduce fever*
   b. maintain intravenous fluid and electrolyte therapy as ordered
   c. maintain oxygen therapy as ordered
   d. institute appropriate safety measures if client is irrational, delirious, or comatose
   e. administer the following medications if ordered:
      1. antipyretics *to reduce fever* (avoid aspirin *because it increases free thyroid hormone levels)*
      2. antithyroid agents (e.g., propylthiouracil, methimazole) and iodine preparations (e.g., sodium iodide) *to suppress production and release of thyroid hormone from the remaining thyroid tissue; propylthiouracil also blocks the peripheral conversion of T_4 to the more potent T_3*
      3. glucocorticoids (e.g., dexamethasone) *to aid the body in handling stress, replenish endogenous glucocorticoids that have probably been depleted by the increased metabolism, and block the peripheral conversion of T_4 to T_3*
      4. adrenergic inhibiting agents (e.g., propranolol) *to reduce the severity of many of the clinical manifestations*
      5. antiatrial fibrillation agents *(atrial fibrillation may occur in thyroid storm as a result of excessive stimulation of the heart).*

2.e. The client will experience resolution of laryngeal nerve damage if it occurs as evidenced by:
1. improved tone and quality of voice
2. gradual resolution of hoarseness
3. absence of dysphagia
4. absence of respiratory distress.

2.e.1. Assess for the following indications of laryngeal nerve damage:
   a. voice changes (e.g., hoarseness; weak, whispery voice; inability to speak)
   b. statements of difficulty swallowing and/or coughing or choking when eating
   c. respiratory distress (see action b.1.c in this diagnosis for signs and symptoms).
2. Implement measures *to reduce the risk of laryngeal nerve damage:*
   a. perform actions *to reduce swelling in the surgical area:*
      1. keep head of bed elevated at least 30°
      2. apply cooling pad or ice packs to neck if ordered
   b. perform actions to reduce the risk of hemorrhage or treat bleeding if it occurs (see actions a.2 and 3 in this diagnosis).
3. If signs and symptoms of laryngeal nerve damage occur:
   a. implement swallowing precautions (e.g., place client in a high Fowler's position when drinking and eating, introduce fluids and foods cautiously, instruct client to avoid putting too much fluid/food in mouth at one time, provide thick rather than thin fluids)
   b. encourage client to avoid unnecessary talking *in order to rest the vocal cords*
   c. implement measures *to facilitate communication* (e.g., ask questions that require a short answer or nod of head, provide materials such as Magic Slate or pad and pencil, answer call signal in person rather than using intercommunication system)
   d. notify physician immediately if signs and symptoms of respiratory distress occur; client is unable to speak; or hoarseness, voice changes, or swallowing difficulties worsen.

Discharge Teaching/Continued Care

3. NURSING DIAGNOSIS: ***DEFICIENT KNOWLEDGE, INEFFECTIVE THERAPEUTIC REGIMEN MANAGEMENT, OR INEFFECTIVE HEALTH MAINTENANCE****

*The nurse should select the diagnostic label that is most appropriate for the client's discharge teaching needs.

Suggested NOC Outcome:
Knowledge: treatment regimen

Suggested NIC Interventions: Health system guidance; Teaching: individual; Teaching: prescribed activity/exercise

Desired Outcomes	**Nursing Actions** *and Selected Purposes/Rationales*
3.a. The client will verbalize an understanding of range of motion exercises of the neck.	3.a.1. Reinforce preoperative teaching about range of motion exercises of the neck. Instruct client to do the exercises as prescribed by physician (exercises are usually begun 2–4 days after surgery and are done 3–4 times/day for a few weeks). 2. Allow time for questions and clarification of information provided.
3.b. The client will state signs and symptoms to report to the health care provider.	3.b.1. Refer to Standardized Postoperative Care Plan, Diagnosis 22, action c (p. 125), for signs and symptoms to report to the health care provider. 2. Instruct client to also report the following signs and symptoms: a. fever above 100° F; feeling unusually anxious or agitated; warm, flushed skin; or nausea and vomiting (may indicate thyroid crisis) b. increased feeling of fullness or tightness in neck c. unexplained weight gain, persistent fatigue, drowsiness, constipation, cold intolerance (indicative of inadequate thyroid hormone replacement or progressive thyroid failure) d. numbness or tingling of toes or fingers or around mouth, muscle twitching or spasms (indicative of hypocalcemia).
3.c. The client will verbalize an understanding of and a plan for adhering to recommended follow-up care including future appointments with health care provider, medications prescribed, dietary recommendations, activity level, and wound care.	3.c.1. Refer to Standardized Postoperative Care Plan, Diagnosis 22 (pp. 125–126), for routine postoperative instructions and measures to improve client compliance. 2. Teach client the rationale for, side effects of, schedule for taking, and importance of taking medications prescribed (e.g., thyroid hormone, calcium supplements, vitamin D). Inform client of pertinent food and drug interactions. 3. If client had a subtotal thyroidectomy: a. explain that thyroid hormone replacement will probably not be given unless symptoms of hypothyroidism develop because the synthetic hormone may delay regeneration of the remaining thyroid tissue b. instruct him/her to maintain an adequate iodine intake (e.g., use iodized salt, eat seafood 1–2 times a week) to promote thyroid hormone production by the remaining thyroid tissue c. instruct him/her to avoid excessive intake of foods that contain thyroid-inhibiting substances (goitrogens) such as turnips, rutabagas, peanuts, and soybeans. 4. Encourage client to participate in a regular exercise program (exercise helps maintain an optimal weight and stimulates remaining thyroid tissue).

Bibliography

See pages 879 and 884–885.

UNIT XVII

Nursing Care of the Client with Disturbances of Musculoskeletal Function

evolve

AMPUTATION

An amputation is the removal of all or part of a limb. Amputation of an upper or lower extremity may be performed to treat conditions such as tumors, uncontrollable infection, or gangrene and may be indicated in situations involving tissue destruction resulting from trauma or thermal injury (e.g. frostbite, electrocution, burns). The majority of amputations, however, are performed on the lower extremities of persons with severe peripheral vascular disease. In these instances, the ischemic limb is removed to prevent life-threatening infection and/or relieve severe, persistent discomfort. The level of amputation (e.g., above the knee, below the knee) is determined by factors such as the adequacy of circulation in the involved extremity; the client's age, general health, and anticipated mobility; and the requirements for proper fit and optimal function of the prosthetic device.

The two types of surgical amputations are open and closed. The open type is performed if the client has an infected limb. The wound is left open, treated until infection resolves, and then closed during a second surgical procedure. An open amputation may also be done if the client has a very high risk for developing a wound or bone infection postoperatively. A closed amputation, which consists of soft tissue flaps sutured over the bone, is the type of amputation that is more frequently performed. The basic techniques for postoperative management of the residual limb following a closed amputation include use of a soft compression dressing or use of a rigid dressing. The technique selected depends on the client's underlying disease process and physiological status and whether the prosthetic fitting will be immediate, early (usually within 10–30 days), or delayed or is not expected to occur (unplanned).

This care plan focuses on the adult client hospitalized for a planned below the knee, closed amputation.* Much of the postoperative information is applicable to clients receiving follow-up care in an extended care facility or home setting.

*If an above the knee amputation is planned, refer to medical-surgical nursing texts for additional nursing diagnoses and related actions that might be appropriate.

OUTCOME/DISCHARGE CRITERIA

THE CLIENT WILL:

- have pain controlled
- have evidence of normal healing of the surgical wound
- achieve expected level of mobility
- have no signs and symptoms of postoperative complications
- demonstrate appropriate ways to prevent contractures, increase strength, and improve mobility
- demonstrate correct transfer and ambulation techniques and proper use of ambulatory aids
- identify ways to maintain health of the remaining lower extremity
- demonstrate the ability to care for the residual limb
- verbalize how to care for the prosthesis and residual limb if a permanent prosthesis is planned
- identify ways to manage phantom limb pain if it occurs
- state signs and symptoms to report to the health care provider
- share feelings and thoughts about the change in body image and effects of the amputation on lifestyle and roles
- identify community resources that can assist with home management and adjustment to changes resulting from the amputation
- verbalize an understanding of and a plan for adhering to recommended follow-up care including future appointments with health care provider, prosthetist, and physical therapist; medications prescribed; and activity level.

NURSING/COLLABORATIVE DIAGNOSES

See p. 771 and Standardized Preoperative and Postoperative Care Plans (pp. 97–126) for additional diagnoses.

PREOPERATIVE

Use in conjunction with the Standardized Preoperative Care Plan.

1. Nursing Diagnosis: *FEAR/ANXIETY*

related to:
a. impending disfiguring surgery;
b. lack of understanding of diagnostic tests, reason for amputation, and planned surgical procedure;
c. anticipated loss of control associated with effects of anesthesia;
d. unfamiliar environment and separation from significant others;
e. financial concerns associated with hospitalization and rehabilitation;
f. anticipated discomfort and effects of amputation on usual lifestyle and roles.

Suggested NOC Outcomes:
Anxiety level; Fear level; Anxiety self-control; Fear self-control

Suggested NIC Interventions: Anxiety reduction; Calming technique; Emotional support; Presence

Desired Outcome	**Nursing Actions** *and Selected Purposes/Rationales* (see pp. 14–16 for additional rationales)
1. The client will experience a reduction in fear and anxiety (see Standardized Preoperative Care Plan, Diagnosis 1 [pp. 97–98], for outcome criteria).	1.a. Refer to Standardized Preoperative Care Plan, Diagnosis 1 (pp. 97–98), for measures related to assessment and reduction of fear and anxiety. b. Implement additional measures *to reduce fear and anxiety*: 1. reinforce physician's explanation about the level of amputation planned including that final determination of the level will be made during the surgical procedure once adequacy of circulation in the operative limb is confirmed 2. if acceptable to client, arrange for a visit with an individual who has successfully adjusted to the loss of a lower limb.

Client Teaching

2. NURSING DIAGNOSIS: ***DEFICIENT KNOWLEDGE***

regarding:
a. the surgical procedure;
b. hospital routines associated with surgery;
c. physical preparation for the amputation;
d. sensations that may occur following surgery and anesthesia;
e. postoperative care and management of the residual limb;
f. postoperative activity and exercises.

Suggested NOC Outcomes: Knowledge: treatment regimen; Knowledge: prescribed activity

Suggested NIC Interventions: Amputation care; Teaching: individual; Teaching: preoperative; Teaching: prescribed activity/exercise

Desired Outcomes	**Nursing Actions** *and Selected Purposes/Rationales*
2.a. The client will verbalize an understanding of the surgical procedure, preoperative care, and postoperative sensations and care.	2.a.1. Refer to Standardized Preoperative Care Plan, Diagnosis 4, actions a.1–4 (pp. 100–101), for information to include in preoperative teaching. 2. Explain that following surgery, the client may experience phantom limb sensation (e.g., tingling, numbness, or itching in phantom limb; feeling that part or all of the amputated limb is still present). Emphasize that phantom limb sensation is typically strongest in the immediate postoperative period and diminishes over time. 3. Provide the following information about postoperative phantom limb pain, including: a. it does not occur in all clients b. it may begin immediately after surgery (especially if the client has been experiencing substantial limb pain preoperatively) but usually starts several weeks postoperatively and disappears gradually over several months to years c. the type of pain experienced varies from client to client and can be similar to pain experienced before the amputation (e.g., stabbing, crushing, cramping, intense burning, and/or electric shock-like sensations) d. it may be triggered by pressure on other body areas e. measures will be implemented to provide effective control of the pain if it occurs. 4. Allow time for questions and clarification of information provided.
2.b. The client will demonstrate the ability to perform recommended activities to prevent postoperative complications.	2.b.1. Refer to Standardized Preoperative Care Plan, Diagnosis 4, action b.1 (p. 101), for instructions on ways to prevent postoperative complications. 2. Provide additional instructions on ways to prevent residual limb contractures resulting from prolonged flexion of the knee or prolonged flexion, hyperextension, abduction, adduction, or external rotation of the hip: a. avoid sitting for long periods b. avoid placing pillows under residual limb c. maintain residual limb in proper alignment d. lie prone several times during the day unless contraindicated (promotes hip extension) e. perform range of motion exercises as instructed. 3. Allow time for questions and clarification of information provided and practice and return demonstration of recommended exercises.
2.c. The client will demonstrate ways to improve strength and facilitate mobility postoperatively.	2.c.1. Instruct client in the following exercises performed to improve strength and facilitate mobility postoperatively: a. range of motion exercises b. strengthening exercises for the upper extremities, chest, residual limb, unaffected lower extremity, and abdominal muscles.

Desired Outcomes	Nursing Actions and Selected Purposes/Rationales
	2. Provide instructions regarding: a. use of overhead trapeze b. transfer techniques c. use of mobility aids (e.g., crutches, cane, walker). 3. Allow time for practice and return demonstration of exercises, transfer techniques, and use of mobility aids.
2.d. The client will verbalize an understanding of the prosthesis and dressings planned.	2.d.1. Reinforce the physician's explanation about the type of prosthesis and dressings planned. 2. If an immediate prosthetic fitting (immediate postoperative prosthesis [IPOP]) is planned, inform client that: a. a rigid dressing (plastic or plaster) will be placed on the residual stump during surgery and the pylon (temporary artificial limb) will attach to the socket that is on the end of this dressing b. in addition to providing a means of securing the pylon, the rigid dressing will help shape the residual limb, reduce edema and support tissue in the surgical area, minimize pain during activity, and promote maturation of the residual limb c. ambulation using the temporary prosthesis usually begins 24–48 hours after surgery and progresses from walking between parallel bars to using ambulatory aids such as a walker, cane, or crutches if needed (ambulatory aids may be needed if client's gait is not steady or only partial weight bearing is allowed as the surgical area heals) d. the rigid dressing will be changed periodically as the residual limb shrinks (the first dressing change usually is done 7–14 days after surgery) e. fitting for a permanent prosthesis will be done when the residual limb size and shape are stable (usually a few months after surgery but may be longer). 3. If there are no plans for an immediate prosthetic fitting, inform client that: a. a soft compression dressing (soft dressing covered by an elastic bandage or sock) will be placed on the residual limb during surgery b. the dressing will help reduce edema and support tissue in the surgical area and shape the stump for future prosthetic fitting if planned c. the elastic bandage or sock will be reapplied if it slips, wrinkles, or loosens d. mobility will be accomplished using a wheelchair, walker, and/or crutches e. fitting for a temporary prosthesis (if planned) will not occur until after the surgical site has healed (usually 3–6 weeks after surgery). 4. Allow time for questions and clarification of information provided.

POSTOPERATIVE

Use in conjunction with the Standardized Postoperative Care Plan.

1. Nursing Diagnosis: ACUTE/CHRONIC PAIN

a. **incisional pain** related to tissue trauma and reflex muscle spasms associated with the amputation, irritation from drainage tube, and stress on surgical area associated with movement;
b. **phantom limb pain** related to altered neural transmission associated with interruption in usual nervous system pathways resulting from the amputation.

Suggested NOC Outcomes:
Pain control; Comfort level

Suggested NIC Interventions: Pain management; Analgesic administration

Desired Outcome	Nursing Actions *and Selected Purposes/Rationales* (see pp. 45–47 for additional rationales)
1. The client will experience diminished pain (see Standardized Postoperative Care Plan, Diagnosis 6 [p. 109], for outcome criteria).	1.a. Refer to Standardized Postoperative Care Plan, Diagnosis 6 (p. 109), for measures related to assessment and management of incisional pain. b. Encourage client to report signs and symptoms of phantom limb pain (e.g., stabbing, cramping, crushing, intense burning, and/or electric shock-like sensations). c. Implement measures *to reduce phantom limb pain if it occurs*: 1. instruct client to apply pressure on residual limb by walking on pylon or pressing limb against a firm surface unless contraindicated 2. consult appropriate health care provider (e.g., physician, pain management specialist) about use of transcutaneous electrical nerve stimulation (TENS), biofeedback, acupuncture, and/or hypnosis 3. encourage participation in diversional activities 4. perform actions to prevent excessive pressure on any area of the body (e.g., position client properly, assist client to turn or reposition self as often as needed) *in order to reduce the risk of triggering or intensifying phantom limb pain* 5. administer the following medications if ordered: a. tricyclic antidepressants (e.g., amitriptyline) *to alter the transmission of pain impulses and/or the client's perception of pain* b. anticonvulsants (e.g., gabapentin, carbamazepine) *to inhibit neurotransmission of pain sensation.*

2. NURSING DIAGNOSIS: ***ACTUAL/RISK FOR IMPAIRED TISSUE INTEGRITY***

related to:
a. disruption of tissue associated with the amputation;
b. delayed wound healing associated with factors such as:
   1. decreased nutritional status
   2. decreased blood supply to wound area resulting from the underlying disease process, edema of the residual limb, and/or excessive or prolonged pressure on operative site (may occur as a result of noncompliance with weight-bearing limitations, improper residual limb wrapping, and/or slippage of the residual limb dressing);
c. irritation of skin associated with contact with wound drainage, pressure from tubings, and use of tape;
d. damage to the skin and/or subcutaneous tissue associated with prolonged pressure on tissues, friction, and/or shearing while mobility is decreased.

Suggested NOC Outcomes:
Wound healing: primary intention; Wound healing: secondary intention; Tissue integrity: skin and mucous membranes

Suggested NIC Interventions: Skin surveillance; Pressure management; Positioning; Wound care; Incision site care; Amputation care

Desired Outcomes	Nursing Actions *and Selected Purposes/Rationales* (see pp. 49–52 for additional rationales)
2.a. The client will experience normal healing of surgical wound (see Standardized Postoperative Care Plan, Diagnosis 10, outcome a [p. 112], for outcome criteria).	2.a.1. Refer to Standardized Postoperative Care Plan, Diagnosis 10, action a (p. 112), for measures related to assessment and promotion of wound healing. 2. Implement additional measures *to promote wound healing*: a. perform actions *to prevent excessive edema* of residual limb: 1. maintain adequate, even pressure on the residual limb (e.g., assist with application of a new rigid dressing if existing one slips or is

Desired Outcomes	**Nursing Actions** *and Selected Purposes/Rationales*
	loose, reapply the elastic bandage or sock of a soft compression dressing if it is wrinkled or slips) 2. elevate the residual limb if ordered (usually ordered for the first 24 hours after surgery and then the limb is placed flat to decrease the risk for hip and knee contractures) 3. instruct client to keep residual limb in an extended rather than dependent position whenever possible (e.g., when in sitting position, use an additional chair to support the limb; keep leg support in a raised position when in wheelchair or recliner; do not hang residual limb over side of bed) b. assess for increasing tightness of the residual limb dressing *(can act as a tourniquet and impede circulation);* assist with reapplication if indicated c. caution client to comply with weight-bearing limitations if prescribed *in order to prevent excessive pressure on wound site.*
2.b. The client will maintain tissue integrity as evidenced by: 1. absence of redness and irritation 2. no skin breakdown.	2.b.1. Inspect the following for pallor, redness, irritation, and breakdown: a. skin areas in contact with wound drainage, tape, and tubings b. back, coccyx, and buttocks c. elbows and remaining heel. 2. Refer to Standardized Postoperative Care Plan, Diagnosis 10, action b.2 (pp. 112–113), for measures related to prevention of tissue irritation or breakdown resulting from contact with wound drainage, tubings, and/or tape. 3. Implement measures *to prevent tissue irritation and breakdown resulting from decreased mobility:* a. assist client to turn at least every 2 hours unless contraindicated b. position client properly; use pressure-reducing or pressure-relieving devices (e.g., pillows, gel or foam cushions, alternating pressure mattress, kinetic bed, air-fluidized bed) if indicated c. instruct client to use overhead trapeze to lift self and shift weight at least every 30 minutes d. gently massage around reddened areas at least every 2 hours e. apply a thin layer of a dry lubricant such as powder or cornstarch to bottom sheet or skin if indicated *to reduce friction* f. lift and move client carefully using a turn sheet and adequate assistance g. limit length of time client is in semi-Fowler's position to 30 minutes *(in this position, client tends to slide down in bed, which can cause skin surface abrasion and shearing)* h. keep client's skin clean i. keep bed linens dry and wrinkle-free j. apply a protective covering such as a hydrocolloid or transparent membrane dressing to areas of the skin susceptible to breakdown (e.g., coccyx, heel, elbows) k. increase activity as allowed and tolerated. 4. Implement measures *to prevent irritation and breakdown of elbows and heel:* a. massage elbows and heel with lotion frequently b. encourage client to use overhead trapeze to move self rather than pushing up with heel and elbows c. provide elbow and heel protectors if indicated. 5. If tissue breakdown occurs: a. notify appropriate health care provider (e.g., wound care specialist, physician) b. perform care of involved area(s) as ordered or per standard hospital procedure.

3. NURSING DIAGNOSIS: *IMPAIRED PHYSICAL MOBILITY*

related to:
a. pain, weakness, and fatigue;
b. depressant effect of anesthesia and some medications (e.g. narcotic [opioid] analgesics);
c. balance difficulties associated with change in the body's center of gravity as a result of loss of a lower limb;
d. inability to control prosthesis;
e. prescribed activity and/or weight-bearing restrictions;
f. fear of falling and compromising surgical wound.

Suggested NOC Outcomes: Balance; Mobility

Suggested NIC Interventions: Exercise therapy: ambulation; Environmental management; Exercise therapy: balance

Desired Outcome	Nursing Actions *and Selected Purposes/Rationales*
3. The client will achieve maximum physical mobility within limitations imposed by the amputation and prescribed activity restrictions.	3.a. Refer to Standardized Postoperative Care Plan, Diagnosis 12 (p. 114), for measures *to increase client's mobility.* b. Implement additional measures *to increase mobility:* 1. perform actions to reduce pain (see Postoperative Diagnosis 1, actions a and c) 2. reinforce physical therapist's instructions on ways to adapt to the body's new center of gravity (e.g., change position slowly) 3. reinforce preoperative instructions about muscle strengthening exercises, transfer and ambulation techniques, and use of ambulatory aids 4. assure client that pylon will provide adequate support during ambulation 5. reinforce prosthetist's instructions about control and use of prosthesis and correct gait technique 6. if only partial weight bearing is allowed or application of a prosthesis is delayed or not planned, assist client with activities to: a. develop standing balance and strength of remaining lower extremity (e.g., knee bends, standing on toes, hopping on the remaining foot while holding on to a chair, balancing on the unoperative leg without support, quadriceps- and gluteal-setting exercises) b. strengthen the residual limb (e.g., quadriceps- and gluteal-setting exercises) c. increase strength of arm and shoulder muscles (e.g., pushups, use of overhead trapeze to move self, flexion and extension of arms holding traction weights or weighted wands, arm pulley exercises) *in order to facilitate use of ambulatory aids* 7. perform actions to prevent falls (see Postoperative Diagnosis 4, actions a and b) *in order to decrease client's fear of injury* 8. assist client with ambulation as soon as allowed (usually 24–48 hours after surgery if client had an immediate prosthetic fitting).

4. NURSING DIAGNOSIS: *RISK FOR FALLS*

related to:
a. weakness and fatigue;
b. dizziness or syncope associated with postural hypotension resulting from peripheral pooling of blood and blood loss during surgery;
c. central nervous system depressant effect of some medications (e.g., narcotic [opioid] analgesics);
d. difficulty with balance, prosthesis control, and transfer and ambulation techniques.

Suggested NOC Outcomes: Falls occurrence; Fall prevention behavior

Suggested NIC Intervention: Fall prevention

Desired Outcome	Nursing Actions *and Selected Purposes/Rationales*
4. The client will not experience falls.	4.a. Refer to Standardized Postoperative Care Plan, Diagnosis 18, action a (p. 120), for measures to prevent falls. b. Implement additional measures *to reduce the risk for falls*: 1. instruct client in and assist with activities to improve standing balance and strength of remaining lower extremity, residual limb, arms, and shoulders (see Postoperative Diagnosis 3, action b.6) 2. reinforce physical therapist's instructions regarding correct transfer and ambulation techniques and proper use of prosthesis and ambulatory aids (e.g., walker, crutches, cane) 3. encourage client to ask for assistance until control of the prosthesis, use of ambulatory aids, and transfer and ambulation techniques are mastered. c. Include client and significant others in planning and implementing measures to prevent falls. d. If client falls, initiate first aid measures if appropriate and notify physician.

5. Collaborative Diagnoses: ***POTENTIAL COMPLICATIONS OF AMPUTATION***

a. **hematoma formation** related to inadequate hemostasis during or following surgical procedure and/or bleeding associated with trauma to the residual limb following surgery;
b. **necrosis of skin flap** related to impaired wound healing and infection if present;
c. **knee and hip contractures on the operative side** related to:
   1. difficulty putting joints through full range of motion associated with decreased mobility, residual limb pain, weakness, and fatigue
   2. prolonged periods of hip flexion associated with increased time in sitting position (especially if prosthesis fitting is delayed or not planned)
   3. improper positioning of residual limb.

Desired Outcomes	Nursing Actions *and Selected Purposes/Rationales*
5.a. The client will not develop a hematoma at the operative site as evidenced by: 1. expected amount of wound drainage 2. no significant increase in swelling and pain in operative area 3. no increase in skin discoloration at surgical site.	5.a.1. Assess for and report signs and symptoms of hematoma formation (e.g., less than expected amount of drainage from wound drain; increased swelling, pain, and/or discoloration in surgical area). 2. Implement measures *to reduce the risk for hematoma formation*: a. maintain patency of drain if present (e.g., keep tubing free of kinks, empty collection device as often as necessary, maintain suction if ordered) b. ensure that residual limb dressing is applied securely *so that adequate pressure is maintained on the vessels in the surgical area in order to control bleeding* c. perform actions *to protect the residual limb from trauma* (e.g., remove pylon from rigid dressing when in bed *[if pylon remains attached, bedding can catch on it and twist the residual limb]*, pad side rails if indicated, assist client with transfer and ambulation as necessary *to reduce the risk for falls*). 3. If signs and symptoms of hematoma formation occur, prepare client for surgical ligation of the bleeding vessels and/or drainage of the hematoma if planned.
5.b. The client will not experience necrosis of the skin flap as evidenced by: 1. skin warm and expected color	5.b.1. Assess for and report signs and symptoms of: a. impaired blood flow in skin flap (e.g., decreased warmth of skin flap, pallor or cyanosis of skin flap, residual limb capillary refill time greater than 3 seconds) b. skin flap necrosis (e.g., pale, cool, darkened skin flap; separation of wound edges; foul odor from flap area).

2. approximated wound edges
3. absence of a foul odor from flap area.

2. Implement measures *to prevent necrosis of the skin flap:*
   a. perform actions to promote wound healing (see Postoperative Diagnosis 2, action a)
   b. perform actions to prevent wound infection (see Standardized Postoperative Care Plan, Diagnosis 17, action b.2 [pp. 118–119]).
3. If necrosis occurs, prepare client for surgical revision of the skin flap if planned.

5.c. The client will not develop knee and hip contractures on the operative side as evidenced by the ability to move joints through their full range of motion.

5.c.1. Assess client for and report development of knee and hip contractures on the operative side (e.g., inability to fully extend knee; inability to extend, adduct, or internally rotate residual limb).
2. Implement measures *to prevent knee and/or hip contractures on the operative side:*
   a. if residual limb elevation is ordered postoperatively, place bed in Trendelenburg position unless contraindicated rather than placing limb on pillows
   b. turn client to prone position several times daily unless contraindicated *in order to promote hip extension*; place a pillow under abdomen and residual limb *to maintain hip extension and stretch flexor muscles*
   c. place trochanter roll or sandbag along outer aspect of thigh on operative side when client is in a supine or Fowler's position *to prevent external rotation of hip*
   d. encourage client to keep knee straight when lying or sitting; avoid use of knee gatch and pillows under knee
   e. limit time that client is in high Fowler's or sitting position (usually no longer than 1 hour at a time)
   f. perform actions to increase client's mobility (see Postoperative Diagnosis 3)
   g. perform actions to reduce pain (see Postoperative Diagnosis 1, actions a and c) *in order to reduce the risk of client flexing residual limb in response to pain.*
3. If contractures develop, assist with rehabilitative efforts to improve range of motion of knee and hip.

6. NURSING DIAGNOSIS: ***DISTURBED SELF-CONCEPT****

related to change in appearance, mobility, usual lifestyle and roles, and level of independence associated with the amputation.

---

*This diagnostic label includes the nursing diagnoses of disturbed body image, low self-esteem, and ineffective role performance.

Suggested NOC Outcomes: Body image; Personal autonomy; Self-esteem; Psychosocial adjustment: life change

Suggested NIC Interventions: Body image enhancement; Grief work facilitation; Self-esteem enhancement; Role enhancement; Counseling; Emotional support; Support system enhancement

Desired Outcome	**Nursing Actions** *and Selected Purposes/Rationales* (see pp. 47–49 for additional rationales)

6. The client will demonstrate beginning adaptation to changes in appearance, mobility, level of independence, body functioning, lifestyle, and roles as evidenced by:
   a. verbalization of feelings of self-worth

6.a. Assess for signs and symptoms of a disturbed self-concept (e.g., verbalization of negative feelings about self, withdrawal from significant others, lack of participation in activities of daily living, refusal to look at or touch the residual limb, lack of plan for adapting to necessary changes in lifestyle).
b. Stay with client during the first dressing change *to provide support as he/she views the residual limb for the first time.*
c. Discuss with client the availability of a natural-looking prosthesis.

Desired Outcome	Nursing Actions *and Selected Purposes/Rationales*
b. maintenance of relationships with significant others c. active participation in activities of daily living d. verbalization of a beginning plan for adapting lifestyle to changes resulting from the amputation.	d. Clarify misconceptions about future limitations on physical activity. Emphasize that a high level of mobility can be achieved with a prosthesis in place and/or use of crutches, walker, or cane. e. Encourage client's participation in activities that can assist him/her to integrate physical changes that have occurred (e.g., exercise, bathing, wrapping residual limb). f. Demonstrate acceptance of client using techniques such as touch and frequent visits. Encourage significant others to do the same. g. Avoid referring to the residual limb as a 'stump' unless that is a term the client prefers. h. Support behaviors suggesting positive adaptation to the amputation (e.g., willingness to care for residual limb, compliance with treatment plan, verbalization of feelings of self-worth, maintenance of relationships with significant others). i. Encourage significant others to allow client to do what he/she is able *so that independence can be re-established and/or self-esteem redeveloped.* j. Encourage client contact with others *so that he/she can test and establish a new self-image.* k. Assist client's and significant others' adjustment by listening, facilitating communication, and providing information. l. Assist client and significant others to have similar expectations and understanding of future lifestyle and to identify ways that personal and family goals can be adjusted rather than abandoned. m. Encourage visits and support from significant others. n. Encourage client to continue involvement in social activities and to pursue usual roles and interests. If previous roles, interests, and hobbies cannot be pursued, encourage development of new ones. o. If acceptable to client, arrange for a visit with an individual who has successfully adjusted to the loss of a limb. p. Provide information about and encourage utilization of community agencies and support groups (e.g., National Amputation Foundation; vocational rehabilitation; family, individual, and/or financial counseling). q. Consult appropriate health care provider (e.g., psychiatric nurse clinician, physician) if client seems unwilling or unable to adapt to changes resulting from the amputation.

Discharge Teaching/Continued Care

7. Nursing Diagnosis: *DEFICIENT KNOWLEDGE, INEFFECTIVE THERAPEUTIC REGIMEN MANAGEMENT, OR INEFFECTIVE HEALTH MAINTENANCE**

*The nurse should select the diagnostic label that is most appropriate for the client's discharge teaching needs.

Suggested NOC Outcomes: Knowledge: fall prevention; Knowledge: prescribed activity; Knowledge: treatment regimen

Suggested NIC Interventions: Health system guidance; Teaching: individual; Teaching: prescribed activity/exercise

Desired Outcomes	Nursing Actions *and Selected Purposes/Rationales*
7.a. The client will demonstrate appropriate ways to prevent contractures, increase strength, and improve mobility.	7.a.1. Instruct client in the following ways to prevent contractures, increase strength, and/or improve mobility: a. performing range of motion exercises of residual limb and other extremities b. lying prone several times a day with pillow under abdomen and residual limb (maintains hip extension and stretches flexor muscles)

c. performing knee bends, standing on toes, balancing on the unoperative leg without support, and performing quadriceps- and gluteal-setting exercises
d. performing pushups, flexion and extension of arms holding weights, and arm pulley exercises (facilitates use of ambulatory aids).
2. Allow time for questions, clarification, and return demonstration.

7.b. The client will demonstrate correct transfer and ambulation techniques and proper use of ambulatory aids.

7.b.1. Reinforce instructions about correct transfer and ambulation techniques, amount of weight bearing allowed, and proper use of ambulatory aids (e.g. crutches, walker, cane).
2. Allow time for questions, clarification, practice, and return demonstration.

7.c. The client will identify ways to maintain health of the remaining lower extremity.

7.c.1. Instruct client in ways to maintain health of the remaining lower extremity:
a. wear a well-fitting shoe to protect foot from pressure and trauma (shoe should be modified by an orthotist to ensure that body weight is evenly distributed when prosthesis is used)
b. perform foot and nail care using appropriate technique
c. avoid breaks in the skin to reduce risk of infection
d. stop smoking
e. avoid sitting with legs crossed and wearing socks, stockings, or garters that are tight in order to reduce the risk of compromising peripheral blood flow
f. adhere to regular follow-up care if diabetes or peripheral vascular disease was a factor leading to the need for amputation.
2. Allow time for questions and clarification of information provided.

7.d. The client will demonstrate the ability to care for the residual limb.

7.d.1. Instruct client in ways to care for the residual limb while dressing is in place:
a. if client has a soft compression dressing (soft dressing covered by an elastic bandage or sock) over the residual limb:
1. demonstrate the technique for rewrapping or changing the elastic bandage or sock; explain that physician may want this to be done routinely during the day and that it should also be done if the dressing slips or the elastic bandage or sock becomes soiled or wrinkled
2. demonstrate the technique for changing the dressing if client is expected to do this following discharge
b. if client has a rigid dressing over the residual limb:
1. stress the importance of removing the pylon when in bed to reduce the risk of twisting the residual limb
2. explain that the dressing should be positioned securely before applying the pylon (a belt may be needed to maintain the proper position of the rigid dressing during ambulation)
3. caution client to adhere to weight-bearing restrictions until the surgical area heals completely.
2. Inform client about expected care of the residual limb once the dressings are no longer needed:
a. the residual limb will need to be inspected daily using a hand mirror if necessary to check for skin irritation and breakdown
b. the residual limb will need to be washed and patted dry daily
c. emollients and powders should not be applied to the residual limb.
3. Allow time for questions, clarification, and return demonstration.

7.e. The client will verbalize how to care for the prosthesis and residual limb if a permanent prosthesis is planned.

7.e.1. Provide the client with information about anticipated care of the prosthesis and residual limb if a permanent prosthesis is planned:
a. after the incision heals, the residual limb should be toughened by massaging it, pushing it against a firm surface, and/or pulling on it with a hand-held towel (a toughened limb is more resistant to irritation and breakdown from the constant pressure exerted on it by the prosthesis)

Desired Outcomes	**Nursing Actions** *and Selected Purposes/Rationales*
	b. a residual limb sock should be worn next to the skin to reduce friction between residual limb and the socket c. only residual limb socks recommended by the prosthetist should be used; socks should be changed daily, laundered gently in cool water with a mild soap, and laid flat to dry d. worn or damaged residual limb socks should be replaced rather than mended e. a prosthetist should examine the prosthesis on a regular basis and monitor the fit of the socket so that repairs and adjustments can be made when necessary (e.g., as the residual limb continues to shrink, if a weight loss or gain of 5 to 10 pounds occurs) f. the socket should be cleansed daily with a damp cloth and dried thoroughly g. care should be taken to keep the leather or metal components of the prosthesis dry h. shoes worn with the prosthesis should be in good repair to maintain a steady, even gait and avoid damage to the prosthesis i. if skin breakdown occurs, the prosthesis should not be worn until the area has been checked by physician and/or prosthetist j. the prosthesis should be applied on arising and worn for the prescribed length of time to prevent residual limb edema k. an elastic sock may need to be worn over the residual limb whenever the prosthesis is removed (the sock helps prevent edema of the residual limb and subsequent difficulty in reapplication of the prosthesis). 2. Allow time for questions and clarification of information provided.
7.f. The client will identify ways to manage phantom limb pain if it occurs.	7.f.1. Instruct client in ways to manage phantom limb pain if it occurs: a. apply intermittent pressure to residual limb by walking on pylon or pressing the limb against a firm surface b. participate in diversional activities c. take medications (e.g., amitriptyline, gabapentin, carbamazepine) as prescribed. 2. Encourage client to consult appropriate health care provider about the use of therapies such as transcutaneous nerve stimulation, biofeedback, acupuncture, and hypnosis to assist in pain control if indicated. 3. Reassure client that phantom limb pain usually disappears but caution him/her that it may take months to years.
7.g. The client will state signs and symptoms to report to the health care provider.	7.g.1. Refer to Standardized Postoperative Care Plan, Diagnosis 22, action c (p. 125), for signs and symptoms to report to the health care provider. 2. Instruct client to report these additional signs and symptoms: a. development of and/or persistent phantom limb pain b. persistent or increased residual limb swelling c. difficulty with full extension of residual limb d. inability to maintain balance e. difficulty controlling prosthesis f. change in color of residual limb (e.g., pallor, cyanosis, duskiness) g. persistent slippage or increased tightness of elastic bandage or sock h. loosening of rigid dressing.
7.h. The client will identify community resources that can assist with home management and adjustment to changes resulting from the amputation.	7.h.1. Provide information about community resources that can assist the client and significant others with home management and adjustment to changes resulting from the amputation (e.g., home health agency; social services; individual, family, and occupational counseling; amputee support groups; National Amputation Foundation). 2. Initiate a referral if indicated.

7.i. The client will verbalize an understanding of and a plan for adhering to recommended follow-up care including future appointments with health care provider, prosthetist, and physical therapist; medications prescribed; and activity level.

7.i.1. Refer to Standardized Postoperative Care Plan, Diagnosis 22 (pp. 125–126), for routine postoperative instructions and measures to improve client compliance.
2. Emphasize the importance of adhering to prescribed weight-bearing restrictions and exercise program.

ADDITIONAL NURSING DIAGNOSIS

*GRIEVING**

related to the loss of a limb and changes in body image and usual lifestyle and roles.

*See Unit II for outcomes, actions, and rationales.

Bibliography

See pages 879 and 885.

evolve

Fractured Hip with Internal Fixation or Prosthesis Insertion

A fractured hip is the term used to describe a fracture of the proximal end of the femur. Hip fractures are classified according to the specific location of the fracture. A common classification system divides hip fractures into three types: femoral neck fractures (also referred to as intracapsular fractures), intertrochanteric fractures, and subtrochanteric fractures (the latter two types are sometimes referred to as extracapsular fractures).

A fractured hip is one of the most common orthopedic injuries in the elderly because of the increased incidence of osteoporosis and falls in the elderly population. Although a fractured hip can be treated by traction, the preferred treatment is surgery because it allows earlier mobility. Surgery involves insertion of a femoral head prosthesis or reduction and internal fixation of the fracture with an intramedullary fixation device, cannulated screws, or a dynamic compression hip screw with a plate assembly. Internal fixation with preservation of the femoral head is the preferred treatment for hip fractures, but the femoral head and neck can be replaced with a prosthetic device (e.g., Austin Moore prosthesis) if an intracapsular fracture has occurred and factors are present that increase the risk for avascular necrosis and/or nonunion. Ideally, surgery is performed within 12–24 hours after the injury, especially if the client has a displaced femoral neck. During the preoperative period, traction is usually applied to stabilize and reduce the fracture and reduce muscle spasms and pain.

This care plan focuses on the elderly adult client who is hospitalized for surgical repair of a hip fracture. Much of the postoperative information is applicable to clients receiving follow-up care in an extended care facility or home setting.

OUTCOME/DISCHARGE CRITERIA

THE CLIENT WILL:

- have evidence of normal healing of the surgical wound
- have clear, audible breath sounds throughout lungs
- have expected level of mobility
- have adequate fracture reduction and healing
- have hip pain controlled
- have no signs and symptoms of infection or postoperative complications
- demonstrate correct transfer and ambulation techniques and proper use of ambulatory aids
- demonstrate the ability to correctly perform the prescribed exercises
- verbalize an understanding of activity and position restrictions necessary to prevent dislocation of the prosthesis or internal fixation device
- identify ways to reduce the risk of falls in the home environment
- share thoughts and feelings about the need to transfer to or remain in an extended care or assisted living facility
- state signs and symptoms to report to the health care provider
- identify community resources that can assist with home management and provide transportation
- verbalize an understanding of and a plan for adhering to recommended follow-up care including future appointments with health care provider and physical therapist, medications prescribed, activity level, and wound care.

NURSING/COLLABORATIVE DIAGNOSES

NURSING/COLLABORATIVE DIAGNOSES

5. Risk for falls p. 778
6. Potential complications p. 778
   a. hypovolemic shock
   b. dislocation of prosthesis or internal fixation device
   c. thromboembolism
   d. fat embolism syndrome (FES)
   e. avascular necrosis
   f. delayed healing of the fractured bone
7. Grieving p. 781

DISCHARGE TEACHING

8. Deficient knowledge, Ineffective therapeutic regimen management, or Ineffective health maintenance p. 782

See Standardized Preoperative and Postoperative Care Plans (pp. 97–126) for additional diagnoses.

PREOPERATIVE

Use in conjunction with the Standardized Preoperative Care Plan.

1. NURSING DIAGNOSIS: FEAR/ANXIETY

related to:
a. severe pain;
b. lack of understanding of traction device and planned surgical procedure;
c. unfamiliar environment and separation from significant others;
d. anticipated postoperative discomfort and loss of control associated with the effects of anesthesia;
e. financial concerns associated with hospitalization;
f. potential embarrassment or loss of dignity associated with body exposure;
g. possibility of changes in usual lifestyle, permanent disability, or death.

Suggested NOC Outcomes: Anxiety self-control; Anxiety level; Fear level; Fear self-control

Suggested NIC Interventions: Anxiety reduction; Calming technique; Emotional support; Presence

Desired Outcome	**Nursing Actions** *and Selected Purposes/Rationales* (see pp. 14–16 for additional rationales)
1. The client will experience a reduction in fear and anxiety (see Standardized Preoperative Care Plan, Diagnosis 1 [pp. 97–98], for outcome criteria).	1.a. Refer to Standardized Preoperative Care Plan, Diagnosis 1 (pp. 97–98), for measures related to assessment and reduction of fear and anxiety. b. Implement additional measures *to reduce fear and anxiety:* 1. perform actions to reduce pain (see Preoperative Diagnosis 2, action d) 2. explain the purpose of traction and how it works 3. reassure client that modern treatment methods for a fractured hip have significantly reduced permanent disability and death rates; inform client that he/she will probably begin ambulation by the 2nd postoperative day.

2. NURSING DIAGNOSIS: ACUTE PAIN: HIP

related to fracture of the bone, tissue trauma, and muscle spasms.

Suggested NOC Outcomes: Comfort level; Pain control

Suggested NIC Interventions: Analgesic administration; Pain management; Environmental management: comfort

Desired Outcome	Nursing Actions *and Selected Purposes/Rationales* (see pp. 45–47 for additional rationales)
2. The client will experience diminished hip pain as evidenced by: a. verbalization of a reduction in pain b. relaxed facial expression and body positioning c. stable vital signs.	2.a. Assess for signs and symptoms of pain (e.g., verbalization of pain, grimacing, reluctance to move, clutching hip or thigh, restlessness, diaphoresis, increased B/P, tachycardia). b. Assess client's perception of the severity of pain using a pain intensity rating scale. c. Assess the client's pain pattern (e.g., location, quality, onset, duration, precipitating factors, aggravating factors, alleviating factors). d. Implement measures *to reduce pain*: 1. perform actions *to reduce fear and anxiety about the pain experience* (e.g. assure client that his/her need for pain relief is understood, plan methods for achieving pain control with client) 2. perform actions to reduce fear and anxiety (see Preoperative Diagnosis 1) *in order to promote relaxation and subsequently increase the client's threshold and tolerance for pain* 3. administer analgesics before activities and procedures that can cause pain and before pain becomes severe 4. perform actions to promote rest (e.g., minimize environmental activity and noise, limit the number of visitors and their length of stay) *in order to reduce fatigue and subsequently increase the client's threshold and tolerance for pain* 5. perform actions *to maintain effective traction on the injured extremity* (client is usually placed in Buck's traction preoperatively *to stabilize and reduce the fracture and reduce muscle spasms and pain*): a. ensure that weights are hanging freely b. do not allow footplate or ropes to rest on end of bed c. keep affected heel off bed d. keep knots away from pulley device e. do not remove traction unless specifically ordered f. do not lift the weights in order to facilitate moving the client or performing other care *(this reduces traction pull and can cause severe muscle spasm)* g. limit head of bed elevation to 20–25° except for meals and toileting *in order to maintain the prescribed traction force* 6. avoid bumping the traction device 7. place a trochanter roll or sandbag firmly against the lateral aspect of injured hip and upper thigh (should extend from iliac crest to midthigh) *in order to maintain leg in proper alignment* 8. consult physician if extremity appears out of alignment; do not attempt to realign extremity *(an attempt to realign the extremity may cause further tissue trauma)* 9. move client carefully, keeping injured extremity well supported 10. if turning is allowed, place pillow between legs before turning *in order to prevent adduction and further strain on the fracture site* 11. provide or assist with additional nonpharmacologic measures for pain relief (e.g., relaxation exercises; diversional activities such as watching television, reading, or conversing) 12. administer analgesics and muscle relaxants if ordered. e. Consult appropriate health care provider (e.g., physician, pharmacist, pain management specialist) if above measures fail to provide adequate pain relief.

3. Nursing Diagnosis:

RISK FOR PERIPHERAL NEUROVASCULAR DYSFUNCTION: FRACTURED EXTREMITY

related to trauma to or excessive pressure on the nerves or blood vessels as a result of the injury; displaced bone fragments; blood accumulation and edema at fracture site; and improper alignment, application of skin traction device, or traction on the injured extremity.

Suggested NOC Outcome:
Tissue perfusion: peripheral

Suggested NIC Interventions: Circulatory care: arterial insufficiency; Circulatory care: venous insufficiency; Lower extremity monitoring; Positioning; Pressure management; Traction/Immobilization care

Desired Outcome	Nursing Actions *and Selected Purposes/Rationales*
3. The client will maintain normal neurovascular function in the injured extremity as evidenced by: a. palpable pedal pulses b. capillary refill time in toes less than 2–3 seconds c. extremity warm and usual color d. ability to flex and extend knee, foot, and toes e. absence of numbness and tingling in leg and foot f. no increase in pain in extremity or buttock.	3.a. Assess for and report signs and symptoms of neurovascular dysfunction in the injured extremity: 1. diminished or absent pedal pulses 2. capillary refill time in toes greater than 2–3 seconds 3. pallor, cyanosis, or coolness of the extremity 4. inability to flex or extend knee, foot, or toes 5. numbness or tingling in leg or foot 6. increased pain in extremity or buttock (new or increased pain that occurs during passive movement is a symptom of compartment syndrome). b. Implement measures *to prevent neurovascular dysfunction in injured extremity:* 1. maintain traction as ordered 2. place a trochanter roll or sandbag firmly against lateral aspect of injured hip and upper thigh (should extend from the iliac crest to midthigh) *in order to help maintain proper alignment* 3. do not attempt to realign injured leg unless specifically ordered (*an attempt to align extremity may cause further trauma to the nerves and blood vessels)* 4. make sure skin traction device (e.g., elastic wraps, foam boot with Velcro strap) is applied properly (if necessary to reapply, obtain assistance *so that one person can maintain traction on the leg during the reapplication process)* 5. make sure that excessive or prolonged pressure is not exerted on Achilles tendon and medial and lateral aspects of knee and ankle 6. do not turn client on injured side unless specifically ordered *(may cause further displacement of fracture and decrease blood flow to area).* c. If signs and symptoms of neurovascular dysfunction occur: 1. assess for and correct improper positioning of the injured extremity and traction device and external cause of excessive pressure 2. notify physician if the signs and symptoms persist or worsen 3. prepare client for surgical intervention (e.g. internal fixation, insertion of hip prosthesis).

POSTOPERATIVE

Use in conjunction with the Standardized Postoperative Care Plan.

1. NURSING DIAGNOSIS: *RISK FOR PERIPHERAL NEUROVASCULAR DYSFUNCTION: OPERATIVE EXTREMITY*

related to trauma to or excessive pressure on the nerves or blood vessels as a result of surgery and the initial injury, blood accumulation and edema in the surgical area, improper alignment of operative extremity, tight or improperly positioned abductor device straps, or dislocation of prosthesis or internal fixation device.

Suggested NOC Outcome:
Tissue perfusion: peripheral

Suggested NIC Interventions: Circulatory care: arterial insufficiency; Circulatory care: venous insufficiency; Positioning; Lower extremity monitoring; Pressure management; Heat/Cold application

Desired Outcome	Nursing Actions *and Selected Purposes/Rationales*
1. The client will maintain normal neurovascular function in the operative extremity (see Preoperative Diagnosis 3, for outcome criteria).	1.a. Assess for signs and symptoms of neurovascular dysfunction in the operative extremity (see Preoperative Diagnosis 3, action a, for signs and symptoms). b. Implement measures *to prevent neurovascular dysfunction in the operative extremity:* 1. maintain extremity in proper alignment

Desired Outcome	Nursing Actions *and Selected Purposes/Rationales*
	2. perform actions to prevent dislocation of prosthesis or internal fixation device (see Postoperative Diagnosis 6, action b.2) 3. make sure that straps on abductor device are not too tight and are not exerting pressure on the popliteal space, lateral calf immediately below the knee, and lateral malleolus 4. apply ice pack or cooling pad to operative hip if ordered *to reduce edema*; remove ice if signs and symptoms of compartment syndrome (e.g., deep, throbbing, unrelenting pain; pain in buttock or thigh with passive movement of the hip or knee) are present. c. If signs and symptoms of neurovascular dysfunction occur: 1. assess for and correct improperly applied or tight straps on abductor device and improper positioning of operative extremity; do not attempt to realign extremity if extreme rotation has occurred 2. notify physician if the signs and symptoms persist or worsen 3. prepare client for closed reduction or return to surgery if planned.

2. Nursing Diagnosis: ***ACUTE PAIN: HIP***

related to tissue trauma and reflex muscle spasms associated with the initial injury, surgery, and strain on the area postoperatively.

Suggested NOC Outcomes: Comfort level; Pain control

Suggested NIC Interventions: Analgesic administration; Pain management; Environmental management: comfort; Heat/Cold application

Desired Outcome	Nursing Actions *and Selected Purposes/Rationales* (see pp. 45–47 for additional rationales)
2. The client will experience diminished hip pain (see Standardized Postoperative Care Plan, Diagnosis 6 [p. 109], for outcome criteria).	2.a. Refer to Standardized Postoperative Care Plan, Diagnosis 6 (p. 109), for measures related to assessment and reduction of pain. b. Implement additional measures *to reduce pain in operative extremity:* 1. adhere to position, activity, and weight-bearing restrictions identified in Postoperative Diagnosis 6, actions b.2.b–g *in order to reduce pain associated with strain on the surgical site* 2. move the operative extremity gently 3. apply ice pack or cooling pad to operative hip if ordered.

3. Nursing Diagnosis: ***IMPAIRED PHYSICAL MOBILITY***

related to:

a. pain and weakness in weight-bearing extremity associated with the fracture and subsequent surgical repair;
b. prescribed activity and weight-bearing restrictions following internal fixation or prosthesis insertion;
c. generalized weakness associated with surgery;
d. depressant effect of anesthesia and some medications (e.g. narcotic [opioid] analgesics, centrally acting muscle relaxants, some antiemetics);
e. fear of falling, moving operative hip improperly, and compromising surgical wound.

Suggested NOC Outcome: Mobility

Suggested NIC Interventions: Exercise therapy: joint mobility; Exercise therapy: muscle control; Exercise therapy: ambulation

Desired Outcome	Nursing Actions *and Selected Purposes/Rationales*
3. The client will achieve maximum physical mobility within prescribed activity and weight-bearing restrictions.	3.a. Refer to Standardized Postoperative Care Plan, Diagnosis 12 (p. 114), for measures to increase client's mobility. b. Implement additional measures *to increase client's mobility:* 1. perform actions to reduce pain (see Postoperative Diagnosis 2)

2. instruct client in and assist with quadriceps- and gluteal-setting exercises *to strengthen muscles needed for ambulation*
3. encourage client to use overhead trapeze to move self *in order to strengthen arm and shoulder muscles needed for proper use of ambulatory aids*
4. reinforce physical therapist's instructions regarding muscle strengthening exercises, transfer and ambulation techniques, and use of ambulatory aids
5. perform actions to prevent falls (see Postoperative Diagnosis 5, actions a and b) *in order to decrease client's fear of injury*
6. assist client with ambulation as soon as allowed (usually by the 2nd postoperative day).

c. Consult appropriate health care provider (e.g., physician, physical therapist) if client is unable to achieve expected level of mobility.

4. NURSING DIAGNOSIS: *RISK FOR INFECTION*

related to:

a. stasis of pulmonary secretions associated with decreased mobility and weak cough effort (an increased risk with elderly clients);
b. wound contamination associated with introduction of pathogens during or following surgery (risk is increased because of close proximity of wound to perineal area);
c. decreased resistance to infection associated with factors such as an inadequate nutritional status and decreased effectiveness of immune system if client is elderly;
d. increased growth and colonization of microorganisms in the urine associated with urinary stasis if mobility is decreased and introduction of pathogens if indwelling catheter is present.

Suggested NOC Outcomes: Immune status; Infection severity

Suggested NIC Interventions: Infection protection; Infection control; Incision site care

Desired Outcome	**Nursing Actions** *and Selected Purposes/Rationales* (see pp. 37–40 for additional rationales)
4. The client will remain free of infection as evidenced by: a. absence of fever and chills b. pulse within normal limits c. normal breath sounds d. usual mental status e. cough productive of clear mucus only f. voiding clear urine without reports of frequency, urgency, and burning g. absence of redness, heat, and swelling around wound h. usual drainage from wound i. no new or increased discomfort in hip j. sedimentation rate and WBC and differential counts returning toward normal range k. negative results of cultured specimens.	4.a. Refer to Standardized Postoperative Care Plan, Diagnosis 17 (pp. 118–119), for measures related to assessment and prevention of infection. b. Assess for and report additional signs and symptoms that may be indicative of wound infection or osteomyelitis: 1. elevated sedimentation rate 2. reports of increased discomfort. c. Maintain patency of wound drainage system if present (e.g. prevent kinking of tubing, keep collection device below surgical wound, keep suction device compressed) *to prevent the accumulation of drainage and subsequent colonization of pathogens in the surgical area.* d. If signs and symptoms of wound infection or osteomyelitis occur: 1. administer antimicrobials as ordered 2. prepare client for drainage of wound if planned.

5. Nursing Diagnosis: RISK FOR FALLS

related to:
a. weakness, fatigue, and postural hypotension associated with the effects of major surgery and physiological changes that may have occurred if client is elderly;
b. central nervous system depressant effect of some medications (e.g., narcotic [opioid] analgesics, centrally acting muscle relaxants, some antiemetics);
c. weakness and pain in weight-bearing extremity associated with the initial injury and surgery on the hip;
d. difficulty with transfer and ambulation techniques.

Suggested NOC Outcome:
Fall prevention behavior;
Falls occurence

Suggested NIC Intervention: Fall prevention

Desired Outcome	**Nursing Actions** *and Selected Purposes/Rationales*
5. The client will not experience falls.	5.a. Refer to Standardized Postoperative Care Plan, Diagnosis 18, action a (p. 120), for measures to prevent falls. b. Implement additional measures *to reduce the risk for falls*: 1. perform actions *to assist client to increase muscle strength*: a. instruct and encourage client to perform isometric quadriceps- and gluteal-setting exercises b. encourage client to use the overhead trapeze to lift self *(strengthens arm and shoulder muscles, which will facilitate use of ambulatory aids)* 2. reinforce physical therapist's instructions regarding correct transfer and ambulation techniques and proper use of ambulatory aids (e.g., walker) 3. administer prescribed analgesics before exercise and ambulation sessions *in order to reduce hip pain and subsequently maximize client's ability to utilize proper transfer and ambulation techniques.* c. Include client and significant others in planning and implementing measures to prevent falls. d. If client falls, initiate first aid measures if appropriate and notify physician.

6. Collaborative Diagnoses: POTENTIAL COMPLICATIONS

a. **hypovolemic shock** related to excessive bleeding associated with fracture of the proximal femur (bones are quite vascular) and intraoperative and postoperative blood loss;
b. **dislocation of prosthesis or internal fixation device** related to improper movement or positioning of operative extremity, noncompliance with weight-bearing limitations, delayed healing of the fracture, or infection of the bone or surrounding tissue;
c. **thromboembolism** related to:
   1. venous stasis associated with increased blood viscosity (can result from deficient fluid volume), decreased mobility, and pressure exerted on blood vessels by abductor device
   2. hypercoagulability associated with increased release of tissue thromboplastin into the blood (occurs as a result of surgical trauma) and hemoconcentration and increased blood viscosity (can occur as a result of deficient fluid volume)
   3. trauma to vein walls during surgery;
d. **fat embolism syndrome** (FES) related to release of fat globules from the bone marrow and injured surrounding tissue into the bloodstream associated with fracture of a long bone and subsequent surgery on the bone;
e. **avascular necrosis** related to an inadequate blood supply to the bone (occurs primarily following intracapsular fractures);
f. **delayed healing of the fractured bone** (with eventual nonunion) related to inadequate reduction and internal fixation of fracture, diminished blood

supply to fracture site, thin or absent periosteum in neck of femur (decreases the healing potential), inadequate nutritional status, preexisting osteoporosis, or development of infection in the fractured bone and/or surrounding tissue.

Desired Outcomes	**Nursing Actions** *and Selected Purposes/Rationales*
6.a. The client will not develop hypovolemic shock (see Standardized Postoperative Care Plan, Diagnosis 20, outcome a [p. 122] for outcome criteria).	6.a. Refer to Standardized Postoperative Care Plan, Diagnosis 20, action a (p. 122), for measures related to assessment, prevention, and management of hypovolemic shock.
6.b. The client will not experience dislocation of the prosthesis or internal fixation device as evidenced by: 1. continued resolution of hip pain 2. ability to maintain operative leg in proper alignment 3. length of operative leg equal to unoperative leg 4. ability to adhere to exercise and ambulation regimen 5. normal neurovascular status in operative leg.	6.b.1. Assess for and report signs and symptoms of dislocation of the hip prosthesis or internal fixation device: a. sudden, severe pain in operative hip b. significant (greater than 10°) external rotation of the operative leg c. operative leg more than 2.5 cm (1 inch) shorter than unoperative leg d. sudden inability to participate in usual exercise and ambulation regimen e. decline in neurovascular status in operative leg. 2. Implement measures *to reduce the risk for dislocation of the prosthesis or internal fixation device:* a. perform actions to promote healing of the fracture (see action e.2 in this diagnosis) b. perform actions *to prevent adduction of the operative extremity:* 1. keep 2–3 pillows or abductor device between legs at all times 2. remind client not to cross legs 3. do not move operative extremity past midline c. maintain the operative extremity in proper alignment d. maintain restrictions on head of bed elevation if ordered (some physicians order a 45–60° maximum elevation for the first few days after surgery) *to reduce hip flexion* e. perform actions *to prevent extreme (beyond 90°) hip flexion:* 1. instruct client not to lean forward to reach objects on end of bed or on floor or to put on slippers, socks, or shoes 2. raise the entire bed to client's midthigh level before he/she gets in or out of bed *in order to reduce the degree of hip flexion that occurs when client sits on edge of bed* 3. provide a high, firm chair (or elevate sitting surface with pillows) and an elevated toilet seat for client's use *in order to reduce degree of hip flexion when client sits down* 4. do not elevate operative leg when sitting in chair f. maintain restrictions on turning (usually allowed to turn on unoperative side only) and always turn client with pillows between legs g. reinforce weight-bearing limitations ordered (partial weight bearing is usually allowed as soon as ambulation is started following prosthesis insertion; weight-bearing restrictions vary following internal fixation depending on the stability of the fracture reduction and fixation) h. perform actions to prevent and treat wound infection and osteomyelitis (see Standardized Postoperative Care Plan, Diagnosis 17, action b.2 [pp. 118–119] and Postoperative Diagnosis 4, actions c and d). 3. If signs and symptoms of dislocation of prosthesis or internal fixation device occur: a. maintain client on bed rest b. prepare client for x-rays of surgical area c. prepare client for closed reduction or surgical repair of the dislocation if planned.

Desired Outcomes	**Nursing Actions** *and Selected Purposes/Rationales*
6.c. The client will not develop a deep vein thrombus or pulmonary embolism (see Standardized Postoperative Care Plan, Diagnosis 20, outcomes c.1 and 2 [pp. 122–123], for outcome criteria).	6.c.1. Refer to Standardized Postoperative Care Plan, Diagnosis 20, actions c.1 and 2 (pp. 122–123), for measures related to assessment, prevention, and treatment of a deep vein thrombus and pulmonary embolism. 2. Implement additional measures *to prevent thrombus formation:* a. make sure that straps on abductor device do not exert excessive pressure on any area b. make sure that antiembolism stockings are applied correctly and that intermittent pneumatic compression device is correctly applied and functioning properly c. encourage client to perform active foot exercises every 1–2 hours while awake; provide adequate analgesia *to promote client compliance* d. administer anticoagulants (e.g., low-dose warfarin, low-molecular-weight heparin) or antiplatelet agents (e.g., aspirin) if ordered e. assist client with ambulation as soon as allowed.
6.d. The client will not experience fat embolism syndrome as evidenced by: 1. usual mental status 2. unlabored respirations at 12–20/minute 3. absence of petechiae 4. Pao_2 within normal limits.	6.d.1. Assess for and report signs and symptoms of fat embolism syndrome (usually occurs within 72 hours after the injury): a. restlessness, apprehension, confusion b. sudden onset of dyspnea c. tachypnea d. elevated pulse and temperature e. petechiae on the chest, neck, or axilla f. low Pao_2 level g. unexpected decrease in Hct and Hgb h. thrombocytopenia. 2. Minimize movement of the fractured extremity during the first few days after the injury *to reduce the risk for fat emboli.* 3. If signs and symptoms of fat embolism syndrome occur: a. maintain client on bed rest and move fractured extremity as little as possible *to prevent further emboli* b. administer oxygen and assist with positive airway pressure techniques (e.g., positive end expiratory pressure) if ordered c. prepare client for chest x-ray or lung scan d. administer intravenous fluids as ordered *to help maintain adequate perfusion to vital organs and prevent shock* e. administer corticosteroids if ordered *to reduce cerebral edema and pulmonary inflammation.*
6.e. The client will not experience avascular necrosis or delayed healing of the fracture as evidenced by: 1. resolution of hip pain 2. expected progression in prescribed physical therapy program 3. radiology reports showing evidence of normal stages of bone healing.	6.e.1. Assess for and report signs and symptoms of avascular necrosis and/or delayed healing of the fracture: a. persistent hip pain b. limited range of motion of operative leg c. inability to make expected progress in physical therapy program d. radiology reports showing delayed healing of fracture. 2. Implement measures *to promote healing of the fracture:* a. maintain operative leg in proper alignment b. maintain restrictions on weight bearing as ordered c. maintain an adequate nutritional status (see Standardized Postoperative Care Plan, Diagnosis 5, action d [p. 108]) d. encourage client to consume foods/fluids high in calcium and vitamin D (e.g., fortified dairy products) e. perform actions to prevent and treat wound infection and osteomyelitis (see Standardized Postoperative Care Plan, Diagnosis 17, action b.2 [pp. 118–119] and Postoperative Diagnosis 4, actions c and d) f. discourage smoking *(evidence strongly suggests that smoking decreases tissue perfusion and may delay bone union)* g. administer the following if ordered: 1. calcium preparations (e.g., calcium carbonate) 2. vitamin D (e.g., calcitriol)

3. medications *to inhibit further bone resorption* (e.g., alendronate, calcitonin).
3. If signs and symptoms of avascular necrosis or delayed healing of the fracture occur:
   a. prepare client for diagnostic tests (e.g., x-ray, CT scan, bone scan, magnetic resonance imaging) if planned
   b. prepare client for surgical intervention (e.g., bone grafting, repeat fixation, prosthesis insertion) if planned.

7. NURSING DIAGNOSIS:

GRIEVING*

related to:
a. physical limitations imposed by the hip fracture and surgery;
b. need for assistance with activities of daily living;
c. possible change in roles and future living situation;
d. possible permanent disability and death.

---

*This diagnostic label includes anticipatory grieving and grieving following the actual losses.

Suggested NOC Outcomes: Grief resolution; Psychosocial adjustment: life change

Suggested NIC Interventions: Grief work facilitation; Emotional support; Presence; Support system enhancement

Desired Outcome	**Nursing Actions** *and Selected Purposes/Rationales* (see pp. 35–37 for additional rationales)
7. The client will demonstrate beginning progression through the grieving process as evidenced by: a. verbalization of feelings about fracturing hip and possible change in roles and living situation b. usual sleep pattern c. participation in treatment plan and self-care activities d. utilization of available support systems.	7.a. Assess for signs and symptoms of grieving (e.g., expression of distress about fracturing hip and the possible change in roles and living situation, change in eating habits, inability to concentrate, insomnia, anger, sadness, withdrawal from significant others, denial of need for possible change in living situation). b. Implement measures *to facilitate the grieving process:* 1. assist client to acknowledge the possible changes *so grief work can begin*; assess for factors that may hinder and facilitate acknowledgment 2. discuss the grieving process and assist client to accept the phases of grieving as an expected response to actual and/or anticipated loss 3. allow time for client to progress through the phases of grieving (phases vary among theorists but progress from shock and alarm to acceptance) 4. provide an atmosphere of care and concern (e.g., provide privacy, be available and nonjudgmental, display empathy and respect) *so client will feel free to express feelings* 5. perform actions *to promote trust* (e.g., answer questions honestly, provide requested information) 6. encourage the verbal expression of anger and sadness about the possible changes; recognize displacement of anger and assist client to see the actual cause of angry feelings and resentment 7. assist client to identify and use techniques that have helped him/her cope in previous situations of loss 8. support realistic hope about successful rehabilitation and resumption of usual roles and level of independence; reassure client that modern treatment methods for a fractured hip have significantly reduced permanent disability and death rates 9. support behaviors suggesting successful grief work (e.g., verbalizing feelings about loss of independence, focusing on ways to adapt to change in mobility, utilizing available support systems) 10. explain the phases of the grieving process to significant others; encourage their support and understanding 11. facilitate communication between the client and significant others; be aware that they may be in different phases of the grieving process

Desired Outcome	Nursing Actions *and Selected Purposes/Rationales*
	12. when appropriate, assist client to meet spiritual needs (e.g. arrange for a visit from clergy). c. Consult appropriate health care provider (e.g., psychiatric nurse clinician, physician) if signs of dysfunctional grieving (e.g., persistent denial of losses, excessive anger or sadness, emotional lability) occur.

Discharge Teaching/Continued Care

8. Nursing Diagnosis: ***DEFICIENT KNOWLEDGE, INEFFECTIVE THERAPEUTIC REGIMEN MANAGEMENT, OR INEFFECTIVE HEALTH MAINTENANCE****

*The nurse should select the diagnostic label that is most appropriate for the client's discharge teaching needs.

Suggested NOC Outcomes: Knowledge: fall prevention; Knowledge: prescribed activity; Knowledge: treatment regimen

Suggested NIC Interventions: Health system guidance; Teaching: individual; Teaching: prescribed activity/exercise

Desired Outcomes	Nursing Actions *and Selected Purposes/Rationales*
8.a. The client will demonstrate correct transfer and ambulation techniques and proper use of ambulatory aids.	8.a.1. Reinforce instructions about correct transfer and ambulation techniques, amount of weight bearing allowed, and proper use of ambulatory aids (a walker is preferable for most elderly clients because it provides the greatest stability). 2. Allow time for questions, clarification, and practice of transfer and ambulation techniques.
8.b. The client will demonstrate the ability to correctly perform the prescribed exercises.	8.b.1. Reinforce instructions on muscle strengthening and range of motion exercises. 2. Explain importance of performing muscle strengthening and range of motion exercises 3–4 times/day. 3. Allow time for questions, clarification, and return demonstration of prescribed exercises.
8.c. The client will verbalize an understanding of activity and position restrictions necessary to prevent dislocation of the prosthesis or internal fixation device.	8.c. Instruct client to adhere to the following activity and position restrictions for at least 2 months (time may vary depending on physician preference) in order to prevent dislocation of prosthesis or internal fixation device: 1. turn only as directed by physician (many physicians allow turning to unoperative side only) 2. keep pillows between legs when lying on back or side and when turning 3. never cross legs 4. do not sit on low chairs, stools, or toilets; place a cushion on low chairs; rent or purchase an elevated toilet seat for home use; and use the high toilets designed for the handicapped when in public facilities 5. do not elevate operative leg higher than hip when sitting 6. sit in chairs with arms and use the arms to raise self off chair 7. support weight on unoperative leg when raising self from a sitting position 8. use assistive devices (e.g., long-handled shoe horn, long-handled grabber) to assist with activities that require flexing hip beyond 90° (e.g., putting on shoes and socks, reaching objects on the floor or in low cupboards or drawers, pulling bed covers up from end of bed) 9. keep operative leg in proper alignment and avoid extreme internal and external rotation of leg

10. do not drive until approved by physician (usu
after surgery)
11. when riding in a car:
    a. sit on a firm pillow or cushion to prevent hip
    than 90°
    b. keep operative leg extended (a sudden impact o
    the dashboard can dislodge the prosthesis)
12. do not resume sexual activity until approved by phy
sexual activity is resumed, avoid positions that involv
rotation of the operative leg, flexing hip beyond 90°, and moving operative leg past the midline
13. avoid lifting heavy objects, excessive twisting and turning of body, walking on uneven surfaces, and activities that place excessive strain on hip (e.g., jogging).

8.d. The client will identify ways to reduce the risk of falls in the home environment.

8.d. If client is to return home, provide the following instructions on how to reduce the risk for falls at home:
1. keep electrical cords out of pathways
2. remove unnecessary furniture and provide wide pathways for ambulation
3. remove scatter rugs
4. provide adequate lighting at all times
5. do not climb stairs until permission is given by physician.

8.e. The client will state signs and symptoms to report to the health care provider.

8.e.1. Refer to Standardized Postoperative Care Plan, Diagnosis 22, action c (p. 125), for signs and symptoms to report to the health care provider.
2. Instruct client to report these additional signs and symptoms:
    a. persistent or increased pain or spasms in operative extremity
    b. loss of sensation or movement in operative extremity
    c. inability to maintain operative extremity in a neutral position
    d. inability to bear weight on operative extremity once weight bearing is allowed
    e. shortening of operative extremity (will probably be noticed as a limp once full weight bearing is resumed).

8.f. The client will identify community resources that can assist with home management and provide transportation.

8.f.1. Provide information about community resources that can assist the client and significant others with home management and provide transportation (e.g. home health agencies, Meals on Wheels, church groups, transportation services).
2. Initiate a referral if indicated.

8.g. The client will verbalize an understanding of and a plan for adhering to recommended follow-up care including future appointments with health care provider and physical therapist, medications prescribed, activity level, and wound care.

8.g.1. Refer to Standardized Postoperative Care Plan, Diagnosis 22 (pp. 125–126), for routine postoperative instructions and measures to improve client compliance.
2. Reinforce the importance of keeping appointments with physical therapist.
3. If client had a hip prosthesis inserted, instruct him/her to inform other health care providers about the hip prosthesis so that prophylactic antimicrobials can be started before any dental work, invasive diagnostic procedures, or surgery is performed.
4. Inform client that the hip prosthesis or fixation device may activate metal detector alarms. Recommend carrying an identification/information card if available.

Bibliography

See pages 879 and 885.

LAMINECTOMY/DISKECTOMY WITH OR WITHOUT FUSION

A laminectomy is the surgical removal of the lamina of a vertebra. It may be performed to allow for removal of a neoplasm or bone fragments that are putting pressure on nerve roots or the spinal cord or to enable a rhizotomy or cordotomy to be performed to treat intractable pain. Most commonly, a laminectomy is performed to gain access to a herniated nucleus pulposus (HNP, "ruptured disk") so that a diskectomy (removal of the herniated portion of the disk) can be accomplished.

Disk herniation is usually the result of trauma (e.g., falls, vehicular accidents) or strain caused by factors such as improper or repeated lifting of heavy objects, twisting, sneezing, or coughing. Age-related degenerative changes in the disks, supporting ligaments, and vertebrae make the disks more prone to rupture. The most common sites of disk herniation are C5–6, C6–7, L4–5, and L5–S1. These areas of the spine are the most flexible and therefore are subjected to a greater amount of movement and strain. Signs and symptoms of lumbar disk herniation can include low back pain which radiates down the buttock, thigh, calf, and ankle on affected side; muscle spasms in lower back; muscle weakness, diminished knee and ankle reflexes, numbness, or tingling in affected lower extremity; constipation; and/or urinary retention. Clinical manifestations of cervical disk herniation can include neck pain which radiates to the shoulder, arm, and fingers on affected side; stiff neck; muscle spasms in neck; and/or muscle weakness, diminished biceps and triceps reflexes, numbness, or tingling in affected upper extremity.

A diskectomy is usually indicated if conservative measures such as rest, heat or cold applications, anti-inflammatory medications, analgesics, muscle relaxants, and local steroid injections fail to control pain or if neurological deficits persist or worsen. Disk removal is usually accomplished by a microdiskectomy or laminectomy and can be performed using an anterior and/or posterior approach. The surgical procedure performed depends on the location and size of the herniated disk and physician preference. If the vertebral column in the surgical area is unstable, a spinal fusion may be performed along with a laminectomy. The surgical immobilization of the unstable area is accomplished using a bone graft (autograft [usually from the iliac crest], allograft, or bone substitute) or implanted fixation devices such as cages, plates, screws, and rods.

This care plan focuses on the adult client admitted for a laminectomy that is being performed to remove a herniated nucleus pulposus. The care of a client hospitalized for a laminectomy with spinal fusion is also discussed. Much of the postoperative information is applicable to clients receiving follow-up care in an extended care facility or home setting.

OUTCOME/DISCHARGE CRITERIA

THE CLIENT WILL:

- have improved neurological function
- have evidence of normal healing of the surgical wound
- have intact skin under stabilization device if one is present
- have pain controlled
- have no signs and symptoms of postoperative complications
- identify ways to prevent recurrent disk herniation
- demonstrate the ability to correctly apply and remove stabilization device if one is required
- verbalize an understanding of ways to maintain skin integrity when wearing a stabilization device
- state signs and symptoms to report to the health care provider
- verbalize an understanding of and a plan for adhering to recommended follow-up care including future appointments with health care provider, medications prescribed, activity level, and wound care.

NURSING/COLLABORATIVE DIAGNOSES

NURSING/COLLABORATIVE DIAGNOSES

5. Potential complications p. 789
   a. respiratory distress
   b. cerebrospinal fluid leak
   c. laryngeal nerve damage
   d. paralytic ileus

DISCHARGE TEACHING

6. Deficient knowledge, Ineffective therapeutic regimen management, or Ineffective health maintenance p. 791

See Standardized Preoperative and Postoperative Care Plans (pp. 97–126) for additional diagnoses.

PREOPERATIVE

Use in conjunction with the Standardized Preoperative Care Plan.

Client Teaching

1. NURSING DIAGNOSIS: ***DEFICIENT KNOWLEDGE***

regarding the surgical procedure, routines associated with surgery, physical preparation for laminectomy and spinal fusion (if planned), sensations that normally occur following surgery and anesthesia, and postoperative care.

Suggested NOC Outcome: Knowledge: treatment regimen

Suggested NIC Interventions: Teaching: preoperative; Teaching: individual

Desired Outcomes	Nursing Actions *and Selected Purposes/Rationales*
1.a. The client will verbalize an understanding of the surgical procedure, preoperative care, and postoperative sensations and care.	1.a.1. Refer to Standardized Preoperative Care Plan, Diagnosis 4, actions a.1–4 (pp. 100–101), for information to include in preoperative teaching. 2. Provide additional information regarding postoperative care: a. if a laminectomy without spinal fusion is planned: 1. explain that progressive activity will probably begin the evening of or morning after surgery 2. reinforce physician's explanation about wearing a soft cervical collar (following a cervical laminectomy) or a back brace or corset (following a lumbar laminectomy) if client is expected to need one while the surgical area heals (some physicians order this stabilization device to provide additional support to the operative area for a few weeks postoperatively if the surgery is fairly extensive and/or the client has a tendency to be too active) b. if a laminectomy with spinal fusion is planned: 1. explain that progressive activity usually begins 1–3 days after surgery depending on physician preference and extensiveness of the surgery 2. reinforce physician's explanation about the type of stabilization device that may be needed while the surgical area heals (e.g., rigid cervical collar or halo brace following a cervical fusion, back brace following a lumbar fusion) c. explain that preoperative pain, muscle weakness, numbness, or tingling in the affected extremity may take weeks to months to lessen or resolve after surgery due to surgical trauma and the time it takes the peripheral nerves to heal. Be aware that the effects of prolonged nerve damage may be irreversible. 3. Allow time for questions and clarification of information provided. 4. Allow time for client to practice putting on and removing stabilization device if available preoperatively.

Desired Outcomes	Nursing Actions and Selected Purposes/Rationales
1.b. The client will demonstrate the ability to perform activities designed to prevent postoperative complications.	1.b.1. Refer to Standardized Preoperative Care Plan, Diagnosis 4, action b.1 (p. 101), for instructions on ways to prevent postoperative complications. 2. Provide additional instructions about ways to prevent postoperative complications: a. instruct client how to logroll and stress the importance of turning in this manner after surgery (the length of time logrolling is necessary increases if a fusion was performed) b. instruct client to avoid extreme flexion, hyperextension, and twisting of the cervical or lumbar spine postoperatively c. demonstrate the correct way to change from a lying to standing position (e.g., keeping spine in proper alignment, utilizing arm and leg muscles) d. reinforce physician's or physical therapist's instructions about exercises to strengthen arm, shoulder, neck, back, leg, and abdominal muscles (increased strength of these muscles decreases strain on the spine) e. demonstrate proper body alignment and good body mechanics and stress the importance of lifelong adherence to these principles. 3. Allow time for questions, clarification, and return demonstration.

POSTOPERATIVE

Use in conjunction with the Standardized Postoperative Care Plan.

1. Nursing Diagnosis: RISK FOR PERIPHERAL NEUROVASCULAR DYSFUNCTION

related to:
a. trauma to the nerves or blood vessels during surgery;
b. blood accumulation and inflammation in the surgical area;
c. dislocation of the bone graft or implanted fixation devices (if a fusion was performed);
d. excessive external pressure on the nerves or blood vessels associated with improper fit or application of stabilization device (e.g., cervical collar, back brace, corset).

Suggested NOC Outcomes: Neurological status: spinal sensory/motor function; Tissue perfusion: peripheral

Suggested NIC Interventions: Neurologic monitoring; Positioning: neurologic; Circulatory care: arterial insufficiency; Circulatory care: venous insufficiency

Desired Outcome	Nursing Actions and Selected Purposes/Rationales
1. The client will have usual or improved peripheral neurovascular function as evidenced by: a. palpable peripheral pulses b. capillary refill time less than 2–3 seconds c. extremities warm and usual color d. ability to flex and extend feet, toes, hands, and fingers e. usual or improved reflexes, muscle tone, and sensation in extremities f. no new or increased pain in extremities.	1.a. Assess for and report signs and symptoms of peripheral neurovascular dysfunction (check upper extremities after surgery on the cervical area and lower extremities after surgery on the lumbar area): 1. diminished or absent peripheral pulses 2. capillary refill time greater than 2–3 seconds 3. pallor, cyanosis, or coolness of extremities 4. inability to flex or extend feet, toes, hands, or fingers 5. diminished or absent reflexes in extremities 6. development of or increase in muscle weakness, numbness, or tingling in extremities 7. development of or increase in pain in extremities. b. Implement measures *to reduce the risk for peripheral neurovascular dysfunction*: 1. perform actions to reduce strain on the surgical area (see Postoperative Diagnosis 2, action b.1) *in order to prevent bleeding and subsequent hematoma formation in the surgical area and to reduce the risk for dislocation of the bone graft or implanted fixation devices (if fusion was performed)*

2. maintain wound suction and patency of wound drain *to reduce the accumulation of blood in the surgical area and subsequently prevent increased pressure on nerves and blood vessels*
3. apply stabilization device properly; notify orthotist if it appears to create excessive pressure on any area
4. administer corticosteroids (e.g., dexamethasone) if ordered *to reduce inflammation in the surgical area.*

c. If signs and symptoms of peripheral neurovascular dysfunction occur:
1. assess for and correct improper body alignment and external cause of excessive pressure (e.g., tight or improperly applied stabilization device)
2. notify physician if signs and symptoms persist or worsen
3. prepare client for surgical intervention (e.g., evacuation of hematoma, repositioning of dislocated bone graft or implanted fixation devices) if planned.

2. NURSING DIAGNOSIS: ACUTE PAIN

related to:
a. tissue trauma and reflex muscle spasms associated with the surgery;
b. removal of bone if an autograft was used to achieve spinal fusion (the bone is usually taken from the client's iliac crest);
c. stretching and compression of sensory nerves associated with blood accumulation and inflammation in the surgical area;
d. irritation from drainage tube (wound drain may be present, especially following a spinal fusion);
e. stress on surgical area associated with movement;
f. release of pressure on compressed spinal nerve root following removal of the herniated nucleus pulposus (improved sensory nerve function can cause a temporary increase in pain in area[s] of previously diminished sensation).

Suggested NOC Outcomes: Pain control; Comfort level

Suggested NIC Interventions: Pain management; Analgesic administration

Desired Outcome	**Nursing Actions** *and Selected Purposes/Rationales* (see pp. 45–47 for additional rationales)
2. The client will experience diminished pain (see Standardized Postoperative Care Plan, Diagnosis 6 [p. 109], for outcome criteria).	2.a. Refer to Standardized Postoperative Care Plan, Diagnosis 6 (p. 109), for measures related to assessment and management of pain. b. Implement additional measures to reduce pain: 1. perform actions *to reduce strain on the surgical area*: a. ensure that client is always positioned with spine in proper alignment b. apply stabilization device if ordered *to provide additional support to surgical area*; if stabilization device loosens, reapply it or tighten straps or screws if allowed or consult orthotist about adjustment of the device *in order to maintain adequate support of the surgical area* c. implement measures *to prevent hyperextension, extreme flexion, and/or twisting of spine* (e.g., instruct and assist client to logroll when turning; put needed items within easy reach; if a cervical laminectomy was performed, place a small pillow or folded pad under client's head rather than a full-size pillow; assist with bathing and dressing as needed) d. if lumbar laminectomy was performed, assist client to maintain a position that results in flattening of the lumbosacral spine (e.g., slight knee flexion when supine, knees flexed while in side-lying position, feet elevated on footstool when sitting in chair) *in order to reduce stretching of the nerves and muscles in the lower back* e. instruct client to avoid sitting or standing for longer than 20–30 minute intervals (some physicians instruct clients to sit only during meals and ambulate only short distances when progressive activity begins)

Desired Outcome	Nursing Actions *and Selected Purposes/Rationales*
	f. instruct client to avoid straining to have a bowel movement (especially after lumbar laminectomy) and vigorous coughing; consult physician about an order for a laxative and antitussive if indicated 2. if appropriate, perform actions *to reduce pressure on bone graft donor site* (e.g., position client so he/she is not lying on site, protect the site with padding if stabilization device is worn over it) 3. administer corticosteroids (e.g., dexamethasone) if ordered *to reduce inflammation in the surgical area.*

3. NURSING DIAGNOSIS: ACTUAL/RISK FOR IMPAIRED TISSUE INTEGRITY

related to:
a. disruption of tissue associated with the surgical procedure;
b. irritation of skin associated with contact with wound drainage, use of tape, and pressure from tubes and/or stabilization device if present.

Suggested NOC Outcomes: Wound healing: primary intention; Tissue integrity: skin and mucous membranes

Suggested NIC Interventions: Skin surveillance; Positioning; Wound care; Pressure management

Desired Outcomes	Nursing Actions *and Selected Purposes/Rationales* (see pp. 49–52 for additional rationales)
3.a. The client will experience normal healing of the surgical wound (see Standardized Postoperative Care Plan, Diagnosis 10, outcome a [p. 112], for outcome criteria).	3.a. Refer to Standardized Postoperative Care Plan, Diagnosis 10, action a (p. 112), for measures related to assessment and promotion of wound healing.
3.b. The client will maintain tissue integrity in areas in contact with wound drainage, tape, tubings, and stabilization device as evidenced by: 1. absence of redness and irritation 2. no skin breakdown.	3.b.1. Inspect the following for signs and symptoms of skin irritation and breakdown: a. areas in contact with wound drainage, tape, and tubings b. area under stabilization device. 2. Refer to Standardized Postoperative Care Plan, Diagnosis 10, action b.2 (pp. 112–113), for measures related to prevention of tissue irritation and breakdown resulting from contact with wound drainage, tape, and tubings. 3. Implement measures *to prevent skin irritation and breakdown under stabilization device:* a. apply stabilization device securely enough to keep it from rubbing and irritating the skin but not too tightly b. position client so that stabilization device is not causing excessive pressure on any area c. assist client to put a cotton T-shirt on under back brace or corset and ensure that the shirt is dry and wrinkle-free d. apply a thin layer of a dry lubricant such as powder or cornstarch to skin under stabilization device *in order to reduce friction* e. pad areas over bony prominences before applying stabilization device f. instruct client to refrain from inserting anything under the stabilization device g. consult physician or orthotist if stabilization device is putting excessive pressure on the skin. 4. If tissue breakdown occurs: a. notify appropriate health care provider (e.g., physician, wound care specialist)

b. perform care of involved area(s) as ordered or per standard hospital procedure.

4. NURSING DIAGNOSIS:

URINARY RETENTION

related to:

a. incomplete bladder emptying associated with horizontal positioning (client may be on bed rest for a few days following a spinal fusion);
b. increased tone of the urinary sphincters and relaxation of the bladder muscle associated with:
   1. indirect sympathetic nervous system stimulation resulting from pain, fear, and anxiety
   2. direct stimulation of the sympathetic nerves that innervate the bladder (can occur as a result of nerve trauma during a lumbar laminectomy and/or pressure on the nerves as a result of inflammation or accumulation of blood in the surgical area following a lumbar laminectomy);
c. relaxation of the bladder muscle and decreased perception of bladder fullness associated with the depressant effect of anesthesia and some medications (e.g., narcotic [opioid] analgesics, centrally acting muscle relaxants).

Suggested NOC Outcome: Urinary elimination

Suggested NIC Intervention: Urinary retention care

Desired Outcome	**Nursing Actions** *and Selected Purposes/Rationales*
4. The client will not experience urinary retention (see Standardized Postoperative Care Plan, Diagnosis 14 [p. 115], for outcome criteria).	4. Refer to Standardized Postoperative Care Plan, Diagnosis 14 (pp. 115–116), for measures related to assessment and management of urinary retention.

5. COLLABORATIVE DIAGNOSES:

POTENTIAL COMPLICATIONS OF LAMINECTOMY

a. respiratory distress related to:
   1. trauma to the phrenic nerve during surgery and/or compression of the phrenic nerve following surgery associated with inflammation or accumulation of blood in the surgical area (can occur with a cervical laminectomy because the phrenic nerve arises at the C3–5 level)
   2. tracheal compression associated with inflammation or accumulation of blood in the surgical area following a cervical laminectomy (particularly if the anterior approach was used)
   3. closure of the glottis associated with paralysis of the vocal cords (can occur as a result of injury to the bilateral recurrent laryngeal nerves during an anterior cervical laminectomy);
b. cerebrospinal fluid leak related to inadvertent damage to and/or incomplete closure of the dura (care is taken during surgery to keep the dura intact; however, it is sometimes necessary to incise dura that extends along the involved nerve);
c. laryngeal nerve damage related to surgical trauma or pressure on the nerve(s) associated with inflammation or accumulation of blood in the surgical area (can occur with an anterior cervical laminectomy);
d. paralytic ileus related to:
   1. impaired innervation of the intestinal tract following a lumbar laminectomy associated with stimulation of sympathetic nerves and/or loss of parasympathetic nerve function in the operative area
   2. the depressant effect of anesthesia and some medications (e.g., centrally acting muscle relaxants, narcotic [opioid] analgesics, some antiemetics).

Desired Outcomes	**Nursing Actions** *and Selected Purposes/Rationales*
5.a. The client will not experience respiratory distress as evidenced by: 1. unlabored respirations at 12–20/minute 2. absence of stridor and sternocleidomastoid muscle retraction 3. usual mental status 4. oximetry results within normal range 5. blood gases within normal range.	5.a.1. Following a cervical laminectomy, assess for and immediately report: a. increased swelling of the neck or bulging of the wound b. statements of difficulty swallowing or choking sensation c. signs and symptoms of respiratory distress (e.g., rapid and/or labored respirations, stridor, sternocleidomastoid muscle retraction, restlessness, agitation) d. abnormal blood gases e. significant decrease in oximetry results. 2. Have tracheostomy and suction equipment readily available following cervical laminectomy. 3. Implement measures *to prevent respiratory distress following a cervical laminectomy*: a. perform actions *to reduce inflammation and/or prevent bleeding and subsequent hematoma formation in the surgical area:* 1. implement measures *to reduce strain on the surgical area* (e.g., keep neck in proper alignment, ensure that cervical collar is applied correctly, instruct and assist client to support neck when moving) 2. elevate head of bed 30–45° unless contraindicated 3. apply ice pack to incisional area as ordered 4. administer corticosteroids (e.g., dexamethasone) if ordered b. maintain wound suction and patency of wound drain *to prevent the accumulation of blood in the surgical area.* 4. If signs and symptoms of respiratory distress occur: a. place client in a high Fowler's position unless contraindicated b. loosen neck dressing or cervical collar if it appears tight c. administer oxygen as ordered d. assist with intubation or emergency tracheostomy if performed e. prepare client for surgical evacuation of hematoma or repair of the bleeding vessel(s) if planned.
5.b. The client will have resolution of cerebrospinal fluid leak if it occurs as evidenced by: 1. absence of cerebrospinal fluid drainage from lower back or neck incision 2. no reports of headache.	5.b.1. Assess for and report signs and symptoms of a cerebrospinal fluid leak: a. clear drainage from the incision b. presence of glucose in wound drainage as shown by positive results on a glucose reagent strip; be aware that drainage containing blood will also test positive for glucose c. yellowish ring ("halo") around bloody or serosanguineous drainage on lower back or neck dressing, sheet, or pillowcase *(CSF dries in concentric circles)* d. reports of headache. 2. Implement measures to reduce strain on the surgical area (see Postoperative Diagnosis 2, action b.1) *in order to promote healing of the dura and subsequent resolution of cerebrospinal fluid leak.* 3. If signs and symptoms of cerebrospinal fluid leak occur: a. maintain activity restrictions as ordered *to reduce stress on the dural tear* b. change dressing as soon as it becomes damp; maintain meticulous sterile technique when changing dressing c. administer antimicrobials if ordered d. assess for and report signs and symptoms of meningitis (e.g., fever; chills; new, increasing, or persistent headache; nuchal rigidity; photophobia; positive Kernig's and Brudzinski's signs) e. prepare client for surgical repair of the torn dura if planned (usually the torn dura heals spontaneously within a few days).
5.c. The client will experience resolution of laryngeal nerve damage if it occurs as evidenced by: 1. improved voice tone and quality	5.c.1. Assess for the following indications of laryngeal nerve damage: a. voice changes (e.g., hoarseness; weak, whispery voice; inability to speak) b. respiratory distress (see action a.1.c in this diagnosis). 2. Implement measures to reduce pressure on the laryngeal nerves (see actions a.3.a and b in this diagnosis).

2. gradual resolution of hoarseness
3. absence of respiratory distress.

3. If signs and symptoms of laryngeal nerve damage occur:
   a. encourage client to avoid unnecessary talking *in order to rest the vocal cords*
   b. implement measures *to facilitate communication* (e.g., provide pad and pencil, flash cards, or Magic Slate; ask questions that require a short answer or nod of head)
   c. reinforce physician's explanation regarding the permanence of voice changes (voice tone and quality usually return to normal as inflammation subsides)
   d. notify physician immediately if signs and symptoms of respiratory distress occur, client is unable to speak, or hoarseness or voice changes worsen.

5.d. The client will not develop a paralytic ileus (see Standardized Postoperative Care Plan, Diagnosis 20, outcome d [p. 123], for outcome criteria).

5.d. Refer to Standardized Postoperative Care Plan, Diagnosis 20, action d (p. 123), for measures related to assessment and management of a paralytic ileus.

Discharge Teaching/Continued Care

6. NURSING DIAGNOSIS: ***DEFICIENT KNOWLEDGE, INEFFECTIVE THERAPEUTIC REGIMEN MANAGEMENT, OR INEFFECTIVE HEALTH MAINTENANCE****

*The nurse should select the diagnostic label that is most appropriate for the client's discharge teaching needs.

Suggested NOC Outcome: Knowledge: treatment regimen

Suggested NIC Interventions: Health system guidance; Teaching: individual; Teaching: prescribed activity/exercise

Desired Outcomes

6.a. The client will identify ways to prevent recurrent disk herniation.

Nursing Actions *and Selected Purposes/Rationales*

6.a.1. Inform client about ways to reduce back and/or neck strain and subsequently reduce the risk of recurrent disk herniation:
   a. lose weight if overweight
   b. support the spine adequately (e.g., sleep on a firm mattress; sit on firm, straight-backed or contoured chairs; wear stabilization device as prescribed)
   c. use proper body mechanics (e.g., bend at the knees rather than waist, push rather than pull heavy objects, carry items close to body)
   d. keep spine in good alignment (e.g., avoid excessive bending or twisting, maintain good posture)
   e. wear flat or low-heeled shoes; avoid wearing high heels
   f. adhere to prescribed, progressive exercise program to strengthen back, neck, shoulders, arms, legs, and abdominal muscles.

2. Provide a dietary consult regarding a weight reduction program if indicated.
3. Refer client to an occupational therapist and/or vocational rehabilitation specialist for assistance in modifying daily routines or pursuing different job opportunities if indicated.
4. Allow time for client to practice proper body alignment when sitting, standing, and walking; proper positioning when resting; and any exercises allowed in immediate postoperative period. Encourage client to think about and plan movements before doing them.

Desired Outcomes	Nursing Actions *and Selected Purposes/Rationales*
	5. Allow time for questions, clarification, and return demonstration of proper body mechanics, positioning, and exercises allowed.
6.b. The client will demonstrate the ability to correctly apply and remove stabilization device if one is required.	6.b.1. Reinforce instructions on the correct way to apply and remove stabilization device (e.g., cervical collar, back brace, corset) if client needs to wear one after discharge. 2. Allow time for questions, clarification, and return demonstration.
6.c. The client will verbalize an understanding of ways to maintain skin integrity when wearing a stabilization device.	6.c.1. If client is to be discharged with a stabilization device, instruct him/her to examine skin daily when device is off (if device should not be removed, demonstrate how to examine underneath it using a mirror and flashlight). 2. Instruct client in ways to maintain skin integrity if a stabilization device needs to be worn: a. apply device properly and maintain spine in good alignment to avoid undue pressure in any area b. wear a cotton T-shirt under back brace or corset and keep shirt dry and wrinkle-free c. apply a thin layer of powder or cornstarch to skin under stabilization device to reduce irritation caused by friction d. avoid inserting anything under the device e. place padding between stabilization device and bony prominences.
6.d. The client will state signs and symptoms to report to the health care provider.	6.d.1. Refer to Standardized Postoperative Care Plan, Diagnosis 22, action c (p. 125), for signs and symptoms to report to the health care provider. 2. Instruct client to report these additional signs and symptoms: a. decreased movement or sensation in extremities b. coolness or bluish color of extremities c. increasing or recurrent numbness, tingling, or pain in surgical area or extremities d. difficulty standing up straight (after lumbar surgery) or keeping neck straight (after cervical surgery) e. persistent and/or severe headache f. drainage of clear or bloody fluid from incision g. persistent hoarseness or difficulty swallowing (following cervical laminectomy) h. reddened or irritated area on skin underneath stabilization device.
6.e. The client will verbalize an understanding of and a plan for adhering to recommended follow-up care including future appointments with health care provider, medications prescribed, activity level, and wound care.	6.e.1. Refer to Standardized Postoperative Care Plan, Diagnosis 22 (pp. 125–126), for routine postoperative instructions and measures to improve client compliance. 2. Reinforce physician's instructions regarding activity (the restrictions will vary depending on extensiveness of surgery, client condition, and physician preference): a. avoid lifting objects weighing more than 5–10 pounds b. progress through exercise program as prescribed c. avoid sitting or standing for longer than 30 minutes at a time (especially after surgery on lumbar area) d. schedule adequate rest periods e. avoid driving a car (causes increased flexion of the spine) and taking long car rides (the vibrations can jar the spine and long periods without significant changes in position can increase stiffness and discomfort) until allowed f. do not participate in contact sports.

Bibliography

See pages 879 and 885.

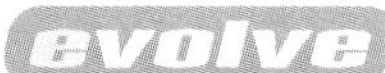

Total Hip Replacement

A total hip replacement (arthroplasty) is a surgical procedure in which the ball and socket components of the hip joint are replaced with prosthetic devices. There are a variety of prosthetic devices available. The prostheses are either cemented in place using an agent called polymethylmethacrylate or are uncemented (cementless). Uncemented prostheses have porous surfaces that permit bone ingrowth to occur and provide biological fixation. A total hip replacement is performed to relieve joint pain that has been resistant to conservative management and/or improve joint mobility in persons with severe arthritis. It may also be performed to treat avascular necrosis of the femoral head, congenital hip deformity, and failure of previous reconstructive hip surgery.

This care plan focuses on the adult client hospitalized for a total hip replacement. Much of the postoperative information is applicable to clients receiving follow-up care in an extended care facility or home setting.

OUTCOME/DISCHARGE CRITERIA

THE CLIENT WILL:

- have evidence of normal healing of the surgical wound
- have clear, audible breath sounds throughout lungs
- have reduced hip pain
- have expected degree of mobility of hip joint
- have no signs and symptoms of infection or postoperative complications
- demonstrate correct transfer and ambulation techniques and proper use of ambulatory aids
- demonstrate the ability to correctly perform the prescribed exercises
- verbalize an understanding of activity and position restrictions necessary to prevent dislocation of the hip prostheses
- identify ways to reduce the risk of falls in the home environment
- state signs and symptoms to report to the health care provider
- identify community resources that can assist with home management and provide transportation
- verbalize an understanding of and a plan for adhering to recommended follow-up care including future appointments with health care provider and physical therapist, medications prescribed, activity level, and wound care.

NURSING/COLLABORATIVE DIAGNOSES

DISCHARGE TEACHING

See Standardized Preoperative and Postoperative Care Plans (pp. 97–126) for additional diagnoses.

PREOPERATIVE

Use in conjunction with the Standardized Preoperative Care Plan.

Client Teaching

1. NURSING DIAGNOSIS: *DEFICIENT KNOWLEDGE*

regarding the surgical procedure, hospital routines associated with surgery, physical preparation for the total hip replacement, sensations that normally occur following surgery and anesthesia, and postoperative care.

Suggested NOC Outcomes: Knowledge: treatment regimen; Knowledge: prescribed activity

Suggested NIC Interventions: Teaching: preoperative; Teaching: prescribed activity/exercise

Desired Outcomes	Nursing Actions *and Selected Purposes/Rationales*
1.a. The client will verbalize an understanding of the surgical procedure, preoperative care, and postoperative sensations and care.	1.a.1. Refer to Standardized Preoperative Care Plan, Diagnosis 4, actions a.1–4 (pp. 100–101), for information to include in preoperative teaching. 2. Provide additional information on specific preoperative care for clients having a total hip replacement: a. explain that the following measures will be performed to reduce the risk of a postoperative hip infection: 1. the operative hip and thigh will be scrubbed with an antiseptic solution (e.g., 2% chlorhexidine) before surgery 2. injections will not be given in the operative extremity 3. existing infections will be treated before surgery; instruct client to report any symptoms of infection (e.g., cough, runny nose, burning on urination) 4. antimicrobials will probably be administered prophylactically before and after surgery b. explain that anticoagulants (e.g., low-molecular-weight heparin, low-dose warfarin, danaparoid) may be administered before surgery to reduce the risk of postoperative thrombus formation; inform client that coagulation studies are usually done before starting these medications, especially if he/she has been taking aspirin or other nonsteroidal anti-inflammatory agents (e.g., ibuprofen). 3. Inform client that an operative site drain and suction device may be present temporarily after surgery and that the blood salvaged in this device may be reinfused if needed. 4. Allow time for questions and clarification of information provided.
1.b. The client will demonstrate the ability to perform activities designed to prevent postoperative complications.	1.b.1. Refer to Standardized Preoperative Care Plan, Diagnosis 4, action b.1 (p. 101), for instructions on ways to prevent postoperative complications. 2. Provide additional instructions about ways to prevent complications following total hip replacement: a. reinforce physician's or physical therapist's instructions on: 1. transfer techniques that can be performed without flexing hip beyond the prescribed limit 2. exercises (e.g., quadriceps- and gluteal-setting, upper extremity strengthening, flexion and extension exercises of feet and ankles) 3. ambulation techniques and proper use of ambulatory aids (weight-bearing limitations are determined by the physician and vary depending on the type of prostheses used) b. instruct client in the correct way to use overhead trapeze and unoperative leg to move self

c. explain the following activity and positioning limitations that need to be adhered to postoperatively to prevent dislocation of the prosthesis(es):
    1. operative extremity will be maintained in an abducted position by a balanced suspension device, abduction wedge, or 2–3 pillows for first few days after surgery
    2. operative leg should be kept in proper alignment and should not be brought toward the midline
    3. if turning is allowed, it should be done only with assistance of trained personnel
    4. hip flexion of 45–60° will be permitted initially and then should not exceed 90° during the rehabilitation phase.

3. Allow time for questions, clarification, and return demonstration.

POSTOPERATIVE

Use in conjunction with the Standardized Postoperative Care Plan.

1. NURSING DIAGNOSIS: RISK FOR PERIPHERAL NEUROVASCULAR DYSFUNCTION: OPERATIVE EXTREMITY

related to trauma to or excessive pressure on the nerves or blood vessels during surgery, blood accumulation and edema in the surgical area, improper alignment of operative extremity, pressure exerted by balanced suspension device or straps on abductor wedge, and dislocation of the prosthesis(es).

Suggested NOC Outcome: Tissue perfusion: peripheral

Suggested NIC Interventions: Circulatory care: arterial insufficiency; Circulatory care: venous insufficiency; Lower extremity monitoring; Positioning; Pressure management; Heat/Cold application

Desired Outcome	**Nursing Actions** *and Selected Purposes/Rationales*
1. The client will maintain normal neurovascular function in the operative extremity as evidenced by: a. palpable pedal pulses b. capillary refill time in toes less than 2–3 seconds c. extremity warm and usual color d. ability to flex and extend knee, foot, and toes e. absence of numbness and tingling in leg or foot f. no increase in pain in extremity.	1.a. Assess for and report signs and symptoms of neurovascular dysfunction in the operative extremity: 1. diminished or absent pedal pulses 2. capillary refill time in toes greater than 2–3 seconds 3. pallor, cyanosis, or coolness of the extremity 4. inability to flex or extend knee, foot, or toes 5. numbness or tingling in leg or foot 6. increased pain in the extremity. b. Implement measures *to prevent neurovascular dysfunction in the operative extremity*: 1. perform actions to prevent hematoma formation (see Postoperative Diagnosis 8, action a.2) 2. make sure that balanced suspension device and straps on abductor wedge are not exerting pressure on the popliteal space, Achilles tendon, and lateral and medial aspects of the knee and ankle 3. maintain extremity in proper alignment 4. perform actions to prevent dislocation of the prostheses (see Postoperative Diagnosis 8, action b.2) 5. apply ice pack or cooling pad to operative hip if ordered *to reduce edema and bleeding in the surgical area.* c. If signs and symptoms of neurovascular dysfunction occur: 1. assess for and correct causes of excessive pressure on operative leg (e.g., tight straps on abductor wedge, improper positioning of balanced suspension device) 2. notify physician if the signs and symptoms persist

Desired Outcome	Nursing Actions *and Selected Purposes/Rationales*
	3. prepare client for closed reduction (e.g. traction) or surgical intervention (e.g., relocation of prosthesis, hematoma evacuation) if planned.

2. Nursing Diagnosis:

ACUTE PAIN: HIP

related to tissue trauma and reflex muscle spasms associated with the surgery, blood accumulation and edema in surgical area, and improper positioning of the operative extremity.

Suggested NOC Outcomes: Comfort level; Pain control

Suggested NIC Interventions: Pain management; Analgesic administration; Environmental management: comfort; Heat/Cold application

Desired Outcome	Nursing Actions *and Selected Purposes/Rationales* (see pp. 45–47 for additional rationales)
2. The client will experience diminished hip pain (see Standardized Postoperative Care Plan, Diagnosis 6 [p. 109], for outcome criteria).	2.a. Refer to Standardized Postoperative Care Plan, Diagnosis 6 (p. 109), for measures related to assessment and reduction of pain. b. Implement additional measures *to reduce pain:* 1. keep operative extremity in proper alignment 2. maintain restrictions on the degree of hip flexion as ordered (a 45–60° maximum may be ordered for first 2–3 days with a maximum of 90° during rehabilitation period) 3. place trochanter roll or sandbag against the operative site for first 24–48 hours after surgery *(pressure on the operative area helps maintain alignment and prevent hematoma formation)* 4. maintain patency of wound drainage system (e.g., prevent kinking of tubing, empty collection device as needed, keep collection device below surgical wound, maintain suction as ordered) *to reduce accumulation of fluid in surgical area* 5. move operative extremity gently 6. if turning is allowed, keep pillows between legs when turning and while in side-lying position *to prevent adduction and resultant strain on surgical site* 7. apply ice packs or cooling pad to operative hip if ordered 8. administer prescribed analgesics before exercise and ambulation sessions.

3. Nursing Diagnosis:

ACTUAL/RISK FOR IMPAIRED TISSUE INTEGRITY

related to:

a. disruption of tissue associated with the surgical procedure;
b. delayed wound healing associated with factors such as decreased nutritional status and inadequate blood supply to wound area;
c. irritation of skin associated with contact with wound drainage, pressure from tubes, and use of tape;
d. excessive or prolonged pressure on tissues from balanced suspension device, straps on abductor wedge, and elastic wraps or stockings;
e. damage to the skin and/or subcutaneous tissue associated with prolonged pressure on tissues, friction, and shearing while mobility is decreased.

Suggested NOC Outcomes: Tissue integrity: skin and mucous membranes; Wound healing: primary intention

Suggested NIC Interventions: Incision site care; Skin surveillance; Positioning; Pressure ulcer prevention; Pressure management; Skin care: topical treatments

Desired Outcomes	Nursing Actions *and Selected Purposes/Rationales* (see pp. 49–52 for additional rationales)
3.a. The client will experience normal healing of the surgical wound (see Standardized Postoperative Care Plan, Diagnosis 10, outcome a [p. 112], for outcome criteria).	3.a. Refer to Standardized Postoperative Care Plan, Diagnosis 10, action a (p. 112), for measures related to assessment and promotion of wound healing.
3.b. The client will maintain tissue integrity as evidenced by: 1. absence of redness and irritation 2. no skin breakdown.	3.b.1. Inspect the following sites for pallor, redness, and breakdown: a. skin in contact with wound drainage, tape, and tubing b. back, coccyx, and buttocks c. elbows and heels d. pressure points on operative extremity in contact with balanced suspension device e. areas in contact with abductor wedge straps f. areas under elastic wraps or stockings. 2. Refer to Standardized Postoperative Care Plan, Diagnosis 10, action b.2 (pp. 112–113), for measures related to prevention of tissue irritation and breakdown in areas in contact with wound drainage, tubings, and tape. 3. Implement measures *to prevent tissue breakdown associated with decreased mobility*: a. position client properly; use pressure-reducing or pressure-relieving devices (e.g., pillows, alternating pressure mattress) if indicated b. instruct client to use overhead trapeze to lift self and shift weight at least every 30 minutes c. gently massage around reddened areas at least every 2 hours d. apply a thin layer of a dry lubricant such as powder or cornstarch to bottom sheet or skin and to opposing skin surfaces (e.g., axillae) if indicated *to reduce friction* e. lift and move client carefully using a turn sheet and adequate assistance f. perform actions to keep client from sliding down in bed (e.g., limit length of time client is in semi-Fowler's position to 30-minute intervals) *in order to reduce the risk of skin surface abrasion and shearing* g. if turning is allowed, turn client every 2 hours (physician may allow client to turn on unoperative side) h. keep client's skin clean i. keep bed linens dry and wrinkle-free j. increase activity as allowed and tolerated. 4. Implement measures *to prevent tissue breakdown associated with excessive pressure caused by balanced suspension device or abductor wedge:* a. make sure metal parts on suspension device are not resting on any area of extremity b. maintain proper alignment of extremity in suspension device c. make sure that straps holding abductor wedge in place are not too tight. 5. Implement measures *to prevent irritation and breakdown on elbows and heels*: a. massage elbows and heels with lotion frequently b. encourage client to use overhead trapeze to move self rather than pushing up with heel and elbows c. provide elbow and heel protectors if indicated. 6. Implement measures *to prevent tissue breakdown under elastic wraps or stockings*: a. remove elastic wraps or stockings at least twice daily, bathe and thoroughly dry skin, and reapply smoothly b. check wraps or stockings frequently and reapply if they have slipped or become wrinkled

Desired Outcomes	**Nursing Actions** *and Selected Purposes/Rationales*

c. if areas of redness develop under wraps or stockings, consult physician before reapplying.

7. If tissue breakdown occurs:
   a. notify appropriate health care provider (e.g., physician, wound care specialist)
   b. perform care of involved areas as ordered or per standard hospital procedure.

4. Nursing Diagnosis: *ACTIVITY INTOLERANCE*

related to:

a. tissue hypoxia associated with anemia (there is usually significant blood loss because the hip is a very vascular area);
b. difficulty resting and sleeping associated with discomfort, position restrictions, fear, and anxiety.

Suggested NOC Outcomes: Activity tolerance; Self-care: activities of daily living

Suggested NIC Interventions: Energy management; Nutrition management; Sleep enhancement; Blood products administration

Desired Outcome	**Nursing Actions** *and Selected Purposes/Rationales* (see pp. 11–12 for additional rationales)
4. The client will demonstrate an increased tolerance for activity (see Standardized Postoperative Care Plan, Diagnosis 11 [p. 113], for outcome criteria).	4.a. Refer to Standardized Postoperative Care Plan, Diagnosis 11 (pp. 113–114), for measures related to assessment and improvement of activity tolerance. b. Implement additional measures *to help resolve anemia and subsequently improve activity tolerance*: 1. encourage client to increase intake of foods high in iron (e.g. organ meats, dried fruits, dark green leafy vegetables, whole-grain or iron-enriched breads and cereals) and vitamin C *(enhances the absorption of iron from plant products)* 2. transfuse blood obtained from intraoperative and postoperative blood salvage device and/or administer packed red blood cells if ordered 3. administer the following medications if ordered: a. iron supplements b. recombinant human erythropoietin (e.g., epoetin alfa) *to stimulate RBC production.*

5. Nursing Diagnosis: *IMPAIRED PHYSICAL MOBILITY*

related to:

a. pain and weakness in weight-bearing extremity associated with surgery on the hip;
b. prescribed activity and weight-bearing restrictions following total hip replacement;
c. generalized weakness associated with surgery;
d. depressant effect of anesthesia and some medications (e.g., narcotic [opioid] analgesics, centrally acting muscle relaxants, some antiemetics);
e. fear of falling, dislodging drainage tube, dislocating prostheses, and compromising surgical wound.

Suggested NOC Outcome: Mobility

Suggested NIC Interventions: Exercise therapy: joint mobility; Exercise therapy: muscle control; Exercise therapy: ambulation

Desired Outcome	Nursing Actions *and Selected Purposes/Rationales*
5. The client will maintain maximum physical mobility within prescribed activity and weight-bearing restrictions.	5.a. Refer to Standardized Postoperative Care Plan, Diagnosis 12 (p. 114), for measures to increase client's mobility. b. Implement additional measures *to increase client's mobility:* 1. perform actions to reduce pain (see Postoperative Diagnosis 2) 2. instruct client in and assist with quadriceps- and gluteal-setting exercises *to strengthen muscles needed for ambulation* 3. encourage client to use overhead trapeze to move self *in order to strengthen arm and shoulder muscles needed for proper use of ambulatory aids* 4. reinforce physical therapist's instructions regarding additional muscle strengthening exercises, transfer and ambulation techniques, and use of ambulatory aids 5. perform actions to prevent falls (see Postoperative Diagnosis 7, actions a and b) *to decrease client's fear of injury* 6. assist client with ambulation as soon as allowed (usually by the 2nd postoperative day). c. Consult appropriate health care provider (e.g., physician, physical therapist) if client is unable to achieve expected level of mobility.

6. NURSING DIAGNOSIS:

RISK FOR INFECTION: OPERATIVE HIP

related to:

a. introduction of pathogens into the wound during or after surgery;
b. hematoma formation (increases the likelihood of infection by providing a good medium for growth of pathogens and compromising blood flow to the area);
c. increased susceptibility to infection associated with decreased effectiveness of immune system if client is elderly and immunosuppression if client has been taking corticosteroids to treat the joint disorder necessitating the surgery (e.g., rheumatoid arthritis);
d. hematogenous seeding of wound from distant sites (e.g., urinary tract).

Suggested NOC Outcomes: Immune status; Infection severity

Suggested NIC Interventions: Infection protection; Infection control; Incision site care; Wound care: closed drainage

Desired Outcome	Nursing Actions *and Selected Purposes/Rationales* (see pp. 37–40 for additional rationales)
6. The client will remain free of infection in the operative hip (see Standardized Postoperative Care Plan, Diagnosis 17, outcome b [pp. 118–119], for outcome criteria).	6.a. Assess for and report the following: 1. continuous drainage of fluid from incision *(may be indicative of a sinus tract)* 2. sloughing or necrosis of skin in the operative area 3. signs and symptoms of wound infection (e.g., chills; fever; altered mental status; redness, heat, and swelling of wound area; unusual wound drainage; foul odor from wound area; persistent or increased pain in operative hip; elevated sedimentation rate). b. Refer to Standardized Postoperative Care Plan, Diagnosis 17, action b.2 (pp. 118–119), for measures related to prevention of wound infection. c. Implement additional measures *to reduce risk for infection in the operative hip:* 1. use strict sterile technique when performing wound care and emptying wound drainage device 2. maintain patency of wound drainage system *to facilitate drainage of exudate and reduce risk of hematoma formation* 3. do not administer injections in operative extremity 4. avoid urinary catheterization but if it becomes necessary, take precautions to prevent urinary tract infection (e.g., use strict sterile technique during catheter insertion, remove catheter as soon as possible); *the presence*

Desired Outcome	Nursing Actions *and Selected Purposes/Rationales*
	of a urinary catheter increases the risk for a urinary tract infection, which can lead to hematogenous seeding of the hip wound 5. administer prophylactic antimicrobials if ordered. d. If signs and symptoms of wound infection occur: 1. administer antimicrobials as ordered 2. prepare client for drainage and irrigation of wound, surgical debridement, and/or revision arthroplasty if planned.

7. NURSING DIAGNOSIS: **RISK FOR FALLS**

related to:

a. weakness, fatigue, and postural hypotension associated with the effects of major surgery and physiological changes that may have occurred if client is elderly;
b. central nervous system depressant effect of some medications (e.g., narcotic [opioid] analgesics, centrally acting muscle relaxants, some antiemetics);
c. weakness and pain in weight-bearing extremity associated with surgery on the hip;
d. difficulty with transfer and ambulation techniques.

Suggested NOC Outcomes: Fall prevention behavior; Falls occurrence

Suggested NIC Intervention: Fall prevention

Desired Outcome	Nursing Actions *and Selected Purposes/Rationales*
7. The client will not experience falls.	7.a. Refer to Standardized Postoperative Care Plan, Diagnosis 18, action a (p. 120), for measures to prevent falls. b. Implement additional measures *to reduce risk of falls:* 1. reinforce preoperative instructions about and assist client with exercises to improve muscle strength, transfer and ambulation techniques, and use of ambulatory aids 2. administer prescribed analgesics before exercise and ambulation sessions *to reduce hip pain and subsequently maximize client's ability to utilize proper transfer and ambulation techniques* 3. perform actions to improve activity tolerance (see Postoperative Diagnosis 4) *in order to reduce fatigue and weakness.* c. Include client and significant others in planning and implementing measures to prevent falls. d. If falls occur, initiate first aid measures if appropriate and notify physician.

8. COLLABORATIVE DIAGNOSES: **POTENTIAL COMPLICATIONS OF TOTAL HIP REPLACEMENT**

a. hemorrhage and/or hematoma formation related to surgical trauma to blood vessels (the hip is a very vascular area) and use of anticoagulants or antiplatelet agents before and after surgery;
b. dislocation of hip prosthesis(es) related to weakness of the hip muscles, improper positioning or movement of the operative extremity, and/or noncompliance with weight-bearing limitations;
c. thromboembolism related to:
   1. trauma to vein walls during surgery
   2. venous stasis associated with decreased mobility, increased blood viscosity (can result from deficient fluid volume), and pressure exerted on veins by balanced suspension device or abductor wedge
   3. hypercoagulability associated with increased release of tissue thromboplastin into the blood (occurs as a result of surgical trauma) and hemoconcentration and increased blood viscosity (can occur as a result of deficient fluid volume);

d. fat embolism syndrome (FES) related to release of fat from the bone marrow into the blood associated with trauma to the bone during preparation for and implantation of the hip prosthesis.

Desired Outcomes	**Nursing Actions** *and Selected Purposes/Rationales*
8.a. The client will not experience hemorrhage or hematoma formation as evidenced by: 1. expected amount of wound drainage 2. no further decrease in RBC, Hct, and Hgb 3. no significant increase in hip pain 4. absence of tense swelling in surgical area.	8.a.1. Assess for and report the following: a. excessive wound drainage (expected loss is 200–500 ml in the first 24 hours, diminishing to less than 100 ml/24 hours by 48 hours after surgery) b. significant decrease in RBC, Hct, and Hgb levels c. signs and symptoms of hematoma formation (e.g., increased pain and tense swelling in buttock and/or thigh). 2. Implement measures *to reduce operative site bleeding and/or prevent hematoma formation:* a. maintain pressure dressing over operative site as ordered b. keep trochanter roll or sandbag placed firmly against operative site for the first 24–48 hours after surgery *to provide additional pressure on surgical site* c. apply ice pack or cooling pad to operative hip if ordered d. maintain patency of wound drainage system if present. 3. If signs and symptoms of excessive bleeding or hematoma formation occur, prepare client for return to surgery to ligate bleeding vessels and/or drain hematoma if planned.
8.b. The client will not experience dislocation of the hip prosthesis(es) as evidenced by: 1. continued resolution of hip pain 2. ability to maintain operative leg in proper alignment 3. ability to adhere to expected exercise and ambulation regimen 4. usual length of operative extremity 5. normal neurovascular status in operative leg.	8.b.1. Assess for and report signs and symptoms of dislocation of the hip prosthesis(es): a. sudden, severe hip pain followed by continued pain and muscle spasms during hip movement b. abnormal rotation of operative leg c. inability to move or bear weight on operative leg d. shortening of operative leg e. decline in neurovascular status in operative leg. 2. Implement measures *to prevent dislocation of the prosthesis(es):* a. maintain bed rest as ordered (may be on bed rest for first 24 hours after surgery) b. perform actions *to prevent adduction of the operative extremity* (if a posterolateral approach was used): 1. maintain extremity in abducted position using balanced suspension device, an abduction wedge, or 2–3 pillows between legs 2. remind client to avoid crossing legs 3. do not move operative extremity past midline 4. turn client only as ordered and always with pillows between legs c. if client had an anterolateral approach, maintain restrictions on abduction d. maintain operative extremity in proper alignment; instruct client to avoid extreme internal and external rotation of operative leg e. maintain restrictions on head of bed elevation if ordered (some physicians order a 45–60° maximum for first 2–3 days after surgery) *to reduce hip flexion* f. perform actions *to prevent extreme (beyond 90°) hip flexion:* 1. instruct client not to lean forward to reach objects on end of bed or on floor or to put on slippers, socks, or shoes 2. raise the entire bed to client's midthigh level before he/she gets in or out of bed *in order to reduce the degree of hip flexion that occurs when client sits on edge of bed* 3. provide a high, firm chair (or elevate sitting surface with pillows) and an elevated toilet seat for client's use *to reduce degree of hip flexion when client sits down* 4. do not elevate operative leg when client is sitting in chair g. reinforce importance of adhering to recommended weight-bearing restrictions (the amount of weight bearing allowed is based on the

Desired Outcomes	Nursing Actions *and Selected Purposes/Rationales*
	type of prostheses inserted; partial weight bearing is usually allowed as soon as ambulation is started) h. instruct and assist client to pivot and bear weight on the unoperative leg when transferring from bed to chair and raising self out of chair. 3. If signs and symptoms of dislocation of the prosthesis(es) occur: a. maintain client on bed rest b. prepare client for x-rays of the surgical area c. prepare client for closed reduction (e.g., traction) or surgical relocation of the prosthesis(es) if planned.
8.c. The client will not develop a deep vein thrombus or pulmonary embolism (see Standardized Postoperative Care Plan, Diagnosis 20, outcomes c.1 and 2 [pp. 122–123], for outcome criteria).	8.c.1. Refer to Standardized Postoperative Care Plan, Diagnosis 20, actions c.1 and 2 (pp. 122–123), for measures related to assessment, prevention, and treatment of a deep vein thrombus and pulmonary embolism. 2. Implement additional measures *to prevent thrombus formation:* a. make sure that antiembolism stockings are applied correctly and that intermittent pneumatic compression device is correctly applied and functioning properly b. assist client with exercises and ambulation as allowed c. perform actions *to reduce risk of compromising venous return:* 1. make sure elastic wraps or stockings are not too tight 2. avoid use of knee gatch or pillows under knees 3. discourage prolonged sitting or standing 4. make sure that balanced suspension device or straps on abductor wedge do not exert excessive pressure on any area d. administer anticoagulants (e.g., low-dose warfarin, low-molecular-weight heparin, fondaparinux, danaparoid) or antiplatelet agents (e.g., aspirin) as ordered.
8.d. The client will not experience fat embolism syndrome as evidenced by: 1. usual mental status 2. unlabored respirations at 12–20/minute 3. absence of petechiae 4. Pao_2 within normal limits.	8.d.1. Assess for and report signs and symptoms of fat embolism syndrome (usually occurs within 72 hours after surgery): a. restlessness, apprehension, confusion b. sudden onset of dyspnea c. tachypnea d. elevated pulse and temperature e. petechiae on the chest, neck, or axilla f. low Pao_2 level g. unexpected decrease in Hct and Hgb h. thrombocytopenia. 2. Move operative extremity gently and avoid excessive movement of the extremity during the first few days after surgery *to reduce the risk for fat emboli.* 3. If signs and symptoms of fat embolism syndrome occur: a. maintain client on bed rest and move operative extremity as little as possible *to prevent further emboli* b. administer oxygen and assist with positive airway pressure techniques (e.g., positive end expiratory pressure) if ordered c. prepare client for chest x-ray or lung scan d. administer intravenous fluids as ordered *to help maintain adequate perfusion to vital organs and prevent shock* e. administer corticosteroids if ordered *to reduce cerebral edema and pulmonary inflammation.*

Discharge Teaching/Continued Care

9. Nursing Diagnosis: ***DEFICIENT KNOWLEDGE, INEFFECTIVE THERAPEUTIC REGIMEN MANAGEMENT, OR INEFFECTIVE HEALTH MAINTENANCE****

*The nurse should select the diagnostic label that is most appropriate for the client's discharge teaching needs.

Suggested NOC Outcomes: Knowledge: fall prevention; Knowledge: prescribed activity; Knowledge: treatment regimen

Suggested NIC Interventions: Health system guidance; Teaching: individual; Teaching: prescribed activity/exercise

Desired Outcomes	Nursing Actions *and Selected Purposes/Rationales*
9.a. The client will demonstrate correct transfer and ambulation techniques and proper use of ambulatory aids.	9.a.1. Reinforce instructions about correct transfer and ambulation techniques and proper use of walker, quad cane, or crutches. 2. Reinforce physician's instructions about amount of weight bearing on operative extremity. 3. Allow time for questions, clarification, and practice of transfer and ambulation techniques.
9.b. The client will demonstrate the ability to correctly perform the prescribed exercises.	9.b.1. Reinforce the physical therapist's instructions on prescribed exercises and the importance of continuing the exercises for the prescribed length of time. 2. Inform client that walking and swimming are good aerobic exercises. 3. Allow time for questions, clarification, and return demonstration of prescribed exercises.
9.c. The client will verbalize an understanding of activity and position restrictions necessary to prevent dislocation of the hip prostheses.	9.c. Instruct client to adhere to the following activity and position restrictions in order to prevent dislocation of the hip prostheses (length of time the restrictions are necessary varies but ranges from 2–6 months): 1. turn only as directed by physician (many physicians allow client to turn to unoperative side only) 2. instruct client to keep pillow between legs when lying on back or side and when turning 3. never cross legs 4. do not sit on low chairs, stools, or toilets; place a cushion on low chairs, rent or purchase an elevated toilet seat for home use, and use the high toilets designated for the handicapped when in public facilities 5. do not elevate operative leg higher than hip when sitting 6. sit in chairs with arms and use the arms to raise self off chair 7. support weight on unoperative leg when raising self from a sitting position 8. use assistive devices (e.g., long-handled shoe horn, long-handled grabber) to assist with activities that require flexing hip beyond 90° (e.g., putting on shoes and socks, reaching objects on the floor or in low cupboards or drawers, pulling bed covers up from end of bed) 9. keep operative leg in proper alignment and avoid extreme internal and external rotation of leg 10. do not drive until approved by physician (usually about 6 weeks after surgery) 11. when riding in a car: a. sit on a firm pillow or cushion to prevent hip flexion of more than 90° b. keep operative leg extended (a sudden impact of the knee against the dashboard can dislodge the prostheses) 12. when sexual activity is resumed, avoid positions that involve extreme rotation of the operative leg, flexing hip beyond 90°, and moving operative leg past the midline 13. avoid lifting heavy objects, excessive twisting and turning of body, and activities that place excessive strain on hip (e.g., jogging, jumping).
9.d. The client will identify ways to reduce the risk of falls in the home environment.	9.d. Provide the following instructions on ways to reduce the risk of falls at home: 1. keep electrical cords out of pathways 2. remove unnecessary furniture and provide wide pathways for ambulation

Desired Outcomes	**Nursing Actions** *and Selected Purposes/Rationales*
	3. remove scatter rugs 4. provide adequate lighting at all times 5. avoid unnecessary stair climbing.
9.e. The client will state signs and symptoms to report to the health care provider.	9.e.1. Refer to Standardized Postoperative Care Plan, Diagnosis 22, action c (p. 125), for signs and symptoms to report to the health care provider. 2. Instruct client to report these additional signs and symptoms: a. persistent or increased pain or spasms in operative extremity b. loss of sensation or movement in operative extremity c. inability to bear weight on operative extremity d. inability to maintain operative extremity in a neutral position e. shortening of operative extremity (will probably be noticed as a limp).
9.f. The client will identify community resources that can assist with home management and provide transportation.	9.f.1. Provide information about community resources that can assist the client and significant others with home management and provide transportation (e.g., home health agencies, Meals on Wheels, church groups, transportation services). 2. Initiate a referral if indicated.
9.g. The client will verbalize an understanding of and a plan for adhering to recommended follow-up care including future appointments with health care provider and physical therapist, medications prescribed, activity level, and wound care.	9.g.1. Refer to Standardized Postoperative Care Plan, Diagnosis 22 (pp. 125–126), for routine postoperative instructions and measures to improve client compliance. 2. Reinforce importance of keeping appointments with physical therapist. 3. Teach client the rationale for, side effects of, schedule for taking, and importance of taking medications prescribed (e.g., iron supplements, anticoagulant). If client is discharged on an anticoagulant (e.g., low-dose warfarin, low-molecular-weight heparin), instruct him/her to follow precautions to prevent bleeding (e.g., avoid injury, use an electric rather than a straight-edge razor) and report bleeding or excessive bruising immediately. 4. Instruct client to inform other health care providers of history of total hip replacement so prophylactic antimicrobials can be started before any dental work, invasive diagnostic procedures, or surgery is performed. 5. Inform client that the prosthetic device may activate metal detector alarms. Recommend carrying an identification/information card verifying presence of device.

Bibliography

See pages 879 and 885.

evolve

TOTAL KNEE REPLACEMENT

A total knee replacement (arthroplasty) is a surgical procedure in which the articular surfaces of the tibia, femur, and patella are replaced with prosthetic devices. It is performed to relieve joint pain that has not been controlled by conservative management and/or improve joint mobility in persons with severe arthritis, congenital knee deformity, hemophilic arthropathy, or severe intraarticular injury.

There are a variety of prostheses available. The type most frequently used is the tricompartmental prostheses that has separate femoral, tibial, and patellar components. Fixation of the prostheses is accomplished by using a cement-like agent called polymethylmethacrylate or, if left uncemented, by bone ingrowth into the porous outer surface on the prostheses.

This care plan focuses on the adult client hospitalized for a total knee replacement. Much of the postoperative information is applicable to clients receiving follow-up care in an extended care facility or home setting.

OUTCOME/DISCHARGE CRITERIA

THE CLIENT WILL:

- have evidence of normal healing of the surgical wound
- have clear, audible breath sounds throughout lungs
- have reduced knee pain
- have expected degree of mobility of knee joint
- have no signs and symptoms of infection or postoperative complications
- demonstrate correct transfer and ambulation techniques and proper use of ambulatory aids
- demonstrate the ability to correctly perform the prescribed exercises
- identify ways to reduce the risk of loosening of the prosthesis(es)
- identify ways to reduce the risk of falls in the home environment
- state signs and symptoms to report to the health care provider
- identify community resources that can assist with home management and provide transportation
- verbalize an understanding of and a plan for adhering to recommended follow-up care including future appointments with health care provider and physical therapist, medications prescribed, activity level, and wound care.

NURSING/COLLABORATIVE DIAGNOSES

Preoperative

1. Deficient knowledge p. 806

Postoperative

1. Risk for peripheral neurovascular dysfunction: operative extremity p. 807
2. Acute pain: knee p. 807
3. Actual/Risk for impaired tissue integrity p. 808
4. Impaired physical mobility p. 809
5. Risk for infection: operative knee p. 810
6. Risk for falls p. 811
7. Potential complications p. 811
   a. dislocation of knee prosthesis(es) or stress fracture of tibia or femur
   b. thromboembolism
   c. fat embolism syndrome (FES)

DISCHARGE TEACHING

8. Deficient knowledge, Ineffective therapeutic regimen management, or Ineffective health maintenance p. 813

See Standardized Preoperative and Postoperative Care Plans (pp. 97–126) for additional diagnoses.

PREOPERATIVE

Use in conjunction with the Standardized Preoperative Care Plan.

Client Teaching

1. Nursing Diagnosis: ***DEFICIENT KNOWLEDGE***

regarding the surgical procedure, hospital routines associated with surgery, physical preparation for total knee replacement, sensations that normally occur following surgery and anesthesia, and postoperative care.

Suggested NOC Outcomes: Knowledge: treatment regimen; Knowledge: prescribed activity

Suggested NIC Interventions: Teaching: preoperative; Teaching: prescribed activity/exercise

Desired Outcomes	**Nursing Actions** *and Selected Purposes/Rationales*
1.a. The client will verbalize an understanding of the surgical procedure, preoperative care, and postoperative sensations and care.	1.a.1. Refer to Standardized Preoperative Care Plan, Diagnosis 4, actions a.1–4 (pp. 100–101), for information to include in preoperative teaching. 2. Provide additional information about specific preoperative care for clients having a total knee replacement: a. explain that the following measures will be performed to reduce the risk of a postoperative knee infection: 1. the operative leg will be scrubbed with an antiseptic solution (e.g., 2% chlorhexidene) before surgery 2. existing infections will be treated before surgery; instruct client to report any symptoms of infection (e.g., cough, runny nose, burning on urination) 3. antimicrobials will probably be administered prophylactically before and after surgery b. explain that anticoagulants (e.g., low-molecular-weight heparin, low-dose warfarin) may be administered before surgery to reduce the risk of postoperative thrombus formation; inform client that coagulation studies are usually done before starting these medications, especially if he/she has been taking aspirin or other nonsteroidal anti-inflammatory agents (e.g., ibuprofen) c. explain that a physical therapist will fit crutches or walker and provide instructions on postoperative physical therapy regimen. 3. Allow time for questions and clarification of information provided.
1.b. The client will demonstrate the ability to perform activities designed to prevent postoperative complications.	1.b.1. Refer to Standardized Preoperative Care Plan, Diagnosis 4, action b.1 (p. 101), for instructions on ways to prevent postoperative complications. 2. Provide additional instructions about ways to prevent complications following total knee replacement: a. reinforce physician's or physical therapist's instructions on: 1. exercises to improve strength and facilitate mobility (e.g., quadriceps- and gluteal-setting, knee flexion, straight leg raising) 2. transfer and ambulation techniques and proper use of ambulatory aids; weight-bearing limitations are determined by the physician and vary depending on the type of prostheses inserted (usually partial weight bearing is allowed initially with progressive weight bearing as tolerated) b. instruct client in the correct way to use overhead trapeze and unoperative leg to move self c. inform client that he/she will need to avoid extreme flexion of the knee for first few weeks after surgery in order to prevent dislocation of the prosthesis(es) d. explain the purpose for the continuous passive motion (CPM) machine and the need to leave the extremity in the machine as ordered e. describe or show client the knee immobilizer and explain purpose for wearing immobilizer. 3. Allow time for questions, clarification, and return demonstration.

POSTOPERATIVE *Use in conjunction with the Standardized Postoperative Care Plan.*

1. NURSING DIAGNOSIS:

RISK FOR PERIPHERAL NEUROVASCULAR DYSFUNCTION: OPERATIVE EXTREMITY

related to trauma to or excessive pressure on the nerves or blood vessels during surgery; blood accumulation and edema in the surgical area; improper alignment of operative extremity; pressure exerted by the dressing, knee immobilizer, or CPM machine; or dislocation of the prosthesis(es).

Suggested NOC Outcome: Tissue perfusion: peripheral

Suggested NIC Interventions: Circulatory care: arterial insufficiency; Circulatory care: venous insufficiency; Lower extremity monitoring; Positioning; Pressure management

Desired Outcome	**Nursing Actions** *and Selected Purposes/Rationales*
1. The client will maintain normal neurovascular function in the operative extremity as evidenced by: a. palpable pedal pulses b. capillary refill time in toes less than 2–3 seconds c. extremity warm and usual color d. ability to flex and extend foot and toes e. absence of numbness and tingling in foot and toes f. absence of foot pain during passive movement of toes and foot g. no increase in pain in extremity.	1.a. Assess for and report signs and symptoms of neurovascular dysfunction in the operative extremity: 1. diminished or absent pedal pulses 2. capillary refill time in toes greater than 2–3 seconds 3. pallor, cyanosis, or coolness of the extremity 4. inability to flex or extend foot or toes 5. numbness or tingling in foot or toes 6. pain in foot during passive motion of toes or foot 7. increased pain in extremity. b. Implement measures *to prevent neurovascular dysfunction in the operative extremity:* 1. apply ice packs or cooling pad to operative knee for the first 24–48 hours after surgery if ordered *to reduce bleeding and edema in surgical area* 2. maintain patency of wound drainage system (e.g., prevent kinking of tubing, empty collection device as needed, keep collection device below wound level, maintain suction as ordered) *to reduce accumulation of fluid in the surgical area* 3. maintain extremity in proper alignment 4. elevate operative leg on pillow (when not in CPM machine) for the first 48 hours after surgery *in order to reduce edema in the surgical area;* place pillows so knee flexion is avoided 5. position leg so that knee immobilizer and CPM machine are not causing excessive pressure on any area 6. loosen straps of knee immobilizer if it appears to be too tight 7. notify physician if dressing appears to be too tight 8. perform actions to prevent dislocation of the prosthesis(es) and stress fracture of the tibia and femur (see Postoperative Diagnosis 7, action a.2). c. If signs and symptoms of neurovascular dysfunction occur: 1. assess for and correct causes of excessive pressure 2. notify physician if the signs and symptoms persist.

2. NURSING DIAGNOSIS:

ACUTE PAIN: KNEE

related to tissue trauma and reflex muscle spasms associated with the surgery, blood accumulation and edema in the surgical area, and improper positioning of the operative extremity.

Suggested NOC Outcomes: Comfort level; Pain control

Suggested NIC Interventions: Pain management; Analgesic administration; Environmental management: comfort; Heat/Cold application

Desired Outcome	Nursing Actions and Selected Purposes/Rationales (see pp. 45–47 for additional rationales)
2. The client will experience diminished knee pain (see Standardized Postoperative Care Plan, Diagnosis 6 [p. 109], for outcome criteria).	2.a. Refer to Standardized Postoperative Care Plan, Diagnosis 6 (p. 109), for measures related to assessment and reduction of pain. b. Implement additional measures *to reduce pain*: 1. maintain operative extremity in proper alignment 2. move the operative extremity carefully 3. apply ice packs or cooling pad to the operative knee for first 24–48 hours after surgery if ordered *to reduce bleeding and edema in the surgical area* 4. elevate operative leg on pillow (when not in CPM machine) for the first 48 hours after surgery *in order to reduce edema in the surgical area;* place pillows so knee flexion is avoided 5. maintain patency of the wound drainage system if present *to prevent accumulation of fluid in the surgical area* 6. remind client to avoid flexing operative knee beyond prescribed limits 7. ensure that knee immobilizer is worn as prescribed *in order to prevent strain on the operative area* 8. administer prescribed analgesics before exercise and ambulation sessions 9. apply ice pack or cooling pad to operative knee for 20–30 minutes before and after exercise and ambulation sessions as ordered.

3. Nursing Diagnosis: ACTUAL/RISK FOR IMPAIRED TISSUE INTEGRITY

related to:

a. disruption of tissue associated with the surgical procedure;
b. delayed wound healing associated with factors such as decreased nutritional status and inadequate blood supply to wound area;
c. irritation of skin associated with contact with wound drainage, pressure from tubes, and use of tape;
d. excessive or prolonged pressure on tissues from compression dressing, knee immobilizer, or CPM machine;
e. damage to the skin and/or subcutaneous tissue associated with prolonged pressure on tissues, friction, and shearing while mobility is decreased.

Suggested NOC Outcomes: Tissue integrity: skin and mucous membranes; Wound healing: primary intention

Suggested NIC Interventions: Incision site care; Skin surveillance; Positioning; Pressure ulcer prevention; Pressure management; Skin care: topical treatments

Desired Outcomes	Nursing Actions and Selected Purposes/Rationales (see pp. 49–52 for additional rationales)
3.a. The client will experience normal healing of the surgical wound (see Standardized Postoperative Care Plan, Diagnosis 10, outcome a [p. 112], for outcome criteria).	3.a. Refer to Standardized Postoperative Care Plan, Diagnosis 10, action a (p. 112), for measures related to assessment and promotion of wound healing.
3.b. The client will maintain tissue integrity as evidenced by: 1. absence of redness and irritation 2. no skin breakdown.	3.b.1. Inspect the following areas for pallor, redness, and breakdown: a. skin in contact with wound drainage, tape, and tubings b. back, coccyx, and buttocks c. elbows and heels d. areas at edges of compression dressing or knee immobilizer e. areas in contact with CPM machine. 2. Refer to Standardized Postoperative Care Plan, Diagnosis 10, action b.2 (pp. 112–113), for measures related to prevention of tissue irritation and

breakdown in areas in contact with wound drainage, tubings, and tape.

3. Implement measures *to prevent tissue breakdown associated with decreased mobility:*
   a. position client properly; use pressure-reducing or pressure-relieving devices (e.g., pillows, alternating pressure mattress) if indicated
   b. instruct client to use overhead trapeze to lift self and shift weight at least every 30 minutes
   c. gently massage around reddened areas at least every 2 hours
   d. apply a thin layer of a dry lubricant such as powder or cornstarch to bottom sheet or skin and to opposing skin surfaces (e.g., axillae) if indicated *to reduce friction*
   e. lift and move client carefully using a turn sheet and adequate assistance
   f. perform actions to keep client from sliding down in bed (e.g., limit length of time client is in semi-Fowler's position to 30 minute intervals) *in order to reduce the risk of skin surface abrasion and shearing*
   g. turn client at least every 2 hours when not in CPM machine; keep pillows between legs and operative knee extended
   h. keep client's skin clean
   i. keep bed linens dry and wrinkle-free
   j. increase activity as allowed and tolerated.
4. Implement measures *to prevent irritation and breakdown on elbows and heels:*
   a. massage elbows and heels with lotion frequently
   b. encourage client to use overhead trapeze to move self rather than pushing up with heel and elbows
   c. provide elbow and heel protectors if indicated.
5. Implement measures *to prevent tissue breakdown in areas in contact with the compression dressing, knee immobilizer, and CPM machine:*
   a. assess for and report tightness of the dressing or reports of a burning sensation under the dressing or knee immobilizer
   b. loosen straps on knee immobilizer if it appears to be too tight
   c. apply cornstarch to skin under immobilizer *in order to reduce friction and subsequent skin irritation*
   d. keep dressing dry
   e. position the operative extremity so that the knee immobilizer and CPM machine are not causing excessive pressure on any area
   f. make sure CPM machine is padded adequately
   g. instruct client to refrain from inserting anything inside the dressing or knee immobilizer.
6. If tissue breakdown occurs:
   a. notify appropriate health care provider (e.g., physician, wound care specialist)
   b. perform care of involved areas as ordered or per standard hospital procedure.

4. NURSING DIAGNOSIS: ***IMPAIRED PHYSICAL MOBILITY***

related to:

a. pain and weakness in weight-bearing extremity associated with surgery on the knee;
b. prescribed activity and weight-bearing restrictions following total knee replacement;
c. generalized weakness associated with surgery;
d. depressant effect of anesthesia and some medications (e.g., narcotic [opioid] analgesics, centrally acting muscle relaxants, some antiemetics);
e. fear of falling, dislocating prostheses, and compromising surgical wound.

Suggested NOC Outcome:
Mobility

Suggested NIC Interventions: Exercise therapy: joint mobility; Exercise therapy: muscle control; Exercise therapy: ambulation

Desired Outcome	Nursing Actions *and Selected Purposes/Rationales*
4. The client will maintain maximum physical mobility within prescribed activity and weight-bearing restrictions.	4.a. Refer to Standardized Postoperative Care Plan, Diagnosis 12 (p. 114), for measures to increase client's mobility. b. Implement additional measures *to increase client's mobility:* 1. perform actions to reduce pain (see Postoperative Diagnosis 2) 2. maintain prescribed degree of flexion and extension on CPM machine and encourage client to keep operative leg in CPM machine for the prescribed length of time *to reduce the risk of scarring in the knee and a subsequent decrease in range of motion* 3. encourage client to perform quadriceps- and gluteal-setting, straight leg raising, and knee flexion-extension exercises as soon as allowed (usually started by the 2nd postoperative day) 4. encourage client to use overhead trapeze to move self *in order to strengthen arm and shoulder muscles needed for proper use of ambulatory aids* 5. reinforce physical therapist's instructions regarding transfer and ambulation techniques and use of ambulatory aids (e.g., crutches, walker) 6. perform actions to prevent falls (see Postoperative Diagnosis 6, actions a and b) *in order to decrease client's fear of injury* 7. assist client with ambulation as soon as allowed (usually by the 2nd postoperative day). c. Consult appropriate health care provider (e.g., physician, physical therapist) if client is unable to make expected progress with knee flexion or if any other joint motion becomes restricted.

5. Nursing Diagnosis: RISK FOR INFECTION: OPERATIVE KNEE

related to:
a. introduction of pathogens into the wound during or following surgery;
b. increased susceptibility to infection associated with decreased effectiveness of immune system if client is elderly and immunosuppression if client has been taking corticosteroids to treat the joint disorder necessitating the surgery (e.g., rheumatoid arthritis);
c. hematogenous seeding of wound from distant sites (e.g., urinary tract).

Suggested NOC Outcomes: Immune status; Infection severity

Suggested NIC Interventions: Infection protection; Infection control; Incision site care; Wound care: closed drainage

Desired Outcome	Nursing Actions *and Selected Purposes/Rationales* (see pp. 37–40 for additional rationales)
5. The client will remain free of infection in the operative knee (see Standardized Postoperative Care Plan, Diagnosis 17, outcome b [pp. 118–119], for outcome criteria).	5.a. Assess for and report the following: 1. continuous drainage of fluid from incision (*may indicate a sinus tract*) 2. sloughing or necrosis of skin in operative area 3. signs and symptoms of wound infection (e.g., chills; fever; altered mental status; redness, heat, and swelling of wound area; unusual wound drainage; foul odor from wound area; persistent or increased pain in knee; elevated sedimentation rate). b. Refer to Standardized Postoperative Care Plan, Diagnosis 17, action b.2 (pp. 118–119), for measures related to prevention of wound infection. c. Implement additional measures *to reduce risk for infection in the operative knee:* 1. use strict sterile technique when performing wound care and emptying wound drainage device 2. maintain patency of the wound drainage device *in order to prevent accumulation of drainage in surgical area* 3. keep CPM machine off the floor when not in use 4. avoid urinary catheterization but if it becomes necessary, take precautions to prevent urinary tract infection (e.g., use strict sterile

technique during catheter insertion, remove catheter as soon as possible); *the presence of a urinary catheter increases the risk for a urinary tract infection, which can lead to hematogenous seeding of the knee wound*
5. administer prophylactic antimicrobials if ordered.

d. If signs and symptoms of wound infection occur:
1. administer antimicrobials as ordered
2. prepare client for surgical debridement and/or revision arthroplasty if planned.

6. Nursing Diagnosis:

RISK FOR FALLS

related to:

a. weakness, fatigue, and postural hypotension associated with the effects of major surgery and physiological changes that may have occurred if client is elderly;
b. central nervous system depressant effect of some medications (e.g., narcotic [opioid] analgesics, centrally acting muscle relaxants, some antiemetics);
c. weakness and pain in weight-bearing extremity associated with surgery on the knee;
d. improper transfer and ambulation techniques.

Suggested NOC Outcomes:
Fall prevention behavior;
Falls occurrence

Suggested NIC Intervention: Fall prevention

Desired Outcome	**Nursing Actions** *and Selected Purposes/Rationales*
6. The client will not experience falls.	6.a. Refer to Standardized Postoperative Care Plan, Diagnosis 18, action a (p. 120), for measures to prevent falls. b. Implement additional measures *to reduce the risk for falls:* 1. reinforce preoperative instructions about and assist client with transfer and ambulation techniques, use of ambulatory aids, and exercises to improve muscle strength 2. administer prescribed analgesics and/or apply ice packs to operative knee before exercise and ambulation sessions *to reduce knee pain and subsequently maximize the client's ability to use proper transfer and ambulation techniques* 3. ensure that client has knee immobilizer on for ambulation sessions *to provide additional support of operative leg.* c. Include client and significant others in planning and implementing measures to prevent falls. d. If falls occur, initiate first aid measures if appropriate and notify physician.

7. Collaborative Diagnoses:

POTENTIAL COMPLICATIONS OF TOTAL KNEE REPLACEMENT

a. **dislocation of knee prosthesis(es) or stress fracture of tibia or femur** related to rotation of or excessive pressure on the knee;
b. **thromboembolism** related to:
1. trauma to vein walls during surgery
2. venous stasis associated with use of a tourniquet on operative leg during surgery; pressure exerted on the veins by the dressing, knee immobilizer, or CPM machine; decreased mobility; and increased blood viscosity (can result from deficient fluid volume)
3. hypercoagulability associated with increased release of tissue thromboplastin into the blood (occurs as a result of surgical trauma) and hemoconcentration and increased blood viscosity (can occur as a result of deficient fluid volume);

c. **fat embolism syndrome** (FES) related to release of fat from the bone marrow into the blood associated with trauma to the bone during preparation for and implantation of the knee prostheses.

Desired Outcomes	Nursing Actions *and Selected Purposes/Rationales*
7.a. The client will not experience dislocation of the knee prosthesis(es) or stress fracture of tibia or femur as evidenced by: 1. continued resolution of knee pain 2. ability to maintain operative leg in proper alignment 3. ability to adhere to planned exercise and ambulation regimen 4. normal neurovascular status in operative leg.	7.a.1. Assess for and report signs and symptoms of dislocation of the knee prosthesis(es) and/or stress fracture of tibia or femur: a. sudden, severe knee pain followed by continued pain and muscle spasms during knee movement b. abnormal rotation of the lower portion of operative leg c. inability to move or bear weight on operative leg d. decline in neurovascular status in operative leg. 2. Implement measures *to prevent dislocation of the prosthesis(es) and stress fracture of the tibia and femur:* a. instruct client to avoid hyperextension, rotation, and acute flexion of knee b. reinforce physician's instructions regarding the amount of weight bearing allowed (usual order is partial weight bearing initially with progressive weight bearing as tolerated) c. reinforce instructions and assist client with gait training and proper use of ambulatory aids d. reinforce the importance of wearing knee immobilizer when ambulating. 3. If signs and symptoms of prosthesis(es) dislocation or stress fracture occur: a. maintain client on bed rest b. prepare client for x-rays of operative leg c. prepare client for closed reduction or surgical intervention (e.g., realignment of prosthesis, internal fixation of fracture) if planned.
7.b. The client will not develop a deep vein thrombus or pulmonary embolism (see Standardized Postoperative Care Plan, Diagnosis 20, outcomes c.1 and 2 [pp. 122–123], for outcome criteria).	7.b.1. Refer to Standardized Postoperative Care Plan, Diagnosis 20, actions c.1 and 2 (pp. 122–123), for measures related to assessment, prevention, and treatment of a deep vein thrombus and pulmonary embolism. 2. Implement additional measures *to prevent thrombus formation:* a. assist client to perform leg exercises and ambulate as soon as allowed b. perform actions *to reduce risk of compromising venous return:* 1. consult physician if dressing appears to be too tight 2. loosen knee immobilizer if it appears to be too tight 3. make sure exercise sling is not exerting pressure on the popliteal space 4. avoid use of the knee gatch or pillows under knees 5. discourage prolonged sitting or standing c. make sure that intermittent pneumatic compression device is applied and functioning properly if ordered d. administer anticoagulants (e.g., low-dose warfarin, fondaparinux, low-molecular-weight heparin) or antiplatelet agents (e.g. aspirin) as ordered.
7.c. The client will not experience fat embolism syndrome as evidenced by: 1. usual mental status 2. unlabored respirations at 12–20/minute 3. absence of petechiae 4. $Pa{O_2}$ within normal limits.	7.c.1. Assess for and report signs and symptoms of fat embolism syndrome (usually occurs within 72 hours after surgery): a. restlessness, apprehension, confusion b. sudden onset of dyspnea c. tachypnea d. elevated pulse and temperature e. petechiae on the chest, neck, or axilla f. low $Pa{O_2}$ level g. unexpected decrease in Hct and Hgb h. thrombocytopenia. 2. Move operative extremity gently and avoid excessive movement of the extremity during the first few days after surgery *to reduce the risk for fat emboli.* 3. If signs and symptoms of fat embolism syndrome occur: a. maintain client on bed rest and move operative extremity as little as possible *to prevent further emboli*

b. administer oxygen and assist with positive airway pressure techniques (e.g., positive end expiratory pressure) if ordered
c. prepare client for chest x-ray or lung scan
d. administer intravenous fluids as ordered *to help maintain adequate perfusion to vital organs and prevent shock*
e. administer corticosteroids if ordered *to reduce cerebral edema and pulmonary inflammation.*

Discharge Teaching/Continued Care

8. NURSING DIAGNOSIS: ***DEFICIENT KNOWLEDGE, INEFFECTIVE THERAPEUTIC REGIMEN MANAGEMENT, OR INEFFECTIVE HEALTH MAINTENANCE****

*The nurse should select the diagnostic label that is most appropriate for the client's discharge teaching needs.

Suggested NOC Outcomes: Knowledge: fall prevention; Knowledge: prescribed activity; Knowledge: treatment regimen

Suggested NIC Interventions: Health system guidance; Teaching: individual; Teaching: prescribed activity/exercise

Desired Outcomes	Nursing Actions *and Selected Purposes/Rationales*
8.a. The client will demonstrate correct transfer and ambulation techniques and proper use of ambulatory aids.	8.a.1. Reinforce instructions about correct transfer and ambulation techniques and proper use of crutches, cane, or walker. 2. Reinforce the importance of adhering to weight-bearing restrictions if prescribed. 3. Allow time for questions, clarification, and practice of transfer and ambulation techniques.
8.b. The client will demonstrate the ability to correctly perform the prescribed exercises.	8.b.1. Reinforce the physical therapist's instructions about prescribed exercises. 2. Reinforce the importance of continuing exercises for the prescribed length of time. 3. Allow time for questions, clarification, and return demonstration of prescribed exercises.
8.c. The client will identify ways to reduce the risk of loosening of the prosthesis(es).	8.c.1. Inform client of the possibility of loosening of the prosthesis (usually does not occur until 2–3 years after surgery). 2. Instruct client to report increasing pain or instability of operative knee (may indicate loosening of the prosthesis). 3. Instruct client regarding ways to minimize risk of loosening of the prosthesis(es): a. adhere to weight-bearing restrictions if prescribed b. avoid unusual twisting of knee c. avoid contact sports d. do not force knee beyond comfortable degree of flexion and avoid kneeling e. avoid placing undue stress on knees (e.g., do not lift and carry heavy objects, maintain ideal body weight, avoid activities such as jogging).
8.d. The client will identify ways to reduce the risk of falls in the home environment.	8.d. Provide the following instructions on ways to reduce risk of falls at home: 1. keep electrical cords out of pathways 2. remove unnecessary furniture and provide wide pathways for ambulation 3. remove scatter rugs 4. provide adequate lighting at all times 5. avoid unnecessary stair climbing.

Desired Outcomes	**Nursing Actions** *and Selected Purposes/Rationales*
8.e. The client will state signs and symptoms to report to the health care provider.	8.e.1. Refer to Standardized Postoperative Care Plan, Diagnosis 22, action c (p. 125), for signs and symptoms to report to the health care provider. 2. Instruct client to report these additional signs and symptoms: a. persistent or increased pain or spasms in operative extremity b. loss of sensation or movement in operative extremity c. inability to bear expected amount of weight on operative extremity d. inability to maintain operative extremity in a neutral position e. instability of operative extremity (feeling of knee "giving out").
8.f. The client will identify community resources that can assist with home management and provide transportation.	8.f.1. Provide information about community resources that can assist client and significant others with home management and provide transportation (e.g., home health agencies, Meals on Wheels, church groups, transportation services). 2. Initiate a referral if indicated.
8.g. The client will verbalize an understanding of and a plan for adhering to recommended follow-up care including future appointments with health care provider and physical therapist, medications prescribed, activity level, and wound care.	8.g.1. Refer to Standardized Postoperative Care Plan, Diagnosis 22 (pp. 125–126), for routine postoperative instructions and measures to improve client compliance. 2. Reinforce the importance of keeping appointments with physical therapist. 3. Teach client the rationale for, side effects of, schedule for taking, and importance of taking prescribed medications (e.g., iron supplement, anticoagulant). If client is discharged on an anticoagulant (e.g., low-dose warfarin, low-molecular-weight heparin), instruct him/her to follow precautions to prevent bleeding (e.g., avoid injury, use an electric rather than a straight-edge razor) and report bleeding or excessive bruising immediately. 4. Instruct client to inform other health care providers of history of total knee replacement so prophylactic antimicrobials can be started before any dental work, invasive diagnostic procedures, or surgery is performed. 5. Inform client that the prosthetic device may activate metal detector alarms. Recommend carrying an identification/information card verifying presence of the device.

Bibliography

See pages 879 and 885.

UNIT XVIII

Nursing Care of the Client with Disturbances of the Breast and Reproductive System

Colporrhaphy (Anterior and Posterior Repair)

Colporrhaphy is the surgical tightening of the vaginal wall and relaxed pelvic muscles. An anterior colporrhaphy is performed to correct a cystocele, which is a herniation of the bladder through weakened supportive fascia of the anterior vaginal compartment. Urethral hypermotility is often present with a cystocele and various techniques for providing urethrovesical angle support during an anterior colporrhaphy can be utilized to correct this problem. A posterior colporrhaphy is performed if weakening of the supporting fascia has resulted in a rectocele (herniation of the rectum into the posterior vaginal wall). If an anterior and posterior colporrhaphy are done at the same time, the surgery is referred to as an anteroposterior (AP) repair. Colporrhaphy is usually performed transvaginally through an incision in the vaginal wall (an incision in the perineum may also be made during a posterior colporrhaphy). An abdominal approach is sometimes used to perform a colporrhaphy depending on the client's diagnosis and need for additional abdominal surgery.

Cystoceles and rectoceles are caused by relaxation of the pelvic floor support system, which is usually associated with changes that occur with childbirth and are exacerbated by aging, loss of estrogen stimulation, and factors such as obesity and chronic abdominal straining (e.g., chronic cough, chronic constipation). Signs and symptoms of a cystocele may include stress incontinence, a feeling of incomplete emptying of the bladder after voiding, and a sensation of fullness or pressure in the pelvic area and/or a feeling that organs are "falling out." Indications that a rectocele may be present are difficult or incomplete emptying of the rectum, constipation, and a heavy or "falling out" feeling in the vagina. Colporrhaphy is indicated when conservative management (e.g., perineal exercises, insertion of a pessary) no longer controls signs and symptoms.

This care plan focuses on the adult client having a transvaginal anterior and posterior repair. The information is applicable to clients having surgery in a hospital or outpatient (e.g., surgical care center) setting.

OUTCOME/DISCHARGE CRITERIA

THE CLIENT WILL:

- have evidence of normal healing of surgical wound
- have adequate urine output
- have surgical pain controlled
- have no signs and symptoms of infection or postoperative complications
- identify ways to decrease the risk of reherniation of the bladder and rectum
- identify ways to relieve surgical site discomfort
- state signs and symptoms to report to the health care provider
- verbalize an understanding of and a plan for adhering to recommended follow-up care including future appointments with health care provider, medications prescribed, and limitations on sexual activity.

NURSING/COLLABORATIVE DIAGNOSES

Postoperative

DISCHARGE TEACHING

See Standardized Preoperative and Postoperative Care Plans (pp. 97–126) for additional diagnoses.

PREOPERATIVE *Refer to the Standardized Preoperative Care Plan.*

POSTOPERATIVE *Use in conjunction with the Standardized Postoperative Care Plan.*

1. Nursing Diagnosis: *ACUTE PAIN*

related to tissue trauma and reflex muscle spasms associated with the surgical procedure.

Suggested NOC Outcomes: Comfort level; Pain control

Suggested NIC Interventions: Pain management; Analgesic administration

Desired Outcome	**Nursing Actions** *and Selected Purposes/Rationales*
1. The client will experience diminished pain as evidenced by: a. verbalization of a decrease in or absence of pain b. relaxed facial expression and body positioning c. ability to sit and walk more comfortably d. increased participation in activities e. stable vital signs.	1.a. Refer to Standardized Postoperative Care Plan, Diagnosis 6 (p. 109), for measures related to assessment and management of postoperative pain. b. Implement additional measures *to reduce pain:* 1. apply ice packs to the perineal area for the first 24 hours postoperatively if ordered 2. instruct client in and assist with sitz baths as ordered 3. encourage client to remain in a flat or semi-Fowler's position rather than a high Fowler's position when in bed *in order to minimize pressure on surgical site.*

2. Nursing Diagnosis: *URINARY RETENTION*

related to:

a. obstruction of the urethral and/or suprapubic catheter(s);
b. impaired urination following removal of catheter(s) associated with:
    1. edema of the bladder neck and urethra resulting from surgical trauma
    2. increased tone of the urinary sphincters resulting from sympathetic nervous system stimulation (can result from pain, fear, and anxiety)
    3. decreased perception of bladder fullness resulting from the depressant effect of anesthesia and some medications (e.g., narcotic [opioid] analgesics)
    4. relaxation of the bladder muscle resulting from the depressant effect of anesthesia and some medications (e.g., narcotic [opioid] analgesics) and stimulation of the sympathetic nervous system (can result from pain, fear, and anxiety).

Suggested NOC Outcome: Urinary elimination

Suggested NIC Interventions: Urinary retention care; Tube care: urinary

Desired Outcome	**Nursing Actions** *and Selected Purposes/Rationales*
2. The client will not experience urinary retention as evidenced by: a. no reports of bladder fullness and suprapubic discomfort	2.a. Assess for and report the following: 1. urinary retention when suprapubic and/or urethral catheter(s) are present (e.g., reports of bladder fullness or suprapubic discomfort, bladder distention, absence of fluid in urinary drainage tubing, output that continues to be less than intake 48 hours after surgery)

b. absence of bladder distention
c. balanced intake and output within 48 hours after surgery
d. voiding adequate amounts at expected intervals after removal of the catheter(s).

2. urinary retention following catheter removal (e.g., reports of bladder fullness or suprapubic discomfort, bladder distention, output that continues to be less than intake 48 hours after surgery, frequent voiding of small amounts [25–60 ml] of urine).

b. Implement measures *to prevent urinary retention:*
   1. perform actions *to maintain patency of urinary catheter(s):*
      a. keep drainage tubing free of kinks
      b. keep collection container below level of bladder
      c. anchor catheter tubing securely *in order to prevent inadvertent removal*
   2. after urethral catheter is removed, open suprapubic catheter (if one is present) as scheduled and if client is unable to void voluntarily
   3. following removal of the catheter(s), refer to Standardized Postoperative Care Plan, Diagnosis 14, actions c and d (pp. 115–116), for measures related to prevention and treatment of urinary retention.

3. Nursing Diagnosis:

RISK FOR CONSTIPATION

related to:
a. decreased gastrointestinal motility associated with decreased activity and the depressant effect of the anesthetic and narcotic (opioid) analgesics;
b. reluctance to defecate associated with fear of pain and reherniation of the bladder and rectum;
c. decreased intake of fluids and foods high in fiber.

Suggested NOC Outcome: Bowel elimination

Suggested NIC Interventions: Constipation/Impaction management; Pain management

Desired Outcome	Nursing Actions *and Selected Purposes/Rationales*
3. The client will not experience constipation (see Standardized Postoperative Care Plan, Diagnosis 15 [p. 116], for outcome criteria).	3.a. Refer to Standardized Postoperative Care Plan, Diagnosis 15 (pp. 116–117), for measures related to assessment and prevention of constipation. b. Implement additional measures *to prevent constipation:* 1. instruct client to request an analgesic prior to attempting to defecate *in order to ease the surgical site pain associated with the increased intra-abdominal and perineal pressure that occur with defecation* 2. consult physician about an order for a laxative if one has not been prescribed.

4. Nursing Diagnosis:

RISK FOR INFECTION

a. **vaginal/perineal wound infection** related to:
   1. wound contamination associated with introduction of pathogens during or following surgery (a high risk with this surgery because of the close proximity of the incisions to the perianal area)
   2. decreased resistance to infection associated with factors such as age and an inadequate nutritional status;

b. **urinary tract infection** related to:
   1. increased growth and colonization of microorganisms associated with urinary stasis
   2. introduction of pathogens associated with the presence of an indwelling catheter.

Suggested NOC Outcomes: Infection severity; Immune status; Wound healing: primary intention

Suggested NIC Interventions: Infection control; Infection protection; Perineal care; Urinary retention care

Desired Outcomes	Nursing Actions *and Selected Purposes/Rationales*
4.a. The client will remain free of wound infection (see Standardized Postoperative Care Plan, Diagnosis 17, outcome b [pp. 118–119], for outcome criteria).	4.a.1. Refer to Standardized Postoperative Care Plan, Diagnosis 17, action b (pp. 118–119), for measures related to assessment and prevention of wound infection. 2. Implement additional measures *to reduce risk of wound infection:* a. instruct client to wipe from front to back following urination and defecation b. assist client with perineal care every shift and after each bowel movement c. if catheter is present, perform catheter care at least twice a day.
4.b. The client will remain free of urinary tract infection (see Standardized Postoperative Care Plan, Diagnosis 17, outcome c [p. 119], for outcome criteria).	4.b.1. Refer to Standardized Postoperative Care Plan, Diagnosis 17, action c (p. 119), for measures related to the assessment, prevention, and management of urinary tract infection. 2. Implement measures to prevent urinary retention when urinary catheter is present (see Postoperative Diagnosis 2, actions b.1 and 2) *in order to prevent urinary stasis and the subsequent risk for urinary tract infection.*

5. Collaborative Diagnoses: POTENTIAL COMPLICATIONS OF COLPORRHAPHY

a. rehерniation of the bladder or rectum related to stress on internal sutures associated with increased intra-abdominal, bladder, rectal, or vaginal pressure;
b. bladder, urethral, or ureteral injury related to accidental tear or ligation during the surgical procedure.

Desired Outcomes	Nursing Actions *and Selected Purposes/Rationales*
5.a. The client will not experience reherniation of the bladder and rectum as evidenced by: 1. absence of stress incontinence 2. no difficulty with evacuation of stool 3. gradual resolution of pelvic pressure.	5.a.1. Assess for signs and symptoms of reherniation of the bladder or rectum (e.g., persistent or increasing stress incontinence, difficulty evacuating stool, or pelvic pressure). 2. Implement measures *to prevent stress on the internal sutures and reduce the risk for reherniation of the bladder and rectum:* a. perform actions to prevent urinary retention (see Postoperative Diagnosis 2, action b) *in order to prevent accumulation of urine in the bladder* b. perform actions to prevent constipation (see Postoperative Diagnosis 3) *in order to prevent distention of the rectum* c. perform actions *to prevent increased intra-abdominal pressure:* 1. instruct client to remain in a flat or semi-Fowler's position rather than a high Fowler's position while in bed 2. instruct client to avoid any activities that may create a Valsalva response (e.g., straining to have a bowel movement, lifting or carrying a heavy object, holding breath while moving in bed, coughing) 3. administer a laxative, antiemetic, and antitussive if ordered *to prevent straining to have a bowel movement and control nausea, vomiting, and persistent cough* d. caution client to avoid prolonged standing and sitting. 3. If reherniation occurs: a. maintain client on bed rest b. prepare client for surgical repair if planned.
5.b. The client will experience healing of bladder, urethral, or ureteral injury if it occurs as evidenced by: 1. gradual resolution of hematuria and backache 2. urine output greater than 200 ml within 6–8 hours after surgery.	5.b.1. Assess for and report signs and symptoms of bladder, urethral, or ureteral injury (e.g., persistent or increasing hematuria or backache, urine output less than 200 ml in first 6–8 hours after surgery). 2. If signs and symptoms of bladder, urethral, or ureteral injury are present: a. continue to monitor output carefully b. prepare client for surgical repair if indicated.

Discharge Teaching/Continued Care

6. NURSING DIAGNOSIS: DEFICIENT KNOWLEDGE, INEFFECTIVE THERAPEUTIC REGIMEN MANAGEMENT, OR INEFFECTIVE HEALTH MAINTENANCE*

*The nurse should select the diagnostic label that is most appropriate for the client's discharge teaching needs.

Suggested NOC Outcomes: Knowledge: disease process; Knowledge: treatment regimen; Knowledge: prescribed activity

Suggested NIC Interventions: Health system guidance; Teaching: individual; Teaching: disease process; Pelvic muscle exercise; Teaching: prescribed activity/exercise

Desired Outcomes	**Nursing Actions** *and Selected Purposes/Rationales*
6.a. The client will identify ways to decrease the risk of reherniation of the bladder and rectum.	6.a.1. Provide the following instructions on ways to minimize pressure on the internal suture lines and decrease the risk of reherniation of the bladder and/or rectum: a. reinforce instructions about avoiding prolonged sitting and standing and any activity that may create a Valsalva response (e.g., straining to have a bowel movement, lifting or carrying heavy objects, coughing) for at least 6 weeks b. instruct client to urinate whenever the urge is felt or at least every 4 hours c. reinforce instructions about how to prevent constipation (e.g., drink at least 8 glasses of water daily, increase intake of foods high in fiber, take stool softeners as prescribed). 2. Instruct client in additional ways to reduce the risk of reherniation of the bladder and rectum: a. do perineal exercises (e.g., stopping and starting urinary stream, alternately contracting and relaxing the gluteal muscles) when healing is complete (usually in 6 weeks) in order to help maintain tone of the pelvic muscles b. adhere to a weight reduction diet and exercise program if overweight.
6.b. The client will identify ways to relieve surgical site discomfort.	6.b. Provide the following instructions regarding ways to relieve discomfort in the surgical area: 1. take a sitz bath 2–3 times/day 2. avoid prolonged sitting and standing 3. sit on a foam pad or pillow 4. take analgesics as prescribed.
6.c. The client will state signs and symptoms to report to the health care provider.	6.c.1. Refer to Standardized Postoperative Care Plan, Diagnosis 22, action c (p. 125), for signs and symptoms to report to the health care provider. 2. Instruct the client to report these additional signs and symptoms: a. foul-smelling vaginal discharge b. heavy, bright red vaginal bleeding or the passage of clots that are thumb-size or larger c. persistent or recurrent stress incontinence, difficulty evacuating stool, or feeling of pressure in pelvic area (may indicate reherniation of bladder or rectum) d. persistent painful intercourse (client should avoid intercourse for approximately 6 weeks) e. presence of urine or stool in vaginal drainage (indicative of fistula formation) f. excessive swelling or pain in perineal area.

Desired Outcomes	**Nursing Actions** *and Selected Purposes/Rationales*
6.d. The client will verbalize an understanding of and a plan for adhering to recommended follow-up care including future appointments with health care provider, medications prescribed, and limitations on sexual activity.	6.d.1. Refer to Standardized Postoperative Care Plan, Diagnosis 22 (pp. 125–126), for routine postoperative instructions and measures to improve client compliance. 2. Instruct client not to have sexual intercourse until permitted by physician (usually 6 weeks). 3. Inform client that loss of vaginal sensation is usually temporary but may persist for several months.

Bibliography

See pages 879 and 885.

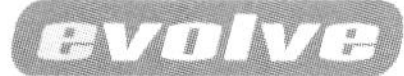

Hysterectomy with Salpingectomy and Oophorectomy

Hysterectomy is the surgical removal of the uterus. It is performed to treat conditions such as malignant and nonmalignant growths in the uterus and cervix, symptomatic endometriosis, uterine prolapse, intractable pelvic infection, irreparable rupture of the uterus, and dysfunctional or life-threatening uterine bleeding. Both the uterus and cervix are removed in a total hysterectomy. A panhysterectomy is the removal of the uterus, cervix, fallopian tubes, and ovaries and is often referred to as a total abdominal hysterectomy with bilateral salpingectomy and oophorectomy (TAH-BSO). A radical hysterectomy also includes a partial vaginectomy and dissection of the pelvic lymph nodes.

A vaginal or abdominal approach can be used to perform a hysterectomy. The approach used depends on factors such as the woman's pelvic anatomy and size of the uterus, whether repairs to the vaginal wall or pelvic floor are needed, the presence of other medical conditions, previous abdominal surgeries, and the diagnosis.

This care plan focuses on the adult client hospitalized for a total abdominal hysterectomy with salpingectomy and oophorectomy.

OUTCOME/DISCHARGE CRITERIA

THE CLIENT WILL:

- have evidence of normal healing of surgical wound
- have clear, audible breath sounds throughout lungs
- have adequate urine output
- have surgical pain controlled
- have no signs and symptoms of postoperative complications
- verbalize an understanding of the effects of surgical menopause
- identify ways to achieve sexual satisfaction
- verbalize an understanding of medications ordered including rationale, food and drug interactions, side effects, schedule for taking, and importance of taking as prescribed
- state signs and symptoms to report to the health care provider
- share feelings about the loss of reproductive ability
- verbalize an understanding of and a plan for adhering to recommended follow-up care including future appointments with health care provider, activity limitations, and wound care.

NURSING/COLLABORATIVE DIAGNOSES

Preoperative

1. Fear/Anxiety p. 824

Postoperative

1. Urinary retention p. 824
2. Potential complications p. 825
   a. bladder or ureteral injury
   b. thromboembolism
3. Disturbed self-concept p. 826
4. Grieving p. 826

DISCHARGE TEACHING

5. Deficient knowledge, Ineffective therapeutic regimen management, or Ineffective health maintenance p. 827

See Standardized Preoperative and Postoperative Care Plans (pp. 97–126) for additional diagnoses.

PREOPERATIVE

Use in conjunction with the Standardized Preoperative Care Plan.

1. Nursing Diagnosis: **FEAR/ANXIETY**

related to:
a. anticipated loss of control associated with the effects of anesthesia;
b. anticipated effects of surgery on femininity and reproductive ability;
c. fear of rejection by partner;
d. unfamiliar environment and separation from significant others;
e. potential embarrassment or loss of dignity associated with body exposure during preoperative care, surgery, and postoperative care;
f. lack of understanding of the surgical procedure and postoperative expectations and care;
g. anticipated surgical findings and postoperative discomfort;
h. financial concerns associated with hospitalization;
i. diagnosis of cancer (if present) and prognosis.

Suggested NOC Outcomes: Anxiety level; Fear level; Anxiety self-control; Fear self-control

Suggested NIC Interventions: Anxiety reduction; Calming technique; Emotional support; Presence; Teaching: preoperative

Desired Outcome	Nursing Actions *and Selected Purposes/Rationales*
1. The client will experience a reduction in fear and anxiety (see Standardized Preoperative Care Plan, Diagnosis 1 [pp. 97–98], for outcome criteria).	1.a. Refer to Standardized Preoperative Care Plan, Diagnosis 1 (pp. 97–98), for measures related to assessment and reduction of fear and anxiety. b. Implement additional measures *to reduce fear and anxiety:* 1. encourage client to verbalize concerns and feelings about loss of ovarian function and reproductive ability; provide feedback 2. discuss alternative methods of becoming a parent (e.g., adoption) if of concern to client 3. assure client she will not suffer needless body exposure during preoperative care, surgery, and postoperative care 4. reinforce physician's explanations about the positive effects of surgery (e.g., removal of malignant and nonmalignant growths, treatment of pain and dysfunctional bleeding).

POSTOPERATIVE

Use in conjunction with the Standardized Postoperative Care Plan.

1. Nursing Diagnosis: **URINARY RETENTION**

related to:
a. obstruction of the urinary catheter;
b. impaired urination following removal of catheter associated with:
   1. decreased perception of bladder fullness associated with the depressant effect of anesthesia and some medications (e.g., narcotic [opioid] analgesics)
   2. increased tone of the urinary sphincters associated with sympathetic nervous system stimulation resulting from pain, fear, and anxiety
   3. relaxation of the bladder muscle associated with:
      a. nerve trauma and/or edema in the bladder area resulting from surgical manipulation
      b. the depressant effect of anesthesia and some medications (e.g., narcotic [opioid] analgesics)
      c. stimulation of the sympathetic nervous system (can result from pain, fear, and anxiety).

Suggested NOC Outcome: Urinary elimination

Suggested NIC Interventions: Urinary retention care; Tube care: urinary

Desired Outcome	**Nursing Actions** *and Selected Purposes/Rationales*
1. The client will not experience urinary retention as evidenced by: a. no reports of bladder fullness and suprapubic discomfort b. absence of bladder distention c. balanced intake and output within 48 hours after surgery d. voiding adequate amounts at expected intervals after removal of catheter.	1.a. Assess for and report the following: 1. urinary retention when catheter is present (e.g., reports of bladder fullness or suprapubic discomfort, bladder distention, absence of fluid in urinary drainage tubing, output that continues to be less than intake 48 hours after surgery) 2. urinary retention following catheter removal (e.g., reports of bladder fullness or suprapubic discomfort, bladder distention, output that continues to be less than intake 48 hours after surgery, frequent voiding of small amounts [25–60 ml] of urine). b. Implement measures *to prevent urinary retention:* 1. perform actions *to maintain patency of urinary catheter:* a. keep drainage tubing free of kinks b. keep collection container below level of bladder c. anchor catheter tubing securely 2. when the catheter has been removed, refer to Standardized Postoperative Care Plan, Diagnosis 14, actions c and d (pp. 115–116) for measures related to prevention and treatment of urinary retention.

2. COLLABORATIVE DIAGNOSES: ***POTENTIAL COMPLICATIONS OF TOTAL ABDOMINAL HYSTERECTOMY***

a. bladder or ureteral injury related to accidental tear or ligation during the surgical procedure;
b. thromboembolism related to:
   1. trauma to the pelvic veins during surgery
   2. venous stasis associated with:
      a. decreased activity
      b. increased blood viscosity (can result from deficient fluid volume)
      c. pelvic congestion resulting from inflammation in the surgical area
      d. abdominal distention (the distended intestine may put pressure on the abdominal vessels)
      e. pressure on the pelvic and calf vessels during surgery if a vaginal approach was used (client is placed in lithotomy position for this approach)
   3. hypercoagulability associated with increased release of tissue thromboplastin into the blood (occurs as a result of surgical trauma) and hemoconcentration and increased blood viscosity (can result from deficient fluid volume).

Desired Outcomes	**Nursing Actions** *and Selected Purposes/Rationales*
2.a. The client will experience resolution of bladder or ureteral injury if it occurs as evidenced by: 1. gradual resolution of hematuria and backache 2. urine output greater than 200 ml within 6–8 hours after surgery.	2.a.1. Assess for and report signs and symptoms of bladder or ureteral injury (e.g., hematuria, backache, urine output less than 200 ml in first 6–8 hours after surgery). 2. If signs and symptoms of bladder or ureteral injury are present: a. continue to monitor output carefully b. prepare client for surgical repair of the bladder or ureter if planned.
2.b. The client will not develop a deep vein thrombus or pulmonary embolism (see Standardized Postoperative Care Plan, Diagnosis 20, outcomes c.1 and 2 [pp. 122–123], for outcome criteria).	2.b.1. Refer to Standardized Postoperative Care Plan, Diagnosis 20, actions c.1 and 2 (pp. 122–123), for measures related to assessment, prevention, and treatment of a deep vein thrombus and pulmonary embolism. 2. Implement additional measures *to prevent thrombus formation:* a. avoid having client in a high Fowler's position b. encourage client to lie flat for short periods at least every 4 hours *to increase blood return from the legs* c. assist client with ambulation as soon as allowed.

3. Nursing Diagnosis:

DISTURBED SELF-CONCEPT*

related to:
a. loss of reproductive organs with subsequent inability to bear children;
b. feeling of loss of femininity and sexuality.

*This diagnostic label includes the nursing diagnoses of disturbed body image, low self-esteem, and ineffective role performance.

Suggested NOC Outcomes: Body image; Self-esteem; Psychosocial adjustment: life change

Suggested NIC Interventions: Body image enhancement; Grief work facilitation; Self-esteem enhancement; Role enhancement; Counseling; Emotional support; Support system enhancement

Desired Outcome	Nursing Actions *and Selected Purposes/Rationales* (see pp. 47–49 for additional rationales)
3. The client will demonstrate beginning adaptation to changes in body image and functioning as evidenced by: a. verbalization of feelings of self-worth and sexual adequacy b. maintenance of relationships with significant others c. active participation in activities of daily living.	3.a. Assess for signs and symptoms of a disturbed self-concept (e.g., verbalization of negative feelings about self, withdrawal from significant others, lack of participation in activities of daily living). b. Implement measures to facilitate the grieving process (see Postoperative Diagnosis 4, action b). c. Inform client that removal of the uterus and cervix should not affect the ability to have sexual intercourse and physiological sexual responses but that surgical menopause created by removal of the ovaries may cause some changes such as decreased libido and painful intercourse. Encourage client to discuss these changes and estrogen replacement therapy with physician. d. Assist client to identify and utilize coping techniques that have been helpful in the past. e. Assist client with usual grooming and makeup habits if necessary. f. Support behaviors suggesting positive adaptation to loss of reproductive organs (e.g., active interest in personal appearance, verbalization of feelings of self-worth, maintenance of relationships with significant others). g. Assist client's and significant others' adjustment by listening, facilitating communication, and providing information. h. Encourage visits and support from significant others. i. If client expresses an interest in the adoption of children, provide names of appropriate agencies. j. Consult appropriate health care provider (e.g., psychiatric nurse clinician, physician) if client seems unwilling or unable to adapt to changes resulting from the surgery.

4. Nursing Diagnosis:

GRIEVING†

related to loss of reproductive ability, early menopause, diagnosis of cancer (if present), and the possibility of premature death.

†This diagnostic label includes anticipatory grieving and grieving following the actual losses.

Suggested NOC Outcomes: Grief resolution; Psychosocial adjustment: life change

Suggested NIC Interventions: Grief work facilitation; Emotional support; Presence; Support system enhancement

Desired Outcome	Nursing Actions *and Selected Purposes/Rationales* (see pp. 35–37 for additional rationales)
4. The client will demonstrate beginning progression through the grieving process as evidenced by: a. verbalization of feelings about the loss of reproductive ability b. usual sleep pattern c. participation in treatment plan and self-care activities d. utilization of available support systems.	4.a. Assess for signs and symptoms of grieving (e.g., expression of distress about having a hysterectomy, change in eating habits, inability to concentrate, insomnia, anger, sadness, withdrawal from significant others, denial of loss). b. Implement measures *to facilitate the grieving process:* 1. assist client to acknowledge the losses *so grief work can begin;* assess for factors that may hinder and facilitate acknowledgment 2. discuss the grieving process and assist client to accept the phases of grieving as an expected response to loss of reproductive ability and usual body functioning 3. allow time for client to progress through the phases of grieving (phases vary among theorists but progress from shock and alarm to acceptance); be aware that not every phase is expressed by all individuals, phases may overlap or recur, the amount of time needed to reach resolution of grief is very individual, and the grieving process may take months to years 4. provide an atmosphere of care and concern (e.g., provide privacy, be available and nonjudgmental, display empathy and respect) *so that client will feel free to express feelings* 5. perform actions *to promote trust* (e.g., answer questions honestly, provide requested information) 6. encourage the verbal expression of anger and sadness about the losses experienced; recognize displacement of anger and assist client to see the actual cause of angry feelings and resentment 7. encourage client to express feelings in whatever ways are comfortable (e.g., writing, drawing, conversation) 8. assist client to identify and utilize techniques that have helped her cope in previous situations of loss 9. support behaviors suggesting successful grief work (e.g., verbalizing feelings about changes in physical functioning, expressing sorrow, focusing on ways to adapt to loss of reproductive function) 10. explain the phases of the grieving process to significant others; encourage their support and understanding 11. facilitate communication between client and significant others; be aware that they may be in different phases of the grieving process 12. provide information about counseling services and support groups that might assist client in working through grief 13. when appropriate, assist client to meet spiritual needs (e.g., arrange for visit from clergy). c. Consult appropriate health care provider (e.g., psychiatric nurse clinician, physician) about referral for counseling if signs of dysfunctional grieving (e.g., persistent denial of losses, excessive anger or sadness, emotional lability) occur.

Discharge Teaching/Continued Care

5. Nursing Diagnosis: ***DEFICIENT KNOWLEDGE, INEFFECTIVE THERAPEUTIC REGIMEN MANAGEMENT, OR INEFFECTIVE HEALTH MAINTENANCE****

*The nurse should select the diagnostic label that is most appropriate for the client's discharge teaching needs.

Suggested NOC Outcomes: Knowledge: treatment regimen; Knowledge: prescribed activity

Suggested NIC Interventions: Health system guidance; Teaching: individual; Teaching: prescribed medication; Teaching: prescribed activity/exercise

Desired Outcomes	**Nursing Actions** *and Selected Purposes/Rationales*
5.a. The client will verbalize an understanding of the effects of surgical menopause.	5.a.1. Reinforce the physician's explanation of surgical menopause and its possible effects (e.g., hot flashes, facial hair growth, decrease in vaginal lubrication, insomnia, fatigue, nervousness, palpitations, depression). 2. Allow time for questions and clarification of information provided.
5.b. The client will identify ways to achieve sexual satisfaction.	5.b.1. Explain the probable effects of the surgery on sexual functioning (e.g., decreased libido, vaginal dryness, painful intercourse). 2. Instruct client in ways to promote sexual satisfaction: a. use a water-soluble lubricant in the vagina to prevent pain during intercourse (the amount of vaginal lubrication decreases as a result of the effects of surgically-induced menopause) b. take hormone replacements (e.g., estrogen) as prescribed c. try different positions for intercourse to determine whether some positions are more comfortable than others. 3. Reinforce physician's instructions regarding when client can resume sexual intercourse (usually 4–6 weeks).
5.c. The client will verbalize an understanding of medications ordered including rationale, food and drug interactions, side effects, schedule for taking, and importance of taking as prescribed.	5.c.1. Explain the rationale for, side effects of, schedule for taking, and importance of taking medications prescribed. 2. If client is discharged on estrogen replacement therapy, instruct to: a. apply patch as prescribed; take oral medication with food or at bedtime to prevent nausea b. be aware that depression; headache; acne; brown, blotchy areas on skin; nausea; and tender breasts are potential side effects of estrogen therapy c. wear a supportive bra if breasts are tender d. stop smoking (smoking may increase the incidence of the thromboembolic side effect of estrogen) e. report the following to the health care provider: 1. side effects that are not controlled or tolerable 2. sudden weight gain and swelling in extremities 3. visual blurring or acuity changes or contact lens intolerance 4. numbness, swelling, pain, or redness of an extremity or sudden onset of chest pain or shortness of breath (indicative of a thromboembolus) f. keep scheduled follow-up appointments with health care provider while on estrogen replacement therapy. 3. Inform client of pertinent interactions between estrogen and other medications she is taking. 4. Instruct client to inform physician of any other prescription and nonprescription medications she is taking and to inform all health care providers of medications being taken.
5.d. The client will state signs and symptoms to report to the health care provider.	5.d.1. Refer to Standardized Postoperative Care Plan, Diagnosis 22, action c (p. 125), for signs and symptoms to report to the health care provider. 2. Instruct the client to report these additional signs and symptoms: a. foul-smelling vaginal discharge (it is normal to have an increased amount of discharge about 2 weeks postoperatively when internal sutures are absorbed) b. heavy, bright red vaginal bleeding or the passage of clots that are thumb-size or larger c. excessive depression or difficulty dealing with changes in body image d. excessive discomfort associated with effects of surgical menopause e. adverse reactions to estrogen replacement therapy (see action c.2.e in this diagnosis).

5.e. The client will verbalize an understanding of and a plan for adhering to recommended follow-up care including future appointments with health care provider, activity limitations, and wound care.

5.e.1. Refer to Standardized Postoperative Care Plan, Diagnosis 22 (pp. 125–126), for routine postoperative instructions and measures to promote client compliance.

2. Reinforce the physician's instructions regarding the need to:
   a. avoid lifting objects over 10 pounds, sitting for long periods, stair climbing, and strenuous physical activity (e.g., vacuuming, aerobics) for 6–8 weeks postoperatively
   b. avoid driving for at least a week after surgery
   c. avoid douching, using tampons, and having sexual intercourse for 4–6 weeks postoperatively.

Bibliography

See pages 879 and 885.

Mastectomy

A mastectomy is the surgical removal of all or part of the breast and is usually performed to treat breast cancer. The type of mastectomy is based on factors such as the location, type, and size of the tumor; the number of tumors; breast size; axillary lymph node status; whether the client has received prior irradiation of the breast; and client preference. The two major types of surgeries performed to treat resectable breast cancer are a modified radical mastectomy and breast-conserving surgery (e.g., lumpectomy, quadrantectomy, partial or segmental mastectomy).

A modified radical mastectomy includes removal of the breast and an axillary node dissection. The pectoral muscles and surrounding nerves are left intact, which allows the client to retain the shape of her breast and avoid the shoulder and arm limitations and skin graft requirements that accompany a radical mastectomy. Leaving the muscles and nerves intact facilitates reconstructive surgery, which may be performed at the time of the mastectomy or delayed for several months depending on physician and client preference and additional treatment planned. The additional treatment (e.g., chemotherapy, hormone therapy, external radiation therapy) that may be considered following a modified radical mastectomy depends on factors such as the immunologic and menopausal status of the client, tumor type and size, and amount of lymph node involvement. Breast-conserving surgery is an option for many women with stage I and II breast cancer. It involves excision of the tumor, a surrounding margin of normal tissue, and an axillary lymph node dissection. It is followed by a course of radiation therapy to eradicate any residual tumor and reduce the risk for tumor recurrence.

Axillary node dissection has traditionally been performed with all invasive breast cancer to stage the tumor. Sentinel node biopsy (lymphatic mapping) is a procedure currently being used to help identify axillary node involvement and avoid unnecessary lymph node dissection. This procedure can be done the day of surgery. If the sentinel node is negative for cancer cells, an axillary dissection is not necessary, which eliminates the need for axillary drains and reduces the risk for lymphedema.

This care plan focuses on the female adult client hospitalized for a modified radical mastectomy. Much of the postoperative information is applicable to clients receiving follow-up care in a home setting.

OUTCOME/DISCHARGE CRITERIA

THE CLIENT WILL:

- have evidence of normal healing of surgical wounds
- have clear, audible breath sounds throughout lungs
- have surgical pain controlled
- have no signs and symptoms of postoperative complications
- identify ways to reduce the risk of trauma to and infection in the arm on the operative side
- identify ways to prevent and treat lymphedema of the arm on the operative side
- demonstrate the ability to care for wound drainage device if present
- demonstrate the ability to perform the prescribed exercises and verbalize an understanding of additional exercises to be done once the incision has healed
- verbalize the importance of and demonstrate the ability to perform a breast self-examination (BSE) on the remaining breast and operative site
- state the factors to consider in selecting a breast prosthesis
- state signs and symptoms to report to the health care provider
- share thoughts and feelings about the change in body image
- identify community resources that can assist with adjustment to the diagnosis of cancer and the loss of a breast
- verbalize an understanding of and a plan for adhering to recommended follow-up care including future appointments with health care provider, medications prescribed, activity level, wound care, and plans for subsequent treatment.

NURSING/COLLABORATIVE DIAGNOSES

Preoperative

1. Fear/Anxiety p. 831
2. Deficient knowledge p. 832

Postoperative

1. Acute pain: chest and arm on operative side p. 833

NURSING/COLLABORATIVE DIAGNOSES

2. Potential complications p. 833
   a. lymphedema of arm on operative side
   b. motor and sensory impairment of the arm and/or shoulder on the operative side
   c. seroma formation
   d. hematoma formation
   e. necrosis of skin flap
3. Disturbed self-concept p. 835
4. Grieving p. 836

DISCHARGE TEACHING

5. Deficient knowledge, Ineffective therapeutic regimen management, or Ineffective health maintenance p. 837

See p. 840 and Standardized Preoperative and Postoperative Care Plans (pp. 97–126) for additional diagnoses.

PREOPERATIVE

Use in conjunction with the Standardized Preoperative Care Plan.

1. Nursing Diagnosis: ***FEAR/ANXIETY***

related to:

a. diagnosis of cancer, treatment plan, and prognosis;
b. anticipated loss of control associated with the effects of anesthesia;
c. anticipated loss of femininity and physical attractiveness and possible change in relationship with significant other associated with the disfiguring effect of the mastectomy;
d. unfamiliar environment and separation from significant others;
e. anticipated surgical findings and postoperative pain;
f. lack of understanding of the surgical procedure and postoperative expectations and care;
g. potential embarrassment or loss of dignity associated with body exposure during preoperative care, surgery, and postoperative assessments and treatments;
h. financial concerns associated with hospitalization and subsequent treatment (if planned).

Suggested NOC Outcomes: Anxiety level; Fear level; Anxiety self-control; Fear self-control

Suggested NIC Interventions: Anxiety reduction; Calming technique; Emotional support; Presence; Teaching: preoperative; Support system enhancement

Desired Outcome	**Nursing Actions** *and Selected Purposes/Rationales*
1. The client will experience a reduction in fear and anxiety (see Standardized Preoperative Care Plan, Diagnosis 1 [pp. 97–98], for outcome criteria).	1.a. Refer to Standardized Preoperative Care Plan, Diagnosis 1 (pp. 97–98), for measures related to assessment and reduction of preoperative fear and anxiety. b. Implement additional measures *to reduce fear and anxiety:* 1. arrange for a Reach to Recovery volunteer to visit client if appropriate 2. if immediate reconstruction is not planned, provide information about the types of prostheses that are available and, if appropriate, the possibility of future breast reconstruction 3. reinforce physician's explanation about the positive effects of the mastectomy on her prognosis.

Client Teaching

2. Nursing Diagnosis: ***DEFICIENT KNOWLEDGE***

regarding the surgical procedure, routines associated with surgery, physical preparation for a mastectomy, sensations that may occur following surgery and anesthesia, and postoperative care.

Suggested NOC Outcomes:
Knowledge: disease process; Knowledge: treatment regimen

Suggested NIC Interventions: Teaching: preoperative; Teaching: individual; Teaching: prescribed activity/exercise

Desired Outcomes	Nursing Actions *and Selected Purposes/Rationales*
2.a. The client will verbalize an understanding of the surgical procedure, preoperative care, and postoperative sensations and care.	2.a.1. Refer to Standardized Preoperative Care Plan, Diagnosis 4, actions a.1–4 (pp. 100–101), for information to include in preoperative teaching. 2. Provide the following information about sensations that may occur after a mastectomy: a. explain to client that it is common to have sensations of pain, numbness, and tingling in the operative area (these sensations usually subside within a year) b. assure client that the sense that both breasts are present (phantom breast sensation) is common c. explain to client that she may feel a change in balance at first, particularly if breasts are large. 3. Allow time for questions and clarification of information provided.
2.b. The client will demonstrate the ability to perform activities designed to prevent postoperative complications.	2.b.1. Refer to Standardized Preoperative Care Plan, Diagnosis 4, action b.1 (p. 101), for instructions on ways to prevent postoperative complications. 2. Provide additional instructions regarding ways to prevent complications following a mastectomy: a. inform the client that she must keep upper arm on operative side close to her body for a few days after surgery (length of time will vary according to physician preference) in order to prevent tension on the suture lines and subsequent hematoma and seroma formation b. explain that exercise of the hand, arm, and shoulder on the operative side is essential in order to facilitate and improve lymphatic and blood circulation, maintain muscle tone, and prevent contractures c. demonstrate recommended postmastectomy exercises (e.g., squeezing a ball, flexion and extension of the fingers and wrist, wall climbing, rope pulley exercises, arm swings, rope turning); inform client that hand and wrist exercises are usually begun the day after surgery with gradual progression to full range of motion exercises of arm and shoulder on operative side when incision has healed d. instruct client on ways to minimize or prevent lymphedema of the arm on operative side: 1. keep arm on operative side elevated on pillows with elbow above heart level and hand higher than elbow in the early postoperative period 2. perform recommended postmastectomy exercises as soon as allowed 3. avoid having B/P measurements, injections, blood draws, and intravenous infusions in arm on operative side (these procedures increase risk of infection or trauma and subsequent lymphedema). 3. Allow time for questions, clarification, practice, and return demonstration of exercises.

POSTOPERATIVE

Use in conjunction with the Standardized Postoperative Care Plan.

1. Nursing Diagnosis:

ACUTE PAIN: CHEST AND ARM ON OPERATIVE SIDE

related to tissue trauma and reflex muscle spasms associated with surgery, irritation from drainage tubes, and strain on the surgical area postoperatively.

Suggested NOC Outcomes: Pain control; Comfort level; Pain: adverse psychological reaction

Suggested NIC Interventions: Pain management; Analgesic administration

Desired Outcome	Nursing Actions *and Selected Purposes/Rationales*
1. The client will experience diminished pain in the chest and arm on the operative side (see Standardized Postoperative Care Plan, Diagnosis 6 [p. 109], for outcome criteria.	1.a. Refer to Standardized Postoperative Care Plan, Diagnosis 6 (p. 109), for measures related to assessment and reduction of pain. b. Implement additional measures *to reduce pain in the chest and arm on the operative side:* 1. place client in a semi-Fowler's position during the immediate postoperative period; elevate the arm on the operative side on pillows, keeping elbow above the level of the heart and hand higher than the elbow *to decrease tension on the incision, promote circulation, and prevent venous congestion in affected arm* 2. do not use arm on the operative side for intravenous therapy, blood draws, injections, and B/P measurements 3. move the operative extremity gently 4. reinforce the importance of adhering to arm and shoulder movement restrictions 5. maintain patency of wound drainage system (e.g., prevent kinking of tubing, empty collection device as needed, maintain suction as ordered, keep collection device below surgical wound) *to prevent fluid accumulation in the operative site* 6. securely anchor drainage tubes and collection device *to reduce strain on the surgical site* 7. if a sling is ordered, apply it to the client's arm before she gets out of bed *to support the arm and reduce strain on the surgical site* 8. instruct client to get out of bed on the unaffected side (*promotes the use of the unaffected arm rather than the arm on the operative side when getting up)* 9. place needed items within easy reach *to prevent excessive arm and shoulder movement.*

2. Collaborative Diagnoses:

POTENTIAL COMPLICATIONS OF MODIFIED RADICAL MASTECTOMY

a. lymphedema of arm on operative side related to interruption in usual lymph flow associated with surgical removal of axillary lymph nodes and channels, edema in the operative area, and infection of or trauma to operative arm;

b. motor and sensory impairment of the arm and/or shoulder on the operative side related to:
   1. transection of or trauma to the nerves during surgery
   2. pressure on nerves associated with lymphedema if it occurs
   3. noncompliance with prescribed exercise program;

c. seroma formation related to delayed or impaired flap adherence associated with irregular shape of chest wall, impaired wound drainage, and excessive movement of operative area with arm and shoulder use;

d. hematoma formation related to inadequate hemostasis during surgery, stress on vessels in operative area, and impaired drainage from the operative area;

e. necrosis of skin flap related to inadequate blood supply in flap or infection of surgical wound.

Desired Outcomes	**Nursing Actions** *and Selected Purposes/Rationales*
2.a. The client will not develop lymphedema of the arm on the operative side as evidenced by: 1. absence or gradual resolution of numbness, tingling, and weakness of the arm 2. absence of pain and feeling of heaviness and tightness in the arm 3. absence of edema in the arm.	2.a.1. Assess for and report signs and symptoms of lymphedema of the arm on the operative side: a. development of or increase in numbness, tingling, or weakness b. pain, sensation of heaviness or tightness c. edema (measure arm on operative side at points 5–10 cm above and below elbow). 2. Implement measures *to prevent lymphedema of arm on operative side:* a. place client in a semi-Fowler's position during the immediate postoperative period; elevate arm on the operative side on pillows, keeping elbow above the level of the heart and hand higher than elbow b. place a sign above bed to remind personnel not to use arm on operative side for intravenous therapy, blood draws, injections, and B/P measurements *in order to decrease risk of infection or trauma and subsequent lymphedema* c. perform actions to prevent wound infection (see Standardized Postoperative Care Plan, Diagnosis 17, action b.2 [pp. 118–119]) d. instruct and assist client to perform postmastectomy exercises as soon as allowed *in order to promote lymphatic drainage.* 3. If signs and symptoms of lymphedema occur: a. apply an elastic pressure gradient sleeve to the affected arm if ordered *to reduce edema* b. assist and instruct client in manual massage of the affected arm and/or use of sequential compression device on affected arm if ordered c. administer antimicrobial agents if ordered *to prevent or treat cellulitis and lymphangitis.*
2.b. The client will have expected motor and sensory function of the arm and shoulder on the operative side as evidenced by: 1. ability to put hand, arm, and shoulder through expected range of motion 2. no reports of new or increased numbness, tingling, or weakness in arm.	2.b.1. Assess for and report signs and symptoms of motor and/or sensory impairment of the arm and shoulder on operative side (e.g., inability to move joints through expected range of motion; reports of new or increased numbness, tingling, or weakness in arm). 2. Implement measures *to prevent arm and shoulder dysfunction:* a. perform actions to prevent lymphedema (see action a.2 in this diagnosis) *in order to reduce pressure on the nerves* b. initiate postmastectomy exercises as soon as allowed c. encourage use of arm on operative side to perform activities of daily living as soon as allowed. 3. If signs and symptoms of impaired arm or shoulder function occur, assist with prescribed physical therapy.
2.c. The client will not develop a seroma at the surgical site as evidenced by: 1. no unusual swelling around incision 2. expected amount of wound drainage in collection device 3. absence of continued drainage from incision.	2.c.1. Assess for and report signs and symptoms of seroma formation (e.g., unusual swelling around incision site, less than expected amount of drainage in collection device, continued drainage from incision). 2. Implement measures *to prevent seroma formation:* a. maintain compression dressing over operative site if one is in place *to promote skin flap adherence so that fluid cannot accumulate in any dead space beneath the flap* b. maintain patency of wound drainage system (e.g., prevent kinking of tubing, empty collection device as needed, keep collection device below surgical wound, maintain suction as ordered) c. place needed items within easy reach *to prevent excessive arm and shoulder movement* d. if a sling is ordered, apply it to client's arm before she gets out of bed *in order to support the arm and reduce strain on the surgical site* e. reinforce importance of adhering to arm and shoulder movement restrictions.

3. If seroma formation occurs:
   a. prepare client for needle aspiration of fluid if planned
   b. assist with application of compression dressing if not already present
   c. administer antimicrobials if ordered.

2.d. The client will not develop a hematoma at the surgical site as evidenced by:
1. no unusual increase in pain, swelling, and skin discoloration in operative area
2. expected amount of wound drainage in collection device.

2.d.1. Assess for and report signs and symptoms of hematoma formation (e.g., increased pain, swelling, and discoloration of operative site; less than expected amount of wound drainage in collection device).
2. Implement measures *to prevent hematoma formation:*
   a. caution client to adhere to arm and shoulder movement restrictions *in order to prevent strain on the surgical site and subsequent bleeding*
   b. maintain compression dressing over operative site if one is in place
   c. maintain patency of wound drainage system (e.g., prevent kinking of tubing, empty collection device as needed, keep collection device below surgical wound, maintain suction as ordered).
3. If signs and symptoms of hematoma formation occur, prepare client for evacuation of hematoma and repair of bleeding vessels if planned.

2.e. The client will not experience necrosis of the skin flap as evidenced by:
1. skin flap warm and expected color
2. approximated wound edges
3. absence of foul odor from flap area.

2.e.1. Assess for and report signs and symptoms of:
   a. impaired blood flow in skin flap (e.g., decreased warmth of skin flap, pallor or cyanosis of skin flap, capillary refill time greater than 2–3 seconds)
   b. skin flap necrosis (e.g., pale, cool, darkened tissue; separation of wound edges; foul odor from flap area).
2. Implement measures *to prevent skin flap necrosis:*
   a. perform actions *to maintain adequate circulation to wound area:*
      1. implement measures to prevent and treat seroma and hematoma formation (see actions c.2 and 3 and d.2 and 3 in this diagnosis)
      2. consult physician about reapplying or loosening the dressing if client reports increased tightness of dressing or if dressing appears too tight
      3. position client on unoperative side or back
      4. encourage client not to smoke *(smoking causes vasoconstriction)*
   b. perform actions to promote healing of surgical incision and prevent wound infection (see Standardized Postoperative Care Plan, Diagnoses 10, action a.2 [p. 112] and 17, action b.2 [pp. 118–119]).
3. If signs and symptoms of skin flap necrosis occur, prepare client for surgical revision of flap.

3. NURSING DIAGNOSIS: ***DISTURBED SELF-CONCEPT****

related to:
a. loss of a breast;
b. temporary dependence on others for assistance with self-care associated with restricted arm movement;
c. possible altered sexuality patterns associated with decreased libido, perceived loss of femininity, and fear of rejection by partner.

*This diagnostic label includes the nursing diagnoses of disturbed body image, low self-esteem, and ineffective role performance.

Suggested NOC Outcomes: Body image; Self-esteem; Psychosocial adjustment: life change

Suggested NIC Interventions: Body image enhancement; Grief work facilitation; Self-esteem enhancement; Role enhancement; Counseling; Emotional support; Support system enhancement

Desired Outcome	Nursing Actions *and Selected Purposes/Rationales* (see pp. 47–49 for additional rationales)
3. The client will demonstrate beginning adaptation to the loss of her breast and integration of the change in body image as evidenced by: a. verbalization of feelings of self-worth and sexual adequacy b. active participation in activities of daily living c. willingness to look at surgical site d. maintenance of relationships with significant others.	3.a. Assess for signs and symptoms of a disturbed self-concept (e.g., verbalization of negative feelings about self, lack of participation in activities of daily living, refusal to look at mastectomy site, withdrawal from significant others). b. Implement measures to facilitate the grieving process (see Postoperative Diagnosis 4, action b). c. Assist the client to identify and use coping techniques that have been helpful in the past. d. Implement measures *to facilitate client's adjustment to the effects of the loss of a breast on her sexuality:* 1. facilitate communication between client and partner; focus on feelings the couple share and assist them to identify factors which may affect their sexual relationship 2. arrange for uninterrupted privacy during hospital stay if desired by the couple. e. If appropriate, involve partner in care of the client's wound *to facilitate partner's adjustment to the change in client's appearance and subsequently decrease the possibility of partner's rejection of client.* f. Assist client with usual grooming and makeup habits. g. Demonstrate acceptance of client using techniques such as touch and frequent visits. Encourage significant others to do the same. h. Stay with client during first dressing change and encourage her to express feelings about appearance of incision and change in body. If the client is reluctant to look at the surgical site, provide support and encouragement to do so before discharge. i. Encourage client's participation in activities that can assist her to integrate the physical change that has occurred (e.g., exercise, grooming, bathing, wound care). j. If breast reconstruction has not been performed: 1. encourage client to discuss possibilities for future reconstruction of breast with physician if desired 2. discuss the variety of prostheses available and ways to obtain one. k. Assist client's and significant others' adjustment by listening, facilitating communication, and providing information. l. Support behaviors suggesting positive adaptation to the loss of a breast (e.g., willingness to look at and care for wound, compliance with exercise program, maintenance of relationships with significant others). m. Reinforce the temporary nature of operative side arm movement restrictions. n. Encourage client contact with others *so that she can test and establish a new self-image.* o. Encourage visits and support from significant others. p. Encourage client to pursue usual roles and interests and to continue involvement in social activities. q. Provide information about and encourage utilization of community agencies and support groups (e.g., Reach to Recovery; sexual, family, and individual counseling services). r. Consult appropriate health care provider (e.g., psychiatric nurse clinician, physician) if client seems unwilling or unable to adapt to the loss of her breast.

4. Nursing Diagnosis: ***GRIEVING****

related to:
a. loss of a breast and subsequent change in body image;
b. potential for premature death associated with the diagnosis of cancer.

*This diagnostic label includes anticipatory grieving and grieving following the actual loss.

Suggested NOC Outcomes: Grief resolution; Psychosocial adjustment: life change

Suggested NIC Interventions: Grief work facilitation; Emotional support; Presence; Support system enhancement

Desired Outcome	Nursing Actions *and Selected Purposes/Rationales* (see pp. 35–37 for additional rationales)
4. The client will demonstrate beginning progression through the grieving process as evidenced by: a. verbalization of feelings about the loss of a breast and diagnosis of cancer b. usual sleep pattern c. participation in treatment plan and self-care activities d. utilization of available support systems.	4.a. Assess for signs and symptoms of grieving (e.g., expression of distress about having cancer and loss of a breast, change in eating habits, inability to concentrate, insomnia, anger, sadness, withdrawal from significant others, denial of loss and diagnosis). b. Implement measures *to facilitate the grieving process:* 1. assist client to acknowledge the changes resulting from loss of her breast and the diagnosis of cancer *so grief work can begin;* assess for factors that may hinder and facilitate acknowledgment 2. discuss the grieving process and assist client to accept the phases of grieving as an expected response to loss of a breast and the diagnosis of cancer 3. allow time for client to progress through the phases of grieving (phases vary among theorists but progress from shock and alarm to acceptance); be aware that not every phase is expressed by all individuals, phases may overlap or recur, the amount of time needed to reach resolution of grief is very individual, and the grieving process may take months to years 4. provide an atmosphere of care and concern (e.g., provide privacy, be available and nonjudgmental, display empathy and respect) *so client will feel free to express feelings* 5. perform actions *to promote trust* (e.g., answer questions honestly, provide requested information) 6. encourage the verbal expression of anger and sadness about the diagnosis of cancer and the loss of a breast; recognize displacement of anger and assist client to see the actual cause of angry feelings and resentment 7. encourage client to express feelings in whatever ways are comfortable (e.g., writing, drawing, conversation) 8. assist client to identify and use techniques that have helped her to cope in previous situations of loss 9. support realistic hope about the effect of surgery on the disease process and the possibility of breast reconstruction if it has not been done 10. support behaviors suggesting successful grief work (e.g., verbalizing feelings about loss of a breast, expressing sorrow) 11. explain the phases of the grieving process to significant others; encourage their support and understanding 12. facilitate communication between the client and significant others; be aware that they may be in different phases of the grieving process 13. provide information regarding counseling services and support groups that might assist client in working through grief 14. when appropriate, assist client to meet spiritual needs (e.g., arrange for visit from clergy) 15. administer antidepressants if ordered. c. Consult appropriate health care provider (e.g., psychiatric nurse clinician, physician) regarding referral for counseling if signs of dysfunctional grieving (e.g., persistent denial of loss, excessive anger or sadness, emotional lability) occur.

Discharge Teaching/Continued Care

5. NURSING DIAGNOSIS: ***DEFICIENT KNOWLEDGE, INEFFECTIVE THERAPEUTIC REGIMEN MANAGEMENT, OR INEFFECTIVE HEALTH MAINTENANCE****

*The nurse should select the diagnostic label that is most appropriate for the client's discharge teaching needs.

Suggested NOC Outcomes: Knowledge: disease process; Knowledge: treatment regimen; Knowledge: treatment procedure(s); Knowledge: health resources

Suggested NIC Interventions: Health system guidance; Teaching: individual; Teaching: disease process; Teaching: prescribed activity/exercise; Teaching: psychomotor skill

Desired Outcomes	**Nursing Actions** *and Selected Purposes/Rationales*
5.a. The client will identify ways to reduce the risk of trauma to and infection in the arm on the operative side.	5.a.1. Provide the following instructions regarding ways to reduce the risk of trauma to and infection in the arm on operative side: a. avoid cuts by pushing cuticles back instead of cutting them and trimming fingernails carefully b. wear heavy work gloves when gardening and rubber gloves when in contact with steel wool, harsh chemicals, abrasive compounds, or water for prolonged periods c. wear insulated gloves when reaching into a hot oven or handling hot items d. use a thimble when sewing in order to avoid pinpricks e. keep pressure off the affected arm (e.g., avoid wearing tight jewelry and clothes with constricting bands, carry heavy objects such as purse or packages with the unaffected arm) f. offer only the unaffected arm for blood pressure readings, injections, blood drawing, and intravenous therapy g. wash any break in the skin on the affected arm with soap and water and cover the area with a protective dressing h. use an electric rather than a straight-edge razor when shaving underarm area i. apply a lanolin hand cream several times/day to prevent drying and cracking of the skin j. use insect repellant when in an area where stinging or biting insects may be located k. avoid prolonged exposure to the sun in order to prevent burns. 2. Instruct client to contact physician immediately if any injury to the arm on the operative side occurs. 3. Instruct client to wear a medical alert bracelet or tag warning others not to draw blood, give injections, insert an intravenous access device, or measure blood pressure in arm on operative side.
5.b. The client will identify ways to prevent and treat lymphedema of the arm on the operative side.	5.b.1. Instruct client in ways to prevent lymphedema of the arm on operative side: a. elevate the affected arm on pillows for 30–45 minutes at least 3 times a day for the prescribed length of time (usually 6–12 weeks) b. sleep on unaffected side or back with affected arm elevated for the prescribed length of time (usually 6–12 weeks) c. adhere to recommended measures for reducing the risk of trauma to and preventing infection in the arm on the operative side (see action a.1 in this diagnosis) d. adhere to the prescribed exercise regimen e. avoid placing the affected extremity in a dependent position for extended periods. 2. Reinforce physician's instructions regarding ways to treat lymphedema if present: a. perform manual massage of the affected arm if prescribed b. wear an elastic pressure gradient sleeve as recommended.
5.c. The client will demonstrate the ability to care for wound drainage device if present.	5.c.1. If the client is to be discharged with wound drain(s) and a suction device, demonstrate how to empty and establish negative pressure in the collection device and provide these additional instructions: a. keep the collection device positioned below the insertion site b. keep the tubing pinned to the dressing and avoid kinks and strain on the tubing

c. empty the collection device at least twice daily or more often if needed
d. keep a record of the amount of drainage (drains will typically be removed once the drainage is less than 20–30 ml in 24 hours).
2. Allow time for questions, clarification, and return demonstration.

5.d. The client will demonstrate the ability to perform the prescribed exercises and verbalize an understanding of additional exercises to be done once the incision has healed.

5.d.1. Reinforce teaching about postmastectomy exercises.
2. Emphasize the need to perform hand and elbow exercises regularly and begin full range of motion exercises of the arm and shoulder once the incision has healed.
3. Allow time for questions, clarification, and return demonstration.

5.e. The client will verbalize the importance of and demonstrate the ability to perform a breast self-examination (BSE) on the remaining breast and operative site.

5.e.1. Explain the reasons for monthly BSE of the remaining breast and operative site.
2. Explore with client ways to remember to carry out BSE. The examination should be done a week after conclusion of menses or on a specific date if postmenopausal.
3. Demonstrate, using a model, film, or chart, how to do a BSE.
4. Allow time for questions, clarification, and return demonstration.

5.f. The client will state the factors to consider in selecting a breast prosthesis.

5.f.1. If acceptable to client, invite a Reach to Recovery volunteer or prosthetist to share information about the various prostheses available.
2. Suggest that client wear a soft, temporary prosthesis until complete healing of the incision has occurred.
3. Encourage the client to take significant other or a close friend with her for the initial fitting of the prosthesis in order to provide emotional support.
4. Emphasize that it is important to select or make a prosthesis that will balance the chest in order to avoid difficulties with posture and subsequent back, shoulder, and neck discomfort.

5.g. The client will state signs and symptoms to report to the health care provider.

5.g.1. Refer to Standardized Postoperative Care Plan, Diagnosis 22, action c (p. 125), for signs and symptoms to report to the health care provider.
2. Instruct client to report these additional signs and symptoms:
a. new or increased sensations of numbness, tingling, heaviness, or tightness in hand, arm, or shoulder on operative side
b. increasing weakness of the affected arm
c. decreased ability to move shoulder or arm on operative side (full range of motion should be regained within 3–6 months)
d. warmth or redness of the affected arm
e. increase in size of arm on affected side (client may be instructed to measure arm circumference weekly at points about 2–4 inches above and below elbow and compare with unaffected arm); inform client that transient edema may occur as she increases use of the affected arm and that this should subside as collateral lymphatic circulation develops
f. increased swelling around incision(s)
g. purulent, foul-smelling drainage from incision site(s) or wound drain insertion site
h. dressings that become saturated with drainage more than once a day
i. unexpected increase in or absence of drainage in collection device.

5.h. The client will identify community resources that can assist with adjustment to the diagnosis of cancer and the loss of a breast.

5.h.1. Provide information about community resources that can assist the client and significant others with adjustment to the diagnosis of cancer and the mastectomy (e.g., American Cancer Society, Reach to Recovery, National Lymphedema Network, National Breast Cancer Coalition, home health agencies, individual and family counselors).
2. Initiate a referral if appropriate.

Desired Outcomes	**Nursing Actions** *and Selected Purposes/Rationales*
5.i. The client will verbalize an understanding of and a plan for adhering to recommended follow-up care including future appointments with health care provider, medications prescribed, activity limitations, exercises, wound care, and plans for subsequent treatment.	5.i.1. Refer to Standardized Postoperative Care Plan, Diagnosis 22 (pp. 125–126), for routine postoperative instructions and measures to improve client compliance. 2. Reinforce physician's explanations and instructions regarding future treatment (e.g., chemotherapy, radiation therapy, hormone therapy such as tamoxifen, breast reconstruction) if planned. 3. Explain the importance of having follow-up breast exams and mammography as prescribed. 4. Reinforce the physician's instructions regarding activity limitations. Instruct client to: a. avoid lifting heavy objects (over 5–10 pounds) until wound has healed (usually about 4–6 weeks) b. avoid driving until approved by physician (usually about 2 weeks). 5. Review physician's instructions regarding exercises (e.g., squeezing a ball, bending and flexing wrist and elbow, hand wall climbing, pulley exercises, rope turning, arm swings, elbow pull-in, scissors). Instructions should include when to start exercises, frequency, and a written description and/or pictures of how to perform them.

Additional Nursing Diagnoses

SELF-CARE DEFICIT

related to impaired physical mobility associated with pain, the depressant effect of anesthesia and some medications (e.g., narcotic [opioid] analgesics, some antiemetics), fear of dislodging tubes and compromising surgical wound, and prescribed arm movement restrictions on the operative side.

*INEFFECTIVE COPING**

related to:

a. perceived loss of femininity and embarrassment associated with loss of a breast;
b. fear of rejection by significant others;
c. fear, anxiety, and feelings of loss of control associated with the diagnosis of cancer, subsequent treatment (e.g., external radiation therapy, chemotherapy, hormone therapy) if planned, and possibility of disease recurrence.

*See Unit II for outcomes, actions, and rationales.

Bibliography

See pages 879 and 885.

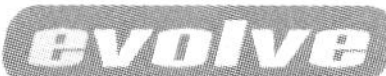

Radical Prostatectomy

A radical prostatectomy is performed to treat cancer of the prostate. The surgery includes removal of the prostate gland, prostatic capsule, seminal vesicles, and part of the vas deferens. In addition, a portion of the bladder neck is sometimes removed prior to the anastomosis of the remaining urethra to the bladder neck. A pelvic lymphadenectomy is usually performed concurrently if the cancer has spread into the pelvic lymph nodes. A radical prostatectomy is accomplished via a retropubic or perineal approach depending on the size and position of the prostate, the anticipated extensiveness of surgery, and physician preference. Occasionally, the client will receive external radiation therapy prior to surgery to reduce the tumor size. If there is evidence of lymph node involvement, a course of external radiation therapy may be done after the client recovers from the surgery.

This care plan focuses on the adult client with cancer of the prostate who is admitted for a radical prostatectomy. Much of the postoperative information is applicable to clients receiving follow-up care in an extended care facility or home setting.

OUTCOME/DISCHARGE CRITERIA

THE CLIENT WILL:

- have adequate urine output
- have normal healing of the surgical wound
- have surgical pain controlled
- have no signs and symptoms of infection or postoperative complications
- demonstrate the ability to perform care related to the urinary catheter and drainage system
- identify ways to manage urinary incontinence if it occurs following catheter removal
- identify ways to manage bowel incontinence if present
- share feelings and concerns about the diagnosis of cancer, the prognosis, and changes in body functioning that may occur as a result of a radical prostatectomy
- state signs and symptoms to report to the health care provider
- verbalize an understanding of and a plan for adhering to recommended follow-up care including future appointments with health care provider, medications prescribed, activity level, wound care, and plans for subsequent treatment.

NURSING/COLLABORATIVE DIAGNOSES

DISCHARGE TEACHING

See Standardized Preoperative and Postoperative Care Plans (pp. 97–126) for additional diagnoses.

PREOPERATIVE

Use in conjunction with the Standardized Preoperative Care Plan.

1. Nursing Diagnosis: FEAR/ANXIETY

related to:
a. diagnosis of cancer, treatment plan, and prognosis;
b. potential embarrassment or loss of dignity associated with body exposure during preoperative care, surgery, and postoperative assessments and treatments;
c. anticipated loss of control associated with effects of anesthesia;
d. lack of understanding of the surgical procedure and postoperative expectations and care;
e. anticipated surgical findings, postoperative pain, and changes in body functioning;
f. unfamiliar environment and separation from significant others;
g. financial concerns associated with hospitalization.

Suggested NOC Outcomes: Anxiety level; Fear level; Anxiety self-control; Fear self-control

Suggested NIC Interventions: Anxiety reduction; Calming technique; Emotional support; Presence; Teaching: preoperative

Desired Outcome	Nursing Actions *and Selected Purposes/Rationales*
1. The client will experience a reduction in fear and anxiety (see Standardized Preoperative Care Plan, Diagnosis 1 [pp. 97–98], for outcome criteria).	1.a. Refer to Standardized Preoperative Care Plan, Diagnosis 1 (pp. 97–98), for measures related to assessment and reduction of fear and anxiety. b. Implement additional measures *to reduce fear and anxiety:* 1. allow time for verbalization of concerns regarding the effects of the radical prostatectomy on body functioning (e.g., sterility, possible impotence, possible urinary and/or bowel incontinence); reinforce physician's explanation that if incontinence occurs, it often resolves over time and that nerve-sparing surgical techniques have greatly reduced the incidence of impotence 2. instruct client to expect the following postoperatively *so that he is not overly concerned when they occur:* a. presence of a urinary catheter (the catheter is usually removed about 1–2 weeks after surgery) b. frequent dressing changes and/or presence of wound drainage collection device for the first 2–4 days after surgery c. possible need for bladder irrigations to keep catheter patent d. presence of some blood in urine (can occur occasionally during the first 1–3 days after surgery) 3. reinforce physician's explanation about the positive effects of surgery (when diagnosed and treated in early stages, prostatic cancer is a highly curable disease) 4. assure client that privacy will be maintained during preoperative care and postoperative assessments and treatments 5. assure client that he will receive thorough instructions about management of the urinary catheter prior to discharge.

POSTOPERATIVE

Use in conjunction with the Standardized Postoperative Care Plan.

1. NURSING DIAGNOSIS:

ACUTE PAIN

related to tissue trauma and reflex muscle spasms associated with the surgery; irritation from drainage tubes; and stress on surgical area associated with movement, sitting (especially following a perineal approach), and straining to have a bowel movement.

Suggested NOC Outcomes: Pain control; Comfort level

Suggested NIC Interventions: Pain management; Analgesic administration

Desired Outcome	Nursing Actions *and Selected Purposes/Rationales*
1. The client will experience diminished pain (see Standardized Postoperative Care Plan, Diagnosis 6 [p. 109], for outcome criteria).	1.a. Refer to Standardized Postoperative Care Plan, Diagnosis 6 (p. 109), for measures related to assessment and management of pain. b. Implement additional measures *to reduce pain:* 1. instruct client to avoid straining to have a bowel movement *in order to prevent increased pressure on operative site;* consult physician about an order for a laxative if indicated 2. if client has a perineal incision, provide a pillow or foam pad for him to sit on if desired.

2. NURSING DIAGNOSIS:

URINARY RETENTION

related to obstruction of the urinary catheter.

Suggested NOC Outcome: Urinary elimination

Suggested NIC Interventions: Tube care: urinary; Bladder irrigation

Desired Outcome	Nursing Actions *and Selected Purposes/Rationales*
2. The client will not experience urinary retention as evidenced by: a. no reports of bladder fullness and suprapubic discomfort b. absence of bladder distention c. balanced intake and output within 48 hours after surgery.	2.a. Assess for and report signs and symptoms of urinary retention (e.g., reports of bladder fullness or suprapubic discomfort, bladder distention, absence of urine in urinary catheter drainage tubing, output that continues to be less than intake 48 hours after surgery). b. Implement measures *to maintain patency of urinary catheter in order to prevent urinary retention:* 1. keep drainage tubing free of kinks 2. keep collection container below level of bladder 3. anchor catheter securely to abdomen or thigh *in order to prevent inadvertent removal* 4. perform bladder irrigations as ordered *to flush out blood clots if present (the clots could obstruct the catheter).* c. Consult physician if signs and symptoms of urinary retention persist.

3. NURSING DIAGNOSIS:

BOWEL INCONTINENCE

related to:

a. unavoidable or inadvertent damage to the anal sphincter or to the pudendal nerve during surgery (this nerve controls the anal sphincter);
b. compression of the pudendal nerve associated with edema in the surgical area;
c. loss of perineal muscle tone associated with surgical incision if a perineal approach was used.

Suggested NOC Outcome: Bowel continence

Suggested NIC Interventions: Bowel management; Pelvic muscle exercise

Desired Outcome	Nursing Actions *and Selected Purposes/Rationales*
3. The client will maintain optimal bowel control as evidenced by absence of or decrease in episodes of incontinence.	3.a. Monitor for episodes of bowel incontinence. b. Implement measures *to reduce the risk of bowel incontinence:* 1. instruct client to perform perineal exercises (e.g., squeezing buttocks together, then relaxing the muscles) regularly when allowed *in order to increase anal sphincter tone and strengthen pelvic floor muscles (helps maintain a normal anorectal angle)* 2. have bedside commode readily available to client and provide easy access to bathroom *in order to reduce delays in toileting.* c. If bowel incontinence occurs, consult physician about initiating a bowel care program *so that client is able to routinely evacuate contents of lower colon and reduce the risk of incontinence.*

4. NURSING DIAGNOSIS: *RISK FOR INFECTION*

a. wound infection related to:
   1. wound contamination associated with introduction of pathogens during or following surgery (especially with a perineal approach because incision is close to the anus)
   2. delayed wound healing associated with factors such as diminished tissue perfusion of wound area (especially if client received external radiation therapy prior to surgery) and decreased nutritional status (if present);

b. urinary tract infection related to:
   1. introduction of pathogens associated with presence of indwelling catheter
   2. increased growth and colonization of microorganisms associated with urinary stasis (can occur with decreased activity and catheter obstruction).

Suggested NOC Outcomes: Immune severity; Infection status; Wound healing: primary intention

Suggested NIC Interventions: Infection protection; Infection control; Wound care; Tube care: urinary

Desired Outcomes	Nursing Actions *and Selected Purposes/Rationales*
4.a. The client will remain free of wound infection (see Standardized Postoperative Care Plan, Diagnosis 17, outcome b [pp. 118–119], for outcome criteria).	4.a.1. Refer to Standardized Postoperative Care Plan, Diagnosis 17, action b (pp. 118–119), for measures related to assessment and prevention of wound infection. 2. If a perineal approach was used, implement additional measures *to prevent wound infection:* a. instruct and assist client to perform good perineal care immediately after bowel movements b. use a double-tailed T-binder, scrotal support, or jockey shorts to secure perineal dressings *(movement of loose dressings can cause skin irritation and subsequent breakdown.)*
4.b. The client will remain free of urinary tract infection as evidenced by: 1. clear urine 2. absence of chills and fever 3. urinalysis showing fewer than 5 WBCs, negative leukocyte esterase and nitrites, and absence of bacteria 4. negative urine culture.	4.b.1. Assess for and report signs and symptoms of urinary tract infection (e.g., cloudy urine; chills; elevated temperature; urinalysis showing a WBC count greater than 5, positive leukocyte esterase or nitrites, or presence of bacteria; positive urine culture). 2. Implement measures *to prevent urinary tract infection:* a. perform actions to prevent urinary retention and subsequent stasis of urine (see Postoperative Diagnosis 2, action b) b. maintain a fluid intake of at least 2500 ml/day unless contraindicated *to promote urine formation and subsequent flushing of pathogens from the bladder* c. maintain sterile technique during bladder irrigations if performed d. perform catheter care as often as needed *to prevent accumulation of mucus and blood around the meatus*

e. keep urine collection container below bladder level at all times *to prevent reflux or stasis of urine*
f. anchor tubing securely *to reduce the amount of in-and-out movement of the catheter (this movement can result in the introduction of pathogens into the urinary tract and can cause tissue trauma, which can result in colonization of microorganisms)*
g. if frequent bladder irrigations are necessary, consult physician about initiation of continuous, closed system irrigation *(frequent intermittent irrigations increase the risk of introduction of pathogens)*
h. increase activity as allowed and tolerated *to decrease urinary stasis.*

3. If signs and symptoms of urinary tract infection are present, administer antimicrobials as ordered.

5. COLLABORATIVE DIAGNOSES:

POTENTIAL COMPLICATIONS OF RADICAL PROSTATECTOMY

a. hypovolemic shock related to:
   1. deficient fluid volume associated with restricted oral intake and excessive fluid loss
   2. hemorrhage associated with surgical trauma to the highly vascular prostate gland, opening of wound (can occur as a result of inadequate wound closure, stress on incision line, and/or poor wound healing), slippage of closures on ligated vessels, and/or disruption of clots at incision site;

b. thromboembolism related to:
   1. trauma to pelvic veins during surgery
   2. venous stasis associated with:
      a. pressure on the pelvic and calf vessels during surgery if client was in lithotomy position (this position is used during a perineal approach)
      b. decreased activity
      c. increased blood viscosity (can result from deficient fluid volume)
      d. abdominal distention (the distended intestine can put pressure on the abdominal vessels)
   3. hypercoagulability associated with increased release of tissue thromboplastin into the blood (occurs as a result of surgical trauma) and hemoconcentration and increased blood viscosity (can occur as a result of deficient fluid volume).

Desired Outcomes	**Nursing Actions** *and Selected Purposes/Rationales*
5.a. The client will not develop hypovolemic shock (see Standardized Postoperative Care Plan, Diagnosis 20, outcome a [p. 122], for outcome criteria).	5.a.1. Assess for and report the following: a. excessive operative site bleeding: 1. excessive bloody drainage on dressings or from drains 2. increased swelling and/or blue-black discoloration in surgical area 3. persistent redness of or blood clots in urine 4. significant decrease in RBC, Hct, and Hgb levels b. difficulty maintaining intravenous or oral fluid intake c. signs and symptoms of hypovolemic shock (see Standardized Postoperative Care Plan, Diagnosis 20, action a.1 [p. 122]). 2. Refer to Standardized Postoperative Care Plan, Diagnosis 20, actions a.2 and 3 (p. 122), for measures to prevent and treat hypovolemic shock. 3. Implement measures *to minimize pressure on the operative area in order to prevent hemorrhage and subsequently reduce the risk of hypovolemic shock:* a. perform actions to prevent urinary retention (see Postoperative Diagnosis 2, action b) *in order to prevent distention of the bladder and subsequent pressure on the suture lines and stress on the newly coagulated blood vessels* b. instruct client to avoid sitting for long periods c. instruct client to avoid straining to have a bowel movement; consult physician regarding an order for a laxative if indicated d. instruct client to return to bed and limit activity for a few hours if urine becomes red when ambulating or sitting in chair.

Desired Outcomes	**Nursing Actions** *and Selected Purposes/Rationales*
5.b. The client will not develop a deep vein thrombus or pulmonary embolism (see Standardized Postoperative Care Plan, Diagnosis 20, outcomes c.1 and 2 [pp. 122–123], for outcome criteria).	5.b. Refer to Standardized Postoperative Care Plan, Diagnosis 20, actions c.1 and 2 (pp. 122–123), for measures related to assessment, prevention, and treatment of a deep vein thrombus and pulmonary embolism. Be aware that prophylactic anticoagulant and antiplatelet medications may be contraindicated *because of the high risk of hemorrhage during and following surgery on the prostate gland.*

6. Nursing Diagnosis: ***DISTURBED SELF-CONCEPT****

related to:

a. temporary presence of urinary catheter (the catheter is usually not removed until 2–3 weeks after surgery);
b. bowel incontinence if present and possible urinary incontinence following removal of the catheter;
c. sterility and absence of ejaculation associated with removal of the prostate gland, seminal vesicles, and a portion of the vas deferens;
d. possibility of impotence (especially following a perineal approach).

*This diagnostic label includes the nursing diagnoses of disturbed body image, low self-esteem, and ineffective role performance.

Suggested NOC Outcomes: Body image; Personal autonomy; Self-esteem; Psychosocial adjustment: life change

Suggested NIC Interventions: Body image enhancement; Grief work facilitation; Self-esteem enhancement; Role enhancement; Counseling; Emotional support; Support system enhancement

Desired Outcome	**Nursing Actions** *and Selected Purposes/Rationales* (see pp. 47–49 for additional rationales)
6. The client will demonstrate beginning adaptation to changes in body functioning as evidenced by: a. verbalization of feelings of self-worth and sexual adequacy b. maintenance of relationships with significant others c. active participation in activities of daily living.	6.a. Assess for signs and symptoms of a disturbed self-concept (e.g., verbalization of negative feelings about self, withdrawal from significant others, lack of participation in activities of daily living, refusal to perform catheter care). b. Implement measures to facilitate the grieving process (see Postoperative Diagnosis 7, action b). c. Discuss with client improvements in bowel, bladder, and sexual function that can realistically be expected. d. Assist client to identify and utilize coping techniques that have been helpful in the past. e. Inform client that when he is discharged, he will be able to connect his urinary catheter to a leg bag and that this bag will allow easier mobility and will not be visible when wearing long pants. f. If client is incontinent of stool and/or if incontinence of urine is an anticipated problem following catheter removal: 1. reinforce the importance of doing perineal exercises when allowed *in order to improve bowel and bladder control* 2. assist him to establish a routine bowel care program *to reduce the risk of bowel incontinence* 3. instruct in ways to minimize incontinence *so that social interaction is possible* (e.g., placing disposable liners in underwear, wearing absorbent undergarments such as Attends). g. Because sterility is expected, discuss alternative methods of becoming a parent (e.g., adoption) if of concern to client. h. If impotence is expected following surgery: 1. reinforce physician's explanation about the temporary or permanent nature of the impotence; if it is expected to be permanent, encourage

client to discuss various treatment options (e.g., medication, vacuum erection aids, penile prosthesis) with physician if appropriate
2. suggest alternative methods of sexual gratification if appropriate
3. discuss ways to be creative in expressing sexuality (e.g., massage, fantasies, cuddling).

i. Support behaviors suggesting positive adaptation to changes that have occurred (e.g., verbalization of feelings of self-worth, compliance with treatment plan, maintenance of relationships with significant others).
j. Assist client's and significant others' adjustment by listening, facilitating communication, and providing information.
k. Encourage visits and support from significant others.
l. Encourage client to pursue usual roles and interests and to continue involvement in social activities.
m. Provide information about and encourage utilization of community agencies and support groups (e.g., sexual, family, or individual counseling).
n. Consult appropriate health care provider (e.g., psychiatric nurse clinician, physician) if client seems unwilling or unable to adapt to changes resulting from the radical prostatectomy.

7. NURSING DIAGNOSIS: ***GRIEVING****

related to impotence and loss of bowel control (if they occur), possible loss of urinary control following removal of the catheter, loss of reproductive ability, the diagnosis of cancer, and possibility of premature death.

*This diagnostic label includes anticipatory grieving and grieving following the actual losses.

Suggested NOC Outcomes: Grief resolution; Psychosocial adjustment: life change

Suggested NIC Interventions: Grief work facilitation; Emotional support; Presence; Support system enhancement

Desired Outcome	Nursing Actions *and Selected Purposes/Rationales* (see pp. 35–37 for additional rationales)
7. The client will demonstrate beginning progression through the grieving process as evidenced by: a. verbalization of feelings about changes in body functioning and diagnosis of cancer b. usual sleep pattern c. participation in treatment plan and self-care activities d. utilization of available support systems.	7.a. Assess for signs and symptoms of grieving (e.g., expression of distress about having cancer and about changes in body functioning, change in eating habits, inability to concentrate, insomnia, anger, sadness, withdrawal from significant others, denial of losses). b. Implement measures *to facilitate the grieving process:* 1. assist client to acknowledge the losses *so grief work can begin;* assess for factors that may hinder and facilitate acknowledgment 2. discuss the grieving process and assist client to accept the phases of grieving as an expected response to actual and/or anticipated losses 3. allow time for client to progress through the phases of grieving (phases vary among theorists but progress from shock and alarm to acceptance); be aware that not every phase is expressed by all individuals, phases may overlap or recur, the amount of time needed to reach resolution of grief is very individual, and the grieving process may take months to years 4. provide an atmosphere of care and concern (e.g., provide privacy, be available and nonjudgmental, display empathy and respect) *so client will feel free to express feelings* 5. perform actions *to promote trust* (e.g., answer questions honestly, provide requested information) 6. encourage the verbal expression of anger and sadness about the losses experienced; recognize displacement of anger and assist client to see the actual cause of angry feelings and resentment 7. encourage client to express feelings in whatever ways are comfortable (e.g., writing, drawing, conversation)

Desired Outcome	Nursing Actions *and Selected Purposes/Rationales*
	8. assist client to identify and utilize techniques that have helped him cope in previous situations of loss 9. if appropriate, support realistic hope that bowel and/or bladder control will improve if he continues to do perineal exercises 10. support behaviors suggesting successful grief work (e.g., verbalizing feelings about losses, focusing on ways to adapt to losses, learning needed skills, developing or renewing relationships) 11. explain the phases of the grieving process to significant others; encourage their support and understanding 12. facilitate communication between the client and significant others; be aware that they may be in different phases of the grieving process 13. provide information about counseling services and support groups that might assist client in working through grief 14. when appropriate, assist client to meet spiritual needs (e.g., arrange for a visit from clergy) 15. administer antidepressants if ordered. c. Consult appropriate health care provider (e.g., psychiatric nurse clinician, physician) regarding referral for counseling if signs of dysfunctional grieving (e.g., persistent denial of losses, excessive anger or sadness, emotional lability) occur.

Discharge Teaching/Continued Care

8. Nursing Diagnosis: ***DEFICIENT KNOWLEDGE, INEFFECTIVE THERAPEUTIC REGIMEN MANAGEMENT, OR INEFFECTIVE HEALTH MAINTENANCE****

*The nurse should select the diagnostic label that is most appropriate for the client's discharge teaching needs.

Suggested NOC Outcomes: Knowledge: disease process; Knowledge: treatment regimen; Knowledge: treatment procedure(s)

Suggested NIC Interventions: Health system guidance; Teaching: individual; Teaching: disease process; Teaching: prescribed activity/exercise; Teaching: psychomotor skill; Pelvic muscle exercise

Desired Outcomes	Nursing Actions *and Selected Purposes/Rationales*
8.a. The client will demonstrate the ability to perform care related to the urinary catheter and drainage system.	8.a.1. Instruct client in care related to the urinary catheter and drainage system including: a. washing the urinary meatus with soap and water at least twice a day b. anchoring the catheter tubing securely to abdomen or thigh c. keeping catheter and urine collection bag tubing free of kinks d. keeping urine collection bag below the level of the bladder e. changing from the leg bag to bedside collection bag when lying down for more than a few hours f. emptying the leg bag and the bedside collection bag g. measuring and recording the amount of urine output if necessary. 2. Allow time for questions, clarification, practice, and return demonstration.
8.b. The client will identify ways to manage urinary incontinence if it occurs following catheter removal.	8.b.1. Provide information about ways to reduce the risk of urinary incontinence following removal of the urinary catheter (incontinence can occur as a result of trauma to urinary sphincters during surgery and/or irritation from the urinary catheter, damage to pelvic nerves during surgery, and/or a temporary decrease in bladder capacity because of the continued decompression of the bladder while the catheter was in place): a. try to urinate every 2–3 hours and when the urge is felt

b. urinate in a standing or sitting position to facilitate complete bladder emptying
c. avoid drinking large quantities of liquid over a short period
d. limit intake of alcohol and caffeine-containing beverages (alcohol and caffeine have a mild diuretic effect and act as irritants to the bladder; these factors may make urinary control more difficult)
e. stop drinking liquids a few hours before bedtime (reduces risk of nighttime incontinence)
f. avoid activities that make it difficult to empty bladder as soon as the urge is felt (e.g., long car rides, lengthy meetings).

2. Reinforce the importance of performing perineal exercises (e.g., stopping and starting stream during voiding; squeezing buttocks together, then relaxing the muscles) regularly when allowed in order to improve urinary control.
3. Inform client that if urinary incontinence occurs following catheter removal, he should:
   a. wash and dry perineal area after each episode of incontinence
   b. wear disposable underwear liners or absorbent undergarments such as Attends if needed
   c. consult physician about treatment options (e.g., biofeedback, insertion of an artificial urinary sphincter) if the problem persists.

8.c. The client will identify ways to manage bowel incontinence if present.

8.c. If client is experiencing bowel incontinence, instruct to:
1. adhere to a routine bowel care program
2. perform perineal exercises (e.g., stopping and starting stream during voiding; squeezing buttocks together, then relaxing the muscles) regularly when allowed in order to improve bowel control
3. wash and dry perineal area after each episode of incontinence
4. wear disposable underwear liners or absorbent undergarments such as Attends if needed.

8.d. The client will state signs and symptoms to report to the health care provider.

8.d.1. Refer to Standardized Postoperative Care Plan, Diagnosis 22, action c (p. 125), for signs and symptoms to report to the health care provider.
2. Instruct client to also report:
   a. urinary or bowel incontinence that persists longer than expected, worsens, or interferes with daily life
   b. persistent, unexpected impotence
   c. difficulty coping with the diagnosis of cancer and/or the effects of the radical prostatectomy on body functioning.

8.e. The client will verbalize an understanding of and a plan for adhering to recommended follow-up care including future appointments with health care provider, medications prescribed, activity level, wound care, and plans for subsequent treatment.

8.e.1. Refer to Standardized Postoperative Care Plan, Diagnosis 22 (pp. 125–126), for routine postoperative instructions and measures to improve client compliance.
2. Reinforce physician's explanations and instructions regarding subsequent treatment (e.g., external radiation therapy) if planned.

Bibliography

See pages 879 and 885.

Transurethral Resection of the Prostate (TURP)

Transurethral resection of the prostate (TURP) is the surgical removal of a prostatic adenoma through the urethra, while leaving the true prostate and its fibrous capsule intact. It may be performed to remove a small cancerous prostatic tumor but most frequently is done to remove a benign prostatic neoplasm that has enlarged enough to block the bladder neck or urethra. The most common cause of a benign neoplasm is benign prostatic hyperplasia (BPH).

BPH is common in men over 50 years of age and results from age-associated changes in androgen levels. Hyperplasia usually occurs gradually and involves the medial portion of the prostate gland which surrounds the urethra. Treatment is indicated when signs and symptoms of prostatism (e.g., urgency, frequency, hesitancy, decreased force of urinary stream, nocturia, post-void dribbling) become problematic or when complications such as recurrent urinary tract infection, urinary retention, hematuria, renal calculi, or hydronephrosis occur.

TURP is the most common surgical method for treating BPH. If the prostate gland is quite large, an open prostatectomy using a suprapubic or retropubic approach may be necessary. Methods such as medication therapy (e.g., doxazosin, tamsulosin, terazosin, finasteride), balloon urethroplasty, laser incision or removal of prostatic tissue, placement of a stent or coil in the prostatic urethra, and thermal therapy may also be used to treat symptomatic BPH. Factors influencing the treatment method selected include the client's age and health status, size of the enlarged prostate, presence of complications, and physician preference and expertise.

This care plan focuses on the adult client with BPH who is undergoing a transurethral resection of the prostate. The information is applicable to client's having surgery in a hospital or outpatient (e.g., surgical care center) setting.

OUTCOME/DISCHARGE CRITERIA

THE CLIENT WILL:

- have adequate urine output
- have bladder spasms controlled
- have no signs and symptoms of infection or postoperative complications
- identify ways to prevent bleeding in the surgical area
- identify ways to regain or maintain control of bladder emptying
- state signs and symptoms to report to the health care provider
- verbalize an understanding of and a plan for adhering to recommended follow-up care including future appointments with health care provider, medications prescribed, and activity level.

NURSING/COLLABORATIVE DIAGNOSES

Preoperative

1. Urinary retention p. 851
2. Deficient knowledge p. 851

Postoperative

1. Risk for excess fluid volume or water intoxication ("TUR syndrome") p. 853
2. Altered comfort: bladder spasms p. 853
3. Impaired urinary elimination p. 854
   a. retention
   b. incontinence following catheter removal
4. Risk for infection: urinary tract p. 856
5. Potential complications p. 856
   a. hypovolemic shock
   b. thromboembolism

DISCHARGE TEACHING

6. Deficient knowledge, Ineffective therapeutic regimen management, or Ineffective health maintenance p. 857

See Standardized Preoperative and Postoperative Care Plans (pp. 97–126) for additional diagnoses.

PREOPERATIVE

Use in conjunction with the Standardized Preoperative Care Plan.

1. NURSING DIAGNOSIS: ***URINARY RETENTION***

related to:
a. obstruction of the urethra and/or bladder neck by the enlarged prostate;
b. loss of bladder muscle tone associated with hypertrophy of the bladder wall (as BPH develops, the detrusor muscle hypertrophies in an attempt to increase its ability to push urine past the bladder neck or urethral obstruction; this hypertrophied muscle has poor contractility).

Suggested NOC Outcome: Urinary elimination

Suggested NIC Interventions: Urinary catheterization; Tube care: urinary

Desired Outcome	**Nursing Actions** *and Selected Purposes/Rationales*
1. The client will experience resolution of urinary retention if it occurs as evidenced by: a. no reports of bladder fullness and suprapubic discomfort b. absence of bladder distention c. balanced intake and output.	1.a. Assess for signs and symptoms of urinary retention: 1. reports of bladder fullness or suprapubic discomfort 2. bladder distention 3. output less than intake. b. Implement measures *to treat urinary retention if present:* 1. insert or assist with insertion of a urethral catheter as ordered (if insertion is difficult because of obstruction of the prostatic urethra or bladder neck, it may be necessary to use a stylet or a firm, specially angled catheter) 2. assist with insertion of a suprapubic catheter if unable to insert a urethral catheter because of obstruction. c. If a urinary catheter is present, implement measures *to maintain patency of the catheter in order to prevent urinary retention:* 1. keep drainage tubing free of kinks 2. keep collection container below level of bladder 3. tape catheter securely to abdomen or thigh *in order to prevent inadvertent removal.* d. Consult physician if signs and symptoms of urinary retention persist despite implementation of above actions.

Client Teaching

2. NURSING DIAGNOSIS: ***DEFICIENT KNOWLEDGE***

regarding surgical procedure, routines associated with surgery, physical preparation for the TURP, sensations that normally occur following surgery and anesthesia, and postoperative care.

Suggested NOC Outcomes: Knowledge: treatment regimen; Knowledge: treatment procedure(s)

Suggested NIC Interventions: Health system guidance; Teaching: preoperative; Teaching: individual; Teaching: procedure/treatment

Desired Outcomes	**Nursing Actions** *and Selected Purposes/Rationales*
2.a. The client will verbalize an understanding of the surgical procedure, preoperative care, and postoperative sensations and care.	2.a.1. Refer to Standardized Preoperative Care Plan, Diagnosis 4, actions a.1–4 (pp. 100–101), for information to include in preoperative teaching. 2. Provide additional information regarding care following a TURP: a. explain that bed rest is usually ordered for 6–18 hours after surgery; activity is then increased gradually (the level of activity allowed depends on physician preference, extensiveness of the resection, and the amount of postoperative bleeding client experiences)

Desired Outcomes	**Nursing Actions** *and Selected Purposes/Rationales*
	b. explain that a urinary catheter will be in place for 24–48 hours after surgery (a urethral catheter with 3 lumens is usually inserted to allow drainage of bladder and simultaneous infusion of irrigation solution if needed) c. describe the procedure and rationale for intermittent and continuous bladder irrigations d. explain that traction may be applied to the catheter for 4–5 hours postoperatively and again as needed so that the catheter balloon puts pressure on the surgical site in order to control bleeding (traction is accomplished by pulling down on the urethral catheter and anchoring it securely to the client's leg so that tension is maintained) e. explain that the following can be expected: 1. red urine that gradually lightens in color (urine color usually goes from bright red to pink within 24–36 hours and to light pink or dark amber within 72 hours) but often temporarily becomes more red when activity increases 2. some blood clots in urine 3. some bloody drainage from urethra f. describe signs and symptoms that can be indicative of bladder spasms (e.g., leakage of urine around catheter, feeling of an urgent need to urinate or defecate, pressure in bladder); stress that these signs and symptoms should be reported to the nurse so that catheter patency can be checked and medication can be given as needed to reduce discomfort g. explain that after the catheter is removed: 1. a mild to moderate burning sensation may be experienced when urinating and that this is expected to decrease with each voiding and resolve within 1–2 days 2. urinary symptoms experienced preoperatively (e.g., urgency, frequency, hesitancy, postvoid dribbling) may still be present or may even increase temporarily postoperatively due to poor bladder muscle tone and/or tissue trauma from the surgery and catheter (these symptoms usually resolve within 2–3 weeks). 3. Reinforce physician's explanation regarding effects of TURP on sexual functioning (after surgery, the client usually experiences retrograde ejaculation as a result of direct trauma to the internal urinary sphincter and/or widening of the bladder neck; normal ejaculatory function usually returns within weeks or months). 4. Allow time for questions and clarification of information provided.
2.b. The client will demonstrate the ability to perform activities designed to prevent postoperative complications.	2.b.1. Refer to Standardized Preoperative Care Plan, Diagnosis 4, action b.1 (p. 101), for instructions on ways to prevent postoperative complications. 2. Provide additional instructions about ways to prevent complications following TURP: a. when oral fluid intake is allowed after surgery, drink one glass of fluid each hour while awake unless contraindicated (helps keep catheter patent and reduces the risk for urinary tract infection) b. avoid activities that can put excessive pressure on the surgical area (e.g., straining to have a bowel movement, attempting to urinate around catheter, pulling on catheter, walking or sitting for too long). 3. Allow time for questions, clarification, and return demonstration.

POSTOPERATIVE *Use in conjunction with the Standardized Postoperative Care Plan.*

1. NURSING DIAGNOSIS:

RISK FOR EXCESS FLUID VOLUME OR WATER INTOXICATION ("TUR SYNDROME")

related to:
a. vigorous fluid therapy during and immediately after surgery;
b. increased secretion of antidiuretic hormone (output of ADH is stimulated by trauma, pain, and anesthetic agents);
c. excessive absorption of irrigation solution via the prostatic veins during and following surgery.

Suggested NOC Outcomes: Fluid overload severity; Fluid balance

Suggested NIC Interventions: Fluid monitoring; Fluid management

Desired Outcome	Nursing Actions *and Selected Purposes/Rationales*
1. The client will not experience excess fluid volume or water intoxication (see Standardized Postoperative Care Plan, Diagnosis 4, outcome b [p. 107], for outcome criteria).	1.a. Refer to Standardized Postoperative Care Plan, Diagnosis 4, action b (p. 107), for measures related to assessment, prevention, and treatment of excess fluid volume and water intoxication. b. Implement measures *to reduce absorption of fluid via the prostatic veins in order to further reduce the risk for excess fluid volume and/or water intoxication:* 1. use normal saline rather than hypotonic solutions for bladder irrigations 2. do not increase frequency of bladder irrigations or speed up continuous irrigation unless indicated.

2. NURSING DIAGNOSIS:

ALTERED COMFORT: BLADDER SPASMS

related to:
a. irritation of the bladder wall associated with tissue trauma during surgery, presence of urinary catheter, rapid infusion of irrigation solution, and distention of the bladder (can occur if urine flow becomes obstructed);
b. increased pressure on the bladder neck and prostatic fossa if traction is applied to the urethral catheter (traction may be applied to pull the catheter balloon into the prostatic fossa in order to put pressure on bleeding vessels).

Suggested NOC Outcomes: Comfort level; Symptom control

Suggested NIC Interventions: Medication administration; Tube care: urinary

Desired Outcome	Nursing Actions *and Selected Purposes/Rationales*
2. The client will experience relief of bladder spasms as evidenced by: a. verbalization of relief of suprapubic discomfort b. no reports of an urgent need to urinate or defecate c. no leakage of urine around the urinary catheter.	2.a. Assess for signs and symptoms of bladder spasms: 1. reports of suprapubic discomfort 2. statements of an urgent need to urinate or defecate 3. leakage of urine around the urinary catheter. b. Implement measures *to decrease the risk of bladder spasms:* 1. maintain patency of the urinary catheter (e.g., irrigate as needed, keep tubing free of kinks) *to prevent distention of bladder* 2. perform actions *to reduce movement of the catheter:* a. anchor catheter securely to client's abdomen or thigh b. instruct client to avoid pulling on and twisting the catheter 3. release traction on the catheter as soon as ordered *to reduce pressure on the bladder neck and prostatic fossa* 4. do not increase frequency of bladder irrigations or speed up continuous irrigation unless bleeding is noted or blood clots or tissue debris are present *(excessive or rapid bladder irrigation can irritate the bladder mucosa)* 5. instruct client to avoid attempting to urinate around the catheter and straining to urinate after catheter is removed *(attempts to forcefully contract bladder can stimulate bladder spasms)*

Desired Outcome	Nursing Actions *and Selected Purposes/Rationales*

6. perform actions to prevent urinary retention following removal of catheter (see Postoperative Diagnosis 3, action a.3) *in order to prevent distention of the bladder.*

c. If bladder spasms occur:
   1. encourage client to take short, frequent walks unless contraindicated *(walking seems to reduce spasms)*
   2. decrease the rate of continuous bladder irrigation if urine is not red and blood clots and tissue debris are not present
   3. administer belladonna and opium (B&O) rectal suppositories if ordered (this combination of an antimuscarinic and narcotic analgesic *reduces spasm of the bladder muscle and the client's perception of discomfort;* it is only prescribed when the urinary catheter is present *because it can cause urinary retention*).

d. Consult physician if above measures fail to control bladder spasms.

3. Nursing Diagnosis: *IMPAIRED URINARY ELIMINATION*

a. **retention** related to:
   1. obstruction of the urinary catheter
   2. difficulty urinating following removal of the catheter associated with:
      a. loss of bladder muscle tone resulting from hypertrophy of the detrusor muscle as BPH developed, overdistention of the bladder preoperatively, and/or decompression of the bladder when the catheter was present
      b. relaxation of the bladder muscle resulting from stimulation of the sympathetic nervous system (can result from surgical site discomfort, fear, and anxiety) and the depressant effect of some medications (e.g., narcotic [opioid] analgesics)
      c. decreased perception of bladder fullness resulting from the depressant effect of some medications (e.g., narcotic [opioid] analgesics)
      d. obstruction of the urethra and bladder neck by blood clots, tissue debris, and/or edema (can occur as a result of surgical instrumentation, irritation from the urethral catheter, and/or pressure from the catheter balloon if traction was applied postoperatively);

b. **incontinence following catheter removal** related to trauma to the urinary sphincter(s) associated with surgical instrumentation, irritation from the urethral catheter, and/or pressure from the catheter balloon if traction was applied postoperatively.

Suggested NOC Outcomes: Urinary continence; Urinary elimination

Suggested NIC Interventions: Urinary incontinence care; Urinary retention care; Bladder irrigation; Tube care: urinary; Pelvic muscle exercise

Desired Outcomes	Nursing Actions *and Selected Purposes/Rationales* (see pp. 59–62 for additional rationales)
3.a. The client will not experience urinary retention as evidenced by: 1. no reports of bladder fullness and suprapubic discomfort 2. absence of bladder distention 3. balanced intake and output within 48 hours after surgery	3.a.1. Assess for and report signs and symptoms of the following: a. urinary retention when catheter is present (e.g., reports of bladder fullness or suprapubic discomfort, bladder distention, absence of urine in urinary drainage tubing, output that continues to be less than intake 48 hours after surgery) b. progressive narrowing of the urethra or bladder neck after catheter removal (e.g., decreasing size of urinary stream, increasing need to strain to empty bladder, increasing urgency) c. urinary retention following removal of catheter (e.g., reports of bladder fullness or suprapubic discomfort, frequent voiding of small amounts [25–60 ml] of urine, bladder distention, output that continues to be less than intake 48 hours after surgery).

4. voiding adequate amounts at expected intervals after removal of catheter.

2. Implement measures *to maintain patency of the urinary catheter in order to prevent urinary retention:*
   a. keep drainage tubing free of kinks
   b. keep collection container below level of bladder
   c. tape catheter securely to abdomen or thigh *in order to prevent inadvertent removal*
   d. perform bladder irrigations as ordered *to flush out blood clots and tissue debris if present.*
3. Following removal of the catheter, implement measures *to prevent urinary retention:*
   a. offer urinal or assist client to bathroom every 2–4 hours if indicated
   b. instruct client to urinate when the urge is first felt *(a hypotonic bladder can easily become distended)*
   c. perform actions *to promote relaxation during voiding attempts* (e.g., provide privacy, have client sit to void, hold a warm blanket against abdomen)
   d. perform actions *that may help trigger the micturition reflex and promote a sense of relaxation during voiding attempts* (e.g., run water, place client's hands in warm water, encourage client to urinate when in shower)
   e. allow client to assume a normal position for voiding unless contraindicated.
4. If signs and symptoms of urinary retention occur after removal of the catheter, consult physician about intermittent catheterization or reinsertion of an indwelling catheter.

3.b. The client will experience urinary continence.

3.b.1. Assess for urinary incontinence after removal of the urinary catheter (catheter is usually removed 1–2 days after surgery).
2. Implement measures *to prevent trauma to the urinary sphincter(s) while the catheter is in place in order to reduce the risk of urinary incontinence following removal of the catheter:*
   a. if urethral catheter traction is ordered to control bleeding, release it as soon as allowed *in order to reduce pressure on and possible damage to the internal urinary sphincter* (traction should not be maintained for longer than 4–5 hours without being released)
   b. anchor catheter securely to client's abdomen or thigh *in order to prevent excessive movement of the catheter.*
3. Following removal of the catheter, implement measures *to reduce the risk of urinary incontinence:*
   a. keep urinal within client's reach and provide easy access to bathroom *in order to reduce delays in toileting*
   b. allow client to assume a normal position for voiding unless contraindicated *in order to promote complete bladder emptying*
   c. instruct client to perform perineal exercises (e.g., stopping and starting stream during voiding; squeezing buttocks together, then relaxing the muscles) regularly *in order to strengthen pelvic floor muscles and improve tone of the external urinary sphincter*
   d. limit oral fluid intake in the evening *to decrease the possibility of nighttime incontinence*
   e. instruct client to limit intake of alcohol and beverages containing caffeine *(alcohol and caffeine have a mild diuretic effect and act as irritants to the bladder; these factors may make urinary control more difficult)*
   f. instruct client to space fluids evenly throughout the day rather than drinking a large quantity at one time *(rapid filling of bladder can result in incontinence if client has decreased urinary sphincter tone).*
4. If urinary incontinence persists, consult physician regarding intermittent catheterization, reinsertion of an indwelling catheter, or use of external collection device (e.g., condom catheter).

4. Nursing Diagnosis:

RISK FOR INFECTION: URINARY TRACT

related to:
a. introduction of pathogens associated with instrumentation of urinary tract during surgery, presence of indwelling catheter, and frequent bladder irrigations;
b. increased growth and colonization of microorganisms associated with urinary stasis resulting from decreased activity and urinary retention if it occurs.

Suggested NOC Outcome: Infection severity

Suggested NIC Interventions: Infection control; Tube care: urinary; Urinary retention care

Desired Outcome	**Nursing Actions** *and Selected Purposes/Rationales*
4. The client will remain free of urinary tract infection (see Standardized Postoperative Care Plan, Diagnosis 17, outcome c [p. 119], for outcome criteria).	4.a. Refer to Standardized Postoperative Care Plan, Diagnosis 17, action c (p. 119), for measures related to assessment, prevention, and treatment of urinary tract infection. b. Implement additional measures *to prevent urinary tract infection:* 1. perform actions to prevent urinary retention (see Postoperative Diagnosis 3, actions a.2 and 3) 2. consult physician about removal of the catheter as soon as the urine is clear and free of blood clots and tissue debris *(risk of urinary tract infection increases the longer the catheter is in place).*

5. Collaborative Diagnoses:

POTENTIAL COMPLICATIONS OF TURP

a. **hypovolemic shock** related to hemorrhage (the prostate gland is very vascular);
b. **thromboembolism** related to venous stasis associated with pressure on the pelvic and calf vessels during surgery (the client is usually in lithotomy position) and decreased activity.

Desired Outcomes	**Nursing Actions** *and Selected Purposes/Rationales*
5.a. The client will not develop hypovolemic shock (see Standardized Postoperative Care Plan, Diagnosis 20, outcome a [p. 122], for outcome criteria).	5.a.1. Assess for and report the following: a. excessive operative site bleeding: 1. bright red drainage (could indicate arterial bleeding) or persistent darker drainage (venous bleeding) and blood clots in urinary catheter 2. persistent redness of and blood clots in urine after removal of the catheter 3. significant decrease in RBC, Hct, and Hgb levels b. signs and symptoms of hypovolemic shock (see Standardized Postoperative Care Plan, Diagnosis 20, action a.1 [p. 122]). 2. Refer to Standardized Postoperative Care Plan, Diagnosis 20, actions a.2 and 3 (p. 122), for measures to prevent and treat hypovolemic shock. 3. Implement additional measures *to prevent or control hemorrhage in order to prevent hypovolemic shock:* a. maintain traction on the urethral catheter as ordered *(provides direct pressure on the bleeding vessels)* b. perform actions *to prevent trauma to and/or unnecessary pressure on the prostatic area:* 1. anchor catheter tubing securely to client's abdomen or thigh *in order to minimize movement of catheter* 2. caution client to avoid pulling on the catheter 3. instruct client to take short rather than long walks and to avoid sitting for long periods 4. instruct client to avoid straining to have a bowel movement; consult physician regarding an order for a laxative if indicated 5. implement measures to prevent urinary retention (see Postoperative Diagnosis 3, actions a.2 and 3) *in order to prevent distention of the*

bladder and subsequent pressure on the newly coagulated blood vessels in the operative area

c. instruct client to return to bed and limit activity for a few hours if urine becomes more red when ambulating or sitting in chair.

5.b. The client will not develop a deep vein thrombus or pulmonary embolism (see Standardized Postoperative Care Plan, Diagnosis 20, outcomes c.1 and 2 [pp. 122–123], for outcome criteria).

5.b. Refer to Standardized Postoperative Care Plan, Diagnosis 20, actions c.1 and 2 (pp. 122–123), for measures related to assessment, prevention, and treatment of a deep vein thrombus and pulmonary embolism. Be aware that prophylactic anticoagulant and antiplatelet medications are usually contraindicated *because of the risk of hemorrhage during and following surgery on the highly vascular prostate gland.*

Discharge Teaching/Continued Care

6. Nursing Diagnosis: ***DEFICIENT KNOWLEDGE, INEFFECTIVE THERAPEUTIC REGIMEN MANAGEMENT, OR INEFFECTIVE HEALTH MAINTENANCE****

*The nurse should select the diagnostic label that is most appropriate for the client's discharge teaching needs.

Suggested NOC Outcomes: Knowledge: disease process; Knowledge: treatment regimen

Suggested NIC Interventions: Health system guidance; Teaching: individual; Teaching: disease process; Teaching: prescribed activity/exercise; Pelvic muscle exercise

Desired Outcomes	**Nursing Actions** *and Selected Purposes/Rationales*

6.a. The client will identify ways to prevent bleeding in the surgical area.

6.a.1. Instruct client in ways to prevent bleeding in the surgical area:
- a. avoid straining during defecation (provide instructions about increasing fluid intake and intake of foods high in fiber if client tends to be constipated)
- b. avoid long walks, prolonged sitting, long car rides, running, climbing stairs quickly, strenuous exercise, sexual intercourse, and lifting objects over 10 pounds for as long as recommended by physician (usually for 2–6 weeks after discharge)
- c. consult physician before resuming preoperative medications such as aspirin and other NSAIDs, warfarin, and clopidogrel (physicians often recommend waiting 1–2 weeks after surgery if possible before resuming these medications).

2. Allow time for questions and clarification of information provided.

6.b. The client will identify ways to regain or maintain control of bladder emptying.

6.b.1. Instruct client in ways to regain or maintain control of bladder emptying:
- a. try to urinate every 2–3 hours and whenever the urge is felt
- b. urinate in a standing or sitting position to facilitate bladder emptying
- c. avoid drinking large quantities of liquids over a short period
- d. limit intake of alcohol and caffeine-containing beverages (alcohol and caffeine have a mild diuretic effect and act as irritants to the bladder; these factors may make urinary control more difficult)
- e. stop drinking liquids a few hours before bedtime (reduces risk of urine retention and nighttime incontinence)
- f. avoid activities that make it difficult to empty bladder as soon as the urge is felt (e.g., long car rides, lengthy meetings) in order to prevent retention and the subsequent risk for incontinence
- g. perform perineal exercises (e.g., stopping and starting stream during voiding; squeezing buttocks together, then relaxing the muscles) 10–20 times/hour while awake until urinary control is regained.

Desired Outcomes	**Nursing Actions** *and Selected Purposes/Rationales*
	2. If client is experiencing urinary incontinence, instruct to: a. wear disposable underwear liners or absorbent undergarments such as Attends if necessary b. consult physician if urinary incontinence persists, worsens, or interferes with daily life so that various options (e.g., biofeedback, insertion of artificial urinary sphincter) can be discussed.
6.c. The client will state signs and symptoms to report to the health care provider.	6.c.1. Refer to Standardized Postoperative Care Plan, Diagnosis 22, action c (p. 125), for signs and symptoms to report to the health care provider. 2. Instruct client to report these additional signs and symptoms: a. persistent burgundy colored or bright red urine (inform client that some blood is expected intermittently for 2–3 weeks after surgery but that urine should become pink to amber after he rests and increases fluid intake for a couple of hours) b. presence of large blood clots or continued passage of smaller clots c. development of or increase in frequency, burning, or pain when urinating d. decrease in urine output or force and caliber of urinary stream e. bladder distention f. unexpected loss of bladder control g. cloudy urine unrelated to orgasm (it is expected that urine will be cloudy after orgasm if client is experiencing retrograde ejaculation) h. persistent or increased bladder spasms.
6.d. The client will verbalize an understanding of and a plan for adhering to recommended follow-up care including future appointments with health care provider, medications prescribed, and activity level.	6.d.1. Refer to Standardized Postoperative Care Plan, Diagnosis 22 (pp. 125–126), for routine postoperative instructions and measures to improve client compliance. 2. Reinforce the physician's instructions regarding the importance of lying down and increasing fluid intake for a few hours if amount of blood or number of blood clots in the urine increases. 3. Explain the importance of having a digital rectal examination and a blood test for prostate-specific antigen (PSA) done each year (cancer of the prostate and recurrent BPH can develop since the entire prostate gland is not removed during a TURP).

Bibliography

See pages 879 and 885.

UNIT XIX

Nursing Care of the Client with Disturbances of the Head and Neck

TOTAL LARYNGECTOMY WITH RADICAL NECK DISSECTION

A total laryngectomy with radical neck dissection is the usual treatment for cancer of the larynx with metastasis to regional lymph nodes and/or adjacent neck structures. A total laryngectomy includes removal of the larynx, the hyoid bone, cricoid cartilage, epiglottis, and 2 to 4 tracheal rings. During the surgery, the pharyngeal opening to the trachea is closed and a permanent tracheostomy is created. The degree of metastasis is a major factor in determining the extensiveness of the neck dissection. A comprehensive radical neck dissection usually involves one side of the neck and includes removal of the tumor, regional lymph nodes and lymphatic channels, submandibular salivary gland, sternocleidomastoid muscle, spinal accessory nerve, and internal jugular vein. Whenever possible, a modified or selective radical neck dissection is performed, leaving the spinal accessory nerve, sternocleidomastoid muscle, and/or internal jugular vein intact. If the remaining tissue does not adequately cover the surgical area, reconstruction is most often accomplished using a myocutaneous flap taken from the pectoralis major, latissimus dorsi, or trapezius muscle.

A tracheoesophageal puncture (TEP) may also be performed at the time of the surgery to create a fistula for the insertion of a voice prosthesis early in the postoperative period. The prosthesis allows for diversion of exhaled air from the trachea into the pharynx when the stoma is occluded. Sound is produced by vibration of the mucosa above the expired air stream and is converted to speech by the client's tongue, lips, teeth, and palate.

This care plan focuses on the adult client with cancer of the larynx hospitalized for a laryngectomy with radical neck dissection. The care plan will need to be individualized according to the extensiveness of the dissection, the amount and type of reconstructive surgery performed, and the physiological and psychological status of the client. If the client has received a preoperative course of radiation therapy, refer to the Care Plan on External Radiation Therapy for nursing care related to side effects the client may be experiencing. **Much of the postoperative information provided in this care plan is applicable to clients receiving follow-up care in an extended care facility or home setting.**

OUTCOME/DISCHARGE CRITERIA

THE CLIENT WILL:

- have an adequate respiratory status
- be able to communicate effectively
- have an adequate nutritional status
- have evidence of normal healing of surgical wounds
- have surgical pain controlled
- have no signs and symptoms of infection or postoperative complications
- demonstrate appropriate stomal care, suctioning, tracheostomy tube care, oral hygiene, and tube feeding techniques
- demonstrate the ability to effectively use and care for an electrolarynx
- demonstrate the ability to care for the tracheoesophageal puncture (TEP) and voice prosthesis if in place
- identify appropriate safety precautions related to the surgery, tracheostomy, and nerve damage (if present)
- identify signs and symptoms to report to the health care provider
- share feelings and thoughts about the effects of the laryngectomy and radical neck dissection on body image and usual lifestyle and roles
- identify community resources that can assist with home management and adjustment to the effects of surgery
- communicate an understanding of and a plan for adhering to recommended follow-up care including future appointments with health care provider and speech pathologist, medications prescribed, exercises, activity level, and wound care.

NURSING/COLLABORATIVE DIAGNOSES

See p. 876 and Standardized Preoperative and Postoperative Care Plans (pp. 97–126) for additional diagnoses.

PREOPERATIVE

Use in conjunction with the Standardized Preoperative Care Plan.

1. Nursing Diagnosis: *FEAR/ANXIETY*

related to:
a. impending surgery that will result in loss of normal speech and a marked change in appearance and body functioning;
b. lack of understanding of diagnostic tests, surgical procedure, and care required for the tracheostomy and voice prosthesis (if planned);
c. anticipated loss of control associated with effects of anesthesia;
d. financial concerns associated with hospitalization;
e. unfamiliar environment and separation from significant others;
f. possible rejection by significant others;
g. anticipated pain, surgical findings, and changes in usual lifestyle and roles;
h. diagnosis of cancer with uncertain prognosis.

Suggested NOC Outcomes: Anxiety level; Fear level; Anxiety self-control; Fear self-control

Suggested NIC Interventions: Anxiety reduction; Calming technique; Emotional support; Presence

Desired Outcome	**Nursing Actions** *and Selected Purposes/Rationales*
1. The client will experience a reduction in fear and anxiety (see Standardized Preoperative Care Plan, Diagnosis 1 [pp. 97–98], for outcome criteria).	1.a. Refer to Standardized Preoperative Care Plan, Diagnosis 1 (pp. 97–98), for measures related to assessment and reduction of fear and anxiety. b. Implement additional measures *to reduce fear and anxiety:* 1. support client's decision to have a total laryngectomy with radical neck dissection; provide realistic hope about the results of cancer treatment 2. reinforce information about ways that verbal communication can occur following a total laryngectomy (e.g., voice prosthesis, electrolarynx [artificial larynx], esophageal speech, computer generated speech)

3. orient to the critical care unit if appropriate
4. discuss and plan with client and speech pathologist a method of communicating during the postoperative period (e.g., hand signals, paper and pencil, picture or word board, computer, Magic Slate, flash cards)
5. if acceptable to client, arrange for a visit with an individual who has successfully adjusted to a laryngectomy.

Client Teaching

2. Nursing Diagnosis: ***DEFICIENT KNOWLEDGE***

regarding the surgical procedure, routines associated with surgery, physical preparation for the laryngectomy and radical neck dissection, sensations that normally occur following surgery and anesthesia, and postoperative care and expectations.

Suggested NOC Outcomes: Knowledge: treatment regimen; Knowledge: prescribed activity

Suggested NIC Interventions: Teaching: individual; Teaching: preoperative; Teaching: prescribed activity/exercise; Teaching: psychomotor skill

Desired Outcomes	Nursing Actions *and Selected Purposes/Rationales*
2.a. The client will verbalize an understanding of the surgical procedure, preoperative care, and postoperative sensations and care.	2.a.1. Refer to Standardized Preoperative Care Plan, Diagnosis 4, actions a.1–4 (pp. 100–101), for information to include in preoperative teaching. 2. Explain the purpose of each part of a tracheostomy tube and how it works. Allow client to handle a tube and use pictures or a model to show where the tube will be inserted and what the stoma will look like when the tube is removed. 3. Provide additional information regarding specific expectations and care after laryngectomy and radical neck dissection: a. length of time the tracheostomy tube will be in place (usually 3–6 weeks depending on physician preference and rate of healing) b. anticipated tracheostomy care c. suctioning procedure and sensations (e.g., pressure) that may be experienced during the procedure d. techniques used to provide moisture to inspired air (e.g., nebulizer, humidifier) e. temporary need for nasogastric or gastrostomy tube feedings; assure client that oral feedings will be initiated as soon as the suture lines have healed and edema has subsided (usually 8–10 days after surgery but may be longer if client has had radiation therapy to the operative area) f. presence and purpose of closed wound drainage system g. involvement in wound care, suctioning, and tube feeding early in the postoperative period h. appearance of neck if a tracheoesophageal puncture (TEP) is planned during this surgery (a stent or catheter will protrude from the stoma and be taped to client's neck; about 5–7 days after surgery, the stent or catheter is removed and the voice prosthesis is inserted) i. different methods of speech production (e.g., esophageal speech, electrolarynx) that can be learned postoperatively if a TEP is not performed or is planned as a subsequent surgery. 4. Allow time for questions and clarification. Provide feedback.
2.b. The client will demonstrate the ability to perform activities designed to prevent postoperative complications.	2.b.1. Refer to Standardized Preoperative Care Plan, Diagnosis 4, action b.1 (p. 101), for teaching related to prevention of postoperative complications. 2. Provide additional instructions on ways to prevent complications associated with a laryngectomy and radical neck dissection: a. demonstrate oral hygiene techniques that will be used postoperatively (e.g., low-pressure power spray, irrigations with saline or hydrogen peroxide and water)

Desired Outcomes | **Nursing Actions** *and Selected Purposes/Rationales*

b. demonstrate exercises (e.g., shoulder flexion, abduction, and external rotation; wall climbing with fingers; pulley exercises) that may be ordered to prevent or treat shoulder and neck dysfunction on the affected side
c. emphasize the need to stop smoking in order to promote healing and reduce the risk for respiratory infection after surgery.

3. Allow time for questions, clarification, practice, and return demonstration of exercises and oral hygiene techniques.

POSTOPERATIVE

Use in conjunction with the Standardized Postoperative Care Plan.

1. Nursing Diagnosis: *INEFFECTIVE AIRWAY CLEARANCE*

related to:

a. obstruction or dislodgment of tracheostomy tube;
b. stasis of secretions associated with:
   1. decreased activity
   2. depressed ciliary function resulting from effects of anesthesia
   3. difficulty coughing up secretions resulting from the depressant effect of anesthesia and some medications (e.g., some antiemetics, narcotic [opioid] analgesics), pain, weakness, fatigue, presence of tenacious secretions (can occur as a result of deficient fluid volume and loss of normal humidification since inspired air no longer passes through the nose and mouth), and inability to raise intrathoracic pressure following removal of the larynx;
c. increased secretions associated with irritation of the respiratory tract resulting from inhalation anesthetics, endotracheal intubation, and presence of tube in trachea;
d. tracheal compression associated with edema and/or bleeding in operative area.

Suggested NOC Outcomes:
Respiratory status: ventilation; Respiratory status: airway patency

Suggested NIC Interventions: Respiratory monitoring; Artificial airway management; Airway suctioning; Positioning

Desired Outcome | **Nursing Actions** *and Selected Purposes/Rationales*

1. The client will maintain clear, open airways (see Standardized Postoperative Care Plan, Diagnosis 3 [p. 105], for outcome criteria).

1.a. Refer to Standardized Postoperative Care Plan, Diagnosis 3 (p. 105), for measures related to assessment and promotion of effective airway clearance.

b. Implement additional measures *to promote effective airway clearance:*
   1. perform actions *to decrease risk of dislodgment of tracheostomy tube:*
      a. obtain adequate assistance when changing tracheostomy tube ties (if assistance is not available, do not remove old ties until new ones are securely in place)
      b. fasten tracheostomy tube ties securely; check frequently to be sure they have not become loose
      c. minimize movement of outer cannula when suctioning or performing tracheostomy care *(movement of the tracheostomy tube can irritate the trachea and stimulate vigorous coughing)*
      d. ensure that dressings placed around the tracheostomy site are made of a nonraveling material *to prevent lint from entering tube and stimulating vigorous coughing*

e. consult physician about an order for an antitussive if client is coughing excessively
2. if tracheostomy tube does become dislodged, perform or assist with immediate replacement according to hospital procedure (an extra tracheostomy tube should be kept at the bedside)
3. perform tracheal suctioning and clean tracheostomy tube as necessary *to remove excessive secretions*
4. instill small amounts (usually 2–5 ml) of sterile normal saline into the tracheostomy when appropriate (e.g. before suctioning, every 2 hours, several times a day, as needed) *to thin secretions that are thick and loosen secretions that are dried*
5. perform actions *to prevent tracheal compression:*
   a. keep head of bed elevated at least 30° *to reduce edema in surgical area*
   b. implement measures to reduce stress on the surgical site (see Postoperative Diagnosis 5, actions a.2.b.2–7) *in order to prevent bleeding and hematoma formation.*

2. NURSING DIAGNOSIS: ***IMBALANCED NUTRITION: LESS THAN BODY REQUIREMENTS***

related to:
a. decreased oral intake associated with:
   1. prescribed dietary modifications
   2. anorexia resulting from factors such as discomfort, weakness, fatigue, depression, and an impaired sense of taste and smell (olfactory stimulation is diminished because client no longer breathes through nose)
   3. fear of choking (especially if choking had been a major symptom preoperatively)
   4. impaired swallowing;
b. inadequate nutritional replacement therapy;
c. increased nutritional needs associated with the increased metabolic rate that occurs during wound healing.

Suggested NOC Outcome: Nutritional status

Suggested NIC Interventions: Nutritional monitoring; Nutrition management; Nutrition therapy; Swallowing therapy; Enteral tube feeding

Desired Outcome	Nursing Actions *and Selected Purposes/Rationales*
2. The client will maintain an adequate nutritional status (see Standardized Postoperative Care Plan, Diagnosis 5 [pp. 107–108], for outcome criteria).	2.a. Refer to Standardized Postoperative Care Plan, Diagnosis 5 (pp. 107–108), for measures related to assessment and maintenance of nutritional status. b. Implement additional measures *to maintain an adequate nutritional status:* 1. administer nasogastric or gastrostomy tube feedings as ordered 2. perform actions *to improve oral intake when allowed* (oral feedings are usually initiated 7–10 days after surgery): a. assure client that there is no longer a connection between his/her esophagus and trachea *(may help reduce client's fear of choking)* b. implement measures to improve client's ability to swallow (see Postoperative Diagnosis 3, action b) c. implement measures *to compensate for impaired sense of taste and smell:* 1. provide extra sweeteners for foods/fluids 2. encourage client to experiment with spices and other seasonings (e.g., lemon, garlic, onion, mint) d. implement measures to facilitate client's psychological adjustment to the effects of the surgery (see Postoperative Diagnoses 8, actions c–r and 9, action b) *in order to reduce depression and improve appetite* e. provide support during mealtime if needed by staying with client and offering encouragement.

3. NURSING DIAGNOSIS: *IMPAIRED SWALLOWING*

related to:
a. edema of surgical area;
b. impaired tongue movement associated with damage to the hypoglossal nerve (can occur as a result of the disease process or surgery);
c. throat and neck discomfort;
d. structural changes in the pharynx (results in difficulty moving food bolus from pharynx into esophagus);
e. dry mouth and viscous oral secretions (can occur as a result of destruction of salivary glands if client had radiation therapy preoperatively, removal of salivary gland during surgery, and/or deficient fluid volume following surgery).

Suggested NOC Outcomes: Swallowing status: oral phase; Swallowing status: pharyngeal phase

Suggested NIC Intervention: Swallowing therapy

Desired Outcome

3. The client will experience an improvement in swallowing as evidenced by:
   a. communication of same
   b. absence of food in oral cavity after swallowing
   c. absence of choking when eating and drinking.

Nursing Actions *and Selected Purposes/Rationales*

(see pp. 54–57 for additional rationales)

3.a. Assess for signs and symptoms of impaired swallowing (e.g., communication of difficulty swallowing, stasis of food in oral cavity, choking when eating or drinking).
b. Implement measures *to improve ability to swallow:*
   1. place client in high Fowler's position for meals and snacks
   2. perform actions *to reduce throat and neck discomfort* (e.g., administer prescribed analgesic before meals)
   3. when oral intake is first allowed, provide thick rather than thin fluids or add a thickening agent (e.g., "Thick-It," gelatin, baby cereal) to thin fluids
   4. assist client to select foods that have a distinct texture and are easy to swallow (e.g., custard, canned fruit, mashed potatoes)
   5. avoid serving foods that are sticky (e.g., peanut butter, soft bread, honey)
   6. moisten dry foods with gravy or sauces (e.g., catsup, sour cream, salad dressings)
   7. if client has impaired tongue movement:
      a. avoid foods that tend to fall apart in mouth (e.g., cake, muffins) and those that consist of small food particles (e.g., rice, peas, corn)
      b. utilize assistive devices (e.g., long-handled spoon) to place food that does not need to be chewed (e.g., gelatin, custard, mashed potatoes) in back of mouth
   8. if client has a dry mouth and/or viscous oral secretions:
      a. perform actions *to stimulate salivation at mealtime:*
         1. provide oral hygiene before meals
         2. provide a piece of hard candy for client to suck on just before meals unless contraindicated
         3. serve foods that are visually pleasing
      b. encourage a fluid intake of 2500 ml/day unless contraindicated
      c. encourage client to use a saliva substitute such as Salivart if indicated
   9. encourage client to avoid milk, milk products, and chocolate *(when combined with saliva, these produce very thick secretions)*
   10. instruct client to avoid putting too much food/fluid in mouth at one time
   11. encourage client to concentrate on the act of swallowing; provide verbal cueing as needed
   12. consult speech pathologist about methods for dealing with impaired swallowing; reinforce recommended exercises and techniques.
c. Consult appropriate health care provider (e.g., speech pathologist, physician) if swallowing difficulties persist or worsen.

4. NURSING DIAGNOSIS: ***IMPAIRED VERBAL COMMUNICATION***

related to surgical removal of the larynx.

Suggested NOC Outcome: Communication

Suggested NIC Intervention: Communication enhancement: speech deficit

Desired Outcome	Nursing Actions *and Selected Purposes/Rationales*
4. The client will successfully communicate needs and desires.	4.a. Implement measures *to facilitate communication:* 1. maintain a patient, calm approach; listen attentively and allow ample time for communication 2. answer call signal in person rather than using the intercommunication system 3. if client is frustrated or fatigued, try to anticipate needs *in order to minimize the necessity of communication attempts* 4. ask questions that require short answers, eye blinks, or nod of head if client is having difficulty communicating and/or is frustrated or fatigued 5. provide materials such as Magic Slate, pad and pencil, computer, and/or picture board; try to ensure that placement of intravenous line does not interfere with client's use of these communication aids 6. reinforce communication techniques prescribed by speech pathologist 7. if a TEP has been performed and the voice prosthesis is in place (usually inserted 5–7 days after surgery), reinforce instructions from speech pathologist about its use 8. assist client to operate an electrolarynx if indicated. b. Post a sign on the door, intercommunication system, and above bed to remind health care personnel that the client is nonverbal. c. Inform significant others and health care personnel of techniques being used to facilitate client's ability to communicate. Stress the importance of consistent use of these techniques. d. Consult appropriate health care provider (e.g., speech pathologist, physician) if client seems reluctant or unable to use communication aids and/or artificial speech devices.

5. NURSING DIAGNOSIS: ***ACTUAL/RISK FOR IMPAIRED TISSUE INTEGRITY***

related to:

a. disruption of tissue associated with the surgical procedure and grafting (if performed);
b. delayed wound healing associated with factors such as:
   1. compromised circulation in wound area resulting from preoperative radiation to tumor site and/or excessive pressure or stress on surgical site
   2. fluid accumulation under skin flaps
   3. inadequate nutritional status;
c. irritation of skin associated with contact with wound drainage, pressure from tubes, and use of tape.

Suggested NOC Outcomes: Wound healing: primary intention; Tissue integrity: skin and mucous membranes

Suggested NIC Interventions: Skin surveillance; Positioning; Wound care; Incision site care

Desired Outcomes	Nursing Actions *and Selected Purposes/Rationales*
5.a. The client will experience normal healing of surgical wounds (see Standardized Postoperative Care Plan, Diagnosis 10, outcome a [p. 112], for outcome criteria).	5.a.1. Refer to Standardized Postoperative Care Plan, Diagnosis 10, action a (p. 112), for measures related to assessment and promotion of wound healing. 2. Implement additional measures *to promote wound healing:* a. use a bed cradle if indicated *to protect donor site from pressure of linens*

Desired Outcomes	**Nursing Actions** *and Selected Purposes/Rationales*

b. perform actions *to reduce stress on and trauma to graft site, suture lines, and/or surrounding tissue:*
   1. position client as ordered (e.g., support head and neck with pillows, elevate head of bed at least 30°) *to maintain head alignment and promote venous and lymphatic drainage*
   2. support client's head and neck during position change until client is able to do so
   3. instruct client to support head and neck with hands when moving in bed and to avoid turning head abruptly, flexing neck, and hyperextending neck
   4. place personal articles and call signal within easy reach *so client does not have to turn or strain to reach them*
   5. maintain patency of wound drainage system *in order to prevent fluid accumulation under the skin flaps*
   6. instruct client to "huff" rather than cough vigorously to promote effective airway clearance *(vigorous coughing can increase stress on the suture line)*
   7. make sure that tracheostomy tube ties are not too tight
   8. loosen adherent dressings with sterile normal saline before removal

c. perform actions to maintain an adequate nutritional status (see Postoperative Diagnosis 2)

d. perform actions to prevent wound infection (see Postoperative Diagnosis 6).

5.b. The client will maintain tissue integrity in areas in contact with wound drainage, tubings, and tape as evidenced by:
1. absence of redness and irritation
2. no skin breakdown.

5.b.1. Refer to Standardized Postoperative Care Plan, Diagnosis 10, action b (pp. 112–113), for measures related to assessment, prevention, and treatment of tissue irritation and breakdown resulting from contact with wound drainage, tubings, and tape.

2. Implement additional measures *to prevent tissue irritation and breakdown in areas in contact with wound drainage, tubings, and tape:*
   a. make sure that tracheostomy tube ties are not too tight
   b. loosen adherent dressings with sterile normal saline before removal
   c. change dressings when damp *to prevent maceration of skin.*

6. Nursing Diagnosis: ***RISK FOR INFECTION: WOUND***

related to:
a. wound contamination associated with introduction of pathogens during or following surgery;
b. increased colonization of microorganisms associated with accumulation of drainage around tracheostomy and beneath flaps (can result from a large dead space and/or obstruction of the wound drainage system);
c. decreased resistance to infection associated with factors such as inadequate nutritional status and diminished tissue perfusion of wound area.

Suggested NOC Outcomes: Immune status; Infection severity; Wound healing: primary intention

Suggested NIC Interventions: Infection protection; Infection control; Tube care; Incision site care; Wound care

Desired Outcome	**Nursing Actions** *and Selected Purposes/Rationales*

6. The client will remain free of wound infection (see Standardized Postoperative Care Plan, Diagnosis 17, outcome b [pp. 118–119], for outcome criteria).

6.a. Refer to Standardized Postoperative Care Plan, Diagnosis 17, action b (pp. 118–119), for measures related to assessment and prevention of wound infection.

b. Implement additional actions *to prevent wound infection:*
   1. perform actions to promote wound healing (see Postoperative Diagnosis 5, action a)
   2. apply an antimicrobial ointment to tracheal stoma and suture lines if ordered

3. perform tracheostomy care as needed *to prevent the accumulation of drainage.*

7. COLLABORATIVE DIAGNOSES:

POTENTIAL COMPLICATIONS OF LARYNGECTOMY AND RADICAL NECK DISSECTION

a. **carotid artery rupture** related to prolonged exposure of the artery during and/or following surgery (causes drying and subsequent destruction of the vessel wall) and weakening of the vessel wall (can occur if client had radiation therapy to the tumor site prior to surgery);
b. **necrosis of the skin flaps** related to:
   1. inadequate blood supply in flaps associated with excessive tension on wound margins, preoperative radiation to wound area, mechanical obstruction of blood flow within the flap, vascular congestion (can result from pressure differences in blood flow to and from flap), and development of hematoma or seroma under flaps
   2. infection of surgical wound;
c. **pharyngocutaneous fistula** related to dehiscence or necrosis of suture line in pharynx associated with wound infection, inadequate nutritional status, tension on suture line, and impaired vascularity of the wound;
d. **thoracic duct fistula** related to injury to the thoracic duct or one of its tributaries during the surgical procedure (can occur if the neck dissection is on the left side);
e. **shoulder and neck dysfunction** related to removal of or damage to the sternocleidomastoid muscle and/or spinal accessory nerve during surgery.

Desired Outcomes	Nursing Actions *and Selected Purposes/Rationales*
7.a. The client will not experience carotid artery rupture as evidenced by: 1. absence of rapidly expanding hematoma on operative side of neck 2. no evidence of profuse bleeding from neck wound 3. stable or improved RBC, Hct, and Hgb levels.	7.a.1. Assess for and report signs and symptoms of: a. impending carotid artery rupture (e.g., slight amount of bright red bleeding from wound [occurs 24–48 hours before rupture], sternal or high epigastric discomfort [often present a few hours before rupture]) b. carotid artery rupture (e.g., rapidly expanding hematoma on operative side of neck; profuse bleeding from neck wound; decreasing RBC, Hct, and Hgb levels). 2. Have suction equipment, gloves, cuffed tracheostomy tube (if one is not already in place), and absorbent dressings at bedside in case of carotid artery rupture. 3. Implement measures *to prevent drying and/or erosion of the carotid artery in order to reduce the risk for carotid artery rupture:* a. perform actions to promote healing of the surgical incision (see Postoperative Diagnosis 5, action a) and prevent wound infection (see Postoperative Diagnosis 6) b. assess for and report pulsation of tracheostomy tube *(indicates tip is in close proximity to carotid artery and may cause undue pressure on and subsequent damage to the carotid artery)* c. maintain tracheostomy tube in midtracheal position at all times d. if the carotid artery is exposed, keep it covered with loosely packed gauze moistened with sterile normal saline solution as ordered. 4. If carotid artery rupture occurs: a. apply firm, prolonged, continuous pressure to bleeding area using absorbent dressings b. position client in high Fowler's position and ensure that tracheostomy cuff is inflated *to reduce the risk for aspiration of blood;* assist with insertion of a cuffed tracheostomy tube if one is not in place c. suction as necessary *to clear airway* d. prepare client for surgical repair of the carotid artery if planned e. administer medications such as intravenous morphine sulfate or lorazepam if ordered *to allay anxiety* (client is typically alert) f. assess for and immediately report signs and symptoms of hypovolemic shock (e.g., restlessness, agitation, or confusion; significant decrease in B/P; rapid, weak pulse; rapid respirations; cool skin; pallor; cyanosis; diminished or absent peripheral pulses; urine output less than 30 ml/hour).

Desired Outcomes	Nursing Actions *and Selected Purposes/Rationales*
7.b. The client will not experience necrosis of skin flaps as evidenced by: 1. skin flaps warm and expected color 2. approximated wound edges 3. absence of foul odor from flap area.	7.b.1. Assess for and report signs and symptoms of: a. impaired blood flow in skin flaps (e.g., paleness or cyanosis of skin flaps; capillary refill time in skin flaps greater than 2–3 seconds) b. skin flap necrosis (e.g., pale, cool, darkened tissue; separation of wound edges; foul odor from flap area). 2. Implement measures to promote wound healing (see Postoperative Diagnosis 5, action a) and prevent wound infection (see Postoperative Diagnosis 6) *in order to prevent skin flap necrosis.* 3. If signs and symptoms of skin flap necrosis occur, prepare client for surgical revision of flap(s) if planned.
7.c. The client will not develop a pharyngocutaneous fistula as evidenced by: 1. absence of redness, edema, and tenderness near incision 2. usual drainage from incision 3. intact skin around incision.	7.c.1. Assess for and report signs and symptoms of a pharyngocutaneous fistula (e.g., redness, edema, and tenderness near incision; drainage of saliva or oral foods/fluids through incision or an opening near incision). 2. Implement measures *to prevent a pharyngocutaneous fistula:* a. perform actions to prevent wound infection (see Postoperative Diagnosis 6) b. perform actions to maintain an adequate nutritional status (see Postoperative Diagnosis 2) c. maintain patency of drain if in place (may be inserted in the pharynx during surgery and left in place for 7–10 days *to allow for controlled drainage of saliva, which subsequently decreases the risk of breakdown of the pharyngeal incision*). 3. If signs and symptoms of a pharyngocutaneous fistula occur: a. withhold oral food and fluid as ordered b. maintain intravenous therapy and tube feedings as ordered until fistula closes c. perform wound care as ordered d. administer antimicrobials if ordered e. prepare client for surgical closure of fistula if planned.
7.d. The client will experience resolution of a thoracic duct fistula if it occurs as evidenced by: 1. usual amount and character of drainage from incision 2. wound drainage negative for chylomicrons.	7.d.1. Assess for and report signs and symptoms of a thoracic duct fistula (e.g., sudden increase in drainage from wound; cloudy, milky-appearing fluid in drain system; wound drainage positive for chylomicrons). 2. If signs and symptoms of a thoracic duct fistula occur: a. apply pressure dressing over fistula site if ordered b. accurately assess amount of fistula drainage c. administer fluid and electrolytes as ordered *to replace those lost via the fistula* d. prepare client for surgical repair of fistula if planned.
7.e. The client will regain optimal shoulder and neck function on affected side as evidenced by: 1. improved range of motion of shoulder 2. ability to maintain shoulder in near-normal position 3. gradual resolution of pain in shoulder and neck.	7.e.1. Assess for and report signs and symptoms of sternocleidomastoid muscle and/or spinal accessory nerve damage on the affected side (e.g., inability to abduct arm, drooping or forward rotation of shoulder, continued pain in neck and shoulder). 2. If shoulder and neck dysfunction occur: a. instruct client to support affected arm in a sling when ambulating and rest it on a chair arm, table, or pillow when sitting b. assist client with self-care activities as needed c. reinforce the need to begin neck and shoulder exercises (e.g., wall climbing with fingers, shoulder swing, pulley exercises, range of motion of neck) as soon as allowed *in order to improve tone and strength of muscles on the affected side* (exercises are usually started 10 days to 6 weeks postoperatively depending on extensiveness of surgery and stage of healing process) d. assure client that partial neck and shoulder function may be regained if exercise program is adhered to.

8. Nursing Diagnosis: **DISTURBED SELF-CONCEPT***

related to:
a. changes in appearance (e.g., disfigurement of neck, presence of tracheostomy, drooling and loss of facial expression if facial nerve is affected, drooping of shoulder if spinal accessory nerve was removed or damaged during surgery, facial edema);
b. alteration in usual body functioning:
   1. loss of ability to speak normally, sing, produce crying and laughing sounds, and whistle
   2. diminished or absent sense of taste and smell and loss of ability to blow nose associated with neck breathing
   3. loss of normal shoulder and neck movement and strength (can occur if the spinal accessory nerve and sternocleidomastoid muscle were removed or damaged during surgery)
   4. impaired swallowing and tongue movement (can occur if the hypoglossal nerve is affected);
c. possible altered sexuality patterns associated with decreased libido, perceived loss of femininity/masculinity and physical attractiveness, and fear of rejection by partner;
d. temporary dependence on others to meet self-care needs;
e. possible lifestyle and role changes.

*This diagnostic label includes the nursing diagnoses of disturbed body image, low self-esteem, and ineffective role performance.

Suggested NOC Outcomes: Body image; Self-esteem; Personal autonomy; Psychosocial adjustment: life change

Suggested NIC Interventions: Body image enhancement; Self-esteem enhancement; Emotional support; Support system enhancement; Role enhancement; Counseling

Desired Outcome

8. The client will demonstrate beginning adaptation to changes in appearance, body functioning, lifestyle, and roles as evidenced by:
   a. communication of feelings of self-worth and sexual adequacy
   b. maintenance of relationships with significant others
   c. active participation in activities of daily living, tracheostomy care, and speech therapy
   d. communication of a beginning plan for adapting lifestyle to changes resulting from the laryngectomy and radical neck dissection.

Nursing Actions *and Selected Purposes/Rationales*

(see pp. 47–49 for additional rationales)

8.a. Assess for signs and symptoms of a disturbed self-concept (e.g., communication of negative feelings about self; withdrawal from significant others; lack of participation in activities of daily living, tracheostomy care, or speech therapy; refusal to look at or touch neck area; lack of plan for adapting to changes in lifestyle).
b. Implement measures to facilitate the grieving process (see Postoperative Diagnosis 9, action b).
c. Implement measures *to facilitate client's adjustment to the effects of changes in appearance and body functioning on his/her sexuality:*
   1. facilitate communication between client and partner; focus on feelings the couple share and assist them to identify factors which may affect their sexual relationship
   2. perform actions *to decrease the possibility of rejection by partner:*
      a. if appropriate, involve partner in care of client's wound and suctioning *to facilitate adjustment to the changes in client's appearance and functioning*
      b. instruct client to suction and clean stoma and cover it with a porous shield just before sexual activity.
d. Implement measures *to reduce drooling if it occurs:*
   1. instruct client to wipe mouth or suction oral cavity frequently (if circumoral paresthesias are present, client may be unaware of drooling)
   2. perform actions to improve client's ability to swallow (see Postoperative Diagnosis 3, action b).
e. Provide privacy for client when eating if indicated *to reduce embarrassment associated with swallowing difficulties.*

Desired Outcome	**Nursing Actions** *and Selected Purposes/Rationales*

f. Remain with client for the first look at the operative area after removal of dressings. Explain that some of the physical changes will not be as severe once edema and redness have subsided and the tracheostomy tube is out. (Facial edema that may occur with a radical neck dissection peaks by the fifth postoperative day and may take 2–6 months to resolve totally.)
g. If client is experiencing impaired movement and strength of neck and shoulder on the affected side, inform him/her that improvement usually occurs if the prescribed exercise regimen is followed and that wearing clothing with shoulder padding can help camouflage a drooping shoulder.
h. Suggest clothing styles and accessories that help camouflage the stoma (e.g., stoma bibs, neck scarves, ties, ascots, clothing with high collars) and accessories that help to draw attention away from the neck area (e.g., hats, belts).
i. Encourage client to pursue available options for regaining speech (e.g., voice prosthesis, esophageal speech, electrolarynx).
j. Encourage client's participation in activities that can assist him/her to integrate physical changes that have occurred (e.g., suctioning, tracheostomy care, tube feeding).
k. Demonstrate acceptance of client using techniques such as touch and frequent visits. Encourage significant others to do the same.
l. Support behaviors suggesting positive adaptation to changes that have occurred (e.g., willingness to participate in wound and tracheostomy care, tube feedings, and suctioning; compliance with treatment plan; communication of feelings of self-worth; maintenance of relationships with significant others).
m. Encourage significant others to allow client to do what he/she is able *so that independence can be re-established and/or self-esteem redeveloped.*
n. Encourage client contact with others *so that he/she can test and establish a new self-image.*
o. If client appears to be rejecting significant others, explain to them that this is a common occurrence (client rejects family and/or spouse before they have a chance to reject him/her). Encourage them to visit often and persist in offering understanding and support for the client.
p. Assist client and significant others to have similar expectations and understanding of future lifestyle and to identify ways that personal and family goals can be adjusted rather than abandoned.
q. Encourage client to pursue usual roles and interests and to continue involvement in social activities. If previous roles, interests, and hobbies cannot be pursued, encourage development of new ones.
r. Provide information about and encourage utilization of community resources and support groups (e.g., Lost Cord [Chord] Club; New Voice Club; American Cancer Society; vocational rehabilitation; sexual, family, individual, and/or financial counseling).
s. Consult appropriate health care provider (e.g., psychiatric nurse clinician, physician) about psychological counseling if client desires or seems unwilling or unable to adapt to changes resulting from the laryngectomy and radical neck dissection.

9. Nursing Diagnosis: *GRIEVING**

related to:
a. changes in appearance and body functioning (e.g., neck breathing; loss of ability to speak normally, sing, blow nose, and audibly laugh and cry; impaired sense of smell and taste; impaired shoulder movement);
b. possible changes in lifestyle and roles;
c. diagnosis of cancer with potential for premature death.

*This diagnostic label includes anticipatory grieving and grieving following the actual losses.

Suggested NOC Outcomes: Grief resolution; Psychosocial adjustment: life change

Suggested NIC Interventions: Grief work facilitation; Emotional support; Presence; Support system enhancement; Spiritual growth facilitation

Desired Outcome	Nursing Actions *and Selected Purposes/Rationales* (see pp. 35–37 for additional rationales)

Desired Outcome

9. The client will demonstrate beginning progression through the grieving process as evidenced by:
   a. communication of feelings about the effects of the laryngectomy and radical neck dissection on appearance, body functioning, lifestyle, and roles
   b. usual sleep pattern
   c. participation in treatment plan and self-care activities
   d. utilization of available support systems.

Nursing Actions *and Selected Purposes/Rationales*

9.a. Assess for signs and symptoms of grieving (e.g., expression of distress about having cancer and about changes in appearance and body functioning, change in eating habits, inability to concentrate, insomnia, anger, sadness, withdrawal from significant others, denial of loss).

b. Implement measures *to facilitate the grieving process:*
   1. assist client to acknowledge the losses *so grief work can begin*; assess for factors that may hinder and facilitate acknowledgment
   2. discuss the grieving process and assist client to accept the phases of grieving as an expected response to actual and/or anticipated losses
   3. allow time for client to progress through the phases of grieving (phases vary among theorists but progress from shock and alarm to acceptance); be aware that not every phase is expressed by all individuals, phases may overlap or recur, the amount of time needed to reach resolution of grief is very individual, and the grieving process may take months to years
   4. provide an atmosphere of care and concern (e.g., provide privacy, be available and nonjudgmental, display empathy and respect) *so client will feel free to express feelings*
   5. perform actions *to promote trust* (e.g., answer questions honestly, provide requested information)
   6. encourage the expression of anger and sadness about the losses experienced; recognize displacement of anger and assist client to see the actual cause of angry feelings and resentment
   7. encourage client to express feelings in whatever ways are comfortable (e.g., writing, drawing)
   8. assist client to identify and use techniques that have helped him/her cope in previous situations of loss
   9. support realistic hope regarding ability to resume usual activities and regain speech
   10. if acceptable to client, arrange for a visit with an individual who has successfully adjusted to the loss of the larynx
   11. support behaviors suggesting successful grief work (e.g., communicating feelings about the loss of speech and changes in body functioning, focusing on ways to adapt to losses, learning needed skills, developing or renewing relationships)
   12. explain the phases of the grieving process to significant others; encourage their support and understanding
   13. provide information regarding counseling services and support groups that might assist client in working through grief
   14. facilitate communication between the client and significant others; be aware that they may be in different phases of the grieving process
   15. when appropriate, assist client to meet spiritual needs (e.g., arrange for a visit from clergy)
   16. administer antidepressant agents if ordered
   17. assist client to identify and use available support systems; provide information about available community resources that can assist client and significant others in coping with effects of the surgery (e.g., New Voice Club, Lost Cord [Chord] Club, American Cancer Society, vocational rehabilitation, International Association of Laryngectomees).

c. Consult appropriate health care provider (e.g., psychiatric nurse clinician, physician) regarding referral for counseling if signs of dysfunctional grieving (e.g., persistent denial of losses, excessive anger or sadness, emotional lability) occur.

Discharge Teaching/Continued Care

10. Nursing Diagnosis: DEFICIENT KNOWLEDGE, INEFFECTIVE THERAPEUTIC REGIMEN MANAGEMENT, OR INEFFECTIVE HEALTH MAINTENANCE*

*The nurse should select the diagnostic label that is most appropriate for the client's discharge teaching needs.

Suggested NOC Outcomes: Knowledge: treatment regimen; Knowledge: personal safety; Knowledge: health resources; Knowledge: treatment procedure(s)

Suggested NIC Interventions: Health system guidance; Teaching: individual; Teaching: prescribed activity/exercise; Teaching: psychomotor skill

Desired Outcomes	**Nursing Actions** *and Selected Purposes/Rationales*
10.a. The client will demonstrate appropriate stomal care, suctioning, tracheostomy tube care, oral hygiene, and tube feeding techniques.	10.a.1. Reinforce instructions about the following if appropriate: a. inserting a new tracheostomy tube in an emergency situation b. cleaning stoma and changing tracheostomy tube ties and dressing c. maintaining skin integrity around stoma (e.g., keep skin clean and dry) d. removing and cleaning the inner cannula of the tracheostomy tube e. tracheal suctioning including instillation of 3–5 ml of normal saline before suctioning if necessary f. increasing moisture content of inspired air (e.g., use humidifier in the room where most time is spent during the day and in the bedroom at night; wear a dampened stoma cover during the day, being sure to moisten it when it dries) g. administering nasogastric or gastrostomy tube feedings h. performing oral care (e.g., irrigation with normal saline or a solution of hydrogen peroxide and water). 2. Allow time for questions, clarification, practice, and return demonstration. 3. Provide client with a list of supplies that he/she will be using and where to obtain them.
10.b. The client will demonstrate the ability to effectively use and care for an electrolarynx.	10.b.1. Reinforce instructions from speech pathologist about use and care of an electrolarynx if appropriate. 2. Allow time for questions, clarification, and return demonstration.
10.c. The client will demonstrate the ability to care for the tracheoesophageal puncture (TEP) and voice prosthesis if in place.	10.c.1. Provide the following instructions about care of the TEP and voice prosthesis if in place: a. clean and reinsert voice prosthesis as instructed by physician or speech pathologist (some models are removed daily and cleaned in a hydrogen peroxide solution while others are left in place and cleaned using an applicator) b. maintain the TEP by inserting a catheter into the site when the prosthesis is out for cleaning or for any other reason (the puncture site will close in 1–2 hours if the catheter or prosthesis is not in place); if unable to insert catheter or prosthesis, call physician or go to the closest medical emergency care facility immediately to have it done c. secure prosthesis strap to skin above stoma with nonallergenic tape d. take antifungal medication (e.g., Mycelex troche) as prescribed to prevent or control growth of *Candida albicans* on the prosthesis (a fungal infection can eventually interfere with function of the valve in the prosthesis)

e. instruct client to report leakage of food/fluids or saliva around the TEP
f. have prosthesis replaced as often as instructed by physician.
2. Emphasize the importance of indicating on medical alert bracelet or tag that a voice prosthesis is in place.
3. Allow time for questions, clarification, and return demonstration.

10.d. The client will identify appropriate safety precautions related to the surgery, tracheostomy, and nerve damage (if present).

10.d. Provide the following instructions regarding appropriate safety precautions related to the surgery, tracheostomy, and nerve damage (may have occurred as a result of the disease or surgery):
1. always keep a tracheostomy tube available for an emergency situation
2. always wear a medical alert bracelet or tag indicating neck breather status
3. reduce the risk of injury in surgical area (the area will remain numb for several months after surgery):
   a. use an electric rather than a straight-edge razor to decrease the risk of cuts in surgical area
   b. avoid extremely hot foods/fluids to decrease risk of burning the oral cavity or esophagus
4. be sure that smoke detectors are installed in the home and are functioning properly to help compensate for impaired sense of smell
5. prevent blockage of stoma and/or entrance of water or particles into stoma:
   a. do not wear constrictive clothing around neck
   b. wear a protective shield over stoma (e.g., crocheted bib, moistened 4 × 4 gauze pad, scarf, ascot) at all times
   c. prevent water from entering stoma (e.g., do not swim unless wearing special snorkel device designed for neck breathers, use a hand-held shower nozzle and direct the spray well below stoma, use stoma guard or shield while bathing)
   d. apply shaving cream by hand rather than spraying directly on face and neck
   e. cover stoma while shaving, trimming facial hair, or getting a hair cut
   f. avoid close contact with animals that shed
6. if shoulder and neck movement are impaired, use caution when driving
7. ensure that significant others are trained in mouth-to-stoma rescue breathing.

10.e. The client will identify signs and symptoms to report to the health care provider.

10.e.1. Refer to Standardized Postoperative Care Plan, Diagnosis 22, action c (p. 125), for signs and symptoms to report to the health care provider.
2. Instruct client to report these additional signs and symptoms:
   a. development of lump(s) in neck and/or persistent choking, difficulty swallowing, feeling of a lump in throat, sore throat, or earache (could indicate recurrence of tumor)
   b. drainage of milky appearing fluid, ingested foods/fluids, or saliva from incision or a nearby opening that develops in the skin (could indicate development of a fistula)
   c. presence of blood or ingested foods/fluids in secretions from stoma
   d. darkening of skin flaps or separation of wound edges
   e. increased weakness of arm on affected side
   f. persistent pain in shoulder or neck on affected side
   g. nausea, vomiting, diarrhea, and/or cramping associated with tube feeding.

10.f. The client will identify community resources that can assist with home management and adjustment to the effects of surgery.

10.f.1. Provide information about community resources that can assist the client and significant others with home management and adjustment to the surgery (e.g., American Cancer Society, home health agencies, counselors, social service agencies, New Voice Club, Lost Cord [Chord] Club, vocational rehabilitation, International Association of Laryngectomees, church groups, American Speech and Hearing Association).
2. Initiate a referral if indicated.

Desired Outcomes	**Nursing Actions** *and Selected Purposes/Rationales*
10.g. The client will communicate an understanding of and a plan for adhering to recommended follow-up care including future appointments with health care provider and speech pathologist, medications prescribed, exercises, activity level, and wound care.	10.g.1. Refer to Standardized Postoperative Care Plan, Diagnosis 22 (pp. 125–126), for routine postoperative instructions and measures to improve client compliance. 2. Caution client to avoid lifting more than 2 pounds with the affected arm until healing occurs and strength improves. 3. Emphasize the importance of adhering to prescribed exercise program to strengthen shoulder and neck muscles on the affected side. 4. Encourage client to follow up with speech rehabilitation if appropriate.

ADDITIONAL NURSING DIAGNOSIS:

INEFFECTIVE COPING*

related to:

a. loss of ability to speak normally and audibly laugh and cry;
b. difficulty mastering new speech techniques;
c. fear of rejection by significant others;
d. fear, anxiety, and/or loss of control associated with changes in appearance and body functioning, the diagnosis of cancer, and possibility of disease recurrence;
e. self-care expectations regarding tube feeding, wound care, tracheostomy care, and speech rehabilitation;
f. guilt associated with the diagnosis of cancer of the larynx if tobacco use was the major cause.

*See Unit II for outcomes, actions, and rationales.

Bibliography

See pages 879 and 885.

Appendix

North American Nursing Diagnosis Association* (NANDA)-Approved Nursing Diagnoses

- Activity Intolerance**
- Activity Intolerance, Risk for
- Adjustment, Impaired
- Airway Clearance, Ineffective**
- Anxiety**
- Anxiety, Death
- Aspiration, Risk for**
- Body Image, Disturbed
- Body Temperature, Imbalanced, Risk for
- Bowel Incontinence
- Breastfeeding, Effective
- Breastfeeding, Ineffective
- Breastfeeding, Interrupted
- Breathing Pattern, Ineffective**
- Cardiac Output, Decreased**
- Caregiver Role Strain
- Caregiver Role Strain, Risk for
- Communication, Readiness for Enhanced
- Communication, Verbal, Impaired
- Conflict, Decisional
- Conflict, Parental Role
- Confusion, Acute
- Confusion, Chronic
- Constipation**
- Constipation, Perceived
- Constipation, Risk for
- Coping, Community, Ineffective
- Coping, Community, Readiness for Enhanced
- Coping, Defensive
- Coping, Family, Compromised
- Coping, Family, Disabled
- Coping, Family, Readiness for Enhanced
- Coping, Ineffective**
- Decisional Conflict
- Denial, Ineffective
- Dentition, Impaired
- Development, Risk for Delayed
- Diarrhea**
- Disuse Syndrome, Risk for
- Diversional Activity, Deficient
- Dysreflexia, Autonomic
- Dysreflexia, Autonomic, Risk for
- Energy Field, Disturbed
- Environmental Interpretation Syndrome, Impaired
- Failure to Thrive, Adult
- Falls, Risk for
- Family Processes: Alcoholism, Dysfunctional
- Family Processes, Interrupted
- Family Processes, Readiness for Enhanced
- Fatigue
- Fear
- Feeding Pattern, Ineffective Infant
- Fluid Balance, Readiness for Enhanced
- Fluid Volume, Deficient**
- Fluid Volume, Deficient, Risk for
- Fluid Volume, Excess**
- Fluid Volume, Imbalanced, Risk for
- Gas Exchange, Impaired**
- Grieving, Anticipatory**
- Grieving, Dysfunctional**
- Growth, Disproportionate, Risk for
- Growth and Development, Delayed
- Health Maintenance, Ineffective
- Health-Seeking Behaviors
- Home Maintenance, Impaired
- Hopelessness
- Hyperthermia
- Hypothermia
- Incontinence, Bowel
- Incontinence, Functional Urinary
- Incontinence, Reflex Urinary
- Incontinence, Stress Urinary
- Incontinence, Total Urinary
- Incontinence, Urge Urinary
- Incontinence, Urge Urinary, Risk for
- Infant Behavior, Disorganized
- Infant Behavior, Disorganized, Risk for
- Infant Behavior, Organized, Readiness for Enhanced
- Infant Death Syndrome, Sudden, Risk for
- Infant Feeding Pattern, Ineffective

*Adapted from NANDA Nursing Diagnoses: Definitions and Classification 2003-2004. Philadelphia: NANDA International, 2003.

**Refer to Unit II for definitions, related factors, risk factors, and defining characteristics for these nursing diagnoses.

- Infection, Risk for**
- Injury, Perioperative-Positioning, Risk for
- Injury, Risk for
- Intracranial Adaptive Capacity, Decreased
- Knowledge, Deficient
- Knowledge, Readiness for Enhanced
- Latex Allergy Response
- Latex Allergy Response, Risk for
- Loneliness, Risk for
- Memory, Impaired
- Mobility, Impaired Bed
- Mobility, Impaired Physical
- Mobility, Impaired Wheel Chair
- Nausea
- Neglect, Unilateral
- Neurovascular Dysfunction, Peripheral, Risk for
- Noncompliance
- Nutrition, Imbalanced: Less Than Body Requirements**
- Nutrition, Imbalanced: More Than Body Requirements
- Nutrition, Imbalanced: Less Than Body Requirements, Risk for
- Nutrition: Readiness for Enhanced
- Oral Mucous Membrane, Impaired**
- Pain, Acute**
- Pain, Chronic
- Parent/Infant/Child Attachment, Impaired, Risk for
- Parenting, Impaired
- Parenting, Readiness for Enhanced
- Parenting, Risk for
- Personal Identity, Disturbed
- Poisoning, Risk for
- Post-Trauma Syndrome
- Post-Trauma Syndrome, Risk for
- Powerlessness
- Powerlessness, Risk for
- Protection, Ineffective
- Rape-Trauma Syndrome
- Rape-Trauma Syndrome: Compound Reaction
- Rape-Trauma Syndrome: Silent Reaction
- Relocation Stress Syndrome
- Relocation Stress Syndrome, Risk for
- Role Performance, Ineffective
- Self-Care Deficit: Bathing/Hygiene
- Self-Care Deficit: Dressing/Grooming
- Self-Care Deficit: Feeding
- Self-Care Deficit: Toileting
- Self-Concept, Readiness for Enhanced
- Self-Esteem, Chronic Low
- Self-Esteem, Situational Low
- Self-Esteem, Situational Low, Risk for
- Self-Mutilation
- Self-Mutilation, Risk for
- Sensory Perception, Disturbed
- Sexual Dysfunction
- Sexuality Pattern, Ineffective
- Skin Integrity, Impaired
- Skin Integrity, Impaired, Risk for**
- Sleep, Readiness for Enhanced
- Sleep Deprivation
- Sleep Pattern, Disturbed**
- Social Interaction, Impaired
- Social Isolation
- Sorrow, Chronic
- Spiritual Distress
- Spiritual Distress, Risk for
- Spiritual Well-Being, Readiness for Enhanced
- Suffocation, Risk for
- Suicide, Risk for
- Surgical Recovery, Delayed
- Swallowing, Impaired**
- Thermoregulation, Ineffective
- Thought Process, Disturbed
- Tissue Integrity, Impaired
- Tissue Perfusion, Ineffective**
- Therapeutic Regimen Management, Effective
- Therapeutic Regimen Management, Ineffective
- Therapeutic Regimen Management, Ineffective Community
- Therapeutic Regimen Management, Ineffective Family
- Therapeutic Regimen Management, Readiness for Enhanced
- Transfer Ability, Impaired
- Trauma, Risk for
- Urinary Elimination, Impaired**
- Urinary Elimination, Readiness for Enhanced
- Urinary Retention**
- Ventilation, Impaired Spontaneous
- Ventilatory Weaning Response, Dysfunctional
- Violence, Other-Directed, Risk for
- Violence, Self-Directed, Risk for
- Walking, Impaired
- Wandering

*Adapted from NANDA Nursing Diagnoses: Definitions and Classification 2003-2004. Philadelphia: NANDA International, 2003.
**Refer to Unit II for definitions, related factors, risk factors, and defining characteristics for these nursing diagnoses.

BIBLIOGRAPHY

General Bibliography

Abrams AC. Clinical drug therapy: rationales for nursing practice (7th ed.). Philadelphia: Lippincott Williams & Wilkins, 2004.

Barkauskas VH, Baumann LC, Darling-Fisher C. Health and physical assessment (3rd ed.). St. Louis: Mosby, 2002.

Bendich A, Deckelbaum RJ (Eds.). Preventive nutrition (2nd ed.). Totowa, NJ: Humana Press, 2001.

Bickley LS, Szilagi PG. Bates' guide to physical examination (8th ed.). Philadelphia: Lippincott Williams & Wilkins, 2003.

Black JM, Hawks JH, Keene AM. Medical–surgical nursing: clinical management for positive outcomes (6th ed.). Philadelphia: W.B. Saunders, 2001.

Braunwald E, Fauci AS, Kasper DL, et al (Eds.). Harrison's principles of internal medicine (15th ed.). New York: McGraw-Hill, 2001.

Carpenito-Moyet LJ. Nursing care plans and documentation (9th ed.). Philadelphia: Lippincott Williams & Wilkins, 2004.

Cavanaugh BM. Nurse's manual of laboratory and diagnostic tests (4th ed.). Philadelphia: F.A. Davis, 2003.

Craven RF, Hirnle CJ. Fundamentals of nursing: human health and function (4th ed.). Philadelphia: Lippincott Williams & Wilkins, 2003.

DeLaune SC, Ladner PK. Fundamentals of nursing: standards and practice (2nd ed.). Clifton Park, NY: Delmar, 2002.

Dillon PM. Nursing health assessment. Philadelphia: F.A. Davis, 2003.

Docterman JM, Bulecheck GM. Nursing Interventions Classification (NIC) (4th ed.). St. Louis: Mosby, 2004.

Doenges ME, Moorhouse MF, Geisler-Murr AC. Nursing care plans: guidelines for individualizing patient care (6th ed.). Philadelphia: F.A. Davis, 2002.

Dudek SG. Nutrition essentials for nursing practice (4th ed.). Philadelphia: Lippincott Williams & Wilkins, 2001.

Estes MEZ. Health assessment and physical examination (2nd ed.). Clifton Park, NY: Delmar, 2002.

Fischbach F. A manual of laboratory and diagnostic tests (7th ed.). Philadelphia: Lippincott Williams & Wilkins, 2004.

Goldman L, Bennett JC (Eds.). Cecil textbook of medicine (21st ed.). Philadelphia: W.B. Saunders, 2000.

Gulanick M, Klopp A, Galanes S, et al. Nursing care plans: nursing diagnosis and intervention (5th ed.). St. Louis: Mosby, 2003.

Guyton AC, Hall JE. Textbook of medical physiology (10th ed.). Philadelphia: W.B. Saunders, 2000.

Hardman JG, Limbird LE (Eds.). Goodman and Gilman's pharmacological basis of therapeutics (10th ed.). New York: McGraw-Hill, 2001.

Holloway NM. Medical–surgical care planning (4th ed.). Philadelphia: Lippincott Williams & Wilkins, 2004.

Ignatavicius DD, Workman ML. Medical–surgical nursing: critical thinking for collaborative care (4th ed.). Philadelphia: W.B. Saunders, 2002.

Jarvis C. Physical examination and health assessment (3rd ed.). Philadelphia: W.B. Saunders, 2000.

Kozier B, Erb G, Berman AJ, Snyder S. Fundamentals of nursing: concepts, process, and process (7th ed.). Upper Saddle River, NJ: Prentice Hall, 2004.

Lewis SM, Heitkemper MM, Dirksen SR. Medical–surgical nursing: assessment and management of clinical problems (6th ed.). St. Louis: Mosby, 2004.

McEvoy GK (Ed.). AHFS drug information. Bethesda, MD: American Society of Health System Pharmacists, 2003.

McKenry LM, Salerno E. Mosby's pharmacology in nursing (Revised 21st ed.). St. Louis: Mosby, 2003.

Metheny NM. Fluid and electrolyte balance: nursing considerations (4th ed.). Philadelphia: Lippincott Williams & Wilkins, 2000.

Moorhead S, Johnson M, Maas M. Nursing Outcomes Classification (NOC) (3rd ed.). St. Louis: Mosby, 2004.

NANDA. Nursing diagnoses: definitions and classification: 2003–2004. Philadelphia: North American Nursing Diagnosis Association, 2003.

Pagana KD, Pagana TJ. Mosby's manual of diagnostic and laboratory tests (2nd ed.). St. Louis: Mosby, 2002.

Phipps WJ, Monahan FD, Sands JK, et al. Medical–surgical nursing: health and illness perspectives (7th ed.). St. Louis: Mosby, 2003.

Porth CM. Pathophysiology: concepts of altered health states (6th ed.). Philadelphia: Lippincott Williams & Wilkins, 2002.

Potter PA, Perry PG. Basic nursing: essentials for practice (5th ed.). St. Louis: Mosby, 2003.

Rakel RE, Bope ET (Eds.). Conn's current therapy (55th ed.). Philadelphia: W.B. Saunders, 2003.

Roth RA, Townsend CE. Nutrition and diet therapy (8th ed.). Clifton Park, NY: Delmar, 2003.

Seidel HM, Ball JW, Dains JE, Benedict GW. Mosby's guide to physical examination (5th ed.). St. Louis: Mosby, 2003.

Smeltzer SC, Bare BG. Brunner and Suddarth's textbook of medical–surgical nursing (10th ed.). Philadelphia: Lippincott Williams & Wilkins, 2004.

Tierney LM, McPhee SJ, Papadakis MA (Eds.). Current medical diagnosis and treatment (42nd ed.). New York: Lange/McGraw-Hill, 2003.

Townsend CM Jr (Ed.). Sabiston textbook of surgery (16th ed.). Philadelphia: W.B. Saunders, 2001.

Warrell DA, Cox TM, Firth JD, Benz EJ (Eds.). Oxford textbook of medicine (4th ed.). Oxford: Oxford University Press, 2003.

Wilson BA, Shannon MT, Stang CL. Nurses drug guide 2004. Upper Saddle River, NJ: Prentice Hall, 2004.

Unit III. Nursing Care of the Elderly Client

Abrams WB, Beers MH, Berkow R. Merck manual of geriatrics (3rd ed.). Whitehouse Station, NJ: Merck & Company, 2000.

American Nurses Association. Scope and standards of gerontological nursing practice (2nd ed.). Washington, DC: American Nurses Publishing, 2001.

Burke MM, Laramie JA. Primary care of the older adult: a multidisciplinary approach. St. Louis: Mosby, 2000.

Cassell CK (Ed.). Geriatric medicine: an evidence-based approach (4th ed.). New York: Springer Publishing, 2002.

DeLaine C, Scammell J, Heaslip V. Continuing professional development: older people. Primary Health Care, 13(1):43–50, 2003.

Ebersole P, Hess P. Geriatric nursing and healthy aging. St. Louis: Mosby, 2001.

Eliopoulos C. Gerontological nursing (5th ed.). Philadelphia: Lippincott Williams & Wilkins, 2001.

Fantl JA, Newman DK, Colling J, et al. Managing acute and chronic urinary incontinence: clinical practice guideline. AHCPR Pub. No. 96-0686. Rockville, MD: Agency for Health Care Policy and Research, Public Health Service, U.S. Department of Health and Human Services, 1996 update.

Hogstell MO. Gerontology: nursing care of the older adult. Clifton Park, NY: Delmar, 2001.

Luekenotte A. Gerontologic nursing (2nd ed.). St. Louis: Mosby, 2000.

Maas ML, Buckwalter KC, Hardy MD, et al. Nursing care of older adults: diagnoses, outcomes, and interventions. St. Louis: Mosby, 2001.

Mayer BH (Ed.). Better elder care: a nurse's guide to caring for older adults. Springhouse, PA: Springhouse, 2002.

McCurren C, Cronin SN. Delirium: elders tell their stories and guide nursing practice. MEDSURG Nursing, 12(5):318–323, 2003.

Mezey MD (Ed.). The encyclopedia of elder care. New York: Springer Publishing, 2001.

Nagel CL, Markie MB, Richards KC, Taylor JL. Sleep promotion in hospitalized elders. MEDSURG Nursing, 12(5):279–288, 2003.

Osterweil D, Brummel-Smith K, Beck JC. Comprehensive geriatric assessment. New York: McGraw-Hill, 2000.

Peate I. Medicines and the older person: principles of good practice. British Journal of Nursing, 12(9):530–535, 2003.

Tallis RC, Fillit HM (Eds.). Brocklehurst's textbook of geriatric medicine and gerontology (6th ed.). New York: Churchill Livingstone, 2003.

Watson RR (Ed.). Handbook of nutrition in the aged (3rd ed.). Boca Raton, FL: CRC Press, 2001.

Unit IV. Nursing Care of the Client Having Surgery

Arbique JC. Stopping UTIs in their tracts. Nursing2003, 33(6): 32hn1–32hn4, 2003.

Byrne B. Deep vein thrombosis prophylaxis: the effectiveness and implications of using below-knee or thigh-length graduated compression stockings. Journal of Vascular Nursing, 20(2):53–59, 2002.

Capriotte T. Preventing nosocomial spread of MRSA is in your hands. MEDSURG Nursing, 12(3):193–196, 2003.

Church V. Staying on guard for DVT and PE. Nursing2000, 30(2):35–42, 2000.

Day MW. Recognizing and managing DVT. Nursing2003, 33(5):37–41, 2003.

Dudek SG. Malnutrition in hospitals. American Journal of Nursing, 100(4):36–42, 2000.

Epley O. Pulmonary emboli risk reductions. Journal of Vascular Nursing, 18(2):61–70, 2000.

Hashmi S, Kelly E, Rogers SO, Gates J. Urinary tract infection in surgical patients. American Journal of Surgery, 186(1):53–56, 2003.

Kleinpell RM. Shock states. Nurseweek, 4(14):20–22, 2003.

Nagel CL, Markie MB, Richards KC, Taylor JL. Sleep promotion in hospitalized elders. MEDSURG Nursing, 12(5):279–288, 2003.

Parini S, Myers F. Keeping up with hand hygiene recommendations. Nursing2003, 33(2):17, 2003.

Stratton MA, Anderson FA, Bussey HI, et al. Prevention of venous thromboembolism. Archives of Internal Medicine, 160(3):334–340, 2000.

Walton J. Helping high-risk surgical patients beat the odds. Nursing2001, 31(3):54–59, 2001.

Unit V. Nursing Care of the Immobile Client

Byrne B. Deep vein thrombosis prophylaxis: the effectiveness and implications of using below-knee or thigh-length graduated compression stockings. Journal of Vascular Nursing, 20(2):53–59, 2002.

Church V. Staying on guard for DVT and PE. Nursing2000, 30(2):34–42, 2000.

Day MW. Recognizing and managing DVT. Nursing2003, 33(5):37–41, 2003.

Epley O. Pulmonary emboli risk reductions. Journal of Vascular Nursing, 18(2):61–70, 2000.

Smith. A comprehensive review of risk factors related to the development of pressure ulcers. Journal of Orthopaedic Nursing, 7(2):94–102, 2003.

Unit VI. Nursing Care of the Client Who Is Dying

Ameling A, Povilonis M. Spirituality, meaning, mental health, and nursing. Journal of Psychosocial Nursing and Mental Health Services, 39(4):14–20, 2002.

Block SD. Assessing and managing depression in the terminally ill patient. Annals of Internal Medicine, 132(3):209–218, 2000.

Brenner ZR, Drenzer ME. Using complementary and alternative therapies to promote comfort at end of life. Critical Care Nursing Clinics of North America, 15(3):355–362, 2003.

Easley MK, Elliott S. Managing pain at the end of life. Nursing Clinics of North America, 36(4):779–794, 200l.

Egan KA, Arnold RL. Grief and bereavement care. American Journal of Nursing, 103(9):42–52, 2003.

Ellershaw J, Ward C. Care of the dying patient: the last hours or days of life. British Medical Journal, 326(7379):30–34, 2003.

Fetters MD, Churchill L, Danis M. Conflict resolution at the end of life. Critical Care Medicine, 29(5):921–925, 2001.

Herman CP. Spiritual needs of dying patients: a qualitative study. Oncology Nursing Forum, 21(91):67, 2001.

Kemp C. Terminal illness: a guide to nursing care (2nd ed.). Philadelphia: Lippincott Williams & Wilkins, 1999.

LaDuke S. Terminal dyspnea and palliative care. American Journal of Nursing, 101(11):26–31, 2001.

Matzo ML, Sherman DW (Eds.). Palliative care nursing: quality care to the end of life. New York: Springer Publishing, 2001.

Palliative care: one vision, one voice. Available at www.palliativecarenursing.net.

Pimple C, Schmidt L, Tidwell S. Achieving excellence in end-of-life care. Nurse Educator, 28(1):40–43, 2003.

Pitorak EF. Care at the time of death. American Journal of Nursing, 103(7):42–52, 2003.

Plaisance L, Ellis JA. Opioid-induced constipation. American Journal of Nursing, 102(3):72–73, 2002.

Poor B, Poirrier GP. End of life nursing care. Sudbury, MA: Jones and Bartlett, 2001.

Radcliffe M. Dealing with death. Nursing Times, 97(21):26, 2001.

Stewart M. Reflecting on the psychological care of patients with a terminal illness. Professional Nurse, 18(7):402–405, 2003.

Werth JL Jr, Gordon JR, Johnson RR Jr. Psychosocial issues near the end of life. Aging and Mental Health, 6(4):402–412, 2002.

Zerwekh J. End-of-life hydration: benefit or burden? Nursing2003, 33(2):32hn1–32hn3, 2003.

Unit VII. Nursing Care of the Client Receiving Treatment for Neoplastic Disorders

Abeloff MD, Armitage JD, Lichter A, Nierderhuber JE (Eds.). Clinical oncology (2nd ed.). New York: Churchill Livingstone, 2000.

American Cancer Society. Available at www.cancer.org.

American Pain Society. Principles of analgesic use in the treatment of acute pain and chronic cancer pain: a concise guide to medical practice (4th ed.). Skokie, IL: American Pain Society, 1999.

Borjeson S, Hursti TJ, Tishelman C, et al. Treatment of nausea and emesis during cancer chemo: discrepancies between antiemetic effect and well-being. Journal of Pain and Symptom Management, 24(3):345–358, 2002.

Brown JK. A systematic review of the evidence on symptom management of cancer-related anorexia and cachexia. Oncology Nursing Forum, 29(3):517–532, 2002.

Buchsel PC, Murph BS, Newton SA. Epoetin alpha: current and future indications and nursing implications. Clinical Journal of Oncology Nursing, 6(5):261–267, 2002.

Cady J. Understanding opioid tolerance in cancer pain. Oncology Nursing Forum, 28(10):1561–1568, 2001.

Cancer Information Network. Available at www.cancernetwork.com.

Chernecky C. Pulmonary complications in patients with cancer. American Journal of Nursing, 101(5):24A, 24E, 24G–H, 2001.

Chu E, DeVita VT Jr. Physicians' cancer chemotherapy drug manual 2003. Sudbury, MA: Jones and Bartlett, 2003.

Cunningham RS (Ed.). Nutrition and cancer. Seminars in Oncology Nursing, 16(2):1–173, 2000.

DeVita VT Jr, Hellman S, Rosenberg SA (Eds.). Cancer principles and practice of oncology (6th ed.). Philadelphia: Lippincott Williams & Wilkins, 2001.

Ghen MJ, Cole F. Nutritional effects of cancer chemotherapy. Natural Pharmacology, 6(3):1, 6–7, 21, 2002.

Haskell CM. Cancer treatment (5th ed.). Philadelphia: W.B. Saunders, 2001.

Holland J. New treatment modalities in radiation therapy. Journal of Intravenous Nursing, 24(2):95–101, 2001.

Janjan N. Radiation therapy: beating side effects. Bottom Line/Health, 17(4):11–12, 2003.

Kufe DW, Pollock RE, Weichselbaum RR, et al (Eds.). Holland and Freis cancer medicine. Hamilton, Ontario: B.C. Decker, 2003.

Kurtz ME, Kurtz JC, Stommel M, et al. Physical functioning and depression among older persons with cancer. Cancer Practice, 9(1):11–18, 2001.

Letizia M. Addressing alopecia: helping patients with cancer deal with hair loss. American Journal of Nursing, 101(40):24, 2001.

Lyne ME, Coyne PJ, Watson AC. Pain management issues for cancer survivors. Cancer Practice, 10(1):S27–S32, 2002.

McCarthy D, Weihofen D. The effect of nutritional supplements on food intake in patients undergoing radiotherapy. Oncology Nursing Forum, 26(5):897–900, 1999.

Mendelson FA, Divino CM, Reis ED, Kerstein MD. Wound care after radiation therapy. Advances in Skin and Wound Care, 15(5):216, 218–224, 2002.

Nail LM. Fatigue in patients with cancer. Oncology Nursing Forum, 29(3):537–546, 2002.

National Cancer Institute. Available at www.nci.nih.gov.

Otto SE. Oncology nursing (4th ed.). St. Louis: Mosby, 2001.

Pierce DN. Use of amifostine (ETHYOL) as a radioprotector. Images, 22(1):7, 28, 2003.

Ratain JM, Tempero M, Skosey C. Outline of oncology therapeutics. Philadelphia: W.B. Saunders, 2001.

Ream E, Richardson A, Alexander-Dann C. Facilitating patients' coping with fatigue during chemotherapy. Cancer Nursing, 25(4):300–308, 2002.

Rogers BB. Mucositis in the oncology patient. Nursing Clinics of North America, 36(4):745–760, 2001.

Sadler GR, Stoudt A, Fullerton JT, et al. Managing the oral sequelae of cancer therapy. MEDSURG Nursing, 12(1):28–36, 2003.

Schnell FM. Chemotherapy-induced nausea and vomiting: the importance of acute antiemetic control. Oncologist, 8(2):187–198, 2003.

Shih A, Misakowski C, Dodd ML, et al. A research review of current treatment for radiation-induced oral mucositis in patients with head and neck cancer. Oncology Nursing Forum, 29(7):1063–1080, 2002.

Swinburne C. Looking good. Nursing Standard, 17(39):16–17, 2003.

Wagler RM, Baum BJ. Prophylactic treatment reduces the severity of xerostomia following radiation for oral cavity cancer. Archives of Otolaryngology: Head and Neck Surgery, 129(2):247–250, 2003.

Watson AC, Coyne PJ. Recognizing the faces of cancer pain. Nursing2003, 33(4):32hn1–32hn8, 2003.

Wickham R, Rehwaldt M, Defer C, et al. Taste changes experienced by patients receiving chemotherapy. Oncology Nursing Forum, 26(4): 697–706, 1999.

Wilkes GM, Ingwersen K, Barton-Burke M. Oncology nursing drug handbook. Sudbury, MA: Jones and Bartlett, 2003.

Wilson RL. Optimizing nutrition for patients with cancer. Clinical Journal of Oncology Nursing, 4(1):23–28, 2000.

Winningham ML, Barton-Burke M (Eds.). Fatigue in cancer: a multidisciplinary approach. Sudbury, MA: Jones and Bartlett, 2000.

Wojtaszek C. Management of chemotherapy-induced stomatitis. Clinical Journal of Oncology Nursing, 4(1):263–270, 2000.

Yarbro CH, Frogge MH, Goodman M, Groenwald S (Eds.). Cancer nursing: principles and practice (5th ed.). Sudbury, MA: Jones and Bartlett, 2000.

Unit VIII. Nursing Care of the Client with Disturbances of Neurological Function

Ackerman P, Kedersha K, Vliet N. Every step of the way: care management of the patient with spinal cord injury. Care Management, 8(3):23–28, 2002.

Adams RD, Victor M. Principles of neurology (7th ed.). New York: McGraw-Hill, 2001.

Baker SK. Stroke: providing the best care: from the ED to rehab. NurseWeek, 7(25):30–32, 2002.

Barker E, Saulino MF. First-ever guidelines for spinal cord injuries. RN, 65(10):32–37, 2002.

Batjer HH, Loftus CM (Eds.). Textbook of neurological surgery. Philadelphia: Lippincott Williams & Wilkins, 2002.

Brown DL, Haley EC. Post-emergency department management of stroke. Emergency Medicine Clinics of North America, 20(3):687–702, 2002.

Bryan J. Milestones in stroke management. Nursing Management, 9(7):15–18, 2002.

Bryant G. When spinal cord injury affects the bowel. RN, 63(2):26–29, 2000.

Church V. Staying on guard for DVT and PE. Nursing2000, 30(2):35–42, 2000.

Elliot S. Ejaculation and orgasm: sexuality in men with SCI. Topics in Spinal Cord Injury Rehabilitation, 8(1):1–15, 2002.

Fellows LS, Miller EH, Frederickson M, et al. Evidence-based practice for enteral feedings: aspiration prevention strategies, bedside detection, and practice change. MEDSURG Nursing, 9(1):27–31, 2000.

Fisher M (Ed.). Stroke therapy (2nd ed.). Boston: Butterworth-Heinemann, 2001.

Frymoyer JW, Wiesel SW (Eds.). The adult and pediatric spine (3rd ed.). Philadelphia: Lippincott Williams & Wilkins, 2003.

Galvan TJ. Dysphagia: going down and staying down. American Journal of Nursing, 101(1):37–42, 2001.

Gibson KL. Caring for a patient who lives with spinal cord injury. Nursing2003, 33(7):36–42, 2003.

Gilroy J. Basic neurology (3rd ed.). New York: McGraw-Hill, 2000.

Hanks RA, Temkin N, Machamer MA, Dikman SS. Emotional and behavioral adjustment after brain injury. Archives of Physical Medicine and Rehabilitation, 80(9):991–997, 1999.

Heinan M. Subtle changes in spinal cord injuries. Clinical Advisor, 6(4):62, 2003.

Hickey JV. The clinical practice of neurological and neurosurgical nursing (5th ed.). Philadelphia: Lippincott Williams & Wilkins, 2003.

Kim J. How do I respond to autonomic dysreflexia? Nursing2003, 33(2):18, 2003.

Klein DG. Management strategies for improving outcome following severe head injury. Critical Care Nursing Clinics of North America, 11(2):209–225, 1999.

Llinas RH, Aldrich E, Wityle R. Update on stroke prevention and treatment. Advanced Studies in Medicine, 3(2):93–101, 2003.

Lower J. Facing neuro assessment fearlessly. Nursing2002, 32(2):58–64, 2002.

Mason DJ. It's all in my head: nurses should know the possible long-term consequences of head injury. American Journal of Nursing, 103(7):61, 2003.

Meng NH, Wang TG, Lien IN. Dysphagia in patients with brainstem stroke. American Journal of Physical Medicine and Rehabilitation, 79(2):170–175. 2000.

Moore LW, Maiocco G, Schmidt SM, et al. Perspectives of caregivers of stroke survivors: implications for nursing. MEDSURG Nursing, 11(6):289–295, 2002.

Newman J. Diagnosis and treatment of stroke. Radiologic Technology, 73(4):305–338, 2002.

O'Connell B, Baker L, Prosser A. The educational needs of caregivers of stroke survivors in acute and community settings. Journal of Neuroscience Nursing, 35(1):21–28, 2003.

Paice JA. Controlling pain: understanding nociceptive pain. Nursing2002, 32(3):74–75, 2002.

Paolucci S, Antonucci G, Pratesi L, et al. Post stroke depression and its role in rehabilitation of inpatients. American Journal of Physical Medicine and Rehabilitation, 80(9):985–990, 1999.

Reichert MCF, Medeiros EAS, Ferraz FAP. Hospital-acquired meningitis in patients undergoing craniotomy: incidence, evolution, and risk factors. American Journal of Infection Control, 30(3):158–163, 2002.

Sadowsky C, Volshteyn O, Schultz L, McDonald JW. Spinal cord injury. Disability and Rehabilitation, 24(13):680–687, 2002.

Siddell PJ, Loeser JD. Pain following spinal cord injury. Spinal Cord, 39(2):63–73, 2001.

Sipski ML, Alexander CJ. Documentation of the impact of spinal cord injury on female sexual function. Topics in Spinal Cord Injury Rehabilitation, 8(1):63–73, 2002.

Somers MF. Spinal cord injury: functional rehabilitation (2nd ed.). Upper Saddle River, NJ: Prentice Hall, 2001.

Stewart-Amidei C, Kunkel J (Ed.). Human responses and neurologic dysfunction. Chicago: American Association of Neuroscience Nurses, 2001.

Sundin K, Jansson L. Understanding and being understood as a creative caring phenomenon: care of patients with stroke and aphasia. Journal of Clinical Nursing, 12(1):107–116, 2003.

Terpstra TL, Terpstra TL. Syndrome of inappropriate antidiuretic hormone secretion: recognition and management. MEDSURG Nursing, 9(2):61–68, 2000.

Terrado M, Russell C, Bowman JB. Dysphagia: an overview. MEDSURG Nursing, 10(5):233–248, 2001.

Turner-Stokes L. Poststroke depression: getting the full picture. Lancet, 361(9371):1757–1758, 2003.

Umphred DA. Neurological rehabilitation (4th ed.). St. Louis: Mosby, 2001.

Victor M, Ropper A. Adams and Victor's manual of neurology. New York: McGraw-Hill, 2002.

Winkler T. Medical issues that impact life care planing for spinal cord injury. Topics in Spinal Cord Injury Rehabilitation, 7(4):21–27, 2002.

Zubkov AY, Lewis AI, Raila FA, et al. Risk factors for the development of post-traumatic cerebral vasospasm. Surgical Neurology, 53(2):126–130, 2000.

Unit IX. Nursing Care of the Client with Disturbances of Cardiovascular Function

Ammon S. Managing patients with heart failure. American Journal of Nursing, 101(12):34–40, 2001.

Bither CJ, Apple S. Home management of the failing heart. American Journal of Nursing, 101(12):41–47, 2001.

Branch WT, Schlant RC, Alexander RW, Hurst JW (Eds.). Cardiology in primary care. New York: McGraw-Hill, 2000.

Braunwald E, Zipes DP, Libby P. Heart disease: a textbook of cardiovascular medicine (6th ed.). Philadelphia: W.B. Saunders, 2001.

Cannon DS. Implantable cardioverter defibrillator trials: what's new? Current Opinion in Cardiology, 17(1):29–35, 2002.

Caplan L. Protecting the brains of patients after heart surgery. Archives of Neurology, 58(4):549–550, 2001.

Capriotti T. Pharmacologic implications of the new JNC 7 blood pressure guidelines. MEDSURG Nursing, 12(5):325–330, 2003.

Chase SL. Hypertensive crisis. RN, 63(6):62–68, 2000.

Chobanian AV, Bakris GL, Black HR, Cushman WC, et al. The Seventh Report of the Joint National Commission on Prevention, Detection, Evaluation, and Treatment of High Blood Pressure: The JNC 7 Report. Journal of the American Medical Association, 289(19):2560–2572, 2003.

Cohen M. The role of low-molecular-weight heparin in the management of acute coronary syndromes. Current Opinion in Cardiology, 16(6):384–389, 2001.

Davis S. How the heart failure picture has changed. Nursing2002, 32(11):36–44, 2002.

Ellenbogen KA, Kay GN, Wilkoff BL. Clinical cardiac pacing and defibrillation (2nd ed.). Philadelphia: W.B. Saunders, 2000.

Fuster V, Alexander RW, O'Rourke RA (Eds.). Hurst's the heart (10th ed.). New York: McGraw-Hill, 2001.

Gravlee G, et al (Eds). Cardiopulmonary bypass principles and practice (2nd ed.). Philadelphia: Lippincott Williams & Wilkins, 2000.

Henke K, Eigsti J. After cardiopulmonary bypass: watching for complications. Nursing2003, 33(3):32cc1–32cc4, 2003.

Irwin RS, Rippe JM (Eds.). Irwin and Rippe's intensive care medicine (5th ed.). Philadelphia: Lippincott Williams & Wilkins, 2003.

Maisel A. B-type natriuretic peptide in the diagnosis and management of congestive heart failure. Cardiology Clinics, 19(4):557–571, 2001.

McErlean ES (Ed.). Unstable angina. Journal of Cardiovascular Nursing, 15(1):1–79, 2000.

McNamara RL, Bass EB, Miller MR, et al. Management of new onset atrial fibrillation. AHRQ Pub. No. 01-E026, Rockville, MD: Agency for Healthcare Research and Quality, 2001.

Miller A, Strvastava P. Angiotensin receptor blockers and aldosterone antagonists in chronic heart failure. Cardiology Clinics, 19(2):195–202, 2001.

Moore WS. Vascular surgery: a comprehensive review (6th ed.). Philadelphia: W.B. Saunders, 2002.

National High Blood Pressure Education Program. The seventh report of the joint national committee on prevention, detection, evaluation, and treatment of high blood pressure. NIH Publication No. 98-4080. Bethesda, MD: National Institutes of Health, 2003.

O'Rourke RA, Huchman JS, Cohen MC, et al. New approaches to diagnosis and management of unstable angina and non-ST segment elevation myocardial infarction. Annals of Internal Medicine, 161(5):674–682, 2001.

Parrillo JE, Dellinger RP. Critical care medicine: principles of diagnosis and management in the adult (2nd ed.). St. Louis: Mosby, 2001.

Reynolds J, Apple S. A systemic approach to pacemaker assessment. AACN Clinical Issues: Advanced Practice Acute Critical Care, 12(1):14–26, 2001.

Rutherford RB. Vascular surgery (5th ed.). Philadelphia: W.B. Saunders, 2000.

Sacks FM, Svetkey LP, Vollmer WM, Appel AJ, et al. Effects on blood pressure of reduced dietary sodium and the Dietary Approaches to Stop Hypertension (DASH) diet. New England Journal of Medicine, 344(1):3–10, 2001.

Topol EJ. Textbook of interventional cardiology (4th ed.). Philadelphia: W.B. Saunders, 2003.

Urden LD, Stacy KM, Lough ME. Thelan's critical care nursing: diagnosis and management (4th ed.). St. Louis: Mosby, 2002.

Wallace CJ. Diagnosing and treating pacemaker syndrome. Critical Care Nurse, 21(1):24–31, 35–37, 2001.

Weber KT. Mechanisms of disease: aldosterone in congestive heart failure. New England Journal of Medicine, 345(23):1689–1697, 2001.

White E. Patients with implantable cardioverter defibrillators: transition to home. Journal of Cardiovascular Nursing, 14(3):42–52, 2000.

Woods SL, Froelicher ESS, Motzer SA. Cardiac nursing (4th ed.). Philadelphia: Lippincott, 2000.

Unit X. Nursing Care of the Client with Disturbances of Peripheral Vascular Function

Aquila A. Deep vein thrombosis. Journal of Cardiovascular Nursing, 15(4):25–44, 2001.

Byrne B. Deep vein thrombosis prophylaxis: the effectiveness and implications of using below-knee or thigh-length graduated compression stockings. Journal of Vascular Nursing, 20(2):53–59, 2002.

Church V. Staying on guard for DVT and PE. Nursing2000, 30(2):34–42, 2000.

Criner JA, Appelt M, Loker C, et al. Rhabdomyolysis: the hidden killer. MEDSURG Nursing, 11(3):58–63, 2002.

Cundy JB. Carotid artery stenosis and endarterectomy. Association of Operating Room Nurses Journal, 75(2):309–310, 312, 314–324, 2002.

Day MW. Recognizing and managing DVT. Nursing2003, 33(5):37–41, 2003.

Epley O. Pulmonary emboli risk reductions. Journal of Vascular Nursing, 18(2):61–70, 2000.

Fahey VA. Vascular nursing (4th ed.). Philadelphia: W.B. Saunders, 2004.

Fort CW. How to combat three deadly trauma complications. Nursing2003, 33(3):58–63, 2003.

Fowler SB. Patient care following carotid endarterectomy. MEDSURG Nursing, 8(1):47–52, 1999.

Hickey JV. The clinical practice of neurological and neurosurgical nursing (5th ed.). Philadelphia: Lippincott Williams & Wilkins, 2003.

Hirsch AT, Criqui MH, Treat-Jacobson D, et al. Peripheral arterial disease detection, awareness, and treatment in primary care. Journal of the American Medical Association, 286(11):1317–1324, 2001.

Krenzer ME. Unplugging the mystery of carotid endarterectomy patient care. Critical Care Nursing Clinics of North America, 11(2):189–208, 1999.

Meister J, Reddy D. Rhabdomyolysis: an overview. American Journal of Nursing, 102(2):75–79, 2002.

Moore WS. Vascular surgery: a comprehensive review (6th ed.). Philadelphia: W.B. Saunders, 2002.

Ridker P, et al. Long-term, low-intensity warfarin therapy for the prevention of recurrent venous thromboembolism. New England Journal of Medicine, 348(15):1425–1434, 2003.

Rutherford RB (Ed.). Vascular surgery (5th ed.). Philadelphia: W.B. Saunders, 2000.

Stordahl NJ, Back MR. The efficacy of carotid endarterectomy: a vascular surgery perspective reducing hospital stay. MEDSURG Nursing, 9(3):113–121, 2000.

Stratton MA, Anderson FA, Bussey HI, et al. Prevention of venous thromboembolism. Archives of Internal Medicine, 160(3):334–340, 2000.

Unit XI. Nursing Care of the Client with Disturbances of Respiratory Function

Agnelli C, Prandoni P, Becattini C, et al. Extended oral anticoagulant therapy after a first episode of pulmonary embolism. Annals of Internal Medicine, 139(10):19–25, 2003.

American Lung Association. Available at www.lungusa.org.

Baddour LM, Gorbach SL. Therapy of infectious diseases. Philadelphia: W.B. Saunders, 2003.

Boyle AH, Locke DL. Update on chronic obstructive pulmonary disease. MEDSURG Nursing, 13(1):42–47, 2004.

Centers for disease control and prevention. Available at www.cdc.gov/health.

Chernecky C. Pulmonary complications in patients with cancer. American Journal of Nursing, 101(5):24A, 24E, 24G–H, 2001.

Chiocca EM. Superior vena cava syndrome. American Journal of Nursing, 30(6):33, 2000.

Chojnowski D. "Gold" standards for acute exacerbation in COPD. Nurse Practitioner, 28(5):26–35, 2003.

Church V. Staying on guard for DVT and PE. Nursing2000, 30(2):35–42, 2000.

Dest V. Lung cancer. RN, 63(5):32–38, 2000.

DeVita VT Jr, Hellman S, Rosenberg SA (Eds.). Cancer: principles and practice of oncology (6th ed.). Philadelphia: Lippincott Williams & Wilkins, 2001.

Dunn N. Keeping COPD patients out of the ED. RN, 64(20):33–37, 2001.

Emtrier M, Porszansz J, Burns M, et al. Benefits of supplemental oxygen in exercise training in nonhypoxemic chronic obstructive pulmonary disease patients. American Journal of Respiratory and Critical Care Medicine, 168(9):1034–1042, 2003.

Enarson DA. Resistance to antituberculosis medications: hard lessons to learn. Archives of Internal Medicine, 160(5):581–582, 2000.

Ferreira I, Brooks D, Lacasse Y, Goldstein R. Nutritional intervention in COPD: a systematic overview. Chest, 119(2):353–363, 2001.

Goodfellow LT, Jones M. Bronchial hygiene therapy. American Journal of Nursing, 102(1):37–43, 2002.

Griner GJ. Symptomatic relief in COPD: considering the full range of outcomes. Advanced Studies in Medicine, 3(SB):S400–407, S424–425, 2003.

Holten KB. How should we manage an acute exacerbation of COPD? Journal of Family Practice, 52(10):780–782, 2003.

Hull RD, Raskob GE, Brant RF, et al. Low-molecular weight heparin vs heparin in the treatment of patients with pulmonary embolism. Archives of Internal Medicine, 160(2):229–236, 2000.

Jones A, Rowe B. Bronchopulmonary hygiene physical therapy and chronic obstructive pulmonary disease. Heart and Lung, 29(2):125–135, 2000.

Knippel SL. Surgical therapies for lung carcinomas. Nursing Clinics of North America, 36(3):517–525, 2001.

Kreamer KM. Getting the lowdown on lung cancer. Nursing2003, 33(11):36–42, 2003.

Lauzardo M, Ashkin D. Phthisiology at the dawn of the new century: a review of tuberculosis and the prospects for its elimination. Chest, 117(5):1455–1473, 2000.

MacNee W, Donaldson K. Exacerbations of COPD: environmental mechanisms. Chest, 117(5)Suppl:396S–397S, 2000.

Mandell GL, Bennett JE, Dolin R. Mandell, Douglas, and Bennett's principles and practice of infectious diseases (5th ed.). New York: Churchill Livingstone, 2000.

Metersky ML. Key points to remember when treating pneumonia in the elderly: a decline in functional status may be the only clue. Journal of Respiratory Diseases, 24(2):61–66, 2003.

Murray JF, Nadel JA (Eds.). Textbook of respiratory medicine (3rd ed.). Philadelphia: W.B. Saunders, 2000.

Parrillo JE, Dellinger RP. Critical care medicine: principles of diagnosis and management in the adult (2nd ed.). St. Louis: Mosby, 2001.

Patel N, Criner G. Community-acquired pneumonia in the elderly: update on treatment strategies. Consultant, 43(6):689–690, 692, 695–697, 2003.

Perin ML. Corticosteroids for cancer pain. American Journal of Nursing, 100(4):15–16, 2000.

Rennard S. New approaches to COPD therapy. Advanced Studies in Medicine, 3(SB):S408–415, S424–425, 2003.

Roman M, Weinstein A, Macaluso S. Primary spontaneous pneumothorax. MEDSURG Nursing, 12(3):161–169, 2003.

Seaton A, Seaton D, Leitch A (Eds.). Crofton and Douglas's respiratory diseases (5th ed.). Oxford: Blackwell Science, 2000.

Shamash J. Catching their breath...chronic obstructive pulmonary disease. Nursing Times, 98(20):14, 2002.

Shields TW, LoCicero J, Ponn RB (Eds.). General thoracic surgery (5th ed.). Philadelphia: Lippincott Williams & Wilkins, 2000.

Stroller JK. Acute exacerbations of chronic obstructive pulmonary medicine. New England Journal of Medicine, 346(13):988–994, 2002.

Tanagho EA, McAninch JW (Eds.). Smith's general urology (15th ed.). New York: Lange/McGraw-Hill, 2000.

Terpstra TL, Terpstra TL. Syndrome of inappropriate antidiuretic hormone secretion: recognition and management. MEDSURG Nursing, 9(2):61–68, 2000.

Turner J, Kelly B. Culture and medicine: emotional dimensions of chronic disease. Western Journal of Medicine, 172(2):124–128, 2000.

Ware LB, Matthay MA. The acute respiratory distress syndrome. New England Journal of Medicine, 342(18):1334–1349, 2001.

Wilkins RL, Stoller JK, Scanlon CL. Egan's fundamentals of respiratory care (8th ed.). St. Louis: Mosby, 2003.

Wisniewski A. Chronic bronchitis and emphysema: clearing the air. Nursing2003, 33(5):46–49, 2003.

Wouters EFM, Creutzberg EC, Scholes AMW. Systemic effects in COPD. Chest, 121(5): Suppl:127S–130S, 2002.

Yarbro CH, Frogge MH, Goodman M, Groenwald SL (Eds.). Cancer nursing: principles and practice (5th ed.). Sudbury, MA: Jones and Bartlett, 2000.

Unit XII. Nursing Care of the Client with Disturbances of the Kidney and Urinary Tract

Brenner BM (Ed.). Brenner and Rector's the kidney (6th ed.). Philadelphia: W.B. Saunders, 2000.

Campbell D. How acute renal failure puts the brakes on kidney function. Nursing2003, 33(10):59–64, 2003.

Chang SS, Baumgartner RG, Wells N, et al. Causes of increased hospital stay after radical cystectomy in a clinical pathway setting. Journal of Urology, 167(1):208–211, 2002.

Colwell JC, Goldberg M, Cramel J. The state of the standard diversion. Journal of Wound Ostomy Continence Nursing, 28(10):6–17, 2001.

DeVita VT Jr, Hellman S, Rosenberg SA (Eds.). Cancer: principles and practice of oncology (6th ed.). Philadelphia: Lippincott Williams & Wilkins, 2001.

Floruta CV. Dietary choices of people with ostomies. Journal of Wound Ostomy Continence Nursing, 28(10):28–31, 2001.

Gillenwater JY, Grayhack JT, Howards SS, Mitchell ME (Eds.). Adult and pediatric urology (4th ed.). Philadelphia: Lippincott Williams & Wilkins, 2002.

Johnson RJ, Feehaley J. Comprehensive clinical nephrology. St. Louis: Mosby, 2000.

Lancaster LE (Ed.). Core curriculum for nephrology nursing (4th ed.). Pitman, NJ: American Nephrology Nurses' Association, 2001.

O'Shea HS. Teaching the adult ostomy patient. Journal of Wound Ostomy Continence Nursing, 28(1):47–54, 2001.

Robbins KC, Cofrancesco DL. Kidney disease: understanding dialysis. NurseWeek, 4(13):20–21, 2003.

Robbins KC, Cofrancesco DL, Griffin E. Kidney disease: early detection can delay progression. NurseWeek, 4(12):19–20, 2003.

Schrier RW (Ed.). Diseases of the kidney and urinary tract (7th ed.). Philadelphia: Lippincott Williams & Wilkins, 2001.

Sprunk E, Alteneder RR. The impact of an ostomy on sexuality. Clinical Journal of Oncology Nursing, 4(2):85–88, 2000.

Turner J, Kelly B. Culture and medicine: emotional dimensions of chronic disease. Western Journal of Medicine, 172(2):124–128, 2000.

Walsh PC, Retik AB, Vaughan ED Jr, et al. (Eds.). Campbell's urology (8th ed.). Philadelphia: W.B. Saunders, 2002.

Yarbro CH, Frogge MH, Goodman M, Groenwald SL (Eds.). Cancer nursing: principles and practice (5th ed.). Sudbury, MA: Jones and Bartlett, 2000.

Unit XIII. Nursing Care of the Client with Disturbances of Hematologic and Immune Function

Bartlett J, Finkbeiner A. The guide to living with HIV infection. Baltimore, MD: Johns Hopkins University Press, 2001.

Beutler E, Coller BS, Lichtman MA, Kipps TJ (Eds.). Williams hematology (6th ed.). New York: McGraw-Hill, 2001.

Bradley-Springer L. HIV infection: what works? American Journal of Nursing, 101:(6):45–50, 2001.

Centers for Disease Control and Prevention (2002). HIV/AIDS Surveillance Report, 13(2):1–44, 2002.

Chettle CC. Sepsis: the body's overreaction to infection can prove deadly. NurseWeek California, 16(4):19–21, 2003.

Coyne PJ, Lyne ME, Watson AC. Symptom management in people with AIDS. American Journal of Nursing, 102(9):48–56, 2002.

Daughtry L, Bankston J, DeShotels J. HIV meds: keeping trouble at bay. RN, 65(2):31–35, 2002.

Dellinger RP. Cardiovascular management of septic shock. Critical Care Medicine, 31(3):946–955, 2003.

Destarac LA, et al. Sepsis in older patients: an emerging concern in critical care. Advances in Sepsis. Available at: www.sepsis.remdica.com. 2002.

Dressler DK. DIC: coping with a coagulation crisis. Nursing2004, 34(5): 58–62, 2004.

Geiter H. Disseminated intravascular coagulopathy. Dimensions of Critical Care Nursing, 22(33):108–116, 2003.

Gracia JS. Taking HAART: how to support patients with HIV/AIDS. Nursing2001, 31(12):36–41, 2001.

Guidelines for the use of antiretroviral agents in HIV-infected adults and adolescents (2002). Panel on Clinical Practices for Treatments of HIV Infection, Department of Health and Human Services. Available at: http://www.hivatis.org.

Hoffman R, Benz EJ, Shattil SJ, et al. Hematology: basic principles and practice (3rd ed.). New York: Churchill Livingstone, 2001.

Keithley JK, Swanson B. Minimizing HIV/AIDS malnutrition. MEDSURG Nursing, 7(5):256–269, 1998.

Mandell GL, Bennett JE, Dolin R. Mandell, Douglas, and Bennett's principles and practice of infectious diseases (5th ed.). New York: Churchill Livingstone, 2000.

McCoy C, Matthews SJ. Drotrecogin alfa (recombinant human activated protein C) for the treatment of severe sepsis. Clinical Therapeutics, 25(2):396–421, 2003.

NIH Guidelines on Opportunistic Infections (2001). Available at: http://www.aidsinfo.nih.gov/guidelines/adultAA_020402.

Parrillo JE, Dellinger RP. Critical care medicine: principles of diagnosis and management in the adult (2nd ed.). St. Louis: Mosby, 2001.

Piliero PJ, Colagreco JP. Clinical practice. Simplified regimens for treating HIV infection and AIDS. Journal of the American Academy of Nurse Practitioners, 15(7):305–312, 2003.

Schulman CS, Hare K. New thoughts on sepsis: the unifier of critical care. Dimensions of Critical Care Nursing, 22(1):20–30, 2003.

Spleen removal. Available at www.health.yahoo.com.

Ungvarski PJ, Flaskerud JH. HIV/AIDS: a guide to primary care management (4th ed.). Philadelphia: W.B. Saunders, 1999.

Wenzel RP. Treating sepsis. New England Journal of Medicine, 347(13): 966–967, 2002.
Williams A. Adherence to HIV regimens: 10 vital lessons. American Journal of Nursing, 101(6):37–44, 2001.

Unit XIV. Nursing Care of the Client with Disturbances of the Gastrointestinal Tract

Ball EM. A teaching guide for continent ileostomy. RN, 63(12):35–40, 2000.
Blackington E. Irritable bowel syndrome: an update on treatment options. Advanced Nurse Practitioner, 8(10):41–70, 2000.
Blam M, et al. Integrating anti-tumor necrosis factor therapy in inflammatory bowel disease: current and future perspectives. American Journal of Gastroenterology, 96(7):1977–1997, 2001.
Bryant D, Fleischer I. Changing an ostomy appliance. Nursing2000, 30(11):51–53, 2000.
Cappola M, Gallus P. Life-threatening upper GI emergencies, part 2. Journal of Critical Illness, 16(8):367–368, 371–373, 2001.
Cash BD. Evidence-based medicine as it applies to acid suppression in the hospitalized patient. Critical Care Medicine, 30(6):Suppl: S361, S373–379, S381, 2002.
Conrad SA. Acute upper gastrointestinal bleeding in critically ill patients: causes and treatment modalities. Critical Care Medicine, 30(6): Suppl: S361, S365–368, S379, 2002.
Dudley-Brown S. Prevention of psychological distress in persons with inflammatory bowel disease. Issues in Mental Health Nursing, 23(4):403–422, 2002.
Elliot D. The treatment of peptic ulcers. Nursing Standard, 16(22):37–42, 2002.
Elliot K. Nutritional considerations after bariatric surgery. Critical Care Nursing Quarterly, 26(2):133–138, 2003.
Farrell JJ, Friedman LS. Evaluating and managing GI bleeding in the elderly: atypical presentations can complicate the workup. Journal of Critical Illness, 18(5):222–236, 2003.
Feldman M, Friedman LS, Sleisenger MH (Eds.). Sleisenger and Fordtran's gastrointestinal and liver disease (7th ed.). Philadelphia: W.B. Saunders, 2002.
Floruta CV. Dietary choices of people with ostomies. Journal of Wound Ostomy Continence Nursing, 28(1):28–31, 2001.
Hahler B. Morbid obesity: a nursing challenge. MEDSURG Nursing, 11(2):85–90, 2002.
Hanauer S. Management of Crohn's disease in adults. American Journal of Gastroenterology, 96(3):635–644, 2001.
Heitkemper M. Irritable bowel syndrome. American Journal of Nursing, 101(1):26–34, 2001.
Kirsner J, Shorter R. Inflammatory bowel disease (5th ed.). Philadelphia: W.B. Saunders, 2000.
Lipsky MS. Gastrointestinal problems. Philadelphia: Lippincott Williams & Wilkins, 2000.
Livingston EH, Fink AS. Cost and future of bariatric surgery. Archives of Surgery, 138(4):383–388, 2003.
Manias E. Pain and anxiety management in the postoperative gastrosurgical setting. Journal of Advanced Nursing, 41(6):585–594, 2003.
Miedema BW, Johnson JO. Methods for decreasing postoperative gut dysmotility. Lancet Oncology, 4(6):365–372, 2003.
Morgan D. Intravenous proton pump inhibitors in the critical care setting. Critical Care Medicine, 30(6):Suppl: S361, S369–372, S379, 2002.
O'Shea HS. Teaching the adult ostomy patient. Journal of Wound Ostomy Continence Nursing, 28(1):47–54, 2001.
Rayhorn N, Rayhorn DJ. Inflammatory bowel disease. Nursing2002, 32(7):34–43, 2002.
Sprunk E, Alteneder RR. The impact of an ostomy on sexuality. Clinical Journal of Oncology Nursing, 4(2):85–88, 2000.
United Ostomy Association. Available at www.uoa.org.
Wilson JA, Clark JJ. Obesity: impediment to wound healing. Critical Care Nursing Quarterly, 26(2):119–132, 2003.

Unit XV. Nursing Care of the Client with Disturbances of the Liver, Biliary Tract, and Pancreas

Arias IM (Ed.). The liver: biology and pathobiology (4th ed.). Philadelphia: Lippincott Williams & Wilkins, 2001.
Bockhold KM. Who's afraid of hepatitis C? American Journal of Nursing, 100(5):26–31, 2000.
Bowers S. Nutrition support for malnourished, acutely ill adults. MEDSURG Nursing, 8(3):145–164, 1999.
Centers for Disease Control and Prevention. Hepatitis C: introduction and background. Available at: www.cdc.gov/nci-dol/diseases/hepatitis/c. 2001.
Cole L. Unraveling the mystery of acute pancreatitis. Nursing2001, 31(12):58–63, 2001.
Dugernier TL, Laterre PF, Wittebole X, et al. Compartmentalization of the inflammatory response during acute pancreatitis. American Journal of Respiratory and Critical Care Medicine, 168(2):148–157, 2003.
Feldman M, Friedman LS, Sleisenger MH. Sleisenger & Fordtran's gastrointestinal disease and liver disease: pathophysiology/diagnosis/management (7th ed.). Philadelphia: W.B. Saunders, 2002.
Fried M, et al. Peginterferon alfa-2a plus ribavarin for chronic hepatitis C virus infection. New England Journal of Medicine, 347(13):975–982, 2002.
Glacken M, Coates V, Kernohan G, Hegarty J. The experience of fatigue for people living with hepatitis C. Journal of Clinical Nursing, 12(2):244–252, 2003.
Harkness GA. Emerging infections. Hepatitis C: the silent stalker: a rapidly mutating virus that's difficult to detect. American Journal of Nursing, 103(9):24–25, 2003.
Hussar DA. New drugs 2003: part III. Nursing2003, 33(8):55–64, 2003.
Iosue K. Chronic hepatitis C: latest treatment options. Nurse Practitioner, 27(4):32–40, 2002.
Kleinpell RM. Shock states. NurseWeek, 4(14):20–22, 2003.
Lauer G, Walker BD. Hepatitis C virus infection. New England Journal of Medicine, 345(1):41–53, 2001.
Mansoor A, Ramsey C, Cheung MD, et al. Differential diagnosis of gallstone-induced complications. Southern Medical Journal, 93(3):261–264, 2000.
Menon KV, Kamath PS. Managing the complications of cirrhosis. Mayo Clinic Proceedings, 75(5):501–509, 2000.
Parini S. Hepatitis C. Nursing2003, 33(4):57–63, 2003.
Qamruddin AO, Chadwick PR. Preventing pancreatic infection in acute pancreatitis. Journal of Hospital Infection, 44(4):245–253, 2000.
Sarbah SA, Younossi ZM. Hepatitis C: an update on the silent epidemic. Journal of Clinical Gastroenterology, 30(2):125–143, 2000.
Schiff ER, Sorrell MF, Maddrey WC (Eds.). Schiff's diseases of the liver (9th ed.). Philadelphia: Lippincott Williams & Wilkins, 2002.
Schlapman N. Spotting acute pancreatitis. RN, 64(11):54–59, 2001.
Sharara AI, Rocky DC. Medical progress: gastroesophageal variceal hemorrhage. New England Journal of Medicine, 345(9):669–681, 2001.
Sherlock S, Dooley J. Diseases of the liver and biliary system (11th ed.). Oxford: Blackwell Science, 2002.
Wair CT, Lok ASF. Treatment of hepatitis B. Journal of Gastroenterology, 37(10):771–778, 2002.

Unit XVI. Nursing Care of the Client with Disturbances of Metabolic Function

American Diabetes Association. Diabetic nephropathy. (Position Statement). Diabetes Care, 26(1):84–98, 2003.
American Diabetes Association: Evidence-based nutrition principles and recommendations for the treatment and prevention of diabetes and related complications. (Position Statement). Diabetes Care, 26(1):51–61, 2003.
American Diabetes Association. Hyperglycemic crisis in patients with diabetes mellitus. (Position Statement). Diabetes Care, 26(1):109–117, 2003.
American Diabetes Association. Implications of the diabetes control and complications trial. (Position Statement). Diabetes Care, 26(1):25–27, 2003.
American Diabetes Association. Insulin administration. (Position Statement). Diabetes Care, 26(1):121–124, 2003.
American Diabetes Association. Preventive foot care in adults with diabetes. (Position Statement). Diabetes Care, 26(1):78–79, 2003.
Beebe C, O'Donnell M. Educating patients with type 2 diabetes. Nursing Clinics of North America, 36(2):375–386, 2001.
Braverman LE (Ed.). Diseases of the thyroid (2nd ed.). Totowa, NJ: Humana Press, 2003.
Braverman LE, Utiger RD (Eds.). Werner and Ingbar's the thyroid (8th ed.). Philadelphia: Lippincott Williams & Wilkins, 2000.
Cole L. Unraveling the mystery of acute pancreatitis. Nursing2001, 31(12):58–63, 2001.
Davidson JK. Clinical diabetes mellitus: a problem-oriented approach (3rd ed.). New York: Thieme, 2000.
DeGroot LJ, Jameson JL (Eds.). Endocrinology (4th ed.). Philadelphia: W.B. Saunders, 2001.

Fain JA. Insulin pumps. Nursing2003, 33(6):51–53, 2003.
Felig P, Frohman LA. Endocrinology & metabolism (4th ed.). New York: McGraw-Hill, 2001.
Flood L, Constance A. Diabetes and exercise safety. American Journal of Nursing, 102(6):47–55, 2002.
Fritschi C. Preventive care of the diabetic foot. Nursing Clinics of North America, 36(2):303–320, 2001.
Gill GV, Pickup JC, Williams G (Eds.). Difficult diabetes. Oxford: Blackwell Science, 2001.
Hess CT. Wound & skin care. Managing a diabetic ulcer. Nursing2003, 33(7):82–83, 2003.
Holstein A, et al. Incidence and costs of severe hypoglycemia. Diabetes Care, 25(11):2109–2110, 2002.
Improving mealtime glucose control by restoring early insulin secretion in type 2 diabetes. Diabetes & Endocrinology Treatment Updates. Available at: http://endocrine.medscape.com/Medscape/En..gy/TreatmentUpdate/2000.
Jungman E. prevention and treatment of diabetic nephropathy in older patients. Drugs and Aging, 20(6):419–435, 2003.
Kumrow D, Dahlen R. Thyroidectomy: understanding the potential for complications. MEDSURG Nursing, 11(5):228–234, 2002.
Larsen PR, Kronenberg HM, Melmed S, Polonsky KS. Williams textbook of endocrinology (10th ed.). Philadelphia: W.B. Saunders, 2003.
Magee MF, Bhatt BA. Management of decompensated diabetes. Diabetic ketoacidosis and hyperglycemic hyperosmolar syndrome. Critical Care Clinics, 17(1):75–106, 2001.
Mensing C, Boucher J, Cypress M, et al. National standards for diabetes self-management. (Position Statement). Diabetes Care, 26(1):149–156, 2003.
Quinn L. Diabetic emergencies in the patient with type 2 diabetes. Nursing Clinics of North America, 36(2):341–360, 2001.
Tkacs NC. Hypoglycemia unawareness: your patients with diabetes won't always know when their blood sugar is low. American Journal of Nursing, 102(2):34–40, 2002.
Watts SA, Anselmo JM, Smith MA. Combating hypoglycemia in the hospital and at home. Nursing2003, 33(3):32hn1–32hn5, 2003.

Unit XVII. Nursing Care of the Client with Disturbances of Musculoskeletal Function

Bailey J. Getting a fix on orthopedic care. Nursing2003, 33(6):58–64, 2003.
Browner BD, Jupiter JB, Levine AM, Trafton PG. Skeletal trauma: basic science, management, and reconstruction (3rd ed.). Philadelphia: W.B. Saunders, 2003.
Canale ST (Ed.). Campbell's operative orthopaedics (10th ed.). St. Louis: Mosby, 2003.
Chan KC, Gill GS. Cemented hemiarthroplasties for elderly patients with intertrochanteric fractures. Clinical Orthopaedics, 371:206–215, 2000.
Chapman MW (Ed.). Chapman's orthopaedic surgery (3rd ed.). Philadelphia: Lippincott Williams & Wilkins, 2001.
Church V. Staying on guard for DVT and PE. Nursing2000, 30(2):34–42, 2000.
Feldt KS, Gunderson J. Treatment of pain for older hip fracture patients across setting. Orthopaedic Nursing, 21(5):63–64, 66–71, 2002.
Ginsberg B. Pain management in knee surgery. Orthopaedic Nursing, 20(2):37–44, 2001.
Maher A, Salmond SW, Pellino TA (Eds.). Orthopaedic nursing (3rd ed.). Philadelphia: W.B. Saunders, 2002.
Nassif JM, Ritter MA, Medling JB, et al. The effect of intraoperative intravenous fixed-dose heparin during total joint arthroplasty on the incidence of fatal pulmonary emboli. Journal of Arthroplasty, 15:16–21, 2000.
Parker MJ. Evidence-based case report: managing an elderly patient with a fractured femur. British Medical Journal, 320:102–103, 2000.
Phantom Pain Options. Available at www.members.fortunecity.com.
Ragucci MV, Leali A, Moroz A, Fetto J. Comprehensive deep vein thrombosis prevention strategy after total knee arthroplasty. American Journal of Physical Medicine and Rehabilitation, 82(3):164–168, 2003.
Reed SJ. Managing phantom limb pain with drugs. Nursing2000, 29(4):32hn1–32hn4, 2000.
Resnick D. Diagnosis of bone and joint disorders (4th ed.). Philadelphia: W.B. Saunders, 2002.
Rutherford RB. Vascular surgery (5th ed.). Philadelphia: W.B. Saunders, 2000.
Samana CM, Vray M, Barre J, Fiessinger J, et al. Extended venous thromboembolism prophylaxis after total hip replacement: a comparison of low-molecular-weight heparin with oral anticoagulants. Archives of Internal Medicine, 162(19):2191–2196, 2002.
Schoen D (Ed.). Adult orthopaedic nursing. Philadelphia: Lippincott Williams & Wilkins, 2000.
Schoen DC (Ed.). NAON core curriculum for orthopaedic nursing (4th ed.). Pitman, NJ: National Association of Orthopaedic Nurses, 2001.
Schuurmans MJ, Duursman SA, Shortridge-Baggett LM, et al. Elderly patients with a hip fracture: the risk for delirium. Applied Nursing Research, 16(2):75–84, 2003.
Stern SH, Wixson RL, O'Connor D. Evaluation of the safety and efficacy of enoxaparin and warfarin for prevention of deep vein thrombosis after total knee arthroplasty. Journal of Arthroplasty, 15(2):153–158, 2000.
Turpie AGG, Gallus AS, Hoek JA. A synthetic pentasaccharide for the prevention of deep vein thrombosis after total hip replacement. New England Journal of Medicine, 344(9):619–625, 2001.

Unit XVIII. Nursing Care of the Client with Disturbances of the Breast and Reproductive System

Baron RH, Fey JV, Raboy S, et al. Eighteen sensations after breast cancer surgery: a comparison of sentinel lymph node biopsy and axillary node dissection. Oncology Nursing Forum, 29(4):651–659, 2002.
Cancer Information Network. Available at www.cancerlinksusa.com.
DeVita VT Jr, Hellman S, Rosenberg SA (Eds.). Cancer: principles and practice of oncology (6th ed.). Philadelphia: Lippincott Williams & Wilkins, 2001.
Erickson VS, Pearson ML, Ganz PA, et al. Arm edema in breast cancer patients. Journal of the National Cancer Institute, 93(2):96–111, 2001.
Held-Warmkessel J. What your patient needs to know about prostate cancer. Nursing2002, 32(12):36–42, 2002.
Holmberg SK, Scott LL, Alexy W, et al. Relationship issues of women with breast cancer. Cancer Nursing, 24(1):53–60, 2001.
Hoskins CN, Haber J. Adjusting to breast cancer. American Journal of Nursing, 100(4):26–31, 2000.
Hull MM. Lymphedema in women treated for breast cancer. Seminars in Oncology Nursing, 16(3): 226–237, 2000.
MacDonald DJ. Women's decisions regarding management of breast cancer risks. MEDSURG Nursing, 11(4):183–186, 2002.
Otto SE. Oncology nursing (4th ed.). St. Louis: Mosby, 2001.
Resnick B, Belcher AE. Breast reconstruction: options, answers, and support for patients making a difficult personal decision. American Journal of Nursing, 102(4):26–33, 2002.
Rondorf-Klym LM, Colling J. Quality of life after radical prostatectomy. Oncology Nursing Forum, 30(2):E24–32, 2003.
Sandau KE. Free TRAM flap breast reconstruction. American Journal of Nursing, 102(4):36–43, 2002.
Therapies for the treatment of benign prostatic hyperplasia. Available at www.cpmcnet.columbia.edu/dept/urology/bphtherapy.
Thomas S, Greifzu SP. Oncology today: breast cancer. RN, 63(4):40–47, 2000.
Walsh PC, Retik AB, Vaughn ED Jr, et al. (Eds.). Campbell's urology (8th ed.). Philadelphia; W.B. Saunders, 2002.

Unit XIX. Nursing Care of the Client with Disturbances of the Head and Neck

Bowers S. Nutrition support for malnourished, acutely ill adults. MEDSURG Nursing, 8(3):145–164, 1999.
DeVita VT Jr, Hellman S, Rosenberg SA (Eds.). Cancer: principles and practice of oncology (6th ed.). Philadelphia: Lippincott Williams & Wilkins, 2001.
Otto SE. Oncology nursing (4th ed.). St. Louis: Mosby, 2001.
Richards BL, Spiro JD. Controlling advanced neck disease: efficacy of neck dissection and radiotherapy. Laryngoscope, 110(7):1124–1127, 2000.
Seikaly H. Xerostomia prevention after head and neck cancer treatment. Archives of Otolaryngology: Head and Neck Surgery, 129(2):247–250, 2003.
Talmi YP, et al. Pain in the neck after neck dissection. Otolaryngology: Head and Neck Surgery, 123(3):302–306, 2000.
Yarbro CH, Frogge MH, Goodman M, Groenwald SL (Eds.). Cancer nursing: principles and practice (5th ed.). Sudbury, MA: Jones and Bartlett, 2000.

INDEX

Note: NANDA-approved nursing diagnoses are highlighted in bold print.